Orthopaedic Manual Physical Therapy

FROM ART TO EVIDENCE

Christopher H. Wise, PT, DPT, OCS, FAAOMPT, MTC, ATC
Doctor of Physical Therapy Program Director
Associate Professor of Physical Therapy
Alvernia University
Reading, Pennsylvania

Owner and President
WISE Physical Therapy LLC
Kutztown, Pennsylvania

F.A. Davis Company • Philadelphia

F.A. Davis Company
1915 Arch Street
Philadelphia, PA 19103
www.fadavis.com

Printed in the United States of America

Last digit indicates print number: 10 9 8 7 6 5 4 3 2 1

Senior Acquisitions Editor: Melissa A. Duffield
Manager of Content Development: George W. Lang
Senior Developmental Editor: Jennifer A. Pine
Art and Design Manager: Carolyn O'Brien

As new scientific information becomes available through basic and clinical research, recommended treatments and drug therapies undergo changes. The author(s) and publisher have done everything possible to make this book accurate, up to date, and in accord with accepted standards at the time of publication. The author(s), editors, and publisher are not responsible for errors or omissions or for consequences from application of the book, and make no warranty, expressed or implied, in regard to the contents of the book. Any practice described in this book should be applied by the reader in accordance with professional standards of care used in regard to the unique circumstances that may apply in each situation. The reader is advised always to check product information (package inserts) for changes and new information regarding dose and contraindications before administering any drug. Caution is especially urged when using new or infrequently ordered drugs.

Library of Congress Cataloging-in-Publication Data

Orthopaedic manual physical therapy : from art to evidence / [edited by] Christopher H. Wise.
    p. ; cm.
Includes bibliographical references and index.
ISBN 978-0-8036-1497-0 — ISBN 0-8036-1497-7
I. Wise, Christopher H., editor.
[DNLM: 1. Manipulation, Orthopedic—methods—United States. 2. Evidence-Based Practice—United States. WB 535]
RM725
615.8'2—dc23
                    2014034975

Foreword

Orthopaedic manual physical therapy (OMPT) has become recognized by the profession of physical therapy as a premier area of clinical specialization. Once part of the practice of our founders, it was shelved during the rise of chiropractic in the 1930s. Chiropractic claims to prevent and cure all diseases through manipulation caused the fledgling physical therapy profession to nearly cease the practice of manual therapy. It survived in a much deemphasized form under such terms as *passive movement*, *articulating*, and *mobilization*. However, in the 1960s, with the advent of physical therapists such as Maitland, McKenzie, and this author, manual therapy once again became an important area of clinical practice. Today, instruction in manual therapy is required within all first professional educational programs in the United States.

National and international organizations now affirm standards of practice and offer forums for the exchange of clinical and scientific knowledge. The Orthopaedic Section of the American Physical Therapy Association was founded by those interested in manual and manipulative therapy as was the International Federation of Orthopaedic and Manipulative Physical Therapy (IFOMPT). The American Academy of Orthopaedic Manual Physical Therapists (AAOMPT) became the first entity to exist outside of the American Physical Therapy Association (APTA) in order to have an organization that could set skill and educational standards for membership. No such opportunity existed within the APTA, and to be a member of IFOMPT such standards are required. The academy has worked closely with the Orthopaedic Section and the APTA to develop operational definitions, standards of practice, and to defend practice via the Manipulation Task Force.

The question could be asked, "What is orthopaedic manual and manipulative physical therapy?" Since its inception, the practice of OMPT has espoused more than simply the mobilizing or manipulating of joints. As Meadows states, OMPT represents "an entire approach to musculoskeletal dysfunction and not just a series of techniques, whose purpose is to mobilize or stabilize a particular joint or spinal segment." As Riddle describes, OMPT is more than just the application of manual techniques and notes that, "manual procedures (may be used) to collect data on patients with musculoskeletal problems." Farrell et al add that OMPT is, "not a specialty that utilizes only passive movement techniques, (but) whose indications are multifactorial evolving from clinical criteria rather than from descriptions of pathology."

That there are so many approaches to OMPT should not be cause for confusion, for many of the differences represent but a minor emphasis on one aspect or another from what has gone before. If a therapist develops a particular interest, skill, or "discovery" they wish to speak up, demonstrate, teach, and write on that particular "discovery." Some in the process have, unfortunately, dammed what has gone before, but most recognize that they share common roots of practice and that their contribution is just that—a contribution.

With the current emphasis on evidence-based practice manual and manipulative practice has fared well. This author feels, however, that some of this research is leading us down the wrong path and that too much influence is being paid to the published literature rather than to patient's wishes and most importantly the expertise of the practitioner—one of the three legs of the stool described by Sackett. Seeking to publish often resorts in asking the simple questions in order to have a published article. The skill of manipulation is in danger of being dumbed down by those who would seek clinical prediction rules regardless of underlying specific impairments. What is required in manual therapy research is to ask the right questions, not the simple ones, and to seek to validate the skills that the masters in this field have developed rather than the gross techniques capable of being taught to the novice. Perhaps for the present we should be talking of evidence-influenced practice rather than evidence-based practice, for there is too little published evidence on which to base practice, and much of it does not stand up to critical scrutiny.

In keeping with its title, Dr. Wise has created a text that provides the reader with a sense of both the art and the science of OMPT, for surely manipulation is an art in search of its science. Well suited for both physical therapy students and clinicians, this text adopts an eclectic approach to OMPT that incorporates detailed descriptions of examination and intervention principles for each anatomic region. This should not confuse readers but rather empower them to see the diversity of practice and the opportunity to discover for themselves which approach best suits their personal style as well as the patients and clients that make up their practice.

The selection of guest authors is excellent and their contributions add to the depth and veracity of the content that is presented. Manual therapy is no longer in the hands of those who led the rebirth of its practice in physical therapy. It has matured, diversified, and in the process it has gained strength. This text captures that essence and will prove to be an invaluable resource for students, clinicians, and researchers who are interested in developing and advancing this area of specialization within the profession of physical therapy.

Stanley V. Paris, PT, PhD, FAPTA
FNZSP (Hon), NZMTA (Hon), IFOMT (Hon),
FAAOMPT (Founding Fellow), MCSP (Eng)
Chancellor, University of St. Augustine for
Health Sciences

Preface

The Purpose of this Book

Mennell exclaimed, "the human hand is the oldest remedy known to man, and historically, no date can be given for its inception."[1] It has only been in recent years, however, that the profession of physical therapy has formally embraced orthopaedic manual physical therapy (OMPT) as an entire approach to the management of musculoskeletal dysfunction. In fact, prior to the early 1990s, formal training in the art and science of OMPT was not routinely included within the educational curricula of physical therapists. Many well-intentioned physical therapists have disregarded the use of these strategies within their clinical practice due to the paucity of literature supporting their veracity or based in an honest attempt to establish distance between the field of physical therapy and other health-related professions. Consequently, a significant number of clinicians have spent a portion of their careers without consideration of these strategies within their diagnostic and intervention armamentarium. It is, therefore, time for a more in-depth exposition of both the art and the science of this unique and important area of specialty practice. The primary objective of this text is to serve as the definitive resource on the principles and practice of OMPT for physical therapist students, instructors, clinicians, and researchers.

About the Title

Orthopaedic Manual Physical Therapy: From Art to Evidence was decided upon following extensive deliberation and debate. Originally targeted to be more inclusive, the text was titled, *Orthopaedic Manual Therapy*. Upon the advice of several of the book's contributors, who espoused the importance of focusing the text on those aspects of manual therapy that have become essential to the practice of physical therapy, the title was changed. This is not to say that all of the content contained herein has been developed, or is exclusively utilized, by physical therapists. After all, the tenets of manual therapy are not specific to any one profession and most strategies have evolved through a gradual process of formative independent and collaborative contribution from a myriad of individuals over the course of many years. The second portion of the title, *From Art to Evidence*, was later added for the specific intent of recognizing, embracing, and communicating the notion that OMPT, in its truest form, is the culmination and amalgamation of both art *and* science. As Salter stated, "Patient care is an art, but the art must be based on science."[2] The writing of this book provided the challenge of coupling science with the artful skill of developing within the reader

what Stoddard described as that, "elusive tissue texture sense."[3]

It is my hope that through deliberate study of these concepts, strict attention to detail, and most importantly, reflective *practice, practice, practice*, the reader will attain a level of proficiency that when applied judiciously will have a profound impact on those whom we serve and subsequently on the profession of physical therapy. It would do the reader well to consider the three pillars of Sackett's model of evidence-based practice when reading this text and when applying its principles.[4] Let the title of this text serve as a reminder of OMPT's perplexing and sometimes conflicting nature as a science that is applied through a variety of art forms and individualized expression.

The Scope of this Book

The scope of this book reflects its objective by presenting a comprehensive review of the principles and practices of the most significant schools of thought that have influenced the practice of OMPT in the United States today. The comprehensive, eclectic, and evidence-based manner in which this book was written facilitates its use in guiding clinical practice.

This book, and the accompanying web-based instructional videos, will attempt to achieve the critical balance between theory and clinical application. Throughout the text, a preoccupation is placed on appreciating concepts in light of the best available evidence with an emphasis on assisting the reader in making connections between theory and practice through a process of critical thinking. This text focuses on supporting the development of the physical therapist student and clinician as a specialist in "applied kinesiology." Despite the strict attention given to every detail of technique performance, the manual procedures presented within this book are deemed to be secondary to the development of astute clinical decision-making skills within the reader.

Philosophic Approach and Pedagogical Features

To accomplish its objectives, this book explicitly and implicitly revolves around four foundational themes:

1. This text approaches OMPT from an *eclectic* perspective that endeavors to equip the reader with an arsenal of clinical tools from which to draw. Developing within the reader an appreciation for the value of each school of thought as it applies to current practice is a major theme

of this text and one that has not been as comprehensively presented elsewhere. This feature is most vividly presented in Part II of this book, where 18 different approaches are expertly presented by the originators of or contributors to each specific school of thought.

2. In recent years, the profession of physical therapy has experienced a healthy paradigm shift toward *evidence-based practice (EBP)*. Orthopaedic manual physical therapy has not enjoyed a long history of evidence to support its efficacy. In developing this resource, it was my intent to present a review of the literature designed to stimulate further inquiry that directly impacts clinical practice. It is my hope that the presentation of these foundational approaches side by side in light of the evidence will advance the cause and the case for the integration of OMPT within the profession of physical therapy. To support this objective, evidence is generously provided throughout the exposition of each approach. Chapter 3 is dedicated to the role of EBP within OMPT, and tools for evaluating and applying evidence to clinical practice are provided. The time-sensitive and ever-evolving nature of the published literature presented within a text of this kind poses several challenges. The literature presented throughout the text provides foundational support for the concepts and practices contained herein; however, the presented literature in many cases is not the most current. The reader is advised to consult other sources for the most recent published evidence.

3. Another foundational philosophical emphasis of this text has been placed on assisting the reader in the development of *sound critical thinking* strategies as they relate to OMPT. With this objective in mind, the reader is empowered with more than just a collection of effective techniques, but rather an entire framework from which to make clinical decisions regarding how best to incorporate OMPT into a comprehensive examination and intervention schema. To facilitate the connection between philosophical constructs and critical thinking, each chapter in Part II is equipped with **Clinical Pillar** boxes, which provide foundational concepts that are integral and germane to each approach. The **Questions for Reflection** boxes enable the reader to engage in a process of critical thinking as information is being presented. The **Notable Quotable** boxes provide thought-reflecting quotes from the originators of each approach that serve to summarize key concepts and inspire. Lastly, summary boxes that review key points presented within the text are placed throughout each chapter to allow the reader to reflect on new concepts.

4. The final philosophical pillar on which this book was developed is its preoccupation with *practical application*. In an effort to avoid the "paralysis of analysis" in which discussion of theory interferes with practical application, this book was written with clinicians, educators, and students in mind. A clear and consistent emphasis has been placed on making connections between theoretical frameworks, proven clinical efficacy, and the clinical performance of

OMPT. The book is organized in a manner that facilitates clinical application. Chapter 2 is dedicated to principles in preparation for OMPT. This chapter includes key concepts designed to facilitate the effective and safe implementation of OMPT procedures. Concepts are presented that attempt to prepare individuals for practice through principles that target the cognitive, affective, and psychomotor domains of learning. Part III of this text is dedicated to the practice of OMPT and is designed to draw from each philosophic approach and provide a template for the clinical application of OMPT. Using a regional approach, each chapter in this section begins with a review of kinematics followed by principles of examination and intervention and concludes with an eclectic and essential skill set of OMPT joint mobilization techniques that provides detailed instruction for optimal performance. To further enhance the psychomotor performance of these OMPT techniques, a web-based instructional resource that provides video demonstration with clear verbal and visual cues is also provided. The conclusion of each chapter in Part II and III of the book contains a **Clinical Case**, which is designed to bring together the principles of exam and intervention previously presented. Following the case, specific questions are included that require critical thinking and serve to ensure that key concepts have been attained. Each chapter within these sections concludes with a **Hands-On** section that provides specific activities that students and educators may use in lab to facilitate learning within each domain.

The Organization of this Book

This book is divided into three main sections:

- **PART I: Perspectives and Principles in Orthopaedic Manual Physical Therapy**
  The first section of this book articulates the foundational concepts that form the underpinnings of OMPT and serves to equip the reader with information paramount to the understanding of concepts presented later in the text. *Chapter 1, Historical Perspectives in Orthopaedic Manual Physical Therapy* is designed to provide the reader with an understanding of the origins of OMPT. *Chapter 2, Principles of Preparation for Orthopaedic Manual Physical Therapy*, addresses fundamental principles related to the safe and effective performance of OMPT. The concept of evidence-based practice is most explicitly covered in *Chapter 3, Principles of Evidence-Based Practice Applied to Orthopaedic Manual Physical Therapy*, which provides practical tools to enhance the reader's ability to critically analyze the OMPT literature and sets the tone for the emphasis on EBP throughout the remainder of the book.

- **PART II: Philosophical Approaches to Orthopaedic Manual Physical Therapy**
  This section consists of 18 chapters, each devoted to a current OMPT approach. Each chapter begins with a brief **historical perspective** section, then progresses to **principles of examination** and **principles of intervention**

sections, which highlight the primary clinical methods germane to each approach. Each chapter concludes with a section entitled *differentiating characteristics* that attempts to identify the unique features of each approach. Each approach is presented in a manner that facilitates clinical application and integration culminating in the presentation of a case study with discussion questions and hands on lab activities.

- **PART III: Practice of Orthopaedic Manual Physical Therapy**

The third section consists of nine chapters, each of which includes an essential skill set of joint mobilization techniques that are eclectic in nature and chosen for their clinical effectiveness and ease of performance. A primary feature of the text are color photographs of each technique, which include anatomic overlays designed to direct the reader to the structural nuances of each articulation. Enhanced with force vector arrows and clearly identified stabilization points, these highly illustrative photos guide technique performance and distinguish this book from others. A detailed description is also provided that will guide the reader and the instructor toward correct technique performance. The accompanying web-based instructional OMPT technique videos complement the text by highlighting key techniques for each anatomic region. The primary feature of these videos is the presentation of each technique in a manner that facilitates the use of sequential partial-task practice (SPTP). Within this teaching strategy, each technique is presented in a step-by-step fashion, concluding with complete performance in real-time. The reader may utilize this skill set as a starting point but is encouraged to routinely modify, enhance, progress, and develop new techniques that most effectively meet the unique needs of each patient.

It's in Your Hands Now

Along with each contributor, I am proud to present to you this "treatise" on the art and science of OMPT, which is the culmination of many long hours of research, critical thinking, and deliberation. My attempt to provide a resource designed to advance the specialization of OMPT has emerged as a direct result of the valuable contributions from these pioneers and leaders of this evolving craft.

A wise man once said, "Education is not the means of showing people how to get what they want. Education is an exercise through which enough people will learn to want what is worth having. No true education can leave out the moral and spiritual dimensions of human life and striving." The challenges of creating a resource that highlights both the theoretical constructs as well as the practical application of the primary schools of thought related to the practice of OMPT have been substantial but worthwhile. This book's success in accomplishing its objective of becoming an essential and invaluable collection of scientific discourse, artful expression, and practical application will only be realized in your hands and through the passage of time.

I invite you to join me on this continuous journey of growth and development. With this book as your trail guide, I hope this resource challenges you...but makes you better, provides answers . . . but raises more questions, dispels myths and incites passion, and at every turn empowers you toward the relentless pursuit of clinical excellence in the service of others. It's in your hands now!

Christopher H. Wise
Reading, Pennsylvania
June 2014

REFERENCES

1. Mennell J. *Back Pain: Diagnosis and Treatment Using Manipulative Techniques.* Boston, MA: Little, Brown; 1960.
2. Salter RB. Textbook of Disorders and Injuries of the Musculoskeletal System. 2nd ed. Baltimore, MD: Williams & Wilkins; 1983.
3. Paris SV, Loubert PV. Foundations of Clinical Orthopaedics, Course Notes. St. Augustine, FL: Institute Press; 1990.
4. Sackett DL. Evidence-based medicine. Spine. 1988; 23:1085-1086.

Contributing Authors

Paul F. Beattie, PT, PhD, OCS, FAPTA
Clinical Associate Professor
Program in Physical Therapy
Department of Exercise Science
School of Public Health
University of South Carolina
Columbia, South Carolina

Stephen John Carp, PT, PhD, GCS
Associate Professor
Director of DPT Admissions
Department of Physical Therapy
Temple University
Philadelphia, Pennsylvania

Jan Dommerholt, PT, MPS, DPT, DAAPM
Adjunct Associate Professor
Performing Arts Medicine Program Instructor
Shenandoah Valley University
Winchester, Virginia

Associate Professor
Universidad CEU Cardenal Herrera
Valencia, Spain

President
Myopain Seminars
Bethesda, Maryland

President
Bethesda Physiocare, Inc
Bethesda, Maryland

Timothy Flynn, PT, PhD, OCS, FAAOMPT
Professor
Rocky Mountain University
School of Health Professions, Doctor of Physical Therapy
    Program
Provo, Utah

Colorado Physical Therapy Specialists
Fort Collins, Colorado

Mary Lou Galantino, PT, PhD, MSCE
Professor of Physical Therapy
The Richard Stockton College of New Jersey

Sharon Giammatteo, PhD, PT, IMT,C
Co-Founder and President
Institute of Integrative Manual Therapy
Co-Founder and President
Connecticut School of Integrative Manual Therapy
Rehabilitation Consultant
Regional Physical Therapy
Bloomfield, Connecticut

Ben Hando, PT, DSc, OCS, FAAOMPT
U.S. Air Force

Gregory S. Johnson, PT, FFCFMT, FAAOMPT
Co-Director & Co-Founder, Institute of Physical Art, Inc.
Vice President, Functional Manual Therapy Foundation
Director, FMT Fellowship Program
Steamboat Springs, Colorado

Vicky Saliba Johnson, PT, FFCFMT, FAAOMPT
President, Institute of Physical Art, Inc.
Director, IPA Orthopedic Residency
Chairman, FMT Foundation
Steamboat Springs, Colorado

Jay B. Kain, PhD, PT, ATC, IMT,C
Director/President
Jay Kain Holistic Healthcare
The Kain Institute–A Center for Body/ Mind Healing
Great Barrington, Massachusetts

Michael L. Kuchera, DO, FAAO
Chair, Osteopathic Manipulative Medicine
Marian University
Indianapolis, Indiana

Johnson McEvoy, PT, BSc, MSc, DPT, MISCP, MCSP
Owner
United Physiotherapy Clinic
Lead Physiotherapist
National Irish Boxing Team

Adjunct Faculty
MSc in Sports Physiotherapy at University College
    Dublin, BSc (Sports Science) at University of Limerick,
    BSc (Athletic Therapy) at Dublin City University

Faculty
Myopain Seminars
Bethesda, Maryland

Philip McClure, PT, PhD, FAPTA
Department Chair and Professor
Department of Physical Therapy
Arcadia University
Glenside, Pennsylvania

Jim Meadows, BSc., PT, FCAMPT
Co-Owner, Institute of Manual Physiotherapy and Clinical
    Training
Colorado Spring, Colorado
Owner, Swodeam Institute
Calgary, AB, Canada

Rachel A. Miller, PT, MS, WCS, CFMT
Owner
Empower Physical Therapy
Exton, Pennsylvania
Associate Faculty, Institute of Physical Art
Steamboat Springs, Colorado

Nancy Parker Neff, PT, DPT, Cert MDT
Formerly Research Associate
Arcadia University
Glenside, Pennsylvania
Formerly Staff Physical Therapist
Aquatic & Physical Therapy Center
Phillipsburg, New Jersey

Stanley V. Paris, PT, PhD, FAPTA, FNZSP
(Hon), NZMTA (Hon), IFOMT (Hon),
FAAOMPT, MCSP
Chancellor of the University of St. Augustine for Health
    Sciences
St. Augustine, Florida

Donald K. Reordan, PT, MS, OCS, MCTA
Jacksonville Physical Therapy
Jacksonville, Oregon

Leslie Davis Rudzinski, PT, OCS, CFMT
Faculty
Institute of Physical Art
Steamboat Springs, Colorado

Orthopedic Mentor
USC Orthopedic Residency Program
Los Angeles, California

Senior Staff
Paulseth and Associates Physical Therapy
Los Angeles, California

Physical Therapist
Malibu Rehabilitation Center
Malibu, California

Kay A.R. Scanlon, PT, DPT, OCS, Dip MDT
Kay Scanlon Physical Therapy
Jenkintown, Pennsylvania

Ronald J. Schenk, PT, PhD, OCS, FAAOMPT, Dip
MDT
Dean of Health and Human Services and Associate Professor
    of Physical Therapy
Daemen College
Amherst, New York

Jim Stephens, PhD, PT, CFP
Movement Learning and Rehab
Havertown, Pennsylvania

Angela R. Tate, PT, PhD, Cert MDT
Research Physical Therapist and Associate Faculty Member
Department of Physical Therapy
Arcadia University
Glenside, Pennsylvania

Clinical Director, Center Coordinator of Clinical Education
Willow Grove Physical Therapy
Willow Grove, Pennsylvania

Heather Walkowich, DPT
The New Jersey Center for Physical Therapy
Riverdale, New Jersey

Kristina M. Welsome, MS PT, DPT, OCS, CFMT,
MTC
Assistant Professor of Clinical Physical Therapy
New York Medical College
Valhalla, New York

Russell Woodman, PT, MS, DPT, FSOM, OCS, MCTA
Professor of Physical Therapy
Quinnipiac University
Hamden, Connecticut

Reviewers

Jacklyn H. Brechter, PT, PhD
Associate Professor and Department Chair
Department of Physical Therapy
Chapman University
Orange, California

Jason Brumitt, MSPT, SCS, ATC, CSCS
Assistant Professor of Physical Therapy
School of Physical Therapy
Pacific University
Hillsboro, Oregon

Terry B. Chambliss, PT, MHS/PT
Assistant Professor of Physical Therapy
University of Evansville
Programs in Physical Therapy
Evansville, Indiana

Staffan Elgelid, PT, PhD, GCFP
Associate Professor
Department of Physical Therapy
Nazareth College of Rochester
Rochester, New York

Jennifer B. Ellison, PhD, PT
Assistant Professor
University of Texas Medical Branch
Department of Physical Therapy
Houston, Texas

Michael A. Geelhoed, PT, DPT, OCS, MTC
Assistant Professor and Director of Clinical Education
The University of Texas Health Science Center at San Antonio
Department of Physical Therapy
San Antonio, Texas

Christopher Geiser, MS, PT, LAT, ATC
Clinical Assistant Professor, Athletic Training Educational Program Director
Department of Physical Therapy
Marquette University
Milwaukee, Wisconsin

Abigail Gordon, PT, DPT
Clinical Assistant Professor
Department of Physical Therapy
Howard University
Washington, District of Columbia

Cheri Hodges, PT, DPT, MAppSc, OCS, FAAOMPT
Assistant Professor
A.T. Still University
Department of Physical Therapy
Mesa, Arizona

Peter A. Huijbregts, PT, MSc, MHSc, DPT, OCS, MTC, FAAOMPT, FCAMT
Assistant Professor
University of St. Augustine for Health Sciences
Department of Online Education
St. Augustine, Florida

Demetra John, PT, PhD
Director of DPT Admissions and Curriculum
University of Illinois at Chicago
Department of Physical therapy
Chicago, Illinois

Kyle B. Kiesel, PT, PhD, ATC, CSCS
Assistant Professor of Physical Therapy
University of Evansville
Department of Physical Therapy
Evansville, Indiana

Bradley Michael Kruse, PT, DPT, OCS, SCS, ATC, Cert. MDT, CSCS
Assistant Professor of Physical Therapy
Clarke College
Department of Physical Therapy
Dubuque, Iowa

Kenneth E. Learman, PT, PhD, OCS, COMT, FAAOMPT
Assistant Professor
Department of Physical Therapy
Youngstown State University
Youngstown, Ohio

Michael T. Lebec, PT, PhD
Assistant Professor of Physical Therapy
Northern Arizona University
Department of Physical Therapy
Flagstaff, Arizona

Peter M. Leininger, PT, PhD, OCS
Program Director
Department of Physical Therapy
The University of Scranton
Scranton, Pennsylvania

Everett B. Lohman III, DPTSc, PT, OCS
Associate Professor
Loma Linda University
Department of Physical Therapy
Redlands, California

Sara F. Maher, PT, DScPT, OMPT
Assistant Professor
Oakland University
Department of Physical Therapy
Rochester, Michigan

Carol A. Maritz, EdD, PT, GCS
Associate Professor of Physical Therapy
Department of Physical Therapy
University of the Sciences in Philadelphia
Philadelphia, Pennsylvania

Eric S. Mason, PT
President
Physiotherapy Works, LLC
Winter Park, Florida

Janna Michelle McGaugh, PT, ScD, OCS, COMT
Assistant faculty
University of Texas Medical Branch (UTMB)
Department of Physical Therapy
Galveston, Texas

David C Morrisette, PT, PhD, OCS, ATC, FAAOMPT
Associate Professor
Medical University of South Carolina
Department of Rehabilitation Sciences
Charleston, South Carolina

Neil Pearson, MSc(RHBS), BScPT, BA-BPHE, CertMDT, Certified Yoga Therapist
Physiotherapist
University of British Columbia
Vancouver, BC Canada

H. James Phillips, PT, PhD, OCS, ATC, FAAOMPT
Associate Professor
Department of Physical Therapy
Seton Hall University
South Orange, New Jersey

Diane H. Pitts, PT, DPT, BS RN
Instructor
Graduate School of Physical Therapy
University of South Alabama
Mobile, Alabama

Daniel R. Poulsen, II, PT, PhD, OCS, ATP
Assistant Professor, Assistant Director of Clinical Education
Department of Rehabilitation Sciences
Texas Tech University Health Sciences Center
Lubbock, Texas

Becky J. Rodda, PT, DPT, OCS, OMPT
Clinical Associate Professor
Physical Therapy Department
University of Michigan –Flint
Flint, Michigan

Proposal Reviewers

Corrie Ann Mancinelli, PT, PhD
Associate Professor
West Virginia University School of Medicine
Department of Human Performance/PT
Morgantown, West Virginia

Steven Raymond Tippett, PhD, PT, SCS, ATC
Associate Professor
Bradley University
Department of Physical Therapy and Health Sciences
Peoria, Illinois

Michael L Voight, DHSc, PT, OCS, SCS, ATC
Professor
Belmont University
School of Physical Therapy
Nashville, Tennessee

Acknowledgments

This book has been in the development stage for more than 10 years! The large expanse of time required for its creation is related in part to the challenge of integrating the thoughts and vision of each contributor into one cohesive theme and is in part due to an attempt to remain true to the book's objective as the definitive resource on OMPT. The concept for the book arose in the spring of 2003, when I was teaching an elective course on OMPT for the first time to third-year physical therapy doctoral students. It became immediately apparent that there was no text that focused on developing students with the ability to make clinical decisions regarding the implementation of an eclectic skill set of manual techniques within the context of a comprehensive physical therapy plan of care. A course manual was developed to supplement the course, which led to the submission of a book proposal and, after many years of writing and re-writing, the eventual completion of what you now hold in your hands.

The hard work and dedication of each contributor to this process and each contributor's passion for advancing the cause of OMPT was an encouragement to me during the long hours of writing and editing. To my past and future students and patients, you have inspired, motivated, and taught me what it is that you *actually* need rather than what it is that *I think* you need. This book was written with you in mind. This project would not have come to completion had it not been for the patience, dedication, commitment to excellence, and did I mention patience, of the F.A. Davis team including Margaret Biblis, Melissa Duffield, and the best Developmental Editor I could have ever hoped for, Jennifer Pine, for her coaching throughout the "birthing process." A very special thanks and all of my love to Jodi, Hilary, Jordyn, Nick, and Jordan for their support of this project, their commitment to the long hours of photos and video, and for their eternal patience. WE did it! There is no meaning in this without you!

Contents in Brief

Table of Contents

PART II
Philosophic Approaches to Orthopaedic Manual Physical Therapy   53

SECTION 1   Traditional Approaches   55
Chapter 4
The Principles and Practice of Osteopathic Manipulative Medicine   55
Michael L. Kuchera, DO, FAAO

Chapter 5
The Cyriax Approach   110
Russell Woodman, PT, MS, DPT, FSOM, OCS, MCTA

Chapter 12
The Functional Mobilization Approach   278

Gregory S. Johnson, PT, FFCFMT, FAAOMPT
Vicky Saliba Johnson, PT, FFCFMT, FAAOMPT
Rachel A. Miller, PT, MS, WCS, CFMT
Leslie Davis Rudzinski, PT, OCS, CFMT
Kristina M. Welsome, MSPT, DPT, OCS, CFMT, MTC

Chapter 13
Soft Tissue Mobilization Mobilization in Orthopaedic Manual Physical Therapy   306

Leslie Davis Rudzinski, PT, OCS, CFMT
Gregory S. Johnson, PT, FFCFMT, FAAOMPT

Perspectives and Principles in Orthopaedic Manual Physical Therapy

Historical Perspectives in Orthopaedic Manual Physical Therapy

Stanley V. Paris, PT, PhD, FAPTA, FNZSP (Hon), NZMTA (Hon), IFOMPT (Hon), FAAOMPT, MCSP

Chapter Objectives

At the conclusion of this chapter, the reader will be able to:

- Identify the history of and key contributing factors in the development of orthopaedic manual physical therapy (OMPT) in the United States.
- List the key figures who were instrumental in forming the foundations for the practice of modern OMPT.
- List important dates on which key events transpired that were critical to the establishment of the specialty of OMPT.
- Identify important organizations that were developed to support the clinical practice of and research in the area of OMPT.

- List key fundamental concepts and operant definitions that have served as the foundation of OMPT that are used extensively throughout this text.
- Identify current trends, opinions, and political issues currently surrounding and influencing the practice of OMPT in the United States.

THE BEGINNING

The Ancient Art of Manipulation

The origins of manual intervention for the relief of discomfort and improved mobility lie within us all. Who has not experienced the relief obtained from the cracking of joints or the stretching of muscles? Drawing back the shoulders, pulling the knees to the chest, stretching the hamstrings, or cracking the joints of the low back, have been innately performed throughout history for the resolution of soft tissue and joint restriction.

The act of walking upon an individual's back is a primitive method of manipulation, predating recorded history. Among the Indian tribes of North America, it was well known that general *bone setting* was skillfully practiced, particularly by the Sioux, Winnebago, and Creek tribes. However, the first recorded description and illustration of joint manipulation and traction techniques were by *Hippocrates* (460–355 BC) (Fig. 1–1). The "father of medicine" wrote at least three works on the bones and joints, including *On Setting Joints by Leverage*, in which he describes a combination of extension

(traction) and pressure (manipulation) exerted on a patient lying prone on a wooden bed.[1] Hippocrates also wrote about a number of techniques, including the reduction of dislocated joints, particularly of the shoulder, which was undoubtedly related to the popularity of wrestling in his time. With regard to spinal manipulation, he wrote, "it's not harmful to either sit on the back during traction or do a shaking movement while easing and sitting down again" (Fig. 1–2). As a result of his many teachings in the area of manual therapy, in addition to his contributions to the practice of medicine, Hippocrates could rightfully be identified as the "father of physical therapy," as well.

NOTABLE QUOTABLE

"It's not harmful to either sit on the back during traction or do a shaking movement while easing and sitting down again."

Hippocrates, 460–355 BC

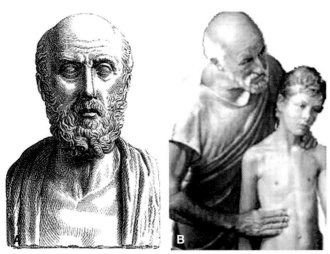

FIGURE 1-1 A. Hippocrates, **B.** Hippocrates healing a child. (Accessed from (a) http://www.med.utu.fi/opiskelu/laatuyksikkohakemus/medical_ethics.html (b) http://blog.bioethics.net/2006/01/, with permission)

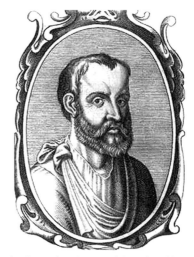

FIGURE 1-3 Claudius Galen. (Accessed from http://www.casebook.org/dissertations/rip-victorian-autopsy.html, with permission)

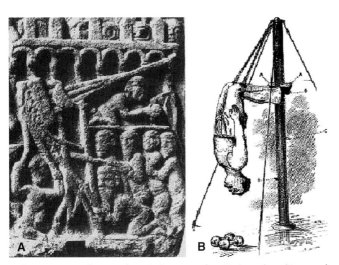

FIGURE 1-2 Ancient traction. **A.** Stone carving, **B.** Inversion. (Accessed from (a) http://www.siege-engine.com/SeussTrebuchet.shtml, (b) traction-http://www.energycenter.com/grav_f/inver_clay.html, with permission)

Claudius Galen[2] (131–202 AD) (Fig. 1–3), a famous Italian surgeon, wrote and illustrated extensively on the topic of manual therapy. In 18 of his 97 surviving theses, he comments on the work of Hippocrates, with illustrations of many of his manipulative techniques. These illustrations frequently adorn texts and treatises dealing with the history of medicine.

The Middle Ages and Renaissance

The Middle Ages represented a decline in medical knowledge throughout the Western world. During this time, the Church became responsible for most healing. For instance, *Saint Lawrence* was named the patron saint for those with backache.

During the Renaissance, the field of medicine was advanced through the work of *Andreas Vesalius* (Fig. 1–4), who in 1543 described the detailed anatomy of the entire human body. Vesalius was the first to outline the anatomy of the intervertebral disc, including differentiation between the annulus and the nucleus.

In 1579, *Ambroise Paré* (Fig. 1–5), famous surgeon to four successive French kings, did much to raise the standard of what has become orthopaedic surgery. For instance, he was the first to attempt trunk support using anterior and posterior metal plates made by armorers. He also used a considerable amount of manipulation, including many of the techniques described by Hippocrates. Paré wrote, "When the vertebrae are dislocated posteriorly and protrude, it is a good idea to put the patient in a prone position on the table. Fasten him to this with ties under his armpits, around the waist and the thighs and after that pull and stretch as much as possible upwards and downwards though without violence."[3]

NOTABLE QUOTABLE

"When the vertebrae are dislocated posteriorly and protrude, it is a good idea to put the patient in a prone position on the table . . . and after that pull and stretch as much as possible."

Ambroise Paré, 1579

THE DAWN OF MODERN MEDICINE

John Hunter (1728–1793) understood the value of movement of joints after injury for the prevention of stiffness and adhesions. Hunter recommended that adhesions, which remain as an end product of inflammation, should be stretched.

John Percivall Pott (1714–1788) has been associated with Pott's disease (known today as tuberculosis of the spine) and to Pott's fracture, the common characteristic break of one or both bones above the ankle (which, incidentally, he sustained when

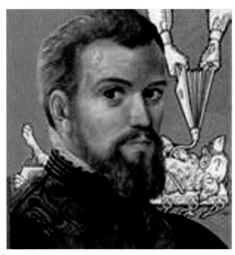

FIGURE 1–4 Andreus Vesalius. (Accessed from: http://clendening.kumc.edu/dc/pc/v.html, with permission)

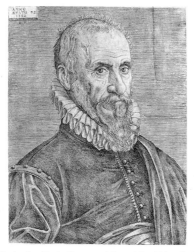

FIGURE 1–5 Ambroise Paré. (Accessed from http://clendening.kumc.edu/dc/pc/pare03.jpg, with permission)

he fell from his horse in 1769). Pott condemned extension exercises and manipulation as useless and dangerous in the management of the spine. Such an opinion, however, must be considered in the context of that time period in which tuberculosis was rampant and, in its early stages, indistinguishable from simple back pain.

In 1741, *Nicholas Andry* (1658–1742) was the first to use the term *orthopaedic*, from the Greek roots *orthos* (straight) and *paidion* (child) when writing his text, *Orthopaedia: or the Art of Correcting and Preventing Deformities in Children* at the age of 81. In the late 18th century, *Hay* described cases of manipulating the semilunar cartilage of the knee, followed by rest in its normal position. In 1784, *Edward Harrison* (1766–1838), a graduate of Edinburgh University, developed a sizable reputation in the use of manual medicine procedures, including manipulation.

In 1817, *James Parkinson* became interested in disorders of the cervical spine as a possible cause of spinal cord disease. This concept did not receive much attention until more

recent times when in 1956 **Lord Brain** and **Marcia Wilkinson** described how advanced stages of cervical spondylosis may result in myelopathy and simulate spinal cord diseases such as multiple sclerosis.[4] By the late 1990s, surgeons had found ways to halt the progress of myelopathy by removing osteophytes and through spinal fusion. Thus, surgery rather than conservative care currently dominates the treatment of this condition.

In 1842, *John Evans Riadore* (?–1861), a London physician practicing manipulation, wrote, "If an organ is insufficiently supplied with nervous energy or blood, its function is decreased, and sooner or later its structure becomes endangered."[5] This statement would be mirrored later in the century by the founder of osteopathy and later by the chiropractic field. In 1864, *Charles Lasègue* (1816–1883) was the first to describe the position in which back pain occurs upon straightening the knee when the leg has already been raised, which has become associated with impairment of the sciatic nerve. His name was later added to a modification of the straight leg raise test.

CLINICAL PILLAR

Since Riadore's proclamation in 1842, the field of medicine has understood that anatomical structures need an adequate neural and vascular supply as a requirement for sustained health and wellness.

Bone Setting

During the 17th and 18th centuries, the practice of *bone setting* was flourishing in Britain. Bone setting was a family affair, passed on from father to son, and occasionally to daughter, and was based on the belief that *little bones* could become out of place. The click that followed manipulation was attributed to the restoration of these little bones to their proper position. The father of *Hugh Owen Thomas* of Oswestry and the designer of the Thomas splint was a bonesetter. That same man was the uncle of *Sir Robert Jones*, the acknowledged father of British orthopaedics and a mentor to *Mary McMillan* (Fig. 1–6), the founder of physical therapy in America. Bonesetters, along with barber surgeons, were the forerunners of orthopaedic medicine and surgery in the United Kingdom. Their practice flourished during the 18th and 19th centuries, with a reduction in the practice of bone setting during the middle of the 20th century when physical therapy and osteopathy assumed a predominant role in the practice of manual interventions.

In 1867, *Sir James Paget* (1814–1899) (Fig. 1–7) gave lectures entitled "Cases That Bone Setters Cure," which were later published in the *British Medical Journal*. He gave the following advice: "learn then, to imitate what is good and avoid what is bad in the practice of bone-setters . . . too long a rest is, I believe, by far the most frequent cause of delayed recovery after injury of joints and not only to injured joints, but to those that are kept at rest because parts near them have been injured."[6]

NOTABLE QUOTABLE

"Learn then, to imitate what is good and avoid what is bad in the practice of bone-setters . . . too long a rest is, I believe, by far the most frequent cause of delayed recovery after injury of joints and not only to injured joints, but to those that are kept at rest because parts near them have been injured."

Sir James Paget, 1867

FIGURE 1-6 Mary McMillan. (Accessed from www.apta.org, with permission)

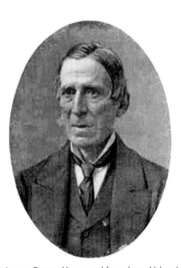

FIGURE 1-7 Sir James Paget. (Accessed from http://clendening.kumc.edu/dc/pc/paget.jpg with permission)

In 1871, **Wharton Hood** published *On Bone-Setting*,[7] the first such book by an orthodox medical practitioner. Hood believed that the snapping sound frequently heard with manipulation was that of adhesions being broken, not that of bones going back into place. Hood's father, also a physician, had been treated effectively by a well-known bonesetter named **Hutton**. This led Hood, the son, to study the topic. By 1870, manipulation was firmly established in contemporary medicine. It was the topic of meetings and papers, and a book had been devoted

to the subject. It is important to note the acceptance of manipulation by the medical community preceded the founding of osteopathy in America by 4 years and chiropractic by 28 years.

In 1882, bone setting was the main topic at the annual meeting of the **British Medical Association's Section on Surgery**. **H. Marsh**[8] and **R. Fox**[9] both considered the term, "manipulation," favorably but instead used the term "bone setting." During the early part of the 20th century, **T.M. Marlin**,[10] **B. Blundell-Bankart**,[11] **H.J. Burrows** and **W.D. Coltart**,[12] and **F.H. Humphris**[13] were among the medical practitioners who were writing on the subject of manipulation.

QUESTIONS *for* REFLECTION

- From what particular discipline did the practice of manipulation first emerge?
- Who should receive credit for bringing the practice of manipulation to the United States?
- Does the practice of manipulation belong to any one specific discipline or ideology?
- Based on these historical perspectives, should the practice of manipulation be exclusive to any one profession or discipline?

Osteopathic Medicine

The discipline of osteopathic medicine and surgery was founded by **Andrew Taylor Still** (1828–1917) (Fig. 1–8) (see Chapter 4). Still was an eccentric nonconformist who had raised considerable wrath among his medical contemporaries who had little time for him or his views. Intending to become a physician like his father, Still attended the **Physicians and Surgeons College of Medicine** in Kansas City. Still's formal medical training coupled with his innovative mind, culminated in the founding of osteopathy on July 22, 1874. In regards to his discovery of this new discipline, Still wrote, "Like a burst of sunshine, the whole truth dawned on my mind."[14] Contrary to the conventional medical philosophy of his day, Still postulated that when joints were restricted in motion because of mechanical locking or other related causes were normalized, certain disease conditions improved.

NOTABLE QUOTABLE

"Like a burst of sunshine the whole truth dawned on my mind. . . ."

Andrew Taylor Still, July 22, 1874 (on the founding of osteopathy)

Taylor stated, "The rule of the artery is absolute, universal, and it must be unobstructed, or disease will result." This statement formed the basis of what became known in osteopathy as the **law of the artery** (Box 1-1). This foundational osteopathic concept has been briefly stated as follows: (1) the body is a unit; (2) structure and function are reciprocally interrelated; and (3) the body possesses self-regulatory mechanisms for

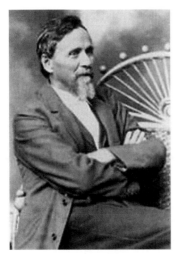

FIGURE 1–8 Andrew Taylor Still. (Accessed from http://www.rocky vistauniversity.org/do.asp, with permission)

Box 1-1 Quick Notes! THE LAW OF THE ARTERY

- The body is a unit.
- Structure and function are reciprocally interrelated.
- The body possesses self-regulatory mechanisms for rational therapies based on an understanding of body unity, self-regulatory mechanisms, and the interrelation of structure and function.

rational therapies based on an understanding of body unity, self-regulatory mechanisms, and the interrelation of structure and function.

As the discipline of osteopathy evolved, it began to embrace current advances in traditional medicine while still maintaining its unique philosophical underpinnings. As a result, by the late 19th century, osteopathy was losing some of its appeal because it no longer claimed to be the panacea for every human ailment. As osteopathy became more aligned with orthodox medical practice, a void was created in the area of manual medicine.

By 1928, osteopathic physicians in the United States achieved equal rights with allopathic physicians in the Armed Forces, and by 1970 they achieved such rights within each state. Today's osteopathic physicians are engaged in maintaining their necessary medical knowledge, and many do not remain active in the practice of manipulative medicine. In many osteopathic hospitals, physical therapists provide the manipulative care and, in some cases, give instruction to osteopaths.

QUESTIONS *for* REFLECTION

Despite their formal training, why have doctors of osteopathy, with some exceptions, largely given over their practice of manipulation?

A branch of osteopathy was originated by ***William Garner Sutherland*** (1873–1954) (Fig. 1–9). In 1966, he marveled at the intricacy and design of the cranial sutures and founded a collection of clinical techniques known as **cranial osteopathy**.[15] Current practitioners of craniosacral technique claim they can detect and treat cranial rhythm dysfunction through gentle touch. Unfortunately, they have been unable to demonstrate reliability in their palpation techniques and have failed to produce sufficient documentation of viable outcomes in published literature. Despite proclamations of treatment effectiveness by its practitioners, in this age of evidence-based practice, cranial osteopathy has undergone much skepticism.

Chiropractic

In 1895, ***Daniel David Palmer*** (1845–1913) (Fig. 1–10), a former green grocer and practicing magnetic healer, founded chiropractic medicine. From the Greek words *cheir* (hand) and *praxis* (done by hand), the discipline of chiropractic had its beginning in the void left by the osteopaths. Some proponents of chiropractic attribute the discovery of manipulation to Palmer. However, Palmer himself makes it quite clear in his book *The Chiropractor's Adjustor* that this was not the case and

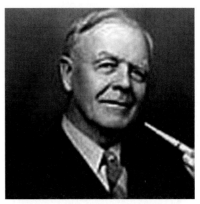

FIGURE 1–9 William Garner Sutherland. (Accessed from http://www.csontmester.hu/kez_tort.html, with permission)

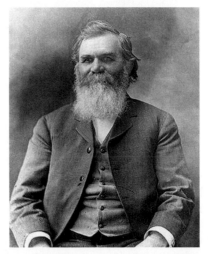

FIGURE 1–10 Daniel David Palmer. (Accessed from http://www.massagenerd.com/_massage_articles_famous_pictures_H.html, with permission)

that indeed he had learned it from a medical practitioner. Palmer stated, "The art of repositioning subluxed vertebra has been practiced for thousands of years. . . . My first acquaintance of this refers to physician *Jim Atkinson*, who practiced in Davenport, Iowa, 50 years ago, and who during his lifetime tried to announce his principles, which are now known as 'chiropractique.'" He also added that his work was a "rediscovery and revival of ancient Hellenic healing practice." Palmer writes, "But I insist on being the first who has repositioned a dislocated vertebra by using the spinous and transverse processes as balance levers . . . and out of this fundamental fact I have founded a science which is decided to revolutionize the art of healing's theory and practice."[16] The foundation of chiropractic manipulation, by the founder's admission, emerged from the medical model. Interestingly, Hippocrates and Galen could both challenge Palmer's assertion as the first to reposition a "dislocated" vertebra.

In 1947, *J. Janse*, *R.H. Houser*, and *B.V. Wells* defined the theoretical basis of chiropractic as follows: (1) that a vertebra may become subluxed; (2) that this subluxation tends to impinge other structures (nerves, blood vessels, and lymphatics passing through the intervertebral foramen); (3) that, as a result of impingement, the function of the corresponding segment of the spinal cord and its connecting spinal and automatic nerves are interfered with and the function of the nerve impulse impaired; (4) that, as a result thereof, the innervation to certain parts of the organism is abnormally altered and such parts become functionally or organically diseased or predisposed; and (5) that adjustment of a subluxed vertebra removes the impingement of the structure passing through the intervertebral foramen, thereby restoring to diseased parts their normal innervation and rehabilitating them functionally and organically.[17] In chiropractic, the above philosophy became known as the **law of the nerve** (Box 1-2).

Although traditional chiropractic theory, whose practitioners are known as **straights,** has declined in more recent years, these concepts persist as the primary teaching emphasis in several existing chiropractic schools. Most chiropractors today may be referred to as **mixers.** A mixer is a chiropractor who mixes traditional chiropractic philosophy with modern physical therapy rehabilitation techniques. In many states, chiropractors may claim that they perform physical therapy procedures, however, chiropractors may not legally promote themselves as physical therapists. Since chiropractic traditionally claimed to be a panacea through the use of spinal adjustments, manipulation was, for many years, the target of orthodox medicine.

In 1975, a conference sponsored by the *National Institute of Neurological Disease and Stroke* was held in Washington, D.C. At the conference, which was titled *The Research Status of Spinal Manipulative Therapy,*[18] chiropractic adopted the term **subluxation** to include virtually every known dysfunction of the spine. If chiropractic was able to prove the existence of the subluxation and its relationship to medical pathology, chiropractors might expect to receive Medicare reimbursement for their services.

Attending this conference as invited participants were *Dr. James Cyriax* (Fig. 1–11) and *Dr. John Mennell*. The American Physical Therapy Association (APTA) had received an invitation, however, President *Stanley Paris* (Fig. 1–12) and Vice President *Sandy Burkhart* of the *Orthopaedic Section* were denied the ability to represent the APTA and listened to the proceedings from a nearby annex. They were indeed vexed when *Scott Haldeman*, speaking for chiropractic, exclaimed that "the absence of physical therapists from this conference clearly shows their lack of interest in this field."

QUESTIONS *for* REFLECTION

- What is the primary difference between the law of the artery and the law of the nerve?
- Does the profession of physical therapy ascribe to either of these philosophies or portions thereof?
- What are the major differences and similarities between physical therapy, chiropractic, and osteopathy in regard to the use of manipulation?

Box 1-2 **Quick Notes! THE LAW OF THE NERVE**

- A vertebra may become subluxed.
- This subluxation impinges upon other structures (nerves, blood vessels, and lymphatics passing through the intervertebral foramen).
- As a result, the function of the corresponding segment of the spinal cord and its connecting spinal and automatic nerves is interfered with and the function of the nerve impulse impaired.
- As a result, the innervation is abnormally altered, leading to functionally or organically diseased structures.
- Adjustment of a subluxed vertebra removes the impingement, thereby restoring normal innervation and rehabilitating them functionally and organically.

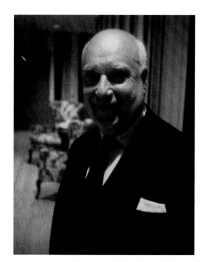

FIGURE 1–11 James Cyriax. (Accessed from http://www.drgoodley.com/site/history.php?id=photoalbum, with permission)

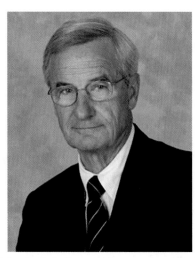

FIGURE 1–12 Stanley Paris. (Accessed from www.usa.edu, with permission)

In 1981, the traditional opposition to chiropractic and other practices considered cultist by the **American Medical Association** and its **Committee on Quackery**, which had also investigated the author of this chapter, was forced to cease. In Chicago, **Chester Wilkes** and others successfully sued the AMA,[19] most notably its Committee on Quackery, on the grounds of restraint of trade. Consequently, today's medical school graduates do not receive AMA-endorsed literature outlining the perceived shortcomings of chiropractic philosophy as had previous generations.

Physical Therapy and Medical Manipulation

It is not possible to speak of manipulation within physical therapy without speaking of manipulation within medicine. Out of the medical model, physical therapy emerged for the purpose of aiding rehabilitation. As such, the history of the two professions is intimately intertwined.

It is difficult to determine when the profession of physical therapy actually began. In Scandinavia, there were a number of groups existing under different names that practiced massage and therapeutic exercise. In Sweden, during the mid-1800s, there were two rival groups: one in rehabilitation and the other in medicine. Both were professional, male-dominated, and required training. However, after a protracted struggle, the medical group became predominant and began admitting less-qualified individuals. Their acceptance of females helped them to gain social and political control of what was to become physiotherapy. Consequently, physiotherapy soon became a female-dominated profession.

In 1899, physiotherapy was founded in England (Box 1-3). It already existed under other names: massage and medical gymnastics or massage and movement. At that time, the two individuals most associated with instruction of manipulation to physical therapists were the fathers and sons, **James** and **John Mennell** and **Edger** and **James Cyriax**. In 1907 James Mennell, MD, aligned himself with the newly formed **Society of Trained Masseuses**, later known as the **Chartered Society of**

Box 1-3 Quick Notes! IMPORTANT DATES IN THE ADVENT OF PHYSICAL THERAPY

- **1899:** Physiotherapy was founded in England.
- James and John Mennell and Edger and James Cyriax were most associated with instruction of manipulation to physical therapists.
- **1921:** Physical therapy established in the United States as the **American Women's Physical Therapeutic Association.**

Physiotherapy. He instructed joint and soft tissue manipulation techniques, and he encouraged his medical colleagues to send patients to "these ladies" by prescription. One such "lady," **Gwen Hislop**, trained with Mennell during World War II and later carried her knowledge to New Zealand after the war.[20] James and John Mennell also published a number of texts on the subject, largely directed toward physical therapists.[21]

In 1921, physical therapy was established in the United States as the **American Women's Physical Therapeutic Association** to "make available efficiently trained women to the medical profession."[22] The need for such trained individuals had been clearly demonstrated during and following World War I. In the second edition of *Massage and Therapeutic Exercise*, Mary McMillan wrote of the four branches of physiotherapy, referring to them as "manipulation of muscle and joints, therapeutic exercise, electrotherapy, and hydrotherapy."[23]

In 1923, speaking to the American Physiotherapy Association, **Robin McKenzie** (Fig. 1–13) advocated that "if we will only pay attention as we should to the study of physiological effects of physiotherapy to the technique of manipulation, to the procedures of massage, and to this question of re-education, we will go far to establish, in its proper relationship, the kinship of Physiotherapy to the general practice of medicine, and we will be able to show up in their true light those pseudo cults which have flourished so luxuriantly because of our neglect."[24] He was, of course, referring to chiropractic and, at that time, no doubt, to osteopathy as well.

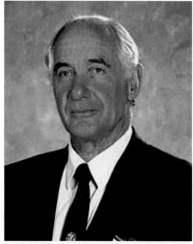

FIGURE 1–13 Robin McKenzie. (Accessed from http://physiomedicine.com/robinmckenzie.aspx, with permission)

Also in 1923, in *Physiotherapy Technique: A Manual of Applied Physics*, *C.M. Sampson* wrote of the physiotherapy staff, "All of the aides were highly trained in massage, manipulation, exercises, etc. and most were trained in one or more departments where electrical treatments were given." He also noted, "No fibrosed joint should be pronounced hopeless until . . . progressively strenuous manipulations have failed."[25]

The 1930s saw the integration of arthrokinematic principles and assessment into clinical practice. Movement had been traditionally described as the spatial relationship of the limbs (or trunk) to the axis of the body. Thus joint movement was described as adduction, abduction, flexion, extension, rotation, etc., with very little attention to the actual movements taking place within the joints themselves, such as roll, glide, and spin. In 1927, *T. Walmsley* began introducing new terminology, known as **arthrokinematics,** which was later adopted by *Gray's British Anatomy*. Walmsley noted, among other observations, that the articular surfaces of joints are incongruous except in one special position (*Walmsley's law*).[26] This special position of joint congruency is now defined as **close packed.** Some years later, *Freddy Kaltenborn,* a Norwegian physiotherapist, saw the significance of the emerging field of arthrokinematics and applied it to the practice of joint manipulation, thus developing an entirely new approach to manipulation that was distinctive to physical therapy. He partnered with *Olaf Evjenth* in establishing what has become known as the *Nordic Approach to OMPT* (Fig. 1–14) (see Chapter 6).

In 1930, *G.W. Leadbetter* published in *The Physiotherapy Review (American)* a discussion of *mechanistic derangements* of the lumbar spine and sacroiliac region: "In cases of unilateral sacroiliac strain which resist the above treatment, one should consider the necessity of manipulation."[27] In 1932, *Humphris* and *Stuart-Webb* defined the mechanical effects of physiotherapy as "massage and manipulation, with exercises active and passive and mechanovibration."[28] *Ghormley* described what he called the *facet syndrome*. He felt that arthritic changes in the facets or a narrowing of the intervertebral foramen as a result of these changes were the etiology of many cases of sciatica.[29] As it turned out, his description of the facet syndrome was one that did not have an operable solution, and it would soon be overshadowed by the discovery of disc protrusions.

On September 30, 1933, and *Joseph S. Barr* and *William Jason Mixter* (Fig. 1–15) presented an epoch-making paper to the annual meeting of the *New England Surgical Society* in Boston. They pointed out a chondroma causing a herniation of the nucleus of an intervertebral disc and suggested surgery as the most reasonable solution. Published in the *New England Journal of Medicine* in 1934, this paper forever changed the way surgeons would look at low back pain,[30] and the "dynasty" of the disc was born.

In 1936, *M.C. Thornhill*, writing in *Physical Therapy*, reported on a presentation by *Troedsson* at the annual session of the *American Congress of Physical Therapy*. The presentation was titled, *Manipulative Treatment for the Lumbosacral Derangement for the Relief of Pain in the Lumbosacral Region*. The presentation was submitted for publication because, to quote Troedsson, "the manipulation can be carried out by the technician, even though the patient may be large and muscular." Also, "until the muscle spasm subsides or some change in the position of the facets takes place, as by manipulation, pains may persist."[31]

This would be the last article on joint manipulation in the journal *Physical Therapy* for the next 30 years, until *Bruce McCaleb*, with the help of John Mennell, published in 1969. Because of the explosive growth of chiropractic in the 1930s, with its claims of manipulation as a panacea, these procedures subsequently slipped into disrepute. During this time, the profession of physical therapy in the United States distanced itself from association with both the term and practice of manipulation.

In 1946, *Sir Morton Smart* wrote extensively concerning adhesions forming within a joint following injury, stating that these adhesions are common even from minor joint injuries. As a surgeon, he spoke of manipulative surgery as the art of moving a joint through all of its ranges. He also wrote on **end feel,** when he stated that adhesions have a "springy feel" similar to muscle spasm and that ligaments do not.[32] In 1948, *Leube* working with

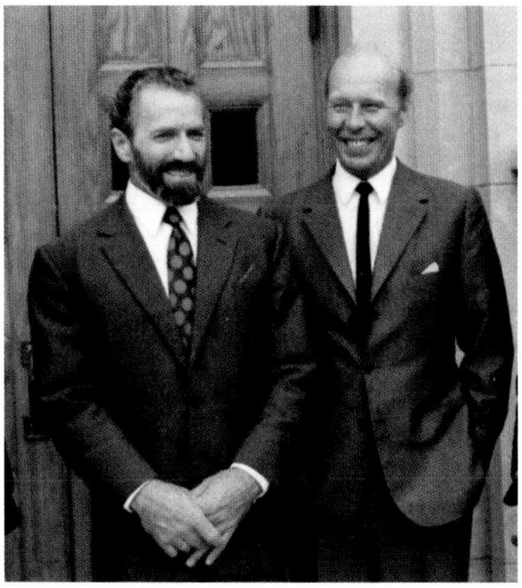

FIGURE 1–14 Olaf Evjenth (left) and Freddy Kaltenborn (right), 1972. (Accessed from http://www.drgoodley.com/site/history.php?id=photoalbum, with permission)

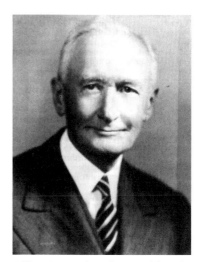

FIGURE 1–15 William Jason Mixter. (Accessed from http://clendening. kumc.edu/dc/pc/mixter.jpg, with permission)

Elizabeth Dicke (Fig. 1–16) of Holland, published a book entitled, *Massage of the Reflex Zones in the Connective Tissue.*[33] In that same year, *James Cyriax* published his theories on practice in the British medical journal, *The Lancet,*[34] and in 1957, he published the third edition of *Textbook of Orthopaedic Medicine* in two volumes.[35] Volume 1 had already become a classic and is valuable to this day for its clarity in differentiating between the soft tissues when examining for dysfunction.

Cyriax envisaged that a sudden onset of back pain was due to a crack and displacement of the annulus that could be manipulated back into place. In contrast, a gradual onset of back pain was due to a protrusion of the nucleus, and this would best be drawn back through the use of traction. It was Cyriax who popularized the term, "end feel" while attempting to distinguish between normal and abnormal tissue. He also trained physiotherapists and advocated for their role in the performance of manipulation (see Chapter 5).

In 1955 at the University of Iowa, *Arthur Steindler*, in his work, *Kinesiology of the Human Body Under Normal and Pathological Conditions*, summarized earlier research and added a great deal of additional arthrokinematic knowledge regarding both joint function and dysfunction.[36] This information would later be used by physical therapists who endeavored to correlate manipulative therapeutic techniques to the principles of joint function. Thus, the new science of arthrokinematics, which had begun with Walmsley and later *M.A. MacConaill*, was to shape much of the future practice of joint manipulation, in particular the approaches espoused by Kaltenborn, Paris, and *Brian Mulligan* (Fig. 1–17).

In 1960, in New Zealand, the *British Medical Association* made the following statement to the *Health Committee*, which was considering a chiropractic bill: "The medical profession readily acknowledges that spinal manipulation is of great value for certain spinal ailments, but emphasizes that these maneuvers should be carried out by properly trained personnel—the orthopaedic surgeon, the specialist in physical medicine, or the physiotherapist under medical direction." In 1961, Fred Kaltenborn began teaching about the mobilization of joints

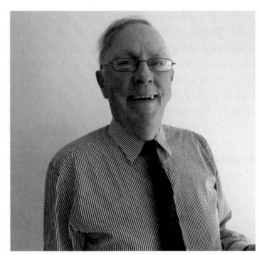

FIGURE 1–17 Brian Mulligan. (Accessed from http://mobilidadefuncional. blogspot.com/2009/10/brian-mulligan-personagem-da-nossa.html, with permission)

based upon a biomechanical model and in 1976 published *Manual Therapy for the Extremity Joints: Specialized Techniques, Tests, and Joint Mobilization*, which has since passed into several editions and languages. His text was the first to relate manipulation to the new knowledge of arthrokinematics.[37] Kaltenborn spent most of the years after 1971 instructing manipulation to physical therapists worldwide (Fig. 1–18). (See Chapter 6.)

In 1962, the *Congress on Manual Medicine* held its first meeting in Nice, France. The congress later became known as the *International Federation of Manual Medicine.* In 1963, the *British Association of Manual Medicine* was formed. At a 1966 meeting of the association, James Cyriax supported physiotherapists continuing to learn manipulation. In 1963, after returning from studies in Europe and North America, S.V. Paris, while on the faculty of the *New Zealand School of Physiotherapy*, published an article in the *New Zealand Medical Journal* titled "The Theory and Technique of Specific Spinal Manipulation." He wrote, "Degeneration will commence in any joint in which there is loss of movement. . . . While this is happening, other joints above and

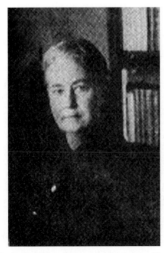

FIGURE 1–16 Elizabeth Dicke. (Accessed from http://www.massagenerd. com/_massage_articles_famous_pictures_E.html, with permission)

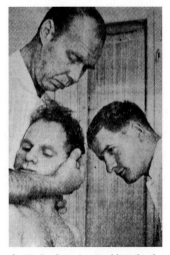

FIGURE 1–18 Stanley Paris observing Freddy Kaltenborn perform cervical manipulation, 1960.

below . . . will have to compensate . . . . They will become hyper-mobile and suffer injury and degeneration." His teachings spoke of the spinal lesion, which later he called **dysfunction.** In 1965, he further developed these ideas in the book, *The Spinal Lesion* (see Chapter 7).[38]

In 1964, ***Geoffrey Maitland*** (Fig. 1–19) of Australia published *Vertebral Manipulation*, in which he refined the art of oscillatory manipulation and used it almost exclusively to treat *reproducible signs*. His approach was to identify either an active or passive movement that was painful, to oscillate that joint, and to test again. If it hurt less, he continued with the oscillations; if there was no change, then he tried a different oscillatory technique that he had observed would be the next most likely to succeed.[39] It is quite possible that Maitland was heavily influenced by ***Robert Maigne*** (Fig. 1–20) of France, who spoke of using manipulation for the relief of pain and who demonstrated repetitive motion to achieve that goal. Conversely, Kaltenborn, Paris, and Mulligan placed their emphasis on the restoration of movement. Maitland's two books *Peripheral Manipulation* and *Vertebral Manipulation* provide a full exposition of his principles and methods.[40] He has instructed extensively

in Australia, where he resided, and in England and Switzerland before his death in 2010 (see Chapter 8).

In 1966, Paris and John Mennell met with ***T.L. Northrup***, the editor of the professional newspaper, ***DO***, resulting in an article by Paris titled "Joint Manipulation: How You (osteopaths) Can Make Manipulation Succeed." This article was directed at gaining support for physical therapists to practice manipulation upon referral from osteopaths.[41]

On October 26, 1966, physical therapists Maitland, ***G. Grieve***, Kaltenborn, and Paris met for the first time in London and discussed setting up an international body to exchange educational ideas and to maintain standards in manual and manipulative therapy (Fig. 1–21). Other therapists present were ***Hickling, Martin-Jones, Dyer,*** and ***Williams***. In all, five countries were represented. Eight years later, as an outgrowth of that meeting, the ***International Federation of Orthopaedic Manipulative Physical Therapists (IFOMPT)*** was formed.

In 1966, ***R. Melzack*** and ***P.D. Wall*** proposed the **gate control** theory of pain, providing an explanation of how large nerve fiber stimulation from joints and muscles can block the transmission and perception of pain. Their theory enabled a better understanding of how such modalities as acupuncture, transcutaneous electrical nerve stimulation (TENS), and other pain-blocking techniques, such as spinal cord implants, could result in pain relief.[42] While manipulation was widely accepted as having psychological and mechanical effects, the gate control theory provided a possible explanation for neurophysiological effects. It would be some years before manipulation was shown to release endorphins, thus accounting for a chemical effect.

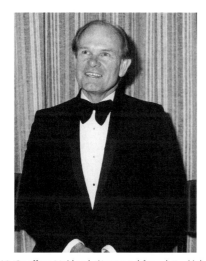

FIGURE 1–19 Geoffrey Maitland. (Accessed from http://physical-therapy. advanceweb.com/Article/Honoring-Our-Giants.aspx, with permission)

CLINICAL PILLAR

The gate control theory proposed by Melzack and Wall in 1966 provided an explanation of how large nerve fiber stimulation from joints and muscles can block the transmission and perception of pain. This theory may also be used to explain the neurophysiological effects provided through manipulation.

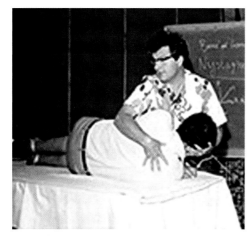

FIGURE 1–20 Robert Maigne, 1971. (Accessed from http://www.drgoodley. com/site/history.php?id=photoalbum, with permission)

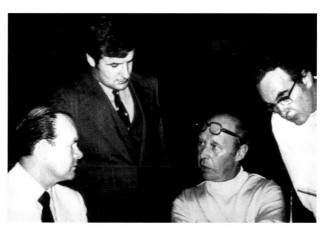

FIGURE 1–21 Inauguration of IFOMPT with Maitland, Paris, Kaltenborn, Grieve, 1974.

In 1966, the **World Confederation for Physical Therapy (WCPT)** was formed in London. Four years later, at the second WCPT Congress in Amsterdam, a group interested in spinal and extremity manipulation and other manual therapy techniques set up a steering committee to form an international body. Paris was chair, and consultants were Kaltenborn, Maitland, and Grieve. Four years later in Montreal, IFOMPT was formed.

In 1967 Mennell and **Janet Travell** (Fig. 1–22), White House physician to President John F. Kennedy and later of trigger point fame, set up the **North American Academy of Manipulative Medicine**. Paris wrote Travell asking for physical therapists to be admitted as members, or at least as associate members. Travell replied that "manipulation was a diagnostic and therapeutic tool that should be reserved for physicians only." Paris then approached the APTA to form a manipulation section but was informed by the then president that there was no place for clinical sections. The only two sections in existence at that time were Education and Private Practice.

Therefore, in August 1968, the **North American Academy of Manipulation Therapy** was founded in Boston, Massachusetts, and chaired by Paris. It represented physiotherapists from Canada and physical therapists from the United States in their efforts to have spinal and extremity joint manipulation further recognized by their profession with additional post-professional education. Within 6 short years, membership would grow to 942.

In 1969, B. McCaleb, a physical therapist influenced by Mennell, published in *Physical Therapy* "An Introduction to Spinal Manipulation," in which he set out the concepts of *joint play* and stated that manipulation was helpful for joint dysfunction. He described the latter as a " partial absence or total absence of joint movement, called a joint lock."[43]

In 1970, John Mennell published "Rationale of Joint Manipulation" in *Physical Therapy*. He outlined his philosophy and stated, "Then you may say, 'But I cannot use manipulative techniques even if I learn them unless they are prescribed.' If you say this you are ignorant of the resolutions which the House of Delegates of the APTA made last year."[44]

In 1974, APTA agreed to the formation of the **Orthopaedic Section of the American Physical Therapy Association** and Paris was named as its first president (Fig. 1–23). As a result, the North American Academy of Manual & Manipulative Therapy was dissolved because it had reached its objective of establishing this specialty section.

Also in 1974, IFOMPT was inaugurated in Montreal, Canada, during the meeting of the World Congress for Physical Therapy under the chairmanship of Paris. There were 13 member nations at the inaugural meeting, and **Richard Erhard** (Fig. 1–24) from the United States was elected president, with **Peter Edgelow,** also of the United States, as secretary. In 1976, **Mariano Rocabado** (Fig. 1–25) of Chile introduced to U.S. physical therapists the role of physical therapy in the diagnosis and management of craniomandibular disorders.

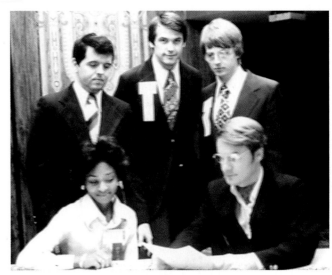

FIGURE 1–23 Inauguration of Orthopaedic Section. Standing: Burkhart, Personius, Gould; Seated: Glover, Paris. 1974

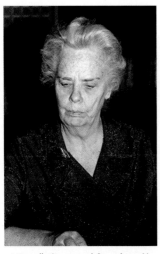

FIGURE 1–22 Janet Travell. (Accessed from http://www.drgoodley.com/site/history.php?id=photoalbum, with permission)

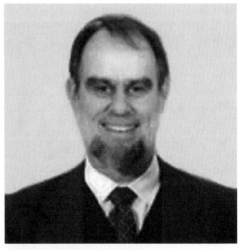

FIGURE 1–24 Richard Erhard. (Accessed from http://www.utimes.pitt.edu/?p=9978, with permission)

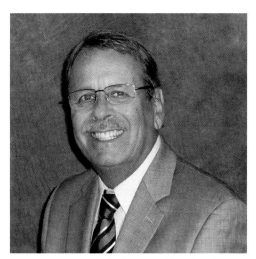

FIGURE 1–25 Mariano Rocabado. (Accessed from http://www.aacfp.org/pdf_files/AACP_2007_Summer_Symposium_Brochure.pdf, with permission)

In 1978, IFOMPT became the first specialty subsection of the WCPT, a status that has since helped member nations gain increasing acceptance for joint manipulation within physical therapy.

In the late 1970s, McKenzie began to popularize the concept of spinal extension for the treatment of low back pain. He felt that the centralization of pain that often follows repetitive motion was due to reducing disc protrusions. His methods have gained wide acceptance, in part because of extensive research that has compared the results of his regimen with others such as Williams' flexion exercises and proponents of the Back School. McKenzie also advocated the use of manipulative techniques, primarily when self-management efforts are insufficient. In 1989, McKenzie cautioned the profession, "I believe we have overvalued the benefits of manipulative therapy, overcomplicated the teaching of manipulative therapy and have applied the technique with inadequate discrimination."[45] (See Chapter 9.)

In 1982, **J.P. Farrell** and **L.T. Twomey**, physical therapists, compared two approaches in conservative treatment and produced a paper often quoted in meta-analyses as having met the rigors of research design. Their study showed that the duration of low back pain symptoms was significantly shorter in patients who received manipulation as compared with those who received standard physical therapy treatment consisting of microwave diathermy, isometric abdominal exercises, and ergonomic instruction; this shortened duration of back pain was also accomplished in fewer treatment sessions.[46]

In 1983, **Richard Deyo**, in an article titled "Conservative Therapy for Low Back Pain," commented on the quality of numerous studies that failed to validate the practices they often advocated. On exercise, he wrote, "The best study was that by Kendall and Jenkins, which demonstrated an advantage of flexion exercises over either general mobilization exercises or extension exercises."[47] Regarding manipulation, Deyo wrote, "Spinal manipulation remains highly controversial, partly because in the United States it is often equated with the practice of chiropractic.

In Great Britain and other Commonwealth countries, however, spinal manipulation by physicians or physical therapists is more common and several clinical trials have been conducted."[48] In 1990 the prestigious **International Society for the Study of the Lumbar Spine**, whose membership is restricted to physicians, surgeons, biomechanists, physical therapists, and chiropractors, published *Lumbar Spine*, in which the only chapter on manipulation was written by a physical therapist.[49]

In the early 1990s, Mulligan, a New Zealand–trained physiotherapist, introduced American physical therapists to the concept of manipulation with movement (see Chapter 10). His premise includes the notion that applying manipulative pressure to the joint or soft tissue during performance of an active movement will greatly facilitate its return to normal function.[50] **Robert Elvey** of Australia explored and developed neural mobilization, which has become popular in current physical therapy practice[51] (see Chapter 19).

In 1991, the **American Academy of Orthopaedic Manual Physical Therapists (AAOMPT)** was founded, with Farrell as the first president. The academy was later accepted for membership in IFOMPT. The AAOMPT established residency standards for manual therapy training in the United States. The president of the APTA is the official liaison to the academy.

In 1993, the House of Delegates of the APTA defined physical therapy, noting that "an exhaustive list of things to be enumerated is not possible but the following should be considered: . . . exercise with and without devices, joint mobilization, manipulation, . . . [and] massage."[52]

NOTABLE QUOTABLE

"An exhaustive list of things to be enumerated is not possible but the following should be considered: . . . exercise with and without devices, joint mobilization, manipulation, . . . massage."

APTA House of Delegates, 1993 (on defining physical therapy)

As a result of a letter-writing campaign, a joint task force formed by AAOMPT, the Orthopaedic Section, and the APTA a strategic plan regarding manipulation-related initiatives was created. This task force remains in effect and has been instrumental in winning nearly 20 of the last 22 chiropractic-related battles. It is clear now that physical therapists have established themselves as competent and effective practitioners whose practice requires the use of these techniques.

The joint task force that was created to support the use of these techniques among physical therapists developed a document in 2004 entitled **Manipulation Education Manual (MEM)**, which was designed to advocate and assist in the implementation of manual therapy instruction, including thrust in the first professional curricula of physical therapists[53] and as such to meet the standards now required for accreditation by the **Commission on Accreditation in Physical Therapy Education (CAPTE)**.

PRESENT DAY PRACTICES AND ATTITUDES

The Osteopathic Manipulation Model

Mainstream osteopathy has, in many environments, reduced its use of manipulation in clinical practice precipitated by the need to remain current in medicine. Consequently, many osteopaths refer patients to chiropractors and physical therapists for these services.

There are, of course, osteopaths who still practice traditional manipulation related to the management of movement restrictions. Two of the more prominent osteopaths, *Fred Mitchell* and *Phillip Greenman*, have placed an emphasis on the perceived position of the vertebra. Michigan State University, which has the largest program in graduate osteopathic manipulation, emphasizes management of positional faults[54] (see Chapter 4). The field of chiropractic has increasingly moved away from the notion of positional faults to a more movement-based paradigm.

The Medical Manipulation Model

Within the medical community, manipulation is represented in the United States by the North American Academy of Manipulative Medicine, which has both osteopathic (doctors of osteopathy) and allopathic (medical doctor) members. Internationally, the *Federation of International Manual Medicine* advocates the use of manipulation techniques. Generally, U.S. medical professionals today refer those in need of manipulation to physical therapists and increasingly to chiropractors and other alternative health-care practitioners.

The Chiropractic Manipulation Model

The chiropractic profession has, by and large, recognized that it is movement of joints, not the position of vertebra, that they must treat. However, all chiropractic schools teach traditional theory, and two, namely *Life University* in Atlanta and California, remain principally traditional, or so-called straight. In April 1997, *Craig Little*, DC, past president of the *American Chiropractic Association's* representative to the *AMA's Health Care Professional's Advisory Committee (HCPAC)*, redefined chiropractic terminology in a letter to *Helene Fearon*, chair of the *Practice Committee of the Orthopaedic Section of the APTA*. He stated that "manipulation" has been redefined as a manual procedure that involves a directed thrust to move a joint past the physiological range of motion, without exceeding the anatomical limit. He further defined "mobilization" as a movement applied singularly or repetitively within or at the physiological range of motion, without imparting a thrust or impulse, with the goal of restoring mobility.

It should be noted that, up until the late 1980s, most chiropractic schools spoke of subluxations and the treatment for these subluxations as adjustments. More recently, chiropractors have begun to use terms that have been traditionally associated with the profession of physical therapy, such as "movement science" and "manipulation."

The Physical Therapy Manipulation Model

Since their inception, physical therapists have included within their armamentarium of clinical practice joint manipulation and mobilization procedures. Initially as massage and therapeutic exercise practitioners, later as reconstruction aides and medically-trained technicians, and now as autonomous professionals with direct patient access, physical therapy has always included the use of skilled passive movement as an important strategy for the amelioration of movement impairments. Since the 1950s, the profession has built on the basic medical sciences, especially in the area of arthrokinematics and neural tension, to devise newer, more relevant treatment techniques and management strategies. Initially these procedures were unique to the discipline of physical therapy but more recently have been adopted by other practitioners. Kaltenborn, Maitland, Grieve, Paris, McKenzie, Elvey, and Mulligan, to name a few, have added to the unique body of knowledge that today constitutes the science and art of physical therapy and manipulation in the musculoskeletal arena. Physical therapists make their diagnosis based not on disease as in the medical model, but rather on functional limitations and pathomechanics. Manipulation consists of both thrust and nonthrust techniques and is routinely accompanied by soft tissue intervention, therapeutic exercise, passive modalities, and patient instruction, among other procedures. This unique area of specialized clinical practice is increasingly referred to as "orthopaedic manual therapy" or, more correctly, *orthopaedic manual physical therapy (OMPT)*. The practice of manipulation by physical therapists has become quite eclectic. Most practitioners have incorporated mechanical, isometric, and oscillatory techniques. For this reason, this text will present an eclectic overview of each of the approaches that have most profoundly influenced the physical therapist's current practice of OMPT.

Throughout the text, the terms joint **manipulation** and joint **mobilization** will be used synonymously and defined as the "skilled passive movement to a joint, ranging from the gentlest oscillations to thrust and including traction." Additionally, AAOMPT has approved the following definition, which has been used in *The Guide to Physical Therapist Practice* and thus adopted by the APTA: "Manipulation and mobilization is the skilled passive movement to a joint and/or the related soft tissues at varying speeds and amplitudes including a small-amplitude, high-velocity therapeutic movement. Manual therapy is defined as a clinical approach utilizing skilled, specific hands-on techniques including, but not limited to, manipulation/mobilization; used by physical therapists to diagnose and treat soft tissue and joint structures for the purpose of modulating pain, increasing range of motion, reducing or eliminating soft tissue inflammation, inducing relaxation, improving contractile and noncontractile tissue repair, extensibility and or stability, facilitating movement, and improving function."[55]

In practice, however, especially within physical therapy in the United States, the term "mobilization" is frequently used to refer to nonthrust techniques and the word "manipulation" to high velocity, low amplitude thrust techniques. This distinction is especially important in the context of the nomenclature used and required by individual state practice acts. This artificial distinction was created during the 1960s when the American Medical Association, through its Committee on Quackery, strongly opposed the practice of chiropractic. By association, they also opposed the word "manipulation." Thus, physical therapists wishing to practice manipulation introduced such terms as "articulation" and later "mobilization."[56] However, with regard to the value of passive motion to the spine, the literature speaks not of mobilization but of manipulation, and it could be argued that we do not serve ourselves well by avoiding this term. It is important for individuals to be aware

of these terms, which vary in meaning, and seek clarification in regards to what specific techniques are being referred to when consulting the literature. Throughout this text, the terms mobilization and manipulation will be used interchangeably to describe the full spectrum of Grade I–V skilled passive movement to joints. Additional descriptors will be provided, as needed, to further clarify the particular technique being discussed. It is recommended that the reader consult the practice act of the state in which he/she practices so that correct terminology may be used when referring to these procedures, particularly in the areas of patient communication and documentation.

REFERENCES

1. Withington ET. *Hippokrates, With an English Translation.* Vol. 3. London: Heinemann; 1944:279-307.
2. Galenus C. *De Locis Affectis.* Vol. 4, Libre 1. *Venice* ; 1625 :6. Renander A, trans. *Om Sjukdomarnas Lokalisation.* Stockholm: Bokbörsen AB; 1960:152-155.
3. Paré A. *Opera.* Liber XV, Cap XVI, Paris; 1582:440-441.
4. Brain L, Wilkinson M. *Cervical Spondylosis and Myelopathy.* Edinburgh: Livingston; 1956.
5. Magner, G. *Chiropractic: Victim's Perspective.* New York, NY: Prometheus Books; 1995: 9.
6. Paget J. Clinical lecture on cases that bone-setters cure. *Br Med J.* 1867;1(314):1-4.
7. Hood W. On the so-called "bone-setting", its nature and results. *Lancet.* 1871;I:336-338, 372-724, 441-443.
8. Marsh H. On manipulation: or the use of forcible movements as a means of surgical treatments. *St. Bart. Hosp. Rep.* 1878;14:205.
9. Fox R. On bonesetting (so-called). *Lancet.* 1882;II:843.
10. Marlin TM. *Manipulative Treatment for the Medical Practitioner.* London: Edward Arnold and Company; 1934.
11. Bankart B. *Manipulative Surgery.* London: Constable and Company Ltd.; 1932.
12. Burrows HJ, Coltart WD. *Treatment by Manipulation.* 2nd ed. London: Eyre Spottiswoode; 1951.
13. Humphris FH. *Physiotherapy: Its Principles and Practice.* New York, NY: The Macmillan Company; 1932:14.
14. Still AT. *Autobiography of Andrew Taylor Still with a History of the Discovery and Development of the Science of Osteopathy.* Kirksville, MO: A.T. Still; 1897.
15. Magoun HI. *Osteopathy in the Cranial Field.* Kirksville, MO: Journal Printing Co.; 1966.
16. Palmer DD. *The Chiropractors' Adjuster.* Portland, OR : Portland Printing House; 1910.
17. Janse J, Houser RH, Wells BV. *Chiropractic Principles and Technique.* Chicago, IL: National College of Chiropractic; 1947.
18. National Institute of Neurological Disorders and Stroke (NINDS). *Monograph No 15: The Research Status of Spinal Manipulative Therapy.* Washington DC: U.S. Department of Health Education and Welfare; 1975.
19. Magner G. The AMA antitrust suit. In: *Chiropractic: The Victim's Perspective.* New York, NY: Prometheus Books; 1995:137.
20. Mennell J. *Physical Treatment by Movement, Manipulation and Massage.* 1st ed. London: J & A Churchill; 1907.
21. Mennell J. Role of manipulation in therapeutics. *Lancet.* 1932;400.
22. Noble IH, Wells EL. Our aim. *Phys Ther Rev.* 1921;1:1.
23. McMillan M. *Massage and Therapeutic Exercise.* Philadelphia, PA: W.B. Saunders: 1921.
24. Granger. Physiotherapy in stiff & painful shoulders. *Phys Ther Review.* 1921.
25. Sampson CM. *Physiotherapy Technique: A Manual of Applied Physics.* St.Louis, MO: C.V. Mosby Company; 1923.
26. Walmsley T. Articular mechanism of diarthroses. *J Bone J Surg.* 10:40-45.
27. Leadbetter GW. The etiology, diagnosis and treatment of lumbo-sacral and sacro-iliac strains. *The Physiotherapy Review* 1930;10:458-460.
28. Humphris FH, Stuart-Webb RE. *Physiotherapy: Its Principle and Practice.* New York, NY: The Macmillan Company; 1932.
29. Ghormley RK. Low back pain: articular facets, etc. *JAMA.* 1933;101: 1773-1777.
30. Mixter WJ, Barr JS. Rupture of the intervertebral disc with involvement of the spinal canal. *N Engl J Med.* 1934;211:210-215.
31. Thornhill MC. Manipulative treatment for the lumbosacral derangement. *Phys Ther.* 1936.
32. Smart M. Manipulation. *Arch.Phys. Med.* 1946;12:730-734.
33. Luebe. *Massage of the Reflex Zones in the Connective Tissue.* 1948.
34. Cyriax, J. Lumbago. *Lancet.* 1948;II:427.
35. Cyriax J. *Textbook of Orthopaedic Medicine.* Vol I. *Diagnosis of Soft Tissue Lesions.* Baltimore, MD: Williams and Wilkins; 1947, and Vol II. *Treatment by Manipulation and Deep Massage.* London: Cassell & Company, 1950.
36. Steindler A. *Kinesiology of the Human Body Under Normal and Pathological Conditions.* Springfield, IL: Thomas; 1955.
37. Kaltenborn F. *Manual Therapy for the Extremity Joints: Specialized Techniques: Tests and Joint Mobilization.* Svendborg, Denmark: Olaf Norlis Bokhandel; 1976.
38. Paris SV. The spinal lesion. *N Z Med J.* 1963;62:371.
39. Maitland G. *Vertebral Manipulation.* 4th ed. London: Butterworth and Company, Ltd.; 1964.
40. Maitland, G. *Peripheral Manipulation.* 2nd ed. London: Butterworth and Company, Ltd.; 1977.
41. Paris SV. Joint manipulation: how you (osteopaths) can make manipulation succeed. *The Osteopathic Physician.* 1971;July.
42. Melzack R, Wall PD. Pain mechanisms: a new theory. *Science.* 1965; 150:971.
43. McCaleb B. An introduction to spinal manipulation. 1969;49:1369-1374.
44. Mennell J. Rationale of joint manipulation. *Phys Ther.* 1970;50:181-186.
45. McKenzie R. A perspective on manipulative therapy. *Physiotherapy.* 1989;75:440-444.
46. Farrell JP, Twomey LT. Acute low back pain: comparison of two conservative treatment approaches. *Med J Aust.* 1982;20:159-164.
47. Kendall PH, Jenkins JM. Exercise for backache: a double blind controlled trial. *Physiotherapy.* 1968;54:154-157.
48. Deyo, R. Conservative therapy for low back pain: distinguishing useful from useless therapy. *JAMA.* 1983;250(8):1057-1062.
49. Paris SV. Manipulation of the lumbar spine. In: Weinstein JN, Wiesel SW, eds. *The Lumbar Spine* . Philadelphia, PA: WB Saunders; 1990:805–811.
50. Mulligan BR. Update on spinal mobilizations with movement. *The Journal of Manual and Manipulative Therapy.* 1977;5:184-187.
51. Elvey RL, Quintner JL, Thomas AN. A clinical study of RSI. *Aust Fam Physician.* 1986;15:1314-1319.
52. American Physical Therapy Association. Guidelines for Defining Physical Therapy Practice Acts; BOD G03-00-16-38. Alexandria, VA: APTA; 2012.
53. APTA Manipulation Task Force. *Manipulation Education Manual.* Alexandria, VA: APTA; 2004.
54. Mitchell MP. *An Evaluation and Treatment Manual of Osteopathic Muscle Energy Procedures.* Valley Park, MO: Mitchell Moran and Pruzzo Associates;1979.
55. American Physical Therapy Association. *Guide to Physical Therapist Practice,* Rev. 2nd ed. Alexandria, VA: APTA; 2003.
56. Paris SV. An introduction to joint manipulation. *J. Canadian Physiotherapy Assoc.* 1968;3:1-4.

Principles of Preparation for Orthopaedic Manual Physical Therapy

Christopher H. Wise, PT, DPT, OCS, FAAOMPT, MTC, ATC

Chapter Objectives

At the conclusion of this chapter, the reader will be able to:

- Operationally define key terms related to the practice of orthopaedic manual physical therapy (OMPT).
- Identify and explain the potential effects of joint mobilization, appreciate the value of each, and understand how each effect may be obtained through technique performance.

- Describe the indications, precautions, and contraindications for the practice of OMPT and how these concepts relate to specific types of OMPT.
- Delineate specific aspects of patient care in OMPT as they apply to each domain of clinical practice as outlined within the Guide to Physical Therapist Practice.

INTRODUCTION

In 1960, Mennell[1] stated that "beyond all doubt, the use of the human hand, as a method of reducing human suffering, is the oldest remedy known to man; historically no date can be given for its adoption." Despite this contention, the practice of orthopaedic manual physical therapy (OMPT) in the United States has only recently entered mainstream clinical practice. Despite an increase in its use, evidence supporting the efficacy of OMPT remains insufficient. Grieve has long expressed the plight of the manual therapist by stating: "We continue to sound as though we know so much, when we know comparatively little. It might be a good thing to admit this. We make much of clinical science, enthusiastically referring to this or that part of the massive mountain of literature which best serves our particular interest. Much of what we do is simply what has been proven on the clinical ship floor to be effective in getting our patients better . . . we do not always know why."[2] Responsible clinicians, researchers, and academicians are equally aware of the value of both the art and the science that supports the practice of OMPT. Salter states, however, that "the care of patients remains as art, but the art must be based on science."[3] Twomey noted, "There is a growing body of evidence that suggests a useful biomechanical model to explain the often dramatic relief that follows such procedures."[4]

The primary objective of this chapter is to serve as an introduction to the principles and practices that govern OMPT. The terms and concepts defined and described in this chapter will provide a theoretical framework upon which the remainder of this text will be developed.

OPERANT DEFINITIONS

The Manipulation Education Manual (MEM),[5] which was developed by the American Physical Therapy Association's (APTA) Manipulation Education Committee in 2004, has correctly identified that the primary consideration regarding the regulations that govern the practice and teaching of manual therapy is *language*. The terminology that is used to define the practice of OMPT varies considerably among physical therapy state practice acts and the rules and regulations of licensing boards. Before pursuing the OMPT strategies set forth within this text, readers are strongly encouraged to become familiar with the details of the practice act of the state in which they practice.

Orthopaedic Manual Physical Therapy

For years, clinicians, researchers, and academicians have attempted to define OMPT. Meadows has defined OMPT as "an entire approach to musculoskeletal dysfunction, and not just a series of techniques." He further notes that the purpose of

OMPT may be to *mobilize* or to *stabilize* a particular joint or spinal segment so other techniques can have an optimal effect (Fig. 2–1).[4] This definition of OMPT highlights the notion that OMPT is, indeed, valuable in stabilizing as well as mobilizing joints. The manual physical therapist is a movement specialist who is trained in the appreciation and restoration of normal movement patterns. They are masters of applied biomechanics and fully understand the intimate *kinetics* and *kinematics* that are acting upon an individual during the performance of functional tasks. Farrell et al note that OMPT is "not a specialty utilizing only passive movement techniques, but rather a specialty whose indications are multi-factorial evolving from clinical criteria rather than from descriptions of pathology."[4] Riddle recognizes the value of OMPT as an evaluative tool that may be used for collecting data on individuals with musculoskeletal impairment.[6]

Mobilization/Manipulation

Maitland defines mobilization as passive movement that is performed with a *rhythm* and a *grade* in a manner in which the patient is able to prevent the technique from being performed.[7,8] Grieve distinguishes the term manipulation from mobilization by defining manipulation as "an accurately localized, single, quick, and decisive movement of small amplitude following careful positioning of the patient."[2] He further notes that the

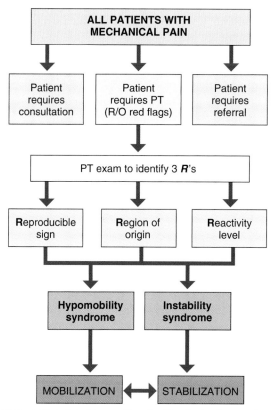

FIGURE 2–1 Clinical decision-making algorithm for implementation of orthopaedic manual physical therapy for mobilization or stabilization in the care of a patient. (Adapted from Wise CH, Gulick DT. *Mobilization Notes: A Rehabilitation Specialist's Pocket Guide.* Philadelphia, PA: FA Davis Company; 2009, with permission.)

manipulation may have a *regional* or more *localized* effect. Paris contends that the terms mobilization and manipulation are identical in meaning and thus can be used interchangeably; they are described as the *skilled passive movement to a joint.*[9]

The document that has been most useful in communicating terminology and establishing the scope of OMPT practice is the **Guide to Physical Therapist Practice (GPTP)**. The GPTP states that "mobilization/manipulation is a manual therapy technique that comprises a continuum of skilled passive movements to joints and/or related soft tissues that are applied at varying speeds and amplitudes, including a small amplitude, high velocity therapeutic movement."[10] The Manipulation Education Committee supports this definition of mobilization and manipulation and advocates the use of these terms interchangeably throughout the *MEM.*[5]

The **Normative Model of Physical Therapist Professional Education: Version 2004,**[11] as well as the **Evaluative Criteria for Accreditation of Education Programs for the Preparation of Physical Therapists,**[12] both support instruction in mobilization/manipulation that ranges from nonthrust to thrust techniques within the first professional educational curricula of physical therapists. The **Practice Affairs Committee of the Orthopaedic Section of the APTA** states that the term manipulation implies a variety of manual techniques that are not exclusive to any specific profession.[13] Throughout this text, the terms mobilization and manipulation will be considered synonymous and will, therefore, be used interchangeably. To avoid confusion, the descriptor **high-velocity low-amplitude thrust,** or **thrust** may be used to describe mobilization techniques that are performed with high velocity and low amplitude at or near the end range of motion. Many advocate for the use of the term manipulation in favor of mobilization and suggest that avoiding this term may not serve the profession of physical therapy well. The term *manipulation*, however, is not included in some state practice acts. Despite this text's emphasis on joint mobilization/manipulation, the reader should be aware that OMPT is, indeed, an entire approach to the management of musculoskeletal dysfunction.

Defining Joint Position

Close-Packed and Open-Packed Positions

Careful prepositioning of a joint prior to mobilization allows the manual physical therapist to achieve the desired outcome in a more efficient and safer fashion. The **close-packed position** is defined as the position in which the least degree of mobility between articular surfaces is available. Conversely, the **open-packed position**, also known as loose-packed, is defined as the position in which the greatest degree of mobility between articular surfaces is available. There are two primary competing criteria that determine whether the joint is considered to be close- or open-packed. The first criterion is *joint congruency.*[9] Paris quotes Walmsley, who identified in 1927 that joint surfaces are generally incongruous, except in one specific position, called the close-packed position.[9] Just as the corrugated pieces of a jigsaw puzzle closely fit together and consequently restrict the degree of play between them, a joint with congruent articular surfaces will display a limited ability for movement. When considering hinge joints, such as the knee and elbow, the close-packed position is considered to be the position of maximum joint congruency and the open-packed position to be the least congruent. In ball and socket joints, such as the glenohumeral and hip joints, the position of maximum joint congruency is actually the open-packed position. The second criterion used to distinguish between open- or close-packed position, is the degree of normal extensibility within the capsuloligamentous complex (CLC) of the joint. Generally, the position of greatest CLC tightness is the close-packed position, with the open-packed position being the position in which the CLC possesses the greatest degree of laxity. At times, disagreement may exist among these two criteria. In the hip, for example, the position of greatest congruency, which is flexion, abduction, and external rotation (FABER) position is considered to be the open-packed rather than the close-packed position because, although it is the position of greatest congruency, it is the position in which the CLC is least restricted and, therefore, the position that affords the greatest degree of mobility (Fig. 2–2). Kaltenborn uses the terms **non-resting position** and **resting position** to refer to close- and open-packed positions, respectively.

The task of determining the actual close- or open-packed position of any given joint is challenging and best accomplished through **joint play** testing. Kaltenborn defines joint play as "a movement that is not under voluntary control yet is essential to the painless performance of active movement."[14] Paris defines joint play as a movement that is not under voluntary control that includes the additional degree of movement that is available at end range.[9]

When attempting to optimally pre-position joints prior to mobilization, the manual therapist must consider the *tri-planar position* of the joint.

Locking Techniques

There are occasions in which a joint is pre-positioned for the purpose of restricting the occurrence of a particular movement. Locking of specific spinal segments, for example, limits movement across those segments and provides a lever for the transfer of mobilizing force into the segments for which

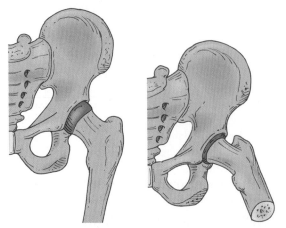

FIGURE 2–2 When the hip is flexed, abducted, and externally rotated, maximal joint congruency is achieved.

the force is intended. Premanipulative locking techniques serve the dual purpose of eliminating mobilization of adjacent segments while also reducing the amount of force required to produce the desired effect.

Facet-opposition locking techniques involve the placement of facet joint surfaces in a maximally opposed position and are said to be in maximal apposition. A common facet-opposition locking technique performed in the mid-cervical spine involves side bending with rotation in the opposite direction which is contrary to normal kinematics (see Chapter 30). The fulcrum created by this position becomes the center of rotation, which leads to gapping of the contralateral facet joints.[15]

Ligamentous-tension locking is described as a soft tissue method of restricting motion across a particular spinal segment. These techniques are predicated upon the concept that when motion is introduced within a spinal segment, movement of that same segment in all other directions will be limited. An example of ligamentous-tension locking is the lumbar rotational technique in which locking of the lower lumbar segments occurs up to the desired segment by flexing the hips (see Chapter 28).[15]

In deciding the optimal joint position for mobilization, the clinician must first consider the objectives of performing the technique and the desired effects. Pre-positioning of the joint at the tissue barrier may be optimal when the goal is to increase the range of motion.[16] Maitland recommends the use of *through-range* and *end-of-range* techniques, as well as the use of *combined movements*, mobilization with *compression*, and *injuring movements*, where the position in which symptoms originally occurred are used.[7,8]

Kaltenborn advocates the use of the non-resting position for the management of subtle joint dysfunctions that cannot be identified in the resting position. These positions are required for stretching of soft tissues; however, mobilization performed in these positions requires greater skill to perform.[14] Patient reactivity and the phase of healing are also important considerations when determining the optimal position for mobilization.

Defining Joint Movement

The amount of joint motion that is available at any given joint may be considered on a continuum that ranges from normal to pathological (Fig. 2–3). Under normal conditions, *active range of motion (AROM)* typically exhibits less mobility than *passive range of motion (PROM)* because full PROM is facilitated through the application of external forces. Beyond passive joint play, injury may occur as either a *sprain or strain* of the joint and its periarticular structures. If additional force is applied, the joint is extended beyond its anatomical confines and a *subluxation or dislocation* is likely to occur.

The term **kinematics** is defined as the study of motion that does not account for the forces responsible for producing or influencing that motion, whereas **kinetics** is the study of movement in relation to forces that are acting upon it.[17,18] Seven kinematic variables may be considered when appreciating joint movement: the type of movement, the location in which the

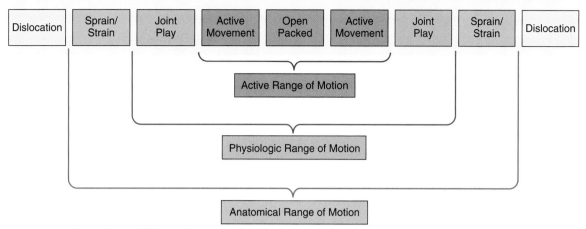

FIGURE 2–3 The continuum of joint motion ranging from normal to pathological movement. (Adapted from Paris, SV, Loubert, PV. *Foundations of Clinical Orthopaedics, Course Notes.* St. Augustine, FL: Institute Press; 1990.)

movement is occurring in space, the movement direction, the quantity of the movement, the speed of the movement, the symptomatic response of the patient to movement, and the quality of the preferred pattern of movement.[18]

Movement of Peripheral Joints

The type of movement that is available at any given joint is either translatory or rotatory (Fig. 2–4). *Translatory*, or linear, movement, which is defined as movement of a body segment in a straight path, rarely occurs in isolation in the body. *Rotatory*, or angular, movement is movement of a segment about an axis. In the human body, this axis is rarely fixed; rather, these axes constantly change during motion. The axis around which segments move throughout their path is sometimes referred to as the **instantaneous center of rotation.** The path circumscribed by the sequential displacement of the joint axis during movement is referred to as the path of the instantaneous center of rotation (PICR) (Fig. 2–5).

Kaltenborn[19] adapted the work of MacConaill[20,21] and supported the notion that a combination of rolling and gliding, termed *roll-gliding*, occurs between joint surfaces during normal movement (Fig. 2–6). **Rolling** is defined as an angular movement that involves approximation of new points on one joint surface with new points on the other joint surface. The direction of rolling is invariably in the direction in which the bone is being displaced. Conversely, **gliding** occurs when joint surfaces are congruent and is defined as a single point on one joint surface repeatedly contacting new points on the other joint surface. This concept has become known as Kaltenborn's **convex-concave rule**[19] and was first described by MacConaill.[20,21] When the convex joint surface moves upon a relatively fixed concave surface, the direction of joint glide is believed to be in the opposite direction to bone displacement. When the concave joint surface moves upon the fixed convex surface, the direction of joint glide is purported to be in the same direction as the bone displacement (Fig. 2–7). Although this arrangement between moving joint surfaces appears to possess good face validity, during actual joint movement many exceptions to the convex-concave rule exist.

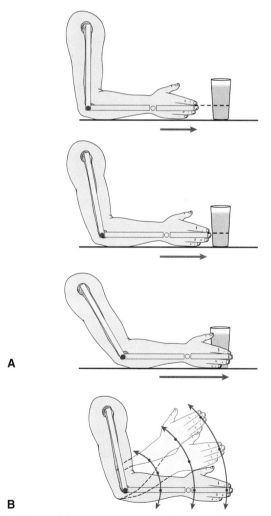

FIGURE 2–4 There are two types of motion available at any given joint. **A.** During translation, each point on a segment moves the same distance at the same time in parallel paths. **B.** During rotation, each point of a segment moves through the same angle, at the same time, at the same distance from the axis of motion. (From Levangie PK, Norkin CC. *Joint Structure and Function: A Comprehensive Analysis.* 4th ed. Philadelphia, PA: FA Davis; 2005, with permission.)

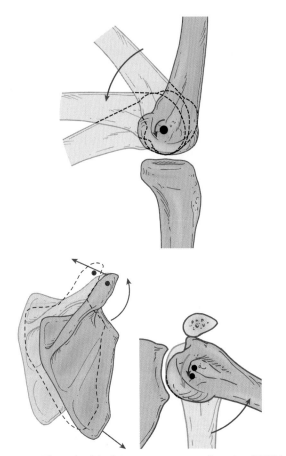

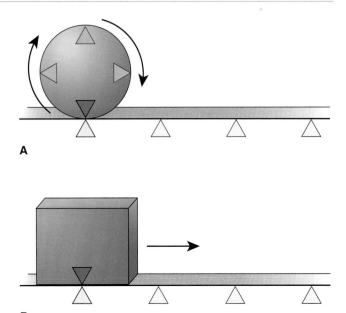

FIGURE 2–6 Combined roll-gliding occurs within all joints during movement. **A.** *Rolling* is defined as an angular movement that approximates new points on one joint surface with new points on the other joint surface. The direction of rolling is invariably in the direction in which the bone is being displaced. **B.** *Gliding* occurs when joint surfaces are congruent and is defined as a single point on one joint surface repeatedly contacting new points on the other joint surface. The direction in which gliding occurs during joint movement is dependent upon whether the convex surface is moving on the concave surface or vice versa.

FIGURE 2–5 The path of the instantaneous center of rotation (PICR) is the path that is circumscribed by the sequential displacement of the joint axis during movement. The PICR denotes the combined rotatory and translatory movements that take place within joints during normal movement.

The term **osteokinematic** may be defined as the gross movement of limbs or body parts relative to one another and relative to environmental references.[9] Others have used the terms *physiologic*[7,8] or *classical*[9,22] to describe these movements. Physiologic movement may be performed either actively or passively by the therapist and are those that are quantified through the use of a goniometer, tape measure, or some other measuring device. Examples of osteokinematic, or physiologic, motion include flexion, extension, and abduction.

The gliding component of normal joint motion is typically referred to as **arthrokinematic** movement, which is defined as the relative motion that occurs between joint surfaces and structures within a joint.[9] These motions, often referred to as **accessory** or **component** movements,[9,22] accompany the gross physiologic motions and are believed to be necessary for full motion to be achieved. Full physiologic knee extension in open chain, for example, requires the accessory motion of anterior glide of the tibia relative to the femur. These smaller, more intimate motions are challenging to evaluate, and examination of accessory movement is often overlooked in clinical practice.

Determination of limitations in accessory motion may be performed directly or indirectly during routine examination.[14,19] The **direct method** of determining restrictions in

joint gliding is employed by the clinician performing passive translatory glides in all directions. During performance of these procedures, the therapist ascertains the relationship between tissue resistance and the patient's report of pain, as well as the quality of resistance at end range, or end-feel, in each direction.[7,8,14,19] The **indirect method** of determining restrictions in joint glide is predicated upon the aforementioned convex-concave rule. As deficits are noted in an individual's physiologic movement, deficits in joint gliding are deduced. The literature reveals acceptable intrarater but unfavorable interrater reliability for assessment of intervertebral accessory movement in the spine.[23] Therapists are more reliable in identifying the impaired spinal segment when pain provocation rather than judgments of stiffness are used.[24]

Segmental Movement of the Spine

Movement of one vertebra relative to an adjacent vertebra is defined as **segmental motion**, whereas gross movements of the spine require *multisegmental motion*. Segmental motion occurs at the **spinal motion segment**, which is defined as the inferior half of the superior vertebra and the superior half of the inferior vertebra and all other structures between them, including muscle, nerve, disc, facet joint, etc. (Fig. 2–8). Each motion segment can move in 12 different directions, involving both linear and angulatory movement. Movement of the spine is determined by both the plane of the synovial zygapophyseal, or facet, joint as well as the cartilaginous intervertebral, or interbody, joints (Fig. 2–9). The position of the spine, region of the

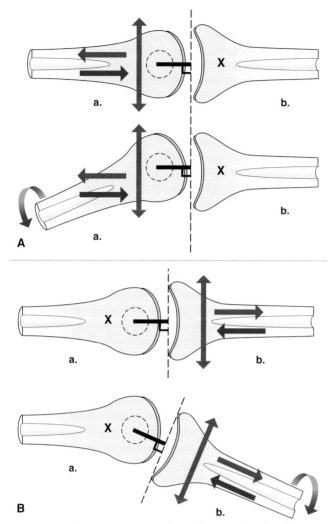

FIGURE 2–7 The convex-concave rule, which states that when the convex joint surface moves upon the concave surface, the direction of joint glide is in the opposite direction to bone displacement. When the concave joint surface moves upon the fixed convex surface, the direction of joint glide is in the same direction as the bone displacement. **A.** Joint mobilization of the (a) convex aspect of a typical synovial joint upon its (b) concave counterpart. The direction of mobilizing forces remains the same when the joint is moved out of the neutral position. **B.** Joint mobilization of the (b) concave aspect of a typical synovial joint upon its (a) convex counterpart. The direction of mobilizing forces changes when the joint is moved out of the neutral position. Dotted Line: Treatment plane of the joint. Red Arrow: Joint Glide, which occurs parallel to the treatment plane of the joint, Green Arrow: Joint Distraction, which occurs perpendicular and away from the treatment plane. Purple Arrow: Joint Compression, which occurs perpendicular and toward the treatment plane.

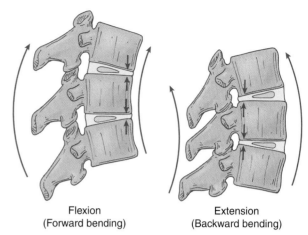

Flexion
(Forward bending)   Extension
(Backward bending)

FIGURE 2–8 Spinal motion segment includes the inferior half of the superior vertebra, the superior half of the inferior vertebra, and all structures in between. (Adapted from Levangie PK, Norkin CC. *Joint Structure and Function: A Comprehensive Analysis.* 4th ed. Philadelphia, PA: FA Davis; 2005, with permission.)

Manual techniques that use accessory movements are those most traditionally identified as joint mobilization. Joint mobilization may also include a combination of both physiologic and accessory movements. In cases of joint mobility restrictions, normal joint rolling is disturbed and is usually associated with impaired joint gliding.[19]

There are three types of mobilization movements that may be employed to address impairments in mobility (see Fig. 2–7). These movements are defined based on their relationship to the treatment plane. The **treatment plane (TP)** is determined by the concave aspect of the joint and is at a right angle to a line drawn from the axis of rotation to the center of the concave articulating surface.[19] It is important to note that the TP is the plane in which joint glide normally occurs during movement, and it may be estimated by envisioning the position of the concave aspect of the joint. For this reason, it is important for manual physical therapists to possess an intimate understanding of joint anatomy and have the capability to visualize the anatomic structures beneath their hands.

Distraction is a mobilization movement that is defined as a passive accessory movement in which force is elicited in a direction that is *perpendicular* and *away* from the TP. With the application of sufficient force, distraction in its purest form has the effect of eliciting tension equally throughout all aspects of the joint's capsuloligamentous complex. Distraction may be used to unweight and relieve pressure upon articular surfaces, to reduce subluxations, to fire capsular mechanoreceptors, to enhance joint nutrition, or to place stretch upon the CLC. Distraction may result in stretching all aspects of the capsule indiscriminately. Distraction is commonly used as an introductory and concluding technique during bouts of mobilization for the purpose of creating a relaxation effect that optimizes the impact of other techniques. As a mobilization movement, **glide** is defined as a passive accessory movement in which force is elicited in a direction that is *parallel* to the TP. Unlike distraction, gliding mobilizations are performed with a distinctly directional preference. Both joint distraction and joint glides

spine, and individual variability must all be considered when appreciating spinal movement.

Defining Joint Mobilization Movements

OMPT procedures that are used to mobilize joints may do so by targeting either the physiologic or the accessory movement of the joint.[7] Manual techniques that use physiologic movements often include a variation of passive range of motion (PROM) or active-assisted range of motion (AAROM).

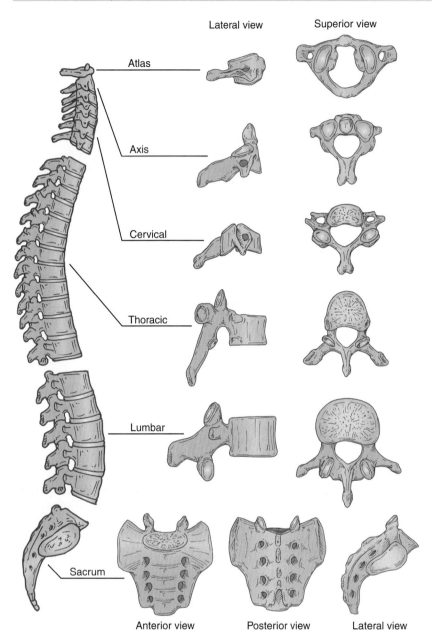

Lateral view   Superior view

Atlas

Axis

Cervical

Thoracic

Lumbar

Sacrum

Anterior view   Posterior view   Lateral view

FIGURE 2–9 Variation in the orientation of the facet joints of the cervical, thoracic, and lumbar spines. Generally, the cervical facet joints are located 45 degrees between the frontal and transverse planes, thoracic are in frontal plane, and the lumbar are in the sagittal plane.

may be performed as either thrust or nonthrust techniques depending on force and amplitude.

Grades of Joint Mobilization

The descriptions of mobilization grades have long been attributed to the work of Geoffrey Maitland[7,8] (Fig. 2–10). Although most commonly used to refer to mobilization that uses accessory movement, these grades may also be used to define the manner in which physiologic mobilization occurs.

Maitland's mobilization grades are often misinterpreted or not fully delineated. When adopting this grading system, it is critical for the manual therapist to appreciate the point in the range of movement in which the first barrier (**Resistance 1 or R1**) and the final barrier (**Resistance 2 or R2**) to movement occurs. Mobilization grades are not arbitrarily assigned but rather are based on their location relative to R1 and R2.

The grade of mobilization may be used to define the *location* in which the mobilization has occurred, the **force** that is required, and the **amplitude** or excursion of movement that is used. A **Grade I** mobilization is defined as a small amplitude mobilization that occurs short of tissue resistance (R1). **Grade II** is a large amplitude movement that is also short of resistance (R1). A **Grade III** mobilization is of large amplitude that occurs at approximately 50%, or halfway, between R1 and R2. A **Grade IV** mobilization is small in amplitude that also occurs at approximately 50% between R1 and R2. A **Grade V** mobilization, also known as a high-velocity thrust mobilization, is of small amplitude and high velocity that occurs at the end of available range of movement. Pluses (+, ++) and minuses (−,− −) are used to further refine the mobilization grades. **Grade III− −** and **Grade IV− −** mobilizations occur at the onset of R1, and **Grades III−** and **Grade IV−** are performed at approximately 25% between R1 and R2. **Grade III+** and **Grade IV+** are

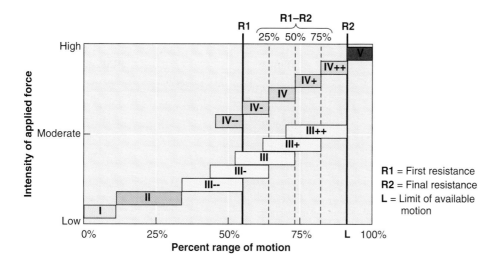

Grade I = Small amplitude, short of **R1**

Grade II = Large amplitude, short of **R1**

Grade III-- = Large amplitude taken to **R1**

Grade III- = Large amplitude taken to 25% **R1-R2**

Grade III = Large amplitude taken to 50% **R1-R2**

Grade III+ = Large amplitude taken to 75% **R1-R2**

Grade III++ = Large amplitude taken to **R2**

Grade IV-- = Small amplitude taken to **R1**

Grade IV- = Small amplitude taken to 25% **R1-R2**

Grade IV = Small amplitude taken to 50% **R1-R2**

Grade IV+ = Small amplitude taken to 75% **R1-R2**

Grade IV++ = Small amplitude taken to **R2**

Grade V = Small amplitude, high velocity at **R2** and beyond

FIGURE 2–10 Mobilization Grades I–V including pluses (+) and minuses (–) based on their position relative to first (R1) and final (R2) resistance. (From Wise CH, Gulick DT. *Mobilization Notes: A Rehabilitation Specialist's Pocket Guide.* Philadelphia, PA: FA Davis; 2009, with permission.)

performed at 75% between R1 and R2, and **Grade III**++ and **Grade IV**++ occur at R2.

End-Feel

James Cyriax[25] popularized the term **end-feel,** which he described as the transmission of a specific sensation to the examiner's hands at the extreme of passive movement (Table 2–1).

Cyriax[25] identified 3 normal end-feels that may be perceived by the manual therapist. Paris and Patla[9,22] define end-feel as the quality of resistance at end range and have identified 5 normal end-feels and 10 abnormal end-feels. The criteria upon which an end-feel is considered to be normal depends on whether the end-feel matches that which is expected for the joint being tested in the direction in which it is normal being tested and is expected to occur at the end range of the tested motion.

Table 2-1	Normal Joint End-Feels as Defined by Cyriax and Paris		
JOINT	**MOTION**	**CYRIAX**[25]	**PARIS et al**[9,22]
Cervical	FB/BB	Capsular	Muscular
	SB	Capsular	Muscular
	Rotation	Capsular	Muscular
Shoulder	Flexion	Capsular	Muscular
	Abduction	Capsular/Hard	Muscular
	Horizontal Adduction	Capsular/Extra-articular	Soft Tissue Approximation
	Scaption	Capsular/Hard	Muscular
	IR/ER	Capsular	Capsular
Elbow	Flexion	Extra-articular	Soft Tissue Approximation
	Extension	Hard	Cartilaginous
Wrist	Pronation/Supination	Capsular	Muscular
	Flexion	Capsular	Cartilaginous
	Extension	Capsular	Cartilaginous
	Radial/Ulnar Deviation	Hard	Ligamentous

Continued

Table 2-1	Normal Joint End-Feels as Defined by Cyriax and Paris—cont'd		
JOINT	**MOTION**	**CYRIAX[25]**	**PARIS et al[9,22]**
Thumb	Flexion/Extension/Abduction	Capsular	Capsular
	Adduction	Extra-articular	Soft Tissue Approximation
Lumbar	FB	Capsular	Muscular
	BB	Capsular	Muscular
	SB	Capsular	Muscular
	Rotation	Capsular	Muscular
Hip	Flex	Capsular/Extra-articular	Muscular (SLR)
	Extension	Capsular	Capsular
	Abduction	Capsular	Capsular
	IR/ER	Capsular	Capsular
Knee	Flexion	Extra-articular	Soft Tissue Approximation
	Extension	Capsular	ligamentous
Ankle	Plantarflexion	Capsular	Capsular
	Dorsiflexion	Capsular	Muscular
	Inversion	Capsular	Ligamentous
	Eversion	Hard	Ligamentous
	Pronation/Supination	Capsular	Capsular
MTP/IP	Flexion	Capsular	Muscular
	Extension	Capsular	Capsular

FB/BB, Forward Bending/Backward Bending; SB, Side Bending; IR/ER, Internal Rotation/External Rotation; SLR, Straight Leg Raise; MTP/IP, Metatarsophalangeal/Interphalangeal.

End-feels may be identified by the manual therapist during passive testing of either physiologic or accessory movement.

End-feel assessment has been criticized for demonstrating less than acceptable reliability. However, the reliability of identifying the pathologic structure improves when pain rather than assessment of resistance to movement is emphasized.[26] Like other examination procedures, considering the results of end-feel testing in light of other examination findings is recommended.

Capsular Pattern

Joints may exhibit motion loss that is said to be capsular or noncapsular in nature (Table 2–2). **Capsular patterns** are said

Table 2-2	Open-Packed and Close-Packed Positions, Concave and Convex Joint Surfaces Defined, and Capsular Patterns of the Extremities				
JOINT	**OPEN-PACKED POSITION**	**CLOSE-PACKED POSITION**	**CONCAVE**	**CONVEX**	**CAPSULAR PATTERN**
Hip	Flexion–30° Abduction –30° Slight ER	Maximal Extension, IR, Abduction	Acetabulum	Femoral head	IR > Extension > Abduction
Radiocarpal	10° Flexion, Slight Ulnar Deviation	Maximal Extension	Radius, Radioulnar Disc	Scaphoid, Lunate, Triquetrum	Restrictions in all directions
Carpometacarpal–2-5	–	–	Base of Metacarpals	Distal carpal row	Restrictions in all directions
Carpometacarpal Thumb Flexion/Extension Abduction/Adduction	Mid-Range Flexion/ Extension, Abduction/ Adduction	Maximal Opposition	Trapezii Trapezii	Metacarpal Metacarpal	Abduction > Extension
Metacarpophalangeal 2–5	Slight Flexion, Slight Ulnar Deviation	Maximal Flexion	Base proximal phalanx	Metacarpal heads	Flexion >other restriction

	Table 2–2 Open-Packed and Close-Packed Positions, Concave and Convex Joint Surfaces Defined, and Capsular Patterns of the Extremities—cont'd				
JOINT	**OPEN-PACKED POSITION**	**CLOSE-PACKED POSITION**	**CONCAVE**	**CONVEX**	**CAPSULAR PATTERN**
MCP Thumb	Slight Flexion	Maximal Extension	Base proximal phalanx	Metacarpal head	—
Interphalangeal; 1-5	Slight Flexion	Maximal Extension	Base phalanx	Head phalanx	—
Humeroulnar	70° Flexion 10° Supination	Full Extension, Full Supination	Ulna trochlear notch	Humerus Trochlea	Flexion > Extension
Radiohumeral	Full Extension, Full Supination	90° Flexion, 5° Supination	Radial Head superior surface	Humerus Capitul	Flexion > Extension
Proximal Radioulnar	70° Flexion, 35° Supination	5° Supination	Ulna radial no	Radial head	Pronation = Supination
Distal Radio-Ulnar	10° Supination	5°Supination	Radius ulnar notch	Ulnar head	Pronation = Supination
Glenohumeral	30°–60° Abduction/ Flexion 30° Horizontal Adduction	Maximal Abduction & ER	Glenoid Fossa	Humeral head	ER > Abduction > IR
Sternoclavicula	Anatomical	Maximal Elevation	Sternum disc	Clavicle–Flexion/ Extension Disc–Protraction/ Retraction	—
Acromioclavicular	Anatomical	Abduction–90° 0° Horizontal Adduction	Acromion	Clavicle	—
Tibiofemoral	25° Flexion	Maximal Extension Maximal ER Tibia	Tibial plateaus	Femoral condyles	Flexion > Extension (9:1)
Proximal Tibiofibular	Resting	—	Tibial postero-lateral facet	Fibular head	—
Distal Tibiofibular	—	—	Tibial facet	Fibular facet	—
Talocrural	10° Plantarflexion	Maximal Dorsiflexion	Distal Tibia/ Fibula	Talus	Plantarflexion > Dorsiflexion
Subtalar			Variable alternating facets	Variable alternating facets	Valgus > Varus
Metatarsophalangeal 2–5	Slight Flexion	Maximal Extension	Phalanx	Metacarpal	Flexion > Extension
Metatarsophalangeal 1	5°–10° Extension	Maximal Extension	Phalanx	Metacarpal	Extension > Flexion

IR, Internal Rotation; ER, External Rotation.

to exist when the capsuloligamentous complex of a joint is restricted, resulting in a characteristic loss of motion specific to that joint. The classic capsular pattern presentation is believed to exist in joints with osteoarthritis. The concept of capsular patterns is controversial and lacks sufficient support in the literature.[27–29]

If a characteristic loss of motion is observed during examination that is suggestive of a capsular restriction, then joint mobilization techniques are indicated. A **noncapsular pattern** denotes a loss of motion that does not follow a characteristic pattern and may be related to isolated capsular restrictions, restrictions in myofascial tissue, or attributed to some other cause. Observation of a capsular pattern provides the manual physical therapist with information regarding the cause of a movement restriction; however, caution must be used in its perceived validity.

OBJECTIVES OF JOINT MOBILIZATION/MANIPULATION

The manual physical therapist's decision to implement nonthrust and thrust manipulation should be made with very clear objectives in mind (Box 2-1). Collectively, the location, speed/rhythm, amplitude, and frequency/duration in which joint mobilization is to be performed creates a stepwise progression of parameters to consider when increasing the specificity of each technique (Fig. 2–11). The criteria for determining the manner in which these variables are performed include (1) level of reactivity/tolerance, (2) desired effect, (3) stage of healing, (4) prior amount of patient/therapist experience and patient compliance, (5) stage of intervention, (6) nature of the restriction, (7) use of other interventions, and (8) the age and health status of the patient.

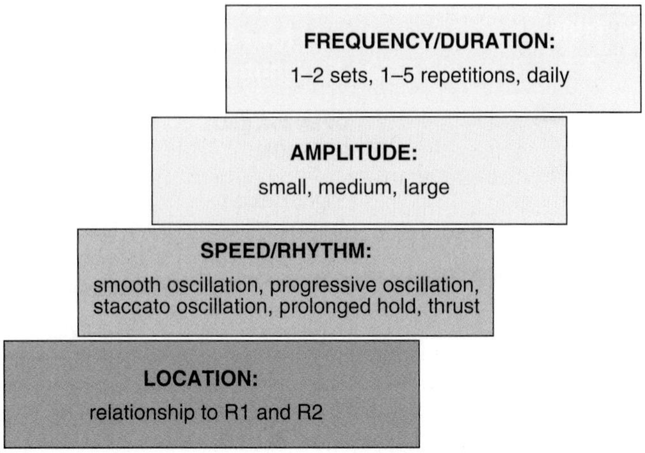

Neurophysiological Effects

Recent evidence suggests that manual interventions may produce neurophysiological effects by stimulating central control mechanisms, namely the descending inhibitory pathways. Evidence suggests that thrust manipulation can have a short-term effect on alpha-motoneuron excitability[30-32], may impact brain function specific to the side of thrust,[33] and may alter pressure pain thresholds (PPTs).[34] These findings provide support for the prospect that the favorable outcomes experienced in response to thrust manipulation may involve neurophysiologic changes.[35]

Box 2-1 EFFECTS OF JOINT MOBILIZATION

NEUROPHYSIOLOGICAL EFFECTS (GRADES I–V)

1. Firing of articular mechanoreceptors, proprioceptors
2. Firing of cutaneous and muscular receptors
3. Altered nociception

MECHANICAL EFFECTS (GRADES III–V)

1. Stretching of joint restrictions
2. Breaking of adhesions
3. Alter positional relationships
4. Diminish/eliminate barriers to normal motion

PSYCHOLOGICAL EFFECTS (GRADES I–V)

1. Confidence gained through improvement
2. Positive effects from manual contact
3. Response to joint sounds

(From Wise CH, Gulick DT. *Mobilization Notes: A Rehabilitation Specialist's Pocket Guide.* Philadelphia, PA: FA Davis; 2009, with permission.)

FREQUENCY/DURATION:
1–2 sets, 1–5 repetitions, daily

AMPLITUDE:
small, medium, large

SPEED/RHYTHM:
smooth oscillation, progressive oscillation, staccato oscillation, prolonged hold, thrust

LOCATION:
relationship to R1 and R2

FIGURE 2–11 The steps to mobilization specificity, which include variables to consider when attempting to improve the specificity of joint mobilization (From Wise CH, Gulick DT. *Mobilization Notes: A Rehabilitation Specialist's Pocket Guide.* Philadelphia, PA: FA Davis; 2009, with permission.)

Mechanical Effects

The *mechanical effects* of joint mobilization/manipulation are expected in response to placing stress through tissues that are restricted. It is presumed that changes in accessory movement will ultimately enhance physiological movement. The effects gleaned from joint mobilization of accessory movement are beyond the capability of the patient and requires the skilled application of extrinsic forces. To achieve a mechanical effect, it may be best for the joint to be pre-positioned at the point of restriction (R2), after which the structure is moved into the **plastic region** of the stress-strain curve where permanent deformation occurs (Fig. 2–12). In such a position, minimal force is required to mechanically influence the barrier.

The rhythm and speed of joint mobilization may be modified to allow smooth, staccato, or progressive oscillations, as well as prolonged holds and thrusts. Maitland[7,8] and Paris,[9] among others, describe a variety of rhythms and speeds that may be altered to enhance the effects of the mobilization technique.

Smooth oscillations are characterized by steady, uninterrupted oscillations that may be performed at either high or low frequency. **Staccato oscillations** are performed with varied

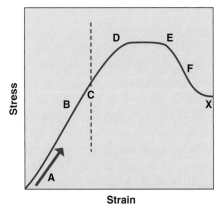

FIGURE 2–12 The stress-strain curve to describe the relationship between the amount of force and temporary and permanent tissue deformation in biological tissues.

amplitude and rhythm in interrupted bursts. Smooth rhythms may be optimal for the patient who is experiencing substantial pain. Because of their unexpected frequency of delivery, staccato rhythms are useful during examination to provide the manual therapist with a good sense of movement in the joint, devoid of patient guarding. **Progressive oscillations** are mobilizations that involve a series of oscillations that go into progressively greater ranges of motion (Fig. 2–13).[7,8]

Psychological Effects

It is incumbent upon all manual physical therapists to understand the power of personal touch. The *psychological effects* of providing OMPT interventions depends largely on the patient's psychoemotional status prior to the interaction. Cook[36] has summarized the work of Main and Watson, who have identified the presence of anxiety, fear, depression, and anger in individuals who are experiencing chronic pain. Increases in self-reported pain, increased sensitivity to painful stimuli, reluctance to movement, learned helplessness, dependency on medication, altered judgment, and a reduction in the desire to improve are often present in the individual who is experiencing chronic pain.[37,38]

Some have suggested that OMPT procedures may have little more than a short-term placebo effect on a patient's presenting condition that is facilitated through providing an intervention that is expected by both the patient and the therapist to have a positive effect.[39] The personal nature inherent to the practice of OMPT may serve as either an invaluable advantage or a detrimental disadvantage regarding the achievement of patient and therapist goals.

Intervention that consists of OMPT has been found to yield better patient satisfaction than intervention that consists of nonmanual procedures, which may be attributed to refocusing the patient into a more positive framework from which to expect improvement.[40–42] In short, patient satisfaction may be as much a factor of who the therapist is as what the therapist does. In addition to learning the skill of manipulative intervention, it is important for the manual physical therapist to create an atmosphere of trust that supports, encourages, and educates the patient regarding expectations.[43]

Regardless of which effect the manual physical therapist is endeavoring to elicit, the therapist must continually engage in a process of examination-intervention-reexamination. Figure 2–14 displays the process by which the manual physical therapist may alter variables based on patient response. Continual reevaluation and collaboration between the therapist and patient allows intervention to be guided by patient response.

INDICATIONS FOR OMPT

Although the indications for the various procedures that constitute manual physical therapy may vary, the primary indication, which applies to all forms, is the *normalization of movement* through manual procedures. When aberrant movement exists, use of OMPT procedures to identify and resolve these conditions should be considered. Box 2-2 summarizes the primary indications for use of joint mobilization techniques for musculoskeletal conditions.

Indications for Soft Tissue Mobilization

The ultimate goal of *soft tissue mobilization (STM)* is the normalization of mobility. Reduced joint mobility may be the result of *myofascial restrictions*, as well as *voluntary muscle guarding*. STM may result in addressing these restrictions and decreasing pain and resistance to movement. More specifically, STM may be used to address **trigger points** within the belly of the muscle, or these techniques may be used to address inflammation, scarring, or adhesions that have taken place in the musculotendinous and tendinous portion of the muscle. *Transverse friction massage (TFM)* is commonly used to eliminate fibrosis and adhesions.[25] These techniques may be extremely beneficial at improving the abnormal *resting tone* of muscle. As myofascial restrictions are addressed, enhanced *muscle performance* is also expected because the muscle is able to function through a greater range of motion.[44]

STM may be important in restoring normal function to the neuromuscular system by eliminating myofascial restrictions

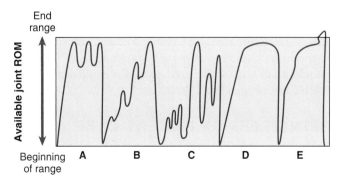

FIGURE 2–13 The rhythm and speed in which joint mobilization is performed may vary depending on the objectives of the intervention and generally consist of a. smooth oscillations, b. staccato oscillations, c. progressive oscillations, d. prolonged holds, and e. high-velocity thrust. (From Paris, SV, Loubert, PV. *Foundations of Clinical Orthopaedics, Course Notes.* St. Augustine, FL: Institute Press; 1990, with permission.)

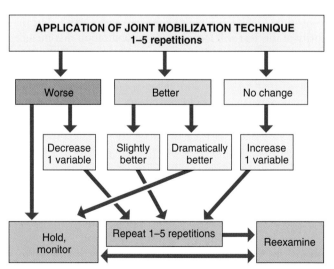

FIGURE 2–14 Clinical decision-making algorithm for guiding variables related to the application of joint mobilization. (From Wise CH, Gulick DT. *Mobilization Notes: A Rehabilitation Specialist's Pocket Guide.* Philadelphia, PA: FA Davis; 2009, with permission.)

that have led to *entrapment neuropathies.*[44] Likewise, STM may be used to enhance cardiopulmonary function through improving thoracic and costal cage mobility and in reducing peripheral edema through *retrograde massage* techniques. These techniques may also be used to reduce inflammatory processes that have occurred within a joint in response to injury. Lymphatic system function may be enhanced through *manual lymph drainage* techniques. See Chapters 13-16 for the philosophy and procedures related to a variety of manual soft tissue approaches.

Indications for Joint Mobilization

Although joint mobilization occupies a large portion of what constitutes OMPT, it is not synonymous with OMPT. The majority of this text will focus on joint mobilization that includes the use of accessory and accessory combined with physiological movement techniques. Joint mobilization techniques may be used to *relieve pain* and enhance *motor function* through facilitation of neurophysiological effects. These techniques may also have the effect of reducing *muscle guarding* that occurs in response to an underlying joint dysfunction. In the presence of *positional faults*, joint mobilization techniques may be used to restore normal articular relationships. (See Box 2-2.)

Indications for Stabilization

Interventions that are used for the purpose of promoting stabilization within a joint are typically provided through nonmanual means (see Chapter 17). In addition to the incorporation of a dynamic stabilization regimen, the manual physical therapist may use joint mobilization techniques to address any adjacent hypomobile segments. In addition, OMPT may take the form

of providing tactile cues during the performance of a stabilization exercise regimen.

CONTRAINDICATIONS AND PRECAUTIONS FOR OMPT

Most restrictions related to the use of OMPT are more relative precautions than strict contraindications. Special care must be exercised when deciding to implement OMPT for the spine, and more specifically, for the cervical spine. The process of patient selection and determining which patients are most likely to benefit and least likely to be harmed by a particular intervention is of paramount importance.

Hurley[45] determined that 88% of physical therapists strongly agree that all available screening tests should be performed prior to performance of Grade V cervical manipulation. Prior to embarking on OMPT for the cervical spine, a *four-tier screening process* is advocated that seeks to identify the presence of any factors that may discourage or prohibit the performance of these techniques (Box 2-3). Because of the inherent risks associated with the performance of these screening procedures, their use is advocated only in cases where intervention is likely to implicate these structures further. The last two tiers of this screening process are recommended only in cases in which the first two tiers have yielded negative findings. It should be noted that these procedures lack sensitivity and specificity. Due to insufficient evidence to support their use, others have attempted to develop criteria for identifying individuals who may be at risk for complications associated with the performance of cervical high velocity thrust manipulation.

Some have suggested use of the simulated manipulation position, in which the cervical spine is placed in a position similar to that in which manipulation is performed, as a screening test. Bowler et al[46] performed a pre-test/post-test single group study on 14 healthy subjects to determine blood flow in both the internal carotid and vertebral arteries in a simulated manipulation position using duplex ultrasound with color Doppler imaging to image the arteries and measure blood flow velocity. The results revealed that there was a significant (p <0.05) reduction in the distal vascular resistance in the vertebral arteries ipsilateral to the side of rotation and the authors concluded that the simulated manipulation position did not adversely affect blood flow through these arteries.[46]

Others have advocated the use of a detailed history that includes identification of risk factors associated with stroke and history of trauma as an important screening tool. The contraindications and relative precautions for implementation of OMPT are listed in Box 2-4.

PRINCIPLES OF PATIENT CARE
Principles of Examination and Evaluation in OMPT

The OMPT Examination

During the process of examination, the manual physical therapist's first responsibility is to determine if the patient's condition is amenable to physical therapy.[47–49] The examination sets the

Box 2-3 THE FOUR-TIER PREMOBILIZATION SCREENING PROCESS FOR THE CERVICAL SPINE

- **Tier 1: Historical Interview:**
  - Rheumatoid arthritis, Down's syndrome, Ehrlos-Danlos syndrome, Marfan's syndrome, lupus erythematosus, ankylosing spondylitis, diffuse idiopathic skeletal hyperostosis (DISH), spondyloarthopathy, cancer (>50 years old, failure to respond, unexplained weight loss, previous history), bone density concerns (osteoporosis, steroid use, chronic renal failure, postmenopausal females)
  - Pregnancy or immediately postpartum, oral contraceptives, anticoagulant therapy
  - Recent trauma, radiculopathy (distal to knee), cauda equina syndrome (+ B/B signs)
  - Intolerance for static postures (Cook, Paris)
  - Acute pain with movement, improved with external support
  - Extension brings on vertigo, nausea, diplopia, tinnitus, dysarthria, and nystagmus
- **Tier 2: Medical Testing and Diagnostic Imaging:**
  - Laboratory values suggesting systemic disease (see Tier 1)
  - Plain film radiography including:
    - *Open-Mouth View:* Visualization of odontoid and C1-C2
    - *Lateral Views and Lateral Stress Views:* Visualization of parallel line relationship and atlanto-dental interface (>3 mm)

- *Oblique Views:* Visualization of defect in pars interarticularis
- Magnetic resonance imaging (MRI), computerized tomography (CT) scans, scintigraphy for identification of subtle pathology
- Doppler ultrasound for detection of vertebrobasilar ischemia (VBI)
- **Tier 3: Clinical Screening Procedures for Segmental Stability:**
  - Sharp-Purser test
  - Aspinall's test
  - Transverse ligament stress test
  - Alar ligament stress test
  - Prone lumbar segmental stability test
  - Anterior lumbar segmental stability test
  - Posterior lumbar segmental stability test
  - Torsional lumbar segmental stability test
  - Prone knee flexion test
  - Axial compression test
  - Passive intervertebral mobility testing (>Grade V)
  - Mobilization prepositioning
  - AROM assessment revealing poor movement quality
  - Palpation revealing step when unsupported and band of hypertrophy
- **Tier 4: Clinical Screening Procedures for VBI**
  - Vertebral artery test
  - Neck torsion test

(From: Wise CH, Gulick DT. *Mobilization Notes: A Rehabilitation Specialist's Pocket Guide.* Philadelphia, PA: FA Davis; 2009, with permission.)

Box 2-4 CONTRAINDICATIONS AND PRECAUTIONS FOR GRADES I–IV JOINT MOBILIZATION

- **Absolute Contraindications:**
  - In the presence of suspected joint hypermobility or instability
  - In the presence of joint inflammation or effusion
  - In the presence of a hard end-feel
  - If medically unstable
  - In the presence of acute pain that worsens with repeated attempts
  - Acute radiculopathy
  - Bone disease or fracture detectable on radiograph
  - Spinal arthropathy (ankylosing spondylitis, diffuse idiopathic skeletal hyperostosis [DISH], spondyloarthopathy)
  - Deteriorating central nervous system pathology
  - Status post-joint fusion
  - Blood clotting disorder
- **Relative Precautions:**
  - Malignancy (>50 years old, failure to respond, unexplained weight loss, previous history)
  - Total joint replacement

- Bone disease not detectable on radiograph (osteoporosis, osteopenia, osteomalacia, osteopetrosis, steroid use, chronic renal failure, postmenopausal females)
- Systemic connective tissue disorders (rheumatoid arthritis, Down's syndrome, Ehrlos-Danlos syndrome, Marfan's syndrome, lupus erythematosus)
- Pregnancy or immediately postpartum, oral contraceptives, anticoagulant therapy
- Recent trauma, radiculopathy (distal to knee or elbow), cauda equina syndrome (+ B/B signs)
- In early healing phase with newly developing connective tissue
- In individuals unable to reliably communicate or respond to intervention (elderly, young children, cognitively impaired, those with language barriers)
- Psychogenic patients exhibiting dependent behaviors, suspected symptom magnification, or irritability
- Long-term use of corticosteroids
- Skin rashes or open wounds in the region being treated
- Elevated pain levels that make palpation and stabilization unreasonable

(From Wise CH, Gulick DT. *Mobilization Notes: A Rehabilitation Specialist's Pocket Guide.* Philadelphia, PA: FA Davis; 2009, with permission.)

tone for the entire course of rehabilitation. It is, therefore, incumbent upon the manual therapist to create an environment that is comfortable yet professional, and one that engenders open communication. The therapist must make every attempt to put the patient at ease through adopting an interactive listening approach, allowing the patient to truly share his or her story.

The therapist must perform the examination without bias and endeavor to make connections between objective data and the patient's condition, only after all data have been obtained.

A minimum of 30 to 45 minutes should be allocated for the examination of most individuals; however, this will vary depending on the therapist's level of experience and the nature of the patient's condition. Since a comprehensive OMPT examination requires skilled use of the hands, this type of examination may be more time intensive than other approaches. In the case of a patient with a complicated presentation, the therapist should not feel compelled to complete the entire examination or initiate intervention on the first day.

The criterion used to determine the depth in which the examination is performed is based upon answering the question, *What data is required to guide the first session?* The manual therapist should not expect to fully understand every nuance of each condition at the time of the initial exam. Furthermore, initiating intervention the first day may be a confounding variable that interferes with the therapist's ability to fully understand the condition, and, therefore, in some cases may not be indicated. Often, the decision regarding how much intervention to provide on the first day depends on the patient's level of tolerance.

The therapist, however, is obliged to educate the patient regarding the findings of the examination and to provide an overview of the anticipated plan of care and prognosis. Instruction in a home exercise program on the first day often serves as the first step toward establishing patient independence. Patients should be informed at the outset of the examination that the initial exam and intervention may induce symptoms. The **twenty-four hour rule** may be applied to both the examination and subsequent interventions. This rule states that the symptoms that occur from any patient encounter should not last longer than 24 hours following the encounter and should only be mild in nature. The patient is asked to pay strict attention, and even document in a journal, the nature and extent of the symptoms in the hours to days following each encounter. Patient tolerance and his or her level of reactivity is critical in determining subsequent care.

The Three Rs of the Examination/Evaluation Process

To provide focus, the manual physical therapist may attempt to identify what is known as the **three Rs** of the examination, which are the (1) reproducible sign, (2) region of origin, and (3) reactivity level. First and foremost, the manual physical therapist seeks to identify the **reproducible sign or symptom**. The purpose of identifying the reproducible sign is to confirm the presence of a mechanical movement disorder and to identify the specific position, movement, or behavior that incites the patient's chief presenting complaint. Upon eliciting a symptom through movement testing, the manual therapist asks the patient, "Is that the pain that brought you in?"

The next *R* that must be determined through the examination/evaluation process is the **region of origin**. When examining a multijoint system of moving parts, it behooves the manual therapist to identify the specific locus of pathology. Identifying the region, or regions, involved in the patient's reproducible sign allows the manual therapist to more efficiently and effectively address the origin of symptoms.

To identify the region of origin, the manual physical therapist begins by having the patient perform single and repeated AROM until the patient's reproducible sign is identified. The therapist then attempts to alter the chief complaint through the application of overpressure and counterpressure. **Overpressure** is applied in the direction in which symptoms were reproduced, and **counterpressure** involves application of forces designed to restrain the symptomatic motion. Alterations in the chief reproducible sign/symptom from specifically applied manual forces provide valuable information regarding the condition's region of origin. If the alleviation of symptoms is noted during the performance of these procedures, the examination may become the intervention.

The third *R* of this evaluative process is **reactivity and relationship** of symptoms to movement. This component of the evaluation allows the therapist to determine the level of irritability and the relationship between the reproducible symptoms and movement. The numeric pain rating scale (NPRS), the amount of time for symptoms to return to baseline, the type of activity that leads to increased symptoms, radiation of symptoms from its site of origin, or the relationship between the onset of symptoms and the range of movement may be used to delineate the patient's level of reactivity. **Low reactivity** consists of pain that is less than 3 on a scale of 1 to 10 or onset of pain at or after end range has been achieved. **High reactivity** is pain that is above 6 with onset that occurs prior to tissue resistance or requires an extended period of time before symptoms return to baseline.[7,8]

The reproducible sign answers the "what" question and allows the therapist to understand what activities or motions are impaired. The region of origin answers the "where" question and allows the therapist to understand the locus of symptom origination. The importance of evaluating the level of reactivity is that it answers the "how" question and assists the therapist in understanding the level of symptom irritability and how aggressively intervention may be provided.

This model of using the patient's symptomatic response to movement in the process of differential diagnosis is useful because it does not require an understanding of pathoanatomy, which is challenging to ascertain without the aid of diagnostic imaging. Furthermore, diagnostic imaging may result in either false-positive findings or true-positive findings that have no correlation to function.[50–52] The symptom-reproduction model provides a means of ensuring immediate clinical relevance by using clinical procedures that can be repeatedly performed as a means of judging the effects of each intervention and showing meaningful change over time.[47–49,53–56]

Principles of Intervention in OMPT

The Role of OMPT Within the Continuum of Care

It may be misinterpreted from reading this text, that OMPT is considered to be the great panacea. Although the specialty of OMPT has enormous promise for enhancing function, it is only one tool within our toolbox of intervention strategies. The principles and practices espoused within this text are the result of efforts that have been clinically demonstrated, but not always empirically proven.

OMPT techniques may be used in *preparation* for other interventions, as the primary *corrective* intervention, or as a *supportive* intervention as follow-up to the primary intervention. The incorporation of active intervention with passive intervention is important for enabling patients to take responsibility for their own care. Within the continuum of care, the use of passive interventions, such as OMPT, are often best used early in the rehabilitation process, with more active interventions used later. Prior to discharge, it is incumbent upon the therapist to provide the patient with the tools needed to maintain progress through active means.

Assessing Tolerance for OMPT Intervention

Particularly during the early-intervention stage, therapists should follow the trial intervention model espoused by Kaltenborn. *Trial interventions* are defined as low-dose interventions designed to assess patient tolerance and confirm the working hypothesis that was established through a process of astute clinical reasoning during the examination and evaluation. These interventions are designed to address one aspect of the patient's condition and are performed in a manner that is approximately 50% to 75% less than what the patient may actually require. The patient's immediate response to these techniques is ascertained, and the patient is asked to monitor symptoms until he or she returns to therapy. The patient's response to the trial intervention determines whether intervention is to be maintained, progressed, or discontinued.

General Recommendations for OMPT Intervention

General recomendations for OMPT, taken from the ***Maitland-Australian Physiotherapy Seminars (MAPS)*** approach,[57-59] which are listed in Box 2-5, may be applied to any of the approaches discussed within this text. Common themes that come from these recommendations are concepts such as using the least force possible and attempting, as best possible, to exercise specificity when performing manual interventions. There is an emphasis on patient assessment as the first step and the most important component of intervention. The process of choosing the individual most likely to benefit from a specific intervention is more important than the actual intervention itself. During intervention, ongoing assessment is used to establish the effectiveness of each technique with new techniques added only after the effects of former techniques have been determined. The process of examination, intervention, and reexamination is conducted repeatedly throughout the course of every intervention session.

Preparation for OMPT Intervention

Therapist Preparation

The manual physical therapist must be aware of the personal physical stresses that result from the performance of manipulative therapy and take every measure to avoid injury. Such interventions demand direct, individualized skilled care that

---

Box 2-5 GENERAL RECOMMENDATIONS FOR PERFORMANCE OF OMPT[57-59]

- Selecting the patients most likely to benefit from a particular technique is more important than the technique itself.
- Begin in the area and direction of greatest restriction.
- Monitor symptoms over the 24-hour period immediately following intervention, and base the next intervention on tolerance.
- If substantial improvement in mobility is noted in response to an intervention, do not be greedy. Wait until the next visit to do more.
- Add a second technique or intervention only after the effects of the first technique have been determined.
- Use as little force as possible to produce the desired effect.
- Use the relationship between pain and resistance to determine aggressiveness.
- Allow individuals to take responsibility for their own care. Initiate active interventions as soon as possible.
- Avoid creation of manual therapy addicts. Do not overuse manual interventions.

- The best way to assess the effect of each technique is to continually reexamine throughout each session by following the process of examination-intervention-reexamination.
- Do not enter into examination with bias. Let the patient's presentation guide your evaluation and plan of care.
- Perform each technique at least twice before abandoning it.
- Do not feel the need to complete the entire examination and initiate intervention on the first day. You need only enough information to educate and advise. The patient's response to intervention on the first day may be confounded by the effects from the examination.
- Use specificity when mobilizing to reduce the effects on adjacent structures. Consider using locking techniques when possible.
- Use the patient's symptomatic response to movement to confirm the clinical relevance of examination findings, as a guide for intervention, and as a dependent variable upon which to confirm the efficacy of chosen interventions.

(From Wise CH, Gulick DT. *Mobilization Notes: A Rehabilitation Specialist's Pocket Guide*. Philadelphia, PA: FA Davis; 2009, with permission.)

requires the sustained and repeated application of forces to individuals of varying body types.

Selecting individuals who are most likely to benefit from chosen interventions takes precedence over decisions regarding specific techniques. The particular manual technique performed is not as important as identifying an appropriate cohort of individuals who are most likely to benefit from manual intervention. The key aspect of manual therapy occurs prior to patient contact through an ongoing process of critical thinking based on clinically-relevant data and patient response. The techniques described in Chapters 22–30 of this text represent an essential skill set of clinically useful techniques designed to assist therapists in embarking upon this area of clinical specialization. However, therapists are encouraged to apply basic principles to the development of new techniques as needs arise. As Maitland stated, "techniques are the brainchild of ingenuity."[7,8]

Prior to embarking on the application of a particular technique, the manual physical therapist should engage in a process of *mental imagery* in which the therapist visualizes ideal performance of each technique. To ensure effectiveness, it is important for the manual physical therapist to engage in diligent and reflective practice.

Therapist Body Mechanics

During mobilization of soft tissues or joints, forces should originate from the therapist's feet, legs, and trunk and not from the upper extremities. The arms are the final component in a multilink system designed to deliver carefully applied forces. To facilitate the proper therapist position, the patient must first be positioned as closely as possible to the therapist to avoid leaning or reaching. Manual physical therapists must adopt efficient postural alignment habitually during examination and intervention so that all of their attention may be directed toward what they perceive through their hands. When performing manual techniques, it is advantageous for the therapist to stand in a **stride-stance position**, with one foot in front of the other and the knees slightly flexed or a **straddle-stance position** in which feet are in line and beyond shoulder-width apart with knees slightly flexed. In this fashion, the therapist's vertical orientation relative to the patient can be controlled through the degree of knee flexion, and the horizontal orientation is controlled through the shifting of body weight from the back to the front foot. Rather than performing trunk rotation, therapists may move their feet to allow them to face the point of contact on the body part that is to be mobilized. Alterations in the amount of applied force occur by transferring body weight and not simply through application of increased arm force. Frequent changes in therapist position are also recommended to more evenly distribute the load across multiple joints. While in the stride-stance or straddle-stance position, the therapist should maintain an erect trunk while performing a drawing in of his or her abdomen to stabilize the spine by transverse abdominis muscle recruitment. Occasionally, when using these positions for an extended period of time, nearly all of the therapist's weight may be placed through the front leg as he or she leans into the table, a position known as the **stride-forward lean position** (see Fig. 2–28).

Regardless of whether standing or sitting techniques are used, the therapist must consider a position with the end of the technique in mind. That is to say, the therapist must be in a position that allows him or her to perform the technique from start to finish in a manner that is safe and effective. While maintaining either the stride-stance or straddle-stance position, the therapist should be prepared to change direction. This may be best accomplished by weight-bearing through the balls of the feet.

Therapist Hand Position

The **hand position** adopted by the therapist is critical for both therapist and patient comfort. The myriad of techniques at the disposal of the therapist often warrants a variety of different hand positions. As a general rule, the therapist's forearm should be placed in the direction in which force is to be applied (Fig. 2–15). The forearm direction, therefore, is often an indicator of the location of the joint's treatment plane. When performing soft tissue mobilization, it may be useful to use either *knuckle* or *elbow pressure* for large areas that require sustained pressure (see Chapter 13). Because these regions are not as sensitive to tactile feedback, it is important for the therapist to monitor patient response when using these contacts. During soft tissue mobilization, it is often best to use the **finger-flexed position**, which maintains the metacarpophalangeal and interphalangeal joints in a slight degree of flexion. Several devices are available to assist in

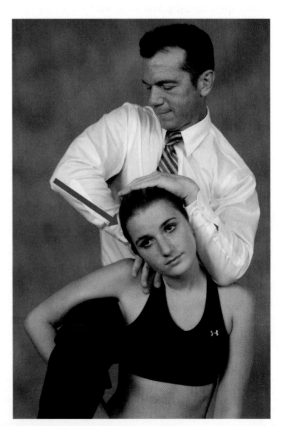

FIGURE 2–15 The position of the therapist's forearm dictates the direction in which forces are applied.

supporting the joints of the fingers and thumb during the performance of soft tissue mobilization (Fig. 2–16). One of the most commonly used hand positions is the **pisiform-contact position**. The area of the hypothenar eminence just distal to the pisiform is placed over the region to be mobilized as the wrist is locked in terminal extension with the fingers extended. This region allows a comfortable contact for the patient and reduces stress through the joints of the fingers and hand that occurs through wrist extension. Another hand position commonly used is the **thumb-over-thumb position** (Fig. 2–17). With this position, the *dumby-thumb* makes contact upon the specific segment to be mobilized while the force-application thumb contacts the dumby-thumb and applies the mobilization force. This position is useful when mobilizing smaller joints such as the sternoclavicular joint, cervical facet joints, or joints of the hand and foot. When mobilizing joints, sometimes **skin-locking techniques** are used (see Chapter 28).

Application of Force

Perhaps the most effective method of protecting the therapist from injury is attending to correct methods of force application. It is recommended that therapists use the *least*

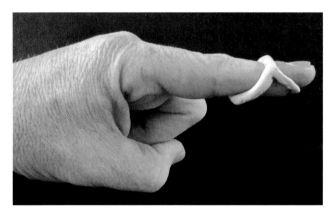

FIGURE 2–16 Protective finger splint for joint mobilization.

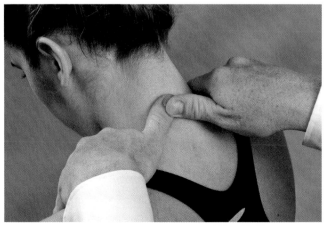

FIGURE 2–17 The thumb-over-thumb position.

amount of force possible to achieve the desired effect. During thrust manipulation, a therapist exerts a force that exceeds the weight of his or her body, which produces deformation in some specified direction.[60] Peak forces delivered during cervical spinal thrust manipulation have been reported to be approximately 100 to 150 N,[61] with forces in other areas of the spine ranging between 400 and 500 N.[62] Studies have found a great degree of variability in the total peak force used among clinicians.[63] Using a pressure pad during performance of a thoracic thrust, Herzog et al[63] identified the average peak force as 238.2 N, the peak local force over the target area as 5 N, and the average rate of force increase as 1,368 N/sec.[63] Additional results revealed that the contact area increases as force increases, calling into question the ability to localize force over the target segment.[63]

It is has been reported that to achieve cavitation in the thoracic spine, an average force of 400 N must be accomplished over a relatively brief period of time. Forand et al compared the forces between male and female chiropractors during thoracic spine thrust manipulation and found that there were no significant differences between gender in the average force provided.[64]

Symons et al attempted to quantify the forces experienced by the vertebral artery during thrust in five cadaver specimens. The results indicated that cervical thrust resulted in an average strain of 6.2% to the vertebral artery at the OA level and 2.1% strain at the C6 level. The values sustained during thrust were lower than those recorded during premanipulative motion testing, including vertebral artery testing.[65] In addition, these results suggest that standard loads used during thrust manipulation are substantially less than that which is able to cause mechanical failure.

Another concept that is valuable in diminishing the amount of force required involves the use of stabilization and locking as described earlier in this chapter. For novice clinicians, it is important to follow the **$1 \times 1 \times 1 \times 1$ rule,** which calls for the manual physical therapist to use one hand to move one joint in one direction at one point in time. That is to say, that when a joint is to be mobilized, one hand should focus on stabilizing as the other mobilizes.

Patient Preparation

Because much of OMPT is passive, it is important that patients understand from the outset that the onus of responsibility for achieving maximal function rests in their hands. Providing a patient with a realistic prognosis that is supported by the findings from the examination and informed by the evidence is important to curtail false expectations. The patient must also be informed of any techniques that may potentially challenge his or her sense of privacy and should be informed regarding appropriate attire. As always, any and all side effects and risks, as well as anticipated benefits, of all procedures must be reviewed, and patients should be given the opportunity to decline any intervention without fear of retribution. Developing a positive and open rapport with each patient prior to the initiation of manual intervention is important to ensure successful outcomes.

After the patient has been informed regarding the plan of care, proper positioning and draping of the patient must be addressed. The factors used to determine the most appropriate position for intervention include the objectives of intervention, patient comfort, the region to be treated, available equipment, the patient's presenting condition, the patient's gender, and the patient's preferences. Positioning the patient comfortably is necessary to ensure maximal relaxation throughout intervention. Having the necessary equipment available and in reach is critical in order to fine-tune each position. The use of pillows, towels, sheets, and bolsters are critical to ensure ideal positioning.

A bolster under the patient's flexed knees when lying supine is often used. In the supine position, the patient's head and neck should be in what has been referred to as the physiologic neutral position,[9] which is about 30 degrees of flexion, unless otherwise indicated. In the prone position, a pillow is often most useful under the abdomen. When mobilization of the thoracic spine is performed with the patient in the prone position, a pillow may be placed lengthwise under the thoracic spine for support. In the prone position, the cervical spine is often subject to increased loads. When this position is required for the performance of OMPT techniques, it is optimal to use a table with a face cutout that places the patient's head and neck in neutral while allowing the patient to breathe comfortably. If such a table is not available, several inexpensive alternatives may be explored. *The Prone Positioning Pillow* (Tumble Forms 2) (Fig. 2–18), found at http://www.sammonspreston.com/Supply/Product.asp?Leaf_Id=920983#, or the *Prone Pillow* (Max-Relax), found at http://www.bannertherapy.com/ProductInfo.aspx?prone-pillow-by-chatt&number=48-100, serve to support the shoulders and cervical spine in neutral and are completely portable.

Having patients wear treatment gowns tied in the back is useful during the performance of most OMPT interventions; however, it is recommended that all body parts receiving manual intervention be completely exposed. This is particularly true when performing soft tissue techniques in which skin contact is critical to the success of the technique. The

gown may be moved aside and held in place by a towel that is tucked in along the border of the gown, thus exposing the region to be treated.

Within this text, we have not included content that addresses more specialized forms of OMPT, such as female-specific internal manual interventions and manual lymph drainage techniques, to name a few. Such interventions require instruction that is beyond the scope of this text.

Equipment and Supplies

Perhaps the most useful piece of equipment for the manual therapist is a medium-sized terry cloth towel. Towels may be used to provide appropriate draping of a body part for patient privacy. When treating the lumbar spine and pelvis, for example, the patient may be asked to unbutton his or her pants. After the patient is lying prone, the towel may be tucked into the waistline of the patient's pants and used to pull them down to the desired level to expose the region. The towel may also be folded over and used to provide padding for patient comfort when mobilizing. A towel may also be rolled up to form a bolster to be used for stabilization or support of a body part. A thin towel or pillow case may also be weaved through the fingers of the therapist during spine techniques to prevent hyperflexion of the fingers. Lastly, a towel may be used as a protective barrier between the patient and therapist to preserve the privacy of the patient and/or therapist.

Another invaluable yet inexpensive piece of equipment is a 3/4- to 1-inch thick, 5- by 7-inch piece of medium-density foam. **Mobilization foam** (Fig. 2–19) is extremely important for improving the comfort of mobilization that is performed over bony prominences or already tender areas. Mobilization foam also serves to enhance contact and disallow sliding over structures to be mobilized. This device is especially useful when mobilizing the glenohumeral joint and the joints of the spine, particularly the cervical region.

Mobilization belts (Fig. 2–20) are also extremely useful devices. Mobilization belts serve to enhance the force-producing

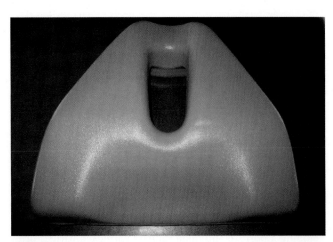
FIGURE 2–18 Prone positioning pillow.

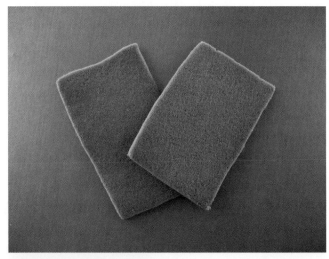
FIGURE 2–19 Mobilization foam.

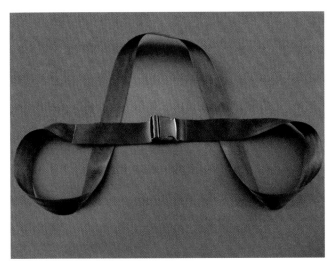

FIGURE 2–20 Mobilization belts.

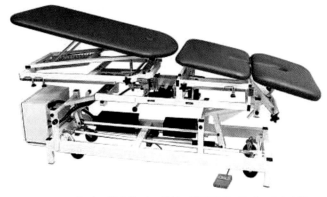

FIGURE 2–21 Cardon Mobilization Table (#R27841, Cardon Rehabilitation Products Inc, Niagara Falls, NY). at: www.cardonrehab.com/Products/Treatment-Tables-Medical-Rehabilitation-Products/Manual-Therapy-Tables/Manual-Mobilization-Rehabilitation-Medical-Treatment-Table.html.

capabilities of the therapist when mobilizing larger joints. These belts should be at least 3 to 6 inches in width and 72 inches in length to ensure a larger surface area for greater patient comfort. They must also be easily adjustable because minor adjustments often need to be made after the belt is in place. Many belts have padding integrated into the belt. These belts work well but are not necessary because a folded towel often serves the same purpose. The belt is typically placed around the therapist's trunk, pelvis, or legs and secured to the most proximal region of the segment to be mobilized. Force is delivered through the belt by the therapist gently leaning or moving away from the patient while stabilizing adjacent regions.

A factor that is not often considered and sometimes is outside of the purview of the treating therapist is the choice regarding the proper *treatment table*. Generally, treatment tables should be stable, easy to clean, well-padded on the top and sides with high-density foam, and at least 28 by 72 inches in size. Ideally, the treatment table should be height-adjustable and include a face hole or additional face cradle attachment to allow for optimal positioning when the patient is prone. Proper table height will vary depending on the size of the patient and therapist and the type of technique to be performed. Generally, the average working height of the table should be at about the tips of the therapist's fingers when they are in an upright standing posture but may be adjusted to as low as the therapist's knees. An additional feature that may also be desirable yet may increase the cost of the table is an electric height adjustment, multi-plane split-table adjustment that allows the therapist to move the patient's trunk or legs in both the sagittal and/or frontal planes. The *Cardon Mobilization Table* (Fig. 2–21) is a highly recommended alternative to the standard nonadjustable plinth. The end section of this table is movable up to 25 degrees in the horizontal plane and can also be rotated 15 degrees around the longitudinal axis on either side. The end section can also be moved back and forth along the longitudinal axis. Each table position may be independently locked. The wide

array of movement capabilities when using this table frees the hands of the therapist to perform all techniques with precision and ease. The controls of the table are accessible from either side, and the electrical Hi-Lo feature adjusts from 21 to 37 inches. The specifications of the table are 80 by 25 inches, 115 V, 60 Hz, 2.2 amps. Although more expensive than the standard table, the Cardon mobilization tables provide the therapist with the ability to easily adjust the table to meet the individual needs of the patient and therapist and is an invaluable adjunct in the practice of OMPT.

When mobilizing soft tissues, massage cream or lubricant may be used to control the degree of glide that occurs between the treating hand of the therapist and the patient's integument. Regardless of the lubricant that is chosen, it should be hypoallergenic, odorless, and dispensed in a manner that is hygienic. The two lubricants recommended for use in most applications of soft tissue mobilization are *Free-Up* (Fig. 2–22) and *Fascia*

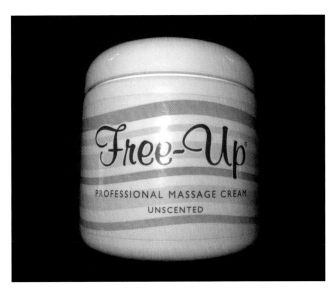

FIGURE 2–22 Free-Up Soft Tissue Mobilization Lubricant (PrePak Products Inc, Oceanside, CA).

Free (Institute of Physical Art Inc., Steamboat Springs, CO). Although many brands of lubricant exist, these two brands are recommended because they do not require frequent reapplication and for their nongreasy, odorless properties.

As described above, stabilization is a critical component of effective joint mobilization. Toward that end, many manual therapists use a **stabilization wedge** (Fig. 2–23) when performing these techniques. The use of the stabilization wedge was originally espoused by Kaltenborn (see Chapter 6). Typically composed of firm rubber with a gutter for pressure relief, stabilization wedges are placed between the treatment table and the body part to be mobilized. These devices enhance performance of stabilization techniques by making the hands of the therapist more available to attend to other aspects of the technique. The use of a wedge is particularly useful when mobilizing the shoulder and spine.

In addition to these standard products, additional items such as **self-mobilization straps** (Fig. 2–24) may also be useful when incorporating these activities into the plan of care for individuals with spinal impairment. Such techniques are espoused by Mulligan and have been described in Chapter 10 of this text.

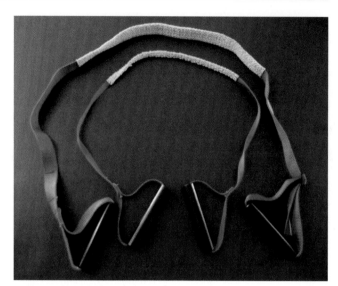

FIGURE 2–24 Self-mobilization straps.

CONCLUSIONS

The purpose of this chapter is to provide the reader with the principles deemed to be most critical to the effective performance of orthopaedic manual physical therapy. Toward that end, the terms used throughout this text have been operationally defined, key theoretical underpinnings related to the practice of OMPT described, and principles related to clinical practice reviewed. This chapter includes important guiding principles that apply to each of the OMPT approaches that follow throughout the remainder of this book. It is recommended that readers familiarize themselves with this chapter before embarking upon the more specific information that is to follow. Readers are reminded that to truly develop the skills required for effective patient care within manual physical therapy, development of psychomotor abilities is required. It is anticipated that with careful study, application of concepts and principles, and practice through guided lab activities and case studies that this textbook will become an invaluable resource for the development of cognitive, affective, and psychomotor skills related to the clinical practice of orthopaedic manual physical therapy.

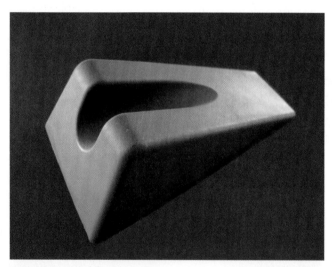

FIGURE 2–23 Stabilization wedge.

REFERENCES

1. Mennell J. *Back Pain: Diagnosis and Treatment Using Manipulative Techniques.* Boston, MA: Little, Brown; 1960.
2. Grieve G. *Modern Manual Therapy of the Vertebral Column.* London, England: Churchill & Livingston; 1986.
3. Salter RB. *Textbook of Disorders and Injuries of the Musculoskeletal System.* 2nd ed. Baltimore, MD: Williams & Wilkins; 1983.
4. Farrell J, Jensen G. Manual therapy: a critical assessment of the role in the profession of physical therapy. *Phys Ther.* 1992;72:843-852.
5. APTA. Manipulation Education Committee. *Manipulation Education Manual.* APTA Manipulation Task Force; 2004.
6. Riddle D. Measurement of accessory motion: critical issues and related concepts. *Phys Ther.* 1992;72:865-887.
7. Maitland GD. *Peripheral Manipulation.* 3rd ed. Woburn, MA: Butterworth-Heinemann; 1991.
8. Maitland GD, Hengeveld E, Banks K, English K. *Maitland's Vertebral Manipulation.* 6th ed. Woburn, MA: Butterworth-Heinemann; 2001.
9. Paris SV, Loubert PV. *Foundations of Clinical Orthopaedics, Course Notes.* St. Augustine, FL: Institute Press; 1990.
10. APTA. *Guide to Physical Therapist Practice.* Rev., 2nd ed. Alexandria, VA: American Physical Therapy Association; 2003.
11. *A Normative Model of Physical Therapist Professional Education: Version 2004.* Alexandria, VA: American Physical Therapy Association; 2004.
12. Commission on Accreditation in Physical Therapy Education. *Evaluative Criteria for the Accreditation of Education Programs for the Preparation of Physical Therapists.* Alexandria, VA: American Physical Therapy Association; 1998.
13. Wainner R. AAOMPT Conference Notes, St Louis, MO: October 19, 2007.

14. Kaltenborn FM. *The Spine: Basic Evaluation and Mobilization Techniques.* 2nd ed. Oslo, Norway: Olaf Norlis Bokhandel; 1993.

15. Paris SV, Irwin M, Yack L. *Advanced Manipulation Including Thrust.* St. Augustine, FL: University of St. Augustine for Health Sciences; 2004.

16. Hsu AT, Hedman T, Chang JH, et al. Changes in abduction and rotation range of motion in response to simulated dorsal and ventral translational mobilization of the glenohumeral joint. *Phys Ther.* 2002;82:544-556.

17. Oatis CA. *Kinesiology: The Mechanics and Pathomechanics of Human Movement.* Philadelphia, PA: Lippincott Williams & Wilkins; 2004.

18. Levangie PK, Norkin CC. *Joint Structure and Function: A Comprehensive Analysis.* 4th ed. Philadelphia, PA: FA Davis Company; 2005.

19. Kaltenborn FM. *Manual Mobilization of the Joints: The Kaltenborn Method of Joint Examination and Treatment, Volume I: The Extremities.* 6th ed. Oslo, Norway: Olaf Norlis Bokhandel; 2002.

20. MacConaill M, Basmajian J. *Muscles and Movement: A Basis for Human Kinesiology.* Baltimore, MD: Williams & Wilkins; 1969.

21. MacConaill M. Joint movement. *Physiotherapy.* 1964;50:363-365.

22. Patla CE, Paris, SV. *E1 Course Notes: Extremity Evaluation and Manipulation.* St. Augustine, FL: Institute of Physical Therapy; 1993.

23. Gonella C, Paris SV. Reliability in evaluating passive intervertebral motion. *Phys Ther.* 1982;62:436-444.

24. Maher C, Adams R. Reliability of pain and stiffness assessments in clinical manual lumbar spine examination. *Phys Ther.* 1994;74:801-811.

25. Cyriax J, Cyriax P. *Cyriax's Illustrated Manual of Orthopaedic Medicine.* Woburn, MA: Butterworth-Heinemann; 1993.

26. Petersen C, Hayes K. Construct validity of Cyriax's selective tension examination: association of end-feels with pain at the knee and shoulder. *J Orthop Sports Phys Ther.* 2000;30:512-521.

27. Hayes K, Petersen C, Falconer J. An examination of Cyriax's passive motion tests with patients having osteoarthritis of the knee. *Phys Ther.* 1994;74:697-707.

28. Bijl D, Dekker J, van Baar M, et al. Validity of Cyriax's concept capsular pattern for the diagnosis of osteoarthritis of hip and/or knee. *Scan J Rheumatol.* 1998;27:347-351.

29. Fritz J, Delitto A, Erhard R, Roman M. An examination of the selective tissue tension scheme, with evidence for the concept of a capsular pattern of the knee. *Phys Ther.* 1998;78:1046-1056.

30. Dishman JD, Bulbulian R. Spinal reflex attenuation associated with spinal manipulation. *Spine.* 2000;25:2519-2524.

31. Dishman JD, Bulbulian R. Comparison of effects of spinal manipulation and massage on motoneuron excitability. *Electromyogr Clin Neurophysiol.* 2001;41:97-106.

32. Dishman JD, Cunningham BM, Burke J. Comparison of tibial nerve H-reflex excitability after cervical and lumbar spine manipulation. *J of Manipulative Physiol Ther.* 2002;25:318-325.

33. Carrick FR. Changes in brain function after manipulation of the cervical spine. *J Manipulative Physiol Ther.* 1998;21:304.

34. Fernandez-De-Las-Penas C, Perez-De-Heredia M, Brea-Rivero M, Miangolarra-Page JC. Immediate effects on pressure pain threshold following a single cervical spine manipulation in healthy subjects. *J Orthop Sports Phys Ther.* 2007;37:325-329.

35. Fernandez-Carnero J, Fernandez-De-Las-Penas C, Cleland JA. Immediate hypoalgesic and motor effects after a single cervical spine manipulation in subjects with lateral epicondylalgia. *J Manipulative Physiol Ther.* 2008; 31:675-681.

36. Cook CE. *Orthopedic Manual Therapy: An Evidence-Based Approach.* Upper Saddle River, NJ: Pearson Education; 2007.

37. Main CJ, Watson PJ. Psychological aspects of pain. *Man Ther.* 1999;4: 203-215.

38. Peters M, Vlaeyen J, Weber W. The joint contribution of physical pathology, pain-related fear and catastrophizing to chronic back pain disability. *Pain.* 2005;115:45-50.

39. Sterling M, Jull G, Wright A. Cervical mobilization: concurrent effects on pain, sympathetic nervous system activity and motor activity. *Man Ther.* 2001;6:72-81.

40. Breen A, Breen R. Back pain and satisfaction with chiropractic treatment: what role does the physical outcome play? *Clin J Pain.* 2003;19:263-268.

41. Curtis P, Carey TS, Evans P, et al. Training in back care to improve outcome and patient satisfaction. Teaching old docs new tricks. *J Fam Pract.* 2000;49:786-792.

42. Goldstein M. Alternative health care: medicine, miracle, or mirage? Philadelphia, PA; Temple University Press: 1999.

43. Cherkin D, Deyo R, Battie M, Street J, Barlow W. A comparison of physical therapy, chiropractic manipulation, and provision of an educational booklet for the treatment of patients with low back pain. *N Engl J Med.* 1998;339:1021-1029.

44. Andrade CK, Clifford P. *Outcome-Based Massage.* Baltimore, MD: Lippincott Williams & Wilkins, 2001.

45. Hurley L, Yardley K, Gross A, Hendry L, McLaughlin L. A survey to examine attitudes and patterns of practice of physiotherapists who perform cervical spine manipulation. *Man Ther.* 2002;7:10-18.

46. Bowler N, Shamley D, Davies R. The effect of a simulated manipulation position on internal carotid and vertebral artery blood flow in healthy individuals. *Man Ther.* 2011;16(1):87-93.

47. Fritz JM, Delitto A, Erhard RE. Comparison of classification-based physical therapy with therapy based on clinical practice guidelines for patients with acute low back pain: a randomized clinical trial. *Spine.* 2003;28: 1363-1371.

48. Delitto A, Cibulka MT, Erhard RE, Tenhula J. Evidence for use of an extension-mobilization category in acute low back syndrome: a prescriptive validation pilot study. *Phys Ther.* 1993;73:216-222.

49. Delitto A, Erhard RE, Bowling RW. A treatment-based classification approach to low back syndrome: identifying and staging patients for conservative treatment. *Phys Ther.* 1995;75:470-489.

50. Frymoyer JW, Newberg A, Pope MH, et al. Spine radiographs in patients with low back pain: an epidemiological study in men. *J Bone Joint Surg Am.* 1984;66:1048-1055.

51. Wiesel S, Tsourmas N, Feffer HL, et al. A study of computer-assisted tomography, I: the incidence of positive CAT scans in an asymptomatic group of patients. *Spine.* 1984;9:549-551.

52. Boden SD, Davis DO, Dina TS, et al. Abnormal magnetic-resonance scans of the lumbar spine in asymptomatic individuals: a prospective investigation. *J Bone Joint Surg Am.* 1990;72:403-408.

53. McClure P. The degenerative cervical spine: pathogenesis and rehabilitation concepts. *J Hand Ther.* 2000;April-June:163-174.

54. Fritz, JM. Use of a classification approach to the treatment of three patients with low back syndrome. *Phys Ther.* 1998;78:766-777.

55. Fritz JM, George S. The use of a classification approach to identify subgroups of patients with acute low back pain: interrater reliability and short-term treatment outcomes. *Spine.* 2000;25:106-114.

56. Delitto A, Shulman AD, Rose SJ, et al. Reliability of a clinical examination to classify patients with low back syndrome. *Phys Ther Prac.* 1992;1:1-9.

57. Maitland Australian Physiotherapy Seminars. *MT-1: Basic Peripheral.* Cutchogue, NY: Cayuga Professional Education; 2005.

58. Maitland Australian Physiotherapy Seminars. *MT-2: Basic Spinal.* Cutchogue, NY: Cayuga Professional Education; 1985.

59. Maitland Australian Physiotherapy Seminars. *MT-3: Intermediate Spinal.* Cutchogue, NY: Cayuga Professional Education; 1999

60. Herzog W. *Clinical Biomechanics of Spinal Manipulation.* New York, NY: Churchill Livingstone; 2000.

61. Kawchuk GN, Herzog W, Hasler EM. Forces generated during spinal manipulative therapy of the cervical spine: a pilot study. *J Manipulative Physiol Ther.* 1992;15:275-278.

62. Conway PJW, Herzog W, Zhang Y, Hasler EM, Ladly K. Forces required to cause cavitation during spinal manipulation in the thoracic spine. *Clin Biomech.* 1993;8:210-214.

63. Herzog W, Kats M, Symons B. The effective forces transmitted by high-speed, low-amplitude thoracic manipulation. *Spine.* 2001;26:2105-2111.

64. Forand D, Drover J, Suleman Z, Symons B, Herzog W. The forces applied by female and male chiropractors during thoracic spinal manipulation. *J Manipulative and Physiol Ther.* 2004;27:49-56.

65. Symons BP, Leonard T, Herzog W. Internal forces sustained by the vertebral artery during spinal manipulative therapy. *J Manipulative Physiol Ther.* 2002;25:504-510.

Principles of Evidence-Based Practice Applied to Orthopaedic Manual Physical Therapy

Paul F. Beattie, PT, PhD, OCS, FAPTA and Philip McClure, PT, PhD, FAPTA

Chapter Objectives

At the conclusion of this chapter, the reader will be able to:

- Define the concept of evidence-based practice (EBP) as proposed by Sackett and colleagues.
- Discuss the importance of using an evidence-based approach to orthopaedic manual physical therapy (OMPT).
- Describe the hierarchy of levels of evidence.

- Recall the primary considerations to be addressed when appraising the strengths and weaknesses of research studies that investigate measures and interventions used in OMPT.

WHY IS THIS CHAPTER IMPORTANT?

If you are like many clinicians, a chapter like this one is readily passed over to get to the *clinically relevant* material that demonstrates actual treatment techniques. However, in today's clinical environment, you can quickly be overwhelmed by the array of possible techniques and approaches to common problems. You may already feel this way if you have attended more than one or two orthopaedic manual physical therapy (OMPT) continuing education courses. Many clinicians will, at this point, simply choose the approach that seems to make the most intuitive sense, or worse, choose the approach advocated by the speaker with the most charm and authority. The real answer to this dilemma, experienced by every conscientious practitioner, is to apply the process and principles of **evidenced-based practice (EBP)**.

WHAT IS EVIDENCE-BASED PRACTICE?

Evidence-based practice can be thought of as a process of using the best available information to assist clinical decisions.[1] In many respects, EBP is what thoughtful, conscientious practitioners have done for years. It simply

has become more systematic and defined in the recent past. The actual process, or steps, involved in EBP are outlined in Box 3-1 and will be discussed in greater detail later in this chapter. EBP has often been erroneously thought of as a recipe for clinical practice that requires a research study to support every action. Clearly this is not practical, thus a more useful way to conceptualize EBP is proposed by Sackett et al[1,2] who describe EBP as a combination of many factors that are used to assist clinical judgments. A simple definition of EBP, therefore, is *using the best available research evidence interfaced with the patient's unique values and circumstances and the clinician's expertise to make clinical decisions.* A fundamental premise of EBP is that research findings assist judgments but do not necessarily mandate them. The insight and skill of the practitioner cannot be ignored. This concept is well-illustrated in the practice of OMPT, which has an interactive form of decision-making; that is, the choice of which procedure to use is often based upon the patient's immediate response to the previous procedure. This phenomenon makes it challenging to design reproducible clinical studies that are able to account for the degree of variation between patients.[3] This is not to suggest that EBP lacks relevance for OMPT. A central core of basic and applied research that addresses mechanisms and outcomes associated with manual therapy is critical for the

Box 3-1 FIVE STEPS TO EVIDENCE-BASED PRACTICE[2]

1. Ask an answerable clinical question.

2. Find the best evidence with which to answer this question.

3. Critically appraise the evidence.

4. Integrate the evidence with clinical expertise and the patient's unique biological features and values to make a clinical decision.

5. Evaluate the effects of applying steps 1 through 4.

advancement of this field. There is a substantial need to distinguish between true and false claims of treatment effectiveness and to determine the factors that identify those patients who are most likely to benefit from care. To achieve these goals, practitioners of OMPT must maximize the use of research findings in a critical manner.[3,4] Historically, the field of OMPT has relied upon an *authoritarian* format of learning. In many ways this is good, but it also leads to *schools of thought* that follow a rigid, often unsubstantiated, protocol approach to evaluation and treatment rather than addressing patients on an individual basis. Expertise is often recognized based on certification and completion of training programs rather than on a record of superior patient outcomes.

QUESTIONS *for* REFLECTION

- Why has the specialty of OMPT not enjoyed a history of evidence to support its efficacy?
- Why have manual physical therapists often relied on authoritarian pronouncements rather than evidence to support their clinical decisions?
- What strategies should clinicians employ to avoid perpetuating this situation?

Consistent with other fields, the base of research evidence addressing OMPT has undergone a gradual but steady growth.[4–11] The reliability and validity of many measures used in manual therapy is now known.[12–14] The emergence of classification systems and clinical prediction rules are assisting the understanding of prognosis and treatment selection,[5,6,15–19] and well-performed intervention studies are supporting the efficacy and effectiveness of many OMPT techniques.[7–11] Although promising data have been presented, there are still many areas of manual therapy that need to be investigated and refined.[9] Innovative applications of research methodology are needed to address this issue.

As the field continues to evolve, there will be large increases in the amount of research findings available. It is important that clinicians are able to critically review relevant research to make the most informed decision regarding patient care.[20–23] The purpose of this chapter is to provide a

fundamental framework of the critical components of research that relate to the diagnostic meaningfulness of OMPT tests and the usefulness of OMPT treatments. This chapter is not intended to be a treatise on research but rather to provide the reader with strategies for incorporating relevant research findings with clinical experience and patient values to optimize the use of manual therapy for evaluation and treatment.

WHEN IS EVIDENCE MOST NEEDED?

Given the rapid growth of information relating to patient care, clinicians are challenged to stay current and to be aware of research findings that may influence their decisions. However, the day-to-day demands of patient care leave most clinicians little time available to find, read, and evaluate the literature. Considering this lack of time, one should prioritize the evaluation of research for those patients for whom the most uncertainty exists regarding the potential risk and benefit of a measure or intervention.[22] Arguably, groups of patients who typically respond favorably to intervention, with few adverse events, do not present the same demand for research evidence as do those who have wide variations in treatment response.[22] For example, most clinicians would agree that performing lumbar manipulation on a young, healthy person with acute, nonradicular low back pain (LBP) is an inexpensive, low-risk procedure that is likely to be helpful for the patient.[6,16] However, the same outcome might not occur in a middle-aged person with severe degenerative disc disease and chronic, work-related low back pain associated with elevated scores on the Fear Avoidance Beliefs Questionnaire.[24] Thus a reasonable question might be, *Under what circumstances is lumbar manipulation likely to be helpful for a patient with chronic work-related LBP that is associated with elevated fear avoidance beliefs?* To address this question, one should strive to obtain the best available evidence.

WHAT IS THE "BEST EVIDENCE"?

Evidence that is used to make clinical judgments comes from many sources including personal experience, intuition, expert opinion, and several different types of research designs. The objective of EBP is to identify the best, or strongest, available evidence to assist in making the relevant clinical decision. Published research findings that have undergone careful peer review are generally considered to be stronger evidence than expert opinion.[1] However, in some instances there is very little meaningful research available, whereas in other cases the volume of research is so vast that it is impractical to completely review.[24] In addition, some published research studies have serious flaws that limit the meaningfulness of the findings.[25,26] Thus, identifying the best evidence is not always a simple task; but it is always an important one.

Conceptually, the best evidence is that which is least likely to be influenced by bias.[22] Consider legal procedures as an example. In courtroom proceedings, the strength of the evidence is typically judged based upon the likelihood of its being affected by bias or error; *hearsay evidence* is more likely to be influenced by bias than is eyewitness evidence. Consistent testimony from multiple eyewitnesses is less likely to be affected by bias compared to testimony from a single eyewitness. DNA testing of human tissue has less error than microscopic examination. Juries are asked to weigh the evidence and make the most logical conclusion. A similar process is used in EBP. A hierarchy of the strength of evidence progresses from authoritarian and personal experience to various types of research design, culminating with the randomized clinical trial (RCT) (Table 3–1). Important information can be derived at any level; however the RCT is likely to be the least biased method to obtain evidence.[22] The reader should be forewarned that the jargon surrounding experimental designs is extensive, and multiple terms and schemes that have overlapping meanings are often used to categorize study designs.

Clinical Experience

Meaningful clinical experience, and the *gestalt* that accompanies this, are critical components of EBP. The wide variation in biological and psychosocial factors[27–32] influencing patient presentation make it very unlikely that the body of research will ever be sufficient to provide an exact formula for patient care. Subtle variations between patients that can be detected by experienced clinicians will always have an important influence on clinical decisions. Thus, even though clinical experience and intuition are considered to be a weak form of knowing, they are nonetheless very important. In instances for which no published research is available to support a clinical decision, experience and intuition are the highest levels of knowing. To be meaningful, clinical experience must be a critical reflection of practice,[33] that is, it is not how much experience one has, but the *quality* of that experience. Experience based upon *this is how we always do it* may be problematic. Experience that develops from self-reflection associated with a consistent, careful evaluation of patients, a logical rationale for treatments, and the use of valid outcome measures is invaluable.[33]

CLINICAL PILLAR

The role of *clinical experience* in EBP is as follows:

- Meaningful clinical experience and intuition are critical components of EBP.

- Experience may detect subtle variations between patients.

- In the absence of published evidence, experience and intuition are the highest level of knowing.

- To be useful, experience must be a critical reflection of practice.

- Clinical experience that develops from self-reflection associated with a consistent, careful evaluation of patients, a logical rationale for intervention, and the use of valid outcome measures is invaluable.

Authoritarian

Within the context of EBP, an *authority* may be a person with an expertise in a given area who provides advice (or mandates) regarding patient care decisions. Although this is considered to be a weak source of evidence, a large portion of medical practice is based on an authoritarian level of knowing. It is noteworthy that, similar to many other fields, the origin and growth of OMPT, until very recently, has been based upon authoritarian levels of knowing provided by leaders in the field such as Cyriax,[34] Maitland,[35] Mennell,[36] and others. Authorities are not necessarily a bad thing. In many instances, the expert level of knowledge provided by these authority figures who act as teachers or consultants has been, and will continue to be, the critical component of clinical decision-making. Unfortunately, in some instances authoritarian levels of knowing can be problematic and may be strongly influenced by bias. For example, an authority figure may have incentive to exaggerate claims of treatment effectiveness in an attempt to increase enrollment in continuing education courses, sales of books, or increase the number of patients seeking care at his or her clinic. If these claims cannot

Table 3–1	Levels of Evidence[81]	
LEVEL	**TYPE OF EVIDENCE**	
1	High-quality systematic reviews, meta-analysis, or randomized clinical trials showing consistent results	
2	Systematic reviews of cohort studies[a] or cohort studies (including lower quality randomized clinical trials) showing consistent results	
3	Systematic reviews of case-control studies[b] or individual case-control studies	
4	Case series or case reports (no control subjects)	
5	Expert opinion and authoritative consensus statements, often based on basic research and "biological plausibility"; clinical experience	

a. Cohort studies involve identifying two groups of patients, one that receives the exposure of interest and one that did not, and *following them forward* for the outcome of interest.

b. Case-control studies use patients who already have a disease (cases) or other outcome of interest and *look back* to see if there are characteristics of these patients that differ from those who don't have the disease.

be substantiated by higher levels of knowing (methodologically sound research), then patients, colleagues, and potential students may be misled into using ineffective and, perhaps, harmful procedures. This may result in wasting time and money and potentially lead to adverse events related to patient care. Therefore, although authoritarian levels of knowing remain vitally important, accurate appraisals of the relevant research are necessary to confirm the meaningfulness of this information. To understand this process it is important to appreciate the strengths and weaknesses of various research designs (Fig. 3–1).

RESEARCH DESIGNS TO ADDRESS ORTHOPAEDIC MANUAL PHYSICAL THERAPY QUESTIONS

Nonexperimental or Quasiexperimental Research Designs (Nonrandom Assignment of Treatment)

Nonexperimental research encompasses many formats and is sometimes called observational research;[37] a treatment may not be involved, or if a treatment is involved, the assignment of a subject to a treatment group is not random. These designs are commonly used to determine reliability and validity of measures, the prevalence, and natural history of a condition, or the outcomes of patients who have similar diagnoses or received similar treatment. Nonexperimental research studies are usually important precursors to randomized designs. They can help to determine relationships between various clinical findings, but

they cannot be used to address causality,[20] that is, the explanation of why a certain outcome has occurred (see Box 3-2).

A fundamental concern with nonexperimental research designs is whether the study was performed prospectively or retrospectively. **Prospective** designs are those in which a specific purpose has been identified and a consistent plan for data collection is used prior to data collection. **Retrospective** studies are designed and performed after data have been collected and are obviously more prone to bias than are prospective designs.

Case Studies

Case studies describe the traits and response to intervention of individual patients. These designs help to formulate, but not test, hypotheses and are a valuable first step in the research process. Well-described case studies can illustrate unique treatment approaches and are especially important when describing patients with uncommon diagnoses.

Case Series

Case series describe a group of patients who have similar characteristics and/or undergo similar interventions. Cases studies and case series designs can be retrospective or prospective and often have longitudinal data collection to describe changes in patient status over time. These designs have been a popular way to describe outcomes in surgical and nonsurgical practices; however, they inherently have many potential sources of bias related to patient selection, treatment application, and measurement. Because they do not use comparison groups, these studies cannot describe causality.

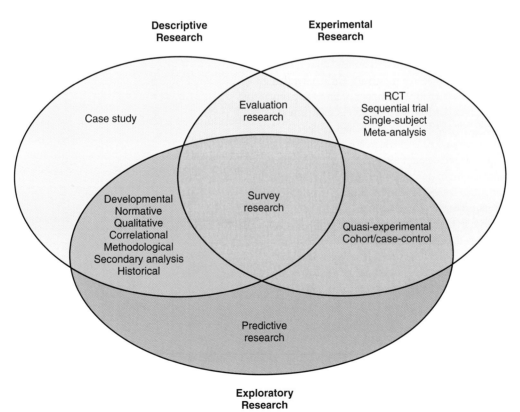

FIGURE 3–1 The three domains of research designs showing overlap between each design. (Adapted from Portney LG, Watkins MP. *Foundations of Clinical Research: Applications to Practice.* 2nd ed. Upper Saddle River, NJ: Prentice Hall Health; 2000.)

Case-Control Designs

These designs retrospectively compare a group of subjects who have a certain condition (cases) to a group of subjects who do not have the condition of interest. These designs are commonly used in epidemiological research and have the advantage of allowing comparisons between groups.[37,38] Thus, they provide a stronger level of evidence than do case study and case series designs. However, because case-control designs do not use random assignment, they can only hypothesize, but not identify, the reason for the differences in outcome between cases and controls.

Experimental Research Designs (Random Assignment of Treatment)

Randomized trials use random assignment of subjects to specific treatment groups and are often called **randomized clinical trials (RCTs).** These designs, although not flawless, allow examiners to test hypotheses and provide the least biased approach to intervention research (see Box 3-3).[22] Subjects are randomly assigned to receive a specific treatment (independent variable), and their outcomes (dependent variables) are compared to similar subjects who are randomly assigned to not receive the treatment (controlled designs) or who receive an alternative treatment of interest (non-controlled designs). Thus, well-performed RCTs can provide evidence of causality for clinical change.[22] If a higher degree of meaningful changes occur over time in the treatment group than occur in other groups who were randomly assigned to not receive the treatment (controls), then one can infer that the treatment caused the change in outcome. RCTs can be difficult to perform, and unfortunately, many of these studies have methodological flaws that limit the meaningfulness of the findings. To address this, researchers have developed rating scales that can be used to quantify the strength of a given RCT. One valuable scale has been described by Maher et al[26] and has been used on the *Physiotherapy Evidence Database* website at the University of Sydney, Australia (Fig. 3–2). This website can be located at http://www.pedro.fhs.usyd.edu.au and is a quick, user-friendly system to identify and determine the rating of relevant RCTs.

HOW DO I USE EVIDENCE IN CLINICAL PRACTICE?

One of the most difficult aspects of EBP is the process by which one incorporates the best available evidence into day-to-day clinical practice. Sackett et al[1] have suggested the five-step process summarized in Box 3-1. In the following section, the first three steps in this process will be described as they relate to identifying an appropriate diagnostic test and determining the potential usefulness of an intervention.

Ask an Answerable Clinical Question

The first challenge of incorporating evidence into practice is to develop a question that can be addressed through a literature search. When developing a research question, it is important to ask, *Is the information likely to matter?* The question should address some area of uncertainty that is likely to have an impact upon improved clinical outcomes, reduced risk to the patient, and/or reduced cost of care. This may result in incorporating a new measure or treatment because it has been shown to be the optimal approach for your intended use; conversely it may also lead to abandoning a previously used measure or treatment. For example, one may ask, *Do the results of this test really provide a meaningful contribution to the way I manage this patient?* If the test is discarded because it is not useful, it may lead to a more efficient use of clinical time and allow clinicians to maximize time used to perform useful procedures.

Relative to measurement, some important questions are as follows: *What test or tests should I use to detect a likely condition? What do the test results tell me? How does this test match up to other tests?* When considering intervention, it is common to ask global questions such as, *What is the likelihood of a specific treatment to be effective relative to cost, risk, and outcome for my patient population?* This issue is of great interest but may be too broad to accurately answer. For example, a common problem with intervention studies is that to control for the effect of the treatment (internal validity), studies often have to use very restricted samples that reduce the generalizability of the findings (external validity). Thus, questions often have to be refined and narrowed to identify research that can address them. Considering this, clinicians must ask if the question is narrow enough to be answerable, yet broad enough to be meaningful.

CLINICAL PILLAR

When determining the usefulness of evidence in clinical practice, ask the following questions:

- Is the information likely to matter?
- Do the results of this test really provide a meaningful contribution to the way I manage this patient?
- What is the likelihood of a specific treatment being effective relative to cost, risk, and outcome for my patient population?
- What test should I use to detect a likely condition, what do the test results tell me, and how does this test match up to other tests?

PEDro Scale

TOTAL SCORE:

1. Eligibility criteria were specified   no ❏   yes ❏

Comments:

2. Subjects were randomly allocated to groups (in a crossover study, subjects were
    randomly allocated in order in which treatments were received)   no ❏   yes ❏

Comments:

3. Allocation was concealed   no ❏   yes ❏

Comments:

4. The groups were similar at baseline regarding the most important prognostic indicators   no ❏   yes ❏

Comments:

5. There was blinding of all subjects   no ❏   yes ❏

Comments:

6. There was blinding of all therapists who administered the therapy   no ❏   yes ❏

Comments:

7. There was blinding of all assessors who measured at least one key outcome   no ❏   yes ❏

Comments:

8. Measures of at least one key outcome were obtained from more than 85%
    of the subjects initially allocated to groups   no ❏   yes ❏

Comments:

9. All subjects for whom outcome measures were available received the treatment or control
    condition as allocated or, where this was not the case, data for at least one key outcome
    was analyzed by "intention to treat"   no ❏   yes ❏

Comments:

10. The results of between-group statistical comparisons are reported for at least one key outcome   no ❏   yes ❏

Comments:

11. The study provides both point measures and measures of variability for at least one key outcome   no ❏   yes ❏

Comments:

Description: The PEDro scale is based on the Delphi list developed by Verhagen and colleagues at the Department of Epidemiology, University of Maastricht *(Verhagen AP et al (1998). The Delphi list: a criteria list for quality assessment of randomised clinical trials for conducting systematic reviews developed by Delphi consensus. Journal of Clinical Epidemiology, 51(12): 1235-41).* The list is based on "expert consensus" not, for the most part, on empirical data. Two additional items not on the Delphi list (PEDro scale items 8 and 10) have been included in the PEDro scale. As more empirical data comes to hand it may become possible to "weight" scale items so that the PEDro score reflects the importance of individual scale items.

Purpose: The purpose of the PEDro scale is to help the users of the PEDro database rapidly identify which of the known or suspected randomised clinical trials (ie RCTs or CCTs) archived on the PEDro database are likely to be internally valid (criteria 2–9), and could have sufficient statistical information to make their results interpretable (criteria 10–11). An additional criterion (criterion 1) that relates to the external validity (or "generalizability" or "applicability" or the trial) has been retained so that the Delphi list is complete, but this criterion will not be used to calculate the PEDro score reported on the PEDro website.

FIGURE 3–2 PEDro criteria are used to rate the methodological quality of a randomized clinical trial and may be applied to other non-RCT intervention studies. (Adapted from Maher C, Sherrington C, Herbert RD, et al. Reliability of the PEDro Scale for rating quality of randomized controlled trials. *PhysTher* 2003;83:713-721.)

Continued

The PEDro scale should not be used as a measure of the "validity" of a study's conclusions. In particular, we caution users of the PEDro scale that studies which show significant treatment effects and which score highly on the PEDro scale do no necessarily provide evidence that the treatment is clinically useful. Additional considerations include whether the treatment effect was big enough to be clinically worthwhile, whether the positive effects of the treatment outweigh its negative effects, and the cost-effectiveness of the treatment. The scale should not be used to compare the "quality" of trials performed in different areas of therapy, primarily because it's not possible to satisfy all scale items in some areas of physiotherapy practice.

Administration of the PEDro scale:

All criteria	**Points are only awarded when a criterion is clearly satisfied.** If on a literal reading of the trial report it is possible that the criterion was not satisfied, a point should not be awarded for that criterion.
Criterion 1	This criterion is satisfied if the report describes the source of subjects and a list of criteria used to determine who was eligible to participate in the study.
Criterion 2	A study is considered to have used random allocation if the report states that allocation was random. The precise method of randomization need not be specified. Procedures such as coin-tossing and dice-rolling should be considered random. Quasi-randomization allocation procedures such as allocation by hospital record number or birth date, or alternation, do not satisfy this criterion.
Criterion 3	*Concealed allocation* means that the person who determined if a subject was eligible for inclusion in the trial was unaware, when this decision was made, of which group the subject would be allocated to. A point is awarded for this criteria, even if it is not stated that allocation was concealed, when the report states that allocation was by sealed opaque envelopes or that allocation involved contacting the holder of the allocation schedule who was "off-site".
Criterion 4	At a minimum, in studies of therapeutic interventions, the report must describe at least one measure of the severity of the condition being treated and at least one (different) key outcome measure at baseline. The rater must be satisfied that the groups' outcomes would not be expected to differ, on the basis of baseline differences in prognostic variables alone, by a clinically significant amount. This criterion is satisfied even if only baseline data of study completers are presented.
Criteria 4, 7–11	*Key outcomes* are those outcomes that provide the primary measure of the effectiveness (of lack of effectiveness) of the therapy. In most studies, more than one variable is used as an outcome measure.
Criterion 5–7	*Blinding* means the person in question (subject, therapist or assessor) did not know which group the subject had been allocated to. In addition, subjects and therapists are only considered to be "blind" if it could be expected that they would have been unable to distinguish between the treatments applied to different groups. In trials in which key outcomes are self-reported (e.g., visual analogue scale, pain diary), the assessor is considered to be blind if the subject was blind.
Criterion 8	This criterion is only satisfied if the report explicitly states *both* the number of subjects initially allocated to groups *and* the number of subjects from whom the key outcome measures were obtained. In trials in which outcomes are measured at several points in time, a key outcome must have been measured in more than 85% of subjects at one of those points in time.
Criterion 9	An *intention to treat* analysis means that, where subjects did not receive treatment (or the control condition) as allocated, and where measures of outcomes were available, the analysis was performed as if subjects received the treatment (or control condition) they were allocated to. This criterion is satisfied, even if there is no mention of analysis by intention to treat, if the report explicitly states that all subjects received treatment or control conditions as allocated.
Criterion 10	A *between-group* statistical comparison involves statistical comparison of one group with another. Depending on the design of the study, this may involve comparison of two or more treatments, or comparison of treatment with a control condition. The analysis may be a simple comparison of outcomes measured after the treatment was administered, or a comparison of the change in one group with the change in another (when a factorial analysis of variance has been used to analyze the data, the latter is often reported as a group $\times$ time interaction). The comparison may be in the form of hypothesis testing (which provides a "p" value, describing the probability that the groups differed only by chance) or in the form of an estimate (for example, the mean or medial difference, or a difference in proportions, or number needed to treat, or a relative risk or hazard ratio) and its confidence interval.
Criterion 11	A *point measure* is a measure of the size of the treatment effect. The treatment effect may be described as a difference in group outcomes, or as the outcome in (each of) all groups. *Measures of variability* include standard deviations, standard errors, confidence intervals, interquartile ranges (or other quantile ranges), and ranges. Point measures and/or measures of variability may be provided graphically (for example, SDs may be given as error bars in a Figure) as long as it is clear what is being graphed (for example, as long as it is clear whether error bars represent SDs or SEs). Where outcomes are categorical, this criterion is considered to have been met if the number of subjects in each category is given for each group.

FIGURE 3–2 (cont'd)

Box 3-3 PROPERTIES OF EXPERIMENTAL RESEARCH DESIGNS

- Use random assignment of subjects to specific treatment groups
- Provide the least biased approach to intervention research
- Provide evidence of causality for clinical change
- May be difficult to perform, and may possess methodological flaws that limit the meaningfulness of the findings

Find the Best Evidence With Which to Answer the Question

With the advent of Internet literature searches, clinicians now have instant access to a large portion of the world's published medical research from a workstation at home or in the clinic. There are an extraordinary number of sites that can be used to identify relevant research studies. One of the most comprehensive and user-friendly websites is *PubMed*, which is maintained by the *National Library of Medicine* (http://www.ncbi.nlm.nih.gov/entrez). This service is free and provides many options and filters to allow refined literature searches. Stratford[39] has described two basic search strategies to find relevant studies on PubMed. The first approach is to identify a systematic review of literature relating to your topic of interest. When multiple RCTs have been performed in a given area, a broader evaluation of the evidence can be identified by providing summaries of the body of literature. Historically, this has been addressed by literature reviews that have qualitatively summarized the body of research. More recently, quantitative reviews of literature, assisted by the development of rating scales, has provided clinicians with **systematic reviews** of many topics that are critical to manual therapy.[7-11,40] The *Cochrane Group* is an international organization that performs systematic reviews of medical literature and generates summary statements that can be of great value for clinicians.[25] These reviews are produced by investigators who identify relevant studies and, using a series of decision rules, create reproducible summaries of the topic of interest. Systematic reviews are considered as secondary analyses and have the advantage of providing a quantitative estimate of the best available evidence. Clinicians should also be fully aware that the specific *rules* used to perform the systematic review may exert a strong influence on the conclusions; therefore, the rules themselves may bias findings, albeit in a systematic way.[41]

In many cases systematic reviews are not available or recent research has not been included in previous reviews. Clinicians should then review the individual studies and critically appraise the strengths, weaknesses, and the likely impact of these studies.

Critically Appraise the Evidence

Considering that research designs vary based upon the intended goal of the study, every study design has inherent strengths and weaknesses. Clinicians who review these studies must decide if the limitations of the study are significant enough to negate the results. The following section discusses research designs that are of central importance to OMPT, that is, those used to investigate diagnostic tests and patient response to manual interventions.

Research Addressing Measurement and Diagnosis

Two basic dimensions in the diagnostic process include a **measurement** and a **judgment**. A measurement requires some form of tool and generates a quantity such as length from a tape measure, degrees from a goniometer, or a percentage score from a questionnaire. A judgment is made by an examiner who rates the quality of one or more patient characteristics, such as passive mobility of a joint. To be meaningful, measurements and judgments must have evidence of reliability and validity (i.e., they are reproducible and provide accurate information that assists in clinical decision making).[42]

Reliability describes the error in a measurement or judgment that occurs in repeated observations made by the same examiner (intrarater) or between different examiners (interrater). Measures or judgments that are reliable have a low degree of error. Conceptually, reliability is the degree to which a finding is reproducible. Measurements or judgments that have not been shown to have adequate reliability should not be used to make clinical decisions.[42] This does not necessarily mean that treatments relating to the measurement should not be used. For instance, a body of research has indicated that precise judgments of lumbar and sacroiliac joint mobility cannot be reliably achieved using manual techniques.[13,14,43,44] Therefore, passive segmental motion testing for the purpose of determining mobility of these joints should not be relied upon for decisions made in the clinical setting.[12,45] However, treatment using lumbar joint mobilization and manipulation by trained clinicians has been shown to be safe, inexpensive, and effective for several patient samples despite the likelihood of disagreement regarding the magnitude of hypomobility.[45] Clinicians may not agree relative to the degree of motion segment mobility, but regardless of this, treating the lumbar spine with manual therapy techniques is often quite effective.

Studies that address reliability must follow several principles. The patient and examiner characteristics must be well-described. A procedure to obtain repeated measures should have a time interval between measures that makes sense; that is, it must be long enough to prevent recall by the examiner and short enough to control for likely changes in the patient's condition. To control for *measurement bias*, the person who obtains the repeated measures must be different from the person who is treating the patient. The researchers must provide numeric estimates of reliability, both as a single measure (point estimate) and a confidence interval (CI) that illustrates the precision of that estimate or the range in which reliability occurs.[42]

A common way to report reliability is by using numeric indices that describe agreement of repeated measures. The **intraclass correlation coefficient (ICC)**[46] is used for continuous measures such as degrees of motion or pain intensity, whereas the **Kappa coefficient (K)**[47] is useful for categorical data such as a positive versus negative test result. An ICC or Kappa value of 1.0 indicates perfect agreement. There are no universally agreed upon cut-off points for determining reliability. This is for the clinician to determine. General guidelines have, however, been described for ICC values by Shrout and Fleiss[46]: ≥0.81 is almost perfect; 0.61 to 0.80 is substantial; 0.41 to 0.60 is moderate; 0.21 to 0.40 is fair; and 0.00 to 0.20 is slight. Landis and Koch[47] have described guidelines for Kappa values as follows: >0.75 is excellent; 0.40 to 0.75 is fair to good; and <0.40 is poor.

Another way to express reliability for continuous measures is to use the **standard error of measurement (SEM)**.[48,49] The SEM allows the degree of error to be expressed in the same units as the measure of interest and is especially valuable when addressing individual patients. Confidence intervals can be generated for the SEM to allow examiners to determine the range of values in which the true score is likely to occur. Those measures with a narrow CI for the SEM provide the most precise estimates.

In addition to addressing reliability, the SEM can be used to calculate the **minimal detectable change (MDC)**, which is a measure that is administered before and after treatment to assess outcome. Although there are several mechanisms described for this process,[50-55] a common way to derive MDC is by multiplying the SEM by the desired CI values (for a 90% CI, multiply by 1.64; for a 95% CI, multiply by 1.96). The resulting value is then multiplied by the square root of 2 to reflect the error associated with the two measures. The resulting MDC indicates how much change is required to be certain that a true change has occurred (i.e., beyond the error). For example, Fritz et al[56] reported that the SEM for the Modified Oswestry Disability Questionnaire was 5.4%. Using this value, they calculated that the MDC was 12.6% (5.4% * 1.64 * √2). Therefore, when obtaining Oswestry measures over time for a given patient, a clinician should be looking for at least a 13% change to be 90% confident that a real change in functional disability has occurred.

If a measure or judgment has been shown to be reliable, it must then be examined for validity to determine the types and strength of information that it provides. *Validity* can be addressed in many forms and is conceptualized as the type of inferences one can make based upon a specific measurement or judgment. **Construct validity** describes the theoretic basis for using a measurement or judgment to make a clinical inference and is typically supported by research evidence.[42] For example, a positive response to a straight leg–raising test has construct validity for inferring the presence of lumbar or sacral spinal nerve entrapment. This construct arose from theory and has been supported by cadaveric and clinical studies.[57] Construct validity is a fundamental property; however, the clinical utility of a test result is increased with evidence of **criterion-referenced validity**, or the comparison of the test result to some outside reference. An important type of criterion-referenced validity for manual therapy evaluation addresses diagnostic accuracy. **Diagnostic accuracy** is determined by comparing the finding in question (usually a positive

or negative clinical test result) to some **gold standard**, or criterion reference, that is an accepted indicator of the diagnosis in question.[58] Studies that assess diagnostic accuracy use several statistical indicators. **Sensitivity** is defined as the number of positive findings/number of people with the condition of interest. Tests with high degrees of sensitivity are generally useful to *rule out* a condition (i.e., a negative test is likely to indicate the absence of the condition). **Specificity** is the number of negative findings/number of people who do not have the condition. Tests with high specificity are generally useful to *rule in* a condition (i.e., a positive test is likely to indicate the presence of the condition). **Positive predictive value** describes the number of true positives/total number of positives. This describes the likelihood that a positive test is truly positive. **Negative predictive value** is the number of true negatives/total number of negative findings. This describes the likelihood that a negative test is truly negative. Positive and negative predictive values are influenced by the prevalence of the condition. For example, false-positive findings are more common when the test is applied to a patient with a low likelihood of having the condition, and negative findings are more common when a test is applied to a patient with high probability of having the condition.[39] Thus, no diagnostic test result should be used in isolation but rather must be considered in light of all other relevant clinical findings.

To provide a richer understanding of a measure, sensitivity and specificity can be combined to calculate **likelihood ratios (LR)**[58,59] (Table 3–2). A LR describes the likelihood that a patient who has the condition of interest would have a certain test result divided by the likelihood that a patient who does not have the condition of interest would have the same test result.[39] The LR for a positive test finding is sensitivity / (1-specificity) and the LR for a negative test result is (1-sensitivity) / specificity. To be useful, positive LRs must be greater than 1.0, and negative LRs must be less than 1.0.[59] Confidence intervals that contain 1.0 indicate that the LRs are not significant. An example of the interpretation of these indices is illustrated by Tong et al[60] who investigated the diagnostic accuracy of findings from the Spurling's test to identify the presence of cervical radiculopathy.

Predictive validity describes the degree to which a finding can be used to predict a future event. Predictive validity is a major requirement of measures used to develop a patient prognosis.[61,62] This can be applied to measures from individual tests or from a single measure derived from several measures such as those described in clinical prediction rules.[15,16] Predictive validity is also a key element in screening tools such as those used during preemployment testing or preseason athletic examinations.[42] Measures used to return injured athletes to competition must have predicative validity to describe the likelihood of reinjury. Predictive validity must be established by longitudinal research designs in which a finding is obtained and the patient is observed over time to determine if the event in question occurs. Similar to diagnostic accuracy, measures of sensitivity, specificity, and likelihood ratios can be determined. In addition, indicators such as *odds ratios* and relative risk can be used.[61,62]

Table 3–2	Measures of Diagnostic Accuracy: Example for Cervical Radiculopathy From Tong and Colleagues[60]	
	FINDINGS FROM GOLD STANDARD (EMG RESULTS)	
	EMG + RADICULOPATHY PRESENT	**EMG – RADICULOPATHY ABSENT**
Clinical Test (+ Spurling's)	A 6 (True-Positive)	B 12 (False-Positive)
Clinical Test (– Spurling's)	C 14 (False-Negative)	D 160 (True-Negative)
	Sensitivity = A /A + C 6/20 = 0.30	Specificity = D / B + D 160/172= 0.93

EMG, electromyogram; LR, likelihood ratios
LR+ = 4.3 = Sensitivity / (1-Specificity)
LR– = 0.75 = (1-Sensitivity) / Specificity

Prescriptive validity is very desirable as it describes the degree to which a certain finding will be influenced by treatment. Prescriptive validity must be established by randomized clinical trials. Treatment-based classification groups represent patients with similar traits who are likely to respond in the same way to treatment.[17]

Research Addressing Intervention

Outcome measures are a fundamental concern when assessing intervention studies.[63,64] If the measures are not reliable or meaningful for the patient, very little inference can be made from the study. Depending on the goal of the study, outcome measures may include assessments of biological events or more clinically relevant measures such as function, pain, cost, or satisfaction with care.[63] As previously discussed, the key measurement property of an outcome measure is its ability to reflect meaningful change over time.[50–55] The MDC scores represent the magnitude of change that must be exceeded to be confident that a meaningful degree of change (i.e., beyond the potential degree of error) has been exceeded.

Construct validity relates to the appropriateness of the overall design to address the question of interest. This implies that the measures, subjects, and manipulation of treatments are suitable.

Internal validity describes the degree to which the observed changes in the dependent variable (outcome of interest) are caused by the independent variable (the treatment). Well-designed RCTs attempt to minimize the influence of factors other than the independent variable (confounding variables) on the outcome of interest. Treatments that have been shown to have a significant effect in controlled studies with high degrees of internal validity are considered to have *efficacy*; that is, when the treatment is applied under very specific conditions, it is likely to have a positive treatment effect.

External validity describes the generalizability of the findings, or to whom the results of a study may be applied. This is a major concern in health-care research because many patients have unique characteristics that may influence their response to treatment. Treatments that have been shown to have a positive effect in studies that have high degrees of external validity are considered to have *effectiveness*, meaning that they are likely to be applicable in real-world settings.

Statistical conclusion validity addresses the possibly of a statistical error that results in a wrong conclusion.[65] A **type I error** occurs when the researcher wrongfully rejects the null hypothesis (i.e., concludes that there is a significant treatment effect when there actually is not). This represents a false-positive finding and is guarded against by setting a minimally acceptable **alpha**, the probability (as measured by a p-value) that any differences observed are due to chance. By convention, the p-value is typically set at $p < 0.05$, meaning that the probability of a difference between measures occurring by chance is 5% or less. If multiple comparisons are made, the likelihood of a random finding increases. This may cause an experiment-wise error. To control for this, researchers often set the alpha lower, that is, $p < 0.01$.

A **type II error** is more common than type I error and occurs when the researcher wrongfully accepts the null hypothesis (concludes that there is no difference when actually there is). This represents a false-negative finding and most typically occurs when studies have small sample sizes, particularly when the differences between group means "look" different based on clinical judgment. This is known as an *underpowered study* and is a major concern in clinical research, where subject recruitment and retention can be a problem. Type II errors are ideally addressed by performing a power analysis that indicates the number of subjects needed in each group before the study begins.[65] Studies with too few subjects are severely limited in their meaningfulness.

In the absence of a type I statistical error, the presence of a statistically significant difference in outcome (usually a p-value <0.05 or 0.01) between groups in an intervention study indicates that there likely is a true difference between the mean scores, but does not indicate how much difference is present. In some cases, particularly with large sample sizes, the difference between groups might be quite small and still be significant. For example, a group of subjects treated by exercise might have significantly lower pain scores than a group treated by manipulation; however, this difference might only be 0.5 out of 10 on a numeric rating scale of pain. This difference, although statistically significant, might be too small to matter to patients. In many cases, this difference may not exceed the lower bound of the confidence interval of the outcome measure MDC, suggesting that the difference may be the result of measurement error and not treatment effect.

Another important measure of difference between groups is known as **effect size**. Effect size provides a ratio value that indicates how much of a difference, in terms of standard deviations, is present between groups. General guidelines for interpreting an effect size are as follows: 0.20 is small; 0.40 is moderate; and >0.80 is large.[66] The main feature of relying on effect size to interpret the magnitude of the treatment effect is that it is not influenced by sample size, whereas *p*-values of statistical tests are dramatically affected by sample size.

Refer to Box 3-4 for a summary of the terms used in this section.

Apply the Evidence to a Specific Clinical Problem

Using a Diagnostic Test

When a research study or systematic review describes a measure, the fundamental question is *Can I apply this measure to my patient in the clinic and expect meaningful results?* This is not always an easy question to answer and requires several steps.[67] Table 3–3 summarizes a series of questions you may ask when reviewing the relevant literature regarding a test. The first concern should be whether the patients sampled during the study share enough characteristics with your patient to expect a similar performance on the test. This is an issue of *external validity* and can be conceptualized as the presence of population-specific measurement characteristics. This means a measure can only be generalized to the same population from which it was tested.[42] A measure that was shown to be reliable when tested on healthy young students may not have the same properties when applied to middle-aged patients with degenerative disc disease. A similar concern relates to the qualifications of the examiners in the research study. People with advanced training and/or certification to perform and interpret a specific manual therapy test may have different reliability than do those who do not possess these skills.

Once it is established that the subjects and the examiner have characteristics similar to those that have been studied, one should consider the rationale for performing the test, that is, one should ask *How will the results of this test influence my management of this patient?* In most medical environments, the cost and risk of a test must be balanced against its diagnostic yield.[68,69] Although most manual therapy tests are inexpensive and of low risk when performed properly on patients who have been adequately screened, ancillary tests such as percutaneous electromyography, spinal radiographs, or magnetic resonance imaging (MRI) may involve a substantial increase in cost and risk to the patient. In certain cases measures and judgments made from lumbar spine radiographs or MRI have low diagnostic accuracy when used to detect or rule out the condition of interest.[70–72] Thus, clinicians must determine if performing a test is likely to increase the detection of a treatment precaution or contraindication that may necessitate referral or consultation or if the test is likely to provide indications for a specific treatment that has not already been identified.

If a clinician believes that a diagnostic test may be indicated for a specific patient, and it can be appropriately performed, a careful review of the validity of the specific findings of the study must be undertaken. If the study is relatively free of bias, one should determine the likelihood of a reliable finding and the strength of the measure to rule in or rule out a given condition.

Applying an Intervention

The major goal of evidence-based practice is to determine the management strategy for an individual patient that provides the best outcome with the least risk. Incorporating the results of well-performed intervention studies is central to this objective. Similar to addressing the concerns of applying a diagnostic test, the key clinical question is, *Can I apply the treatments investigated in this study to my patient and expect the same results?* As previously described, the four basic dimensions that need to be considered when appraising the value of an intervention study are construct validity, external validity, internal validity, and the meaningfulness of the differences between treatment groups. A checklist to address these dimensions is described in Table 3–4.

An additional concern relates to the degree to which using a certain intervention is superior to using a different intervention. Recently, researchers have addressed this issue using a measure called the **number needed to treat (NNT)**.[73,74] The

---

Box 3-4 THE TERMINOLOGY OF EBP

- **Construct validity**: Describes the theoretic basis for using a measurement or judgment to make a clinical inference and relates to the appropriateness of the overall design to address the question of interest
- **Criterion-referenced validity:** The comparison of the test result to some outside reference
- **Diagnostic accuracy:** Determined by comparing the finding in question to some gold standard
- **External validity:** Describes the generalizability of the findings, or to whom the results may be applied
- **Internal validity:** The degree to which the observed changes in the dependent variable are caused by the independent variable
- **Minimal detectable change (MDC)**: A measure used before and after treatment to assess how much change is required to be certain that a true change has occurred

- **Negative predictive value:** Describes the likelihood that a negative test is truly negative
- **Positive predictive value:** Describes the likelihood that a positive test is truly positive
- **Predictive validity:** Describes the degree to which a finding can be used to predict a future event
- **Prescriptive validity:** Describes the degree to which a certain finding will be influenced by treatment
- **Reliability**: The degree to which a finding is reproducible
- **Sensitivity:** Useful to *rule out* a condition (i.e., a negative test is likely to indicate the absence of the condition)
- **Specificity:** Useful to *rule in* a condition (i.e., a positive test is likely to indicate the presence of the condition)
- **Type I error:** Represents a false-positive finding
- **Type II error:** Represents a false-negative finding

Table 3–3	A Checklist to Use When Reviewing Research Findings That Address Clinical Measures		
CRITICAL CONCERNS		**YES**	**NO**
Are the patients that were studied similar enough to my patient to allow me to perform the test and apply the results?	Age, clinical picture, comorbidities Indications for test: Pretest likelihood of the condition being present Risk of applying test		
Do I have similar enough characteristics to the examiners to apply the test correctly?	Training Equipment		
Is the test result likely to influence the way I treat my patient?	Identify a contraindication or precaution for treatment Need to refer or consult Identify an indication for treatment		
Are the results of the study valid?	Control for measurement bias Meaningful gold standard measured by a blinded examiner Adequate sample size		
Are the test results reliable?	Point estimates and CIs for reliability coefficient and standard error of measure		
What do the test results tell me? Can I make a meaningful judgment from a positive or negative test? *Diagnostic accuracy*: Increase the likelihood of the presence or absence of a condition? *Predictive validity*: Predict outcome *Prescriptive validity*: Identify the likelihood of treatment response from a specific intervention	Sensitivity Specificity Predictive values (+) and (−) LRs with CIs		

Each category should be answered yes to provide meaningful research support for using the measure in question.

Table 3–4	A Checklist to Use When Reviewing Research Findings That Address Intervention Studies		
CONCERN	**DESCRIPTION**	**YES**	**NO**
External validity: Is the study sample similar enough to my patient to expect similar results following the intervention?	Age, clinical picture, comorbidities Stage of condition Contraindications and precautions Psychosocial factors		
Do I have similar enough characteristics to the examiners to perform the intervention?	Training Equipment		
Internal validity: Is the reported outcome likely to be caused by the treatment?	True randomized group assignment Equal application of treatment within the intervention group Adequate subject follow-up Reliable outcome measures Control for measurement bias Control for type I and type II statistical error		
Is the treatment effect meaningful enough to use the intervention?	Outcome measure is meaningful to patient Mean difference is significant and exceeds minimal detectable change score Effect size is large enough to be meaningful and is comparable, or better, than other similar interventions		

Each category should be answered yes to provide meaningful research support for using the measure in question.

NNT describes the number of patients you would need to treat with one intervention before you can be sure that one patient improved who would not have improved without that intervention.[73] For example, a NNT of 3 would indicate that three patients would need to be treated with the intervention of interest before one patient had better outcomes than he or she would have if treated with a different intervention. The NNT of 3 does not predict which patient will have superior outcomes or how great the differences will be, only that after three patients have been treated one patient will have benefited more from the intervention than if he or she had not had it.[73]

CLINICAL PILLAR

The major goal of EBP is to determine the management strategy for an individual patient that will provide the best outcome with the least risk.

Evaluate the Effects of Applying the Evidence to Clinical Practice

Applying research evidence to practice is only meaningful if it results in improved clinical practice. To properly evaluate this, you must decide upon the outcomes that are of concern and use meaningful measures to assess these. These measures are a component of the initial question that was asked and could include estimates of pain or functional status, patient satisfaction, or cost of care.

CONCLUSIONS

In this chapter, we have discussed many of the components that must be addressed to use evidence in the practice of OMPT. Evidence-based practice is a complex process that often involves transferring data observed from group designs to individual patients.[75] Careful reflection is required to identify when evidence is most needed and by what procedures it can be implemented and evaluated.[22] In some cases, research evidence can be difficult to accept. Outcome studies that address OMPT interventions often have favorable results; however, the mechanism by which manual therapy is associated with these results may be much different from that which is generally believed. For example, arguments have been made regarding the role of displacement of the sacroiliac joint (SIJ) in regional back pain.[76] A large body of research, however, concludes that for most subjects displacement of the SIJ is minimal and is not likely to be detected by examiners—nor is it likely to be changed by manipulation.[43,77,78] However, clinical studies that have employed SIJ manipulation have reported favorable treatment outcomes.[79]

Based upon these findings, one could conclude that properly applied manipulation is likely to be a useful treatment, but its mechanism of action may be much different from that which was previously thought. This observation could lead to exciting new research inquiries that may, in turn, lead to the development of more effective interventions.[9]

CLINICAL PILLAR

To use evidence most effectively, the clinician must do the following:

● Use careful reflection to identify when evidence is most needed and by what procedures it can be implemented and evaluated

● Be open to considering how evidence may support the use of certain interventions but suggest alternative mechanisms for their efficacy

---

There are many challenges in applying research evidence to medical care.[1,21–23] The potential for heterogeneity of treatment responses between patients[75] illustrates the potential for clinical variation that has led Upsur[80] to describe EBP as "making rules in a world of uncertainty." Thus, it is unlikely that systems will evolve to allow evidence-based recipes for care. Clinicians will always need to integrate the best research evidence with the unique circumstances of individual patients. Ignoring research evidence, however, will result in stagnation of the field and potential propagation of myths and ineffective treatments that would be catastrophic for the specialty of OMPT. Herbert et al[22] have concluded that "evidence-based practice is not perfect but it is the best system we have."

NOTABLE QUOTABLE

Evidence-based practice is "making rules in a world of uncertainty."

R.E. Upsur, 2005

NOTABLE QUOTABLE

"Evidence-based practice is not perfect but it is the best system we have."

H.D. Herbert et al, 2001

REFERENCES

1. Sackett DL. Evidence-based medicine. *Spine.* 1988;23:1085-1086.
2. Sackett DL, Haynes RB, Guyatt GH, et al. *Clinical Epidemiology: A Basic Science for Clinical Medicine.* Boston, MA: Little, Brown; 1991.
3. Fitzgerald K, McClure P, Beattie PF, et al. Issues in determining the efficacy of manual therapy. *Phys Ther.* 1994;74:227-233.
4. DiFabio R. Efficacy of manual therapy. *Phys Ther.* 1992;72:853-864.
5. Delitto T, Cibulka M, Erhard R. Evidence for the use of an extension-mobilization category in acute low back syndrome. A prescriptive-validation pilot study. *Phys Ther.* 1993;73:216-228.
6. Flynn T, Fritz J, Whitman J, et al. A clinical prediction rule for classifying patients with low back pain who demonstrate short-term improvement with spinal manipulation. *Spine.* 2002;27:2835-2843.
7. Lisi AJ, Holmes EJ, Ammendolia C. High-velocity low-amplitude spinal manipulation for symptomatic lumbar disk disease: a systematic review of the literature. *J Manipulative Physiol Ther.* 2005;28:429-442.
8. Rademeyer I. Manual therapy for lumbar spinal stenosis: a comprehensive physical therapy approach. *Phys Med Rehabil Clin N Am.* 2003;1:103-110.
9. Smith AR, Jr. Manual therapy: the historical, current, and future role in the treatment of pain. *Scientific World Journal.* 2007;2:109-120.
10. vanTudler MW, Koes BW, Bouter LM. Conservative treatment of acute and chronic nonspecific low back pain: a systematic review of randomized controlled trials of the most common interventions. *Spine.* 1997;22:2128-2156.
11. van der Wees PJ, Lenssen AF, Hendriks EJ, et al. Effectiveness of exercise therapy and manual mobilisation in ankle sprain and functional instability: a systematic review. *Aust J Physiother.* 2006;52:27-37.
12. Fritz JM, Whitman JM, Childs JD. Lumbar spine segmental mobility assessment: an examination of validity for determining intervention strategies in patients with low back pain. *Arch Phy Med Rehab.* 2005;86:1745-1752.
13. Maher C, Adams R. Reliability of pain and stiffness assessments in clinical manual lumbar spine examination. *Phys Ther.* 1995;74:801-811.
14. McCombe PF. Reproducibility of physical signs in low-back pain. *Spine.* 1989;14:908-918.
15. Beattie P, Nelson RM. Clinical prediction rules: what are they and what do they tell us? *Aust J Physiother.* 2006;52:157-163.
16. Childs J, Fritz J, Flynn T, et al. A clinical prediction rule to identify patients with low back pain most likely to benefit from spinal manipulation: a validation study. *Ann Inter Medicine.* 2004;141:920-928.
17. Delitto A, Erhard RE, Bowling RW: A treatment-based classification approach to low back syndrome: identifying and staging patients for conservative treatment. *Phys Ther.* 1995;75:470-485.
18. Fritz JM, Delitto A, Erhard RE. Comparison of classification-based physical therapy with therapy based on clinical practice guidelines for patient with acute low back pain. *Spine.* 2003;28:1363-1372.
19. Wang WT, Olson SL, Campbell AH, et al. Effectiveness of physical therapy for patients with neck pain: an individualized approach using a clinical decision-making algorithm. *Am J Phy Med Rehab.* 2003;82:203-218.
20. Elwood JM. The importance of causal relationships in medicine. In: Elwood JM. *Causal Relationships in Medicine: A Practical System for Critical Appraisal.* New York, NY: Oxford Press; 1988:3-9.
21. Haynes B, Haines A. Barriers and bridges to evidence based clinical practice. *BMJ.* 1998;317:273-276.
22. Herbert RD, Sherrington C, Maher C, et al. Evidence-based practice-imperfect but necessary. *Physiother Theory Prac.* 2001;17:201-211.
23. Straus SE, Sackett DL. Using research findings in clinical practice. *BMJ.* 1998;317:339-342.
24. Waddell G. *The Back Pain Revolution.* 2nd ed. London, UK: Churchill-Livingstone; 2004.
25. vanTulder M, Furlan A, Bombardier C, et al. Updated method guidelines for systematic reviews in the Cochrane Collaboration Back Review Group. *Spine.* 2003;28:1290-1299.
26. Maher C, Sherrington C, Herbert, RD, et al. Reliability of the PEDro Scale for rating quality of randomized controlled trials. *Phys Ther.* 2003 83:713-721.
27. Beattie P. The relationship between symptoms and abnormal magnetic resonance images of lumbar intervertebral discs. *Phys Ther.* 1996;76:601-608.
28. Feuerstein M, Beattie P. Biobehavioral factors affecting pain and disability in low back pain. *Phys Ther.* 1995;75:267-280.
29. Riipinen M, Neimisto L, Lindgren KA, et al. Psychosocial differences as predictors for recovery from chronic low back pain following manipulation, stabilizing exercises and physician consultation or physician consultation alone. *J Rehab Med.* 2005;37:152-158.
30. Turner JA, Franklin G, Fulton-Kehoe D, et al. Worker recovery expectations and fear-avoidance predict work disability in a population-based workers' compensation back pain sample. *Spine.* 2006;31:682-689.
31. Verbunt JA, Seelen HA, Vlaeyen JW, et al. Fear of injury and physical de-conditioning in patients chronic low back pain. *Arch Phys Med Rehabil.* 2003;84:1227-1232.
32. vanTulder M, Assendelft W, Koes B, et al. Spinal radiographic findings and nonspecific low back pain. *Spine.* 1997;22:427-434.
33. Shepard KF, Jensen GM. Physical therapist curricula for the 1990s: educating the reflective practitioner. *Phys Ther.* 1990;70:566-573.
34. Cyriax J. *Textbook of Orthopedic Medicine. Vol. 1: Diagnosis of Soft Tissue Lesions.* London, UK: Balliarre Tindall; 1981.
35. Maitland GD. *Vertebral Manipulation.* 4th ed. Boston, MA: Butterworth; 1984.
36. Mennel J. *The Science and Art of Joint Manipulation.* London, UK: Churchill; 1952.
37. Mann CJ. Observational research methods. Research design II: cohort, cross-sectional, and case-control studies. *Emerg Med J.* 2003;20:54-60.
38. Bombardier C, Kerr HS, Shannon HS, et al. A guide to interpreting epidemiologic studies on the etiology of back pain. *Spine.* 1994;19:2047S-2056S.
39. Stratford P. Applying results from diagnostic accuracy studies to enhance clinical decision-making. *Physiother Theory Prac.* 2001;17:153-160.
40. Gross AR, Kay T, Hondras M, et al. Manual therapy for mechanical neck disorders: a systematic review. *Man Ther.* 2002;3:131-149.
41. Ferreira PH, Ferreira ML, Maher CG, et al. Effect of applying different "levels of evidence" criteria on conclusions of Cochrane Reviews of interventions for low back pain. *J Clin Epidemiol.* 2002;55:1126-1129.
42. Rothstein JM, Echternach J. *Primer on Measurement:An Introductory Guide to Measurement Issues.* Alexandria, VA: American Physical Therapy Association; 1993.
43. van der Wurff P, Meyne W, Hagmeijer RH. Clinical tests of the sacroiliac joint. *Man Ther.* 2000;5:89-96.
44. Binkley J, Stratford PW, Gill C. Inter-rater reliability of lumbar accessory motion mobility testing. *Phys Ther.* 1995;75:786-792.
45. Flynn TW. Move it and move on. *J Orthop Sports Phys Ther.* 2002;32:192-193.
46. Shrout PE, Fleiss JL. Intraclass correlations: uses in assessing rater reliability. *Psychol Bull* 1979;86:420-428.
47. Landis JR, Koch GG. The measurement of observer agreement for categorical data. *Biometrics.* 1977;33:159-174.
48. Diamond JJ. A practical application of reliability theory to family practice research. *Fam Prac Res J.* 1991;11:357-362.
49. Roddy TS, Olson SL, Cook KF, et al. Comparison of the University of California-Los Angeles Shoulder Scale and the Simple Shoulder Test with the Shoulder Pain and Disability Index: single administration reliability and validity. *Phys Ther.* 2000;80:759-768.
50. Liang MH. Longitudinal construct validity: establishment of clinical meaning in patient evaluation instruments. *Medical Care.* 2000;28:632-642.
51. Schmitt JS, Di Fabio RP. Reliable change and minimum important difference (MID) proportions facilitated group responsiveness comparisons using individual threshold criteria. *J Clin Epidemiol.* 2004;57:1008-1018.
52. Stratford P, Binkley J, Solomon P, et al. Assessing change over time in patients with low back pain. *Phys Ther.* 1994;74:528-533.
53. Stratford P, Binkley J, Solomon P, et al. Defining the minimum level of detectable change for the Roland-Morris Questionnaire. *Phys Ther.* 1996;76:359-365.
54. Haley SM, Fraggala-Pinkham M. Interpreting change scores of tests and measures used in physical therapy. *Phys Ther.* 2006;86:735-743.
55. de Vet HC, Terwee CB, Ostelo RW, et al. Minimal changes in health status questionnaires: distinction between minimally detectable change and minimally important change. *Health Qual Life Outcomes.* 2006;22:54.
56. Fritz JM, Irrgang JJ. A comparison of a modified Oswestry Low Back Pain Disability Questionnaire and the Quebec Back Pain Disability Scale. *Phys Ther.* 2001;81:776-788.
57. Supik LF, Broom MJ. Sciatic tension signs and lumbar disc herniation. *Spine.* 1994;1066-1069.
58. Riddle DL, Stratford PW. Interpreting validity indexes for diagnostic tests: an illustration using the Berg Balance Test. *Phys Ther.* 1999;79:939-948.
59. Jaeschke R, Guyatt GH, Sackett DL. Users guide to the medical literature, III: how to use an article about a diagnostic test, B: what are the results and will they help me in caring for my patients? *JAMA.* 1994;271:703-770.
60. Tong HC, Haig AJ, Yamakawa K. The Spurling Test and Cervical Radiculopathy. *Spine.* 2002;27:156-159.
61. Fletcher RW, Fletcher SW. Prognosis. In: Fletcher RW, Fletcher SW. *Clinical Epidemiology: The Essentials.* 4th ed. Philadelphia, PA: Lippincott Williams & Wilkins; 2005:105-124.

62. Straus SE, Richardson WS, Glasziou P, et al. Prognosis. In: Straus SE, Richardson WS, Glasziou P, et al. *Evidence-Based Medicine*. 3rd ed. New York, NY: Elsevier-Churchill-Livingstone; 2005:101-114.

63. Beattie P. Measurement of health outcomes in the clinical setting: applications to physiotherapy. *Aust Physiother Theory Prac*. 2001;17:173-185.

64. Quinn L, Gordon J. *Functional Outcomes: Documentation for Rehabilitation*. St Louis, MO: Saunders; 2003:99.

65. Ottenbacher KJ, Barrett KA. Statistical conclusion validity of rehabilitation research. *Am J of Phys Med Rehabil*. 1990;69:102-107.

66. Ottenbacher KJ, Barrett KA. Measures of effect size in the reporting of rehabilitation research. *Am J of Phys Med Rehabil*. 1989;68:82-88.

67. Stratford P, Binkley J. Applying the results of self-report measures to individual patients: an example using the Roland-Morris questionnaire. *J Orthop Sports Phys Ther*. 1999;29:232-239.

68. Deyo R. Understanding the accuracy of diagnostic tests. In: Weinstein J, et al, eds. *Essentials of the Spine*. New York, NY: Raven Press; 1995:55-69.

69. Sackett DL, Haynes RB. The architecture of diagnostic research. *BMJ*. 2002;324:539-541.

70. Beattie P, Meyers SM. Lumbar magnetic resonance imaging: general principles and diagnostic efficacy. *Phys Ther*. 1998;78:738-753.

71. Beattie P, Meyers S, Stratford P, et al. Associations between patient report of symptoms and anatomic impairment visible on lumbar magnetic resonance. *Spine*. 2000;25:819-828.

72. Buirski G, Silberstein M. The symptomatic lumbar disc in patients with low-back pain. Magnetic resonance imaging appearances in both symptomatic and control population. *Spine*. 1993;18:1808-1811.

73. Dalton GW, Keating JL. Number needed to treat: a statistic relevant to physical therapists. *Phys Ther*. 2000;80:1214-1219.

74. Laupacis A, Sackett DL, Roberts RS. An assessment of clinically useful measures of the consequences of treatment. *N Eng J Med*. 1998;318:1728-1733.

75. Kravitz RL, Duan N, Braslow J. Evidence-based medicine, heterogeneity of treatment effects, and the trouble with averages. *Milbank Q*. 2004;82:661-687.

76. DonTigny RL. Function and pathomechanics of the sacroiliac joint. A review. *Phys Ther*. 1985;65:35-44.

77. Walker JM. The sacroiliac joint: a critical review. *Phys Ther*. 1992;72:903-916.

78. Scholten PJM, Schultz AB, Luchico CW, et al. Motion and loads within the human pelvis: a biomechanical study. *J Orthop Res*. 1988;6:840-850.

79. Cibulka MT. The treatment of the sacroiliac joint component to low back pain: a case report. *Phys Ther*. 1992;72:917-922.

80. Upsur RE. Looking for rules in a world of exceptions: reflections on evidence-based practice. *Perspect Biol Med*. 2005;48:477-489.

81. Sackett DJ, Strause SE, Richardson WS. *Evidenced Based Medicine: How to Practice and Teach EBM*. 3rd ed. New York, NY: Elsevier; 2005.

PART II

Philosophic Approaches to Orthopaedic Manual Physical Therapy

The Principles and Practice of Osteopathic Manipulative Medicine

Michael L. Kuchera, DO, FAAO

Chapter Objectives

At the conclusion of this chapter, the reader will be able to:

- Recognize the historic and ongoing contributions of osteopathic medicine with respect to various other manual therapy systems.
- Understand the philosophy underlying the osteopathic approach to the treatment of musculoskeletal conditions.
- Recognize the importance of incorporating manual treatment in the context of complete care and of incorporating complete care in the context of manual treatment.
- Design and apply manual approaches using the interrelationship between structure and function, somatovisceral interactions, and the mental-emotional linkage to the physical body.
- Recognize and classify biomechanical and other somatic clues to differential diagnoses found in the neuromusculoskeletal system.
- Understand that somatic clues to diagnosis found in the neuromusculoskeletal system are potentially indicative of visceral or systemic problems.

- Understand the osteopathic examination concepts and methods leading to the identification of somatic dysfunction.
- Understand and competently apply the concepts and methods used to integrate positional diagnostic clues with active and/or passive motion testing.
- Identify six documented somatic dysfunction diagnoses that are commonly found in patients with chronic low back pain that are amenable to manual intervention.
- Understand the concepts of direct and indirect method manipulations in general and the concept of myofascial release specifically, and then demonstrate the ability to competently perform these techniques.
- Understand the principles of muscle energy and demonstrate a basic level of competence in performing reciprocal inhibition, postisometric relaxation, and rhythmic resistive duction variations with this activating force.
- Understand the principles of counterstrain and demonstrate a basic level of competence in performing this technique.

HISTORICAL PERSPECTIVES IN OSTEOPATHIC MANIPULATIVE MEDICINE

Major Osteopathic Contributors to the Evolution of Manual Systems

The Birth of Osteopathic Medicine

Osteopathic medicine is the fastest growing health-care profession in the United States today.[1] *Osteopathy* was

introduced by an allopathic physician, **Andrew Taylor Still, MD**, who in 1874 came to the conclusion that allopathy and homeopathy were ineffective as practiced by the medical doctors of that period. Still studied the structure and function of the neuromusculoskeletal system to become a *lightning bonesetter* and putatively integrated the science of *spinal irritation*[2,3] to link his therapeutic manual treatments to more systemic care that went beyond the management of neuromusculoskeletal conditions.

Between his introduction of osteopathy in 1874 and the opening of the American School of Osteopathy in Kirksville, Missouri, in 1892, Still developed the philosophical underpinnings and manual skills that were to be his lasting contribution to a worldwide health-care movement. Still also came to the conclusion that the neuromusculoskeletal, or **somatic**, system, comprising 60% of the body mass, was the *machinery of life*. He concluded that inefficiency of this system may lead to the onset of disease.

QUESTIONS *for* REFLECTION

- Define the term somatic system.
- Why is the somatic system referred to as the "machinery of life"?
- How does inefficiency of the somatic system lead to the onset of disease?
- What is the role of the physical therapist in treating disease?

Still charged his graduates "to find health . . . [because] anyone can find disease." As Still explained in his early writings, "The Osteopath seeks first physiological perfection of form, by normally adjusting the osseous frame work, so that all arteries may deliver blood to nourish and construct all parts. Also that the veins may carry away all impurities dependent upon them for renovation. Also that the nerves of all classes may be free and unobstructed while applying the powers of life and motion to all divisions, and the whole system of nature's laboratory."[4]

NOTABLE QUOTABLE

"The Osteopath seeks first physiological perfection of form, by normally adjusting the osseous frame work, so that all arteries may deliver blood . . . veins may carry away all impurities . . . nerves . . . may be free. . . ."

Andrew Taylor Still

From its inception, Still's system was less about manual technique than it was about applying anatomy, physiology, and the skills of a *master mechanic* to improve the body's ability to self-heal. "It is my object in this work to teach principles as I understand them, and not rules. I do not instruct the student to punch or pull a certain bone, nerve or muscle for a certain disease, but by a knowledge of the normal and abnormal, I hope to give a specific knowledge for all diseases." That said, he left his students descriptions of technique in his writings.[5,6] Manual interventions, known as Still techniques, have been reconstructed by Still's successor, ***Richard van Buskirk, DO, FAAO***.[7]

CLINICAL PILLAR

From its inception, Still's system was less about manual technique than it was about applying anatomy, physiology, and the skills of a "master mechanic" to improve the body's ability to self-heal.

Most modern nonosteopathic disciplines have borrowed more heavily from the manual techniques developed or taught by osteopathic practitioners than from the underlying philosophy upon which these techniques are based. The detailed evolution of the osteopathic approach is beyond the scope of this chapter. Table 4-1 provides an overview of the chronology, key innovators, and implications of this approach.

A Brief History of Osteopathic Research
Early Osteopathic Research

The earliest osteopathic research was published in 1898. The second roentgenographic unit west of the Mississippi River was purchased by the American School of Osteopathy (ASO) and was used by ***William Smith, MD, DO*** (1862–1912) to study basic structure-function relationships.[8]

In an attempt to independently support Still's clinical observations, several other observational studies that were

Table 4–1	Historical Evolution of Osteopathic Technique/Approach[1]		
TIME PERIOD	**INNOVATION**	**OSTEOPATHIC INNOVATOR**	**COMMENTS AND/OR IMPLICATIONS**
1874–1892	Development and codification of the osteopathic philosophy	Still	Would lead to a separate second school of medicine in the USA acknowledged in modern medicine to play an important role in focusing emphasis on a host-oriented, generalist approach in which the musculoskeletal system is prominently featured in diagnosis and in treatment[2]
1892–1918	Development of osteopathic academic institutions and oversight	Still, Littlejohn	From 1892 until his death in 1917, Still influenced direction; however, students established the precursor of the American Osteopathic Association (AOA) in 1897 for oversight of educational quality in the USA. Littlejohn laid groundwork for European version of osteopathy.
1900–1925	Balancing the equation structure-function = anatomy-physiology; balancing the equation allopathic and osteopathic approach	Littlejohn (1901); osteopathic students/AOA	Steps needed to avoid dogma and cult standing: (While Still said "keep it pure," faculty, students, and AOA integrated expanding medical advances. Flexner Report (1910) strengthened osteopathic college curricula)

Table 4–1   **Historical Evolution of Osteopathic Technique/Approach[1]—cont'd**

TIME PERIOD	INNOVATION	OSTEOPATHIC INNOVATOR	COMMENTS AND/OR IMPLICATIONS
1915–1920	Origins of direct and indirect techniques; spinal mechanics and principles	Ashmore (1915); Fryette (1917)	Despite osteopathic manipulative therapy (OMT) options, much of the profession chooses to emphasize teaching and performing direct high-velocity low-amplitude (HVLA techniques).
1923 and 1935	Function rather than position	Downing (1923) and McConnell (1935)	
1920s	Lymphatic approach	Millard, Miller, Chapman, Galbreath	Reemphasizing and recommitting to role of palpatory diagnosis and manual treatment to promote health by enhancing functions of breathing, removal of waste products, and improvement of vascular flow
1930s–1950s	Postural approach	Hoskins, Beilke, Schwab, Pearson, Heilig	Extensive research but not published in literature available outside osteopathic profession so general patient care impact not felt until 1980s; postural research reopens with Irvin, Kuchera, Pope
1930s; 1970s to current	Chapman's reflexes; autonomic approach	Chapman (through Owens)	Evolution from neuroendocrine (Owens 1930/40s) to neurolymphatic (Kimberly, 1940s–1970s) to autonomic (Kuchera and Kuchera, 1980s/current) interpretation *In the mid-1960s, chiropractor G. Goodheart combined the muscle testing of Kendall and Kendall to test the osteopathic Chapman's reflexes with eventual evolution into "applied kinesiology"*[3]
1939–1959	Osteopathy in the cranial field; balanced ligamentous/membranous tension; functional technique	Sutherland (1939); Lippincotts (1942); Hoover (1949)	Returned osteopathic profession's full spectrum of treatment techniques by teaching and emphasizing indirect techniques
1940s1961	Muscle pumps, rhythmic resistive duction, muscle energy (ME) techniques	Ruddy; Mitchell (1940/1950s)	Mitchell credits Ruddy (an ENT surgeon who used his muscle pump technique to move venous-lymphatic fluids in his patients) with the basic premise that became ME. Ruddy published his long-time method in 1961.[4]
1945–1975	Lost Generation – Osteopathy kept alive with research in autonomic and postural importance.	Denslow; Korr (PhD); Cathie; Heilig	Denslow trained in research design in 1938, and the Kirksville College committed faculty and equipment to validate palpatory diagnostic characteristics relative to physiologic activity; results in identifying objective physiological basis for somatic dysfunction; defines the "facilitated segment" and an understanding of axoplasmic flow
1955	Percussion vibratory technique	Fulford	
1964	Strain-counterstrain	Jones	*Originally "spontaneous release by positioning,"[5] Jones's technique is adopted by physical therapists and others under many names, including the general public's "Fold and Hold"*[6]
1973	Compensatory fascial patterning	Zink	
1977	Facilitated positional release	Schiowitz	
1997	Integrated neuromusculoskeletal release	Ward	
1969–Current	Rapid rebirth of osteopathic schools in the USA		The founding of Michigan State University College of Osteopathic Medicine would increase the number of osteopathic schools graduating doctors of osteopathy from 5 in 1970 to 15 in 1980 to 21 in 2000; there are now 26 open or opening colleges of osteopathic medicine in the USA.

Continued

Table 4-1	Historical Evolution of Osteopathic Technique/Approach[1]—cont'd		
TIME PERIOD	**INNOVATION**	**OSTEOPATHIC INNOVATOR**	**COMMENTS AND/OR IMPLICATIONS**
Revival of past (1980s–current)	Visceral technique revived	Still to Barral	
Revival of past (1990s–current)	Still technique revived: from Still and Back	Bowles to van Buskirk	

[1]Kuchera ML, Kuchera WA. *Osteopathic History, Philosophy and Somatic Influences in Health and Disease.* Columbus, OH: Greyden Press; 1997.
[2]Kuchera ML, Kuchera WA. *Current Challenges to M.D.s and D.O.s.* New York, NY: Josiah Macy, Jr. Foundation; 1996.
[3]Frost R. *Applied Kinesiology: A Training Manual and Reference Book of Basic Principles and Practices.* Berkeley, CA: North Atlantic Books; 2002.
[4]Ruddy TJ. Osteopathic manipulation in eye, ear, nose, and throat disease. *AAO Yearbook.* 1962;133-140.
[5]Jones LH. Spontaneous release by positioning. *The D.O.* 1964;4:109-116.
[6]Anderson DL. *Muscle Pain Relief in 90 Seconds The Fold and Hold Method.* Hoboken, NJ: John Wiley & Sons; 1994.

designed to modify somatic dysfunction and reflexively alter visceral function were conducted in Kirksville from 1898 to 1901. At the ASO, research involved manually stimulating and inhibiting the spinal and vagal regions of dogs, with subsequent anatomical analysis of heart, lung, and spinal tissues. Studies of electrocardiograms after manipulation of patients reported the effects of inhibition and stimulation resulting from manipulation of the spine.[1]

Basic Science Research on Somatic Dysfunction and the Facilitated Segment

In 1938, the foundation for the modern period of osteopathic research was ushered in by the osteopathic college in Kirksville. The college provided the resources needed for training *J. Stedman Denslow, DO,* in research methodology and electromyographic (EMG) techniques. Denslow's carefully controlled research demonstrated that objective EMG changes, consistent with reflexive muscle activity, were present in the area of the osteopathic "lesion." He published outside the profession in the *Journal of Neurophysiology,* documenting the basis of the facilitated segment and the effect of biomechanical stressors, such as posture, on the central excitatory state.[9] In 1949, he was nominated and elected as the first doctor of osteopathy member of the *American Physiological Society.*

Perhaps, the most notable addition to the dedicated Kirksville research team was *Irvin M. Korr, PhD,* who, after World War II, joined the faculty as professor and chairman of the division of physical sciences. Korr, Denslow, and the research team that they assembled continued to explore the nature of the facilitated segment, publishing in several refereed journals,[10] including the *American Journal of Physiology.*[11] Korr later chaired an international multidisciplinary conference and edited its proceedings, entitled *The Neurobiological Mechanisms in Manipulative Therapy.*[12]

The Kirksville team documented that palpatory changes were accurate measures of physiologic parameters that could be verified by EMG, electrical skin resistance, thermographic, sweat gland activity, red reflex, and other objective measurements. They also provided a physiologic basis to help explain the diagnostic efficacy of the osteopathic palpatory examination and the therapeutic benefits reportedly achieved by using osteopathic manipulative therapy (OMT).

Osteopathic Clinical Research Involving OMT

Research on the efficacy of OMT in clinical situations has largely been performed in a less systematic manner than the basic scientific research. From 1960 until the advent of electronic search engines, the only referenced peer-reviewed osteopathic periodical has been the *Journal of the American Osteopathic Association.* Read mainly by individual osteopathic physicians trained for clinical service, which often took place in small rural communities, studies tended to have little impact or influence on directing the evidence base outside the osteopathic profession. A partial compilation of the wealth of postural research conducted by the osteopathic profession can be found in the 1983 AAO yearbook, *Postural Balance and Imbalance* .[13]

Evidence-Based Summary and Current Directions in Osteopathic Research

While traditional explanations propose that OMT acts to cause mechanical, neurophysiologic, biochemical, and psychological effects, newly proposed mechanisms of action that range from mechanical transduction of genes[14] to the release of endothelial nitric oxide synthase (eNOS)[15] are now being explored.

Mechanically, OMT is purported to help restore normal positional bony and postural relationships, restore ergonomic and muscular balance, and reduce disc protrusion. Neurophysiologically, OMT can be used in a specific fashion to alter the relationship between central processes and peripheral mechanoreceptor, proprioceptor, and/or nociceptor input. Various sites of action for different techniques have been identified, ranging from central mechanisms in the *substantia gelatinosa* of the posterior spinal horn to peripheral levels, such as *Golgi tendon organs* or receptors associated with intrafusal and extrafusal muscle fibers. Manipulation is also thought to enhance the release of endorphins and eNOS, cause an increase in the water content of collagenous and cartilaginous structures, and stimulate glucosaminoglycan synthesis, thereby increasing the pain threshold and cellular transport while providing blood flow to and drainage from targeted tissues and lubrication of joint surfaces.

QUESTIONS *for* REFLECTION

- What type of effects may be anticipated from osteopathic manipulative therapy (OMT)?
- What are the mechanisms by which OMT exerts its effects?

SCIENCE AND ART WITHIN A PHILOSOPHICAL FRAMEWORK

Osteopathy is described as an integration of science, philosophy, and art in the search for health.[16] A.T. Still made this integration clear from the beginning, stating, "My objective is to make the osteopath a philosopher, and place him on the rock of reason."[17] But he also noted that the level of the osteopathic practitioner's art had to be sufficient to implement philosophy and science. "Your duty as a master mechanic is to know that the engine is kept in so perfect a condition that there will be no functional disturbance to any nerve vein or artery that supplies and governs the skin, the fascia, the muscle, the blood or any fluid that should freely circulate to sustain life and renovate the system from deposits that would cause what we call disease."[18]

Osteopathic Philosophical Tenets

Osteopathy embraces four tenets that, when considered as a whole, define its approach.[19] These four tenets are as follows: *(1) the body is a unit; (2) the body has self-healing, self-regulating mechanisms; (3) structure and function are interrelated; and (4) rational osteopathic treatment is based on applying these first three tenets to the individual patient.* Examples of topics commonly given to illustrate the fourth tenet are offered in Table 4-2.

Integrating Philosophy, Science, and Art in a Patient-Centered Osteopathic Approach

When a somatic dysfunction, defined as a dysfunction of the neuromusculoskeletal system, serves as a clue or as a contributing factor to underlying pathology, the clinician must determine whether it is a *primary cause*, a *secondary consequence*, a *precipitating element*, or a *perpetuating factor*. The reductionist approach in identifying and studying an isolated somatic dysfunction may

Table 4-2 Examples of Applying the Osteopathic Tenets

TENET, TOPIC, OR PRINCIPLE INVOLVED	CLINICAL EXAMPLES OR COMMENTS APPLICATION IN DIAGNOSIS AND/OR TREATMENT OF:
The Body Is a Unit	
Physical Unity: Pan-somatic postural changes in multiple regions	Impact of a pronated foot or short lower extremity on spinal postural patterns above, or of cranial base dysfunction on these patterns below
Physical Unity: Specific dysfunctional patterns within the biomechanically related body unit are predictable in both occurrence and location.	Impact of overuse or dysfunction in one muscle creating overuse or dysfunction in functionally related (myotatic) muscles or in compensatory structures
Physical Unity: Tensegrity	Hypomobility in one area causing hypermobility in another; plays a role in the postural changes above
Triune Unity: Physical pain in mental depression	Chronic somatic pain leads to mental-emotional-spiritual depression. Such depression leads to somatic pain magnification
Triune Unity: Pyschoneurophysiology	Emotional-physical-mental stressors may reduce immune functions
Structure and Function Are Reciprocally Interrelated	
Function → Structure: Wolff's Law	Calcium is laid down structurally along functional lines of stress; role in functional causes of degenerative changes, bony remodeling, etc.
Function → Structure: Functional demands on developing structure shape the eventual structure and its potential function.	Ranges from understanding and/or affecting eventual shape and function of cranial sutures in pediatrics to preventing osteoarthritis of the hip on the long leg side of individuals with uneven leg lengths

Continued

Table 4-2	Examples of Applying the Osteopathic Tenets—cont'd
TENET, TOPIC OR PRINCIPLE INVOLVED	**CLINICAL EXAMPLES OR COMMENTS APPLICATION IN DIAGNOSIS AND/OR TREATMENT OF:**
Structure and Function Are Reciprocally Interrelated—cont'd	
Function → Structure: Biomechanically/ergonomically compromised function or heavy functional demand may initiate pathways leading to pain, inflammation, and subsequent structural change.	Implications in overuse syndromes, patient education in exercise or activities of daily living; postural treatment
Structure → Function: Muscle type determines response to functional demands	The structure of so-called postural (antigravity) muscles makes them respond with hypertonicity when functionally stressed; their antagonists are structured and reflexly hardwired to respond with pseudoparesis (weak) behavior and decreased tone
Structure → Function: Physiologic motions of the spine	Functional spinal motion patterns will behave predictably on the basis of articular shape (e.g., a thoracic vertebral unit side bending and rotating to the same side when fully flexed and returning to a normal position in the absence of somatic dysfunction)
Structure → Function: Joint structures that are structurally altered owing to inflammation or pathology function differently leading to differential diagnosis of somatic dysfunctional patterns versus pathologic capsular patterns of motion	Dysfunctional patterns are different from patterns when structure is altered. Somatic dysfunction patterns show restriction in one direction but freedom in the paired opposite motion. Capsular patterns with rheumatological disorders show restriction in a number of paired opposite motions.
The Body Has Self-Healing and Homeostatic Mechanisms	
Compensation occurs to maximize function within an existing structure.	Homeostatic responses in postural disorders often compensate in alternating motions; trauma often prevents normal compensatory patterns
Swelling initiates cellular-level connections to open end lymphatics; motion permits fluid exchange where osmotic pressures alone would be incapable of tissue exchange.	Part of the basis of the respiratory-circulatory model to introduce motion and regional pressure changes and to maximize breathing in accomplishing these effects
Reflex mechanisms exist to protect the body.	Ranges from decreasing inappropriate influence of nociception or segmentally related afferent information from receptors stimulated by dysfunctional rather than pathological conditions
The sympathetic system evolved to be a quickly reactive system to alert and prepare the body for "fight, flight, and preservation"; prolonged activation of this system disrupts the general adaptive response (homeostasis)	Part of the basis for identifying somatic dysfunction that causes segmental facilitation acting as a neurologic lens for stressors within the body unit to maintain artificially heightened sympathetic activity

be ineffective or impossible. Radin remarked, "Functional analysis, be it biological, mechanical or both, of a single tissue will fail to give a realistic functional analysis as, in all complex constructs, the interaction between the various components is a critical part of their behavior."[20]

CLINICAL PILLAR

When a somatic dysfunction, defined as a dysfunction of the neuromusculoskeletal system, serves as a clue or as a contributing factor to underlying pathology, the clinician must determine whether it is a **primary cause,** a **secondary consequence,** a **precipitating element,** or a **perpetuating factor.**

PRINCIPLES OF EXAMINATION

Practically speaking, the complete osteopathic examination relative to each aspect of the history and physical begins with looking at function and dysfunction of the patient, etiologically examining progressively smaller somatic units, and then mapping the role these units play into the integrated total body context.

General Principles of the Osteopathic Manipulative Medicine Examination for Somatic Dysfunction

The term **somatic dysfunction,** was first coined by the osteopathic profession in 1961 to replace the provincial term *osteopathic lesion.* Defined as "impaired or altered function of related components of the somatic (body framework) system: skeletal, arthrodial, and myofascial structures, and related vascular, lymphatic and neural elements,"[21] somatic dysfunction embraces a wide range of relevant clinical findings and conditions. Furthermore, the term *somatic dysfunction*, is recognized as a valid and codeable diagnostic term in the *International Classification of Diseases, 9th edition, Clinical Modification (ICD-9-CM).*[22]

The palpable characteristics of somatic dysfunction may be caused by structural or functional aberrations in various somatic tissues associated with recognized pathophysiological processes. These palpable characteristics are interpreted by various health-care practitioners to be associated through their anatomical, central nervous system (CNS), or autonomic connections with a particular joint or joints, myofascial structure, subcutaneous tissue or fascia, viscera, or condition.[23]

There are several basic principles that govern the diagnosis and management of a somatic dysfunction by an osteopathic practitioner. First, diagnostic testing for somatic dysfunction consists of simple, reproducible palpatory and provocative procedures. The four major diagnostic criteria for somatic dysfunction include (1) *sensation change* including pain or tenderness, (2) *tissue texture change*, (3) *asymmetry*, and (4) *restriction of motion*. These objective findings may be summarized by the mnemonic **STAR**, as shown in Box 4-1.

Somatic dysfunction can be subdivided by its physiologic characteristics (e.g., acute, chronic); its anatomical location (e.g., cervical, lumbosacral); and/or the specific pattern of anatomical and physiologic characteristics (e.g., acute psoas syndrome, latent sternocleidomastoid myofascial trigger point, etc.). The severity of somatic dysfunction can be graded as 1 (mild), 2 (moderate), or 3 (severe).[24]

Primary somatic dysfunction typically responds well to various manipulative medicine approaches; however, secondary somatic dysfunction may respond equivocally to these approaches alone. The failure to consider somatic dysfunction in diagnosis and treatment risks overlooking an important underlying pathophysiologic process that plays a role in a significant number of patient complaints.

Skill and Knowledge Set for the Osteopathic Manipulative Medicine Examination

Diagnostic testing for somatic dysfunction consists of simple, reproducible palpatory and provocative examinations. Such examinations can be taught to a wide range of health-care practitioners; however, interpreting them in the manner of an osteopathic practitioner requires additional training. Manual therapy (by therapists) or manual treatment (by physicians)

cannot be considered professional without the clinician's ability to first identify, quantify, and describe the somatic dysfunction and to recognize the indications and contraindications for such care. Osteopathic manipulative medicine (OMM) examination in the United States requires the skills of a broadly trained physician to establish an adequate differential diagnosis and fully weigh the variety of available treatment options.

STAR Criteria for Acute and Chronic Somatic Dysfunction

Professional diagnostic palpation is an acquired skill that requires time, patience, and practice. It may be defined as "the application of variable manual pressures to the surface of the body for the purpose of determining the shape, size, consistency, position, inherent motility, and health of the tissues beneath."[25] The art of interpreting diagnostic palpation also requires an extensive knowledge base of normal anatomy and physiology. Other requirements include the ability to recognize host variability and pathophysiologic connections and manifestations. Therefore, early palpatory evidence of underlying pathophysiologic change requires a higher level of palpatory skill than that required in palpation of a salient pathological state, such as a tumor.[26]

CLINICAL PILLAR

Diagnostic palpation

- is an acquired skill requiring time, patience, and practice.
- is the application of variable manual pressures to the surface of the body for the purpose of determining the shape, size, consistency, position, inherent motility, and health of the tissues beneath.
- requires an extensive knowledge base of normal anatomy and physiology, the ability to recognize host variability, and pathophysiological connections and manifestations.
- requires a higher level of skill for palpatory evidence of underlying pathophysiological change, therefore, than that required in palpation of a salient pathological state.

Diagnostic, time-efficient palpation for somatic dysfunction combines screening and scanning surveys of the entire body framework and those specific region(s) indicated by historical and physical findings. Focused layer palpation is then directed at any suspected or identified sites of significance.

In osteopathic practice, palpation begins with assessment of successively deeper body anatomical layers. The site of palpation is selected according to knowledge of pain and referred pain mechanisms, structural interconnectedness, and the developing differential diagnosis. At each of these sites, palpators are guided by STAR findings, which can be interpreted as a diagnosis of somatic dysfunction, but may indicate the need for additional testing (Table 4-3).

Box 4-1 THE FOUR DIAGNOSTIC CRITERIA FOR SOMATIC DYSFUNCTION

1. Sensation change (including pain or tenderness)
2. Tissue texture change
3. Asymmetry
4. Restriction of motion

Table 4–3	Additional Testing for Identification of Somatic Dysfunction

GENERAL SCREENING PROCEDURE	EXAMPLE OF SCREENING ABNORMALITY AND INTERPRETATION RELATIVE TO THE DIAGNOSIS OR TREATMENT OF SOMATIC DYSFUNCTION
Observation of General Appearance and Movement (With or Without Added Palpation)	
General Habitus	Obesity may suggest biomechanical/postural strain on skeletal, arthrodial, myofascial structures.
General Facial Screen During Interview	Abnormal facial appearance may indicate genetic or acquired neuromusculoskeletal condition: • Flat facial expression may indicate pathology (Parkinson's) or functional diagnosis (depression) • Asymmetrical facial movement may indicate central disorder (stroke) or peripheral disorder (facial nerve palsy) • Shape of the head and face may indicate underlying functional or structural cranial disorder to be correlated with birth history, cranial nerve function, cerebral function, reflex function, postural alignment, presence of small hemipelvis, etc.
Static Posture	• Altered spinal postural curves in one or more of the cardinal planes may suggest increased and/or asymmetrical biomechanical strain on certain skeletal, arthrodial, and myofascial structures. • Postural asymmetry has been linked to segmental facilitation (highest at postural crossover sites) and myofascial trigger-point somatic dysfunction. • The presence of aberrant postural alignment may direct a scanning examination of the junctional areas of the spine and postural crossover sites or a local examination of specifically stressed ligaments and muscles.[1] Often, comparing key landmarks in the scanning examination for postural asymmetry is performed simultaneously with this postural observational screening test.
Gait	Beyond recognizing pathologic gaits, the gait analysis portion of the musculoskeletal screening examination provides information about the presence and impact of underlying somatic dysfunction. • Observe gait for forward head position, a straight lumbar spine, decreased hip flexion during single support phase, flexed knee in midstance, failure of heel lift, and visible foot pronation during the single support phase. Each of these compensatory motions is a screening **gait marker**[2] whose presence warrants further examination. • Gait analysis should assess length, pattern, and symmetry of stride; arm swing; heel strike; toe off; tilting of the pelvis; and shoulder compensatory movements. Additional clues may be obtained by observing the wear patterns of the patient's shoes. • Antalgic gait may indicate pain and/or neuromusculoskeletal dysfunction; other specific gaits provide a positive screen for certain other neuromusculoskeletal system pathologies. • Variability in stride is the best predictor of falls in the elderly (source of traumatic dysfunction); widened stance with shortened stride indicates a fear of falling.
Gross Motion (active–directed)	• Gross spinal motion observation easily screens total range of motion of the cervical, thoracic, and lumbar regions in flexion, extension, side bending, and rotation. It becomes even more informative if, at the end of active regional motion observation, the physician continues the passive motion in the direction of the test. This scans for restriction of motion in that particular region and for possible etiologies for the restriction by evaluating and assessing the characteristic quality of the restrictive barrier. • Fully raising both upper extremities from the anatomical position in the coronal plane and turning the backs of the hands together quickly provides functional motion screening of the upper extremities (especially the shoulder girdle). • While standing with feet flat on the floor and with arms extended, a complete squat down and subsequent return screens lower extremity foot, ankle, knee, and hip joints for strength and mobility a well as proprioceptive information. • Asymmetrical motion during either seated or standing flexion test indicates dysfunction localized to one side of the pelvis. Comparison of the two tests can assist in determining whether major restrictors involve the pelvic structures or whether function is affected by structures below the pelvis. The screening "stork" (Gillett) test and/or the scanning ASIS Compression Test may replace or supplement these flexion tests.
Gross Motion (passive motion)	• Examination of the lower extremities using a modification of Patrick's FABERE (flexion, abduction, external rotation, and extension) test screening pain and/or limited range of motion to detect hip or sacroiliac dysfunction/pathology.

Table 4-3	Additional Testing for Identification of Somatic Dysfunction—cont'd

GENERAL SCREENING PROCEDURE	EXAMPLE OF SCREENING ABNORMALITY AND INTERPRETATION RELATIVE TO THE DIAGNOSIS OR TREATMENT OF SOMATIC DYSFUNCTION
Observation of General Appearance and Movement (With or Without Added Palpation)—cont'd	
Gross Motion (inherent)	• Comparing side-to-side symmetry during a full respiratory cycle (especially while gently palpating over the anterior upper chest and anterolateral lower rib cage) may screen gross motion of the chest cage. • Observation of passive respiration provides insight into diaphragmatic and thoracic cage function. Normally, effective passive inhalation by a supine patient should create visible anterosuperior movement of the chest and abdomen all the way down to the pubic region.
Observation of Ectodermal Tissues: Preface to Layer-by-Layer Scanning Examination	
Hair	Hair distribution and pattern may suggest metabolic, endocrine (e.g., hypothyroidism), or sympathetic disorder.
Skin	Poor skin turgor in nicotine abuse suggests poor connective tissue health[3–5] and may prognosticate a lesser response to otherwise successful strategies for reestablishing neuromusculoskeletal health.
Nails	Nail pitting, ridging, and discoloration may indicate rheumatological, respiratory-circulatory, or autonomic pathologies important in care of the musculoskeletal system; nicotine abuse may also be observed here.

[1]Kuchera ML, Kuchera WA. General postural considerations. In: Ward RC, ed. Foundations for Osteopathic Medicine, (1997). Baltimore, MD: Williams &Wilkins; 1997: 969-977.
[2]Dananberg HJ. Lower back pain as a gait-related repetitive motion injury. In: Vleeming A, Mooney V, Snijders CJ, Dorman TA, Stoeckart R, eds. Movement, Stability and Low Back Pain: The Essential Role of the Pelvis. New York, NY: Churchill-Livingstone; 199:253-267.
[3]Amoronso PJ, et al. Tobacco and Injuries: An Annotated Bibliography. U.S. Army Research Laboratory Technical Report ARL-TR-1333. U.S. Army Research Laboratory; 1997.
[4]Naus A, et al. Work injuries and smoking. Industrial Med Surg. 1966;35:880-881.
[5]Reynolds KL, Heckel HA, Witt CE, et al. Cigarette smoking, physical fitness, and injuries in infantry soldiers. Am J Prev Med. 1994;19:145-150.

Integrating History and General Physical Findings

After ruling out conditions requiring emergent care, integration of the history with physical examination findings is critical. Extensive knowledge of regional and systemic structure and function related to the chief complaint is important. With this knowledge, using palpation can provide information that narrows the presumptive diagnoses.

The resulting presumptive diagnosis informs decisions regarding additional testing, need for referral, and subsequent treatment. Palpatory data also provide input concerning indications and contraindications and guides subsequent medical, surgical, and/or manipulative prescriptions.[16] With time, most manual practitioners come to recognize common patterns that increase the efficiency of patient management.

Essentials of Differential Diagnosis

Failure to consider the various etiologies of somatic dysfunction limits the process of differential diagnosis and disregards the underlying pathophysiologic processes that may be involved in the primary complaint. Nocireflexive neural afferent activity that results from somatic and/or visceral problems is capable of initiating facilitation in the CNS. Regardless of its origin, the resulting somatic dysfunction may act as a clue to identifying the underlying visceral dysfunction (viscerosomatic reflex), as a perpetuating somatic contributor to visceral dysfunction (somatovisceral reflex), or as one of

several structures to treat to decrease the afferent load within the CNS (Fig. 4-1).

If somatic dysfunction originates from direct tissue injury, palpable STAR characteristics would be consistent with a diagnostic classification of **primary somatic dysfunction**. Here, the somatic dysfunction site usually corresponds with the biomechanical history, site of specific trauma, or area of compensation.

Somatic dysfunction arising from a viscerosomatic or somatosomatic reflex would be classified as **secondary somatic dysfunction**. In the absence of a biomechanical history, moderate to severe somatic dysfunction correlates with a wide range of visceral conditions.[27–31] Conversely, irritation of upper thoracic spinal joint receptors has been shown to evoke numerous reflex alterations, including paravertebral muscle spasm and alterations in endocrine, respiratory, and cardiovascular function.[32]

Recurrent Patterns of Somatic Dysfunction and Missed Perpetuating Factor Clues

The presence of recurrent somatic dysfunction despite appropriate care may indicate the need for reconsideration. In some cases, there may be a missed underlying diagnosis. Because there is a difference between recurrent, randomly distributed somatic dysfunction and a specific recurrent pattern of somatic dysfunction, the answer to this question is often found in the location of the dysfunction (Table 4-4). In such cases, manual procedures alone may be insufficient.

CLINICAL PILLAR

Recurrent somatic dysfunction despite appropriate care may indicate a missed underlying diagnosis. There is a difference between recurrent, randomly distributed somatic dysfunction and a specific recurrent *pattern* of somatic dysfunction. The answer is often found in the location of the dysfunction. In such cases, manual procedures alone may be insufficient.

Techniques for Conducting and Recording the Osteopathic Examination

Screening Tests and Procedures

A relevant **screening examination** for the neuromusculoskeletal system answers the question, *Is there a problem that deserves additional evaluation?*[25] As in most health-care professions, osteopathic screening tests include static observations (Table 4-5). They also incorporate observation of asymmetry and gross restrictions of active or passive motion, gait, and breathing.

Regional Scanning and Local Palpatory Tests and Procedures

A **scanning examination** is "an intermediate detailed examination of specific body regions which have been identified by findings emerging from the initial screen; the scan (for somatic dysfunction) focuses on segmental areas for further definition or diagnosis."[25] A scanning examination answers the questions, What part of the region and what tissues within the region may be significantly dysfunctional?[25]

All osteopathic scanning examinations will seek to identify one or more of the STAR findings. Combinations of these findings constitute the diagnostic criteria for local or regional somatic dysfunction, but in isolation, these findings may alert the clinician to evaluate for the presence of other underlying

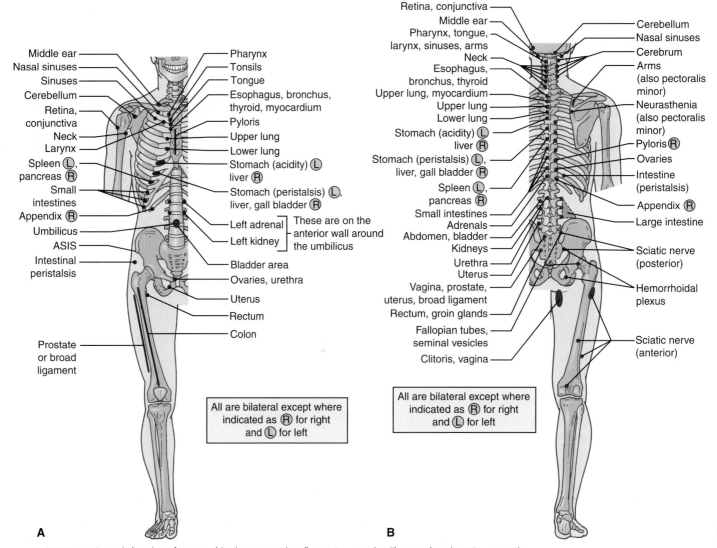

FIGURE 4–1 Somatic location of osteopathic viscerosomatic reflexes. **A** = anterior Chapman's points; **B** = posterior Chapman's points.

Table 4-4	**Recurrent Somatic Dysfunction**

RECURRENT–NONPATTERNED SOMATIC DYSFUNCTION

Nutritional, metabolic, and endocrine inadequacies preclude the body from using nutritive building blocks or impair physiologic pathways necessary for neuromusculoskeletal function.	• Travell and Simons note the importance and balance of vitamins B_1, B_6, and B_{12} as well as folic acid, vitamin C, calcium, iron, and potassium in the health of myofascial tissues.[1] There appears to be empirical benefit in nutritionally supplementing patients with the myofascial tissue building blocks, glucosamine, and chondroitin sulfate.[2] • They also note the clinical relevance of conditions such as hypothyroidism and hypoglycemia that interfere with muscular energy metabolism. Tests for thyroid function, fasting blood sugar, serum vitamin levels, or other blood chemistry profiles may therefore be helpful in diagnosis. • Cigarette smoking interferes with myofascial tissue oxygenation and metabolism and is therefore a perpetuating factor for somatic dysfunction and soft tissue healing.[3–6] • Treatment may require pharmacologic or dietary strategies as well as patient education.
Psychological factors may arise from chronic pain and dysfunction and, in turn, may also perpetuate pain and somatic dysfunction.	Thus suspicion and special questioning may be required to identify those factors interfering with optimum function of the individual. Treatment of underlying anxiety or depression may be required before complete resolution of somatic dysfunction can be accomplished.
Infections and infestations are capable of causing muscle ache and perpetuating myofascial somatic dysfunction.	Such a diagnosis might be initiated by the presence of eosinophilia or an elevated white count. Antibiotics, dental care, or other pharmacological intervention for chronic infection may be required before the musculoskeletal findings can be addressed satisfactorily.

RECURRENT–PATTERNED SOMATIC DYSFUNCTION

Mechanical and postural stressors are a major consideration in both osteopathic practices and other manual health-care professions.	Gravitational stress is magnified in a number of postural and structural disorders such as leg length inequality, small hemipelvis, obesity, and accentuation of sagittal plane postural curves.[7] Acute overload or overwork fatigue[3] can be aggravated by prolonged exposure to ill-fitting furniture, poor and/or excessive habitual body mechanics, obesity, immobility, repetitive occupational motions, or inappropriate gait mechanics owing to pronated or Morton's foot deformity. Direct muscular constriction or trauma as well as joint micro- and macrotrauma are precipitating and perpetuating factors for somatic dysfunction. Assessing whole-body postural alignment, analysis of standing postural radiographs, or assessing ergonomic factors in the home or workplace may augment diagnosis. Treatment may require adjunctive use of foot or pelvic orthotics, postural and/or proprioceptive reeducation, use of assistive devices, and modification of activities of daily living.
Visceral disease or dysfunction should be a consideration in the differential diagnosis of recurrent, patterned somatic dysfunction.	Some of these viscerosomatic reflex patterns, such as those associated with acute appendicitis and gallstones, are widely known and described in a number of texts. Other patterns are less generally known and are described in surgical[9] or pain[10] texts written for specialists in those fields; osteopathic primary care practitioners and osteopathic manipulative medicine. Osteopathic specialists are taught to routinely consider and integrate such patterns. Regardless of practice type or degree, the finding of specific recurrent patterns of somatic dysfunction in the distribution or combination should prompt the astute practitioner to consider visceral dysfunction as part of the complete differential diagnosis. A compilation describing the specific role of somatic dysfunction in visceral problems is found in *Osteopathic Considerations in Systemic Dysfunction*.[11]
Recurrent posturing or repetitious motions	Recurrent patterns of somatic dysfunction may arise from recurrent posturing or repetitious motions associated with habit or occupation. With this in mind, history and an ergonomic evaluation often provide insights to diagnosis and treatment.

SPECIAL CASES: RECURRENT SOMATIC DYSFUNCTION–NOT NECESSARILY PATTERNED

Trauma in certain predisposed individuals	• Constitutional congenital predisposition: hypermobility, Ehlos-Danlos, etc. • Certain preexisting pathologies
Trauma in certain regions	• Regional congenital predisposition: sacralization, lumbarization, congenital scoliosis • Traumatically weakened structure: prior surgery, fracture, torn support structures, etc. • Vectors of force may change structural or piezoelectric alignment along a pathway that thereafter responds differently from the way it did before the trauma but in a fashion consistent with the new anatomical-physiologic characteristics of the tissue.

Continued

Table 4–4	Recurrent Somatic Dysfunction—cont'd

SPECIAL CASES: RECURRENT SOMATIC DYSFUNCTION–NOT NECESSARILY PATTERNED

Coexisting radiculopathy or proximal neural entrapment neuropathy have been implicated in decreasing axoplasmic flow needed to provide trophic factors required in the periphery.	This postulated mechanism may contribute to the so-called double-crush phenomenon,[12] leading to increased incidence and symptomatology from more distal somatic dysfunction and neural entrapments. This could also account, in part, for the 10% of patients with carpal tunnel syndrome who are found to have a primary cervical radiculopathy.[13] Such diagnoses can usually be made clinically but may require special imaging or neuroelectrodiagnostic studies to localize an anatomical cause or physiologic consequence. Treatment may require integration of pharmacological, physical therapeutic, and/or surgical elements.

[1]Simons DG, Travell JG, Simons LS. *Travell and Simons' Myofascial Pain and Dysfunction: The Trigger Point Manual.* Vol. 1. *Upper Half of Body.* Baltimore, MD: Lippincott, Williams & Wilkins; 1999:186-220.
[2]Deal CL, Moskowitz RW. Nutraceuticals as therapeutic agents in osteoarthritis. The role of glucosamine, chondrotin sulfate, and collagen hydrosalt. *Rheum Dis Clin North Am.* 2000;25: 75-95.
[3]Amoroso PJ, Reynolds KL, Barnes JA, et al. *Tobacco and Injuries: An Annotated Bibliography.* Natick (MA): US Army Research Institute of Environmental Medicine Technical Report TN96–1; 1996
[4]Naus A, et al. Work injuries and smoking. *Industrial Med Surg.* 1966;35:880-881.
[5]Reynolds KL, Heckel HA, Witt CE, et al. Cigarette smoking, physical fitness, and injuries in infantry soldiers. *Am J Prev Med.* 1994;19:145-150.
[6]Treiman GS, Oderich GS, Ashrafi A, Schneider PA. Management of ischemic heel ulceration and gangrene: an evaluation of factors associated with successful healing. *J Vasc Surg.* 2000;31:1110-1118.
[7]Kuchera ML. Gravitational stress, musculoligamentous strain, and postural alignment. *Spine: State of the Art Reviews.* 1995;9:463-490.
[8]Smith LA, ed.. An Atlas of Pain Patterns: Sites and Behavior of Pain in Certain Common Disease of the Upper Abdomen. Springfield, IL: C.C. Thomas; 1961.
[9]Cousins MJ. Visceral pain. In: Andersson S, Bond M, Mehta M, Swerdlow M, eds. *Chronic Non-Cancer Pain: Assessment and Practical Management.* Lancaster, UK: MTP Press; 1987.
[10]Kuchera ML, Kuchera WA. *Osteopathic Considerations in Systemic Dysfunction.* 2nd ed., rev. Columbus, OH: Greyden Press; 1994.
[11]Hurst LC, Weissberg D, Carroll RE. The relationship of the double crush to carpal tunnel syndrome (an analysis of 1000 cases of carpal tunnel syndrome). *J Hand Surg.* 1995;10B: 202-204.
[12]Upton AR, McComas AJ. The double crush in nerve entrapment syndromes. *Lancet.* 1973;ii:359-362.

Table 4–5	General Osteopathic Screening Procedures

GENERAL SCREENING PROCEDURE	EXAMPLE OF SCREENING ABNORMALITY AND INTERPRETATION RELATIVE TO THE DIAGNOSIS OR TREATMENT OF SOMATIC DYSFUNCTION
Observation of General Appearance and Movement (With or Without Added Palpation)	
General Habitus	Obesity may suggest biomechanical/postural strain on skeletal, arthrodial, myofascial structures
General Facial Screen During Interview	Abnormal facial appearance may indicate genetic or acquired neuromusculoskeletal condition: • Flat facial expression may indicate pathology (Parkinson) or functional diagnosis (depression). • Asymmetrical facial movement may indicate central disorder (stroke) or peripheral disorder (facial nerve palsy). • Shape of the head/face may indicate underlying functional or structural cranial disorder to be correlated with birth history, cranial nerve function, cerebral function, reflex function, postural alignment, presence of small hemipelvis, etc.
Static Posture	• Altered spinal postural curves in one or more of the cardinal planes may suggest increased and/or asymmetrical biomechanical strain on certain skeletal, arthrodial, and myofascial structures. • Postural asymmetry has been linked to segmental facilitation (highest at postural crossover sites) and myofascial trigger point somatic dysfunction. • The presence of aberrant postural alignment may direct a scanning examination of the junctional areas of the spine and postural crossover sites or a local examination of specifically stressed ligaments and muscles.[1] Often comparing key landmarks in the scanning examination for postural asymmetry is performed simultaneously with this postural observational screening test.
Gait	Beyond recognizing pathologic gaits, the gait analysis portion of the musculoskeletal screening examination provides information about the presence and impact of underlying somatic dysfunction. • Observe gait for forward head position, a straight lumbar spine, decreased hip flexion during single support phase, flexed knee in midstance, failure of heel lift, and visible foot pronation during the single support phase. Each of these compensatory motions is a screening **gait marker**[2] whose presence warrants further examination.

| Table 4-5 | General Osteopathic Screening Procedures—cont'd |

GENERAL SCREENING PROCEDURE	EXAMPLE OF SCREENING ABNORMALITY AND INTERPRETATION RELATIVE TO THE DIAGNOSIS OR TREATMENT OF SOMATIC DYSFUNCTION
Observation of General Appearance and Movement (With or Without Added Palpation)—cont'd	
	• Gait analysis should assess length, pattern, and symmetry of stride, arm swing, heel strike, toe off, tilting of the pelvis, and shoulder compensatory movements. Additional clues may be obtained by observing the wear patterns of the patient's shoes. • Antalgic gait may indicate pain and/or neuromusculoskeletal dysfunction; other specific gaits provide a positive screen for certain other neuromusculoskeletal system pathologies. • Variability in stride is the best predictor of falls in the elderly (source of traumatic dysfunction); widened stance with shortened stride indicates a fear of falling.
Gross motion (active—directed)	• Gross spinal motion observation easily screens total range of motion of the cervical, thoracic, and lumbar regions in flexion, extension, side bending, and rotation. It becomes even more informative if, at the end of active regional motion observation, the physician passively continues the passive motion in the direction of the test. This scans for restriction of motion in that particular region and for possible etiologies for the restriction by evaluating and assessing the characteristic quality of the restrictive barrier. • Fully raising both upper extremities from the anatomical position in the coronal plane and turning the backs of the hands together quickly provides functional motion screening of the upper extremities (especially the shoulder girdle). • While standing with feet flat on the floor and with arms extended, observing a complete squat down and subsequent return screens lower extremity foot, ankle, knee, and hip joints for strength and mobility while also gleaning proprioceptive information. • Asymmetrical motion during either seated or standing flexion test indicates dysfunction localized to one side of the pelvis. Comparison of the two tests can assist in determining whether major restrictors involve the pelvic structures or whether function is affected by structures below the pelvis. The screening "stork" (Gillett) test and/or the scanning ASIS Compression Test may replace or supplement these flexion tests.
Gross motion (passive motion)	• Examination of the lower extremities using a modification of Patrick's FABERE (flexion, abduction, external rotation, and extension) test screening pain and/or limited range of motion to detect hip or sacroiliac dysfunction/pathology
Gross motion (inherent)	• Comparing side-to-side symmetry during a full respiratory cycle (especially while gently palpating over the anterior upper chest and anterolateral lower rib cage) may screen gross motion of the chest cage. • Observation of passive respiration provides insight into diaphragmatic and thoracic cage function. Normally, effective passive inhalation by a supine patient should create visible anterosuperior movement of the chest and abdomen all the way down to the pubic region.
Observation of Ectodermal Tissues: Preface to Layer-by-Layer Scanning Examination	
Hair	Hair distribution and pattern may suggest metabolic, endocrine (e.g., hypothyroidism), or sympathetic disorder.
Skin	Poor skin turgor in nicotine abuse suggests poor connective tissue health[3-5] and may prognosticate a lesser response to otherwise successful strategies for reestablishing neuromusculoskeletal health.
Nails	Nail pitting, ridging, discoloration may indicate rheumatological, respiratory-circulatory, or autonomic pathologies important in care of the musculoskeletal system; nicotine abuse may also be observed here.

[1]Kuchera ML, Kuchera WA. General postural considerations. In: Ward RC, ed. *Foundations for Osteopathic Medicine*. Baltimore, MD: Williams & Wilkins; 1997:969-977.
[2]Dananberg HJ. Lower back pain as a gait-related repetitive motion injury. In: Vleeming A, Mooney V, Snijders CJ, Dorman TA, Stoeckart R, eds. *Movement, Stability and Low Back Pain: The Essential Role of the Pelvis*. New York, NY: Churchill-Livingstone; 1997:253-267.
[3]Amoronso PJ, et al. *Tobacco and Injuries: An Annotated Bibliography*. U.S. Army Research Laboratory Technical Report ARL-TR-1333. U.S. Army Research Laboratory; 1997.
[4]Naus A, et al. Work injuries and smoking. *Industrial Med Surg.* 1966;35:880-881.
[5]Reynolds KL, Heckel HA, Witt CE, et al. Cigarette smoking, physical fitness, and injuries in infantry soldiers. *Am J Prev Med.* 1994;19:145-150.

pathophysiologic diagnoses. Local diagnostic testing for the remaining STAR characteristics are performed to gather the final information needed to formulate an individualized manual medicine prescription.

Most osteopathic practitioners initially scan regions with a quick survey of sensitivity and tissue texture abnormalities (Table 4-6). Typical scanning tests include *skin drag, red reflex induction, skin rolling, and layer-by-layer progressive pressure* over sequential structures between the skin and the bone (Fig. 4-2).

Layer palpation is also effective in identifying various myofascial points. Three specific types of myofascial points merit specific mention: myofascial **trigger points (TrPs)**, empirically mapped by Travell and Simons[33,34]; myofascial **tender points** used in Jones' system of strain–counterstrain[35]; and myofascial *reflex points* empirically mapped by Chapman[36].

After scanning for tissue texture abnormalities and changes in sensitivity, osteopathic practitioners typically scan for static asymmetry of key landmarks (Fig. 4-3) and for active or passive changes in motion characteristics (Table 4-7).

The chief complaint and its onset can be helpful in identifying the underlying joint motions involved in the somatic dysfunction. For example, in the thoracic and lumbar regions, where sagittal plane position modifies the pattern of coupled motion,[37] two types of somatic dysfunction can be differentiated: **Type I somatic dysfunction** occurs when the patient is in the neutral position, and side bending and rotation occur to opposite sides, usually in groups. In **type II somatic dysfunction,** which occurs with significant flexion or extension, rotation and side bending occur at a single segment and to the same side.

CLINICAL PILLAR

In the thoracic and lumbar regions, two types of somatic dysfunction can be differentiated:

- *Type I somatic dysfunction* occurs when the patient is in the neutral position and side bending and rotation occur to opposite sides, usually in groups.

- *Type II somatic dysfunction* occurs with significant flexion or extension, and rotation and side bending occur at a single segment and to the same side.

Table 4–6	Tissue Texture Scanning Tests

TISSUE TEXTURE ABNORMALITY SCANNING TESTS

Skin drag: The fingers pass over the skin with varying degrees of pressure depending upon the information sought. Positive skin drag testing is demonstrated by asymmetrical responses in sensitivity, temperature, sweat gland activity, hyperesthesia, drag or ease, and/or the reddening-blanching pattern of the skin.
- The lightest pressure is used to sense minor variations in skin temperature or sweat gland activity.
- In the paraspinal regions, increased resistance to lightly dragging the pads of the fingers along the skin in a stroking fashion denotes relative cutaneous humidity; less resistance denotes dryness.
- Significant changes can also be visually monitored in the friction-induced **red reflex pattern** produced by heavier stroking with the finger pads

Skin rolling: A fold of skin and subcutaneous tissue is held between each thumb and index finger and the fold rolled forward. A positive finding is either the provocation of local tenderness and pain in a dermatomal distribution and/or a palpatory sense of tightness of the skin and loss of resiliency in the related subcutaneous structures. Generally touted as a scanning test, skin rolling can be very segmentally specific.[1]
- Observe for induration or resistance to roll
- Observe for *peau d'orange* appearance
Small tender nodules may also be identified in or on the deeper fascia using this test.

Layer palpation: Involves progressively increasing pressure over muscles, ligaments, vertebral processes, joint lines, or other clinically relevant structures in each region. A positive test involves palpable tissue texture abnormalities, subjective tenderness, and pain provocation, either over the local structure or in conjunction with a referred sensitivity phenomenon.
- Pressure on one site may be locally tender or may elicit a pain/dysesthesia referral pattern consistent with that structure.
- In the case of muscle, contraction or inhibition are palpable reactions to pressure, providing clinically valuable information.
- In the spinal region, this test, applied to the supraspinal ligaments and over each transverse process, identifies vertebral units requiring further examination.

Quality of End Feel: Various terms are used to describe the tissue-texture component assessed at the end of passive motion testing. Barrier end feel quality may be assessed at a variety of sites.
- Assess for an "empty" end feel, indicating ligamentous tear/laxity
- Assess for a pattern of opposing freedom-restriction, indicating somatic dysfunction
- Assess for a pattern of multiple opposite direction restrictions, indicating a capsular pattern (joint inflammation or pathology)
- Assess for abrupt versus less-abrupt restriction in one direction helpful in differentiating joint from muscular restrictions

[1]Greenman PE. *Principles of Manual Medicine*. Baltimore, MD: Williams & Wilkins; 1996.

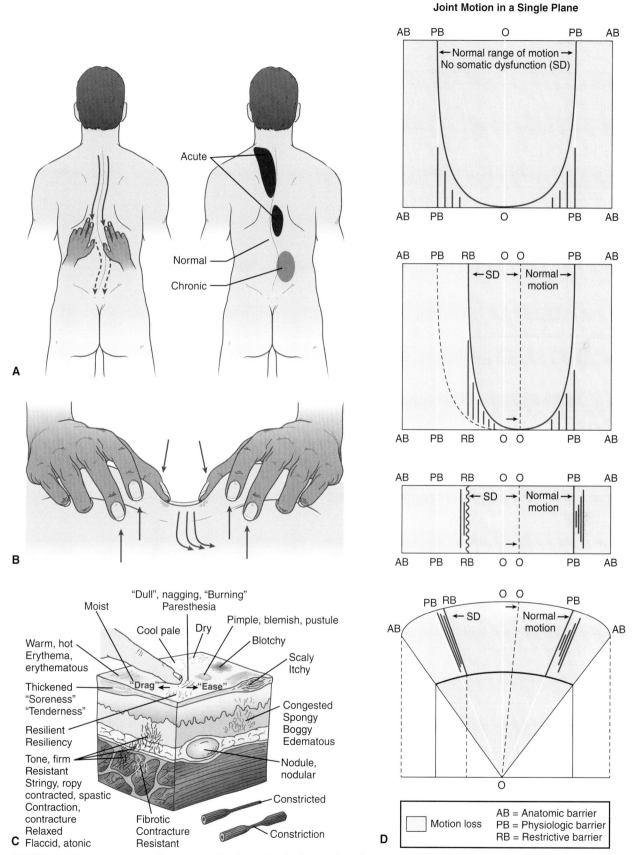

FIGURE 4–2 Tissue texture scanning tests. **A.** Skin drag and red reflex. **B.** Skin rolling. **C.** Layer-by-layer palpation. **D.** Quality of end feel (barriers).

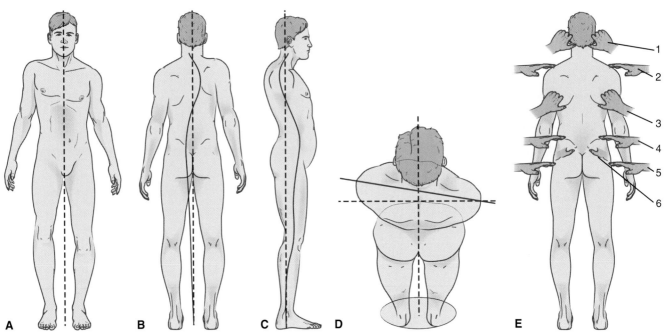

FIGURE 4–3 Asymmetry. **A.** and **B.** Coronal plane posture. **C.** Sagittal plane posture. **D.** Horizontal/transverse plane posture. **E.** Bony landmarks: E1 = occipital condyles; E2 = acromioclavicular joint; E3 = scapular angle; E4 = iliac crest; E5 = greater trochanter; E6 = posterior superior iliac spine.

Table 4–7	Scanning Tests Identifying Static-Dynamic Asymmetry

EXAMPLES OF COMMON SCANNING TESTS FOR ASYMMETRY OF STATIC LANDMARKS (ALSO SEE INDIVIDUAL REGIONAL ASSESSMENT)

Upright Postural Landmark Symmetry: Clues to regional involvement will combine observation/palpation of symmetry of key representative landmarks in seated and/or standing positions.

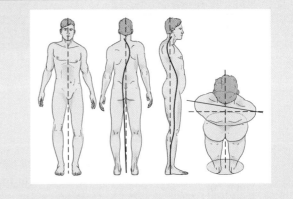

- Coronal plane dysfunctional scan: Visual comparisons (often assisted by palpatory landmark identification) of upright symmetry/levelness of the ears, mastoid processes, acromioclavicular joints, infralateral angles of the scapulae, iliac crests, posterior superior iliac spine (PSIS), greater femoral trochanters, joint line of the knees, and the foot arch are performed and recorded, including site of apices of curves and sites where the postural lines and the gravitational midline cross over. Often the space around the body, including how close the upper extremity is to the pelvis or whether one extremity hangs lower than the other, provides valuable information about the region involved.
- Sagittal plane dysfunctional scan: Using observation, the degree and apices of regional kyphotic and lordotic curves are noted and recorded.
- Horizontal plane dysfunctional scan: Using observation with or without palpatory assistance, the degree to which one of each of the following paired structures is anterior or posterior: anterior superior iliac spines (ASISs), lower ribs, acromioclavicular joints, mastoid processes, orbits, and ears.

Supine Landmark Symmetry: Clues to regional involvement with potentially significant somatic dysfunction include palpatory levelness of paired medial malleoli, ASISs, iliac crests, arms extended overhead (using the thumbs), intercostal spacing and sides of the squamous portion of the occiput.

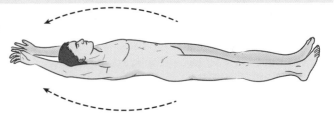

Table 4–7	Scanning Tests Identifying Static-Dynamic Asymmetry—cont'd

EXAMPLES OF COMMON SCANNING TESTS FOR ASYMMETRY OF STATIC LANDMARKS (ALSO SEE INDIVIDUAL REGIONAL ASSESSMENT)

Prone Landmark Symmetry: Clues to regional involvement with potentially significant somatic dysfunction include palpatory levelness of the PSISs, iliac crests, depth of sacral sulci, inferolateral angles of the sacrum, and ischial tuberosities, as well as the lumbar vertebral transverse and spinous processes.

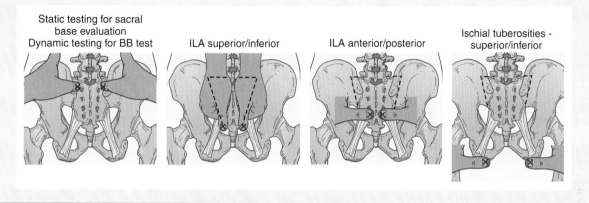

EXAMPLES OF COMMON SCANNING TESTS FOR RANGE OF MOTION (ALSO SEE INDIVIDUAL REGIONAL ASSESSMENT)

Transition zone scan (Fascial pattern testing): Craniocervical junction, cervicothoracic junction, thoracolumbar junction, and lumbopelvic junction are sequentially held and the fascial tissues of each junctional region are manually engaged to test rotation, side bending/translation, and flexion-extension preferences. Each area is rotated and/or translated to the point at which the tissues begin to tighten. Fascial drag and ease are noted. Asymmetrical motion characteristics in any region are considered a positive test result.

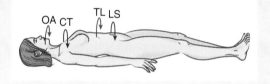

- Often the pattern of restriction from region to region provides as much insight into the underlying dysfunction as the individual regional restriction. Patterns have been described by Zink[1] and others.
- **Alternating regional fascial patterns** are usually compensatory and may be relatively asymptomatic.
- **Nonalternating fascial patterns** from one transition zone to the next are said to be **noncompensated** and are often traumatically induced and/or symptomatic.[2]

Vertebral motion scans: A positive scan for vertebral somatic dysfunction reveals restriction in one direction and freedom of motion in the opposite direction. Zygapophyseal tenderness is often elicited on the restricted side.[3] Significant regional asymmetrical restriction or tenderness identified in this manner should be examined more completely on a local (segmental) basis.

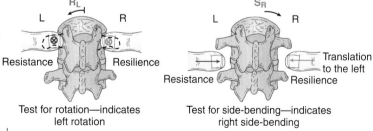

Test for rotation—indicates left rotation

Test for side-bending—indicates right side-bending

- Alternating side-to-side pressures over vertebral transverse processes provide a quick scan of rotational asymmetry within the same vertebral unit and compared to adjacent units.
- Alternating left-right translational pressures provide a quick scan for side bending motion symmetry within the same vertebral unit and compared to adjacent units.

Continued

Table 4-7	Scanning Tests Identifying Static-Dynamic Asymmetry—cont'd

EXAMPLES OF COMMON SCANNING TESTS FOR RANGE OF MOTION (ALSO SEE INDIVIDUAL REGIONAL ASSESSMENT)

Springing motion scans: Used for regional or segmental motion, typically, the heel of the hand or a thumb/digit is gently positioned, depending on the amount of area to be tested. Gradual pressure is applied, compressing soft tissues that overly the deeper tissues being evaluated. A springing force is then gently applied seeking to assess the quality of the end feel barrier. A **positive springing** test is recorded if the tissues have an abrupt rather than a physiologic resilient end feel. Elicited pain may augment the interpretation of regional or segmental springing. Spring tests include:

- **Interspinous spring test:** Scan for restricted backward bending of a vertebral unit
- **Supine costal spring test:** Scan for restricted rib motion.
- **Sacral spring test:** Scan for restricted anterior motion of an upper sacral pole or base
- **ASIS compression test:** Scan to lateralize motion restriction to one hemipelvis (pubic or sacral dysfunction)

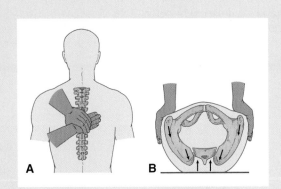

Inherent global motion scans: Both hands are placed over as much of a region as possible and inherent motions (including those of respiration) are palpated for symmetry. Typically, if asymmetry is palpated, the side with less amplitude is considered to have restricted motion, although hypermobility of the opposite side must be considered.

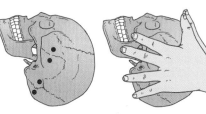 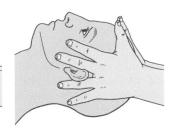

- **Spinal or extremity hold scans:** During inhalation, all spinal curves straighten, the sacral base moves posteriorly, paired structures externally rotate, ribs elevate anteriorly and/or laterally; the opposite occurs with exhalation.
- **Vault hold scans:** A scanning examination of the cranial vault palpates for an inherent motion named the CRI (cranial rhythmic impulse). Characteristics important in this model include symmetry, rate, amplitude, and perception of "vitality."[4] Flexion of midline structures is accompanied by external rotation of paired structures; extension with internal rotation.

[1]Zink JG, Lawson WB. An osteopathic structural examination and functional interpretation of the soma. *Osteopathic Ann.* 1979;**7**:433-440.
[2]Kuchera ML. Diagnosis and treatment of gravitational strain pathophysiology: research and clinical correlates (part I and II). In: Vleeming A, ed. *Low Back Pain: The Integrated Function of the Lumbar Spine and Sacroiliac Joints.* Proceedings of the 2nd Interdisciplinary World Congress, November 9–11, 1995, University of California, San Diego; 1995: 659-693.
[3]Paterson JK, Burn L. *An Introduction to Medical Manipulation.* Lancaster, UK: MTP Press; 1985: 144.
[4]Drengler K, King H. Interexaminer reliability of palpatory diagnosis of the cranium. *J Am Osteopath Assoc.* 1998;98:387.

Using local examination tests, the osteopath seeks to determine whether the motion is normal for that individual. If abnormal, then the pattern of motion, coupled with other STAR findings, permits determination of whether the problem represents somatic dysfunction, pathology, or a combination of both. If the diagnosis is somatic in origin, the pattern of findings will help determine if the dysfunction is physiologic or nonphysiologic, type I or type II, acute or chronic, and mild, moderate, or severe in nature.

Somatic dysfunction patterns are different from the capsular patterns of rheumatologic pathology and do not have the empty end feel of joints with ligamentous damage. A synopsis

of the normal physiologic motions of various arthrodial structures and the combination of patterns making up somatic dysfunction of these joints is included in Table 4-8.

Formerly, the osteopathic profession made a distinction between naming the arthrodial *osteopathic lesion* by its position or by its permitted motion. For example, a vertebral unit that was side bent left and rotated right (named for its asymmetrical position) would need to be motion tested to see if it was restricted in side bending to the right and rotating to the left. Currently, these designations have become synonymous because motion testing has been recognized as the gold standard.

Table 4–8	**Articular Somatic Dysfunction by Region**	
SELECTED SEGMENT/JOINT	**PHYSIOLOGIC MOTION PRESENT**	**SOMATIC DYSFUNCTION NAME/PATTERN**
Cranium–sphenobasilar symphysis (SBS)–spheno-occipital relationship	Perception with vault hold: symmetrical, equal amplitude cranial rhythmic impulse (CRI) described as flexion and extension with good vitality	• Compression of SBS: Symmetrical low amplitude, poor vitality CRI • SBS Flexion—Flexion CRI amplitude greater than that of extension; paired bones of head externally rotated leading to round shape to head, wide dental arch and flat palate, etc. • SBS Extension—Extension CRI amplitude greater than that of flexion; paired bones internally rotated; narrow dental arch and high palate, etc. • SBS Torsion (Right or Left)—Sphenoid and occiput appear rotated in opposite direction around common antero-posterior (AP) axis. • SBS Side Bending-Rotation (Right or Left)—Sphenoid and occiput appear rotated in opposite directions around paired vertical axes and the same direction around an AP axis. • SBS Lateral Strain (Right or Left)—Sphenoid and occiput appear rotated in the same direction around paired vertical axes. • SBS Vertical Strain (Superior or Inferior)—Sphenoid and occiput appear rotated in the same direction around paired transverse axes.
Other cranial bones and articulations in the cranium	• Midline structures flex and extend. • Paired structures externally rotate during flexion phase and internally rotate during extension phase. • The occiput has the most effect on the temporal bones. • The sphenoid most has the most effect on the facial bones.	Example: External rotation of the right temporal bone (prefers to externally rotate on an axis along its petrous portion during flexion phase of the CRI and is restricted moving toward internal rotation during the extension phase); accompanied by an apparent flared ear and retrusion of the mandible on the same side
Occipitoatlantal (OA or CO) articulation	Regardless of the sagittal plane position, coupled motion of the occiput, if introduced, will result in side bending and rotating in opposite directions.	Somatic dysfunctions: • OA flexion or OA extension • OA F[1] $S_L R_R$ or OA F $S_R R_L$ • OA N $S_L R_R$ or OA N $S_R R_L$ • OA E $S_L R_R$ or OA E $S_R R_L$ • Counterstrain points
Atlantoaxial (AA or C1)	For all intents, the only motion of concern in dysfunction of this joint is rotation.	Somatic dysfunction of AA: • R_L or R_R • Counterstrain points
C2–7	Regardless of the sagittal plane position, coupled motion of the typical cervical spinal joints, if introduced, will result in side bending and rotation in the same directions.	Somatic dysfunctions C2–7: • Flexion or extension • F $S_L R_R$ or F $S_R R_L$ • N $S_L R_R$ or N $S_R R_L$ • E $S_L R_R$ or E $S_R R_L$ • Anterior or posterior counterstrain points
T1–L5	Depending upon the sagittal plane position, coupled motions in the thoracic and lumbar regions, if introduced, will vary: • Type I (Fryette I): In the "easy neutral" position, side bending to one side automatically induces rotation to the opposite side (these motions are "coupled"). Such motions are	Somatic dysfunctions of T1–L5: • Flexion or extension • F $S_L R_L$ or F $S_R R_R$ (usually single vertebral unit) • N $S_L R_R$ or N $S_R R_L$ (usually a group of several vertebral units, although the apex is typically most pronounced)

Continued

Table 4–8	Articular Somatic Dysfunction by Region—cont'd	
SELECTED SEGMENT/JOINT	**PHYSIOLOGIC MOTION PRESENT**	**SOMATIC DYSFUNCTION NAME/PATTERN**
	usually part of a multisegmental compensatory pattern. • Type II (Fryette II) motion: Side bending and rotation occur to the same side when the vertebral unit facets are engaged, as in extreme forward or backward bending. (These motions are "coupled.") Such motions usually occur first to one segment in the region, providing adequate "slack" in the system that the remainder of the spinal curve will follow type I mechanics.	• E $S_L R_L$ or E $S_R R_R$ (usually single vertebral unit) • Counterstrain points for anterior or posterior thoracic or lumbar segments

Pelvis:
• Pubic rami
• Sacrum on ilium
• Ilium on sacrum
	The pubic symphysis is a synchondrosis that should allow slight yielding within the pelvic ring; it has a viscoelastic response to shearing and rotation (along an axis running perpendicular to the joint line).
	There are three transverse sacral axes proposed:
	1. Superior transverse axis: Associated with respiratory and craniosacral motions leading to nutation and counternutation (nutation is craniosacral extension and counternutation is craniosacral flexion)
	2. Middle transverse axis: Associated with the sacrum flexing and extending on the innominates
	  • The range from slight extension to a moderate amount of flexion causes the sacral base to rotate forward.
	  • Flexing further toward 90 degrees causes the sacrum to rotate posteriorly
	3. Inferior transverse axis: Associated with one or both innominates rotating around the sacrum
	  There are proposed to be vertical sagittal (and/or parasagittal) axes leading to pure sacral rotations
	  • The sacrum can rotate to the right or left Oblique sacral axes are described (left and right), although they are probably representative of combinations of transverse and vertical axes.
	  • Side bending left usually engages a so-called left oblique axis for side bending to the right engaging a right oblique axis.
	  L5 and the sacral base usually rotate in opposite directions (called lumbosacral torsions).
	  • Forward torsions occur in neutral positions when side bending-rotation is initiated
	  • Backward torsions occur in nonneutral positions when the patient is significantly flexed at the time of compression (flexed toward 90 degrees).
		Somatic dysfunctions of the pubic symphysis (usually traumatic)
		• Pubic shear (superior or inferior)
		• Pubic shear (anterior or posterior)
		• Pubic compression
		• Pubic gapping
		Somatic dysfunctions of the sacrum
		• Traumatic: Right or left sacral shear (inferior or superior; also called unilateral sacral flexion or extension, respectively)
		• Sacral base rotation (anterior or posterior)
		• Sacral margin posterior (left or right)
		• Left rotation on a left oblique axis; if L5 is $S_L R_R$, then this is also called a left sacral torsion or a left forward torsion (can interchange L and R for similar diagnosis)
		• Left rotation on a right oblique axis; if L5 is also rotated left, then this is a backward torsion (can interchange L and R for similar diagnosis)
		Somatic dysfunctions of the ilium/innominate
		• Traumatic: right or left innominate shear (superior or inferior)
		• Innominate rotation anteriorly (right or left)
		• Innominate rotation posteriorly (right or left)
		• Inflare innominate (right or left)
		• Outflare innominate (right or left)
		Counterstrain points for pelvis and pelvic muscles

Table 4-8	Articular Somatic Dysfunction by Region—cont'd	
SELECTED SEGMENT/JOINT	**PHYSIOLOGIC MOTION PRESENT**	**SOMATIC DYSFUNCTION NAME/PATTERN**
Ribs (R1–12)	Upper typical ribs tend to move more in the midclavicular line around a semitransverse axis (pump handle motion), whereas lower typical ribs tend to move more in the midaxillary line around a semi-AP axis (bucket bale motion). Ribs 11 and 12 move in a more pincer-like motion, moving down and out with inhalation and up and in with exhalation. Rib 1 has a synchondrosis in front.	Common somatic dysfunctions include: • 1st rib elevated or depressed posteriorly • 1st rib elevated or depressed anteriorly • Inhalation or exhalation rib 2–12 • Counterstrain points for elevated or depressed ribs Traumatic compressions, torsions, and subluxations may also affect rib function
Sternoclavicular (SC) and acromio clavicular (AC) joints	The two ends of the clavicle move in opposite directions around an axis approximately one-third of the way from the SC to the AC joint; a shoulder shrug up causes the lateral clavicle to move up and the medial clavicle to move down; a shoulder shrug anterior causes the lateral clavicle to move anterior and the medial clavicle to move posterior	AC somatic dysfunction (single or combined): • Superior or Inferior • Anterior or posterior AC somatic dysfunction (single or combined): • Inferior or superior • Posterior or anterior
Glenohumeral (GH) shoulder joint	This joint has circumduction, major motions of flexion and extension, external rotation with anterior glide of the humeral head, internal rotation with posterior glide of the humeral head, abduction with inferior glide, and adduction with superior glide.	GH somatic dysfunction (single or combined) includes: • Flexion or extension • External rotation with anterior glide or internal rotation with posterior glide • Abduction + inferior glide or adduction + superior glide
Ulnohumeral (UH) and radiocarpal (RC) joints	These two joints physiologically are related through the interosseous membrane between radius and ulna; the movement is "parallelogram" in the sense that abduction of the forearm at the elbow is accompanied by adduction of the hand at the wrist.	Ulnohumeral and radiocarpal somatic dysfunction (single or combined in the pairing associated with parallelogram motions) include the following: • Ulna abducted with medial glide or adducted with lateral glide at the UH joint • RC joint: adduction with lateral glide or abduction with medial glide
Femoroacetabular joint	The major motion of this joint is in flexion and extension; however, the motion of external rotation is linked to the minor motion of anterior glide while the motion of internal rotation is linked to posterior glide; there are also abduction and adduction motions.	Hip joint somatic dysfunction includes: • Flexion or extension • External rotation with anterior glide or internal rotation with posterior glide • Abduction or adduction
Knee (femorotibial joint)	The tibia (on femur) may flex with posterior glide, extend with anterior glide; abduct with medial glide or adduct with lateral glide; externally rotation with anteromedial glide or internally rotate with posterolateral glide.	Knee joint somatic dysfunction includes: • Flexion with anterior glide or Extension with posterior glide • Abduction with medial glide or Adduction with lateral glide • External rotation with anteromedial glide or internal rotation with posterolateral glide
Fibula	When the fibular head glides posteriorly (actually posteromedial), then the lateral malleolus glides anteriorly *et vv*	Somatic dysfunction is named at the fibular head end. • Fibular head anterior (left [L] or right [R]) • Fibular head posterior (left or right)
Ankle (talocrural joint)	The talus in a plantar flexed position with anterior glide is much less stable than a dorsiflexed with posterior glide position.	Somatic dysfunction of the ankle includes • plantar flexion with anterior glide (R or L) or • dorsiflexion with posterior glide (R or L)

Continued

Table 4-8	Articular Somatic Dysfunction by Region—cont'd	
SELECTED SEGMENT/JOINT	**PHYSIOLOGIC MOTION PRESENT**	**SOMATIC DYSFUNCTION NAME/PATTERN**
Talocalcaneal (subtalar) joint	The joint shape also has a gliding with slight twist with movement of the talus on the calcaneus posterolaterally during supination and anteromedially during pronation.	Somatic dysfunction of the talocalcaneal (TC) joint includes • posterolateral TC (left or right) • anteromedial TC (left or right)
Cuboid-navicular-2nd cuneiform	Part of the arch system(s) of the foot; minor gliding motion of each is permitted to allow the foot to conform to the shape of the ground, etc.	Somatic dysfunction is a dropping of one or more of these bones (the cuboid and navicular each drop and pivot slightly with the edge of the bone that is nearest the middle of the foot dropping further than the edge nearest the respective sides of the foot)
Other tarsals, metatarsals, carpals, metacarpals, and phalanges	Major motions are well known; each, however, is also capable of minor gliding motions with passive motion testing.	Somatic dysfunction often is found in the minor gliding motion of the joint (e.g., one somatic dysfunction of the PIP of the right index finger might be abduction with medial glide); somatic dysfunctions with trauma also commonly have a degree of compression or traction in these peripheral joints

1. F = flexion; N = neutral; S_L = side bending left; S_R = side bending right; R_R = rotation right; R_L = rotation left.

QUESTIONS *for* REFLECTION

- How are somatic dysfunctions of the spine identified within the osteopathic approach?
- What are the advantages and limitations of using this approach?
- How does this differ from the method that a physical therapist may use?

Therefore, it is recognized that a segment that is asymmetrically positioned would have motion limitations in the directions that are opposite that position (Box 4-2). That is to say, the **positional diagnosis** (i.e., the asymmetric position of the segment) is opposite that of the **movement diagnosis** (i.e., the direction in which the segment is currently restricted). In the example above, a positional diagnosis of side-bent left and rotation right would have the movement diagnosis, or be limited in moving into, side bending right and rotation left.

Box 4-2 Quick Notes

- **Positional diagnosis (PD):** Asymmetrical position that the segment is currently in
- **Movement diagnosis (MD):** Direction in which the segment is currently restricted, which is opposite that of the PD
- **Position of treatment (PT):** Direction in which motion is to be restored, which is the same as the MD

As previously noted, rotation and/or lateral translation tests may be performed at each spinal level as a scan or used for specific diagnosis of individual vertebral units. To test for the rotational component of somatic dysfunction, the clinician should place the palpating fingers over the left and right articular pillars/transverse processes of the vertebral unit in question. Either the patient's active rotation or the examiner's induction of passive rotation should be used as the examiner palpates and assesses the quality of the end feel of any barrier to motion (Fig. 4-4).

A practitioner gains additional palpatory information if this procedure is repeated with the spine in both forward-bent and backward-bent positions. In the *lateral translation test*, assessing side-bending capabilities, the physician places fingertips over the posterolateral aspects of the articular facets. The force is localized to one segmental level, and translation is checked in each direction. It is important to note that translation to the left creates side bending to the right. This test can also be performed with the spine in flexion and then repeated in extension. Restriction in left translation (restricted right side bending) at C5 on C6 that is worse when performed in extension and coupled with a restriction in right rotation may be recorded as a C5 flexed (F), rotated left (RL), side bent left (SL) somatic dysfunction or, using the Fryette format of documentation, $C5\ FR_LS_L$ (abbreviated as *FRS left*). It is important to note that a segment that is found to be positioned in flexion in the sagittal plane is identified when the segment is tested in extension, as described in the previous example. Conversely, a positional diagnosis of extension is best identified when the segment is tested in flexion.

Joint Motion in a Single Plane

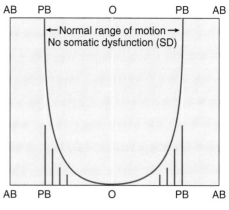

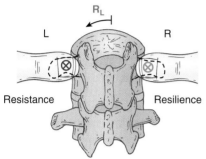

Test for rotation—indicates left rotation

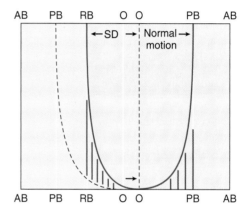

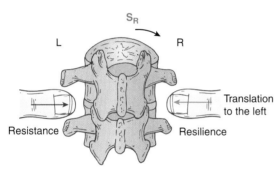

Translation to the left

A   Test for side-bending—indicates right side-bending

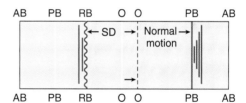

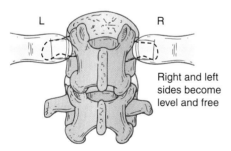

Right and left sides become level and free

FR$_R$S$_R$: Patient moves into flexion

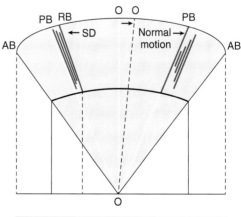

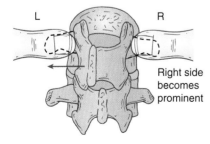

Right side becomes prominent

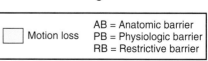

	AB = Anatomic barrier
Motion loss	PB = Physiologic barrier
	RB = Restrictive barrier

B   FR$_R$S$_R$: Patient moves into extension   **C**

FIGURE 4–4 Motion testing of a vertebral unit. **A.** Passive. **B.** Active. **C.** Barrier type is determined by the quality of the end feel for each plane of motion tested. Motion in one plane modifies motion in the remaining two planes.

QUESTIONS *for* REFLECTION

- What is the value of performing the lateral translation test for segmental mobility in neutral, then in flexion, then in extension?
- What is the best position to identify a positional diagnosis of extension or a positional diagnosis of flexion?

Recording and Grading Somatic Dysfunction

A grading system for somatic dysfunction was developed[24] to standardize the osteopathic palpatory examination. Somatic dysfunction, if found, is essentially rated as mild (1), moderate (2), or severe (3) based upon the STAR characteristics (Table 4-9).

Table 4–9	Standardized Severity Rating for Somatic Dysfunction[1]
0	No somatic dysfunction, or only background level changes
1	Minor STAR; more than background levels
2	STAR is obvious (especially R and T); ± symptoms
3	Symptomatic; R and T very easily found. This is the key lesion.

Kuchera, M. L., Kuchera, W. A., *Osteopathic Musculoskeletal Examination of the Hospitalized Patient*. American Osteopathic Association, 1998.

Region-Specific Osteopathic Examination for Somatic Dysfunction

Compensatory, reflex, and central mechanisms dictate that a change in one region creates dysfunctions in adjacent regions. A single somatic dysfunction (segmental or regional) is unlikely to be the sole cause or consequence of most clinical presentations. Table 4-10 and Table 4-11, for example, depict common combinations of somatic dysfunction associated with common clinical conditions.

Head and Craniocervical Junction

Anatomical relationships of the head and craniocervical junction are capable of significant pain referral as well as autonomic and cranial nerve dysfunction (Fig. 4-5). Furthermore, palpatory diagnostic findings in this section are particularly relevant to common musculoskeletal disorders such as headache, postural imbalance, and temporomandibular joint (TMJ) dysfunction. Furthermore, management of secondary somatic dysfunctions may improve the physiologic homeostatic mechanisms important in healing.[38]

CLINICAL PILLAR

- Anatomical relationships of the head and craniocervical junction are capable of significant pain referral as well as autonomic and cranial nerve dysfunction.
- Many structures of the head are pain-sensitive or are capable of pain referral.

Table 4–10	Examples of Multiple Somatic Dysfunctions in Head and Upper Thoracic Regions Involved With Somatic or Visceral Complaints

COMMON CLINICAL CONDITIONS

EXAMPLES OF POSSIBLE ASSOCIATED MULTIREGIONAL SOMATIC DYSFUNCTION COMPLEXES

Common Headache
a. Left occipitomastoid suture
b. Occipitoatlantal = S_RR_L[1]
c, d. C2–3 = E R_RS_R[2]
e. Travell points for upper end of the semispinalis muscle
f. Travell points for suboccipital muscle

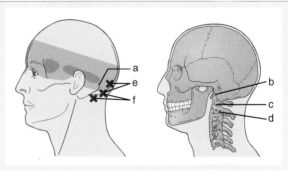

Sternocleidomastoid Headache
a. Right occipitomastoid suture
b. Travell right Sternocleidomastoid (SCM) trigger points (TrP) and pain pattern
c. Jones AC7 point
d. Temporomandibular joint dysfunction

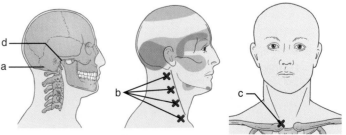

Table 4–10	Examples of Multiple Somatic Dysfunctions in Head and Upper Thoracic Regions Involved With Somatic or Visceral Complaints—cont'd

COMMON CLINICAL CONDITIONS

EXAMPLES OF POSSIBLE ASSOCIATED MULTIREGIONAL SOMATIC DYSFUNCTION COMPLEXES

Patient with Reactive Airway
a. Cranial extension head
b, d. Left rib 2–3 somatic dysfunction (SD)
c. Fullness of left supraclavicular region
d. Chapman's point tender reference to the bronchus
e. C2 Tender to Contact (TTC)
f. Left T1–3 TTC

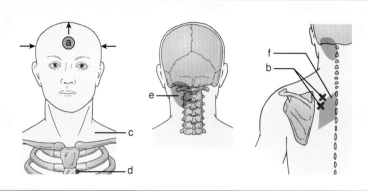

1. Side bending right, rotation left.
2. Extension, rotation right, side bending right.

Table 4–11	Examination for Somatic Dysfunction of the Sacroiliac Articulation

STEP	PATIENT POSITION	EXAMINATION	RESULTS AND POSTULATED INTERPRETATION
1	Standing	Evaluate anatomical landmarks, standing flexion test	A positive standing flexion test means dysfunction in the lower extremity and/or pelvis on that side.
2	Seated	Perform seated flexion test	Will specifically determine whether there is a sacroiliac dysfunction, and if so, which side (but not which arm) of the sacroiliac joint is dysfunctional
3	Supine	Perform anterior superior iliac spine (ASIS) compression test; positional assessment of ASISs, pubic tubercles, and medial malleoli	Helps determine the etiology of the problem and whether it is purely sacral or a mixed problem, incorporating iliac and pubic dysfunction
4	Prone	Palpate for tissue texture changes, motion testing of the sacrum, motion testing of L5, ligamentous tension testing	Helps the physician discover which axis is involved, find what portion of the SI joint is restricted, determine L5 motion and position, and evaluate pelvic ligamentous tensions

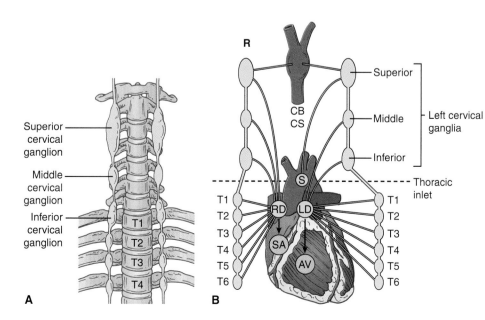

FIGURE 4–5 A. Cervical collateral ganglia relationships to cervical and upper thoracic somatic structures. **B.** Innervation of the heart. RD = right deep cardiac plexus; LD = left deep cardiac plexus; S = superficial plexus; SA = sinoatrial node; AV = atrioventricular node; CB and CS = carotid body and carotid sinus.

Headache is the most common pain-presenting complaint in the United States. Osteopathic practitioners use palpation extensively in the differential diagnosis of this condition and consider manual treatment quite frequently as an adjunctive modality to many of its causes.[39]

Many structures of the head are pain sensitive or are capable of pain referral. Pain may result from afferent referral originating from the eyes, ears, sinuses, temporomandibular joint, teeth, pharynx, respiratory tract, heart, and the upper gastrointestinal tract, as well as musculoskeletal referral from the cervical region. Pain-sensitive intracranial structures include the venous sinuses, the arteries of both the pia-arachnoid and the dura mater, and the dura itself. Extracranial structures such as the skin, myofascial structures, regional articulations, arteries, and cranial periosteum are also pain sensitive. Nociception may be transmitted along cranial nerves V, VII, IX, and X, as well as the C2,3 cervical nerve roots. Secondary somatic dysfunction may result from muscular splinting and positional compensations used to reduce pain.[34] The craniocervical junction is influenced by the occipital condyles, atlas, axis, and the muscular and connective tissues that govern their function. The palpatory scan of the suboccipital region requires individualized testing of all three craniocervical joints.[40]

Evidence suggests that 91% of patients had an occiput (C0) or atlas (C1) articular somatic dysfunction and 56% had TrPs in the semispinalis capitis muscle predominantly ipsilateral to the symptomatic side.[33,34] In individuals with retro-orbital headaches, common findings include an upper semispinalis capitis trigger point (Fig. 4-6) on the palpably anterior portion of a rotated C1 somatic dysfunction.[41]

Segmental motion scanning for C0 dysfunction is often accomplished passively using the lateral translation test. Palpating digits placed in the suboccipital triangle sense the end feel to right and left translation of the occiput with respect to the atlas (Fig. 4-7). This test can be easily translated into specific segmental motion in all three planes. An active scan is positive

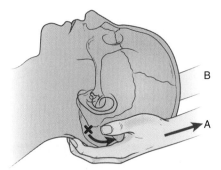

Cephalad test pull for side-bending is applied on one side at a time. A pulls first followed by B.

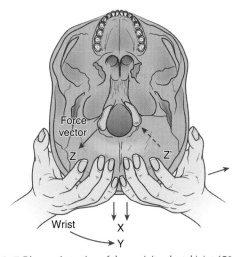

FIGURE 4–7 Diagnostic testing of the occipitoatlantal joint (C0). Regardless of flexion (bilateral X motion preference), extension, or neutral sagittal position, OA side bending in one direction is linked to rotation in the opposite direction. For example, a right index finger posterolateral draw (Z) to the first palpable resistance (with left index gliding anteromedial [Z'] and right wrist moving medial [Y] with slight supination) will assess side bending right with rotation left barriers.

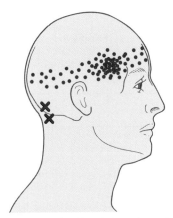

FIGURE 4–6 Referred retro-orbital headache with myofascial somatic dysfunction in upper semispinalis capitis and atlantoaxial articular somatic dysfunction (rotated to side opposite the headache). (From Simons DG, Travell JG, Simons LS. *Travell and Simons' Myofascial Pain and Dysfunction: The Trigger Point Manual.* Vol. 1. *Upper Half of Body.* Baltimore, MD: Williams &Wilkins; 1999.)

for C0 dysfunction if the chin deviates from the midline to either side in subjects without TMJ dysfunction.

Scanning for C1 somatic dysfunction may be accomplished by fully forward bending the entire cervical spine followed by rotating the head. Asymmetrical motion indicates a positive test, which suggests the need for segmental evaluation of C1 (Fig. 4-8).

Segmental examination for occipitoatlantal (OA) somatic dysfunction recognizes that these joints are placed so as to converge anteriorly (Fig. 4-7). In a forward-bent OA dysfunction, the occiput will allow forward bending but is restricted when backward bending is attempted, whereas the opposite is true for a backward-bent OA dysfunction. In coupled plane somatic dysfunction, side bending and rotation occur to opposite sides.[42] In an OA side-bent left and rotated right somatic dysfunction, the occiput is restricted when side bending to the right and rotation to the left are attempted. Because of the two condylar joints, motion characteristics of OA somatic dysfunction can be localized further to the right and/or the left occipitoatlantal articulation according to the dominant sensitivity, tissue texture abnormality, and restriction of motion. Thus in the example of

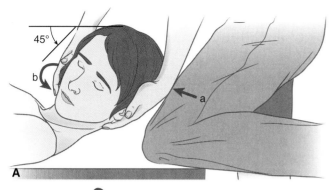

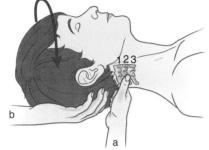

B Segmental C1 test where a. stabilizes C2 while b. produces right rotation

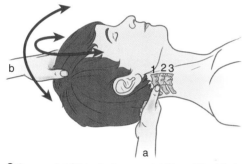

C Segmental C0 test where a. stabilizes C1 while b. produces forward/backward nod or side nod.

FIGURE 4–8 Motion tests for superior cervical segments. **A** = Gross scanning for atlantoaxial (AA or C1) somatic dysfunction. This cannot be performed in all patients in whom pain, potential pathology (as in severe rheumatoid arthritis), or guarding prevent safe or accurate findings. a = flex to lock out motion below the AA; b = observe/palpate range and symmetry of superior cervical segment (normal = 25–45 degrees). **B** = Segmental C1 test stabilizing C2 spine; **C** = Segmental C0 test stabilizing C1 transverse processes.

coupled motion as described above ($OA\ S_R R_L$), there may be an anterior left occiput, a posterior right occiput in relation to the atlas, or both.

Segmental motion examination of the atlantoaxial joint (AA) is best accomplished by stabilizing the axis with one hand. This is accomplished by grasping the posterior spine of C2 between the thumb and index finger of one hand; the occiput is cupped in the other hand with the fingers in the suboccipital groove and resting over the posterior arch of the atlas (Fig. 4-8).

The C2 nerve root has direct attachments to the vagus nerve and is a common palpatory site of secondary somatic dysfunction. This results from vagal visceral afferent stimuli arising from dysfunction of certain upper respiratory, cardiac,

and/or upper gastrointestinal structures (see Fig. 4-9). The segmental examination of C2-C3, as discussed below, is conducted in the same manner as all typical cervical vertebral units in the lower cervical area.

In interpreting palpatory findings in this region, a wealth of clinical evidence, including a 5-year double-blind study of 5,000 hospitalized patients,[43] suggests that the differential diagnosis of palpatory findings in this region should include secondary somatic dysfunction from sinus, respiratory, cardiac, and gastrointestinal disorders.[16,44] Paterson provides a synopsis of eye, nose, and throat symptoms resulting from cervical dysfunction and notes that in the absence of contraindications, manipulation is the treatment of choice.[45] It is presumed that when cervical somatic dysfunction is eliminated by manipulation, precipitating visceral factors that are still present will no longer trigger the referred headaches.[27,46]

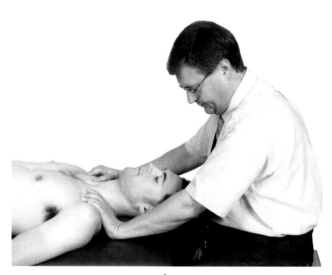

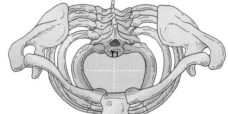

Anatomical thoracic outlet

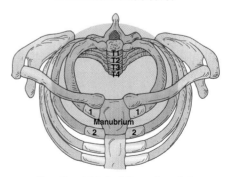

Functional (clinical) thoracic outlet

FIGURE 4–9 Superior thoracic inlet regional diagnosis. Combined influence of T1–4, ribs 1–2, manubrium, and all myofascial attachments.

Lower Cervical, Cervicothoracic, and Superior Thoracic Inlet

The typical cervical spine extends from C2 through C6 or C7. Taken together with the cervicothoracic junction, this region contains sympathetic ganglia whose cell bodies originate in the upper thoracic region. Osteopathic practitioners agree with the ***International Headache Society (IHS)*** in recognizing that the cervical spine must be included in classification schema.[47] According to the IHS, inclusion criteria for cervicogenic headaches include several of the STAR characteristics used to diagnosis cervical somatic dysfunction.

From a pathophysiologic perspective, cervical somatic dysfunction has been implicated in reducing the transport of centrally produced trophic substances to the tissues of the upper extremities.[48] This may predispose the upper extremities to an increased risk of developing symptomatic entrapment neuropathies and other regional disorders. The area is also subject to secondary somatic dysfunction.

The application of pressure posteriorly over spinous processes or articular pillars is commonly used to scan for segmental cervical dysfunction.[34,46] Jones's nomenclature for these tender points is standardized and considered during counterstrain techniques. Differentiation between cervical somatic dysfunction and nerve root pathophysiology cannot be made by palpation alone.

More specific tissue texture scanning in the lower cervical region may be indicated. Common coexisting dysfunctions may include the following: trapezius TrPs with C2 and/or C3 articular somatic dysfunction and C4 hypermobility,[34] splenii cervicis TrPs with articular C4 and/or C5 dysfunction,[34] levator scapulae TrPs with articular somatic dysfunction anywhere between C3 and C6.[34]

Palpation of C2 to C7 segmental motion is most easily accomplished by using the passive segmental rotation and lateral translation tests described previously. To test rotation, support the supine patient's head with the fingers contacting the posterior surfaces of the articular pillars. In the neutral position, rotate each vertebral unit along the plane of its posterior cervical facets (roughly toward the patient's opposite eye) bilaterally, assessing the end feel in each direction. Additional palpatory information is gained when repeated in both forward-bent and backward-bent positions.

For the lateral translation test, the physician contacts the lateral portion of the cervical articular pillar with fingertips while supporting the head. While localizing force to one level, translation is assessed in each direction. The test can also be performed with the neck held in flexion and then repeated in extension.

The cervicothoracic junction and superior thoracic inlet are extremely important from an autonomic and circulatory perspective. The superior thoracic inlet is in close relationship with the superior thoracic outlet, and dysfunction of one affects the function of the other (Fig. 4-9). Recall that differential diagnostic considerations in this region include viscerosomatic and somatovisceral reflexes.

Thoracic Spine and Thoracic Cage

The wide distribution of sympathetic fibers originating from the cell bodies located in the lateral horn of the thoracic region coupled with the anatomical relationship between the sympathetic chain ganglia and the heads of each rib (Fig. 4-10) closely associate thoracic cage somatic dysfunction with visceral and somatic problems throughout the body (Fig. 4-11). With every respiratory cycle, numerous muscle groups and approximately 146 articulations in the thoracic cage are called upon to move. Therefore, the differential diagnosis must include common somatic problems such as costochondritis, other chest wall syndromes, somatic clues of viscerosomatic and somatovisceral reflex phenomena, and a wide range of pathologic and infectious processes. Likewise, dysfunctions in the thoracic cage can be expected to influence function in the cervicothoracic and thoracolumbar junctional areas. In addition to palpatory diagnosis, appropriate history and physical examination to rule out pathologic change in the thoracic cage or of the viscera referring to the region is required (Fig. 4-12). Segmental motion diagnosis requires assessment of end feel in all planes. The "thoracic rule of threes" (Fig. 4-13) is useful in guiding hand placement. Once finger placement is assured, segmental motion can be assessed actively or passively.

One test unique to the thoracic region is the *shingle test of Kuchera*.[16] Medial pressure with one thumb is applied on the lateral side the spinous process of the thoracic level in question with a counterforce imposed by the other thumb on the spinous process of the vertebra below. The clinician's thumbs and the pressures are then reversed. In the thoracic region, where the facets lie relatively in a coronal plane, opposite rotations induced at adjacent segments cancel one another, and only side bending occurs to the side of the superior thumb (Fig. 4-14). In the shingle test of Kuchera, the freer end feel determines the direction of side bending.

Specific passive motion testing of each of three planes in the thoracic region can be most easily accomplished with the

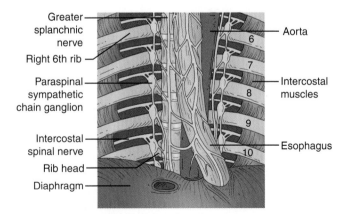

FIGURE 4–10 Distribution of sympathetic fibers originating from the cell bodies located in the lateral horn of the thoracic region coupled with the anatomical relationship between the sympathetic chain ganglia and the heads of each rib.

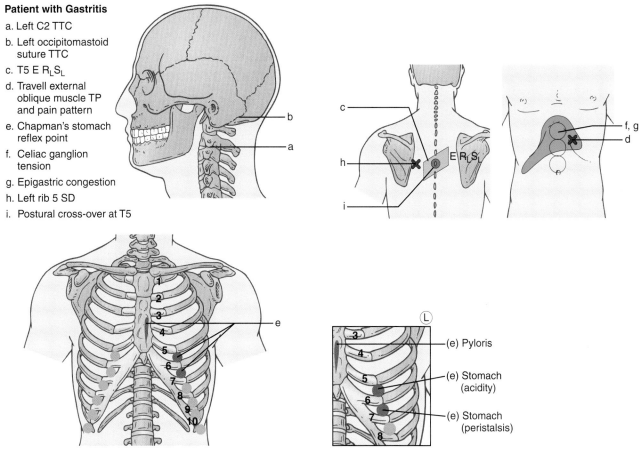

Patient with Gastritis

a. Left C2 TTC

b. Left occipitomastoid suture TTC

c. T5 E R$_L$S$_L$

d. Travell external oblique muscle TP and pain pattern

e. Chapman's stomach reflex point

f. Celiac ganglion tension

g. Epigastric congestion

h. Left rib 5 SD

i. Postural cross-over at T5

FIGURE 4–11 Examples of the pattern of multiple somatic dysfunctions associated with primary (viscerosomatic) or secondary (somatovisceral) gastritis.

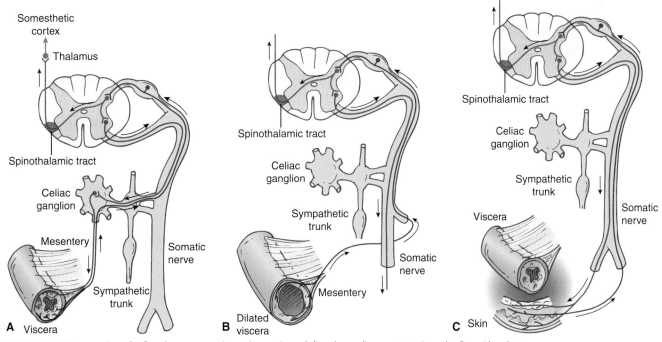

FIGURE 4–12 Progression of reflex changes seen in a primary visceral disorder or disease. **A** = Visceral reflex with palpatory tension over appropriate collateral ganglion; **B** = Viscerosomatic reflex with palpatory findings (especially tissue texture change) in segmentally related paraspinal and Chapman's sites; **C** = Peritoneocutaneous reflex associated with tissues adjacent to inflamed or ruptured viscus.

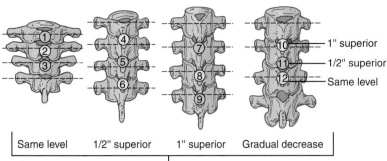

Same level | 1/2" superior | 1" superior | Gradual decrease

Distance of transverse process from spinous process

FIGURE 4–13 "Rules of Three" relationship of thoracic transverse processes to spinous processes.

patient seated or prone. Alternating pressure over the transverse processes of each segment is applied, and rotation end feel is assessed. Translation or passively induced side bending is applied to assess the quality of that barrier at each thoracic vertebral unit (Fig. 4-15). The third plane of motion is assessed by passively testing interspinous approximation and separation. If there is vertebral unit somatic dysfunction, the quality of each barrier is restrictive in one direction and physiologic in the opposing direction. The combination of restrictive barriers determines whether type I or type II dysfunction is present, and the combination of tissue texture changes determines whether it is acute or chronic.

CLINICAL PILLAR

- Segmental motion testing and the combination of restrictive barriers is used to diagnose the presence of a type I or type II dysfunction.

- The combination of tissue texture changes identified during the palpation examination, determines whether the condition is acute or chronic.

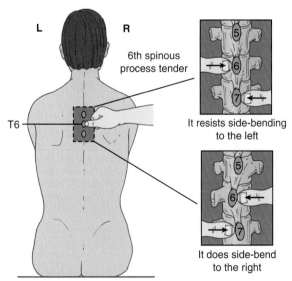

FIGURE 4–14 Shingle method of W. Kuchera for thoracic side bending. Opposing pressures on sequential thoracic vertebrae cancel out rotation permitting side bending assessment.

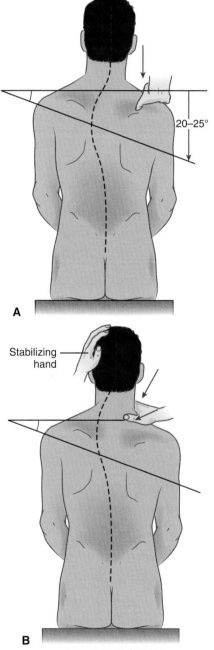

FIGURE 4–15 A = Acromion drop test screens for upper thoracic somatic dysfunction. **B** = Modification to specifically test upper thoracic side bending.

Dynamic thoracic motion examination involves monitoring change in the relationship of transverse process pairs during active forward and backward bending motion from a neutral starting point. This method helps identify which of two possible type II somatic dysfunction diagnoses is present; both typically involve a single vertebral unit, and both involve unidirectional side bending and rotation to the same side.

Type II Somatic Dysfunction

The **extended, rotated, and side-bent (ERS)** somatic dysfunction is diagnosed when the transverse process on one side becomes more prominent with forward bending and more symmetric with backward bending. The opposite findings are palpated in a **flexed, rotated, and side-bent (FRS)** somatic dysfunction.

Type I Somatic Dysfunction

Type I somatic dysfunctions typically involve three or more adjacent vertebral units. These dysfunctions are identified in the neutral spinal position (Box 4-3). Dynamic motion testing in type I somatic dysfunction may result in a slight change in the asymmetry of transverse processes, but significant symmetry is not achieved with either forward or backward bending.

Ribs identified in the screening or scanning processes can be individually named according to their structural and respiratory characteristics. Structural, traumatically induced rib dysfunction diagnoses include anterior or posterior subluxed ribs, torsioned ribs, and anteroposterior or laterally compressed ribs.

Box 4-3 DIFFERENTIATION OF SPINAL POSITIONAL DIAGNOSES

Type I Somatic Dysfunction:
- Restriction in group (three or more)
- Side Bending (SB) in one direction and Rotation (ROT) in the opposite direction
- Identify in **neutral** and named by side of **SB**
- *Neutral, rotated right, side-bent left (NRS left or NSL):* Transverse process prominent on right in neutral
- *Neutral, rotated left, side-bent right (NRS right or NSR):* Transverse process prominent on left in neutral

Type II Somatic Dysfunction:
- Involves one or two segments
- Restriction of **SB** and **ROT** to same side
- *Extended, rotated, and side-bent (ERS):* Transverse process on one side becomes more prominent with forward bending and more symmetric with backward bending.
- *Flexed, rotated, and side-bent (FRS):* Transverse process on one side becomes more prominent with backward bending and more symmetric with forward bending.

Anterior or Posterior Subluxed Ribs

In this condition, the ribs exhibit hypermobility and are palpably displaced anteriorly or posteriorly along the axis of motion between the costovertebral and costotransverse articulations.

Torsioned Ribs

These ribs are often seen in conjunction with thoracic rotation (affecting ribs on both sides) and should return to bilateral symmetry when the thoracic spine returns to a symmetrical position. With T4 rotation to the right on T5, for example, rib 5 on the right would demonstrate **external torsion** along its long axis, resulting in palpable prominence at the superior border of the rib angle and the inferior border of the sternal end. **Internal torsion** of the left fifth rib would be present with sharper inferior border palpated posteriorly and a sharper superior border palpated anteriorly.

Anteroposterior or Laterally Compressed Ribs

This condition may result from an anteroposterior or a laterally directed trauma, leading to sustained rib deformation. A palpable prominence will be respectively noted in either the midaxillary line or both anteriorly and posteriorly.

More commonly found are rib 2 to 10 dysfunctions that can be named according to their respiratory characteristics (Fig. 4-16). These diagnoses include inhalation or exhalation costal somatic dysfunction and pump-handle and/or bucket-handle costal somatic dysfunction.

Inhalation or Exhalation Costal Somatic Dysfunction

Costal symmetry and motion with respiration should be assessed bilaterally on both anterior and lateral chest walls.

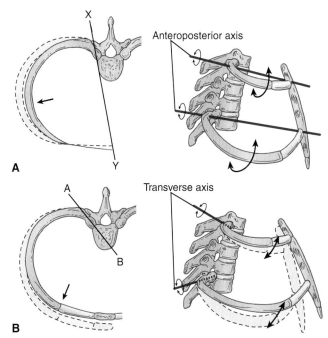

FIGURE 4–16 Respiratory characteristics of rib dysfunction. **A** = Bucket bale (lower ribs): Check motion midaxillary line; **B** = Pump handle (upper ribs): Check motion midclavicular line.

Palpating digits straddle each pair of ribs being tested, and the patient is instructed to take a full breath in and out. During one phase of the respiratory cycle, the rib with restricted motion will stop moving before the rib on the normal side. The costal dysfunction is named for the respiratory component that is permitted, thus suggesting that the rib is unable to move in the opposite direction. An inhalation right 5th rib dysfunction, for example, will have palpatory findings in which both fifth ribs rise in inhalation, but during continued exhalation, the right 5th rib stops moving while the left continues to move inferiorly. Note that the 11th and 12th ribs, without an anterior sternal attachment, have more of a pincer or caliper motion that exhibits a posterolateral motion during inhalation and an anteromedial motion during exhalation. In general, inhalation rib dysfunctions often involve several ribs. Conversely, exhalation rib dysfunction often arises in patients with a persistent cough wherein a localized spasm of an intercostal muscle typically results in an exhalation dysfunction of a single rib. In Jones's counterstrain system, anterior (depressed) rib points often correspond with exhalation ribs whereas posterior (elevated) rib points often correspond with inhalation ribs.

Pump-Handle and/or Bucket-Handle Costal Somatic Dysfunction

The axis of respiratory motion is influenced by a number of factors, including the angle between the body of the thoracic vertebra and the transverse processes (Fig. 4-16).[16] Each rib has a mixture of pump-handle motion (assessed on the anterior chest wall) and bucket-handle motion (assessed on the lateral aspects of the chest wall) (Box 4-4). The upper ribs typically have a higher percentage of pump-handle motion, whereas the lower typical ribs have a higher percentage of bucket-handle-type motion. Motion loss to either springing or to a portion of the respiratory cycle noted anteriorly is described as pump-handle dysfunction; motion loss noted laterally is consistent with bucket-handle dysfunction.

Thoracolumbar Junction, Inferior Thoracic Outlet, and Lumbar Spine

Common musculoskeletal and visceral disorders found to have significant somatic dysfunction in this area include quadratus lumborum TrPs; psoas syndrome; viscerosomatic referral from the kidneys, gastrointestinal, and genitourinary tract; and signs and/or symptoms of hypertension, dysmenorrhea, or constipation. Additionally, the importance of this area by virtue of its association with the thoracic diaphragm make it a major consideration for somatic dysfunction in the presence of reduced diaphragm mobility.

In supine patients, regional thoracolumbar motion is evaluated by exerting rotational and translational pressures over the lower rib cage (Fig. 4-17d) to the point where the fasciae first begin to resist. The physician evaluates for asymmetrical motion characteristics of resiliency (ease) and resistance (drag) in side bending and rotation.

A number of other regional screening and scanning examinations identify the need for the specific segmental diagnosis of thoracolumbar and lumbar somatic dysfunction. The

---

Box 4-4 TYPES OF SOMATIC RIB DYSFUNCTIONS

- **Anterior or posterior subluxed ribs:** Ribs exhibit hypermobility and are palpably displaced anteriorly or posteriorly along the axis of motion between the costovertebral and costotransverse articulations.
- **Torsioned ribs:** Seen in conjunction with thoracic rotation. With rotation to the right of T4 on T5, rib 5 has *external torsion* on the right and *internal torsion* on the left.
- **Anteroposterior or laterally compressed ribs:** Result of anteroposterior or laterally directed trauma leading to sustained rib deformation. A palpable prominence is noted in midaxillary line or both anteriorly and posteriorly.
- **Inhalation costal somatic dysfunction:** With an inhalation right fifth rib dysfunction, both fifth ribs rise in inhalation. but the right fifth rib stops moving while the left continues inferiorly during exhalation. It often involve several ribs.
- **Exhalation costal somatic dysfunction:** With an exhalation right fifth rib dysfunction, both fifth ribs lower in exhalation but the right fifth rib stops moving while the left continues superiorly during inhalation. Often arises from persistent cough and spasm of intercostals muscle.
- **Pump-handle and/or bucket-handle costal somatic dysfunction:** Motion loss to either springing or to a portion of the respiratory cycle noted anteriorly is described as pump-handle dysfunction; motion loss noted laterally is consistent with bucket-handle dysfunction.

---

most commonly used screening tests include the hip drop test (Fig. 4-17a), trunk side bending, trunk rotation, Schober's test (Fig. 4-17b), and the prone lumbar springing test.

In lumbar somatic dysfunction, the quality of each barrier is restrictive in one direction and physiological in the opposing direction; the combination of restrictive barriers determining whether type I or type II dysfunction is present. Alterations in spinal motion are the most prominent consideration in the differential diagnosis of somatic dysfunction. The capsular pattern in the lumbar region involves marked but symmetrical limitation of side bending accompanied by lesser limitation of both flexion and extension. The sagittal plane capsular barriers arising from degenerative and inflammatory processes (such as ankylosing spondylitis) create a positive Schober's test (Fig. 4-17b).

For passive segmental motion evaluation[49] (Fig. 4-4a), the end feel in all planes is assessed. Specific passive triplanar motion testing is most easily accomplished in the lumbar region with the patient seated or prone. Alternating pressure over the transverse processes assesses the end feel of the barrier to rotation at that level. Note that the transverse processes in this region are located essentially in the same horizontal plane as the spinous process of the same vertebra. Translation or

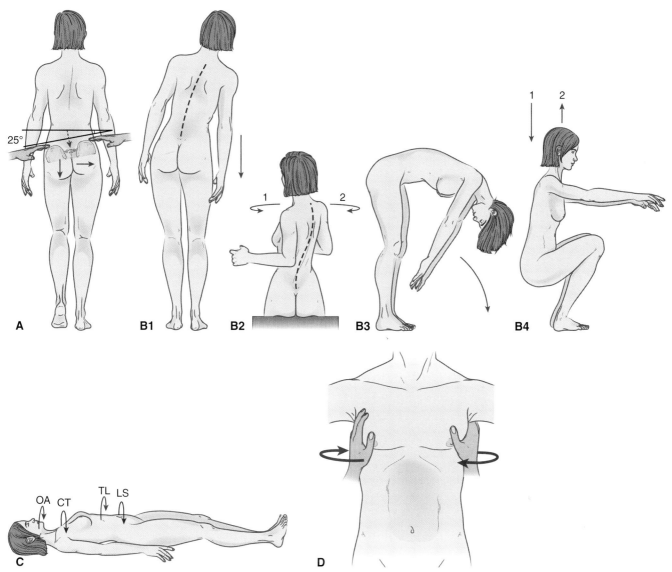

FIGURE 4–17 Regional motion testing. **A** = Hip drop test; **B1** = Side bending range of motion (ROM); **B2** = rotational ROM; **B3** = flexion ROM; **B4** = deep squat; **D** = regional (fascial) ROM at transition zones with detail motion testing for rotation to the right of the inferior thoracic outlet (thoracolumbar region).

passively induced side bending is applied to assess the quality of that barrier at the same vertebral level. Passively testing interspinous approximation or separation permits assessment of the sagittal plane of motion.

In applying the dynamic motion-testing method,[49] the transverse processes are palpated in neutral, extended (sphinx position), and forward-bent positions (Fig. 4-4b). As in the thoracic region, two different type II somatic dysfunction diagnoses are possible in this region: ERS and FRS. The diagnosis of a type I somatic dysfunction typically involves three or more adjacent vertebral levels, and testing may change the asymmetry of transverse processes slightly, but symmetry is not achieved with either forward or backward bending.

Pelvis and Lumbopelvic Junction

The pelvis and lumbopelvic junction contain more musculoskeletal congenital anomalies than any other body region. Sacroiliac articular somatic dysfunction commonly coexists in

patients with myofascial points in the quadratus lumborum.[34] Innominate dysfunction typically accompanies both latissimus dorsi and quadratus lumborum TrPs.[34] Pubic and innominate dysfunctions are commonly associated with abdominal TrPs.[50] TrPs in the iliocostalis lumborum are associated with pelvic obliquity secondary to the muscle's insertional aponeurosis onto the sacral base that in turn leads to sacroiliac dysfunction.[33] In this latter case, the positive seated flexion test will be worse than the standing flexion test.[51]

Finally, it should be noted that the sacral base extends the impact of local dysfunction far beyond the lumbopelvic area. Unleveling of the sacral base is well documented to be a precipitating and perpetuating cause of muscle imbalance and myofascial TrPs throughout the entire body[52] as well as a cause of recurrent patterns of somatic dysfunction.[53,54] In addition, segmental facilitated spinal dysfunction arising in compensation for an unlevel sacral base is capable of creating a wide range of visceral and systemic symptomatology (Fig. 4-18).

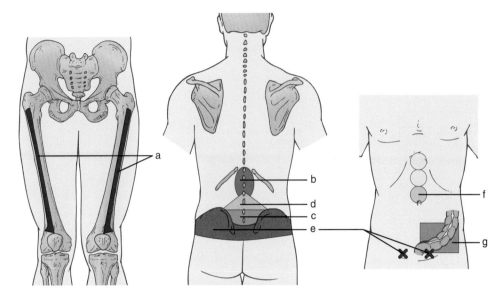

Patient with Irritable Bowel Dysfunction

a. Bilateral iliotibial band tenderness and TTC (Chapman's)

b. Thoracolumbar SD and TTC

c. Left SI TTC

d. Post. Chapman's, lumbar TTC, (low-back pain)

e. Lower rectus abdominis muscle TP and pain pattern

f. Inferior messenteric ganglion TTC

g. Sigmoid loop palpable

FIGURE 4–18 Examples of pattern of multiple somatic dysfunctions associated with primary (viscerosomatic) or secondary (somatovisceral) irritable bowel syndrome.

QUESTIONS _for_ REFLECTION

• Why is an unleveling of the sacral base believed to be a factor in creating a wide range of visceral and systemic symptomatology and precipitating and perpetuating the cause of muscle imbalance and myofascial TrPs throughout the entire body, as well as to be a cause of recurrent patterns of somatic dysfunction?

• How might the clinician reliably identify an unlevel sacral base, and what manual interventions might be used to restore its normal position?

Dermatomal pain is widely recognized in both distribution and quality. Conversely, _sclerotomal_ pain is little known and is characteristically described as deep and dull, or arthritic in nature. _Myotomal_ involvement can lead to muscle cramps and/or TrPs; individual muscles may test weak or be in spasm. Ligamentous pain tends to be sclerotomal; severe myofascial TrPs often demonstrate characteristics of both myotomal and sclerotomal patterns (Fig. 4-19).

QUESTIONS _for_ REFLECTION

• What are the primary characteristics of _dermatomal_, _sclerotomal,_ or _myotomal_ involvement?

• What procedures might be used to identify the presence of each?

Pain and/or dysesthesia can be caused by either neurological or somatic structures in patients with lumbar disc disease, spondylolisthesis, and severe lumbar degenerative changes. To better understand the importance of assessing each of the possible somatic structures involved in the differential diagnosis

of this region, see Figure 4-20. Note the similarity in the distribution of an S1 radiculopathy caused by a herniated disc, a gluteus minimus myofascial trigger point caused by hip dysfunction, and posterior sacroiliac ligament strain caused by sacroiliac shear somatic dysfunction.

A lumbopelvic regional restriction may be scanned in supine position by gently rotating the pelvis on the lumbar spine. Gently grasping both sides of the pelvis just below the iliac crests and translating the pelvis right and left assesses the point at which the fasciae first begin to resist side bending.

Trigger points in the quadratus lumborum are noted to be one of the most commonly overlooked muscular sources of low back pain and are often responsible, through satellite gluteus minimus TrPs, for the pseudo-disc syndrome and the failed surgical back syndrome (Fig. 4-21).[55] They were also the most commonly involved muscle TrPs (32%) in soldiers with musculoskeletal complaints.[56] TrPs may respond to a variety of manual techniques directed to the muscle itself, including massage, tapotement, and postisometric muscle energy manipulative treatment.[57,58]

CLINICAL PILLAR

Trigger points in the quadratus lumborum are noted to be one of the most commonly overlooked muscular sources of low back pain and are often responsible, through satellite gluteus minimus TrPs, for the pseudo-disc syndrome and the failed surgical back syndrome.

The most commonly used screening and scanning tests have already been described and include _tests for lateralization_, including flexion tests[16] (standing and/or seated), which are also called the _Piedaullu test_ or _lock sign_, and the _ASIS compression test_. Direct _dynamic tests_ for general restriction of

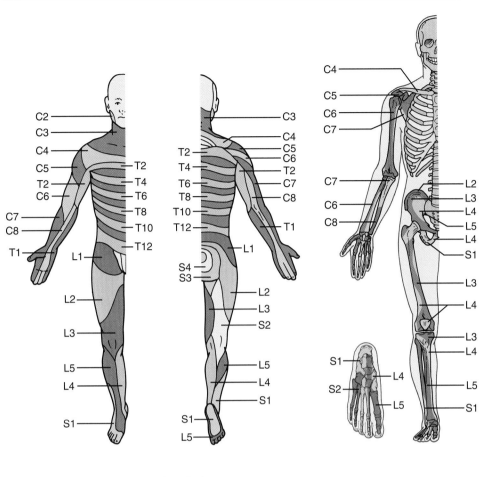

FIGURE 4–19 Sensory change patterns. 1A. Dermatome. 1B. Sclerotome. Myotomal patterns are not depicted here.

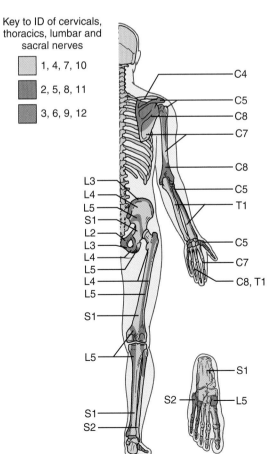

Key to ID of cervicals, thoracics, lumbar and sacral nerves

1, 4, 7, 10

2, 5, 8, 11

3, 6, 9, 12

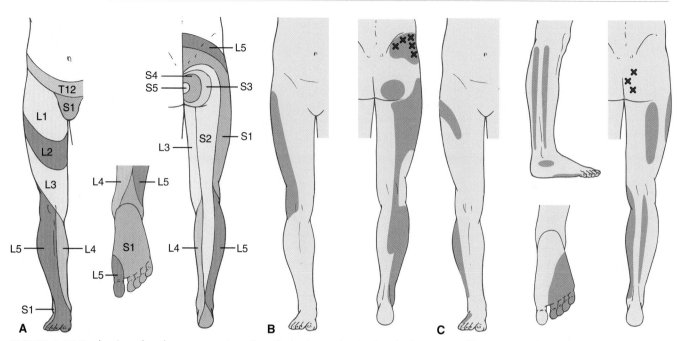

FIGURE 4–20 Overlapping referred sensory symptoms from the lumbosacral region into the lower extremities. Compare sites of **A** = S1 dermatome dysesthesia from herniated L5 disc; **B** = gluteus minimus trigger point myotomal cramping pain; and **C** = posterior sacroiliac sclerotomal deep pain due to sacral shear somatic dysfunction.

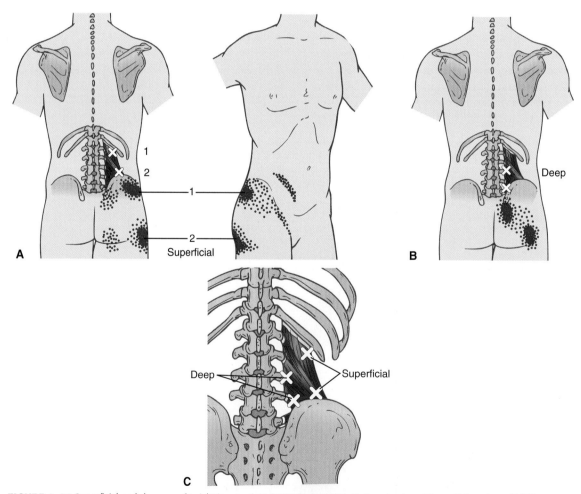

FIGURE 4–21 Superficial and deep myofascial trigger points (MTrPs). **A.** and **B.** Referred pain patterns. **C.** Location of MTrPs. (Reprinted with permission from Simons, DG, Travell JG, Simons LS. *Travell and Simons' Myofascial Pain and Dysfunction: The Trigger Point Manual.* Vol. 1. *Upper Half of Body.* Baltimore, MD: Lippincott, Williams & Wilkins; 1999.)

sacroiliac motion may include the *one-legged stork test* (also called *Gillet's test*), indirect passive examination using *long-sitting tests (yo-yo sign), hip rotation tests,* and/or the *SI gapping test.* A variety of *pelvic ligamentous stress tests*[32] (Fig. 4-22) may also be included, which consist of the *cranial shear test, pelvic distraction and compression tests, SI gapping test* (also known as the *thigh thrust SI stress test,* the *posterior pelvic pain provocation test,* the *FADE test,* and the *POSH test*), *sacral thrust test, Gaenslen's test, Yeoman's test,* and/or variations of *Patrick's (FABER) test.* Generic identification of sacroiliac dysfunction has been shown to be significant in the patient using a single finger to identify the region of discomfort (known as the *Fortin finger test*).[54] *Local motion screening tests* may be used, which involve springing of various areas of the pelvic girdle in conjunction with positional changes.

Sacroiliac Joint

In the widely adopted osteopathic models, three major systems have had a significant impact on the nomenclature now commonly employed to describe sacroiliac joint dysfunction (SIJD). Each of these historic systems examine sacral motion related to a different anatomical structure. In the *Strachan (high velocity low amplitude) model,*[55,56] diagnosis of the sacrum is named largely with respect to its motion, or restriction, relative to the innominates. In the *Mitchell (muscle energy) model,*[57] a series of postulated sacral axes are coupled with diagnoses of sacral torsions to reflect sacral motion, or restriction, relative to the lumbar spine and the mechanics of gait. In the *Sutherland (craniosacral) model,*[58] motion, or restriction, of the sacrum is described relative to the cranium. Regardless of the model

selected, each diagnosis of somatic dysfunction implies freedom in one direction of motion around an axis with restriction in the opposite direction. For a more complete discussion of these models, the reader is directed to the chapter on the sacrum and pelvis in the standard text, **Foundations for Osteopathic Medicine**.[59]

The goal of local palpatory examination is to compile enough specific information about tenderness, key landmark asymmetry, sites and characteristics of restricted motion, and evidence of tissue texture change to extrapolate a tentative diagnosis. The guidelines[64] provided in Table 4-12 help with this interpretation. A suggested series of local palpatory tests for ascertaining the symmetry of sacral landmarks and the quality of motion available is depicted in Figure 4-23. Sacral somatic dysfunction diagnoses include the following postulated axes about which associated somatic dysfunctions exist.

Box 4-5 OSTEOPATHIC MODELS FOR IDENTIFYING SACROILIAC JOINT DYSFUNCTION

- *Strachan (high-velocity low-amplitude) model*: Diagnosis of the sacrum is named largely with respect to its motion, or restriction, relative to the innominates.
- *Mitchell (muscle energy) model*: A series of postulated sacral axes are coupled with diagnoses of sacral torsions to reflect sacral motion, or restriction, relative to the lumbar spine and the mechanics of gait.
- *Sutherland (craniosacral) model*: Motion, or restriction, of the sacrum is described relative to the cranium

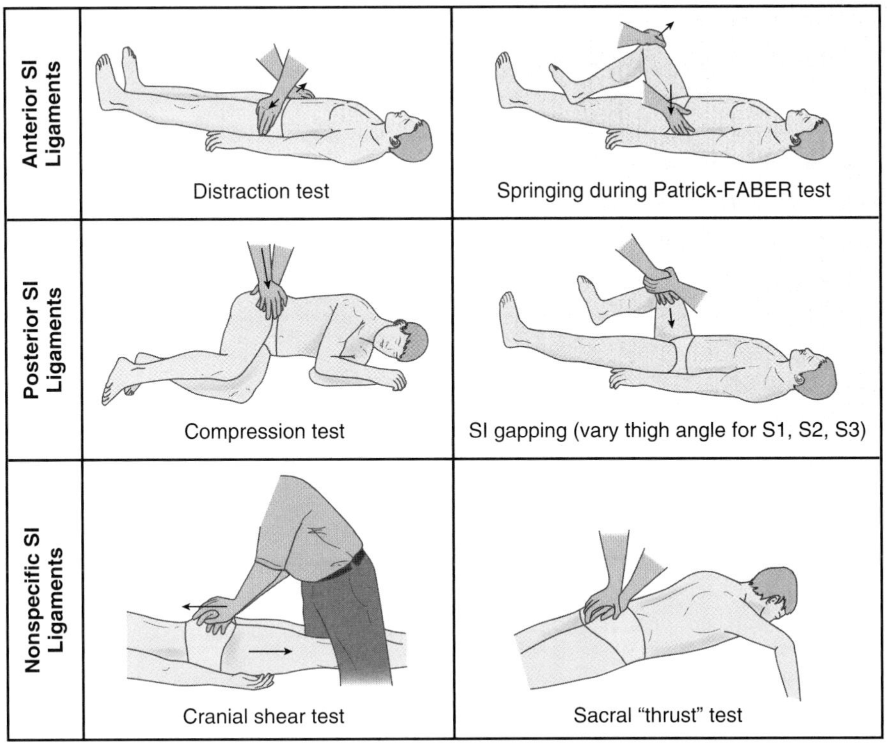

FIGURE 4-22 Pelvic ligamentous stress tests.

Anterior SI Ligaments: Distraction test | Springing during Patrick-FABER test

Posterior SI Ligaments: Compression test | SI gapping (vary thigh angle for S1, S2, S3)

Nonspecific SI Ligaments: Cranial shear test | Sacral "thrust" test

Table 4-12 Constellation of Static and Dynamic Findings of Common Sacral Somatic Dysfunctions

STATIC AND DYNAMIC FINDINGS	SACRAL BASE ANTERIOR (BILATERAL SACRAL FLEXION)	LEFT ROTATION ON A LEFT OBLIQUE AXIS	RIGHT ROTATION ON LEFT OBLIQUE AXIS	SACRAL MARGIN POSTERIOR ON THE LEFT	LEFT SACRAL SHEAR (LEFT LATERAL "UNILATERAL" SACRAL FLEXION)
Static Findings Palpated Over the Sacrum	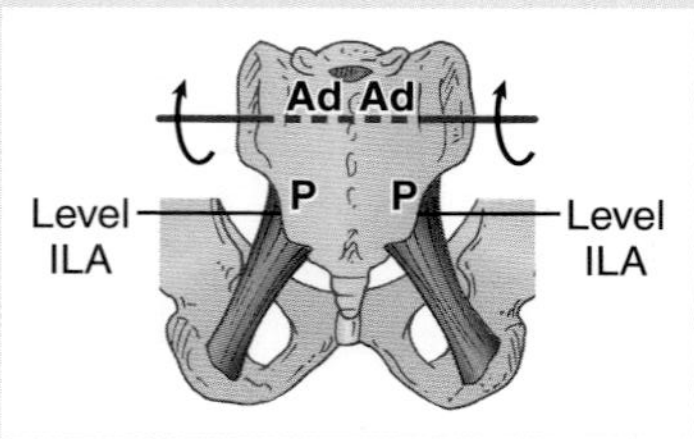	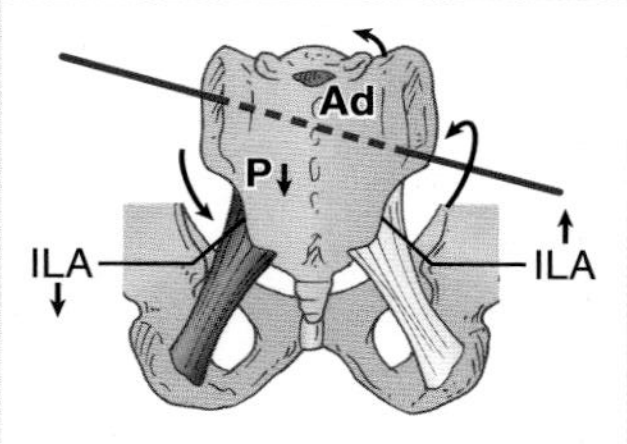	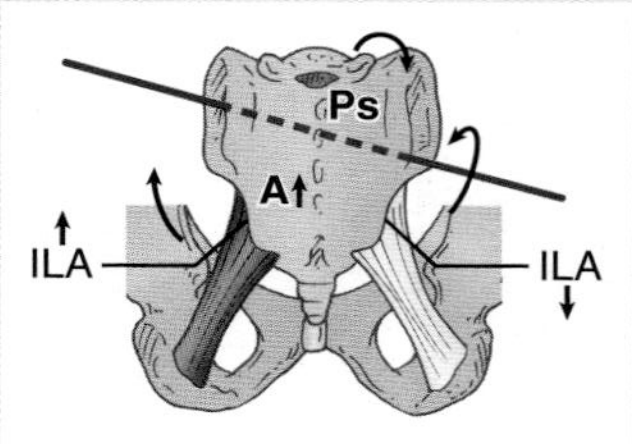	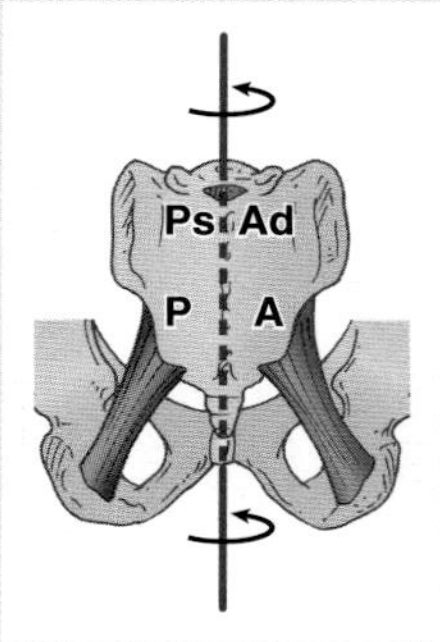	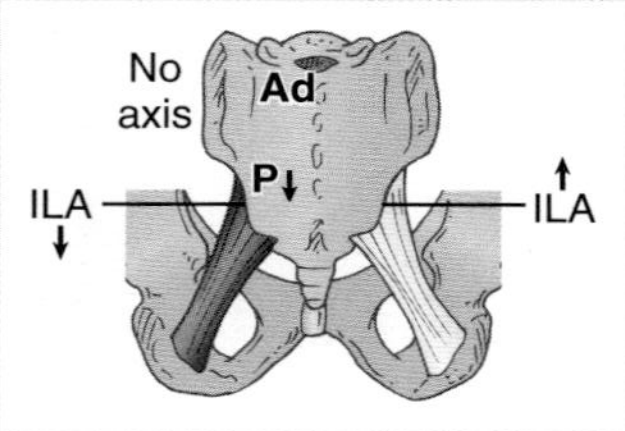
Lateralization Tests	N/A	Right commonly reported (Theoretically either left upper or right lower pole or both could be restricted.)	Right commonly reported (Theoretically either left upper or right lower pole or both could be restricted.)	Left	Left
Sphinx Test (backward bending test)	N/A Remains symmetrical	More symmetrical than previously	Less symmetrical than previously	Less symmetrical than previously	More symmetrical than previously
Motion Testing or "Rattle" of the Four Poles	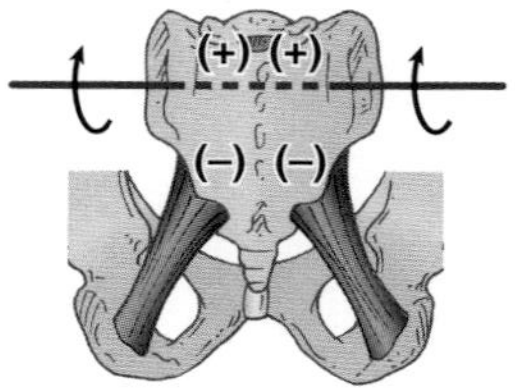	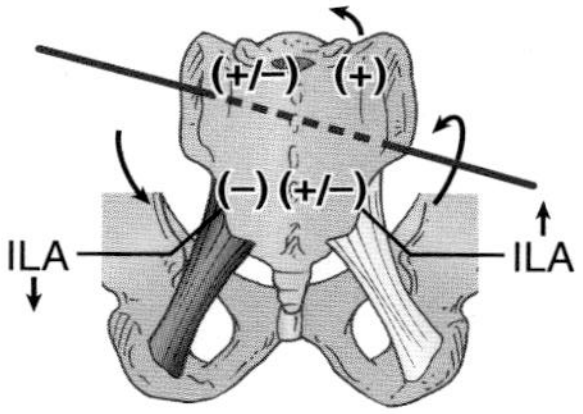	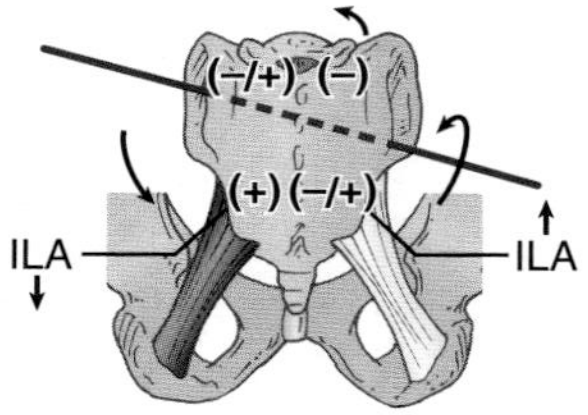	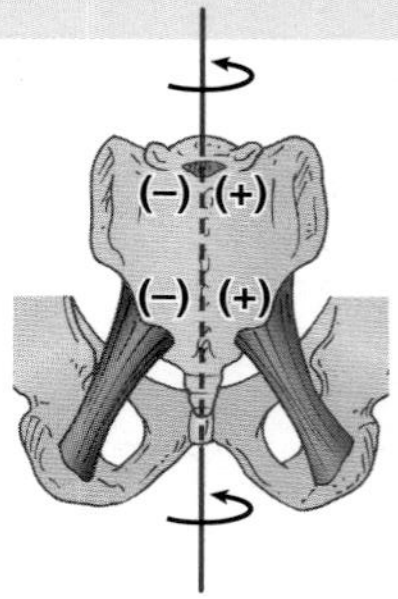	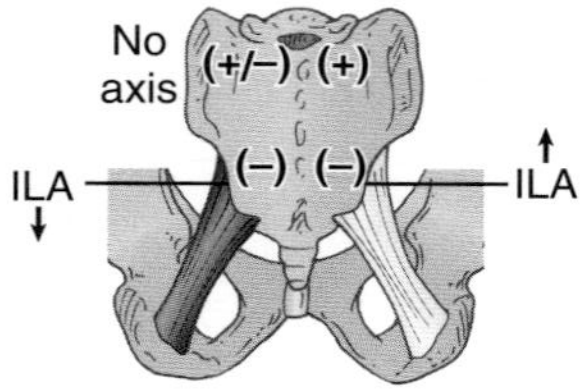

d = deep
s = shallow

A = anterior
P = posterior

↑ = superior
↓ = inferior

(+) = moves
(−) = restricted

(+/−) = some motion
ILA = Inferior lateral angle

normal ligament

tight ligament

loose ligament

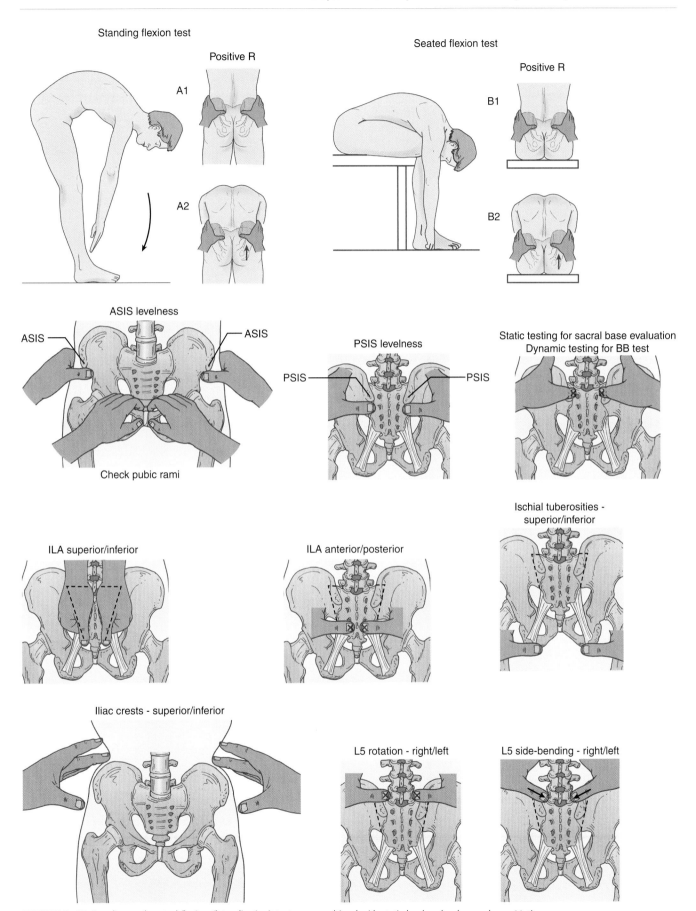

FIGURE 4–23 Standing and seated flexion (lateralization) tests are combined with static landmarks shown above. Motion testing of the sacroiliac joint (or a sphinx test) completes the diagnostics.

- *Bilateral sacral flexion and extension somatic dysfunction:* The sacral base is anterior (bilateral sacral flexion somatic dysfunction) or the sacral base is posterior (bilateral sacral extension somatic dysfunction) about the *middle transverse axis (S2 level).*
- *Left or right rotation on left oblique axis somatic dysfunction:* The presence of a left or right rotation about the *left oblique axis (upper left S1 to lower right S3).*
- *Left or right rotation on right oblique axis somatic dysfunction:* The presence of a right or left rotation about the *right oblique axis (upper right S1 to lower left S3).*
- *Left or right sacral margin posterior somatic dysfunction:* The presence of a left or right sacral margin posterior somatic dysfunction about the *sagittal or parasagittal axis.*
- *Left or right sacral shear somatic dysfunction:* The presence of a left or right sacral shear somatic dysfunction that is *traumatically induced, with no axis* (Fig. 4-24).

It is important to move beyond static landmark assessment and integration of functional tests of motion in making a diagnosis. While several sacral diagnoses may present with the same static sacral landmarks upon palpation, variations in motion characteristics provide differential diagnosis upon which the most appropriate intervention is predicated (Table 4-13).

The Extremities

The osteopathic physician's first diagnostic steps when examining the extremities is to ensure that pain and/or dysfunction in an extremity was not due to critical extremity pathology (e.g., deep vein thrombosis in the calf) or referred as part of one of the local, systemic, or visceral "red-flag" diagnoses (e.g., myocardial infarction arm pain, compartment syndrome with loss of pulse, etc.). To this end, osteopathic palpatory findings may augment standard tests to influence the suspicion of a particular diagnosis. The following case examples were selected to illustrate how an osteopathic approach might augment the diagnostic approach to extremity symptoms not originating in the extremity (Table 4-14).

The examination of extremity joints for the somatic dysfunctions listed in Table 4-9 is an extension of interpreting the traditional tests of the joints and ligaments. In this fashion, the palpable characteristics in testing motion can be interpreted as too loose, too tight, or just right. If "too loose," with an "empty" end feel, a damaged support structure is suspected. If "too tight" in one direction and "just right" in the other, somatic dysfunction is suspected, whereas being "too tight" in one or more paired motions may indicate a pathologic capsular pattern.

Finally, the generalized and relatively unique osteopathic examination for systemic homeostasis with regard to the spinal autonomic and central respiratory-circulatory systemic factors are added to the more traditional local examination of those neural, vascular, and lymphatic elements that are related to somatic dysfunction in the extremities. Special attention is paid to the tissue texture changes comparing

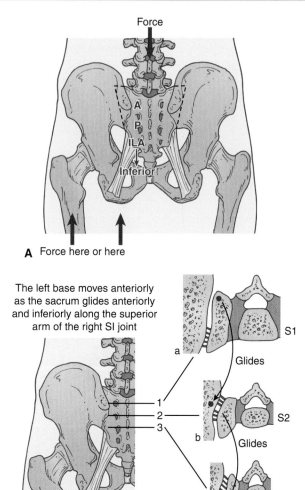

A Force here or here

The left base moves anteriorly as the sacrum glides anteriorly and inferiorly along the superior arm of the right SI joint

The apex of the sacrum moves posteriorly and inferiorly as the sacrum moves along the inferior **B** arm of the SI joint

FIGURE 4–24 Mechanism creating an inferior sacral shear. In the sacral shear, one sacral margin nutates along the L-shaped joint, giving rise to its alternate name, "unilateral sacral flexion."

any sense of swelling or thickening in the lymphatic-rich sites associated with the extremity being examined. The addition of palpatory diagnosis in this fashion expands the differential diagnosis and the potential avenues of treatment for common extremity problems (Fig. 4-25). A few examples of an osteopathic approach illustrating differential diagnosis in the extremities would include those selected in Table 4-15.

PRINCIPLES OF OSTEOPATHIC MANIPULATIVE MEDICINE INTERVENTION

Both the *Osteopathic Core Curriculum of the Educational Council on Osteopathic Principles*[60] and the consensus document on osteopathic practice published by the *World Health Organization*[61] discuss five models commonly used

Table 4–13 Summary of the Importance of Not Only Recording Findings but Also Performing Motion Tests for Accurate Diagnosis

STATIC AND DYNAMIC FINDINGS	LEFT ROTATION ON A LEFT OBLIQUE AXIS	ANTERIOR SACRUM RIGHT	POSTERIOR SACRUM LEFT (ONLY IN STRACHAN MODEL)	LEFT FORWARD TORSION	LEFT ROTATION ON A RIGHT OBLIQUE AXIS
Static Findings Palpated Over the Sternum	Same -			Same	
Lateralization Tests	+Right	+Right with texture change over right pole	+Left with tissue change over the left upper pole	+Right	Left
Sphinx Test (backward bending test)	More symmetrical	More symmetrical		More symmetrical	Less symmetrical
Motion Testing					
Restriction of Gapping	N/A	Left upper and lower; right lower	Left upper; right upper and lower	Left upper and lower	Left upper and lower

d = deep
s = shallow
A = anterior
P = posterior
(+) = moves
(−) = restricted
↑ = superior
↓ = inferior
(+/−) = some motion
ILA = Inferior lateral angle
normal ligament
tight ligament
loose ligament

Table 4–14	Osteopathic Considerations in Secondary and Referred Symptoms

EXAMPLES/CASES	INTEGRATION OF OSTEOPATHIC CONSIDERATIONS IN THE DIAGNOSIS
Consideration: Referred From a Visceral Structure?	
Pain radiation/referral into the left arm	The first concern is to rule out cardiac-related pathology. The requisite electrocardiogram (ECG) and cardiac enzymes may be supplemented by the doctor of osteopathy palpating for cardiac-related tissue texture changes. In cardiac problems, STAR characteristics are found in the T1–6 region, Chapman's reflex points in the second intercostal space and TrPs in the pectoralis major (which has the same pain pattern, but which also occurs in 60% of patients with coronary artery disease and angina).[1–3]
Pain referral to the right shoulder	One possible consideration would be referral secondary to irritation of the right hemidiaphragm as in gallbladder disease. In addition to history, physical, and imaging data, the doctor of osteopathy might also palpate C3–5 and diaphragmatic attachments in addition to palpating the gallbladder site (Murphy's) and viscerosomatic reflexes, such as Chapman's in the right sixth intercostal space as well.
Consideration: Referred in a Sclerotomal Fashion From a Bony, Arthrodial, or Ligamentous Structure?	
Knee pain	For the doctor of osteopathy the differential diagnosis of a deep, dull, achy pain referred to the knee could include a range of diagnoses from slipped capital epiphysis of the hip or metastatic prostatic lesion in the body of the L4 vertebra to pathology/severe dysfunction of the pubic symphysis.
Hip pain	For the doctor of osteopathy who would also look for hip pathology, knowing that common somatic referrals are commonly misdiagnosed as greater trochanteric bursitis would widen the differential and encourage palpation of the iliolumbar ligament and quadratus lumborum for tissue texture changes or trigger points. In addition, a complete osteopathic approach would look for postural strain, lumbosacral instability, and certain somatic dysfunctions (such as an inferior sacral shear) known to stress these pain generators.[4]
Consideration: Secondary to a Neurological Compression Affecting a Nerve Root or Plexus?	
Cervical radiculopathy with dysesthesia, weakness, and pain in a C7 distribution	In this case, after determining that the patient's symptoms are associated with cervical osteoarthritic spurs, the patient's posture was evaluated. It was determined that this patient's cervical hyperlordosis (caused by increased postural curves in all regions) was aggravating symptoms.
Lumbar radiculopathy with dysesthesia, weakness, and pain in an L5 distribution	The doctor of osteopathy recognized that trigger points (TrPs) in the hamstrings could provide a false-positive straight leg raise test by limiting the range of motion prior to initiating pain down the leg; however, the test remained positive after inactivating the trigger points. In this electromyogram-positive case, magnetic resonance imaging showed a large posterolateral L4 herniated disc. Additional palpatory findings determined in this case that the patient's symptoms were supplemented/magnified by secondary myofascial trigger points in the gluteus minimus, creating both myotomal TrP referral into the lower extremity as well as recurrent sacroiliac somatic dysfunction (with posterior sacroiliac [SI] ligament sclerotomal referral into the lower extremity).
Alternating thumb-sided and 5th digit-sided dysesthesia with finger swelling	The patient in this case had been told that her pattern of symptoms was not possible. It was recognized by the doctor of osteopathy as being the commonly seen scalene TrP pattern alternating referred TrP pain and scalene entrapment of the lower trunk of the brachial plexus. The condition was further complicated by 1st rib and clavicular somatic dysfunction on the same side. No pectoralis minor involvement was noted, but there was congestive, tender fullness in the posterior axillary fold. Adson maneuver improved after a trial of osteopathic manipulative treatment of the somatic dysfunctions found.
Consideration: Secondary to a Systemic or Metabolic Problem?	
Stocking distribution foot numbness	It was confirmed that this patient had diabetic peripheral polyneuropathy, but further palpatory examination suggested that symptoms were complicated by thoracolumbar segmental facilitation causing increased sympathetic tone and subsequent vasoconstriction to the lower extremities.
Median entrapment neuropathy (carpal tunnel symptoms)	Diagnostic work-up revealed this EMG-positive diagnosis was actually secondary to hypothyroidism. While waiting for medical control, the patient experienced relief with treatment of palpable latent and active myofascial TrPs in the pronator teres and wrist/finger flexor muscles and a home stretching exercise for these and thumb muscles. No surgery was needed in this case.

[1]Kuchera ML, Kuchera WA. *Osteopathic Considerations in Systemic Dysfunction.* 2nd ed. rev. Columbus, OH: Greyden Press; 1994.
[2]Nicholas AS, DeBias DA, Ehrenfeuchter W, et al. A somatic component to myocardial infarction. *Br Med J.* 1985;291:13-17.
[3]Simons DG, Travell JG, Simons L. S. *Travell and Simons' Myofascial Pain and Dysfunction: The Trigger Point Manual.* Vol. 1. *Upper Half of Body.* Baltimore, MD: Lippincott, Williams & Wilkins; 1999:832-833.
[4]Kuchera, M. L. Gravitational stress, musculoligamentous strain, and postural alignment. *Spine: State of the Art Review.* 1995; 9:463-490.

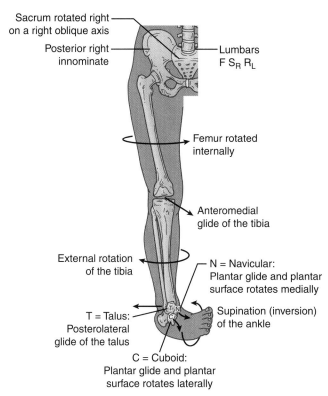

Sacrum rotated right on a right oblique axis

Posterior right innominate

Lumbars
F S$_R$ R$_L$

Femur rotated internally

Anteromedial glide of the tibia

External rotation of the tibia

N = Navicular: Plantar glide and plantar surface rotates medially

Supination (inversion) of the ankle

T = Talus: Posterolateral glide of the talus

C = Cuboid: Plantar glide and plantar surface rotates laterally

FIGURE 4–25 Somatic dysfunction pattern seen in the more common supination ankle sprain.

by osteopathic practitioners in patient care. These five models include the *respiratory-circulatory model*, the *biomechanical-structural model*, the *metabolic-nutritional model*, the *neurological model*, and the *behavioral-biopsychosocial model*.

Algorithms in Establishing an Osteopathic Manipulative Medicine Treatment Approach

Osteopathic physicians incorporate treatment choices, manual or otherwise, by applying diagnostic algorithms within one or more of the aforementioned models. Differential diagnosis is followed by an assessment of indications and contraindications and a consideration of possible treatments in the context of their risk-to-benefit ratio. This process is particularly true when more mechanical diagnoses are being considered.[62] As an example of such an algorithm for the management of a patient with chronic pain, see Figure 4-26.[39]

The role of the osteopathic tenets and the acquisition and demonstration of the safe and effective use of manual skills is part of the training and testing of all osteopathic physicians in the United States. These elements are also part of the core competencies expected in osteopathic postgraduate programs. That being said, not all osteopathic physicians use OMM in their practices. This makes it difficult sometimes for patients

Table 4–15	Integrating Extremity Somatic Dysfunction and Symptoms

SYMPTOM–SOMATIC DYSFUNCTION	DISCUSSION OF INTEGRATING OSTEOPATHIC DIFFERENTIAL DIAGNOSIS
Foot drop[1]: A variety of somatic dysfunctions supplement the differential diagnosis of this condition that could also be related to pathology such as an L5 radiculopathy.	
Piriformis tension, trigger point (TrP), syndrome	• Entrapment leading to footdrop is especially true in the anatomical variant in which the peroneal portion of the sciatic nerve passes through the belly of this muscle. (This variant occurs in 11% of Caucasian patients and 33% of patients of Asian descent.) • There is an increased risk of TrP secondary to sacroiliac shear dysfunction. • This postural muscle may be increased in tension with contralateral psoas spasm.
Posterior fibular head dysfunction	• This articular somatic dysfunction may cause pressure on the common peroneal nerve similar to symptoms arising from a crossed leg palsy placing external pressure on this same site. • Increased risk with supination stress or position at the ankle owing to anterior pull through the anterior talofibular ligament
Myofascial trigger points(MTrPs) in tibialis anterior and/or peroneus muscles	• As phasic muscles, MTrPs will reduce strength predisposing to footdrop. • Reflex weakness owing to TrPs in these muscles will be accentuated by tight gastroc-soleus complex (or TrPs).
Recurrent ankle sprains[2]: A variety of somatic dysfunctions increase the risk of recurrent ankle sprains (usually supination type) after experiencing one previously. Many are initiated during the initial trauma but are not rehabilitated with programs focused on the anterior talofibular ligament alone.	
Posterolateral glide of the talocalcaneal joint	• Posterolateral glide of the talocalcaneal joint is often part of the original supination sprain. • Without treatment after a supination ankle sprain, this dysfunction predisposes the ankle to supination. • As the functional joint that acts as the lower extremity's main "shock absorber" for accumulated impact loading, dysfunction increases forces transferred into the ankle.
Plantar flexion of the talus with anterior glide	• Plantar flexion of the talus with anterior glide also occurs during the typical supination ankle sprain. • This dysfunction places the narrow portion of the talus (which is wider anteriorly) into the wide part of the ankle mortis, which is not as stable as the dorsiflexed position. • Ankles in this less stable position are more likely to be resprained.

Continued

Table 4-15	Integrating Extremity Somatic Dysfunction and Symptoms—cont'd

SYMPTOM–SOMATIC DYSFUNCTION	DISCUSSION OF INTEGRATING OSTEOPATHIC DIFFERENTIAL DIAGNOSIS
Interosseous membrane strain	• Interosseous membrane strain if not corrected early in the sprain process (coupled with other somatic dysfunction and MTrPs in the leg) limits lymphatic drainage with the consequence that when the traumatic swelling is finally resorbed, the proteins from the edema fluid are left behind to create fibrotic change. • The resultant thickened tissues are more likely to be sprained again.
Posterior fibular head somatic dysfunction	• Posterior fibular head somatic dysfunction may occur as the anterior talofibular ligament pulls the distal fibula anteriorly. • This somatic dysfunction may cause pressure on the common peroneal nerve leading to weakness in dorsiflexion and positioning of the ankle in the less stable plantar flexed position. • Ankles in this less stable position are more likely to be resprained.
Somatic dysfunctions associated with footdrop causes	• See all of the footdrop causes above that place the ankle in the less stable position. • Additionally, the pain pattern of MTrPs in the peroneus brevis simulates the pain pattern of an ankle sprain.
Proprioceptive dysfunction	• One of the theories associated with recurrent ankle sprains blames inappropriate proprioception, which are known consequences of trigger point activity and muscle imbalance.

Patellar tracking dysfunction with chondromalacia patellae: A variety of somatic dysfunctions and/or biomechanical conditions may increase the Q angle at the knee and/or accentuate muscle imbalance in thigh muscles, each leading to tracking disorders of the patella and subsequent chondromalacia patellae.

Anteromedial glide at the talocalcaneal joint	• This somatic dysfunction predisposes to a **pronated/flat foot** that biomechanically will increase the Q angle from below. • A pronated foot predisposes to this talocalcaneal somatic dysfunction. • There may also be secondary dropped tarsal bones that in turn alter gait and magnify symptoms.
Abduction with medial glide of the tibia	• This dysfunction positions the knee as in **genu valgus.** • Genu valgus predisposes to abduction with media glide somatic dysfunction.
Internal rotation with posterior glide at the femoroacetabular joint	• This dysfunction positions the hip in the direction of coxa vara. • Coxa vara increases the Q angle from above.
MTrPs in the vastus medialis	• Trigger points in the vasti can cause the knee to buckle or give away spontaneously. • Tight hamstrings will reflexly accentuate the weakness in the vastus muscles.
Somatic dysfunction with segmental facilitation between T11 and L2	• Segmental facilitation may increase sympathetic tone to the lower extremity affecting the ability of the patella to repair cartilage subjected to wear and tear • Nociception from chondromalacia patellae and other somatic dysfunction in the lower extremity can increase segmental facilitation between T11 and L2

Carpal tunnel syndrome (CTS) with median entrapment neuropathy at the wrist: A number of systemic and biomechanical conditions predispose to compromise of the median nerve at this site with others that amplify the symptoms. There are hormonal, neurotrophic, congestive, ergonomic, and compressive causes of CTS with significant concomitant skeletal, arthrodial, and myofascial dysfunctions.

Cervical somatic dysfunction or other conditions	• Considered a contributing factor to the development or perpetuation of CTS; so-called "double-crush" phenomenon (neurotrophic basis)
Thoracic inlet and/or first rib somatic dysfunction	• Involvement of the first rib affects the scalene muscle; TrPs in the scalenes may cause entrapment of the lower trunk of the brachial plexus (neurotrophic basis), and the pain pattern classically shifts from median to ulnar side of the hand. • This dysfunction decreases lymphaticovenous drainage from the upper extremity (congestive basis).
Somatic dysfunction with segmental facilitation between T2 and T8	• This region represents the sympathetic supply to the upper extremity; somatic dysfunction may increase sympathetic tone and decrease blood flow to the region. • Felt to play a role in interactions associated with causalgia/reflex sympathetic dystrophy/complex regional pain syndromes of the upper extremity
Myofascial trigger points in the scalenes, pronator teres, wrist and finger flexors, and/or opponens pollicis	• Overlapping pain patterns; treatment of these TrPs has been shown to be effective in decreasing or eliminating CTS symptoms in mild-moderate CTS[3] • Stretching osteopathic manipulative therapy /exercise has been shown to physically open the carpal tunnel.[4]

[1]Kuchera ML, Kuchera WA. Lower extremities. In: Ward RC, ed. *Foundations for Osteopathic Medicine.* Baltimore, MD: Williams & Wilkins; 1997:969-977.
[2]Kuchera WA, Kuchera ML. *Osteopathic Considerations in Systemic Dysfunction.* 2nd ed., 2nd rev. Columbus, OH: Greyden Press; 1994.
[3] Foley M, Silverstein B, Polissar N. The economic burden of carpal tunnel syndrome: Long-term earnings of CTS claimants in Washington State. *Am J of Industrial Medicine.* 2007;10:1002.
[4]Sucher BM, Hinrichs RN. Manipulative treatment of carpal tunnel syndrome: biomechanical and osteopathic intervention to increase the length of the transverse carpal ligament. *J Am Osteopath Assoc.* 1998;98:679-686.

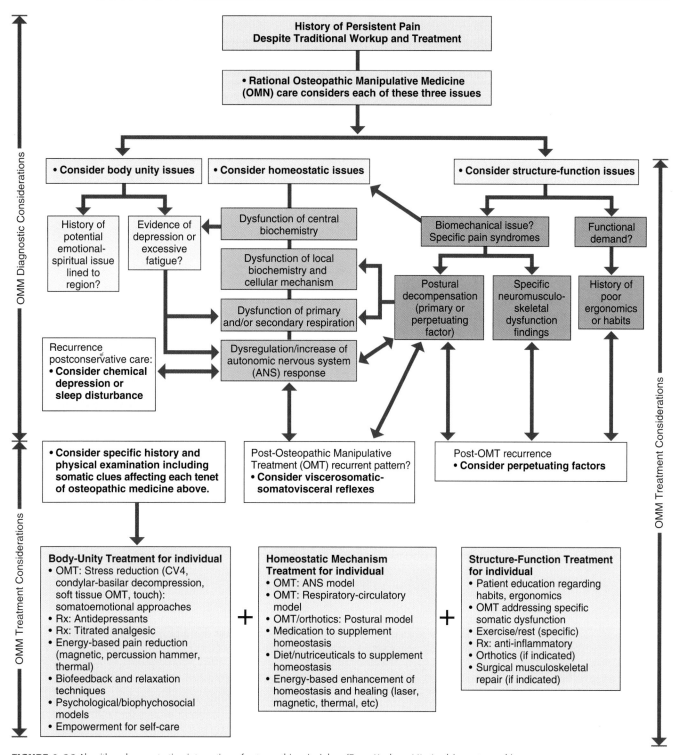

FIGURE 4–26 Algorithm demonstrating integration of osteopathic principles. (From Kuchera ML. Applying osteopathic principles to formulate treatment for patients with chronic pain. *J Am Osteop Assoc.* 2007;107:ES28–ES38.)

and other practitioners to discern the difference between an American doctor of osteopathy and an American medical doctor.

The Osteopathic Manipulative Prescription

The *osteopathic manipulative prescription (OMP)*[63] is best directed by an osteopathic practitioner working toward definitive goals. To do this properly, a working diagnosis derived from the previously discussed historic, physical, and palpatory findings is

essential. Common OMP-related questions and clinical experiences are outlined in Table 4-16.

The Osteopathic Manipulative Medicine Spectrum: Taxonomy, Indications, Contraindications, and Exemplars

The taxonomy involved in osteopathic manipulative treatments is based on the direction(s) used in positioning or

Table 4–16	Clinical Experiences Modifying Musculoskeletal Medicine Manipulative Treatment

QUESTION/OPTION	CLINICAL EXPERIENCE (GENERALITIES AND GUIDELINES ONLY)
Selection of direct or indirect method	• Indirect or direct techniques are of no value to a physician who lacks the skill to use that technique.[1] • Indirect techniques may be especially helpful in somatic dysfunction manifesting acute, edematous tissue texture changes. • Direct techniques may be especially helpful in somatic dysfunction with chronic changes such as fibrosis.
How much force should be used in a high-velocity low-amplitude **(HVLA) thrust?**	"Enough to affect a physiologic response (increased joint mobility, produce a vasomotor flush, produce palpable circulatory changes in periarticular tissues, and/or provide pain relief) but not enough to overwhelm the patient."[2]
Parameters modifying dose or frequency in OMM.[1]	• The sicker the patient, the less the dose. • Pediatric patients can be treated more frequently. • Geriatric patients require a longer interval between treatments to respond. • Acute cases should have a shorter interval between treatments initially.
General guidelines for treatment order based upon regional effects?	• In the chest cage, generally treat somatic dysfunction in this order: thoracic vertebrae, ribs, sternum. • In the pelvis, generally treat nonphysiologic somatic dysfunctions (shears) before other dysfunctions. • For very acute somatic dysfunction, it may be necessary to treat secondary or peripheral areas first to allow access to the acute site. • In lymphatic goals, open fascial drainage pathways before enhancing the effects of diaphragmatic or augmented lymphatic pumps; local effleurage or other local tissue drainage is best done after other lymphatic techniques designed to achieve tissue drainage.
What side effects alert the clinician to modify the OMM?	• If the patient reports a flare-up of discomfort for more than 24 hours, modify the dosage, choice of activating method, and/or duration of treatment as needed. • In set-up and activating phases, it is best to avoid certain positions that aggravate otherwise intermittent radiculopathic signs (cervical or lumbar spine) in patients with spinal degenerative joint disease (DJD) or herniated nucleus pulposus. • Care must be paramount if HVLA is selected in a patient suspected to harbor significant osteoporosis; often forward-bending pressures should be avoided as well.
Guidelines: How long to treat?	• Caring, compassionate novices often err on the side of overdosage. • Chronic conditions usually require chronic treatment; one rule of thumb suggests that it may take as many treatment sessions as years of dysfunction.
Risk-to-benefit issues	• An appropriate assessment and diagnostic examination before, during, and after OMM permits accurate risk-to-benefit decision making regarding indications, relative contraindications, and absolute contraindications. • Manipulative treatment is among the safest treatments that a physician can administer (serious adverse response report 1:400,000 to 1:1,000,000).[3]

[1]Kappler RE, Kuchera WA. Diagnosis and plan for manual treatment: a prescription. In: Ward RC, ed. *Foundations for Osteopathic Medicine*. 2nd ed. Baltimore, MD: Lippincott, Williams & Wilkins; 2002:574-579.

[2]Kimberly P. Forming a prescription for osteopathic manipulative treatment. *J Am Osteopath Assoc.* 1980;79:512.

[3]Kuchera ML, DiGiovanna EL, Greenman PE. Efficacy and complications. In: Ward RC, ed. *Foundations for Osteopathic Medicine*. 2nd ed. Baltimore, MD: Lippincott, Williams & Wilkins; 2002: 1143-1152.

carrying out the technique, the force and speed employed, and the proposed underlying mechanism of action or the intent of the practitioner (Table 4-17).

Often the therapeutic goal of OMT is to remove somatic dysfunction or a portion of the somatic dysfunction complex, such as pain. On occasion, the goal may be to enhance homeostasis with a technique such as lymphatic pump or rib-raising OMT. In many cases the clinical goal may be accomplished by a number of methods or activating forces; however, the choice of which OMT technique to use or the order in which a series of techniques should be applied may need to be varied to fit the clinical situation.

Osteopathic techniques are classified as either "direct" or "indirect." In *direct method techniques*, the setup engages the somatic dysfunction barrier and an activating force is applied that moves through the barrier to reestablish motion. In *indirect method techniques*, the setup requires moving away from the barrier to a specific site ('balance point') where various physiologic or inherent mechanisms cause the somatic dysfunction barrier to dissipate.

Table 4-17	Spectrum of Osteopathic Technique

Osteopathic manipulative medicine (OMM): The application of osteopathic philosophy, structural diagnosis, and use of OMT in the diagnosis and management of the patient.

Osteopathic manipulative therapy (OMTh): The therapeutic application of manually guided forces by an osteopath (nonphysician) to improve physiological function and homeostasis that has been altered by somatic dysfunction.

Osteopathic manipulative treatment (OMT): The therapeutic application of manually guided forces by an osteopathic physician (US Usage) to improve physiologic function and/or support homeostasis That has been altered by somatic dysfunction.

OMM, OMTh, and OMT all employ a variety of techniques including the following:

TECHNIQUE AS RELATED TO OMT	DEFINITION[1]
Active method	Technique in which the person voluntarily performs an osteopathic practitioner-directed motion
Articulatory treatment, (archaic); **articulatory treatment system (ART)**	A low-velocity/moderate- to high-amplitude technique in which a joint is carried through its full motion with the therapeutic goal of increased range of movement. The activating force is either a repetitive springing motion or repetitive concentric movement of the joint through the restrictive barrier.
Balanced ligamentous tension (BLT)	1. According to Sutherland's model, all the joints in the body are balanced ligamentous articular mechanisms. The ligaments provide proprioceptive information that guides the muscle response for positioning the joint, and the ligaments themselves guide the motion of the articular components.[1] First described in "Osteopathic Technique of William G. Sutherland," which was published in the *1949 Year Book of Academy of Applied Osteopathy.* See also *ligamentous articular strain.*
Chapman reflex[2,3]	1. A system of reflex points that present as predictable anterior and posterior fascial tissue texture abnormalities (plaque-like changes or stringiness of the involved tissues) assumed to be reflections of visceral dysfunction or pathology. 2. Originally used by Frank Chapman, DO, and described by Charles Owens, DO.
Combined method **Combined treatment** (archaic).	1. A treatment strategy in which the initial movements are indirect; as the technique is completed, the movements change to direct forces. 2. A manipulative sequence involving two or more different osteopathic manipulative treatment systems (e.g., Spencer technique combined with muscle energy technique). 3. A concept described by Paul Kimberly, DO.
Compression of the fourth ventricle (CV-4)	A cranial technique in which the lateral angles of the occipital squama are manually approximated, slightly exaggerating the posterior convexity of the occiput and taking the cranium into sustained extension.
Counterstrain (CS)	1. A system of diagnosis and treatment that considers the dysfunction to be a continuing, inappropriate strain reflex, which is inhibited by applying a position of mild strain in the direction exactly opposite to that of the reflex. This is accomplished by specific directed positioning about the point of tenderness to achieve the desired therapeutic response. 2. Australian and French use: Jones technique, (correction spontaneous by position), spontaneous release by position. 3. Developed by Lawrence Jones, DO.
Cranial treatment (CR)	See *osteopathy in the cranial field.*
CV-4	Abbreviation for compression of the fourth ventricle. See *osteopathic manipulative treatment, compression of the fourth ventricle.*
Dalrymple treatment	See *pedal pump.*
Direct method (D/DIR)	An osteopathic treatment strategy by which the restrictive barrier is engaged and a final activating force is applied to correct somatic dysfunction.
Exaggeration method	An osteopathic treatment strategy by which the dysfunctional component is carried away from the restrictive barrier and beyond the range of voluntary motion to a point of palpably increased tension.
Exaggeration technique	An indirect procedure that involves carrying the dysfunctional part away from the restrictive barrier, then applying a high-velocity/low-amplitude force in the same direction.
Facilitated oscillatory release technique (FOR)	1. A technique intended to normalize neuromuscular function by applying a manual oscillatory force, which may be combined with any other ligamentous or myofascial technique. 2. A refinement of a long-standing use of oscillatory force in osteopathic diagnosis and treatment as published in early osteopathic literature. 3. A technique developed by Zachary Comeaux, DO.
Facilitated positional release (FPR)	A system of indirect myofascial release treatment. The component region of the body is placed into a neutral position, diminishing tissue and joint tension in all planes, and an activating force (compression or torsion) is added. 2. A technique developed by Stanley Schiowitz, DO.

Continued

Table 4-17	Spectrum of Osteopathic Technique—cont'd

TECHNIQUE AS RELATED TO OMT	DEFINITION[1]
Fascial release	See *myofascial release*.
Fascial unwinding	A manual technique involving constant feedback to the osteopathic practitioner who is passively moving a portion of the patient's body in response to the sensation of movement. Its forces are localized using the sensations of ease and bind over wider regions.
Functional method	An indirect treatment approach that involves finding the dynamic balance point and one of the following: applying an indirect guiding force, holding the position or adding compression to exaggerate position and allow for spontaneous readjustment. The osteopathic practitioner guides the manipulative procedure while the dysfunctional area is being palpated to obtain a continuous feedback of the physiologic response to induced motion. The osteopathic practitioner guides the dysfunctional part so as to create a decreasing sense of tissue resistance (increased compliance).
Galbreath treatment[4,5]	See *mandibular drainage technique*.
Hepatic pump	Rhythmic compression applied over the liver for purposes of increasing blood flow through the liver and enhancing bile and lymphatic drainage from the liver.
High-velocity, low-amplitude technique (HVLA)	An osteopathic technique employing a rapid, therapeutic force of brief duration that travels a short distance within the anatomical range of motion of a joint and that engages the restrictive barrier in one or more planes of motion to elicit release of restriction. Also known as thrust technique.
Hoover technique	1. A form of functional method. 2. Developed by H.V. Hoover, DO. See also *osteopathic manipulative treatment, functional method*.
Indirect method (I/IND)	A manipulative technique in which the restrictive barrier is disengaged and the dysfunctional body part is moved away from the restrictive barrier until tissue tension is equal in one or all planes and directions.
Inhibitory pressure technique	The application of steady pressure to soft tissues to reduce reflex activity and produce relaxation.
Integrated neuromusculoskeletal release (INR)	A treatment system in which combined procedures are designed to stretch and reflexly release patterned soft tissue and joint-related restrictions. Both direct and indirect methods are used interactively.
Jones technique	See *counterstrain*.
Ligamentous articular strain technique (LAS)	1. A manipulative technique in which the goal of treatment is to balance the tension in opposing ligaments where there is abnormal tension present. 2. A set of myofascial release techniques described by Howard Lippincott, DO, and Rebecca Lippincott, DO. 3. Title of reference work by Conrad Speece, DO, and William Thomas Crow, DO.
Liver pump	See *hepatic pump*.
Lymphatic pump	1. A term used to describe the impact of intrathoracic pressure changes on lymphatic flow. This was the name originally given to the thoracic pump technique before the more extensive physiologic effects of the technique were recognized. 2. A term coined by C. Earl Miller, DO.
Lymphatic treatment	Techniques used to optimize function of the lymphatic system. See *lymphatic pump*. See also *pedal pump* and *thoracic pump*.
Mandibular drainage technique	Soft tissue manipulative technique using passively induced jaw motion to effect increased drainage of middle ear structures via the eustachian tube and lymphatics.
Mesenteric release technique (mesenteric lift)	Technique in which tension is taken off the attachment of the root of the mesentery to the posterior body wall. Simultaneously, the abdominal contents are compressed to enhance venous and lymphatic drainage from the bowel.
Muscle energy technique	1. A system of diagnosis and treatment in which the patient voluntarily moves the body as specifically directed by the osteopathic practitioner. This directed patient action is from a precisely controlled position against a defined resistance by the osteopathic practitioner. 2. Refers to a concept first used by Fred L. Mitchell, Sr, DO, originally called muscle energy treatment. See also *postisometric relaxation* and *reciprocal inhibition*.
Myofascial release (MFR)	A system of diagnosis and treatment first described by Andrew Taylor Still and his early students that engages continual palpatory feedback to achieve release of myofascial tissues. • **direct MFR,** a myofascial tissue restrictive barrier is engaged for the myofascial tissues and the tissue is loaded with a constant force until tissue release occurs • **indirect MFR,** the dysfunctional tissues are guided along the path of least resistance until free movement is achieved

Table 4-17	Spectrum of Osteopathic Technique—cont'd

TECHNIQUE AS RELATED TO OMT	DEFINITION[1]
Myofascial technique	Any technique directed at the muscles and fascia. See also *osteopathic manipulative treatment, myofascial release.* See also *soft tissue technique.*
Myotension	A system of diagnosis and treatment that uses muscular contractions and relaxations under resistance of the osteopathic practitioner to relax, strengthen or stretch muscles, or mobilize joints.
Osteopathy in the cranial field (OCF)	1. A system of diagnosis and treatment by an osteopathic practitioner using the primary respiratory mechanism and balanced membranous tension. 2. Refers to the system of diagnosis and treatment first described by William G. Sutherland, DO. 3. Title of reference work by Harold Magoun, Sr, DO.
Passive method	Based on techniques in which the patient refrains from voluntary muscle contraction.
Pedal pump	A venous and lymphatic drainage technique applied through the lower extremities; also called the pedal fascial pump or Dalrymple treatment.
Percussion vibrator technique	1. A manipulative technique involving the specific application of mechanical vibratory force to treat somatic dysfunction. 2. An osteopathic manipulative technique developed by Robert Fulford, DO.
Positional technique	A direct segmental technique in which a combination of leverage, patient ventilatory movements, and a fulcrum are used to achieve mobilization of the dysfunctional segment. May be combined with springing or thrust technique.
Postisometric relaxation (PIR)	See *muscle energy technique.* Immediately following an isometric contraction, the neuromuscular apparatus is in a refractory state, during which enhanced passive stretching may be performed. The osteopathic practitioner may take up the myofascial slack during the relaxed refractory period.
Progressive inhibition of neuromuscular structures (PINS)	1. A system of diagnosis and treatment in which the osteopathic practitioner locates two related points and sequentially applies inhibitory pressure along a series of related points. 2. Developed by Dennis Dowling, DO.
Range-of-motion technique	Active or passive movement of a body part to its physiologic or anatomical limit in any or all planes of motion.
Reciprocal inhibition	See also *muscle energy technique.* The inhibition of antagonist muscles when the agonist is stimulated.
Soft tissue (ST)	A system of diagnosis and treatment directed toward tissues other than skeletal or arthrodial elements.
Soft tissue technique	A direct technique that usually involves lateral stretching, linear stretching, deep pressure, traction and/or separation of muscle origin and insertion while monitoring tissue response and motion changes by palpation. Also called myofascial treatment.
Spencer technique[6]	A series of direct manipulative procedures to prevent or decrease soft tissue restrictions about the shoulder. See also *articulatory treatment (ART)*
Splenic pump technique	Rhythmic compression applied over the spleen for the purpose of enhancing the patient's immune response. See also *lymphatic pump.*
Spontaneous release by positioning	See *counterstrain.*
Springing technique	A low-velocity/moderate-amplitude technique in which the restrictive barrier is engaged repeatedly to produce an increased freedom of motion. See also *articulatory treatment system.*
Still technique	1. Characterized as a specific nonrepetitive articulatory method that is indirect rather than direct. 2. A system of diagnosis and treatment attributed to A.T. Still. 3. A term coined by Richard Van Buskirk, DO, PhD.
Strain-counterstrain	1. An osteopathic system of diagnosis and indirect treatment in which the patient's somatic dysfunction, diagnosed by (an) associated myofascial tender point(s), is treated by using a passive position, resulting in spontaneous tissue release and at least 70% decrease in tenderness. 2. Developed by Lawrence H. Jones, DO, in 1955. See *counterstrain.*
Thoracic pump	1. A technique that consists of intermittent compression of the thoracic cage. 2. Developed by C. Earl Miller, DO
Thrust technique (HVLA)	See *high-velocity/low-amplitude technique (HVLA).*

Continued

Table 4-17	Spectrum of Osteopathic Technique—cont'd

TECHNIQUE AS RELATED TO OMT	**DEFINITION[1]**
Toggle technique	Short lever technique using compression and shearing forces.
Traction technique	A procedure of high or low amplitude in which the parts are stretched or separated along a longitudinal axis with continuous or intermittent force.
v-spread	Technique using forces transmitted across the diameter of the skull to accomplish sutural gapping.
Ventral techniques	See *visceral manipulation.*
Visceral manipulation (VIS)	A system of diagnosis and treatment directed to the viscera to improve physiologic function. Typically, the viscera are moved toward their fascial attachments to a point of fascial balance. Also called ventral techniques.

[1]Education Council on Osteopathic Principles. Glossary of osteopathic terminology. In: Ward RC, ed. *Foundations for Osteopathic Medicine.* 2nd ed. Baltimore, MD: Lippincott, Williams & Wilkins; 2002:881-907.

[2] Owens C. *An Endocrine Interpretation of Chapman's Reflexes* (reprint). Indianapolis, IN: American Academy of Osteopathy; 1963.

[3]Lippincott R. Chapman's reflexes. *The Osteopathic Profession.* 1946;May:18-22.

[4]Galbreath WO. Acute otitis media, including its postural and manipulative treatment. *J Am Osteopath Assoc.* 1929;28:377-379.

[5]Pratt-Herrington D. (2000) Galbreath technique: a manipulative treatment for otitis media revisited. *J Am Osteopath Assoc.* 2000;100:635-639.

[6]Knebl JA, Shores JH, Gamber RG, Gray WT, Herron KM. Improving functional ability in the elderly via the Spencer technique, an osteopathic manipulative treatment: a randomized, controlled trial. *J Am Osteopath Assoc.* 2002;102:387-396. www.jaoa.org/cgi/reprint/102/7/387. Accessed December 3, 2013.

The **exaggeration method** is essentially an exaggerated indirect method wherein the setup moves in the direction of freedom, past the balance point, to the normal physiologic barrier opposite the motion loss barrier. At this point, an activating force is applied. This method was used more commonly in the early years of the osteopathic profession than it is now, although this is often the first step in the reemerging *Still technique* sequence.[7]

Physiological response method techniques depend upon careful patient positioning and movement to obtain a therapeutic result by creating conditions in which tissues must move in certain physiologically predetermined directions. The lumbosacral junction, for example, may be positioned in the sagittal and coronal planes to limit physiologic motion of the sacrum to a single desired rotatory response. Motion induced actively or passively would then cause the sacrum to move in the specific direction needed to restore its normal motion characteristics.

It is not uncommon for multiple techniques to be used during the course of a single manipulative session. For example, the technique may start with a direct method technique, whereupon the regional soft tissues are moved to maintain the indirect balance point. This form of *myofascial release (MFR)* (see Chapter 14), which is also referred to as "myofascial unwinding" because of its appearance, best fits a *combined method technique* classification. These methods are summarized in Box 4-6.

Once a method is selected, there are a number of possible activating forces that may be employed. Activating forces[25] may include the following: **high-velocity low-amplitude (HVLA)** or thrust[64]; **low-velocity, moderate-amplitude (LVMA,** springing or articulation)[65]; various applications of patient-assisted **muscle energy techniques (MET)** (especially postisometric relaxation, reciprocal inhibition, or rapid rhythmic resistive

Box 4-6 TYPES OF OSTEOPATHIC TECHNIQUES

- *Direct method techniques*: Set-up engages the barrier, and an activating force is applied that moves through the barrier to reestablish motion.
- *Indirect method techniques*: Set-up requires moving away from the barrier to a specific site (balance point), where various physiologic mechanisms cause the barrier to dissipate.
- *Exaggeration method techniques:* Set-up moves in the direction of freedom, past the balance point, to the normal physiologic barrier opposite the motion loss, at which point an activating force is applied.
- *Physiological response method techniques:* Technique depends upon careful patient positioning and movement designed to create conditions in which tissues move in certain physiologically predetermined directions.

duction)[66]; **respiratory cooperation or force** (inhalation causing spinal curves to straighten and extremities to externally rotate; exhalation causing spinal curves to accentuate and extremities to internally rotate); **inherent forces** or the body's tendency toward balance and homeostasis; **patient cooperative reflex activities** (including eye movements and activation of other specific muscles in specific directions and/or at a specific time). These methods are summarized in Box 4-7.

Pairing a method and an activating force creates a technique; grouping such techniques has resulted in an extensive osteopathic treatment armamentarium (Table 4-18). An understanding of the osteopathic nomenclature found in the *"Glossary of Osteopathic Terminology"*[25] is useful in negotiating the evidence-based literature.

Box 4-7 TYPES OF OSTEOPATHIC ACTIVATING FORCES

- *High-velocity low-amplitude (HVLA):* Thrust
- *Low-velocity moderate-amplitude (LVMA):* Springing or articulation
- *Muscle energy techniques (MET):* Postisometric relaxation, reciprocal inhibition, or rapid rhythmic resistive duction
- *Respiratory cooperation or force:* Inhalation causing spinal curves to straighten and extremities to externally rotate; exhalation causing spinal curves to accentuate and extremities to internally rotate
- *Inherent forces*: Body's tendency toward balance and homeostasis
- *Patient cooperative reflex activities*: Eye movements and activation of other specific muscles in specific directions and/or at a specific time

Examples of Documented Clinical Osteopathic Manipulative Medicine Outcomes

OMM is integrated for the purpose of *physicians treating people, not just symptoms*, a trait that the ***American Osteopathic Association*** emphasizes heavily. Most modern research designs emphasize measurements and outcomes in treating a disease or a symptom. As in physical therapy, this research emphasis makes it difficult to design studies for the osteopathic profession where "seeking health" through addressing individualized treatment is based upon unique host factors (see Chapter 3).

DIFFERENTIATING CHARACTERISTICS
Semantic Distinction

"Manipulation" is a generic word that in medicine historically denotes the use of "therapeutic application of manual force."[2] **Manipulative treatment,** in contradistinction to **manual therapy,** is one attempt to make a semantic distinction between physician-applied "treatment" rather than a therapist-applied technique. As described in Chapter 2, in some circles, "manipulation" is specifically reserved as a term for high-velocity thrust techniques, but in other circles it remains a generic term for all forms of hands-on therapeutic interventions. The chiropractic profession refers to its manipulative techniques as "chiropractic adjustments," which are not to be confused with the manual medicine techniques performed by German physicians, known as *chiropraktiker*s, who incorporate *chiropraxis*.

Osteopathic physicians in the United States employing OMT attempted, through specific nomenclature, to convey that guiding osteopathic principles and practices (OPP) with subsequent therapeutic goals were an integral part of the manual techniques they deliver. The difference between a physical therapist applying a counterstrain technique and an osteopathic physician performing OMT using that same counterstrain technique lay in the physician-level differential diagnosis that may include diagnosis of disease and pathology.

In the United States, differences in the delivery of manual techniques by practitioners with different professional education and degrees also extend to the coding arena. Thus, different billing codes are found in the *CPT* literature to differentiate OMT performed by physicians (MD or DO) from adjustments performed by chiropractors or OMPT by physical therapists.

Naming of Treatments and Osteopathic Practitioners (U.S. and International)

In the United States, the practice of osteopathy, osteopathic medicine, and/or osteopathic surgery is limited to osteopathic physicians and surgeons who have graduated from a college of osteopathic medicine accredited by the ***American Osteopathic Association***. The American DO degree represents the synonymous designation "doctor of osteopathy" or "doctor of osteopathic medicine." No other credential or school is accepted for this practice in any state, and by law, no one but a U.S.-trained and graduated doctor of osteopathy can legally advertise that they have an "osteopathic" practice (even if they have attained the full knowledge base and apply both the osteopathic philosophy and approach).

Table 4–18	Osteopathic Terminology Compared to Terminology Used in Other Discplines	
OSTEOPATHIC NAME	**EQUIVALENT OR NOT**	**NAME IN ANOTHER PROFESSION**
OMT = Osteopathic manipulative treatment	Not	OMT = Orthopedic manual therapy
Osteopathic medicine	Not	Manual medicine
Counterstrain	Same	Strain-Counterstrain; fold & hold
High-velocity, low-amplitude (HVLA)	Same	Thrust; mobilization with impulse
Osteopathy in the cranial field	Varies	Craniosacral Therapy
Manipulation (USA)	Not always	Manipulation (Europe)
DO (USA) = Doctor of osteopathy equivalent to DO (USA) = Doctor of osteopathic medicine	Not	DO (International) = Diplomat of osteopathy

The U.S. schools of osteopathic medicine integrate the osteopathic perspective and core skills for the palpation and treatment of somatic dysfunction throughout the predoctoral education of all physicians in training, regardless of their eventual specialty. Osteopathic principles and practices education continues with pertinent core principles and training in residency and recertification training.

Internationally, physicians wishing to practice in an osteopathic manner may first obtain core postgraduate training in manual medicine skills and then add OPP skills to an evolving perspective gained through reading and professional interactions with osteopathic colleagues. In a limited number of countries, such manual/musculoskeletal medicine physicians (MD) may formally study and adopt the osteopathic approach through a formalized college degree program (United Kingdom) or in extensive, formalized postgraduate educational modules (Germany). Furthermore, evidence-based osteopathic elements have also been integrated into a variety of physician-specialty algorithms for the care of musculoskeletal disorders by those practicing disciplines such as physical medicine and rehabilitation, musculoskeletal medicine, or orthopaedic medicine.

Internationally trained physicians (MD) who study manual medicine may or may not be exposed in their studies to the osteopathic approach. In many countries outside the United States, nonphysicians who study the osteopathic philosophy and manual techniques may be granted a non-U.S. D.O. degree, with the designation "diplomat of osteopathy." Use of the same letters for "doctor" and "diplomat" has been a source of confusion to the public and legislators alike. This is especially true in Canada, where osteopathic practitioners trained in both U.S. or non-U.S. systems coexist. The variability in education and naming prompted the formation of an *Osteopathic International Alliance* and a consultation with the *World Health Organization* to publish a consensus document on these issues.

The Role of Osteopathic Manipulative Medicine in Osteopathic Medicine Today

The osteopathic technique examples in this chapter illustrate how to correctly apply general principles to correct single somatic dysfunctions palpated and deemed clinically relevant. These and other manual techniques can be integrated and used as valuable adjunctive tools in the complete management of patients with a wide variety of complaints. They have been shown to be capable of playing a role in reducing pain and improving function within the neuromusculoskeletal system as well as in supporting certain self-healing mechanisms.

An integrated osteopathic treatment regimen is most commonly prescribed within the context of its risk-to-benefit therapeutic ratio. It is deemed to be adjunctive or primary to the care of the patient (or even contraindicated) by physicians who have undertaken additional hours learning palpatory diagnosis and can make this determination based upon the entirety of the clinical context, the host factors involved, and the range of approaches available. Such extensive training also extends to skills needed to safely and effectively administer manual techniques and integrated regimens to remove somatic dysfunction.

The form that the treatment protocol may take, the goals selected, and the choice of techniques used to accomplish those goals are part of the science, philosophy, and art of the attending physician and the clinical specialty context in which he or she is practicing. For the osteopathic approach, the osteopathic philosophy is, by definition, a requisite and central component, whereas the use of osteopathic manipulative treatment is the most outward and visible sign of its application.

CLINICAL CASE

History of Present Illness

A 45-year old farm-hand presented to the clinic with the chief complaint of chronic back pain for 3 years. He reported that the pain was deep, nagging, and constant on the right side, with periods of acute exacerbation into the right hip, groin, and down the back of the leg to just above the knee. Full symptoms would occur with prolonged walking or standing and would last several weeks; he was unable to lift more than 25 pounds without aggravating symptoms. His back took several hours to relax fully after lying down even on "good" days.

Pain onset had occurred while carrying a small bale of hay in front of his body. He had stepped in an unseen pothole, stumbled, and fell. The next day he noted full-blown symptoms that lasted several months. Between and during episodes, he had only partial relief with 800 mg of ibuprofen; attempts at physical therapy had reportedly aggravated his constant nagging pain.

Over the next 3 years, he saw several physicians because of three to four significant recurrences of the pain radiation per year. Negative electromyographic, radiographic, and magnetic resonance imaging studies, coupled with negative reflex changes and nonspecific, nonradicular pattern of weakness upon muscle testing over this period left him without a specific diagnosis. He was unable to work on the farm and stated that he had the impression that doctors thought he was "malingering" or lazy. He became increasingly depressed, which placed a strain on his relationships.

Past Medical History, Social History

The patient denied smoking or illicit drug use. A review of his nonmusculoskeletal systems was noncontributory.

Structural Observation

Findings revealed a slim white male. Somatic dysfunction included reduced lumbar lordosis.

Neurological Assessment

Deep tendon reflexes, pathologic reflexes, straight leg-raising test, Lloyd's kidney punch, and Chapman's reflex screen were negative.

Mobility Testing

Flexion tests and iliac crest heights suggested a possible "short leg syndrome." The common compensatory pattern of Zink[67] was violated by the lumbopelvic junction, and the pelvic floor was tight.

Special Tests

There was a questionable result from the right Trendelenburg test.

Palpation

Upon palpation, a left iliacus tender point, tenderness over the right iliolumbar and posterior sacroiliac ligaments, right sacral shear, as well as tenderness and hypertonicity over the right piriformis was identified.

Intervention

Treatment consisted of springing technique to the right sacral shear, counterstrain to the iliacus and piriformis tender points, and indirect balanced ligamentous tension to articular regions from the thoracolumbar to sacral regions. The fascial patterns were treated with HVLA toward symmetry, and both abdominal and pelvic diaphragms were treated with indirect and direct myofascial release respectively. Post-OMT iliac crest heights and flexion tests were normal. He left with instructions to drink lots of fluid, switch to acetaminophen as needed, avoid jumping or lifting until his next visit, and to return in 1 week for follow-up.

Upon return, he noted that both acute and nagging pains were relieved for nearly 4 days, but thereafter his nagging pain had recurred mildly. A recurrence of the sacral shear (approximately 40% of original) and piriformis muscle dysfunctions were noted and retreated with OMT. Two weeks later, he returned with no symptoms and no recurrence of pain. He was told to make an appointment for 1 month, but to cancel if he remained symptom-free. He called 1 month later, without pain and able to function completely at home.

1. Why is it important to include a combination of both articular and myofascial interventions for the treatment of a patient such as this? For this patient, which collection of techniques would you use first, myofascial soft tissue techniques or techniques designed to enhance articular mobility?

2. Describe the sacral shear syndrome. Briefly discuss its etiology, clinical presentation, and OMT management techniques.

Using the descriptions and figures of techniques found in this chapter, perform the techniques that were used in the care of this patient on your partner.

HANDS-ON

Perform the following activities in lab with partner.

1 Perform general palpatory diagnosis procedures of the thoracolumbar paravertebral soft tissues and osseous structures in an attempt to identify the following features:
a. Sensitivity (tenderness)
b. Tissue texture change
c. Asymmetry
d. Restriction/alteration in range of motion

2 Perform specific palpatory diagnosis procedures of both the osseous and soft tissue structures of the following regions:
a. Ankle
b. Sacrum
c. Midthoracic vertebral unit
d. Typical cervical vertebral unit
e. Occipitomastoid suture

3 Perform the following osteopathic manipulative treatment techniques on your partner:
a. Direct method: Postisometric relaxation muscle energy activating force incorporating the oculocervicogenic reflex (e.g., occipitoatlantal joint)
b. Direct method: High-velocity low-amplitude activating force (e.g., lumbar vertebral unit)
c. Direct method: Soft tissue-activating forces with or without inhibition, stretching-kneading, and direct myofascial release (e.g., quadratus lumborum)
d. Combined method (Still technique): Articulatory activating force (e.g., radiocarpal joint)
e. Indirect method: Myofascial release inherent activating force with respiratory release enhancement maneuver (e.g., upper thoracic vertebral unit)
f. Indirect method: Balanced ligamentous tension inherent activating force (e.g., talocalcaneal joint)
g. Indirect method: Counterstrain technique (e.g., sternocleidomastoid points)

REFERENCES

1. Gevitz N. *The DOs: Osteopathic Medicine in America.* 2nd ed. Baltimore, MD: Johns Hopkins University Press; 2004.
2. Radcliffe C. *Diseases of the Spine and of the Nerves.* Philadelphia, PA: Henry C. Lea; 1871:58-70.
3. Gevitz N. *The DOs: Osteopathic Medicine in America.* Baltimore, MD: Johns Hopkins University Press; 1982.
4. Still AT. *Philosophy of Osteopathy.* Kirksville, MO: American Academy of Osteopathy; 1899:27-28.
5. Still AT. *Autobiography of Andrew T. Still, with a History of the Discovery and development of the Science of Osteopathy, Together with an Account of the Founding of the American School of Osteopathy.* Kirksville, MO: Author; 1897.
6. Still AT. *Osteopathy, Research and Practice.* Kirksville, MO: Journal Printing Co; 1910.
7. VanBuskirk R. *Applications of a Rediscovered Technique of Andrew Taylor Still.* 2nd ed. Indianapolis IN: American Academy of Osteopathy; 1999.
8. Smith W. Skiagraphy and the circulation. *J Osteopathy.* 1899;3:356-378.
9. Denslow JS, Hassett CC. The central excitatory state associated with postural abnormalities. *J Neurophysiol.* 1942;5:393-402.
10. Peterson B, ed. *The Collected Papers of Irvin M. Korr.* Colorado Springs, CO: Academy of Osteopathy; 1979.
11. Denslow JS, Korr IM, Krems AD. Quantitative studies of chronic facilitation in human motoneuron pools. *Am J Physiol.* 1947;50:229-238.
12. Korr IM, ed. *The Neurobiological Mechanisms in Manipulative Therapy.* 3rd ed. New York, NY: Plenum Press; 1978.
13. Peterson B, ed. *Postural Balance and Imbalance. 1983 AAO Yearbook.* Newark, OH: American Academy of Osteopathy Press; 1983.
14. Dodd JG, Good MM, Nguyen TL, et al. In vitro biophysical strain model for understanding mechanisms of osteopathic manipulative treatment. *J Am Osteopath Assoc.* 2006;106:157-166.
15. Salamon E, Zhu W, Stefano GB. Nitric oxide as a possible mechanism for understanding the therapeutic effects of osteopathic manipulative medicine (review). *Int J Mol Cell Med.* 2004;14:443-449.
16. Kuchera WA, Kuchera ML. *Osteopathic Principles in Practice.* 2nd ed. Columbus, OH: Greyden Press; 1994.
17. Truhlar RE. *Doctor A.T. Still in the Living: His Concepts and Principles of Health and Disease.* Cleveland, OH: Author; 1950:123.
18. Still AT. *Philosophy of Osteopathy.* Colorado Springs, CO: American Academy of Osteopathy; 1977. http://www.interlinea.org/atstill/eBookPhilosophyofOsteopathy_V2.0.pdf. A
19. Special Committee on Osteopathic Principles and Osteopathic Technic, Kirksville College of Osteopathy and Surgery. Interpretation of the osteopathic concept prepared by committee at Kirksville. *J Osteopath.* 1953;60:7-10.
20. Vleeming A, Snijders CJ, Stoeckart R, Mens JMA. The role of the sacroiliac joints in coupling between spine, pelvis, legs and arms. In: Vleeming A, Mooney V, Snijders CJ, Dorman TA, Stoeckart R, eds. *Movement, Stability and Low Back Pain: The Essential Role of the Pelvis.* New York, NY: Churchill-Livingstone; 1997:53-71.
21. Education Council on Osteopathic Principles. Glossary of osteopathic terminology. In: Ward RC, ed. *Foundations for Osteopathic Medicine.* 2nd ed. Baltimore, MD: Lippincott, Williams & Wilkins; 2003.
22. World Health Organization. *International Classification of Diseases, 9th revision, Clinical Modification* (ICD-9-CM). 3rd ed. Geneva, Switzerland: World Health Organization; 1979.
23. Gilliar WG, Kuchera ML, Giulianetti DA. Neurologic basis of manual medicine. *Phys Med Rehabil Clin N Am.* 1996;7:693-714.
24. Sleszynski SL, Glonek T, Kuchera WA. Standardized medical record: a new outpatient osteopathic SOAP note form: validation of a standardized office form against physician's progress notes. *J Am Osteopath Assoc.* 1999;99(10):516-529.
25. Education Council on Osteopathic Principles. Glossary of osteopathic terminology. In: Ward RC, ed. *Foundations for Osteopathic Medicine.* 2nd ed. Baltimore, MD: Lippincott, Williams & Wilkins; 2002.
26. Mitchell F Jr. The training and measurement of sensory literacy in relation to osteopathic structural and palpatory diagnosis. *J Am Osteopath Assoc.* 1976;75:881.
27. Steele KM. Treatment of the acutely ill hospitalized patient. In: Ward RC, ed. *Foundations for Osteopathic Medicine.* Baltimore, MD: Williams & Wilkins; 1997:1037-1048.
28. Beal MC. Viscerosomatic reflexes: a review. *J Am Osteopath Assoc.* 1985;85:53-68.
29. Smith LA, ed. *An Atlas of Pain Patterns: Sites and Behavior of Pain in Certain Common Disease of the Upper Abdomen.* Springfield, IL: CC Thomas; 1961.

30. Patriquin DA. Viscerosomatic reflexes. In: Patterson MM, Howell JN, eds. *The Central Connection: Somatovisceral/Viscerosomatic Interaction. 1989 International Symposium.* Athens, OH: American Academy of Osteopathy; 1992;4-18.

31. Wyke BD. The neurologic basis of thoracic spinal pain. *Rheum Phys Med.* 1970;10:356.

32. Greenman PE. *Principles of Manual Medicine.* 2nd ed. Baltimore, MD: Williams & Wilkins; 1996:18-36.

33. Travell JG, Simons DG. *Myofascial Pain and Dysfunction: The Trigger Point Manual.* Vol. 2. Baltimore, MD: Williams & Wilkins; 1992.

34. Simons DG, Travell JG, Simons LS. *Travell and Simons' Myofascial Pain and Dysfunction: The Trigger Point Manual.* Vol. 1. *Upper Half of Body.* Baltimore, MD: Lippincott, Williams & Wilkins; 1999.

35. Jones L, Kusunose R, Goering E. *Jones' Strain–Counterstrain.* Jones Strain-Counterstrain. Philadelphia, PA: American Academy of Osteopathy; 1995.

36. Owens C. *An Endocrine Interpretation of Chapman's Reflexes* (reprint). Indianapolis, IN: American Academy of Osteopathy; 1963.

37. Fryette HH. Physiologic movements of the spine. *JAOA.* 1917;18:1-2.

38. Kuchera ML. Diagnosis and treatment of gravitational strain pathophysiology: research and clinical correlates (part I and II). In: Vleeming A, ed. *Low Back Pain: The Integrated Function of the Lumbar Spine and Sacroiliac Joints.* Proceedings of the 2nd Interdisciplinary World Congress, November 9-11, 1995: San Diego, CA: University of California; 1995:659-693.

39. Kuchera ML. Applying osteopathic principles to formulate treatment for patient with chronic pain. *J Am Osteop Assoc.* 2007;107:ES28-ES38.

40. Kappler RE. Cervical spine. In: Ward RC, ed. *Foundations for Osteopathic Medicine* Baltimore, MD: Williams & Wilkins ; 1997:541-546.

41. Jaeger B. Are "cervicogenic" headaches due to myofascial pain and cervical spine dysfunction? *Cephalalgia.* 1989;9(suppl 3):157-164.

42. Kapandji IA. *The Physiology of Joints.* New York, NY: Churchill-Livingstone; 1970.

43. Kelso AF. A double-blind clinical study of osteopathic findings in hospital patients–progress report. *J Am Osteopath Assoc.* 1971;70:570-592.

44. D'Alonzo GE, Krachman SL. Respiratory system. In: Ward RC, ed. *Foundations for Osteopathic Medicine.* Baltimore, MD: Williams & Wilkins; 1997:441-458.

45. Paterson JK, Burn L. *An Introduction to Medical Manipulation.* Lancaster, UK: MTP Press; 1985:77.

46. Maigne R. Manipulation of the spine. In: Basmajian JV, ed. *Manipulation, Traction and Massage.* 3rd ed. Baltimore, MD: Williams & Wilkins; 1985:99.

47. Olesen J. Classification and diagnostic criteria for headache disorders, cranial neuralgias and facial pain. *Cephalalgia.* 1988;8(suppl 7):1-96.

48. Upton AR, McComas AJ. The double crush in nerve entrapment syndromes. *Lancet.* 1973;ii:359-362.

49. Kuchera ML. Gravitational stress, musculoligamentous strain, and postural alignment. *Spine: State of the Art Review.* 1995;9:46-490.

50. Kuchera ML, Kuchera WA. Postural considerations in coronal and horizontal planes. In: Ward RC, ed. *Foundations for Osteopathic Medicine.* Baltimore, MD: Williams & Wilkins; 1997:983-997.

51. Good MG. Diagnosis and treatment of sciatic pain. *Lancet.* 1942;ii:597-598.

52. Lewit K. Muscular pattern in thoraco-lumbar lesions. *Manual Med.* 1986;2:105-107.

53. Kimberly P, Funk SF, eds. *Outline of Osteopathic Manipulative Procedures: The Kimberly Manual.* Millennium ed. Marceline, MO: Walsworth; 2000.

54. Fortin JD, Falco FJE. The Fortin finger test: an indicator of sacroiliac pain. *Am J Orthop.* 1997;24:477-480.

55. Strachan WF. A study of the mechanics of the sacroiliac joint. *J Am Osteopath Assoc.* 1938;43:576-578.

56. Walton WJ. Osteopathic diagnosis and technique. In: *Sacroiliac Diagnosis.* St. Louis, MO: Matthews Book Co;1966:187-197. (Reprinted in 1970 and distributed by the American Academy of Osteopathy, Indianapolis, IN.)

57. Mitchell FL. Structural pelvic function. In: 1965 *American Academy of Osteopathy Yearbook. Vol 2.* Indianapolis, IN: American Academy of Osteopathy; 1965.

58. Magoun HI. *Osteopathy in the Cranial Field.* Indianapolis, IN: The Cranial Academy; 1976.

59. Heinking KP, Kappler RE. Pelvis and sacrum. In: Ward RC, ed. *Foundations for Osteopathic Medicine.* 2nd ed. Baltimore, MD: Lippincott, Williams & Wilkins; 2002:762-783.

60. Heinking K, Jones J, Kappler R. Pelvis and sacrum In: Ward RC, *Foundations for Osteopathic Medicine.* Baltimore, MD: Williams & Wilkins; 1997.

61. World Health Organization. Benchmarks for Training in Traditional/Complementary and Alternative Medicine and Benchmarks for Training in Osteopathy. Geneva, Switzerland: WHO Press; 2010.

62. Carey TS, Motyka TM, Garrett JM, Keller RB. Do osteopathic physicians differ in patient interaction from allopathic physicians? An empirically derived approach. *JAOA.* 2003;103:313-318.

63. Kimberly PE. Formulating a prescription for osteopathic manipulative treatment. *J Am Osteopath Assoc.* 1980;79:506-513.

64. Kappler RE, Jones JM. Thrust (high-velocity/low-amplitude) techniques. In: Ward RC. *Foundations for Osteopathic Medicine.* 2nd ed. Baltimore, MD: Lippincott, Williams & Wilkins; 2002:852-880.

65. Patriquin DA, Jones JM. Articulatory techniques. In: Ward, RC. *Foundations for osteopathic medicine.* 2nd ed. Baltimore, MD: Lippincott, Williams & Wilkins; 2002:834-851.

66. Ehrenfeuchter WC, Sandhouse M. In: Ward RC. *Foundations for Osteopathic Medicine.* 2nd ed. Baltimore, MD: Lippincott, Williams & Wilkins ; 2002: 881-907.

67. Zink JG, Lawson WB. An osteopathic structural examination and functional interpretation of the soma. *Osteopathic Ann.* 1979;7:433-440.

The Cyriax Approach

Russell Woodman, PT, MS, DPT, FSOM, OCS, MCTA

Chapter Objectives

At the conclusion of this chapter, the reader will be able to:

- Cite the three primary intervention strategies used within the Cyriax approach to orthopaedic manual physical therapy.
- Identify when each intervention is most appropriate and provide rationale for the use of each.
- Understand the nature of referred pain and how symptoms can change based on which structure is compressed.
- Define the pressure phenomenon and the release phenomenon.
- List the questions believed to be pertinent during the subjective examination.
- List the major components of the objective examination.

- Define selective tissue tension (STT) testing and the three major components that comprise this testing.
- Describe the four possible responses to STT testing and the structure that each implicates.
- Define end-feel and identify the major end-feels as described by Cyriax.
- Define capsular (full articular) and noncapsular (partial articular) patterns and describe how each may be used in diagnosis.
- Describe the purpose and value of palpation during the examination.
- List the five questions that may be used to determine the specific soft tissue lesion at fault for the patient's symptoms.

HISTORICAL PERSPECTIVES

James Cyriax (1904–1985) was born in London, England, the son of Edgar and Annyuta Kellgren, who were both physicians. Cyriax qualified to practice medicine in 1928 after attending *University College School* in Gonville, *Caius College* in Cambridge, and *St. Thomas Medical College* in London. He commenced his practice at St. Thomas Hospital in 1929. Early in his career, Cyriax observed that orthopaedic surgical diagnosis was based almost entirely upon palpation and radiographic findings that often proved to be fairly accurate. Conversely, the diagnosis of soft tissue lesions appeared to present a greater challenge to the physician. Cyriax concluded that the discipline of orthopaedic medicine lacked a well-developed system for diagnosis of such disorders as **tendinosis, ligamentous sprains,** and **capsulitis.** Over the subsequent 12 years, Cyriax developed a system of examination and intervention that was designed to address nonsurgical, soft tissue lesions.

In his private practice on Wimpole Street in London, Cyriax collaborated with physical therapists in the development of this new approach. From its inception, a major component of this approach was the concept of **selective tissue tension (STT),** which is designed to aid in the identification of specific soft tissue lesions. Cyriax's intervention approach focused primarily on the use of three types of nonsurgical procedures. These intervention procedures are **manipulation (high-velocity thrust),** and **deep friction massage (DFM),** *traction,* and *injection.* Cyriax believed that most, if not all, musculoskeletal impairments could be effectively managed through the use of one, or a combination, of these three procedures.

NOTABLE QUOTABLE

"To be effective, treatment must be an appropriate countermeasure for the condition diagnosed, and this is as much a concern of the doctor as the physiotherapist . . . the relationship between physician and physiotherapist becomes complimentary. Between the two of them, nearly all patients can be dealt with on the spot."

James Cyriax

PHILOSOPHICAL FRAMEWORK

The Cyriax approach to orthopaedic manual physical therapy (OMPT) is based on the premise that all pain has a source. It is incumbent on the examiner to identify the source of pain and apply an intervention that will effectively treat the source.[1] The Cyriax Approach to OMPT is based on a theoretical framework that attempts to identify the locus of pathology through an appreciation of the nature and location of the patient's presenting symptoms. This framework leads to a conclusive pathoanatomical differential diagnosis that guides subsequent intervention. The primary tenets of the Cyriax approach will now be described.

Referred Pain

Cyriax asserted that referred pain may arise from a central disorder that will give rise to central or bilateral symptoms. **Central disorders** are defined as space-occupying lesions within the spinal canal (Fig. 5-1). Both tumors and disc lesions are examples of space-occupying lesions. Cyriax believed that the disc was the most common initiator of mechanical pain emanating from the spine. In addition, he believed that spinal ligaments and zygapophyseal joints (facet joints) may also serve as potential sources. Ombregt and colleagues[2] supported this belief by identifying that lesions of the supra- and interspinous ligaments have the potential to cause central low back pain, and the iliolumbar ligament may contribute to the onset of unilateral low back and groin pain. Dreyfuss et al[3] has described patterns of pain induced by the distention of the thoracic zygapophyseal joints. The zygapophyseal joint has also been shown to be a contributor to the onset of cervicogenic headaches (Fig. 5-2).[4]

QUESTIONS *for* REFLECTION

- What anatomical structures may be responsible for the referral of symptoms?
- How might the structure involved influence the nature of the patient's symptoms?
- How might the manual therapist differentiate between compression of the dural sheath, dura mater, spinal cord, nerve root, nerve trunk, and peripheral nerve?

Pain Is Referred Unilaterally and Does Not Cross Midline

Most frequently, individuals seen in physical therapy have unilateral pain. Although such symptoms may be the result of a spinal mechanical problem (Figs. 5-3 and 5-4), the examiner must rule out the possibility that the patient has an upper or lower extremity musculoskeletal lesion. Cyriax was among the first to formally recognize the fact that a lesion on one side of the body cannot refer pain across the midline to the contralateral side of the body. Therefore, the spine or the ipsilateral

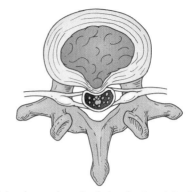

FIGURE 5–1 Lumbar nuclear disc lesion (prolapse) leading to a *central disorder*, which is compressing the dura mater resulting in central pain.

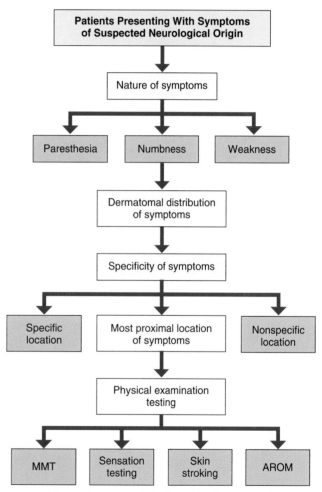

FIGURE 5–2 Algorithm for identifying the origin of neurological symptoms secondary to compression.

limb should be considered as the locus of pathology when treating a patient with unilateral symptoms.

Pain Is Referred Distally

When considering patterns of referred pain, it is important to note that symptoms generally migrate from a more proximal

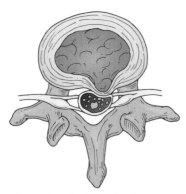

FIGURE 5–3 Lumbar nuclear disc lesion (prolapse) compressing the dura mater on the right, resulting in right-sided low back pain.

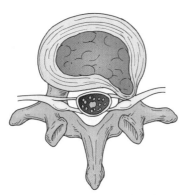

FIGURE 5–4 Lumbar nuclear posterior-lateral disc lesion (prolapse) compressing the dural sheath of the nerve root on the right, resulting in unilateral right leg pain.

to a more distal location. A soft tissue problem of the shoulder, for example, is more likely to refer pain distally into the arm than proximally toward the neck. Therefore, if a patient complains of pain in the shoulder, the examiner must clear the neck and shoulder as the potential source of the symptoms.

The segment to which most tissues refer pain is based on its embryological derivation. Cyriax articulated this theory in great detail.[5] Figure 5-5 illustrates a 4-week-old embryo. The embryo's limbs develop from its **mesodermic somites.** The shoulder joint capsule and skin covering the lateral aspect of the shoulder and extending to the radial styloid of the wrist develop from the fifth cervical segment. The greater the insult, the more distally the pain can be referred.

The Dura Mater Refers Pain Extrasegmentally

The only tissue that is believed to refer pain in a manner that is not based on its embryological derivation is the *dura mater.* The dura mater is capable of referring pain into more than one dermatomal distribution. Therefore, it is said that the dura mater refers pain **extrasegmentally**. One explanation for this phenomenon is the extensive overlap of consecutive sinuvertebral nerves innervating the anterior aspect of the dura mater.[2] A cervical disc lesion that protrudes posteriorly, for example, may compress the anterior aspect of the dura mater, producing pain that is referred to the head, laterally to the shoulder, and caudally as far as the inferior angle of the

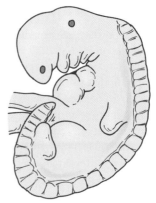

FIGURE 5–5 A 4 week-old human embryo. The embryo's limbs develop from its mesodermic somites. The shoulder joint capsule and skin covering the lateral aspect of the shoulder and extending to the radial styloid of the wrist develop from the fifth cervical segment. An injury to the shoulder joint capsule can, therefore, refer pain deeply within the arm as far distally as the lateral aspect of the wrist.

scapula. In such cases, the symptoms will typically not extend distally into the arms.

Cyriax also noted that the dura mater is sensitive to stretch. Under normal conditions, the dura mater moves cephalically with neck flexion and caudally with such movements as knee flexion combined with hip extension (tension on the femoral nerve) or straight leg raising (tension on the sciatic nerve). A space-occupying condition, such as a large disc lesion, may impede dural mobility. In such cases, placing tension on the femoral or sciatic nerve will produce symptoms.[6] Diagnosis of dura mater involvement is challenging because the dura mater may mimic other conditions. For example, a cervical disc lesion compressing the dura mater will often refer tenderness to the region of the upper trapezius.

Pressure on Dural Sheaths

The dural sheaths, an extension of the dura mater, surround each nerve root and are approximately 2 centimeters long. The dural sheaths refer pain *segmentally*. For example, pressure on the dural sheath of the third lumbar nerve root has the potential of referring *pain* as far distally as the anterior aspect of the leg (Fig. 5-6).

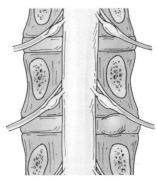

FIGURE 5–6 Lumbar disc lesion (prolapse) compressing the dural sheath of the nerve root, which refers pain segmentally. If the disc lesion impinges the dural sheath with enough pressure, an ischemic reaction may occur as the small capillaries bringing nutrition to the sheath are compromised, producing erosion of the sheath and eventual pressure on the bare nerve root.

When pressure is applied to the portion of the nerve root that is not covered by the dural sheath, *paresthesia rather than pain* is typically reported. This scenario is referred to as the **compression phenomenon**. The short length of the dural sheath makes the bare nerve root susceptible to pressure from an osteophyte at the facet joint or uncovertebral joint.

If a disc lesion impinges the dural sheath with enough pressure, an ischemic reaction may occur as the small capillaries bringing nutrition to the sheath are compromised. As the sheath erodes, the disc lesion will eventually compress the bare nerve root (Fig. 5-7). In such cases, the patient will report less pain and more paresthesia. Stroking the skin over the paresthetic region may create a cascade of paresthesias.

The onset of paresthesia is clinically significant because a disc lesion large enough to produce such symptoms may alter nerve conduction, resulting in a loss of sensation or strength. In such cases, these individuals are not likely to benefit from OMPT, and surgical intervention may be indicated.

Pressure on the Nerve Trunk

Pressure on the nerve trunk typically produces paresthesia after the pressure has been released. Frequently, stroking the skin over the paresthetic region or performance of active motion of the involved extremity will produce a cascade of paresthesias. This scenario is called the **release phenomenon**. The classic example of the release phenomenon occurs in costoclavicular thoracic outlet syndrome. Typically, patients with this syndrome feel fine during the day but are awakened in the middle of the night by paresthesias. During the day, the nerve trunk is compressed between the clavicle and the first rib. Upon retiring for the evening and assuming the reclined position, the clavicle no longer exerts pressure against the nerve trunk. The release of these compressive forces results in paresthesia.

Brismee[7] evaluated the specificity of the *modified Cyriax release test*. This test is designed to initiate the release phenomenon by opening the costoclavicular space through elevation of the clavicle. The patient is seated as the examiner passively lifts the shoulder girdle while documenting the amount of time it takes for the release phenomenon to occur. In patients with suspected thoracic outlet syndrome, the release test demonstrated a specificity of 97.4% when the paresthesias occurred within 1 minute of initiating the test.[7]

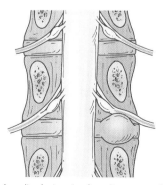

FIGURE 5–7 Lumbar disc lesion (prolapse) compressing the bare nerve root, typically producing paresthesia as opposed to pain. The shortened length of the dural sheath makes the bare nerve root susceptible to pressure from various structures, including disc lesions and osteophytes.

Pressure on Small Peripheral Nerves

Pressure on small peripheral nerves may result in pain, paresthesia, and/or numbness. The primary symptom, however, is often numbness. The patient is usually able to describe the exact location of symptoms. A patient with carpal tunnel syndrome at the wrist, for example, may state that the symptoms are present on the palmer aspect of the lateral three and a half fingers.

Pressure on the Spinal Cord

Pressure on the spinal cord may result from a disc lesion, tumor, or osteophyte. Compression of the spinal cord will produce extrasegmental bilateral paresthesias occupying an area innervated by more than one nerve root. Neither stroking the skin nor moving the extremity increases the paresthesia. An appreciation of the manner in which symptoms may be referred from compressed neurological structures is critical as the manual therapist endeavors to identify the specific source of pathology (Table 5-1).

PRINCIPLES OF EXAMINATION
General Principles

Diagnostic imaging such as computed tomography (CT) scan and magnetic resonance imaging (MRI) often reveal "lesions" that are not the specific cause of the patient's complaints.[8,9] The results of such tests should be considered in light of a thorough clinical examination. The examiner obtains the patient's history, assesses function, then makes inferences about which component of the musculoskeletal system is responsible for the patient's chief complaint. The patient's cooperation is an absolute necessity, as both examiner and patient must take responsibility for identifying the cause of the symptoms.

CLINICAL PILLAR

In the specialty area of OMPT, the approach is always indirect. There is no practical way to view and assess the internal structures directly. The examiner must, therefore, ask the proper questions, assess function, then make inferences about which component of the musculoskeletal system is responsible for the patient's chief complaint. The patient's cooperation is an absolute necessity, as both examiner and patient must take responsibility for identifying the cause of the symptoms.

The Subjective Examination

Knowledge of the natural course of pathological conditions is paramount in allowing the manual therapist to glean valuable information from the patient's subjective report. An accurate interpretation of a detailed patient history can frequently identify the cause of pain for the therapist.

Once the examiner has ascertained the nature and location of the patient's symptoms, the next step is to ask, "How did your pain begin?" Further information regarding the nature of the

Table 5-1	Primary Neurological Symptoms From Compression and Their Suspected Structural Origin					
NEUROLOGICAL SYMPTOM	SPINAL CORD LESION	DURA MATER LESION	DURAL SHEATH LESION	NERVE ROOT LESION	NERVE TRUNK LESION	PERIPHERAL NERVE LESION
Unilateral symptoms		X	X	X	X	X
Bilateral symptoms	X	X				
Extrasegmental pain/ paresthesia	X	X				
Sensitivity to tension		X	X			
Tenderness at distal site		X				
Distal paresthesia	X	X	X	X	X	X
Segmental pain vs. paresthesia			X			
Segmental paresthesia vs. pain				X		
Deep paresthesia				X		
Paresthesia from superficial stroking				X		
Paresthesia postpressure release					X	
Specific numbness						X

dysfunction can be obtained by asking, "What activities increase and decrease your pain?"

In the natural course of events, a loose body in a peripheral joint or a disc lesion at the spine can shift in location. This concept can aid in diagnosis. The mechanism by which Cyriax believed a high-velocity thrust technique to be effective relates to the ability of these techniques to move the injured fragment of tissue to a painless location.

QUESTIONS *for* REFLECTION

What is your initial working hypothesis regarding the origin of your patient's symptoms for each of the following subjective examination findings?

- Rapid and insidious onset of shoulder pain, usually lasting no longer than 6 weeks
- Moderate shoulder pain present for several months
- Cervical trauma with radiating symptoms into digits 2–4
- Gradual onset of elbow pain
- Sudden onset of low back pain during lifting, which is exacerbated with movement and coughing and better in non–weight-bearing
- Symptoms not altered by movement or position
- Inconsistency between the degree of reported pain and the patient's movement patterns
- Pain that shifts from the posterior aspect of the knee to the medial aspect of the knee

The Objective Examination

The examiner begins the physical examination through careful inspection of posture and skin. The process of selective tissue tension testing is germane to the Cyriax approach. This testing uses range of motion (ROM) and resistance testing within a symptom-reproduction model. Examination of movement includes an appreciation of a restricted joint's end-feel, painful arc, and capsular or noncapsular pattern. Palpation serves as an important component of the examination that helps to refine the diagnosis. Diagnostic imaging may also be used as an adjunct. At the conclusion of the examination, the manual physical therapist hopes to identify the specific pathoanatomic structure or structures involved in the patient's disability (Box 5-1).

Inspection

Within this framework, postural inspection and tissue tension testing are critical. For example, in the shoulder, weak upward scapular rotator musculature and/or tight scapular downward rotator musculature may result in a static postural scapular position of downward rotation. Insufficient upward rotation may contribute to impingement of the rotator cuff and surrounding soft tissues (Fig. 5-8). This scenario may manifest itself as a painful arc (Fig. 5-9). Inspection of the patient's resting scapular position prior to movement may, therefore, be useful in informing subsequent intervention.

In the region of the foot and ankle, a common postural abnormality is excessive subtalar joint pronation (Fig. 5-10). Excessive pronation as a compensation for rearfoot or forefoot

Box 5-1 THE MAJOR ASPECTS OF THE CYRIAX OBJECTIVE EXAMINATION AND THEIR PURPOSES

Inspection
- Identify the possibility of a biomechanical cause of a soft tissue lesion
- Identify by skin inspection inflammation (red), a venous disorder or hematoma (blue), or an arterial disorder (pallor)
- Identify muscle wasting, swelling, or bony deformity

Selective Tissue Tension Testing
- Identify the specific pathological structure responsible for the patient's presenting symptoms
- PROM: Identify noncontractile, inert lesions
- AROM: Identify contractile lesions and use to guide isometric examination
- Isometric Resistance: Identify the integrity of contractile tissue, neurological structures, and the interface between musculotendinous structures and their bony attachments

Movement Examination
- Identify the end-feel
- Identify the relationship between symptoms and end-feel (phases)
- Identify a painful arc
- Identify capsular and noncapsular patterns

Palpation
- Provide information to refine the differential diagnosis

Diagnostic Imaging
- An adjunct to the thorough physical examination that precedes it, providing additional data to refine the diagnosis

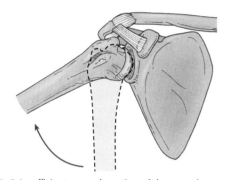

FIGURE 5–8 Insufficient upward rotation of the scapula caused by poor muscle function or glenohumeral joint tightness may contribute to impingement of the rotator cuff and surrounding soft tissues as the humeral tuberosities approximate the coracoacromial arch. Inspection of the patient's resting scapular position prior to movement may be useful in determining the biomechanical origin of symptoms and may inform subsequent intervention.

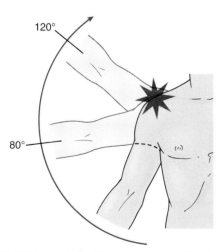

FIGURE 5–9 Impingement of soft tissues may occur at the shoulder resulting in a painful arc as the pathological soft tissue structures approach the coracoacromial arch. Pain is typically produced between 80 and 120 degrees of glenohumeral elevation.

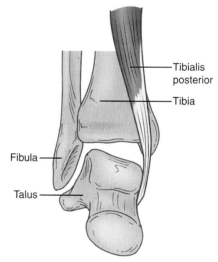

FIGURE 5–10 Posterior view of the ankle during pronation. Excessive pronation as a compensation for rearfoot, or forefoot varus, increases stress to the tibialis posterior musculotendonismusculotendinous unit, among other structures. Symptoms of overuse are seen at the distal attachment of the tendon. Observation of overpronation upon inspection directs intervention toward reducing the effects of overuse and the biomechanical cause of the patient's complaints.

varus, increases stress to the tibialis posterior musculotendinous unit, among other structures.

Skin inspection should also be performed during this phase of the examination. Skin that appears *red* in color is indicative of inflammation, *blue* is often a sign of a venous disorder or hematoma, and *pallor* suggests the presence of an arterial disorder. In certain cases, muscle wasting, swelling, or bony deformity may also be visible.

Selective Tissue Tension Testing

STT testing is, perhaps, the most recognized aspect of Cyriax's approach to musculoskeletal examination. STT is designed to identify the specific pathological structure responsible for the patient's presenting symptoms.[10,11] STT consists of *active range-of-motion testing*, *passive range-of-motion testing*, and *midrange isometric resistance testing*.

STT testing uses a symptom reproduction model; therefore, the results of STT testing depend heavily on the skill of the therapist in eliciting specific stresses of suspected tissues and the ability of the patient to provide relevant and accurate information throughout testing. The examiner precedes testing with the following statement, "I am going to be performing a series of tests. After each of these tests, I will be asking you if the test either reproduces or diminishes the pain that brought you here. Stretching sensations are to be expected and considered to be a normal response to testing." (Fig. 5-11)

Active Range-of-Motion Testing

Active range-of-motion (AROM) testing is a functional test to examine the patient's willingness to move. It is valuable for assessing improvement in function throughout intervention. AROM may be limited by pain, stiffness, and/or muscle weakness. AROM is also useful in identifying a painful arc or the presence of hypermobility.

Passive Range-of-Motion Testing

When performing passive range-of-motion (PROM) testing, there are three critical pieces of information that the examiner hopes to ascertain. First, the examiner must determine whether the motion reproduces or diminishes the patient's presenting symptoms. Next, the **end-feel**, or quality of resistance at end

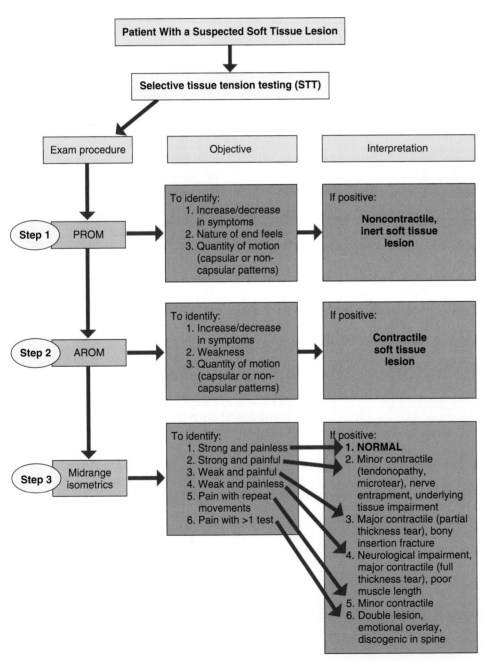

FIGURE 5–11 The process of selective tissue tension (STT) testing in a patient with a suspected soft tissue lesion.

range, for each motion must be determined. Finally, the quantity of available motion must be identified as normal, excessive, or limited. PROM testing is also used to ascertain if a patient has lost range of motion in the *capsular or noncapsular pattern* of the joint. The concepts of end-feel and capsular versus noncapsular patterns will be discussed individually in subsequent sections.

Isometric Midrange Resistance Testing

Lastly, isometric muscle testing is performed to assess the integrity of the contractile tissue, neurological structures, and the interface between musculotendinous structures and their bony attachments. When possible, isometric resistance testing is performed in midrange to minimize stress to the joint or painful stretch to the noncontractile, inert soft tissues. Figures 5-12 and 5-13 present the process of STT testing for elbow ROM and isometric resistance testing. At the conclusion of isometric testing, the examiner seeks to identify one of four possible responses that immediately implicates one or several specific structures as the origin of symptoms.

Strong and Painless
Strong and painless is the anticipated result for a musculotendinous unit that is free from pathology. This finding suggests that

the muscle, innervation, and bony attachments being tested are normal and that the origin of the patient's presenting symptoms is a *-noncontractile*, or **inert**, structure.

Strong and Painful
This finding suggests that a *minor contractile lesion* is present, such as a tendonopathy. Given the fact that testing reveals a strong response from the muscle, a partial or full-thickness tear is not suspected. The examiner must also keep in mind that, at certain locations, nerves pass through the muscle belly. A muscle contraction may painfully compress the nerve, revealing a nerve entrapment pathology.

Midrange isometric testing may also reveal a strong and painful result in a case where the muscle contraction painfully compresses underlying tissue. Isometric hip abduction will reproduce pain that may be associated with *greater trochanteric bursitis*.

Weak and Painful
Isometric muscle testing that results in a weak and painful response suggests the presence of a *major contractile lesion* that not only produces symptoms, but also impacts the force-producing capability of the musculotendinous unit. This response may occur in the case of a partial-thickness tear or secondary to a severe tendonopathy, which elicits pain that inhibits muscle

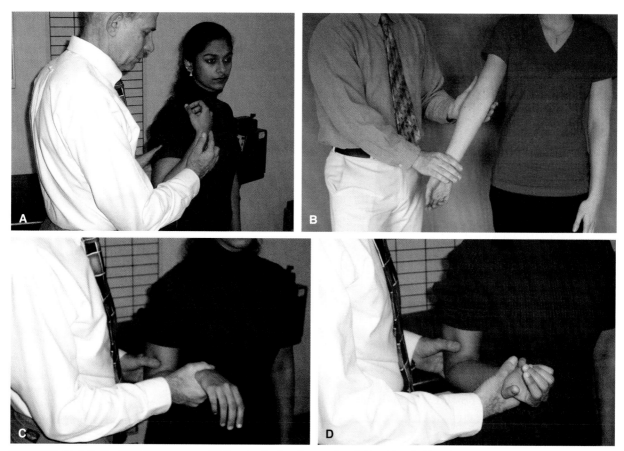

FIGURE 5–12 A–D. The PROM component of STT testing for the elbow. Early arthritis is identified by a limitation in the capsular pattern. Flexion is usually more limited than extension. The end-feels become hard. Pronation and supination are limited in long-standing arthritis. Normal extension has a hard end-feel. In patients with a loose body at the elbow, the end-feel becomes springy. A lesion at the tenoperiosteal insertion of the biceps will produce pain on passive pronation. **A.** Passive elbow flexion. **B.** Passive elbow extension. **C.** Passive forearm pronation. **D.** Passive forearm supination.

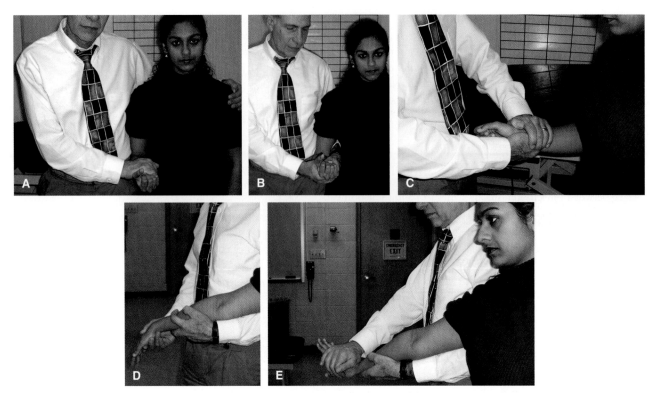

FIGURE 5–13 A–E. The resisted isometric component of STT testing for the elbow. Resisted flexion incriminates the biceps or brachialis. Pain on resistive extension suggests a triceps lesion. Resisted pronation will incriminate the pronator teres or is suggestive of golfer's elbow. Resisted supination will produce pain along with elbow flexion if the biceps is involved. Pain on resisted wrist flexion is indicative of golfer's elbow. Pain on resisted wrist extension is indicative of tennis elbow. **A.** Resisted elbow flexion. **B.** Resisted elbow extension. **C.** Resisted pronation/supination. **D.** Resisted wrist flexion. **E.** Resisted wrist extension.

contractility. Such a response may also reveal the presence of a fracture at one of the muscle's bony attachments.

Weak and Painless

A *neurological deficit* may be present in a patient presenting with a weak and painless response to isometric testing. A weak and painless response may also occur in response to a **full-thickness tear** of the musculotendinous unit. Although tearing of contractile structures is a painful experience, an attempt to contract the torn muscle will not increase the patient's pain because increased tension through a completely torn muscle is not possible.

Painful Only After Repetitive Muscle Contraction

When a minor contractile lesion exists, the pain may only be elicited upon repeated contractions of the muscle. A long distance runner with tibialis posterior tendonopathy, for example, may have anterior lower leg pain only after running several miles. To implicate the involved structures in the clinical setting, the examiner may consider placing the athlete on the treadmill until his or her pain is produced. Following activity, isometric resistance testing is more likely to identify the tissue(s) at fault.

During testing, it is important to appreciate that muscles often have dual functions and more than one action. To clarify the results of isometric testing, the examiner must have full knowledge of the combined function of each muscle operating about a joint (Fig. 5-14). Adequate stabilization is provided

during muscle testing to minimize undesirable participation of adjacent muscles.

Movement Examination

End-Feel

End-feel is defined as the quality of resistance at the end range of passive movement. Since the inception of OMPT, individuals have attempted to define both normal as well as abnormal end-feels for selected joints. Cyriax was, perhaps, the first to popularize and carefully describe both normal and abnormal end-feels for each joint (Table 5-2). The manual physical therapist's skill in evaluating end-feel is critical in identifying the cause of an observed movement disorder and will assist in determining the course of intervention. Although descriptions of end-feel vary between approaches, many similarities exist.

An abnormal end-feel suggesting the need for intervention is identified if the end-feel for the particular joint or motion being tested is not consistent with that which is expected or if the end-feel is reached prior to end range. For example, soft tissue approximation end-feel is expected for knee flexion; however, if this end-feel is identified at midrange or if the end-feel is hard rather than soft, pathology is suspected that must be further explored (Box 5-2).

Soft Tissue Approximation or Soft End-Feel

This end-feel occurs when tissue on one side of the joint compresses tissue on the other. Examples of tissue approximation

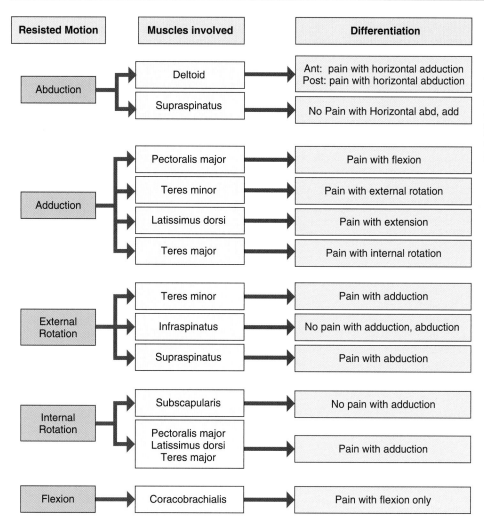

Resisted Motion	Muscles involved	Differentiation
Abduction	Deltoid	Ant: pain with horizontal adduction Post: pain with horizontal abduction
	Supraspinatus	No Pain with Horizontal abd, add
Adduction	Pectoralis major	Pain with flexion
	Teres minor	Pain with external rotation
	Latissimus dorsi	Pain with extension
	Teres major	Pain with internal rotation
External Rotation	Teres minor	Pain with adduction
	Infraspinatus	No pain with adduction, abduction
	Supraspinatus	Pain with abduction
Internal Rotation	Subscapularis	No pain with adduction
	Pectoralis major Latissimus dorsi Teres major	Pain with adduction
Flexion	Coracobrachialis	Pain with flexion only

FIGURE 5–14 Algorithm for determining the pathologic structure at the shoulder using the isometric resistance portion of STT testing. During STT, the examiner uses PROM, AROM, and midrange isometric resistance to make this determination in conjunction with other aspects of the examination. Submaximal isometric resistance is applied with the joint in the midrange open-packed position. A muscle is implicated if pain and/or weakness are noted during testing.

end-feel include ankle plantar flexion as the heel compresses the Achilles tendon against the tibia, horizontal adduction of the shoulder as the humerus and surrounding tissue compresses the pectoral musculature, and knee flexion as the hamstring muscle mass contacts the gastrocnemius-soleus complex.

Bone-to-Bone or Hard End-Feel

Hard end-feel is characterized by movement that reaches an abrupt stop. Hard end-feel may occur under normal conditions, as in elbow extension. The hard end-feel that occurs in elbow extension is typically caused by the olecranon process of the ulna engaging the olecranon fossa of the humerus, but it may be due to tension on the anterior joint capsule. Abnormally, a hard end-feel can occur secondary to a contracture of tissue, malunion of a fracture, or ossification in a joint or muscle caused by trauma. Perception of an abnormal hard end-feel serves as a contraindication to OMPT and suggests a poor prognosis.

Elastic or Capsular End-Feel

An elastic end-feel is reminiscent of a piece of rubber being stretched. It is most frequently experienced upon performance of rotational movements in the cervical spine, shoulder, or hip. Under normal conditions, an elastic end-feel is attributed to stretching of the joint capsule and is therefore referred to more specifically as a *capsular end-feel.*

Springy End-Feel

This type of end-feel is considered to be pathological and indicates the presence of an internal derangement, such as a piece of intra-articular cartilage caught between two bony surfaces. Springy end-feel is sometimes described as producing a "bouncy" or "rebound" sensation.

Spasm End-Feel

This type of end-feel is considered to be a protective, involuntary mechanism to guard against painful motion or to protect an underlying instability. As the examiner moves the joint, the muscle contracts to prevent further irritation or damage to the underlying tissues.

Empty End-Feel

Much like spasm end-feel, empty end-feel is also considered to be protective in nature. As the painful joint is brought through a range of motion, the patient requests that the examiner cease the test. The end-feel is called *empty* because the examiner does not perceive tissue tension that prohibits further motion.

Neurogenic Hypertonic End-Feel

Identification of this end-feel involves a cogwheel rigidity sensation as the joint is moved. Such an end-feel is noted in the presence of a central nervous system disorder, such as Parkinson's disease. In the absence of such a disorder, however, this end-feel

Table 5-2	Normal End-Feels as Defined by Cyriax for Each Joint and Motion	

JOINT	MOTION	NORMAL END-FEEL
Neck	FB/BB	Elastic
	SB	Elastic
	Rotation	Elastic
Shoulder	Flexion	Elastic
	Abduction	Elastic/hard
	Horizontal adduction	Elastic/soft
	Scaption	Elastic/hard
	IR/ER	Elastic
Elbow	Flexion	Soft
	Extension	Hard
Forearm	Pronation/supination	Elastic
Wrist	Flexion	Elastic
	Extension	Elastic
	Radioulnar development	Hard
Thumb	Flexion/extension	Elastic
	Abduction	Elastic
	Adduction	Soft
Finger	Flexion	Soft
	Extension	Elastic
LB	FB/BB	Elastic
	SB	Elastic
	Rotation	Elastic
Hip	Flexion	Elastic/soft
	Extension	Elastic
	Abduction	Elastic
	Adduction	Elastic/soft
	IR/ER	Elastic
Knee	Flexion	Soft
	Extension	Elastic
Ankle	Plantar flexion	Elastic
	Dorsiflexion	Elastic
	Inversion	Elastic
	Eversion	Elastic
	Pronation/supination	Elastic
Toes	Flexion	Elastic
	Extension	Elastic

FB/BB, forward bending/backward bending; SB, side bending; IR/ER, internal rotation/external rotation; LB, left bending.

Soft signifies a limitation due to the approximation of soft tissues. Elastic signifies the stretching of the joint capsule and is also referred to as capsular end-feel. Hard signifies bone-to-bone contact. Each is considered normal for a specific motion at end range and may be considered pathological if the end-feel is inconsistent with a specific motion or if it occurs early in the range.

may suggest a significant emotional overlay to the patient's complaint of pain.

The Relationship Between Pain and End-Feel (Phases)

During the objective examination, it is important for the manual physical therapist to ascertain the relationship between pain and end-feel. Identifying whether pain is reproduced before, at, or after the end-feel has been reached is an important

Box 5-2 TYPES OF END-FEELS AND THEIR INTERPRETATION

1. ***Soft tissue approximation, soft end-feel:*** Tissue on one side of the joint compresses tissue on the other normally (i.e., knee flexion)

2. ***Bone-to-bone, hard end-feel:*** Abrupt stop caused by bone-to-bone contact normally (i.e., elbow extension)

3. ***Elastic end-feel:*** Stretching of join capsule normally or abnormally if early in range, at which time referred to as capsular end-feel (i.e., shoulder external rotation)

4. ***Springy end-feel:*** Rebound-type sensation indicating the presence of an internal derangement, such as a piece of intra-articular cartilage caught between two bony surfaces (i.e., knee, hip)

5. ***Spasm end-feel:*** A protective, involuntary mechanism to guard against painful motion indicating severe arthritis, displacement, or joint destruction (i.e., knee, hip)

6. ***Empty end-feel:*** Pain or fear of pain causes patient to resist further motion and request that the examiner ceases the test without perception of tissue tension

7. ***Neurogenic hypertonic end-feel:*** Cogwheel rigidity as the joint is moved noted in the presence of a central nervous system disorder or it suggests emotional overlay

consideration in this approach. The concept of determining the relationship between pain and end-feel was defined using the term *phases* by Cyriax.

There are three possible phases for the therapist to consider when examining a joint for the relationship between pain and end-feel. **Phase one** is characterized by pain that is reproduced or exacerbated *after* the end-feel has been reached. The joint is, therefore, determined to be minimally irritable. For this joint, traditional range of motion and stretching interventions are indicated.

Phase two is characterized by pain that is reproduced or exacerbated at the *same time* that the end-feel is reached. This joint is therefore considered to be moderately irritable and more challenging to manage with standard ROM and stretching interventions. This patient may require anti-inflammatory medication to help control symptoms. This patient may also respond to the judicious administration of joint mobilization oscillatory techniques, which are discussed in detail elsewhere in this text.

Phase three consists of pain that is reproduced or exacerbated at some point *before* end-feel is reached. The joint is therefore considered to be severely irritable. This patient may require a bout of palliative measures for a period of time before the therapist is able to commence mobilization techniques (Fig. 5-15).

Painful Arc

A **painful arc** is defined as a point, or points, within a range of motion in which a patient experiences discomfort. An individual may experience a painful arc when pressure-sensitive structures

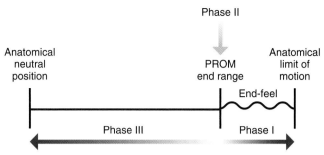

FIGURE 5–15 Relationship between phases and end-feel.

become compromised between two bony surfaces or when a minor mechanical problem exists at an intervertebral joint. Cyriax hypothesized that in the spine a painful arc may be due to the displacement of a small fragment of disc that is momentarily pressed against the dura mater (Fig. 5-16).

Capsular Versus Noncapsular Patterns

A **capsular pattern** occurs when restrictions in movement occur as a result of restrictions within the **capsuloligamentous complex (CLC)** of the joint. Although controversy exists among researchers regarding these patterns, capsular patterns have been described for each joint. These patterns are typically expressed by stating the most restricted motion first, followed by the next most restricted motion and so on. For example, ER > ABD > IR indicates that external rotation is more limited than abduction, which is more limited than internal rotation. Limitations in range of motion that do not display characteristics of a capsular pattern are considered to be noncapsular and require another course of intervention. Ombregt[2] provides excellent descriptions of passive testing that may be used to specifically identify the presence of a capsular pattern.[2]

QUESTIONS *for* REFLECTION

- What are the potential causes of a capsular (full articular) and noncapsular pattern?
- How would your plan of care differ if there was a capsular pattern as opposed to a noncapsular pattern present?

At a synovial joint, a lesion of either the fibrous capsule or synovial membrane results in a predictable pattern of reduced motion (Table 5-3). In the acute phase, this loss of motion is believed to be a protective mechanism that occurs in an attempt to avoid pain. In the chronic phase, this lesion may lead to a contracture of the connective tissue. This condition is often referred to as *capsulitis, synovitis,* or *arthritis*. Evidence related to osteoarthritis of the knee using selective tissue tension testing supports the capsular pattern concept.[12]

Ombregt[2] recommends referring to this predictable loss of motion in the spinal joints as **full articular pattern**.[2] When the full articular pattern is present, the examiner must determine the cause of the observed motion loss. Additional testing may be required to ascertain the origin of motion loss, since the

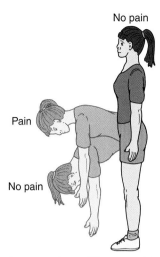

FIGURE 5–16 Displacement of a small fragment of the disc may result in a painful arc caused by momentary compression on dura mater.

existence of a more serious condition may require a medical referral. Within this approach, the terms *capsular pattern* and *full articular pattern* may be used interchangeably.[2]

For a noncapsular pattern, Ombregt[2] advocates use of the term **partial articular pattern.** Loss of motion in a noncapsular pattern may be due to a ligamentous adhesion, internal derangement, or extra-articular lesion. Ligamentous adhesions result from injured ligaments that are subjected to prolonged immobilization. For example, a sprain to a dorsal wrist ligament will produce a partial articular pattern that selectively impairs wrist flexion while preserving full wrist extension (Fig. 5-17).

Palpation

Within the Cyriax approach, *palpation* is often successfully used to refine the diagnosis that has emerged from the process of STT testing. Palpation for bony tenderness is considered to be extremely helpful in determining the need for diagnostic imaging.[13] Nevertheless, the examiner must be careful to avoid the common mistake of making a diagnosis based on palpation alone.

CLINICAL PILLAR

During the examination, palpation may be used to identify the following:

1. Tenderness
2. Pulses
3. Temperature
4. Swelling
5. Thickened synovial membrane
6. Muscular gap
7. Bone
8. Crepitus

Table 5–3	Capsular (Full Articular) Patterns for the Upper Extremities, Lower Extremities, and the Spine as Defined by Cyriax

ARTICULATION	CAPSULAR PATTERN
Temperomandibular	Loss of mandibular depression
Cervical and thoracic spine	BB > ROT = SB > FB
Lumbar spine	BB > SB > FB
Shoulder	ABD > ER > IR
Sternoclavicular and acromioclavicular	Pain at extremes of range
Elbow	FLEX > EXT, variable
Radioulnar	Pronation and supination are full range but painful
Wrist	FLEX = EXT>Radial, ulnar deviations
First carpometacarpal	ABD = EXT
Metacarpophalangeal, interphalangeal	FLEX > EXT
Sacroiliac	Pain with distraction
Hip	FLEX = IR > ABD > EXT > ER
Knee	FLEX > EXT
Tibiofibular	Pain with biceps femoris contraction and when ankle mortise is distracted (i.e., during dorsiflexion)
Ankle	Plantar flexion > dorsiflexion
Subtalar	Inversion > eversion
Midtarsal	ADD = IR > other movements
First metatarsophalangeal	EXT > FLEX
Second through fifth metatarsophalangeal and interphalangeal	EXT = FLEX or EXT > FLEX

">" indicates that the preceding motion is more limited than the next motion. BB, =backward bending; FB, forward bending; SB, side bending; ROT, rotation; ER, external rotation; IR, internal rotation; ABD, =abduction; ADD, =adduction; FLEX, =flexion; EXT, extension.

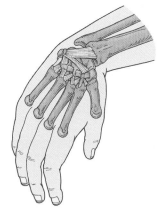

FIGURE 5–17 Sprain to a dorsal wrist ligament will produce a partial articular pattern that selectively impairs wrist flexion while preserving full wrist extension. Wrist flexion may produce pain because this motion places tension on the dorsal ligaments of the wrist.

The temperature of the tissue being palpated may provide information regarding the stage of the condition and the type of tissue involved. A structure that is warm to the touch is suggestive of a recent injury, inflammation, or infection. A structure that is cold to the touch indicates an arterial compromise, and may be associated with a diminished arterial pulse. The presence of *local swelling* is indicative of an injury to the joint or bursa. More *generalized edema* can be a sign of poor venous return or a compromised lymphatic system.

Palpation may also be used to identify the presence of *inflammatory arthritic conditions*. Rheumatoid arthritis, gout, or psoriatic arthritis may produce joint capsular thickening that can be easily palpated at extremity joints.

A *subluxed bone* is often palpable, as is an *osteophyte* that occurs in response to severe arthritic conditions or neoplasm. A step deformity due to a spondylolisthesis of the spine is palpable, particularly when the region is in an unsupported, weight-bearing position (Fig. 5-18).

Joint crepitus may indicate the presence of joint erosion. Tendinous crepitus occurs in cases of tenosynovitis as the tendon attempts to glide within its sheath. Crepitus may occasionally be found in the case of a muscular lesion or in a bursa that is recovering from inflammation.

Evaluation

Differential Diagnosis of a Mechanical Dysfunction and Internal Derangement

Within this approach, a **mechanical dysfunction** is a term that is often used to define a lesion of the spine that will present as

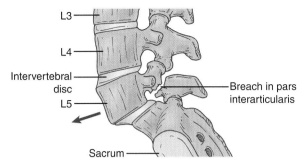

FIGURE 5–18 Isthmic spondylolisthesis consists of a break in the pars interarticularis resulting in a forward slippage of the vertebra.

a loss of motion in a partial articular pattern. Cyriax used the term **internal derangement** to refer to peripheral joint lesions such as loose bodies or subluxed bones, which will cause a loss of motion in a partial articular pattern.

A patient with a long-standing full articular pattern who develops an internal derangement will present with a concomitant partial articular pattern. For example, a patient with osteoarthritis of the spine with a long-standing loss of cervical extension and an equal loss of cervical rotation and side bending (full articular pattern) may develop an internal derangement with subsequent alteration in his or her movement pattern that reveals a greater loss of motion in one or more directions (partial articular pattern). Treatment that is directed toward the more recent primary impairment should attempt to return the newly acquired partial articular pattern back to the preexisting full articular pattern, after which, the full articular pattern may be addressed.

Differential Diagnosis of Soft Tissue Lesions

One of the greatest contributions of the Cyriax approach to OMPT lies in the differential diagnosis of soft tissue lesions. To reach a differential diagnosis regarding the specific soft tissue structure at fault, the therapist should ascertain the answer to specific diagnostic questions. The answer to these diagnostic questions serves to guide intervention, which will vary depending on the suspected structure at fault.

NOTABLE QUOTABLE

"Few conditions are as common as soft-tissue lesions; not many ailments respond so readily to treatment. Yet all too often their care is regarded as a matter of indifference or, little better, as the province of the narrow and complex specialty beyond ordinary reach."

James Cyriax

If passive testing is more painful than midrange isometric resistance testing, then a lesion in the noncontractile inert tissue is suspected. Painful PROM testing with the presence of either a full articular pattern or partial articular pattern confirms the presence of an inert lesion. The cause of the observed movement aberration, however, will be different depending on which pattern is present. Full articular patterns

may be the result of the shortening of the joint's fibrous capsule or synovial membrane from fibrosis following injury or from prolonged immobility secondary to pain or fear of pain during movement. Often the presence of these findings, particularly in peripheral joints, are the sequelae of joint osteoarthritis.

To confirm the most likely cause for the observed capsular pattern, the examiner may use the results of the subjective history, including the onset, nature, and severity of the patient's reported symptoms. A detailed palpation examination of the involved joint and testing for end-feel will also provide confirmation of the suspected origin.

A mechanical problem, such as a disc lesion may produce a movement pattern that is noncapsular in the spine. When considering the origin of noncapsular patterns in peripheral joints, it is imperative that the examiner have an understanding of common conditions that are most likely to occur at each specific joint. Additional procedures, including a detailed history, palpation, and end-feel examination, are often important to determine the cause of a noncapsular pattern.

If resistance testing in midrange produces symptoms and passive range of motion testing is pain free, then a contractile lesion is suspected. Resistance testing in midrange places inert structures on slack and selectively isolates contractile structures. To confirm the presence of a contractile lesion, stretching of the structure may also produce symptoms.

PRINCIPLES OF INTERVENTION

The Cyriax approach to OMPT places a significant emphasis on the use of three specific, nonsurgical intervention procedures in the care of musculoskeletal impairment. This approach is best known for its refinement in the application of *deep friction massage*, *injectable medication*, and *manipulation and traction*. Cyriax believed that most musculoskeletal impairments could be effectively managed through use of one or a combination of these three intervention strategies (Table 5-4).

Intervention for Lesions of Contractile Tissue

For a contractile lesion, the specific type of intervention to be used depends on the location of the lesion within the contractile unit. For most contractile tissue lesions, deep friction massage is the primary intervention of choice. While case studies have been published describing the efficacy of DFM, scientific evidence regarding the efficacy of DFM is still lacking.[14] Some suggest that DFM acts as a local anti-inflammatory agent or anesthetic agent. Others believe that DFM softens inflamed scar tissue or improves the alignment of the collagen fibers within soft tissue.[15] Davidson et al[16] demonstrated that compression at the healing site of a tendinous lesion stimulates fibroblastic proliferation.[16] These findings support the belief that microtears of the tendon are the primary culprit for the pain and disability that results from tendinosis.

When implementing *deep friction massage (DFM)* the following guidelines should be followed:

1. Diagnostic movements and palpation must identify the tissue at fault and the *exact location* on that tissue.

2. The therapist's fingers and the patient's skin must *move simultaneously* to avoid injury to skin.

3. DFM must be given *perpendicular* to the tissue fiber.

4. DFM must be given with sufficient *sweep* to ensure that the whole lesion is treated.

5. DFM must be given *deeply* and administered within the patient's tolerance. Tolerance will improve during the massage.

6. Patient must adopt a posture that *exposes* the tissue to be treated.

7. If the lesion lies in a belly of the muscle, the muscle belly must be put on *slack.* This will aid in the separation of the muscle fibers during the massage.

8. Tendons with a sheath must be put on *stretch* to ensure maximum success of the massage.

9. Generally, *6–12 sessions, 20 minutes each* on alternate days is required.

Contraindications of deep friction massage include:

1. Inflammation caused by infection

2. Traumatic arthritis of the elbow

3. Bursitis

4. Rheumatoid arthritis

5. Pressure on nerves

Stratford[17] challenged the efficacy of DFM for extensor carpi radialis tendonitis.[17] This study, however, did not adhere to the recommended guidelines for application of DFM. The intervention was not performed for the recommended 15 to 20 minutes. Furthermore, lesions at the origin, as was the case in this study, are actually best treated by the use of steroid injections.[18]

The specific region to which DFM is applied is found through meticulous palpation. It is important when performing DFM that the therapist's fingers and the patient's skin move as one unit to avoid skin breakdown and to ensure that the forces are reaching the site of the lesion. The applied friction forces must be introduced in a perpendicular direction relative to the fibers composing the affected structure.[16] In addition to proper direction, friction forces must also be applied with the proper breadth and depth. The applied friction forces must be adequately applied across the entire lesion. Friction forces must be applied deeply enough to ensure that the target tissue is being reached. As a general rule, DFM is applied for up to 10 minutes after the numbing effect has been achieved at a minimum interval of 48 hours. This time period is adequate to allow the reduction in hyperemia caused from the procedure.[19]

When performing DFM to a muscle belly, the involved muscle must be placed in a slackened position. DFM can then "tweeze" the muscle fibers to ensure normal glide of these fibers during muscle contraction. For recent injuries, this positioning helps prevent fibroblasts from proliferating perpendicular to the site of the injury. Tendons with a sheath are placed in a position of stretch to ensure that the sheath is kept immobile. The applied forces are then better able to reduce the roughened surfaces between the tendon and its sheath.

DFM is often considered to be very painful. Pain, however, is often the result of incorrect technique. If applied correctly, DFM often produces the fairly rapid onset of numbness. The

Table 5-4	Recommended Interventions for Selected Lesions as per the *Cyriax Approach to OMPT*		
TYPE OF LESION	**DEEP FRICTION MASSAGE (DFM)**	**MANIPULATION, TRACTION**	**INJECTION, IONTOPHORESIS**
General Contractile Tissue Lesion	XX		X
Tenoperiosteal Junction Lesion			XX
Musculotendinous Lesion	XX		X
Muscle Belly Lesion	XX		X
Ligamentous Tissue Lesion	XX (Acute, chronic)	X (Chronic)	
Spinal disc Lesion		XX	
Loose Bodies in Peripheral Joint Lesion		XX	
Bursitis			XX
Capsular pattern Lesion		X (Nonthrust)	X (Arthritis)

X indicates intervention that may be used in the care of this lesion. **XX** indicates primary intervention to be used in the care of this lesion.

mechanism by which pain relief is achieved through DFM is subject to debate. Some believe its effects are the result of modulation of nociceptive impulses at the level of the spinal cord as described in the gate control theory. Cyriax has postulated that the effects are the result of increased destruction of pain-causing metabolites. Another mechanism for pain relief is believed to be due to diffuse noxious inhibitory controls that release endogenous opiates.[19]

Although considered to be the primary intervention for soft tissues lesions, DFM may also be used in combination with other interventions. DFM may be used as a means of preparing tissues for manipulation in an effort to optimize outcomes. Nagrale et al[19] compared the application of phonophoresis with exercise to DFM and use of the Mills manipulation and found that Cyriax's approach is the superior of the two treatment methods.[19]

CLINICAL PILLAR

Cyriax Approach to the Management of Lateral Epicondylitis

1. Deep Friction Massage

- Position patient with elbow supinated, 90 degrees of flexion.
- Identify anterolateral aspect of epicondyle and region of tenderness.
- Apply DFM with thumb tip in posterior direction to teno-osseous junction.
- Maintain pressure with fingers on other side of elbow for counterpressure.
- Apply DFM for 10 minutes after numbing to prepare for Mills manipulation.

2. Mills Manipulation

- Perform immediately after DFM if elbow has full extension PROM.
- Patient sitting in chair with backrest, therapist stands behind.
- Patient's shoulder in 90 degree abduction, internal rotation, forearm pronation, and supported by therapist's elbow.
- Therapist's thumb in space between patient's thumb and index.
- Fully flex wrist and pronate forearm.
- Move hand of supporting arm to posterior elbow and with full wrist flexion and forearm pronation, extend elbow until slack taken up.
- Apply minimal amplitude, high-velocity thrust by side bending away and pushing downward with the hand over the patient's elbow.
- Perform only once per intervention session.

DFM is contraindicated in the presence of ossified or calcified tendons, bacterial infections of the tendon, and in the presence of ulcers or blisters that traverse the location of the soft tissue lesion. In addition, DFM is not recommended in cases of bursitis and neuritis. Therefore, it is critical that the manual physical therapist be able to accurately distinguish between bursitis and tendonopathy.

Lesions of the *tenoperiosteal junction* are most effectively treated by steroid injections. If the tendon is superficial, iontophoresis with dexamethasone is a viable alternative. If residual symptoms persist after injection, DFM is often effective in facilitating the healing process, but it is not usually the best first line of intervention. Lesions at the *musculotendinous junction* are best managed with DFM. The majority of lesions within the *muscle belly* can be managed with DFM or an anesthetic injection delivered directly to the region of pathology.

The success of interventions designed to manage a contractile unit lesion is dependent on the willingness of the patient to avoid strenuous activity of the involved region until the pain is relieved. If stretching is to be performed, careful attention must be given to avoid an exacerbation of symptoms. In cases of tendonopathy, DFM is most effective when performed for 15 to 20 minutes two to three times per week. With an acute strain, DFM is most effective when performed 5 minutes daily for the prevention of scar tissue deposition. In this case, DFM is performed perpendicular to the alignment of the muscle fibers. In addition, 5 minutes of gentle muscle contraction with electrical stimulation daily may assist in the promotion of healing. Muscle strains that are first seen 1 month or more after injury are typically treated with 20 minutes of DFM three times a week to isolate the painful adhesion that has developed within the muscle belly (Figs. 5-19 and 5-20).

Intervention for Lesions of Ligamentous Tissue

During the acute stage of grade one or two sprains, it is recommended to apply 5 minutes of daily DFM with carefully graded active or passive range-of-motion exercises. The role of exercise in this process is to keep the junction between the injured ligament and the underlying bone mobile to prevent the development of adhesions. In the presence of ligamentous adhesions, 20 minutes of DFM is recommended, followed by a high-velocity thrust technique that is designed to eliminate

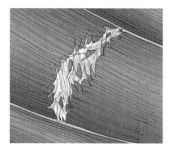

FIGURE 5–19 Injury to muscle may create scar tissue that develops in the muscle and consists of fibers that are both longitudinal and transverse to the fibers of the muscle belly.

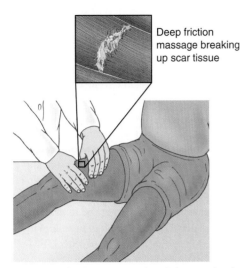

FIGURE 5–20 Deep friction massage (DFM) for a strained quadriceps muscle belly for the purpose of breaking up scar tissue. When performing DFM, the therapist must be sure to elicit force transversely across the fibers of the muscle at the appropriate depth.

the adhesion. This process often requires one to three sessions to achieve optimal results.

Intervention for Disc Lesions of the Spine

Cyriax believed that mechanical problems of the spine were primarily caused by lesions of the intervertebral disc. When diagnosing disc lesions, Cyriax made a distinction between *nuclear disc lesions* and *annular disc lesions*. The distinction between the type of disc lesion is based primarily on the patient's subjective history.

To denote a nuclear disc lesion, Cyriax used the term, **soft disc lesion**. The pathogenesis of this condition involves the nucleus (soft material) gradually becoming displaced. In the case of a prolapse, the nucleus pulposus is displaced within the confines of the annulus fibrosis, causing a distortion of the annular rings of lamellae (see Fig. 5-1). In the case of a contained herniation, radial tears develop in the annulus and a portion of the nucleus displaces to the extent of the tear but remains contained within the disc (Fig. 5-21). A nuclear soft disc lesion is believed to have a gradual onset of symptoms, taking several

minutes or hours to occur. These lesions often occur in response to prolonged sitting in a flexed posture.

Cyriax referred to the annular disc lesion as a **hard disc lesion**. A fissure beginning at the innermost portion of the annulus develops with gradual extrusion of nuclear material along the path of the fissure. An annular disc lesion is believed to occur instantaneously. Activities that involve rapid movements with poor body mechanics are often the mechanism of injury for an annular disc lesion. Although the annulus is compromised, as long as the nuclear material remains contained, nonsurgical management is usually effective (Fig. 5-22). Many have supported the notion that the intervertebral disc is a common source of spine-related symptoms.[6,20–22]

The Cyriax approach strongly advocates the use of spinal high-velocity thrust manipulation for mechanical problems of the spine. He believed that thrust techniques are able to move the annular disc material back into its normal position, leading to a reduction in pain and disability. Mobilization/manipulation techniques typically used within this approach include *grade A, B, or C distraction using short or long lever rotation, grade A, B, or C straight extension, unilateral extension, and extension with leverage*. Grades A and B are used to define mobilization that is performed at different points within a range of motion, and grade C is used to define a high-velocity thrust procedure.[23] Maitland mobilization was used by experienced physical therapists in the United Kingdom 40.4% of the time, Maitland mobilization and Cyriax manipulation was used 40.4% of the time, and Cyriax manipulation was used 19.1% of the time. Subjects who received a combination of OMPT and interferential therapy received a greater degree of Cyriax manipulation techniques (29.2%) than did those in the manual therapy only group. Regardless of the type of manual therapy used, subjects improved at discharge and 12 month follow-up, with no difference between groups except that those receiving a combination of Maitland mobilization and Cyriax manipulation required more therapy than did those receiving Cyriax manipulation alone (mean difference = 1.47).[23]

Cyriax also believed in the use of spinal mechanical traction as an extremely effective procedure in specific cases of *nuclear disc lesions*. He theorized that the static intervertebral forces provided by traction create a negative pressure within the intervertebral space, which is effective at drawing the nuclear protrusion back into its normal position.

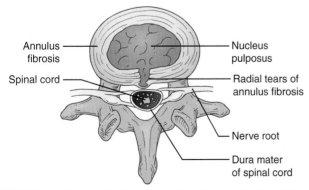

FIGURE 5–21 Herniated lumbar nuclear disc lesion resulting in radial tears of the annulus.

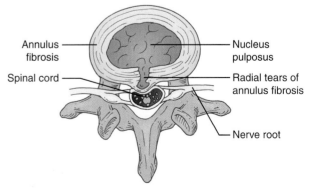

FIGURE 5–22 Lumbar annular disc lesion compressing the dura mater resulting in central pain.

Intervention for Loose Bodies Within Peripheral Joints

One of the most gratifying aspects of the Cyriax approach relates to the recommended intervention regimen for intra-articular loose bodies within peripheral joints. Loose bodies may occur secondary to advanced osteoarthritis most commonly at the hip or knee, yet may also be seen at the elbow and ankle. The intervention of choice is specific **nonthrust mobilization or high-velocity thrust manipulation** (see the Clinical Pillar on joint manipulation). These procedures are believed to be effective by relocating the painful loose body to a painless region within the joint. A recurrence may be expected, which would require subsequent intervention. If manual therapy was unsuccessful, arthroscopic surgery may be indicated. Figure 5-23 displays a high-velocity thrust manipulation for a loose body of the hip.

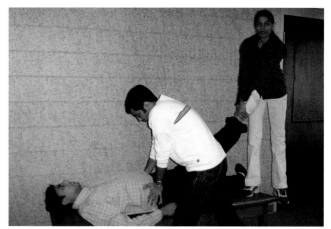

FIGURE 5–23 High-velocity thrust manipulation for loose body of the hip. Long-axis traction is applied by the therapist as an assistant holds the pelvis. The therapist leans back and gradually steps off the table. While the therapist applies traction, the patient's leg is slowly extended during repeated rotation. Generally, the manipulation is more effective if the rotation and final thrust is performed in the pain-free direction. For example, if on examination the patient had painful hip internal rotation, the manipulation is first attempted with rotation into external rotation. The technique is completed by providing a sharp thrust toward one extreme of rotation. The final thrust is provided in the direction that is found to be most beneficial for improving range. A series of three thrusts is usually provided. Reexamination is provided after each thrust to evaluate change.

CLINICAL PILLAR

During joint *manipulation*, the therapist should remember the following:

1. Use for capsular contracture, adhesions, and to reduce a displacement.

2. For *contracture*, use *slow*, steady movement over several sessions *(shoulder, hip)*.

3. For rupture of *adhesions*, use sharp *jerk (knee, ankle)*.

4. For reduction of *displacement*, apply and maintain manual *traction*.

5. Take the joint to the *end range* of movement during repeated *rotations*.

6. Apply *overpressure*.

7. *Reexamine* the joint.

Intervention for Bursitis

Depending on the location of the lesion, bursitis may impact movement of the associated joint ranging from a loss of motion that is in a noncapsular pattern to an insignificant loss of motion. An acute bursitis of the subacromial bursa of the shoulder, for example, will produce a gross loss of abduction with a moderate loss of rotation. Conversely, bursitis of the olecranon bursa will not restrict elbow motion because of the bursa's extra-articular location. Bursitis that is not secondary to infection or hemorrhage is most effectively treated by steroid or anesthetic injection.

Intervention for Capsular Patterns (Full Articular Pattern)

If capsular patterns are present in the spine, the therapist must differentiate between arthritis, fracture, or bone tumor. If they are identified in a peripheral joint, the cause is most likely arthritis. The type of arthritis must then be determined. **Septic**

arthritis requires antibiotic therapy. **Traumatic arthritis,** or monoarticular steroid-sensitive arthritis, will often benefit from a steroid injection. Traumatic arthritis refers to joint inflammation secondary to trauma.

Monoarticular steroid-sensitive arthritis occurs spontaneously without any signs of rheumatological involvement and is a diagnosis of exclusion. It most commonly occurs at the shoulder, elbow, hip, knee, or ankle and often resolves spontaneously over several months or years. The intervention of choice for this condition is steroid injection. [2]

Traumatic arthritis of the shoulder typically requires an aggressive range-of-motion program. For the first month following the onset of traumatic arthritis of the elbow, stretching is contraindicated. Posttraumatic hemorrhaging into the brachialis muscle may increase if the elbow is stretched into extension too early. In such cases, the risk and severity of heterotopic bone formation, or **myositis ossificans,** is increased.[24]

DIFFERENTIATING CHARACTERISTICS

The Cyriax approach to OMPT has its origins in the medical model and was born out of dissatisfaction with current methods used to differentially diagnose soft tissue lesions. Cyriax's major contribution to our current body of knowledge is the use of an examination process that seeks to specifically identify the origin of suspected soft tissue lesions. The Cyriax approach to OMPT emphasizes the use of three primary interventions for the management of musculoskeletal conditions. The use of deep friction massage, injectable medication, and/or manipulation and traction is judiciously applied only after a thorough examination that attempts to identify the specific anatomical origin of the patient's presenting symptoms has been performed.

Cyriax introduced the concept of selective tissue tension testing, which has become the primary feature of this approach's examination process. The Cyriax passive movement examination focuses on identification of end-feel, or the quality of resistance at end range, and the nature of movement loss, known as the full, or partial, articular pattern. Cyriax has contributed to the body of knowledge in defining seven different end-feels (soft, hard, elastic, springy, spasm, empty, neurological hypertonic) that may be identified at any given joint. In addition, Cyriax has described characteristic losses of motion at a joint that are representative of the culpable structure. As in other approaches, palpation is used to further refine the differential diagnosis. Through astute examination, which includes STT testing, end-feel testing, and an appreciation of movement patterns and losses of movement, the manual therapist is able to specifically differentiate a contractile lesion from a noncontractile lesion. The choice of intervention is dictated by the pathoanatomical diagnosis.

Unlike other OMPT approaches in common use that base diagnosis on clinically recognizable impairments, the Cyriax approach demands specific identification of the pathological structure(s) that are responsible for the patient's symptoms. This approach is more closely aligned with the traditional medical model in which the diagnosis of disease is based on the search for the anatomical cause.

Cyriax's recommended intervention strategies are based on an understanding of pathological, histological processes. For example, Cyriax's DFM attempts to influence fibroblastic activity that occurs in response to immobility and/or inflammatory processes in the tendon. Cyriax's rationale for the use of high-velocity thrust techniques in the spine departs from our current understanding. The Cyriax approach operates under the belief that thrust procedures have the ability to relocate loose bodies in peripheral joints or reduce discogenic lesions in the spine, which subsequently reduce pain and improve mobility.

As the father of orthopaedic medicine, James Cyriax's philosophy regarding the examination and intervention of musculoskeletal impairment has had a profound effect on the current practice of OMPT. As an advocate of physical therapy and a contributor to the popularization of OMPT in the United States, James Cyriax holds an important place, among others, as a major contributor to the specialty area of OMPT.

EVIDENCE SUMMARY

[Christopher H. Wise, PT, DPT, OCS, FAAOMPT, MTC, ATC]

Selective Tissue Tension Testing

Most of the literature on STT testing has failed to report the effectiveness of using this system in its entirety. Franklin et al[25] attempted to investigate the construct validity of STT testing in nine subjects with exercise-induced minor hamstring lesions. After performance of eccentric isokinetic hamstring exercise, PROM remained unchanged; however, resistance testing produced hamstring pain. Pain upon palpation increased 48 and 72 hours postexercise. There was a reduction in AROM, with the least amount of motion occurring at 48 hours postexercise.[25] According to Cyriax, a minor lesion of this kind should present with STT test results that include a change in AROM and should be strong and painful. The results of this study call into question the validity of using STT testing to identify minor contractile lesions.

Pellecchia et al[10] examined the intertester reliability of the Cyriax examination, which included a detailed history, preliminary examination, and STT testing in the diagnosis of 21 cases of shoulder pain. Two experienced therapists demonstrated 90.5% agreement identifying the same classification in 19 of 21 cases of shoulder pain (kappa = 0.875). Both therapists also classified the same four cases as not fitting the Cyriax model. The authors concluded that this method of examination is a highly reliable method of examining painful shoulders.[10]

To determine the level of agreement between an expert examiner and three other examiners in diagnosing individuals with painful shoulders using STT testing, Hanchard et al[26] demonstrated good agreement between the expert and other examiners in 93% of the cases. Agreement was fair-moderate for bursitis, good for rotator cuff lesions and other diagnoses, and good to very good for capsulitis.[26]

The current best evidence on STT testing suggests that these examination procedures may be reliable and valid in diagnosing soft tissue lesions in individuals with existing pathology, particularly of the shoulder. However, STT testing may be ineffective in the diagnosis of minor contractile lesions. The two studies[10,26] that demonstrated favorable results were performed on symptomatic patients compared to poor outcomes that were found in a cohort of individuals with minor exercise-induced lesions.[25]

End-Feel

The magnitude of applied force required to obtain an end-feel may vary depending on the direction of translation. Anterior translation has been found to require more force than inferior translation in nonimpaired shoulders. [27]

Chesworth et al[28] attempted to simultaneously evaluate the intrarater and interrater reliability of two experienced manual therapists in the use of movement diagrams and end-feel classification of external rotation in a group of 34 patients with shoulder pathology. Components of the movement diagram as well as evaluation of end-feels showed high reliability.[28]

It is generally believed that determination of joint mobility is best considered when both pain and resistance to further movement at end range is considered.[29] Petersen and Hayes[30] studied the relationship between pain and both normal and abnormal end-feels at the knee and shoulder. The results revealed that abnormal end-feels are indicative of dysfunction in 40 subjects with knee pain and 46 subjects with shoulder pain.[30] Abnormal pathological end-feels were associated with more pain than normal end-feels at the knee and shoulder for all motions.[30] The authors concluded that end-feels are useful in identifying tissue pathology.[30]

Along with other examination procedures, identification of an empty end-feel and noncapsular pattern may be used as screening tools to identify the presence of a medical condition that requires a referral. An empty end-feel, suggestive of a painful condition, in conjunction with a noncapsular pattern, suggestive of nonarticular limitations, may be used to effectively screen for conditions that are outside the purview of physical therapy and require further medical testing.[31]

Consideration of pain reproduction during end-feel testing, as opposed to relying on the quality of the resistance at end range alone, seems to provide the most relevant data. Additional examination procedures should be considered in light of findings from end-feel testing, and future studies that investigate the reliability of Cyriax's classification system as well as experimental studies that seek to identify the outcomes of interventions based on end-feel classification should be conducted.

Capsular Pattern

In the case of a 39-year-old female patient with insidious onset of hip pain, both end-feel examination and examination for capsular/noncapsular patterns were used to successfully screen this patient who required a referral leading to the eventual diagnosis of a non-Hodgkin's lymphoma of the hip.[31]

In five individual cases, Greenwood et al[32] used the concepts of noncapsular patterns and the *sign of the buttock* as screening tools to differentiate between low back pain and pain caused from hip pathology that required a medical referral.[32] On examination, identification of a noncapsular pattern at the hip in conjunction with a positive sign of the buttock is suggestive of hip pathology, the cause of which lies beyond the scope of physical therapy.[32]

Winters et al[33] sought to determine if a cluster analysis using variables related to medical history and physical examination could be used to classify shoulder complaints in 101 patients. Three meaningful and stable clusters arose that were distinguished primarily by the prevalence of various limitations in ROM. However, no specific patterns of motion limitations were found, making a more detailed classification for diagnosis of shoulder pathology challenging.[33] It was proposed that determining patterns of motion loss may be more useful in identifying the degree of inflammation or irritation as opposed to aiding in the establishment of the exact anatomical location of the disorder. This calls into question the Cyriax classification of shoulder dysfunction, which is based, in part, on distinct deficits in ROM. Hayes et al[34] were unable to identify a proportional definition of a capsular pattern in a group of patients with osteoarthritis of the knee. They concluded that the validity of the passive components for identifying patients with osteoarthritis of the knee is questionable.[34]

To investigate the evidence in support of the PROM component (capsular pattern, pain-resistance sequence) of the Cyriax STT testing scheme for patients with knee dysfunction, Fritz et al[35] studied 152 subjects with unilateral knee pain from 15 different centers. They explored the ratio of motion loss of extension to loss of flexion during PROM in patients with and without evidence of arthritis and evaluated the relationship between inflammatory status and the pain-resistance sequence and between chronicity and the pain-resistance sequence. To study this, they recorded ROM, pain-resistance sequence (pain before, during, or after achieving end range), and assessment of inflammation according to the cardinal signs. The results indicated that the capsular pattern for the knee had sensitivity of 74.7% and specificity of 76.7% with a likelihood ratio of 3.20.[35] A subject with a capsular pattern, therefore, was 3.2 times more likely to have arthritis of the knee. Motion loss within a capsular pattern explained 26.4% of variability in the presence or absence of arthritis, confirming the association between arthritis and a capsular pattern.[35] Chronicity and inflammatory status explained 5.3% and 12.3% of the variability in the pain-resistance sequence, respectively.

Deep Friction Massage and Manipulation

Several studies have attempted to explain the morphological changes and therapeutic benefit from use of DFM. Davidson et al[16] attempted to characterize morphological and functional changes in the Achilles tendon of the rat following enzyme-induced injury and subsequent transverse friction massage using an instrument for the application of forces. In addition to revealing poor collagen fiber orientation and the presence of fibroblasts in injured tissue, electron microscopic examination showed rough endoplasmic reticulum, which is a feature of fibroblasts actively making collagen in the groups where friction massage was applied.[16] These findings suggest that friction massage may promote healing through increased fibroblast recruitment.

Most of the clinical studies designed to investigate the effects of DFM on patient populations have been performed using DFM among other forms of intervention. Guler-Uysal and Kozanoglu[36] compared the effects of using a Cyriax approach, which included DFM and manipulation, versus an approach that included heat and diathermy in 40 patients with adhesive capsulitis. Results revealed that 19 patients in the Cyriax group and 13 in the alternate therapy group reached 80% of normal ROM by the second week.[36] Improvement in ROM and a decrease in pain with motion were better in the Cyriax group after the first week of therapy.[36] Verhaar et al[18] compared the effects of local corticosteroid injections with a combination of DFM and manipulation in the management of 106 lateral epicondylitis patients. The OMPT group received 12 interventions over 4 weeks, including DFM and Mills manipulation by experienced therapists.[18] At 6 weeks, the injection group demonstrated an increase in grip strength that was greater than in the OMPT group, and 22 of 53 in the injection group were pain free compared with only 3 in the OMPT group.[18] Although the injection group did better than the OMPT group at 6 weeks, 1 year follow-up revealed no difference between groups.[18] In the study by Nagrale et al,[19] Mills manipulation and DFM was more effective than cortisone phonophoresis in the treatment of tenoperiosteal lateral epicondylitis.[19]

Hurrell and Woodman[14] described the use of DFM in conjunction with scapular taping, scapular stabilization exercises, and neural glides in the care of a patient diagnosed with supraspinatus tendonitis. Results revealed that this patient was able to return to her previous level of functional activity after 18 sessions of physical therapy.[14]

Morphological changes in the targeted soft tissue have been observed in response to DFM. Although several studies exist to support the combined use of DFM and manipulation and the use of these procedures in conjunction with other interventions, at present, there is insufficient evidence to support their sole use in the management of musculoskeletal lesions. To date, to our knowledge, there are no randomized controlled trials to support the use of these interventions.

ACKNOWLEDGMENT

We give special thanks to Jessica Canhao for her contributions to the art in this chapter.

CLINICAL CASE

History of Present Illness: A 65-year-old female states that she has developed a gradual onset of right hip and thigh stiffness and pain. Walking increases the pain. On a bad day, it is difficult to get out of the sitting position. Coughing and sneezing do not increase the pain.

Observation: When ambulating, the patient is observed to have reduced weight bearing on the right, which creates a limp.

ROM: Passive range of motion of right hip internal rotation is severely limited. Flexion, abduction, and extension are moderately limited. External rotation and adduction are within normal limits. All movements have a capsular end-feel. The limited movements reproduce the patient's pain. The pain is only reproducible when overpressure is exerted at end range.

Strength: All muscle tests at the hip are strong and painless.

1. In this case, if passive motion testing was painful with overpressure at end range and resistance testing was strong and painless, what type of lesion would be suspected? What additional information would you need to know to confirm your diagnosis?
2. For the hip, what is the typical capsular (full articular) pattern as defined by Cyriax? If this patient demonstrated a capsular pattern at the hip, based on the remainder of the examination, what structure is the likely cause of the capsular pattern?
3. Given the data from this case, if the patient demonstrated a noncapsular pattern, what would be the likely cause?
4. What information in this case is suggestive of a noncontractile lesion?
5. Based on your diagnosis, select an intervention regimen based on the Cyriax approach to OMPT that may be used in this case. Perform these interventions on a partner.

History of Present Illness: A 50-year-old male states that a few weeks ago he painfully twisted his neck when looking out his car window. The onset of pain was sudden. Originally, he had pain down his arm and into his middle three fingers. Now the pain is almost gone, but he reports pins and needles at the left side of the neck, extending down the arm and into the hand.

Observation: The patient has difficulty actively moving his neck and voluntarily braces.

AROM: Active cervical extension, left rotation, and side bending are about 50% limited. The patient states that these movements increase his pins and needles.

PROM: Passive extension has a bone to bone end-feel, left rotation has a spasm end-feel, and left side bending has a springy end-feel. All of these movements increase the paresthesia.

Strength: Isometric resistive left shoulder adduction, elbow extension, and wrist flexion are weak and painless. Sensation is slightly diminished in the left middle three fingers.

Reflexes: The left triceps reflex is depressed.

Special Tests: Stroking the patients arm and fingers increases the "pins and needles." Moving the digits does not increase the pins and needles.

Radiographs: Radiographs are negative.

1. Based on the results of the movement examination, does this patient have a capsular or noncapsular pattern?
2. Based on Cyriax's classification of spinal intervertebral disc lesions, would you classify this patient's disc lesion as an annular (hard) or nuclear (soft) disc lesion and why?
3. Based on the patient's reported symptoms at the time of onset, what structure is likely being compressed and at what level?
4. This patient reports a change in symptoms from arm pain to pins and needles. Explain anatomically what has likely occurred to produce such a change.
5. Based on the list of muscles that are weak and painless and the location of diminished sensation, what is the suspected level of compression?

HANDS-ON

With a partner, perform the following:

1 Using the checklist below, perform selective tissue tension testing on your partner's elbow and document your findings. Because of its relationship to the elbow, be sure to include wrist muscle testing during your examination. Switch partners and perform STT testing on your partner's shoulder.

ISOMETRIC TESTING	STRONG/PAINLESS	STRONG/PAINFUL	WEAK/PAINLESS	WEAK/PAINFUL
Elbow Flexion				
Elbow Extension				
Elbow Supination				
Elbow Pronation				
Wrist Extension				
Wrist Flexion				

2 On a partner, test the end-feel for each joint and complete the following table. Compare your partner's end-feel with the expected normal end-feel for each specific joint. Perform end-feel examinations on one other person and note any differences between individuals. Note the type of end-feel as defined by Cyriax as well as the place in the range of motion where the end-feel occurs.

JOINT	MOTION	NORMAL END-FEEL	OBSERVED END-FEEL SUBJECT 1	OBSERVED END-FEEL SUBJECT 2
Shoulder				
Elbow				
Wrist				
Metacarpophalangeal				
Hip				

3 On your partner, palpate the common wrist extensor tendon just distal to the lateral epicondyle. According to Cyriax's guidelines, perform deep friction massage on your partner. Repeat the same procedure on the long head of the biceps tendon as it lies within the bicipital groove of the humerus. During performance of DFM, be sure to follow Cyriax's guidelines using proper depth and direction.

REFERENCES

1. American Physical Therapy Association. *Code of Ethics and Guide for Professional Conduct.* 2nd ed. Fairfax, VA: American Physical Therapy Association; 2003.
2. Ombregt L, Bisschop P, ter Veer H, eds. *A System of Orthopaedic Medicine.* 2nd ed. Philadelphia, PA: Churchill Livingstone; 2003.
3. Dreyfuss P, Tibiletti C, Dreyer SJ. Thoracic zygapophyseal joint pain patterns. *Spine.* 1994;19:807-811.
4. Slipman CW, Lipetz JS, Plastaras HB, Yang ST, Meyer AM. Therapeutic zygapophyseal joint injections for headaches emanating from the C 2-3 joint. *Amer J Phys Med Rehab.* 2001;80:182-188.
5. Cyriax J. *Textbook of Orthopaedic Medicine, Volume One.* 8th ed. London: Bailliere Tindall; 1982.
6. Xin SQ, Zhang QZ, Fan DH. Significance of the straight-leg-raising test in the diagnosis and clinical evaluation of lower lumbar intervertebral-disc protrusion. *J Bone Joint Surg Am.* 1987;69:517-522.
7. Brismee JM. Rate of false positive using the Cyriax release test for thoracic outlet syndrome in an asymptomatic population. *J Man Manip Ther.* 2004;12:73-81.
8. Sutterlin CE, Gutentag I, Martinez CR, Rechtine GR. False-positive diagnosis of an odontoid fracture by CT scan. *J Orthop Trauma.* 1989;3:348-351.
9. Yinggang Z, Liew SM, Simmons E. Value of magnetic resonance imaging and discography in determining level of cervical discectomy and fusion. *Spine.* 2004;29:2140-2145.
10. Pellecchia GL, Paolino J, Connell J. Intertester reliability of the Cyriax evaluation in assessing patients with shoulder pain. *J Orthop Sports Phys Ther.* 1996;23:34-38.
11. Zimny NJ. Clinical reasoning in the evaluation and management of undiagnosed chronic hip pain in a young adult. *Phys Ther.* 1998;78:62-72.
12. Fritz JM, Delitto A, Erhard RE, Roman M. An examination of the selective tissue tension scheme, with evidence for the concept of a capsular pattern of the knee. *Phys Ther.* 1998;78:1046-1056.
13. Philbin T, Donley B. When do you x-ray ankle sprains in patients with acute ankle injuries? *Cleveland Clinic Journal of Medicine.* 2000;67:405-406.
14. Hurrell JE, Woodman RM. Diagnosis and intervention for a patient with shoulder and scapula pain. *Phys Ther Case Reports.* 1999;2:175-187.
15. DeBruijn R. Deep transverse friction: its analgesic effect. *Int J Sports Med.* 1984;5:35-36.
16. Davidson CJ, Ganion LR, Gehlsen GM, et al. Rat tendon morphologic and functional changes resulting from soft tissue mobilization. *Med Sci Sports Exerc.* 1997;29:313-319.
17. Stratford PW. The evaluation of phonophoresis and friction massage as treatments for extensor carpi radialis tendonitis: a randomized trial. *Physiother Canada.* 1989;41:93-98.
18. Verhaar JAN, Walenkamp GHIM, Van Mameren H, Kester ADM, Van Der Linden AJ. Local corticosteroid injection versus Cyriax-type physiotherapy for tennis elbow. *J Bone Joint Surg Am.* 1996;78:128-132.
19. Nagrale AV, Herd CR, Ganvir S, Ramteke G. Cyriax physiotherapy versus phonophoresis with supervised exercise in subjects with lateral epicondylalgia: a randomized clinical trial. *J Man Manip Ther.* 2009;17:171-178.
20. Thelander U. Straight leg raising test versus radiological size, shape are of lumbar disc hernias. *Spine.* 1992;17:395-399.
21. Kosteljantez MN, Bang F, Schmidt-Olsen S. The clinical significance of straight-leg raising (Laseague's sign) in the diagnosis of prolapsed lumbar disc. Interobserver variation and correlation with surgical finding. *Spine.* 1988;13:393-395.
22. Vucetic N, Svensson O. Physical signs in lumbar disc hernia. *Clin Ortho Rel Res.* 1996;333:192-201.
23. Hurley DA, McDonough SM, Baxter GD, Dempster M, Moore AP. A descriptive study of the usage of spinal manipulative therapy techniques within a randomized clinical trial in acute low back pain. *Man Ther.* 2005;10:61-67.
24. Huss CD, Puhl JJ. Myositis ossificans of the upper arm. *Amer J Sports Med.* 1980;8:419-424.
25. Franklin M, Conner-Kerr T, Chamness M, et al. Assessment of exercise-induced minor muscle lesions: the accuracy of Cyriax's diagnosis by selective tension paradigm. *J Orthop Sports Phys Ther.* 1996;24:122-129.
26. Hanchard NCA, Howe TE, Gilbert MM. Diagnosis of shoulder pain by history and selective tissue tension: agreement between assessors. *J Orthop Sports Phys Ther.* 2005;35:147-153.
27. Borsa PA, Sauers EL, Herling DE, Manzour WF. In vivo quantification of capsular end-point in the nonimpaired glenohumeral joint using an instrumented measurement system. *J Orthop Sports Phys Ther.* 2001;31: 419-431.
28. Chesworth BM, MacDermid JC, Roth JH, Patterson SD. Movement diagram and "end-feel" reliability when measuring passive lateral rotation of the shoulder in patients with shoulder pathology. *Phys Ther.* 1998;78:593-601.
29. Maher C, Adams R. Reliability of pain and stiffness assessments in clinical manual lumbar spine examination. *Phys Ther.* 1994;74:801-811.
30. Petersen CM, Hayes KW. Construct validity of Cyriax's selective tension examination: association of end-feels with pain at the knee and shoulder. *J Orthop Sports Phys Ther.* 2000;30:512-527.
31. Browder DA, Erhard RE. Decision-making for a painful hip: a case requiring referral. *J Orthop Sports Phys Ther.* 2005;35:738-744.
32. Greenwood MJ, Erhard RE, Jones DL. Differential diagnosis of the hip vs. lumbar spine: five case reports. *J Orthop Sports Phys Ther.* 1998;27:308-315.
33. Winters JC, Groenier KH, Sobel JS, Arendzen HH, Jongh BM. Classification of shoulder complaints in general practice by means of cluster analysis. *Arch Phys Med Rehabil.* 1997;78:1369-1374.
34. Hayes KW, Petersen C, Falconer J. An examination of Cyriax's passive motion tests with patients having osteoarthritis of the knee. *Phys Ther.* 1994;74:697-707.
35. Fritz JM, Delitto A, Erhard RE, Roman M. An examination of the selective tissue tension scheme, with evidence for the concept of a capsular pattern. *Phys Ther.* 1998;78:1046-1061.
36. Guler-Uysal F, Kozanoglu E. Comparison of the early response to two methods of rehabilitation in adhesive capsulitis. *Swiss Med Weekly.* 2004;134:353-358.

CHAPTER
6

The Nordic Approach

Christopher H. Wise, PT, DPT, OCS, FAAOMPT, MTC, ATC

Chapter Objectives

At the conclusion of this chapter, the reader will be able to:

- Discuss the important contributions of Freddy Kaltenborn to the specialty of orthopaedic manual physical therapy (OMPT).
- Describe the contribution of Olaf Evjenth to the Nordic approach.
- Discuss the major foundational principles upon which the Nordic approach is established and the other approaches to OMPT that have been most influential in its development.
- Define the primary philosophical framework upon which this approach has been grounded.
- Define the terms used to describe joint positioning within this approach.

- Describe the concept of joint roll-gliding and the convex-concave theory.
- Define the term "treatment plane" and how this concept can be used when mobilizing joints.
- Define the Kaltenborn grades of joint mobilization.
- Discuss the concept of trial treatment and how this may be used in the OMPT management of a patient.
- Describe what "tests of function" are and how they can be used during the OMPT examination.
- Define the Kaltenborn classification of end-feels.
- Match the type of mobilization grade with its indication.
- Identify the factors that distinguish the Nordic approach from other OMPT approaches.

HISTORICAL PERSPECTIVES

The *Nordic approach* to orthopaedic manual physical therapy (OMPT) emerged in the 1940s when its founder, *Freddy Kaltenborn*, became frustrated with the ineffectiveness of current physical therapy interventions in the management of spinal disorders. Although there have been many contributors, Kaltenborn is recognized as the founder of the Nordic approach to OMPT. Kaltenborn's career began as a physical educator in Germany in 1945. In 1949, he became a physical therapist in Norway, at which time he became aware of the limitations of massage, mobilization, and active and passive movement in the care of his patients. Kaltenborn soon turned to the principles and strategies that were being used by two prominent physicians of the day, *Dr. James Mennell* and *Dr. James Cyriax*.

NOTABLE QUOTABLE

"What I especially like about [this approach] is the marriage of functional anatomy to clinical practice."

Michael A. MacConaill, 1980

In the early 1950s, Kaltenborn traveled to London where he studied under Mennell and Cyriax and subsequently brought the principles that he had gleaned back to Norway. In 1954, Kaltenborn taught his first course on Cyriax's approach to manual therapy. In 1955, Cyriax's visit to Norway led to the formation of the *Norwegian Manipulation Group*. This group of physical therapists applied Cyriax's concepts to the development of a specialized manual therapy approach.

In 1958, an osteopath, *Alan Stoddard*, began to work with Kaltenborn in the development of these new concepts. At the time, Stoddard was using specific osteopathic techniques in the management of spinal conditions and was introducing them to the profession of physical therapy. Between 1958 and the early 1960s, Kaltenborn continued to collaborate with both Cyriax and Stoddard as he attempted to blend both approaches into one unified concept. Kaltenborn also began to interject his own theories into this newly evolving system. His greatest early contribution to the specialty area of OMPT was the emphasis that he placed on biomechanical principles as they related to examination and intervention.

In 1973, a physical therapist by the name of *Olaf Evjenth* brought an emphasis on muscle stretching, strengthening, and coordination into the approach. Evjenth added methods of assessing performance to the examination process and introduced symptom alleviation testing as a method for the localization of lesions. The collaboration between Kaltenborn and Evjenth spawned a new comprehensive and eclectic manual therapy approach. Over the years, the Nordic approach to OMPT has also become known as the *Kaltenborn-Evjenth concept*. The hallmark of this approach, which continues to evolve, is its emphasis on joint kinematics and the eclectic nature of its principles and techniques (Fig. 6-1).[1]

The Nordic approach was first presented worldwide in 1973. In 1974, Kaltenborn and *Geoffrey Maitland*, among others, founded the *International Federation of Orthopaedic Manipulative Physical Therapists (IFOMPT)* (see Chapter 1). The concepts and techniques described within this chapter are based almost entirely upon Kaltenborn's two texts on mobilization of the spine and mobilization of the extremities.[1,2]

PHILOSOPHICAL FRAMEWORK

The Nordic approach is unique in its philosophical orientation largely because concepts from a myriad of other approaches have been incorporated into this system. The principles used within this approach have been derived from sources both within and outside of the profession of physical therapy. At the philosophical core of this approach lies a preoccupation with the biomechanical principles that govern movement. These principles include an appreciation for the **convex-concave theory**, the use of *rotational motion* and *translatory gliding* in examination and intervention, the *grading of movement*, and the use of the *trial treatment* to determine efficacy. During examination, pain, joint dysfunction, and soft tissue changes are identified and evaluated in combination.[2]

Foundational Principles and Operational Definitions

When examining the motion characteristics of a joint or when using mobilization techniques to resolve movement impairments and restore full function, the Nordic approach advocates the use of three-dimensional joint positioning and grading.

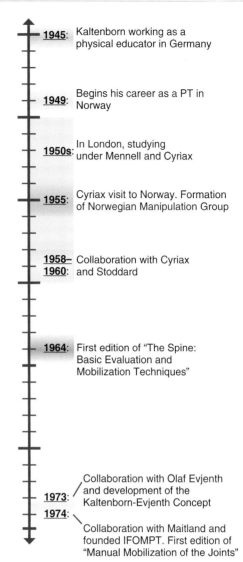

FIGURE 6-1. F.M. Kaltenborn's professional timeline.

The **zero position** is a term that is used synonymously with anatomical position. All range-of-motion measurements are taken from the zero starting position. The **resting position** is defined as the **open-packed position**, in which the periarticular structures have their highest degree of laxity allowing for the greatest range of joint mobility. During examination, the therapist attempts to achieve the resting position of the joint in all three planes, at which time the degree of mobility is evaluated in all directions. The resting position varies greatly among individuals and is best identified by recruiting motion in each of the three cardinal planes with subtle repositioning while assessing the degree of mobility in each plane. The position that allows the greatest ease of movement in all three planes is the resting position for that joint. This position encourages muscle relaxation and is often the patient's position of optimal comfort (Fig. 6-2, Table 6-1).

When it is impossible, difficult, or impractical to achieve the true resting position, the therapist places the joint in the position in which the least amount of tension is elicited and where the patient reports the least discomfort. This position

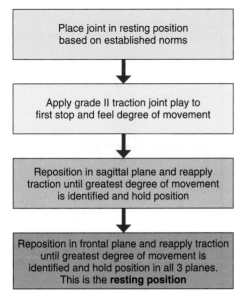

FIGURE 6–2. Sequence of procedures for finding the three-dimensional resting position of a joint.[3]

is known as the **actual resting position.** The **non-resting position** is defined as any position that is outside of the resting position. There is less joint mobility in this position, and more skill is required to perform techniques with the patient in this position. Subtle dysfunctions may only be seen and treated in these non-resting positions. A specific example of the non-resting position is the **close-packed position.** In the close-packed position, the joint capsule and ligaments are maximally

tensed and there is maximal congruency of articular surfaces. In this position, joint mobility is considered to be most limited.[1,3]

The Spinal Motion Segment

The Nordic approach to OMPT requires the manual physical therapist to possess an intimate knowledge of joint kinematics. The **spinal motion segment** is defined as a three-joint complex that includes the facet joints and the intervertebral disc. Although each aspect of the motion segment serves a distinct role, each component is functionally interdependent. Spinal motion requires coordination among all of the component parts of the motion segment.[1]

Bone Rotations and Translations

To restore normal movement patterns, the manual physical therapist must possess a thorough understanding of bone rotations and translations, as well as corresponding *joint movements* that occur under normal conditions. **Bone rotational movement** is used to refer to movement that occurs around an axis, whereas **bone translational movements** are linear motions that occur parallel to an axis in one particular plane. Bone rotational movements that are classified as *standard*, or *uniaxial*, are motions that occur around one axis in one plane, and they are often referred to as **anatomical movements.** Bone rotational movements that occur simultaneously around more than one axis in more than one plane are called combined, or **multi-axial movements.** This type of motion is often referred to

Table 6–1	Resting and Non-Resting Positions of Selected Synovial Joints Along With Each Joint's Inherent Convex-Concave Relationships and Suspected Capsular Patterns as Described by Kaltenborn				
JOINT	**RESTING POSITION (OPEN-PACKED)**	**NON-RESTING POSITION (CLOSE-PACKED)**	**CONCAVE**	**CONVEX**	**CAPSULAR PATTERN**
TibioFemoral	25° Flexion	Maximum Extension Maximum Tibia External Rotation	Tibial plateaus	Femoral condyles	Flexion > Extension (9:1)
Superior Tibia/Fibula	Resting	—	Posterolateral Tibial facet	Fibular head	—
Inferior Tibia/Fibula	—	—	Tibial facet	Facet fibula	—
Talocrural	10° Plantarflexion	Maximum Dorsiflexion	Distal Tibia/ Fibula	Talus	Plantarflexion > Dorsiflexion
Subtalar			Variable alternating facets	Variable alternating facets	Valgus > Varus
Metatarsophalangeal 2–5	Slight Flexion	Maximum Extension	Phalanx	Metacarpal	Flexion mostly limited
Metatarsophalangeal 1	5°–10° Extension	Maximum Extension	Phalanx	Metacarpal	Extension mostly limited

Every synovial joint has a position in which the periarticular structures demonstrate the greatest degree of laxity, thus allowing the greatest degree of joint play. This position, known as the resting or open-packed position, is often the position of maximal comfort. The non-resting position is any position that is other than the resting position, of which the closed-packed position is one. In this position, periarticular structures are maximally taut, and there is maximal contact between the articular surfaces of the joint. In this position, joint play is maximally reduced, thus making joint mobilization challenging. Novice therapists are encouraged to position the joint in the resting position prior to mobilization.

as **functional movement** because it represents the manner in which joints traditionally move.

Combined movements may be further subdivided into **coupled** or **noncoupled movements.** Coupled movements are motions that are mechanically forced to occur together.[1,3] For example, midcervical side bending and rotation occur ipsilaterally. These coupled movements are mechanically forced to occur together regardless of the starting position and are based on the structure of the joints.[1] Noncoupled movements describe motions that do not invariably occur together, but rather may occur together depending on the condition. For example, in the thoracolumbar spine, side bending and rotation are considered to be noncoupled movements**.**

Noncoupled movements may be used during intervention in an attempt to lock or inhibit motion in joints adjacent to the targeted region. For example, C4-C7 may be pre-positioned in side bending to the right to reduce forces through these segments as a mobilization force for rotation to the left is initiated at C3-C4. In addition to standard and combined rotational movements, bone movements may also be considered to undergo translational movements that are linear movements occurring parallel to an axis in either the *sagittal*, *longitudinal*, or *frontal plane*.

Joint Roll-Gliding and Translatory Joint Play

Joint movement, also known as accessory, or arthrokinematic, movement accompanies bone movement. Joint **roll-gliding** occurs during bone rotational movements, and **translatory joint play** occurs during bone translatory movements. Roll-gliding is a combined movement that occurs within the joint in response to bone rotations. Rolling predominates when joint surfaces are less congruent, and gliding predominates when joint surfaces are more congruent. **Rolling** is defined as new points on one surface coming into contact with new points on another surface. Rolling typically occurs in the same direction as bone movement (Fig. 6-3). **Gliding** occurs when the same point on one surface comes in contact with new points on another surface (Fig. 6-4).

The direction in which glide occurs is dependent upon what is known as the Kaltenborn *convex-concave theory*. This concept is based on the relationship between rotations of bone and their corresponding joint glides.[3] When the convex aspect of

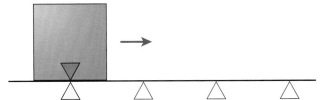

FIGURE 6–4. Glide occurs when the joint is congruent and the same point on one surface contacts new points on opposing surface. The direction of joint glide depends on the concave-convex theory.

the joint rotates on the concave aspect, then glide occurs in the direction that is opposite to the movement of the bone, or osteokinematic motion. In this case, mobilization to restore glide must be in the opposite direction from the osteokinematic motion (Fig. 6-5). The opposite is true when the concave aspect of the joint rotates on the convex aspect. Glide and subsequent mobilization occurs in the same direction as the osteokinematic motion (Fig. 6-6).

The restoration of normal joint glide must be accomplished for normal mobility to be restored. To restore normal mobility

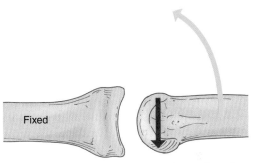

FIGURE 6–5. The Kaltenborn convex-concave theory. The yellow curved arrow indicates the direction of osteokinematic motion. The red arrow indicates the direction of arthrokinematic joint glide. When the convex aspect of the joint moves on the fixed concave aspect, joint glide is in the direction opposite the osteokinematic motion. In such cases, joint mobilization should include joint glide in the direction opposite the osteokinematic motion. For example, glenohumeral elevation should improve with inferiorly directed joint glide mobilizations.

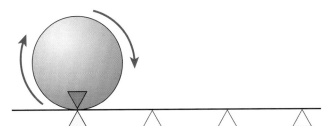

FIGURE 6–3. Roll occurs when friction is high and surfaces are incongruent, concave is at least as large as convex surface, new points on one surface meet new points on the opposing surface, and it always occurs in same direction as osteokinematic motion.

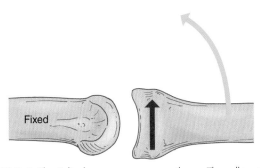

FIGURE 6–6. The Kaltenborn convex-concave theory. The yellow curved arrow indicates the direction of osteokinematic motion. The red arrow indicates the direction of arthrokinematic joint glide. When the concave aspect of the joint moves on the fixed convex aspect, joint glide is in the same direction as osteokinematic motion. In such cases, joint mobilization should include joint glide in the same direction as osteokinematic motion. For example, open chain knee extension should improve with anteriorly directed joint glide mobilizations.

to a glenohumeral joint with restrictions into forward elevation, where the convex aspect of the joint is moving on the concave, joint glide mobilization that is inferiorly directed is
indicated. Conversely, to restore normal mobility to a knee
joint with restrictions into open chain knee extension, where
the concave aspect of the joint is moving on the convex, joint
glide mobilization that is anteriorly directed is indicated (see
Table 6-1).

Translatory joint play occurs in conjunction with bone
translatory movement. The Nordic approach places the examination and restoration of normal joint play in high regard.
Joint play is defined as the small amount of motion available
at end range of all movements and is not under voluntary control. Joint play movements are easiest to produce and palpate
in a joint's resting position. These movements are considered
to be essential to the performance of active movement and in
the prevention of injury.

The Treatment Plane

To understand joint play, it is imperative that the manual physical therapist is first able to visualize the Kaltenborn **treatment
plane** of the joint in question. The treatment plane passes
through the joint and is positioned at a right angle to a line
that runs from the axis of rotation of the convex aspect of the
joint to the deepest portion of the concave aspect of the joint.
Simply defined, the treatment plane is delineated by a line
drawn across the concave aspect of the joint.

The translatory joint play movements used within this approach are traction, compression, and glide, which accompany
bone translatory movement. Each type of joint play movement
is defined according to its relationship to the treatment plane.
Traction occurs perpendicular to the treatment plane in a direction that is away from the joint. **Compression** occurs perpendicular to the treatment plane in a direction that is toward
the joint. **Glide** occurs parallel to the treatment plane.

Based on the fact that the treatment plane is determined
by the concave aspect of the joint, when the concave aspect
moves, so does the treatment plane. Consequently, the direction of applied traction, compression, and gliding forces must
also change in direction when the concave aspect of the joint
is moved out of the neutral position. The manual physical

therapist must be careful to appreciate even minor changes in
joint position and alter the direction in which forces are applied accordingly (Fig. 6-7a,b).

Hypomobility within a joint usually involves a restriction
in normal joint glide. The goal of manual physical therapy is
to evaluate the presence of impaired joint glide through either
the **direct** or the **indirect method**. The direct method uses the
glide test and is the preferred method because it provides the
most accurate information regarding end-feel and the extent
and nature of the gliding restriction. The glide test involves
passive translation of the joint in all directions for the purpose
of identifying specific limitations. The indirect method uses
the Kaltenborn convex-concave theory to deduce the direction
of decreased joint gliding based on whether the moving portion
is the convex or concave aspect of the joint, as previously
described. This approach is useful for joints with a small degree
of motion, in cases of severe pain, or for novice therapists who
have difficulty with perceiving motion using the glide test.
The indirect method is most often used; however, the manual
physical therapist must be aware of the limitations of using this
method and is encouraged to use the glide test in all directions
when routinely examining joint movement.

Grades of Mobilization

For the purpose of documentation and repetition of a technique on subsequent visits, it is important for the manual physical therapist to assign grades to the mobilizations being
performed. The ability to perform graded mobilization on a
joint is dependent on the therapist's skill in determining when
tissues that cross the joint are in either a *slackened* or *tightened*
position. These movements are best identified with the joint
in its resting position.

Within this approach, there are three distinct grades in
which mobilization techniques may be applied (Fig. 6-8).
Grade I techniques consist of small amplitude motions without joint separation. These techniques are designed to produce joint *loosening* and are typically used for pain modulation
through the firing of joint mechanoreceptors. With Grade I
techniques, there is no significant separation of joint surfaces.

During **Grade II** mobilization, a *tightening* of periarticular
structures occurs as the slack is taken up in the tissues about the
joint. Grade II techniques are used effectively for pain modulation and mobilization of the joint in the absence of shortened
connective tissues. The **slack zone (SZ)** is located at the beginning of Grade II movement. Within the SZ, there is minimal
resistance to movement. Within the **transition zone (TZ)**, tissues become taut and more resistance is appreciated. The **first
stop** is where marked resistance is felt toward the end of the
Grade II motion. For stretching to occur, the joint must be
brought beyond the first stop. Grade II mobilizations are used to
test joint play traction and glide, relieve pain, and increase motion.

Once the tissues are brought beyond the TZ, **Grade III**
mobilization occurs. These techniques involve enough force
to *stretch* the tissues crossing the joint. Grade III mobilizations
are typically used to test end-feel and to increase the range of
joint motion.[1,3]

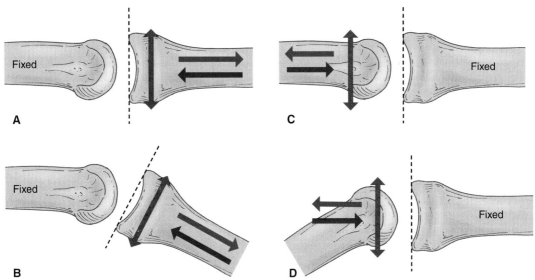

FIGURE 6–7. A. Joint mobilization of the concave aspect of a typical synovial joint upon its convex counterpart. **B.** The direction of mobilizing forces changes when the joint is moved out of the neutral position. **C.** Joint mobilization of the convex aspect of a typical synovial joint upon its concave counterpart. **D.** The direction of mobilizing forces remains the same when the joint is moved out of the neutral position. Dotted line indicates the treatment plane (TP) determined by the concave aspect of the joint and is at a right angle to a line drawn from the axis of rotation to the center of the concave articulating surface. Red arrow indicates the direction of joint glide that is parallel to the TP. Green arrow indicates the direction of joint distraction that is perpendicular and away from the TP. Purple arrow indicates the direction of joint compression that is perpendicular and toward the TP. (From: Wise CH, Gulick DT. *Mobilization Notes: A Rehabilitation Specialist's Pocket Guide.* Philadelphia, PA: F.A. Davis Company; 2009, with permission.)

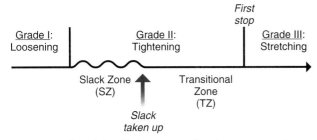

FIGURE 6–8. The relationship between grades of movement and resistance (From: Kaltenborn FM. *Manual Mobilization of the Joints: The Kaltenborn Method of Joint Examination and Treatment. Volume I: The Extremities.* 6th ed. Oslo, Norway: Olaf Norlis Bokhandel; 2002, with permission.)

PRINCIPLES OF EXAMINATION
Guiding Concepts

Within the Nordic approach to OMPT, the three primary objectives of the examination process include identification of the physical diagnosis, defining the indications and contraindications to manual physical therapy, and establishing a baseline for measuring progress. The physical diagnosis is based on joint biomechanics. Unlike the medical diagnosis, which rules out serious pathology that mimics musculoskeletal dysfunction, the physical therapy diagnosis focuses on a more detailed biomechanical assessment and the structures that may be contributing to the patient's functional limitations. The eclectic nature of this approach becomes evident as we explore the primary components of the examination process. The examination process is based on a model of *somatic dysfunction* that assumes an interdependent relationship between signs and symptoms. In the presence of musculoskeletal dysfunction, a clear relationship between signs and symptoms typically suggests that the condition will respond well to manual intervention. A condition that lacks such a correlation may indicate that the patient's presenting symptoms are originating from a structure outside the musculoskeletal system.

Somatic dysfunction typically presents as impairment of the musculoskeletal system, along with a myriad of impairments in related systems such as the neurovascular, lymphatic, and cardiopulmonary systems. The manual physical therapist uses the musculoskeletal system as a window into the specific nature of the many structures that may be contributing to the constellation of impairments that characterizes the somatic dysfunction. It is presumed that a skilled manual physical therapist may have the ability, through careful palpation and identification of subtle alterations in movement quality, to identify the exact nature of the somatic dysfunction before a medical diagnosis can be made.

The manual physical therapist also uses the examination process to identify the indications and contraindications to intervention. Indications are based primarily on the biomechanically based physical diagnosis rather than on the medical diagnosis. The presence of hypomobility through identification of restricted joint play and abnormal end-feel are the two primary indicators that suggest the use of mobilization techniques. Excessive joint play requires the use of stabilization techniques. General contraindications relate primarily to concomitant health concerns that reduce the body's tolerance for mechanical forces, such as *neoplasms* and various congenital abnormalities. Screening tests are used to identify any antecedent conditions that may serve as contraindications to specific mobilization techniques.

The third objective of the examination process is to establish a baseline for the purpose of measuring progress. The manual physical therapist seeks to identify changes in the patient's condition through the identification of a **dominant sign.** A dominant sign is a reproducible physical examination finding that relates to the patient's reported chief complaint. For example, the presence of headaches may correlate with the dominant sign of restricted suboccipital mobility, which when tested reproduces the exact nature of the patient's headaches. Continual reexamination of the relationship between the patient's chief complaint and the dominant physical signs interspersed with intervention throughout the course of a single therapy session will serve to guide the manual physical therapist.

Distinguishing the manifestations of somatic dysfunction is necessary in order to administer the most appropriate plan of care. Following careful examination, the manual physical therapist determines if the locus of pathology is in the joint or related soft tissue, if the joint is *hypomobile* or *hypermobile*, and whether or not intervention should be directed toward pain control or biomechanical dysfunction.

When an individual presents with shoulder pain, reduced motion, and functional limitations of the shoulder, it is imperative that the therapist first differentiate between degenerative changes within the glenohumeral, acromioclavicular, or sternoclavicular joints versus supraspinatus tendonopathy, among other things. The second diagnostic decision attempts to identify the presence of hypo- or hypermobility. This distinction is often challenging because hypermobility may mimic hypomobility through voluntary or involuntary muscle guarding. In the case of shoulder pathology, the manual physical therapist will use traction, glide, and compressive passive movements to delineate the movement characteristics of the joint. The patient's level of irritability during the examination procedures will determine whether intervention should be directed toward pain control or whether the underlying biomechanical tissue can be treated directly. In addition to the patient's history, the manual physical therapist may determine the focus of intervention through correlating the onset of symptoms with the range of motion. An individual with pain that occurs early in the range before tissue resistance is experienced can be classified as being irritable and may require intervention that is focused primarily on pain control, compared to an individual with pain only at end range who may tolerate intervention that is directed toward the biomechanical dysfunction at fault.

Once the objectives of the examination have been met, the manual physical therapist attempts to confirm the initial physical diagnosis of somatic dysfunction by using a **trial treatment** approach. A low-risk intervention procedure is chosen and implemented based on the therapist's physical

diagnosis. Immediately after the intervention has been rendered, the patient is reexamined in an attempt to identify a change in the patient's chief complaint or dominant sign. If there is no change or there is a worsening in any of these parameters, further evaluation and use of a different trial treatment is warranted. The hallmark of this approach is the ongoing nature of the examination process that occurs at the time of each subsequent session; it is not viewed as a single event but rather a series of events that leads to the continual refinement of the physical diagnosis (Fig. 6-9).

QUESTIONS *for* REFLECTION

What would you choose to do next if your patient responded to their initial low-risk *trial treatment* as follows?

- Experienced a 50% improvement in range of motion.
- Experienced pain that increased from a 3/10 to 7/10 level.
- Experienced no change in the quantity of motion or symptoms.
- Experienced only slight changes in the quantity of motion and symptoms.
- Experienced an increase in symptoms that lasted 48 hours following the intervention.

The Patient History

During the patient history, it is incumbent on the manual physical therapist to identify the mechanical characteristics of the patient's presenting complaints. The specific mechanical factors, such as movement pattern or position, that produces the onset of symptoms must be identified so that they can be further explored during the physical examination. To provide the most relevant information to the manual physical therapist, it is recommended that the examination be scheduled during the symptomatic period. In so doing, the impact of examination procedures on the patient's symptoms can be better evaluated.

NOTABLE QUOTABLE

"To comfort always, to alleviate often, to cure sometimes: These are the three aims of the healer."

Michael A. MacConaill, 1980

The Physical Examination

The primary objective of the physical examination is to correlate the physical signs with the patient's presenting symptoms. The presence of a relationship between the patient's complaints and the findings of the physical examination suggests that the condition is mechanical in origin and will likely respond to manual intervention. The components of the physical

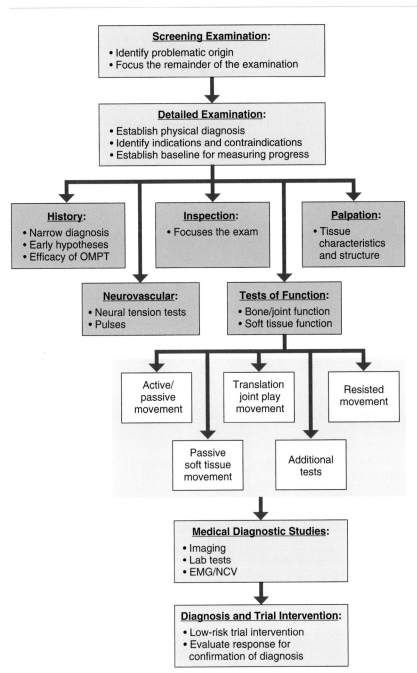

FIGURE 6–9. Nordic approach to OMPT examination scheme.[1]

examination include *inspection, palpation, neurological and vascular tests,* and *tests of function.*

The *palpation* component of the examination progresses from superficial to deep structures, with comparisons made between palpation findings in weight-bearing compared to non-weight-bearing postures. Palpation during activity and performing tests of function provides useful information as well. Palpation during passive movement testing is of particular value. Palpation of positional faults is deemed unreliable and invalid in the absence of confirmatory movement findings. The challenge of palpating bony landmarks and identifying positional faults reliably suggests that the therapist should place a greater level of confidence in the results of movement testing.

Neurological and vascular testing is part of the standard examination process. The examination often begins with neurological scans that quickly alert the therapist of the possible presence of neurological involvement. Tests designed to assess neural mobility are often used and are routinely performed in both weight-bearing and non-weight-bearing positions. Neural mobility is also tested in the positions in which the patient expresses symptoms. In addition to performing the typical myotomal strength testing, the manual physical therapist is also encouraged to test muscle fatigability, or endurance. Vascular testing is also performed in weight-bearing and non-weight-bearing positions. Screening maneuvers, such as the vertebral artery test, is advocated prior to performance of rotational techniques to the cervical spine during examination and intervention. The results of neurological testing are not considered in isolation but rather are viewed in relation to the results from other portions of the examination.

QUESTIONS *for* REFLECTION

What is the value of performing *neurological* and *vascular tests* in weight-bearing and non-weight-bearing positions? How might the change in position alter the results of these tests?

A key differentiating concept of this approach is what is known as *tests of function*. During this aspect of the examination, the manual physical therapist seeks to assess the quality and quantity of motion while also monitoring the patient's symptomatic behavior. The therapist pays particular attention to whether or not the patient's reported symptoms influence movement. Localization of a lesion is possible if the therapist is able to either provoke or alleviate symptoms with a particular maneuver. Tests of function can be divided into bone/joint function tests and soft tissue function tests.

Bone/Joint function testing can be further subdivided into active movements, which examine rotations of joints and passive movements, including examination of rotations and translations and the use of localization tests. During bone/joint active movement testing, standard, uniaxial motions are performed, followed by combined or multiaxial motions. During bone/joint function testing, both the quantity and quality of motion is observed. Active range of motion for both standard and combined movements is tested, followed by passive range of motion with overpressure. Typically, examination of passive range begins where active movement stops; therefore, the range of passive motion with overpressure should be greater than the range of active movement. It is important to test motion slowly through the entire range until the first stop is appreciated. For smaller joints, the manual physical therapist may test range using rapid oscillations first, after which more careful examination may be performed. The presence of hypo- or hypermobility is considered pathological only if it is associated with symptoms and a pathological end-feel. Careful examination must be performed in all directions because a joint may be hypomobile in one direction and hypermobile in another direction (Fig. 6-10). Following manual examination, joint range of motion may be graded using the following classification system: Grade 0–2 indicates hypomobility; Grade 3 indicates normal range of motion; and Grade 4–6 indicates hypermobility (Fig. 6-11).

QUESTIONS *for* REFLECTION

What region would be implicated if, during *joint function testing* using active range of motion, cervical flexion produced symptoms but cervical flexion with the upper cervical spine in extension neither produced nor increased symptoms?

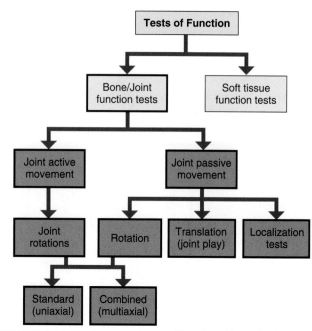

FIGURE 6–10. Nordic approach tests of function with emphasis on bone/joint function testing.[3]

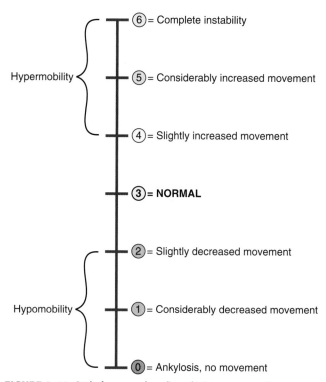

FIGURE 6–11. Scale for manual grading of joint movement.[3]

Along with quantifying joint movement, the quality of movement must also be considered. The ability to feel movement quality in a joint serves to identify slight alterations that lead to a correct diagnosis. To test movement quality, the therapist first observes active, then passive, movement until the first stop. It is important to consider quality early in the range since subtle abnormalities may be realized long before the first stop is experienced. **End-feel** is the sensation imparted to the therapist's hands at the limit of available range after the first stop during passive movement. End-feel can be evaluated during passive rotations and translations and must be done carefully and slowly so as to differentiate normal or physiologic from pathological end-feels. Examination of end-feel can be performed during standard and combined rotatory movements or during translational joint play movements. End-feel is tested slowly and carefully from the first stop to the final stop (Fig. 6-12).

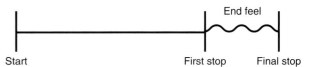

FIGURE 6–12. The relationship between end-feel and first and final stop. (From: Kaltenborn FM. *Manual Mobilization of the Joints: The Kaltenborn Method of Joint Examination and Treatment. Volume I: The Extremities.* 6th ed. Oslo, Norway: Olaf Norlis Bokhandel; 2002, with permission.)

CLINICAL PILLAR

End-feels are considered to be normal if the following is true:

- They occur at an end range that is considered to be normal for the joint being tested.
- They demonstrate characteristics that are considered to be normal for the joint being tested.
- They are pain free.

QUESTIONS *for* REFLECTION

- Why must the manual therapist be sure to examine both movement *quality* as well as movement *quantity*?
- What type of information can be obtained through the careful examination of movement *quality* that cannot be found with examination of movement *quantity* alone?
- Why do many therapists preferentially focus on examination of movement *quantity* without consideration of movement *quality*?

In a normally functioning joint, the therapist carefully applies more force once the first stop has been met and experiences one of three types of physiologic end-feels. Each of these

normal end-feels are symptom free and display varying degrees of elasticity. A **soft end-feel** is the result of soft tissue approximation or stretching. This type of end-feel is not believed to be present in the spine. An example of soft tissue end-feel is elbow flexion or hip flexion. A **firm end-feel** is the result of capsular or ligamentous stretching. An example of a firm end-feel is spinal forward bending and hip rotation. A **hard end-feel** is experienced during elbow extension when there is normally occurring bone-to-bone contact (Table 6-2).

Although variations exist between individuals, each joint is expected to have a particular type of end-feel that should occur at the very end range of passive movement. A dysfunctional joint may have normal range but may present with an abnormal end-feel. Likewise, a joint may have a fairly normal end-feel that occurs too early in the range. The latter case may be and would nonsymptomatic, and would therefore be considered normal. In the case of hypermobility, the final stop is later in the range and a softer end-feel is present. An **empty end-feel** occurs in response to significant pain or spasm. Other pathologic end-feels may be attributed to shortened connective tissues, joint swelling, scar tissue, and muscle spasm.

Passive joint rotations include examination of both standard, anatomical movements and combined, functional movements. Passive joint translation, or joint play, is examined through the use of traction, compression, and gliding in all directions. Joint play may be tested by moving one aspect of the joint on its fixed counterpart or by application of oscillations without stabilization while the joint space is palpated. During testing, the manual physical therapist attempts to gain an

Table 6–2	Normal and Abnormal End-Feels for Upper and Lower Extremity Movements According to Kaltenborn		
JOINT	**MOVEMENT**	**NORMAL END-FEEL**	**ABNORMAL END-FEEL**
Neck	FB/BB	Soft	Bone-to-bone = osteophytes
	SB	Sof	
	Rotation	Soft	
Shoulder	Flexion	Elastic	Empty = subacromial bursitis
	Abduction	Firm	Hard capsule = frozen shoulder
	Horizontal Adduction	Soft	Muscle guarding = anterior shoulder dislocation
	Scaption	Firm	
	IR/ER	Firm	
Elbow	Flexion	Soft	Boggy = Joint Effusion
	Extension	Hard	
Forearm	Pronation/supination	Firm	
Wrist	Flexion	Firm	Empty = sprain/strain
	Extension	Firm	
	Rad/ulnar development	Hard	

Table 6-2	Normal and Abnormal End-Feels for Upper and Lower Extremity Movements According to Kaltenborn—cont'd		
JOINT	**MOVEMENT**	**NORMAL END-FEEL**	**ABNORMAL END-FEEL**
Thumb	Flexion/extension	Firm	Empty = sprain/strain
	Abduction	Firm	
	Adduction	Soft	
Finger	Flexion	Soft	
	Extension	Elastic	
LB	FB/BB	Soft	Empty = sprain/strain
	SB	Soft	
	Rotation	Soft	
Hip	Flexion	Soft	
	Extension	Firm	
	Abduction	Firm	
	Adduction	Soft	
	IR/ER	Firm	
Knee	Flexion	Soft	Springy block = meniscus derangement
	Extension	Firm	
Ankle	Plantar flexion	Firm	Tissue stretch = tight muscle
	Dorsiflexion	Soft	
	Inversion	Firm	
	Eversion	Hard	
	Pronation/supination	Elastic	
Toes	Flexion	Elastic	
	Extension	Elastic	

FB, forward bending; BB, backward bending; SB, side bending; ER, external rotation; IR, internal rotation.

appreciation of related symptoms and the motion characteristics of the joint (Fig. 6-13).

Traction tests that elicit symptoms in the resting position may be modified to include three-dimensional positioning, after which traction tests are performed and assessed for greater comfort. If compression testing increases symptoms and traction alleviates symptoms, an articular lesion is suspected. In such cases, additional tests that produce compression, such as resistance testing, may be avoided or three-dimensional positioning for greater comfort may be attempted. Gliding tests are most valuable for determining the direction in which the joint is restricted. In the spine, gliding translations are performed to compare the mobility of adjacent segments. Although subtle changes in segmental mobility vary throughout the spine, there should not be an abrupt change in mobility of adjacent segments.

QUESTIONS *for* REFLECTION

- What is the physiologic mechanism by which *resisted tests* produce joint compression?
- Based on this concept, how might resisted tests be used to identify the presence of articular lesions?
- Based on this concept, when would it be inappropriate to use resisted tests?
- What might be performed prior to considering the use of resisted tests?

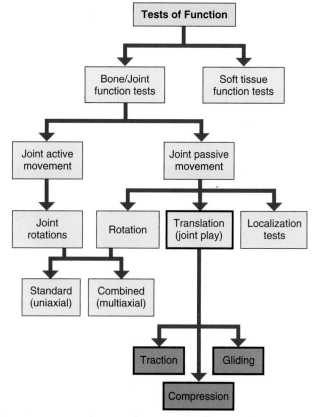

FIGURE 6–13. Nordic approach to tests of function with the addition of joint passive translation (joint play) tests.[3]

Joint function testing may also reveal the presence of a painful arc or capsular pattern. Differentiation between articular and extra-articular dysfunction may be determined by undergoing the process of testing for contractile and noncontractile lesions as espoused by Cyriax[4] (see Chapter 5). This process involves using active, passive, and resisted movements. To more definitively rule out the presence of a noncontractile joint lesion, the Nordic approach advocates the use of *traction-alleviation* and *compression-provocation* testing as a complement to these procedures (Fig. 6-14, Table 6-3). Collectively, these procedures are known as passive localization tests.

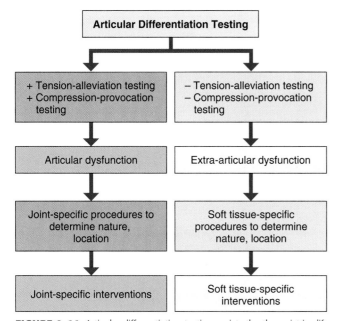

FIGURE 6–14. Articular differentiation testing assists the therapist in differentiating between a noncontractile articular lesion and an extra-articular lesion. It is recommended that articular differentiation testing precedes noncontractile vs. contractile testing to avoid the confounding information that may result from these tests in the case of subtle contractile lesions or when significant inflammation is present.[3]

Passive localization tests are used to identify the specific location of the lesion, to identify the direction that is symptomatic, and to measure the degree of restriction. To localize the lesion through passive movement, **symptom provocation tests**, which use joint compression and movement that is in a symptom-provoking direction, may be incorporated. Consequently, **symptom alleviation tests** use joint traction and movement in a direction that attempts to alleviate symptoms. These tests are most effectively used when the symptomatic joint is positioned as close as possible to the point of symptom onset. In this position, specific movements can then be used to either provoke or alleviate the symptoms. In so doing, the therapist is able to identify the specific location and direction of dysfunction (Figs. 6-15, 6-16).

CLINICAL PILLAR

Symptoms are easier to provoke or alleviate if the affected joint is positioned as close as possible to the point at which symptoms commence.

Soft tissue function testing also includes the use of both active and passive movements. *Resisted tests* are used to examine the status of the contractile elements. These tests may include traditional manual muscle testing procedures or functional maneuvers that involve multi-plane motions. Prior to performance of resistance testing, it is important to rule out the underlying joint as a source of symptoms. Examination of **soft tissue passive movement** can be performed using physiological soft tissue movements and accessory soft tissue movements. During **physiological soft tissue movement testing**, the muscle is moved into the maximally lengthened position, and careful assessment of end-feel may differentiate the presence of muscle shortening as opposed to restricted joint movement. These tests may also be used to examine neural tension and mobility. **Accessory soft tissue movement testing** is performed by

Table 6–3	Differentiating Between a Noncontractile and a Contractile Lesion	
EXAMINATION PROCEDURE	**NONCONTRACTILE DYSFUNCTION**	**CONTRACTILE DYSFUNCTION**
Active Movement	• Commensurate with passive movement • Symptoms provoked in same direction as passive movement • Symptoms provoked at same point in the range as passive movement • Restricted in the same direction and at the same point in the range as passive movement	• Conflicting with passive movement • Symptoms provoked in opposite direction as passive movement • Restricted in the opposite direction as passive movement
Passive Movement	• Commensurate with active movement • Symptoms provoked in same direction as active movement • Symptoms provoked at same point in the range as active movement • Restricted in the same direction and at the same point in the range as active movement	• Conflicting with active movement • Symptoms provoked in opposite direction as active movement • Restricted in the opposite direction as active movement

Continued

Table 6–3	Differentiating Between a Noncontractile and a Contractile Lesion—cont'd	
EXAMINATION PROCEDURE	**NONCONTRACTILE DYSFUNCTION**	**CONTRACTILE DYSFUNCTION**
Passive Joint Play	• Produce symptoms • Reveal restrictions	• Normal movement and symptom free
Resisted Movement	• No weakness present • Symptom free	• Weakness present • Increase symptoms

Examination procedures modified from Cyriax's selected tissue tension testing used to differentiate between noncontractile and contractile lesions. The Nordic approach advocates the use of traction-alleviation and compression-provocation testing first, to rule out the presence of a joint dysfunction.[3]

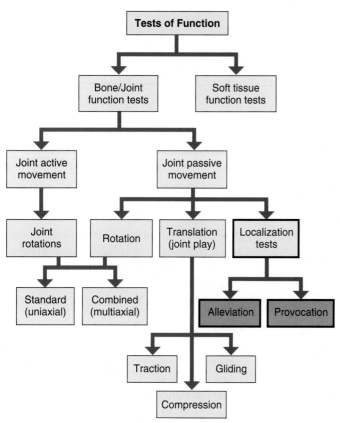

FIGURE 6–15. Nordic approach to tests of function with the addition of passive localization tests.[3]

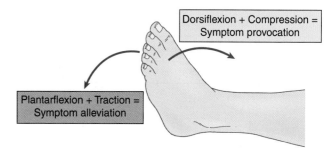

FIGURE 6–16. Direction of symptom alleviation and provocation tests suggesting talocrural joint dysfunction.

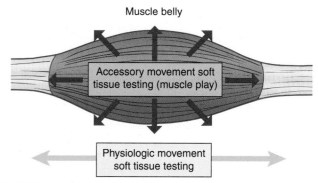

FIGURE 6–17. Direction of soft tissue passive movement testing. *Physiological movement soft tissue testing* is performed when the muscle is moved into the maximally lengthened position in a direction that is parallel to the muscle fibers, and assessment of end-feel differentiates the presence of muscle shortening as opposed to restricted joint movement. *Accessory movement soft tissue testing* is performed in transverse, oblique, and parallel directions in relation to the orientation of the muscle fibers for the purpose of evaluating mobility and to identify the presence of scarring, edema, and adhesions within and between muscles.

passively moving soft tissues in all directions. **Muscle play** is a type of accessory movement that serves to identify the presence of scarring, edema, and adhesions within and between muscles. These tests are performed by passively moving the musculotendinous unit in transverse, oblique, and parallel directions in relation to the orientation of the muscle fibers for the purpose of evaluating mobility (Figs. 6-17, 6-18).

PRINCIPLES OF INTERVENTION
General Overview

The Nordic approach to OMPT relies on the results of the detailed biomechanical examination that has identified specific regions of either hypomobility or hypermobility. However, when the nature of the dysfunction does not allow for intervention

that is biomechanically based, such as in the case of pain or spasm, intervention may be directed toward the alleviation of symptoms. This approach's intervention regimen routinely includes the use of additional procedures in conjunction with manual techniques. The specific use and sequencing of these adjunctive procedures are often quite useful in preparing a region for manual therapy or for maintaining gains following the application of manual techniques. To gauge progress and the results of intervention, reexamination at the beginning and end of each intervention session is recommended. Chosen interventions should not result in symptoms that persist beyond the day in which the intervention was rendered.

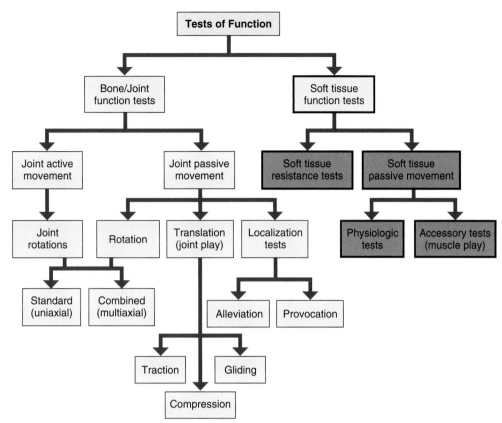

FIGURE 6–18. Nordic approach to tests of function with the addition of soft tissue function tests.[3]

QUESTIONS *for* **REFLECTION**

For the list of impairments below, consider the following:

- What *interventions* in addition to manual interventions might you use?
- How might you *integrate* both manual and nonmanual interventions into a comprehensive plan of care?
- How would you *sequence* your chosen interventions?
- How would you evaluate patient *tolerance*, *a positive response*, and *a negative response* to your chosen interventions?
- How would you *progress* or *regress* each patient through your integrated plan of care?

1. Pain before end range of forearm supination
2. Grade I hypomobility intervertebrally at L1-L4
3. Grade V hypermobility intervertebrally at C6-T1
4. Poor movement quality with full range of motion for shoulder elevation
5. Reduced muscle play over surgical scar at lateral epicondyle
6. Pain and reduced motion, with a dominant sign of flexion in weight-bearing at the knee
7. Reduction in wrist extension with normal end-feel and joint

Indications and Contraindications

Intervention is based on the identified physical diagnosis that is obtained through a detailed, ongoing examination process. Although useful, the medical diagnosis is not required in order for the therapist to intervene. The primary indication for the use of manual physical therapy within this approach is the discovery of an abnormal end-feel. Manual techniques are often necessary in order to identify the presence of abnormal end-feels and joint play restrictions in a joint. A joint may be found to be hypomobile, yet have a normal end-feel. In such cases, the presence of mechanical restrictions that are effecting mobility are not suspected and manual intervention is, therefore, not indicated. It is presumed that the cause of the identified hypomobility is nonmechanical in origin, thus rendering any attempt at manual therapy ineffective. Within this approach, the provocation of symptoms discovered throughout the examination takes a secondary role to identification of biomechanical findings. Grade III mobilizations are indicated for the patient who presents with hypomobility, abnormal end-feel, and symptoms that are less irritable. Grade I and II mobilizations are implemented when the symptoms are more irritable, or acute, in nature.

Contraindications to the use of manual physical therapy within this approach are primarily assigned to the use of Grade III mobilization techniques. Grade III techniques are contraindicated in the presence of decreased joint play with a hard

---

CLINICAL PILLAR

Hypomobility or *hypermobility* are considered pathological only if they are associated with symptoms and an aberrant end-feel.

end-feel that occurs in the hypomobile direction. Such findings suggest the presence of a pathological bony block. Increased joint play with soft end-feel in the hypermobile direction is suggestive of joint laxity for which stabilization, not mobilization, techniques would be indicated. Pain and protective spasm during the performance of Grade III techniques suggests the presence of an irritable condition at which time the grade of mobilization must be reduced. Other contraindications to manual physical therapy are similar to those used in other approaches and include the presence of neoplasms, coagulation disorders, collagen-vascular disorders, acute inflammation, autonomic disturbances, massive degenerative changes, and various congenital abnormalities (Fig. 6-19).

QUESTIONS *for* REFLECTION

- How might the belief that a joint may be hypomobile in one direction and hypermobile in another direction impact the manual therapy examination and intervention regimen?

- How might a joint present with a normal end-feel in one direction and a pathologic end-feel in another direction?

- In reference to these concepts, what special considerations must the manual therapist keep in mind?

Intervention for the Reduction of Symptoms (Grade I-IISZ Pain-Relief Traction-Mobilization)

Interventions designed to relieve symptoms may be used in the presence of hypomobility, hypermobility, and nerve root involvement. Although the biomechanical findings take precedence, the individual's reported symptoms are directly treated

when the level of pain interferes with the ability of the manual physical therapist to identify the antecedent biomechanical cause, when end-range of movement cannot be tolerated, and in the presence of suspected inflammation, intervertebral disc pathology, and when increased muscle activity is present about the symptomatic joint (Table 6-4).

The initial trial intervention of choice when directly treating an individual's symptoms is identified as **Grade I-Grade II traction-mobilizations, within slack.** Although the effects of these techniques are considered to be short term, they are effective in controlling pain and promoting muscle relaxation. These techniques may impact range of motion through the introduction of low-level movement that serves to alter joint inflammation and reduce pain. These techniques are applied through the slow distraction of joint surfaces in the resting or actual resting position. The starting position is maintained briefly between each repetition. For optimal results, the manual physical therapist must intermittently readjust the three-dimensional actual resting position of the joint as changes take place. During repositioning, mobilization is halted until an optimal position of comfort can be obtained, after which the techniques are resumed. When treating symptoms, tissue stretching is avoided by occupying the within-slack range short of the transition zone. The manual physical therapist should expect a reduction in symptoms if these techniques are truly indicated and are performed correctly. If these techniques increase symptoms or prove to be ineffective, the therapist should attempt to adjust patient position, alter the distraction force, correct an underlying positional fault, or in some cases, discontinue the technique. Vibrations and oscillations may also be used for managing symptoms and may be interspersed with stretch mobilizations to minimize discomfort. Other interventions may also be indicated in conjunction with manual therapy in the management of symptoms. Such interventions may include modalities for pain and edema and/or immobilization.

CLINICAL PILLAR

The use of joint mobilization techniques for relief of symptoms must be performed within the *slack zone*, prior to the *first stop* and *transition zone*.

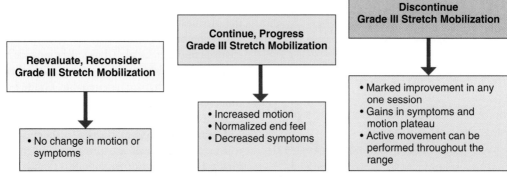

FIGURE 6–19. Clinical decision-making for Grade III stretch mobilization techniques.[3]

Table 6–4	Nordic Approach Mobilization Techniques and Their Primary Indications

Level of Aggressiveness

Low → High

INDICATION FOR MOBILIZATION	GRADE I–IISZ PAIN-RELIEF TRACTION	GRADE I–IISZ-TZ–RELAXATION-TRACTION	GRADE III STRETCH-TRACTION	GRADE III STRETCH-GLIDE	MANIPULATION	STABILIZATION, SUPPORT, ADJACENT MOBILIZATION
Pain and Symptoms	X					
Muscle Spasm		X				
Nerve Root Findings		X	X			
Hypomobility			X	X	X	
Hypermobility						X

SZ, slack zone; TZ, transition zone.

Intervention for Nerve Root Findings (Grade I-IISZ-TZ Relaxation-Traction Mobilization and Grade III Stretch-Traction Mobilization)

During examination of patients with nerve root involvement, certain portions of the biomechanical examination may be deferred or modified to allow for better patient tolerance. A thorough neurological examination which places the patient in positions that provoke their neurological symptoms are often used by the manual therapist to delineate the exact nature of the patient's symptoms. **Grade I-Grade II traction-mobilizations, within-slack (Grade I-IISZ-TZ Relaxation-Traction Mobilization)** are the initial techniques of choice for individuals presenting with these findings. These techniques are believed to improve vascular flow, which facilitates drainage of metabolites from inflamed nerve tissue. As when treating symptoms, intermittent joint repositioning and constant reexamination of the patient's response is critical. If the examination reveals the presence of hypomobility, which is associated with the nerve root findings, **Grade III stretch-traction mobilization** with three-dimensional positioning may be used based on patient tolerance. Such techniques are believed to alter positional relationships, which may have an impact on the presenting neurological symptoms. Rotational mobilization techniques may exacerbate symptoms in the presence of suspected nerve root involvement and must, therefore, be avoided in the early stages of rehabilitation.

Intervention for Hypomobility (Grade III Stretch-Traction and Stretch-Glide Mobilization)

Grade III stretch mobilizations are effective in restoring joint play when hypomobility is associated with an abnormal end-feel that relates to the patient's symptoms. The relationship between restrictions in motion and abnormal end-feels to the patient's presenting symptoms are the chief indication for the use of stretch mobilizations. These mobilizations are performed by first experiencing resistance to movement followed by engagement of the restricted tissue. Once the tissue is engaged, stretching is typically sustained for a minimum of *7 seconds* up to *1 minute* or longer, based on patient tolerance. To maximize effects, mobilization should be performed in a cyclic manner for *10 to 15 minutes*. Returning to the neutral position is not required between mobilizations. Typically, the amount of time over which the stretch is applied is more critical than the amount of force used. Except in chronic cases, improvement should occur immediately. If there is failure to make progress, reconsider the patient's position, the direction of forces, the magnitude of forces, and whether this technique is truly indicated. When applying stretch mobilizations, it is important to examine the degree of mobility in all directions and to specifically apply techniques in only those directions that prove to be limited.

NOTABLE QUOTABLE

"[The Nordic] System stresses the role of the patient in reestablishing and maintaining normal mobility, in preventing recurrence, and in improving musculoskeletal health."

Freddy Kaltenborn, 1993

The least aggressive of the Grade III stretch mobilizations is the **Grade III stretch-traction mobilization.** This technique seeks to improve motion in directions that are both parallel (joint glide) as well as perpendicular (joint distraction) to the treatment plane. Specific **Grade III stretch-glide mobilizations** are ideally performed first in the direction of greatest restriction. However, in the case of a highly irritable condition, mobilization in less restricted and less symptomatic directions may be performed first for better patient tolerance.

Stretch-glide mobilizations attempt to introduce translatory motions to the joint that are parallel to the joint's treatment plane while disallowing the rolling component that is associated with normal motion. This is best achieved by the therapist pre-positioning the joint by taking up the slack in the restricted direction by using rotational movements, after which small translatory stretch-glide mobilizations are performed. As motion improves, the therapist takes up the slack by advancing the starting position to the new limit of range. It is recommended that novice therapists use stretch-traction techniques in the resting position. These techniques may be progressed into stretch-glide mobilizations in the resting position followed by mobilization in the direction in which movement is restricted.

CLINICAL PILLAR

Consider the use of *Grade III stretch mobilizations* when the following occurs:

- Hypomobility is associated with an abnormal end-feel.
- Hypomobility is related to the patient's presenting symptoms.
- There are no contraindications.

CLINICAL PILLAR

Joint rolling movements produce compressive forces. In the absence of gliding, these movements may produce damage to the joint.

Upon reexamination, if range is improved and end-feel is normalized, then these techniques may be continued. Marked improvement during any one session should be an indication to discontinue the intervention so as to avoid exacerbation. If there is no appreciable change in response to these procedures, reevaluate the patient position, technique aggressiveness, and the efficacy for manual therapy in general. These techniques should be discontinued when gains have plateaued and when the patient can actively move through the acquired range independently.

CLINICAL PILLAR

Results from performance of *Grade III stretch mobilizations* are as follows:

- They are immediate.
- They last only after several sessions.
- They produce a change in the patient's dominant signs and symptoms.

During stretch-glide mobilizations, a *Grade I traction* force may be used to reduce compressive forces to the joint and subsequently reduce the potential for increased symptoms. Within the Nordic approach, Grade III stretch-traction and glide mobilizations in conjunction with specific three-dimensional pre-positioning are deemed to be safer and just as effective as general rotational techniques in the spine and are therefore preferred. Adjunctive interventions such as application of heat, soft tissue mobilization, and muscle relaxation techniques are considered to be useful in enhancing the effects of the chosen manual therapy joint mobilizations.

Intervention for Hypermobility (Specific Training of the Deep Stabilizing Musculature, External Support, and Joint Mobilization for Adjacent Regions)

Joint hypermobility may lead to positional faults because of the inability of a joint to remain within its normal anatomical confines. Careful accessory motion testing is required in order for the manual therapist to identify the existence of underlying joint hypermobility in an apparently hypomobile joint. Once identified, management of hypermobility involves three distinct intervention strategies. Specific training of the deep stabilizing musculature around the joint occurs initially through controlled contractions facilitated through tactile cueing from the manual therapist and progressed to independently controlled contractions during functional tasks (see Chapter 17). External support, in the form of taping and bracing, may be required early in the process until adequate muscle performance can be achieved and may continue to be used as a secondary support indefinitely. Joint mobilization for adjacent regions of hypomobility is also indicated in the presence of hypermobility. The objective is to reduce the forces and the need for excessive motion at a particular joint by providing a greater opportunity for loads to be distributed across all joints that are contributing

NOTABLE QUOTABLE

"Patient education takes time, but often saves time in the end as it leads to active participation by the patient and clearer communication between patient and [therapist]."

Freddy Kaltenborn, 1993

QUESTIONS *for* REFLECTION

- How might a *hypermobile* joint present with apparent *hypomobility*?
- What *voluntary* and *involuntary* processes might contribute to the masking of underlying joint hypermobility?
- In such situations, how might a manual therapist go about identifying the presence of hypermobility?

to a given motion. When treating patients with hypermobility, instruction in methods to reduce daily stressors is also considered to be vital.

Application of Techniques

As previously noted, for examination and the most basic mobilization techniques, placing the joint in the resting or actual resting position is recommended. In this position, muscular influences around the joint are reduced. The resting position for each joint in different patients may vary; therefore, careful examination and repeated trials may be necessary to identify the proper, three-dimensional position for that specific joint prior to performance of mobilization (Box 6-1). During performance of mobilization techniques, it is imperative that the manual therapist assumes an ergonomically sound position to avoid injury (Box 6-2)

Hand placement during mobilization involves movement of one hand with the patient's body while the other hand remains stable for palpation and fixation. To ascertain both the quality and quantity of movement, the therapist should use the least amount of force possible. For specific passive motion tests and mobilization, one finger on the stable hand palpates while the remainder of the hand stabilizes motion at adjacent segments. In the spine, motion palpation takes place at the interspinous space or at the side of the spinous processes. For end-feel testing and mobilization, the stabilizing hand increases contact pressure to provide fixation of neighboring segments (Box 6-3). Fixation is particularly important when performing Grade III stretch techniques. Fixation can be further enhanced by using locking techniques and external fixating devices such as wedges and belts.

QUESTIONS *for* REFLECTION

- Why are *rotational mobilizations* considered to be dangerous in the presence of suspected spinal disc involvement, nerve root irritation, and/or vertebral artery compromise?
- What is the physiologic effect of producing rotation on each of these structures?

When performing examination and mobilization techniques, the manual therapist attempts to produce movement that is specific to the joint in question. Following each repetition, the joint is returned to its initial resting position (Box 6-4). To more accurately reflect the motion characteristics of the joint, therapists produce motion using their hands as well as their body to allow better control. Strict adherence to the use of sound ergonomic principles in the performance of manual techniques and the use of external support devices is an important component of this approach.

Box 6-1 RECOMMENDED PATIENT POSITION

- **Standing:** The patient and the manual therapist should be separated and parallel to each other.
- **Sitting:** Feet should be supported on the floor to provide stability.
- **Prone:** Place a pillow under the patient's abdomen and/or thorax to achieve the resting position of the spine. Head piece should have a cutout to avoid cervical rotation, and the head may be lowered slightly.
- **Side-lying position**: Hips and knees flexed to provide stability and to approximate normal curves observed in standing. A pillow under the waist may control side bending.
- **Supine:** Head supported by table or pillow, and legs abducted and relaxed in hook-lying position using pillow under the knees.

The manual therapist must be prepared to make frequent modifications of these recommended positions to accommodate the individual needs of the patient.

Box 6-2 RECOMMENDED THERAPIST POSITION

- Be as close as possible to the patient throughout the entire technique.
- Maintain a wide base of support.
- Maintain flexed hips and knees.
- Maintain a natural lumbar lordosis.
- Adjust table height to ensure efficient and effective body mechanics.

Box 6-3 RECOMMENDED HAND PLACEMENT

- One hand moves with the patient's body throughout the technique.
- One hand remains stable for palpation, stabilization, or fixation.
- Both hands monitor the quality and quantity of movement.
- The less hand contact, the more sensitive the therapist's hands are for monitoring movement quality.
- Excessive pressure masks feedback, distorts movement, and allows unwanted movement of adjacent joints.
- The therapist must develop the ability to use either hand for each task.
- When learning new techniques, therapists must be sure to practice using both hands on either side of the patient.
- Therapists should be prepared to modify their hand placement for better patient comfort by avoiding uncomfortable bony prominences and moving aside sensitive structures.

Box 6-4 RECOMMENDED PROCEDURE FOR OMPT

- Produce movement primarily in the targeted segment, avoiding movement in adjacent structures.
- Start with the segment in the resting position.
- Movement is produced and controlled by the therapist's hands and body, which moves around an axis of motion in the targeted segment.
- Unweight aspects of the patient's body in order to reduce friction from the table.
- Allow the patient to assist performance of a passive movement actively.

CLINICAL PILLAR

When practicing mobilization techniques with asymptomatic subjects, *Grade II within-slack mobilizations* are recommended so as to avoid injury.

Measuring Progress and Documentation

Changes in a patient's condition is assessed by monitoring changes in the most *dominant symptom* and comparing these changes with routine screening tests and the patient's *dominant signs*. If the patient's functional status is not normalizing and there is no change in the patient's symptoms, then further examination is required.

CLINICAL PILLAR

The skilled manual therapist has the ability to continuously appreciate the subtle changes that occur in response to intervention and immediately modify the intervention based on these changes.

When identifying intervertebral segmental motion, the movement is always described in terms of the cranial vertebra in relation to the caudad vertebra of the motion segment. Therefore, when describing a specific motion segment, the cranial vertebra is identified to denote the motion segment. The **star diagram** may be used to provide a visual description of spinal motion. This method of recording motion uses a combination of long and short lines and arrows. This diagram provides information regarding both the quality and quantity of spinal motion at a glance and expedites the often laborious task of documenting spinal motion (Fig. 6-20).

DIFFERENTIATING CHARACTERISTICS

The most distinguishing feature of the Nordic approach to OMPT is the strict adherence to *biomechanical principles* in

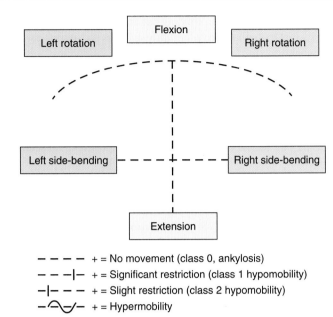

FIGURE 6–20. The star diagram for documentation of spinal motion. Ankylosis (class 0) is recorded with a circle marked around the center cross of the star. Hypomobility (class 1 or 2) is recorded with short lines that cross dashed lines at points that indicate the degree of movement from neutral. Hypermobility (class 4, 5, 6) is recorded with curved line placed over the dashed line. Treatment direction can be recorded with an arrow placed at the end of the dashed line showing the movement direction. (From: Kaltenborn FM. *The Spine: Basic Evaluation and Mobilization Techniques.* 2nd ed. Oslo, Norway: Olaf Norlis Bokhandel; 1993, with permission.)

both diagnosis and intervention. The Nordic approach emphasizes the use of biomechanics in the analysis and management of musculoskeletal impairment to localize symptomatic structures. Traction, gliding, and occasionally compression forces, in relation to normal biomechanics and joint structure, is used extensively during the examination and intervention process. The convex-concave theory guides the therapist in determining the direction of joint glide that is indicated in the presence of impairment. Joint play is divided into grades of movement and is determined by considering the relationship between end-feel and range of motion. Three-dimensional joint positioning and an appreciation of standard and combined movements are important concepts that must be considered. This approach also devotes a considerable degree of attention to the concept of hypermobility as a pathological entity.

Within this approach, multiple intervention strategies are often included within any one intervention session. This combination of technique approach often includes using soft tissue mobilization, joint mobilization, self-management techniques, strengthening and coordination techniques, and instruction in biomechanics and ergonomics. Using a combination of intervention strategies is believed to be optimal for addressing all of the potential contributors to an individual's presenting dysfunction.

Foundational to this approach, is the use of the trial treatment, which assists the therapist in determining the efficacy of a chosen intervention. This approach espouses the concept that diagnosis is confirmed or refuted through the use of a low-risk trial treatment. The patient's response to intervention over the period between sessions assists in determining the appropriateness of the intervention provided and the accuracy of the diagnosis. Future intervention is modified according to the patient's response to the trial treatment. Since its inception, many other approaches to OMPT have also adopted the concept of the trial treatment for diagnosis and for guiding intervention.

CLINICAL PILLAR

The *24-hour rule* states that symptoms produced as a result of manual intervention should not persist beyond the day on which the intervention was rendered.

Lastly, this approach places an emphasis on the use of *ergonomic principles* as it relates to proper therapist mechanics when performing techniques. Adherence to the strict performance of techniques that are ergonomically sound assists in reducing stress to the therapist and ensures the proper performance of each technique. The emphasis on ergonomic principles has led to the development of several external devices that may be used to enhance the effectiveness and ease with which manual interventions are performed. Such instruments include the first *pneumatic high-low adjustable table*, *fixation belts*, and *wedges*, among others.

NOTABLE QUOTABLE

"Many challenges confound the conduct of useful research in the manual therapies. . . . For researchers with a pioneering spirit, creativity, and determination, this is an exciting new arena for study."

Freddy Kaltenborn, 1993

CONCLUSION

The contributions of Freddy Kaltenborn and Olaf Evjenth to the development of the Nordic approach to OMPT has had an important impact on the advancement of this area of specialty practice. This system's emphasis on sound biomechanical principles has been effective in establishing the manual physical therapist as a clinical scientist and movement specialist and has supported the development of OMPT practice as a specialty of "applied kinesiology." Although the specific manual techniques of this approach may not vary greatly from other systems, the emphasis on clinical decision-making and the intimate interaction between intervention and patient response has been well-defined and subsequently applied to other approaches. The Nordic approach's preoccupation with understanding the kinematics that lie beneath the presenting movement impairment and the relentless pursuit of procedures designed to restore normal mobility has formed the basis of many subsequent paradigms a variety of paradigms within OMPT. The impact of Kaltenborn's life and work on the practice of OMPT will forever be remembered. His legacy will live on in those who seek to understand and ameliorate the presence of impairments in mobility.

CLINICAL CASE

Patient History

HPI: The patient is a 65-year-old male with complaint of low back pain (LBP) occurring gradually over the past 2 weeks and appearing to be related to his present work duties, which involve prolonged awkward positions while painting. His symptoms consist of central lumbosacral pain that is at a 4/10+ level of intensity on average and of the constant, dull ache variety with intermittent complaint of right lower extremity (LE) pain and paresthesia into the posterior aspect of his thigh to the knee when painting overhead. He notes that these symptoms are affecting his job performance. He notes having significant difficulty with sleeping and that his best position is sitting. He has experienced similar complaints in the past; however, this time his symptoms are much worse. He wishes to return to gainful employment, but is unsure if he will be able to assume the positions required of his job. At present, no diagnostic imaging has been done. His Oswestry score is 60%.

Past Medical History: Unremarkable with the exception of intermittent LBP.

Physical Examination

Inspection: In standing, the patient presents with swayback posture, bilateral anterior pelvic rotation, rounded shoulders and forward head.

Neurological and Vascular Tests: Deep tendon reflexes (DTR) reveal right (R) patellar tendon = 1+; all else within normal limits (WNL). Light touch sensation is intact and symmetrical at bilateral lower extremities. Babinski is negative.

Bilateral dorsiflexion musculature reveals fatigue upon 15 repetitions of repeated resistance testing. Dorsal pedal pulse is WNL bilaterally.

Special Tests: Straight leg raising (SLR) R is positive at 45 degrees, and L is negative; slump test R is positive, and L is negative; quadrant sign R is positive, and L is negative.

Palpation: Hyperactivity and tenderness over quadratus lumborum L > R, hamstrings bilaterally, right piriformis, and psoas trigger points. L3-L4 motion segment reveals a left rotated positional fault.

Joint Function Tests

Standard Active Movements: Flexion = 75%, with relief of symptoms; Extension = 10% with increased right LE paresthesia; side bending R = 10%, with increased right LE paresthesia; side bending L = 75%, with reduction in symptoms; rotation R = 75%; rotation L = 10% with increased pain and paresthesia.

Combined Active Movements: Central LBP, bilateral posterior thigh paresthesia into the feet, and decreased mobility with combined extension and side bending bilaterally.

Passive Translations (Joint Play): *Posterior-Anterior Gliding:* T12-L1 = Grade 3; L1-L2 = Grade 2; L3-L4 = Grade 1; L4-L5 = Grade 2; L5-S1 = Grade 5. **Spinal Traction Testing** in the resting position reveals reduction of LBP from 4 to 2/10+ level of intensity, with elimination of bilateral lower extremity paresthesia. Compression not tested. *End-feel testing:* reveals L3-L4 = firm end-feel noted at first stop in midrange, L5-S1 = soft end-feel.

Passive Localization Tests: *Provocation Tests:* Positive for left rotation of L3 and for posteroanterior (PA) glide of L4 with patient in prone press-up position. **Alleviation Tests:** Positive for right rotation of L3 and for PA glide of L3 with patient in prone press-up position.

Soft Tissue Function Tests: *Resisted Tests:* 5/5 strength throughout bilateral lower extremities with the exception of bilateral quadriceps (L3), which is 4/5. **Muscle Length Tests:** Significant restrictions in bilateral hamstrings and rectus femoris musculature. **Muscle Play Tests:** Multi-planar restrictions at bilateral quadratus lumborum R > L.

1. Based on this presentation, what is your biomechanically based physical diagnosis? Explain your rationale and the process of coming to this conclusion.
2. What is this patient's dominant symptom/sign, and how does it relate to his movement patterns and end-feels? How will the dominant symptom/sign influence your plan of care?
3. How would the results of *joint function testing*, namely joint play and end-feel, impact your physical diagnosis and your plan of care for this patient?
4. How would the results of *soft tissue function testing* impact your physical diagnosis and your plan of care for this patient?
5. Based on the results of *passive localization testing* for symptom provocation and alleviation, what functional movements or positions would you expect to be problematic for this patient, and what functional movements or positions would you expect to provide symptom relief? Given this information, what manual therapy techniques would be most appropriate for this patient at this time?

6. Based on the results of *joint and soft tissue function testing*, would you emphasize soft tissue or joint manual therapy techniques, or would you integrate both into your plan of care? Explain how you might optimally integrate both types of manual therapy into your plan of care. How might other forms of intervention such as therapeutic exercise and physical modalities be integrated into the plan of care for this patient?
7. Draw a *star diagram* that accurately depicts the findings of your active range-of-motion testing?
8. What additional information would you like to have before initiating intervention?
9. Identify three specific manual therapy techniques that you would implement at the time of this patient's first visit to physical therapy. Describe each in detail (i.e., grade, position, direction, duration, etc.) and perform them on your partner. Be sure to adhere to strict technique performance, which includes correct hand placement, therapist position, and patient position, and incorporate appropriate ergonomic principles. (See "Principles of Intervention" section.)

HANDS-ON

Perform the following activities in lab with a partner:

1 Visualize the treatment plane of two upper extremity and two lower extremity joints and perform both traction and glide mobilizations on the joint as dictated by the treatment plane specific to that joint.

2 Using the proposed grading system (0–6), choose an extremity joint and grade joint play motions in all planes of motion for both traction and glide. Are you able to identify hypomobility in one plane of motion with normal or hypermobility in another plane? Are there differences in mobility when comparing side to side?

3 Choose a joint and compare the amount of joint play available between the **resting position** (open-packed) and the **non-resting position** (close-packed) of the joint. Choose another partner and compare findings between individuals for the same joints.

4 On your partner's shoulder, identify the **slack zone (SZ), the transition zone (TZ),** and the **first stop** of the joint. Verify your findings by having another student attempt to identify the same. Subjects should provide feedback to the examiner on how each zone feels different from the others.

5 Perform end-feel testing for elbow extension, hip flexion, and shoulder external rotation. Evaluate the quality of resistance at end range and where in the range the resistance is felt. Appreciate the differences in normal end-feels between each of these motions.

6 Observe your partner perform a spinal mobilization technique and critique hand placement of the mobilizing hand, fixating hand, therapist body position, and patient position based on a strict ergonomically sound model.

7 Allow your partner to portray the patient described in the case scenario above. Ask your partner the three most important questions that might be useful in determining the future course of intervention. Describe how you will use the dominant symptom and your physical diagnosis to determine the plan of care.

8 Choose one spinal technique and one extremity technique from the "Principles of Intervention" section and perform each technique using the following methods: (1) Grade I and II traction-mobilization within slack, (2) Grade III stretch-traction mobilization, (3) Grade III stretch-glide mobilization.

9 Switch partners and perform these techniques on one other person. Teach your chosen techniques to one other person and provide them with feedback regarding his or her performance.

10 If possible, video your performance of these techniques. Self-assess your performance of the chosen techniques by writing down three areas of deficiency and three areas of proficiency when using these techniques. Focus on such factors as therapist position, patient position, hand placement, force direction, instruction to the patient, etc. Critique the performance of others in a similar fashion.

REFERENCES

1. Kaltenborn FM. *The Spine: Basic Evaluation and Mobilization Techniques.* 2nd ed. Oslo, Norway: Olaf Norlis Bokhandel; 1993.
2. Farrell JP, Jensen GM. Manual therapy: a critical assessment of role in the profession of physical therapy. *Phys Ther.* 1992;72:843-852.
3. Kaltenborn FM. *Manual Mobilization of the Joints: The Kaltenborn Method of Joint Examination and Treatment. Volume I: The Extremities.* 6th ed. Oslo, Norway: Olaf Norlis Bokhandel; 2002.
4. Cyriax, J. *Textbook of Orthopaedic Medicine, Volume One.* 8th ed. London: Bailliere Tindall; 1982.

CHAPTER 7

The Paris Approach

Christopher H. Wise, PT, DPT, OCS, FAAOMPT, MTC, ATC

Chapter Objectives

At the conclusion of this chapter, the reader will be able to:

- Discuss the important contributions of Stanley V. Paris to the specialty of orthopaedic manual physical therapy (OMPT).
- Discuss the major foundational principles upon which the Paris approach is established and the other approaches to OMPT that have been most influential in its development.
- Describe the Paris approach's view of pain and its role in examination and intervention.
- Define dysfunction and differentiate it from disease.

- Identify Paris's classification of motion and the value in identifying each during the clinical examination.
- Discuss the value of palpation and the three distinct ways in which palpation is used to guide intervention within this approach.
- Describe the factors that influence patient outcomes.
- Identity common dysfunctions along with their pathogenesis, sequelae, and recommended intervention.
- Demonstrate basic proficiency in the performance and grading of passive intervertebral mobility (PIVM)

HISTORICAL PERSPECTIVES

Stanley V. Paris graduated from the New Zealand School of Physiotherapy at the University of Otago in 1958, after which he joined his father in private practice. He was appointed as a physical therapist to the New Zealand Olympic Team for the 1960 and 1968 Olympic Games. In 1966, Paris came to the United States where he was on the faculty at Boston University and was staff physical therapist at Massachusetts General Hospital. Soon after his immigration to America, Paris became involved in the teaching of orthopaedic manual physical therapy (OMPT) courses to therapists in the United States. At that time in the United States, the principles and practices of OMPT had not yet found their way into mainstream physical therapy. Paris established the *Institute of Graduate Physical Therapy* and, along with a cohort of skilled clinicians, began to teach a series of continuing education courses across the country. These courses, which emphasized hands-on training, were designed to culminate in manual therapy certification (MTC). Paris's efforts to make these innovative concepts accessible have contributed greatly to the popularization of OMPT in the United States. These courses have continued to develop and expand over the years, with several certifications now offered. Paris completed his PhD in 1984, using his

research on lumbar spine neuroanatomy, which identified previously undiscovered neural pathways. Paris was the first president of the *Orthopaedic Section of the American Physical Therapy Association (APTA)*, was the founding chairman and later president of the *International Federation of Orthopaedic Manipulative Physical Therapists (IFOMPT)*, and was a founding member of the *American Academy of Orthopaedic Manual Physical Therapists.* Paris is a Catherine Worthingham Fellow of the APTA and is a Mary McMillan lecturer. Paris's institute is now the *University of St. Augustine for Health Sciences,* which currently offers five majors in the health-related professions and is accredited by the *Commission on Accreditation in Physical Therapy Education.* It is the first privately owned university of its kind in the country, graduating approximately 200 entry-level physical and occupational therapists annually from its campuses in St. Augustine and Boca Raton, Florida, and San Diego, California. Paris's passion and vision for OMPT and the profession of physical therapy has profoundly impacted practice in the United States and abroad. His contributions range from his endeavors in education, research, and clinical practice to his efforts in shaping the political landscape. For his significant and continuous efforts, Paris is sometimes referred to as the "father" of OMPT in the

United States, where he continues to teach, practice, administrate, and embrace with vigor the newly emerging challenges that face the profession and practice of OMPT (Fig. 7-1).[1]

PHILOSOPHICAL FRAMEWORK
General Philosophy

The *Paris approach to OMPT* is considered to be an eclectic approach that is foundationally based on a detailed understanding of functional anatomy and biomechanics. The major tenets of this approach may be identified within other paradigms; however, the systematic and explicit manner in which these concepts are defined, articulated, and combined are unique to this approach. Within the Paris approach, injury to the joint is referred to as a **dysfunction**, which is defined as a state of altered mechanics manifesting itself as either an increase (hypermobility) or decrease (hypomobility) in the expected amount of motion, or as aberrant motion (i.e., poor motion quality) (Box 7-1). The primary role of the manual physical therapist is to diagnose and manage dysfunction. Conversely, the role of the physician is to diagnose and treat disease.

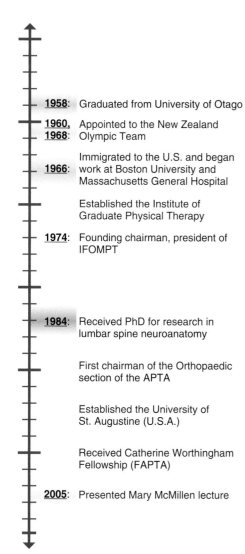

FIGURE 7–1 S.V. Paris's biographical timeline.

1958: Graduated from University of Otago

1960, 1968: Appointed to the New Zealand Olympic Team

1966: Immigrated to the U.S. and began work at Boston University and Massachusetts General Hospital

Established the Institute of Graduate Physical Therapy

1974: Founding chairman, president of IFOMPT

1984: Received PhD for research in lumbar spine neuroanatomy

First chairman of the Orthopaedic section of the APTA

Established the University of St. Augustine (U.S.A.)

Received Catherine Worthingham Fellowship (FAPTA)

2005: Presented Mary McMillen lecture

Box 7-1 DEFINITION of DYSFUNCTION

A state of altered mechanics manifesting itself as:

1. **Hypermobility:** Requires stabilization and mobilization of adjacent regions
2. **Hypomobility:** Requires mobilization
3. **Aberrant motion:** Requires neuromuscular reeducation

NOTABLE QUOTABLE

"The future of physical therapy lies not so much with detection and treatment of disease but with the evaluation, documenting, and treating of dysfunction."

Stanley V. Paris

Alterations in the quantity or quality of movement may lead to premature degenerative changes within the joint. In the case of hypomobility, the indicated intervention is thrust and nonthrust manipulation/mobilization, whereas hypermobility requires both stabilization, including posture reeducation and exercise, as well as manipulation of any neighboring hypomobilities. Therefore, within this approach, the scope of OMPT encompasses both manipulation as well as stabilization. These interventions are directed toward the **pathoanatomical origin** of the dysfunction, and an appreciation of joint mechanics is deemed to be a critical component in understanding dysfunction.[1-5]

CLINICAL PILLAR

The primary role of the manual physical therapist is to diagnose and manage dysfunction. Manual interventions are directed toward the *pathoanatomical origin* of the dysfunction, and an appreciation of joint mechanics is deemed to be a critical component in understanding dysfunction.

Perhaps one of the most unique features of this approach is the emphasis that is placed on understanding deficits in function over the patient's pain-related symptoms. Within this approach, pain is viewed as a subjective entity that may be influenced by a multitude of nonorganic factors and subject to events outside the control of either the patient or the therapist.[1] The entity of pain may be confounding because it includes aspects from the physical, emotional, and psychological domains (Fig. 7-2). The manual physical therapist is trained to influence the physical component of one's health and, therefore, should primarily focus on this domain. Dysfunction is the cause of the pain, and thus it is not possible for pain to precede dysfunction. Management directed toward the patient's subjective report of pain may lead the therapist on a

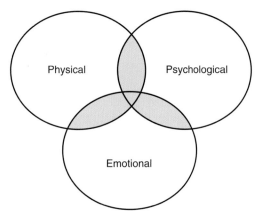

FIGURE 7–2 The three domains of pain. Shaded region represents the crossover among each of the domains. The manual physical therapist's primary influence is related to the physical domain. Because of its multidimensional nature, pain does not provide a reliable measure of a dysfunction's severity, nature, location, and overall improvement and thus should be de-emphasized as a useful gauge of progress.[1]

never-ending chase that guides the therapist away from addressing the true origin of symptoms. The primary goal of the therapist is in the management of dysfunction and not in the management of pain itself. Because dysfunction is viewed as the origin of pain-related symptoms, resolution of the dysfunction through OMPT will eliminate the patient's complaint of pain. If the symptoms do not resolve in the midst of changes in objective measures, then the patient's condition is nonorganic and thus outside the purview of the manual physical therapist. Therefore, within this approach, resolution of pain is not explicitly documented as a specific goal or listed within the plan of care. Manual intervention is directed toward treating the dysfunction and not the pain, and the patient interview is constructed so as to ascertain deficits and improvement in function versus levels of pain over time. The only exception to this principle occurs when the patient's level of pain is so acute that it interferes with direct intervention toward the pain-causing dysfunction; it then must be addressed. Thus, pain is directly treated only when it interferes with correction of the primary dysfunction.[1,2]

QUESTIONS *for* REFLECTION

- Within the Paris approach, why is pain not relied upon as the primary indicator for intervention and the primary gauge to denote progress?
- How would you describe the use of pain during examination and intervention within this approach?

In practice, this philosophy requires the manual physical therapist to astutely observe and document objective signs related to the presence of joint dysfunction and then skillfully work at resolving these aberrations through carefully performed techniques. These objective signs are based on identification of abnormal joint kinematics, and the medical

diagnosis is not required to provide adequate intervention. This approach relies heavily on the skill of the therapist in executing specific mobility testing in order to identify the dysfunction and to provide subsequent intervention.

NOTABLE QUOTABLE

"The past is never past but continues and is very active in every form and at every manifestation of the present."

Achille Castiglioni

Foundational Principles

Within this approach, movement is classified within one of three distinct categories. **Classical movements** are considered to be synonymous with osteokinematic movement. They consist of active movements, which are used to evaluate joint range and muscle function, and passive movements, which are used to determine the nature of the resistance at end range. **Accessory movements** are those motions available within a joint that may accompany the classical movements or those that may be passively produced apart from the classical movement. Accessory movements are necessary for normal kinematics and subsequent joint function. **Component movements** are one type of accessory movement that takes place within a joint to enable a particular active movement to occur. Full, pain-free motion cannot occur in a joint without a normal degree of component motion. Examination of a joint's component motion assists with detecting dysfunctions that may interfere with normal active motion. **Joint play** is considered to be one type of accessory movement that is not under voluntary control. These movements only occur in response to external forces that take place at the terminal range of normal joints. **Manipulation movements** are described as *skilled passive movements to joints*. Within this approach, the term "manipulation" is used synonymously with "mobilization" to define therapeutic maneuvers that are directed toward restoring accessory motion to a joint.[6] Manipulation may take the form of **distraction** techniques, **nonthrust** techniques, or **thrust** techniques (Fig. 7-3).[1,2] As defined by Kaltenborn,[7,8] distraction techniques involve the separation of two joint surfaces perpendicular to the plane of the joint. Distraction may be used to unweight the joint, stretch the joint capsule, and to reduce a dislocation. Nonthrust techniques include oscillations as described by Maitland,[9,10] as well as stretch and progressive oscillation, combining oscillation with stretch. Nonthrust is used to mechanically elongate connective tissues and to fire muscle and joint receptors. Thrust techniques involve a sudden, high-velocity, short-amplitude motion that is delivered at the pathological limit of an accessory motion. These techniques are used to reduce positional faults, release an adhesion, or fire joint receptors.

Joint mobilization produces an increase in the firing of mechanoreceptors and nerve endings that are located within the capsule and ligaments of the joint. Firing of these receptors

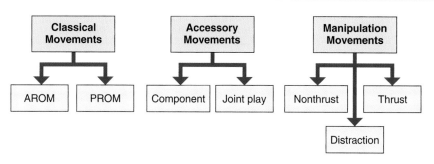

FIGURE 7–3 Paris's classification of movement types.[1]

is believed to reduce nociception and encourage muscle relaxation. Evidence supporting the impact of joint mobilization on adjacent muscle function has been documented in the literature.[11] Although mobilization may produce neurophysiologic effects, it is the mechanical effects of joint mobilization that are considered to be of greatest value within this approach. Therefore, joint mobilization is primarily performed for the purpose of increasing the extensibility of connective tissue structures about a joint and for restoration of normal positional relationships. Grade I and II mobilizations are typically used to target the neurophysiologic effects; however, Grade III and IV, stretch, and progressive oscillation mobilizations are required in order to produce direct mechanical effects. The mechanical effects are considered greatest if stretching at end range is performed in either a sustained or rhythmical fashion (Box 7-2).

PRINCIPLES OF EXAMINATION
General Goals and Considerations

The goals of the first patient visit focus on identification of the joint dysfunction that is sufficient enough to allow advice and instruction in self-treatment. It is important during the first visit to explain the examination findings to the patient; however, initiation of intervention is often not necessary, may confound the interpretation of the patient's response to the examination, and, therefore, it may be best to initiate

treatment when the patient returns for their next visit. The therapist must continually be aware of patient tolerance and reactivity during the first visit and all subsequent visits. A complete understanding of normal joint mechanics is necessary for the therapist to provide the most appropriate intervention. It is important for the therapist to recognize that bias may hinder good decision-making.[1–5]

QUESTIONS *for* REFLECTION

- Within the Paris approach, describe the goals for the first patient visit.
- What is the primary objective, what must be accomplished during this visit, and what can wait until the next visit?

Components of the Examination
Patient History

Although pain is de-emphasized, it must be evaluated. This evaluation routinely occurs through standard means, including the numeric pain scale and other self-assessment questionnaires. Pain may provide misleading information about which the manual therapist should be aware. Typically, pain is the result of dysfunction, and rarely does it function as a warning of impending dysfunction. The degree of reported symptoms is not always proportional to the severity of the condition, and a reduction in a patient's reported pain does not always indicate improvement in the identified dysfunction. As mentioned, pain is affected by nonphysical factors, many of which are outside the scope of physical therapy practice. It is also important to note that pain does not always follow specific dermatomes and therefore offers no information regarding its origin. For these reasons, the therapist must proceed cautiously when evaluating pain.

Box 7-2 EFFECTS OF JOINT MOBILIZATION/ MANIPULATION

1. **Psychological effects:** Produced through the laying on of hands and associated joint audibles

2. **Neurophysiologic effects:** An increase in the firing of mechanoreceptors and nerve endings that are located within the capsule and ligaments of the joint. Firing of these receptors is believed to reduce nociception and encourage muscle relaxation. The goal of Grade I and II manipulation.

3. **Mechanical effects:** An increase in the extensibility of connective tissue structures about a joint and for restoration of normal positional relationships. The goal of Grade III, IV and V manipulation.

NOTABLE QUOTABLE

"Few, if any, rules for therapy are more than 90% correct. If one does not understand the fundamentals, one does more harm in the 10% of instances to which the rules do not apply than one does good in the 90% to which they do apply."

Fuller Albright

As with most other systems, the Paris approach includes a detailed series of questions that are to be asked during the history and interview. It is important to note that the patient interview is focused toward questions of function. Instead of asking whether certain activities produce symptoms, patients are asked which activities are possible. As progress is made, patients express changes in their functional abilities, thus providing objective evidence of improvement.[1-5]

Active Range of Motion

Active range of motion is performed for cardinal plane motions, which are defined as **nonfunctional movements** and **functional movements**. They occur in oblique planes and simulate the motions that patients normally perform (Table 7-1). Side bending of the cervical spine with the head facing forward in the frontal plane is deemed a nonfunctional movement because it is not a movement that typically occurs outside of a physical therapy evaluation. However, side bending of the cervical spine while rotation ipsilaterally toward the shoulder is considered to be functional side bending. Examining the difference between these two types of motions assists the therapist in understanding where the locus of dysfunction lies. If the patient has normal functional side bending, but is lacking full nonfunctional side bending, then the restriction is likely to be in the suboccipital region as evidenced by the inability of this region to produce contralateral rotation (Fig. 7-4). This example serves to reveal how a detailed understanding of biomechanics will assist in focusing intervention.[1,2] Throughout active movement testing, the therapist is constantly concerned with identifying both the quantity and quality of motion as well as any provocation of symptoms noted upon testing. Although

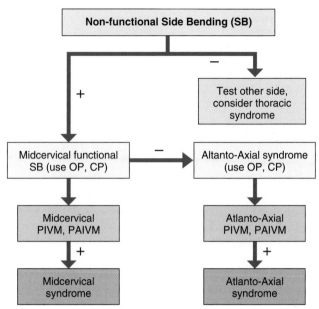

FIGURE 7–4 Algorithmic approach to differentiating between midcervical and suboccipital regional mobility restrictions. + = reproducible symptom and/or mobility restriction; CP = counterpressure; OP = overpressure; SB = side bending; PAIVM = passive accessory intervertebral mobility; PIVM = passive intervertebral mobility.[1,2]

examination of quantity is vital, this approach emphasizes examination of movement quality as well. Two joints may each present with a normal range of motion, yet each may have very different characteristics related to movement quality. It is often these differences in quality that assist the therapist in providing the most appropriate intervention.

Table 7-1	Components of Cervical Spine Functional and Nonfunctional Side Bending	
CERVICAL REGION	**FUNCTIONAL SIDE BENDING**	**NONFUNCTIONAL SIDE BENDING**
Suboccipital Motion	• None	1. Side bending right: • C1-C2 rotation to the left 2. Side bending left: • C1-C2 rotation to the right 3. Rotation right: • O-C1 side bending to the left 4. Rotation left: • O-C1 side bending to the right
Midcervical Motion	1. Side bending right: • Accompanied by rotation right • Right downglide • Left upglide • Closing on right • Opening on left 2. Side bending left: • Accompanied by rotation left • Left downglide • Right upglide • Closing on left • Opening on right	1. Side bending right: • Same as functional 2. Side bending left: • Same as functional

Functional side bending requires pure midcervical motion, whereas nonfunctional side bending requires both midcervical and suboccipital motion.

Selective Tissue Tension Testing

Following performance of standard neurovascular procedures and special tests, **selective tissue tension (STT) testing** is performed. Cyriax[12] espoused that when a healthy muscle contracts isometrically, it should be both strong and pain free. STT seeks to selectively facilitate an isometric contraction of the muscle in question and, in so doing, identify the muscle's strength and any provocation of symptoms. The principles and process of STT testing are delineated in detail in Chapter 5 of this text. Formal **manual muscle testing**, as described elsewhere in the literature, is also performed for any muscles deemed as weak upon screening.[13]

Palpation

Finally, within this approach the manual physical therapist embarks on three distinctly different types of palpation testing. These include palpation for condition, palpation for position, and palpation for mobility. **Palpation for condition** includes the palpation of structures in an attempt to identify the level of involvement or status of various tissues in the region of dysfunction. By palpating the skin, subcutaneous tissue, muscle, and joint, the manual therapist attempts to identify the presence of tightness, tenderness, altered temperature, altered texture, and the presence of trigger or tender points. If soft tissue tightness or tenderness is found within a muscle, the therapist attempts to identify the underlying cause of muscle guarding. A muscle that is undergoing **involuntary muscle guarding** will display a reduction in the degree of guarding when the joint is supported. This form of guarding may be the result of injury to the muscle or it may be occurring in response to underlying joint dysfunction. A muscle with **chemical muscle guarding** presents as having a heaviness or bogginess to the touch related to chemical responses to injury. **Voluntary muscle guarding** involves an increase in muscle tone owing to pain or fear of pain and is primarily revealed during active movement. A muscle that is *adaptively shortened* presents as having normal tone with significant restrictions in its ability to lengthen during motion (Fig. 7-5).

Palpation for position is an attempt to identify the presence of positional faults, or altered relationships between adjacent bony structures about a joint (Fig. 7-6). Within this approach, there is a preferential attention to the observance

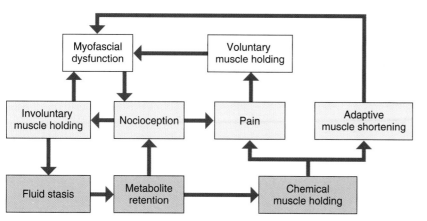

FIGURE 7–5 The pathogenesis of muscle dysfunction syndromes.[1]

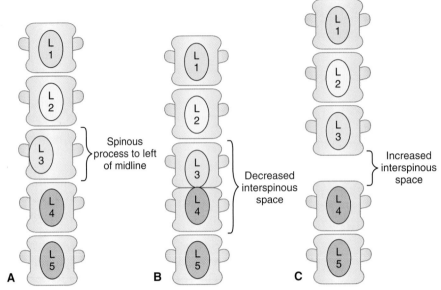

FIGURE 7–6 Palpation for position. Palpation of spinous processes and their corresponding interspinous spaces (ISS) provides information regarding the position of one vertebra relative to the adjacent vertebrae. Palpation for position is performed using the pinch test, in which the therapist pinches each adjacent spinous process and considers its position relative to the vertebra above and below. Palpation for positional faults alone is inadequate for identification of joint dysfunction because of the high occurrence of bony anomalies. Within this approach, palpation for mobility is the best indicator of joint dysfunction. **A.** L3 is rotated to the right as evidenced by the spinous process that is displaced to the left of midline. **B.** L3 is "extended" on L4 as evidenced by a reduction in the ISS between L3 and L4, with normal spacing between L2-L3 and L4-L5. **C.** L3 is "flexed" on L4 as evidenced by an increase in the ISS between L3 and L4, with normal spacing between L2-L3 and L4-L5.[1-4]

of altered movement patterns as opposed to positional relationships. The presence of a positional fault is deemed to be an issue only if such faults produce an alteration in the expected patterns of normal movement. This feature is in contrast to other approaches that use positional diagnoses as a critical factor in determining joint dysfunction. Because of issues related to the ability of the therapist to reliably identify the presence of positional faults and because anatomical anomalies often mimic positional faults, the manual physical therapist is advised to consider positional faults only in light of the motion characteristics of the joint (Box 7-3).

Box 7-3 CLASSIFICATION OF INTERVENTION

1. **Palliative interventions**: Designed to provide relief of symptoms and readily used in the case of an acute condition

2. **Preparatory interventions**: Engage the involved tissues so that they will respond more favorably to the primary intervention that is to follow

3. **Corrective interventions**: The reason why patients seek care; the interventions that facilitate achievement of the primary objectives as established during the examination

4. **Supportive interventions**: Used following corrective techniques for the purpose of maintaining the gains just achieved and reducing any negative secondary effects of such changes

Palpation for mobility is focused on the use of **passive intervertebral mobility testing (PIVM)** to ascertain the degree of accessory motion within a joint and to identify end-feels, or the quality of resistance at end range. PIVM testing has been found in the literature to possess good intrarater, yet poor interrater, reliability.[14] PIVM testing involves the introduction of passive motion across a joint while palpating for the motion's quantity and quality, as well as end-feel (Fig. 7-7). In addition, the therapist identifies any provocation of symptoms from the selected measures. Measures of passive accessory movement of the spine have been found to be most reliable when symptom provocation, rather than segmental mobility, is used as the primary criterion.[15] The quantity of motion is graded using a 0 to 6 scale, with 0 being equal to complete ankylosis, or no movement, and 6 being equal to instability. A grade of 3 is considered to be normal (Table 7-2).

NOTABLE QUOTABLE

"By continuous practice and thinking hard through the fingers, in other words concentrating upon the senses observed through the fingertips, it is possible to develop that elusive quality of the manipulative skill—tissue tension sense."

Alan Stoddard

Cyriax[12] is often credited with formalizing the concept of end-feels, which are of greatest value when examining the extremity articulations. Chesworth et al[16] demonstrated significant agreement for pain and moderate agreement for resistance

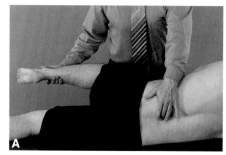
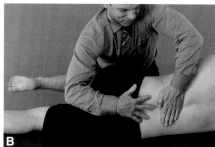
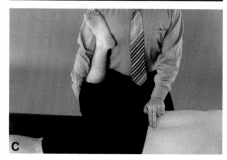
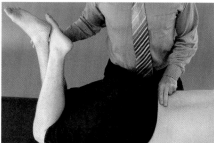
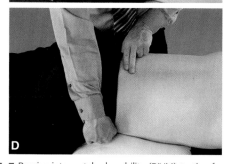

FIGURE 7–7 Passive intervertebral mobility (PIVM) testing for **A.** forward bending, **B.** backward bending, **C.** side bending, and **D.** rotation. Movement is elicited in the spine via the legs during palpation of the interspinous space.[2–4]

Table 7–2	Accessory Motion Grading System	
GRADE	**DESCRIPTION**	
0	Ankylosis	
1	Considerable restriction	
2	Slight restriction	
3	Normal	
4	Slight increase	
5	Considerable increase	
6	Unstable	

A grade is assigned based on the results of PIVM testing.[1–4]

(Table 7-3).[1] Before testing for end-feels, it is important for the therapist to understand that if the passive range of motion of a joint is not greater than its active range, there will be an abnormal end-feel. End-feels exist beyond the control of muscular influences and are, therefore, considered to be tests of joint function. End-feels are often referred to as barriers.[19] Examination of end-feel is considered to be the best method for determining normal versus abnormal joint play.

During both active movement testing and PIVM testing, the therapist attempts to identify whether restrictions in motion are either capsular or noncapsular in nature. Cyriax[12] has also addressed issues related to the use of capsular and noncapsular patterns in determining etiology (see Chapter 5).

Table 7–3	Paris's Classification of Normal and Abnormal End-Feels[1,5]	
END-FEEL	**EXAMPLE/DESCRIPTION**	
Normal End-Feels		
Soft tissue approximation	Elbow, knee flexion	
Muscular	Straight leg raise, shoulder abduction	
Ligamentous	Varus stress test	
Cartilaginous	Elbow extension	
Capsular	Elbow hyperextension	
Abnormal End-Feels		
Capsular	Tight resistance to creep	
Adhesions, scarring	Sudden, sharp arrest in one direction	
Bony block	Sudden, hard stop short of normal range	
Bony grate	Rough, grating	
Springy rebound	Slight bounce back	
Pannus	Soft crunchy squelch	
Loose	Ligamentous laxity	
Empty	Not mechanically limited	
Painful	Pain before reaching end range	
Muscle	Abnormal elastic resistance	

when testing end-feels at the shoulder. Other authors have concurred that intrarater and interrater reliability for shoulder end-feels are substantial.[17,18] Paris has expanded Cyriax's classification of end-feels, with 5 normal end-feels and 10 abnormal end-feels

If the joint capsule is involved in the observed joint restriction, then the pattern of limitation that emerges should be consistent for that joint. With a **capsular pattern**, active and passive motions are often painful and restricted in the same directions and often exhibit the same degree of restriction. Pain is often associated with approaching the end of the available range. In the case of a capsular pattern, resisted movements typically do not produce pain. These capsular patterns of motion restrictions are in contrast to motion loss that is due to myofascial restrictions. Such patterns are referred to as **myofascial patterns**.[1,2,5]

Within the Paris approach to OMPT, the most skilled part of patient management is not intervention but rather examination. At the conclusion of the examination, the therapist should have identified the key objective: the physical features that are contributing to the patient's dysfunction. These features must relate directly to the patient's level of physical disability and not be based upon the patient's symptom behavior. Restoring function is deemed to be the preferred goal of manual physical therapy intervention.

Notable Quotable

"While science takes time, the clinician needs to know today!"

Stanley V. Paris

PRINCIPLES OF INTERVENTION
Factors that Influence Outcomes

Within this approach to OMPT, there are several inherent themes that serve as the basis for clinical decision-making. Some authors contend that lifting injuries are more common in the United States compared to other countries, suggesting the presence of *secondary gain.*[1] When the potential for secondary gain is present, it behooves the therapist to be suspicious of the patient's history. Evidence suggests that the longer an individual is out of work, the more likely he or she is to stay out of work, and early, effective intervention that returns the individual to gainful employment is the goal.[20] Many individuals experience resolution of their symptoms without receiving care.[21] However, patients with symptoms that remain after approximately 2 weeks, or patients who are experiencing a re-exacerbation of a preexisting problem, are appropriate candidates for physical therapy. Due to the great potential for reoccurrence,[21] manual physical therapists must be sure to continue intervention until functional maximum benefit has been achieved and not discontinue therapy simply because symptoms have subsided.

The value of considering the *stage of healing* for any given injury is important.[1] It is believed that what is done by the therapist within the *first 2 weeks* following an injury is most critical. At *3 months* after onset, it is likely that, in most cases, the patient has now adopted a more chronic component to their dysfunction. Early intervention is therefore paramount in determining prognosis. In consideration of the stages of healing following an injury, it is important that the manual therapist avoid manipulation to improve range within the *first 10 days* following an injury to allow for healing from the inflammatory process. However, manipulation to improve range is indicated in the presence of a displacement. *Lower grade mobilizations* to provide pain relief only are indicated to avoid interruption of the healing process.

It is important for therapists and medical practitioners to appreciate the fact that the results of diagnostic imaging are not always conclusive. Visualization of pathology on an image does not necessarily indicate that the observed pathology is the cause of the patient's symptoms; therefore, such an observation should be appreciated, but not considered to be the primary factor in arriving at a differential diagnosis.[22-24]

Prior to embarking on a course of intervention, it is critical that the manual physical therapist gain an appreciation of the stage of healing as it relates to the patient's presenting dysfunction. Favorable outcomes may be as much a factor of proper patient selection and timing as it is a factor of therapist skill. Within this approach, five stages for the process of recovery and healing have been outlined. The **immediate stage** exists within the first few minutes following the onset of the condition. During this phase, appropriate action could be taken to provide immediate correction of the condition or lessen its effects. The **acute stage** is characterized by a progressive increase in signs and symptoms. During this stage, it is critical that the therapist provide intervention only if it will aid in the reparative process. In the **subacute stage**, patients experience a plateau in signs and symptoms. Although intervention may provide intermittent relief for the patient in this stage, care must be taken so as not to interfere with the natural course of healing. The condition becomes more stable in the **settled stage**, and the therapist is better able to appreciate the effects of intervention. During this stage, the patient is able to handle moderate stresses, including manipulation. The term **chronic stage** is typically applied to static conditions with a history of usually greater than 3 months. It is important for the therapist to appreciate that chronic conditions often involve a considerable degree of behavioral changes that lack a direct correlation to true organic pathology. When attempting to ascertain the patient's stage of recovery, it is important to consider the degree of symptom irritability, or reactivity, as opposed to basing this determination solely on the amount of time since onset.

Although not unique to this approach, there are three levels of reactivity that serve to direct the manual therapist in his or her choice of intervention. **High reactivity** is characterized by pain that occurs prior to end range. **Moderate reactivity** is present when pain occurs simultaneous with achieving end range. **Low reactivity** is indicated when there is no pain at end range or when pain occurs with overpressure only. The type of manual technique, grade of technique, sequencing of techniques, and decisions regarding the use of other procedures will all be governed by the patient's observed level of reactivity (Fig. 7-8). The patient's level of reactivity may change on a daily basis, thus requiring intervention to be adjusted accordingly.

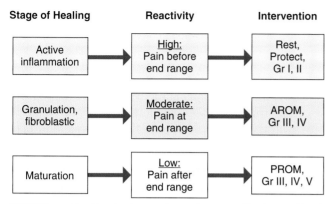

Stage of Healing	Reactivity	Intervention
Active inflammation	High: Pain before end range	Rest, Protect, Gr I, II
Granulation, fibroblastic	Moderate: Pain at end range	AROM, Gr III, IV
Maturation	Low: Pain after end range	PROM, Gr III, IV, V

FIGURE 7–8 Matching the intervention to the stage of healing and level of reactivity.[1]

In the acute stage, providing palliative intervention at the time of the initial visit is justified. However, initiating a trial intervention on the first day may be more than what is reasonably tolerated by the patient and may confound the results of the examination. Providing home exercises and educating the patient may be sufficient. Similar to the *Nordic approach* to OMPT (see Chapter 6), this approach also ascribes to the *trial treatment* concept.[7,8] In addition, it is important to introduce only one procedure or technique at a time so that the effects of each procedure can be adequately evaluated. The manual therapist must constantly observe patient tolerance to interventions, learning which procedures have the greatest effect and adjusting interventions to consistently meet the needs of the patient.

QUESTIONS for REFLECTION

- What are the primary factors believed to effect outcomes?
- What impact does the stage of healing and level of reactivity have on outcomes?
- How might the concept of the trial treatment be used to guide intervention?

Sequencing the delivery of chosen interventions is as important as the choice of intervention itself. Within this approach, interventions may be classified as either palliative, preparatory, corrective, or supportive. **Palliative interventions** are designed to provide relief of symptoms and are readily used in the case of an acute condition. Such procedures may include rest, ice, or electric stimulation. **Preparatory interventions** are used to engage the involved tissues so that they will respond more favorably to the primary intervention that is to follow. Massage, moist heat, and Grade I and II oscillations are examples of interventions used to prepare the structures for **corrective interventions**, which are often the reason why patients seek care. These are the interventions that facilitate achievement of the primary objectives as established during the examination. Manipulation to eliminate

restrictions, exercise to improve strength and endurance, and transverse friction massage to eliminate adhesions are all included within this domain. **Supportive interventions** are those interventions used following corrective techniques for the purpose of maintaining the gains just achieved and reducing any negative secondary effects of such changes. Supportive techniques include patient education, home exercises, and modalities to relieve postactivity soreness (Box 7-3).

Common Dysfunctions and Their Principles of Intervention

In this section, a myriad of common dysfunctions will be covered using nomenclature that is, in some cases, unique to this approach. Because of the high priority given to identifying the nature of the dysfunction and the implications for chosen interventions, an understanding of these dysfunctions is foundational to patient care. These concepts are not designed to be all inclusive, nor is it suggested that these syndromes occur in isolation. A common confounding variable of patient care occurs when multiple dysfunctions are present simultaneously.

NOTABLE QUOTABLE

"Orthopaedic surgery is preventable."

Stanley V. Paris

Dysfunction of Synovial Joint Origin

Synovial joints may develop a synovitis and/or hemarthrosis, restrictions, painful entrapment, mechanical locking, or degenerative arthrosis. Synovitis differs from hemarthrosis in that synovitis involves swelling that is gradual in onset, as opposed to hemarthrosis, in which swelling occurs within minutes following insult. Synovitis is typically warm to the touch and elicits a moderate amount of pain, whereas hemarthrosis is hot to the touch with a significant degree of pain present. Because it is difficult to determine which condition is present, especially in the case of spinal dysfunction, it is recommended that the manual physical therapist engage the patient in a period of rest including modalities to manage the swelling followed by mobilization of the joint after approximately 10 days to ensure that the healing process has not been disrupted. Synovial joint restrictions often occur in response to a resolving synovitis or hemarthrosis. Typically, these lesions are not painful; however, limited motion is present. Restrictions are best managed through the use of Grade III and IV oscillations and thrust techniques. Painful entrapment of the synovial joint occurs in response to an awkward movement performed in a rapid fashion, such as a quick turn of the cervical spine. The patient often presents with an inability to return the neck to the neutral, or fully erect, position. Intervention includes distraction to release the impingement followed by isometric recruitment of capsular muscles to retrieve the facet joint capsule from impingement.

Mechanical locking is typically the result of a loose body or degeneration of joint surfaces. Patients typically present relatively pain-free but with restricted motion that is sudden in onset. Intervention techniques include thrust manipulation, which is often in the direction of the restriction to release the mechanical block, much like closing a stuck drawer in order to release it.

Degenerative processes related to the joint and the structures about the joint are referred to as *osteoarthritis* or *osteoarthrosis*, depending on whether or not active joint inflammation is present. Degenerative processes typically involve both intra- and extra-articular structures. Intervention includes specific techniques designed to improve both classical and component movements.[1,25]

Dysfunction of Muscular Origin

Within this approach, there are five main types of muscular dysfunctions that have been delineated. Muscle spasm of orthopaedic origin occurs rarely in response to a pinching of sensitive tissue such as the facet joint capsule or because of reflexive activity from a facilitated segment. A facilitated segment refers to a spinal segment that is dysfunctional, resulting in an increase in neurological input to all structures innervated by the nerves exiting that segment. Paris has summarized previous work and has identified that each structure of the spine is innervated by at least three segmental nerves.[26–31] Therefore, symptoms of various kinds and in various locations may be, in part, related to a spinal segment that is dysfunctional and in need of correction. Management consists of correcting the underlying cause, which may include release of the capsule or postural correction. The term "muscle spasm" is most appropriate for describing conditions of neurological origin.

Involuntary muscle guarding is defined as a state of increased tone that may be observed or palpated, usually suggesting the presence of an underlying lesion. This condition may be observed within the paravertebral musculature of the lumbar spine despite the fact that the patient is in a relaxed position or may be identified as a *heaviness* in an extremity on attempts at passive movement. It is important for the manual therapist to identify the underlying cause in order to eliminate the subsequent holding. Chemical muscle guarding is often the result of prolonged involuntary holding. A reduction in fluid flow and retention of metabolites and tissue fluids may occur in response to abnormal muscle activity. The manual physical therapist may perceive firmness or fullness within the muscle belly along with a loss of extensibility. These symptoms are not typically influenced by changes in position but should resolve in response to heat-reducing modalities, in addition to soft tissue massage to facilitate an increase in blood flow and stretching. Voluntary muscle guarding is produced by the patient who is actively resisting movement because of the perception of pain or the fear of pain. Patients typically present with pain upon movement with observable splinting of the

extremity. Once movement is deemed to be favorable, pendular activities, Grade I and II mobilizations with oscillations, and pain-relieving modalities are indicated. Finally, myofascial restrictions or **adaptive shortening** may result from any of the aforementioned conditions (Fig. 7-5). Because of prolonged immobility, muscles and their connective tissue structures adaptively shorten, leading to restricted movement that eventually impacts the joint over which the muscles lie. Muscle and joint pain along with loss of function typically occurs. Intervention typically consists of heat and sustained stretching at end range.[1]

Dysfunction of Neurological Origin

This approach to manual therapy considers what is termed **nerve entrapment syndromes.** These syndromes are often caused by degenerative, postural, or myofascial restrictions. Symptoms often consist of paresthesia or pain that is nonspecific and intermittent and is affected by movement and position. The classic neurological signs may also be present, which include a change in sensation, reflexes, and myotomal strength. Intervention typically involves addressing the insulting factor, such as correcting posture or stretching tight muscle and nerve-gliding activities.

Dysfunction Secondary to Overuse

Overuse syndromes are common dysfunctions of the musculoskeletal system when the stress introduced to tissues is greater than the ability of the tissues to respond through repair or by an increase in their strength. These conditions involve three levels of progression. The first level includes discomfort that is experienced several hours after activity. This is deemed to be normal and may be reduced by incorporating appropriate rest periods, using massage, and stretching after the activity. The second level occurs when pain comes on during, or immediately after, activity. Examination for the presence of dysfunction that may be affecting performance and evaluation of technique must be considered. The third level involves pain that is present even at rest, indicating tissue damage. Rest is indicated for these individuals, along with cross-training and pharmacological aids. A specific type of overuse syndrome involves postural aberrations. **Postural syndromes** occur from prolonged positions that place undue stress on anatomical tissues. As with other overuse syndromes, dysfunction that results from prolonged poor posture is often insidious and takes a long time to occur. Intervention strategies focus on correction of poor posture, stretching of muscles that may have developed tightness, and activities designed to improve muscle endurance. Patient education is vital to long-term outcomes.

It is important to note that the interdependency of anatomical structures, which is particularly true when managing spinal conditions, often results in dysfunctions that involve more than one structure. Erhard states that the lumbopelvic complex is "a system of inter-dependent joints and dysfunction in any one joint will cause dysfunction in the others."[32] Paris uses the term lesion complex dysfunction to delineate this point.[1]

Describe the etiology, typical examination findings, and proposed intervention for the following dysfunctions:

1. Synovitis
2. Hemarthrosis
3. Painful entrapment
4. Mechanical locking
5. Osteoarthrosis
6. Muscle spasm
7. Involuntary/voluntary muscle holding
8. Chemical muscle holding
9. Adaptive shortening
10. Nerve entrapment
11. Overuse syndrome
12. Postural syndrome

Mobilization/Manipulation Theory and Practice

As defined by Paris, *mobilization* and *manipulation* are terms that may be used synonymously to describe the skilled, passive movement to a joint.[1-5] Within this approach, joint mobilization is used to preferentially restore accessory motion.

Nonthrust mobilization techniques are those techniques that are performed with lower velocity within the available range of motion. These techniques include **prolonged stretch** or **oscillatory** movements and are the most frequent mobilizations used by manual therapists. General nonthrust mobilizations do not involve locking of adjacent regions and are, therefore, less specific. These techniques may involve a steady stretch at end range or an overstretch beyond end range. These techniques are not preferred because nonspecific mobilization may have the effect of producing motion in the regions that may already be hypermobile while failing to introduce motion in the region of hypomobility (see Fig. 2-13).

Nonthrust specific mobilization techniques involve procedures designed to address the specific motion limitations that have been identified during the examination. For example, if there is a limitation in shoulder external rotation, specific mobilization directed toward reducing restrictions within the posterior capsule would be indicated. The specificity of these techniques may be accomplished through application of mobilizing force and stabilizing counterforce across the joint in question or through the use of locking techniques. Specific **stretch without locking mobilizations** techniques are applied at the end range for the purpose of moving the joint capsule into the plastic region of deformation, thus improving available motion. An example may include performing a dorsal glide of the radiocarpal joint to improve wrist mobility without locking intercarpal and radioulnar joints owing to the limited motion introduced into these regions. Specific **progressive oscillation without locking mobilizations** involve a progressive series of three to five medium-amplitude oscillations that

begin at midrange and gradually move toward end range. These techniques are commonly performed in the spine and are often used for their neurophysiologic effects. These oscillations may also be performed in a graded fashion. The grades used to provide these oscillations have been defined by Maitland[9,10] and are described in detail in Chapter 8 of this text. Specific **isometric without locking mobilizations** may also be used, which involve using specifically localized isometric muscle contractions to mobilize joints. These techniques are often referred to as **muscle energy techniques (MET)** (see Chapter 4).

Specific mobilization may also be performed with locking. Locking procedures are used to increase the stiffness of regions adjacent to the target segment to reduce the forces experienced by these regions. Due to its multisegmental nature, the use of locking procedures is particularly valuable when mobilizing the spine. In the presence of hypomobility, it is not uncommon for adjacent hypermobility to exist, for which manipulation would be contraindicated. Locking, therefore, increases specificity by directing the mobilizing forces to the specific regions of hypomobility. Locking techniques may take the form of either **ligamentous tension locking** procedures or **facet joint opposition locking** procedures. The former involves movement of the joints into a position that engages the ligaments, whereas facet opposition locking is accomplished by moving joints in a manner that produces apposition of articular surfaces. These maneuvers are fully described in Chapter 2, and techniques involving their use are described in Chapter 18.

- Describe the purpose of using *locking techniques* when performing mobilization.
- What are the major differences between *ligamentous tension locking* and *facet opposition locking* techniques?
- Which locking technique provides greater specificity?

Within the therapeutic arsenal of the manual physical therapist lies high-velocity thrust mobilization or manipulation. It is a common misconception that thrust manipulation requires a significant increase in force to achieve results. Although increased forces may be necessary, careful prepositioning of the joint often disallows the need for a substantial increase in the quantity of force. Prepositioning will reduce the amplitude, or distance, over which the thrust will take place, thus reducing the risk of injury. Thrust techniques may be performed in the direction of glide, which is parallel to the plane of the joint, or as a distraction technique, which is performed perpendicular to the plane of the joint. This approach adopts a more judicious use of thrust manipulation than do most other approaches. Thrust techniques are not considered to be a primary intervention strategy but may be used when appropriate to infiltrate intra-articular mechanical restrictions. Instruction in the performance of spinal thrust manipulation is advocated only after competence has been demonstrated in the performance of nonthrust. An overview of the practice of thrust manipulation is provided in detail in Chapter 18.

As previously mentioned, during mobilization procedures that involve joint glide, graded oscillations as defined by Maitland[9,10] are most commonly used. However, when the manual physical therapist chooses to provide separation, or distract, joint surfaces, the grading system espoused by Kaltenborn[7,8] is used. *Grade I* distraction is when the joint is barely unweighted. *Grade II* is when the slack in the joint capsule has been engaged. *Grade III* occurs when the capsule and ligaments are stretched (Fig. 7-9). As with mobilization glides, distraction mobilizations also have many variations. **Rhythmic distraction**, which is performed with alternate periods of rest, is designed to *"gate"* the patient's perception of pain. **Adjustive distraction** typically involves the use of high-velocity thrust for the purpose of repositioning sub-luxed or dislocated joints. These techniques are not routinely used in the clinic, but are important for therapists engaged in the care of athletes. Paris has defined the concept of **positional distraction**. Most valuable when treating the spine, this technique involves careful patient positioning that provides maximal triplanar opening of an intervertebral foramen for the purpose of reducing nerve root pressure. The use of pillows or straps allows maintenance of this position for a period of time that the patient may independently perform several times each day. This technique may be useful in combination with modalities before or after corrective interventions as a method of controlling symptoms. In addition to the manual distraction techniques described, the manual therapist may be greatly aided by the use of *mechanical distraction, or traction*. Spinal traction tables can be performed in a traditional single or a multiplanar fashion. Triplanar traction tables have been developed by both Paris and Kaltenborn that seek to position the patient to facilitate

distraction at both the level and side in which spinal dysfunction exists (Box 7-4).

DIFFERENTIATING CHARACTERISTICS

The Paris approach to OMPT may best be viewed as an eclectic approach that emphasizes the need for identification of joint dysfunction through a thorough understanding of joint kinematics and function. The perception of pain is the result of an accumulation of factors that occurs as a direct result of underlying dysfunction. The role of the manual physical therapist is to identify the inciting dysfunction based on an understanding of movement rather than the position of the involved joint(s). Dysfunction may present itself as hypomobility,

---

Box 7-4 TYPES OF MOBILIZATION/MANIPULATION

1. **Prolonged stretch or oscillation nonthrust techniques**: General nonspecific, nonthrust techniques that involve sustained stretch or oscillations at end range or overstretch beyond end range

2. **Stretch without locking nonthrust techniques**: Applied at end range for the purpose of moving the joint capsule into the plastic region of deformation, thus improving available motion; often performed at extremity joints where adjacent joints have limited mobility and do not require locking

3. **Progressive oscillation without locking nonthrust techniques**: Progressive series of three to five medium-amplitude oscillations that begin at midrange and gradually move toward end range that may be performed in a graded fashion.

4. **Isometric without locking nonthrust techniques**: Involve the use of specifically localized isometric muscle contractions for the purpose of mobilizing joints; often referred to as muscle energy techniques (MET)

5. **Stretch or oscillation with locking nonthrust techniques**: Ligamentous tension or facet opposition locking with stretch or oscillation to improve specificity

6. **Rhythmic distraction**: Performed with alternate periods of rest and designed to gate the patient's perception of pain

7. **Adjustive distraction**: Involves the use of high-velocity thrust for the purpose of repositioning subluxed or dislocated joints

8. **Positional distraction**: Involves careful patient positioning that provides maximal opening of an intervertebral foramen for the purpose of reducing nerve root pressure; use of pillows or straps allow maintenance of this position for a period of time, and patient may independently perform the distraction several times each day

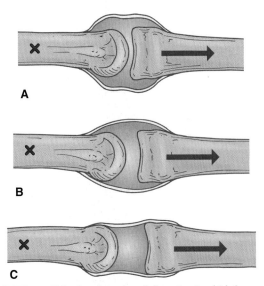

FIGURE 7–9 Kaltenborn's grades of distraction in which force occurs within the long axis of the bone. **A.** Grade I distraction in which the joint surfaces are unweighted. **B.** Grade II distraction in which the slack in the joint capsule is taken up. **C.** Grade III distraction in which the capsule and ligaments are stretched.[1]

hypermobility, or some form of aberrant movement. Therefore, the examination must include a thorough, detailed appreciation for movement quantity, quality, as well as any provocation of symptoms that may occur during movement. Because of its presumably subjective nature, the patient's report of pain is de-emphasized as a valid means of documenting the severity, nature, or location of the dysfunction and is discouraged as a means to demonstrate progress or describe outcomes.

In much the same fashion as Kaltenborn (see Chapter 6), this approach places great emphasis on the manual therapist as movement specialist who seeks to appreciate deficits in either classical or accessory movement. Identification of dysfunction is obtained through the use of a detailed process of examination leading to the strict performance of mobilization techniques. The manner and specificity in which techniques are performed is highlighted. As opposed to some approaches, where therapists are encouraged to develop and modify techniques in the moment, the Paris approach advocates the use of strictly performed procedures that specifically mandate patient and therapist position, hand placement, and mobilizing force. The manual therapist is encouraged to be aware of not only the mechanical, but also the neurophysiological and psychological impact of manual intervention. Progress toward patient-centered functional goals is documented through an observance of improved movement patterns and function.

Stanley V. Paris's approach to OMPT has served to further the cause of manual physical therapy in the United States and abroad. His well-organized system of continuing education courses leading to certification, in addition to the creation of graduate education programs, has established this approach as foundational to the practice of OMPT in this country. The Paris approach to OMPT embodies the important connection between basic science and clinical practice, and in its truest form it may best be considered as the premier applied kinesiological approach to musculoskeletal impairment. Based on a detailed understanding of kinematics, therapists everywhere are reclaiming their role as movement specialists. The attention to detail and specificity by which examination and intervention procedures are conducted with an emphasis on functional progress serve as foundational principles that may be applied to other manual and nonmanual approaches in the management of musculoskeletal impairment.

CLINICAL CASE

History of Present Illness (HPI)

Mr. Johnson comes to physical therapy today noting an incident that occurred 2 weeks ago involving twisting to the left and forceful hyperextension secondary to being struck with a large steel beam while at work. He intermittently reports tingling into the posterior aspect of his right leg. He notes that since his injury, he has been inactive and spends much of his time sitting and playing video games.

Observation: Antalgic gait
Neurological: Deep tendon reflex (DTR) all 2+, LT sensation intact and symmetrical bilateral lower extremity (LE)
Strength: 4/5 strength in proximal hip musculature with pain
Palpation: Tender to the touch over left midbuttock region with increased LE symptoms upon palpation; significant involuntary guarding noted at bilateral paravertebral musculature. The right quadratus lumborum and piriformis reveals increased tissue tone and tenderness, with trigger points noted. Decreased interspinous space is noted between L4 and L5 and the L4 spinous process is displaced to the right relative to the spinous process above and below.
PIVM: Hypomobility noted upon testing of forward bending (FB), side bending (SB) to the left, and rotation (ROT) to the right at L4-5.
AROM: In standing: FB=25% of normal range with deviation to the right and stiffness which improves with repeated movements, BB=75% of normal range with pain at end range with overpressure, SB right=WNL with pain at end range, Left=10% with pain and restriction, ROT Right=10% with pain and restriction, Left=WNL with pain at end range.

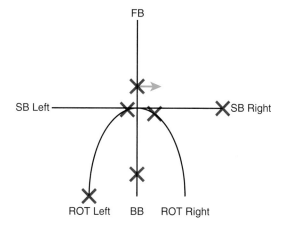

1. Based on your examination findings, what is your current clinical hypothesis regarding Mr. Johnson's condition?
2. List in order of value from most important to least important three physical examination procedures/tests that you would use to differentially diagnose this patient. Perform each procedure on your partner.
3. Based on the information presented and your suspected findings from further testing, describe three to five interventions that you would use with this patient.
4. Describe the value of *passive intervertebral mobility* testing in diagnosis and treatment of this patient. How can PIVM testing be used to document progress and confirm improvement?
5. Summarize the results from palpation testing. What is meant by palpation for condition, position, and mobility, and how do these findings contribute to the diagnosis and guide subsequent intervention?
6. What is the capsular pattern of the lumbar spine? What segment and side do you suspect are problematic in this patient given the results of both AROM and PIVM testing? What manual interventions may be used to address these restrictions? Practice them on your partner.

HANDS-ON

With a partner, perform the following activities:

1 Palpate the interspinous spaces of adjacent vertebrae in the lumbar spine. Palpate these same regions on a partner. Attempt to identify each level of the lumbar spine and have another partner confirm your findings.

2 While palpating the interspinous spaces in prone as instructed above, attempt to introduce movement into the spine by moving your partner's lower extremity into hip abduction (see Fig. 7-7). First concentrate on your ability to introduce movement through the leg and then concentrate on feeling the movement as it arrives at your palpating finger. See if you are able to sequentially elicit movement at L5-S1, followed by L4-L5, and so on.

3 On your partner's ankle, perform a classical motion assessment in all planes followed by an assessment of accessory motion in all planes. During the movement examinations, identify the quantity, quality, and any provocation of symptoms. What are the two types of classical motion, and what are the two types of accessory motion that may be tested? What type of information does classical versus accessory motion testing provide, and how would this information serve to guide intervention?

4 What questions might you ask your partner that focus on function as opposed to level of pain? How might you restructure the patient interview process to focus more on functional status and improvement?

5 With your partner sitting, observe as he or she performs nonfunctional followed by functional side bending of his or her cervical spine actively. Use Figure 7-4 to guide your examination. Based on your findings, seek to identify the area of primary restriction (midcervical or suboccipital). Confirm your findings by performing PIVM testing on the cervical spine.

6 On your partner's thoracolumbar spine in prone, practice your *palpation for condition* by closing your eyes, and attempting to identify areas of increased tissue texture, tone, and temperature. Are there differences from side to side? Are there differences between individuals? Seek to identify areas of increased tension without your partner's feedback and then confirm if the identified region is symptomatic or tender to the touch.

7 On your partner's lumbar spine in prone, practice your *palpation for position* by using the "pinch test" of the spinous processes for identification of positional faults. Have another partner confirm your findings.

8 Place your patient in a position of triplanar *positional distraction* for each of the following regions: (a) C5-C6 on the right, (b) T7-T8 on the left, (c) L4-L5 on the right. Consider the use of pillows or straps to maintain these positions. Consider what other interventions you might combine with these positions. Consider for what conditions these positions may be most effectively used.

9 On your partner's lumbar spine, follow the principles of *ligamentous tension locking* to localize forces to the midlumbar segments. Then, follow the principles of *facet opposition locking* to localize forces to the upper cervical spine. What is the value of using locking techniques when mobilizing the spine? Which type of locking seems to provide the firmest lock and therefore is the most effective?

REFERENCES

1. Paris SV, Loubert, PV. *Foundations of Clinical Orthopaedics, Course Notes.* St. Augustine, FL: Institute Press; 1990.
2. Paris SV. *S1 Introduction to Evaluation and Manipulation of the Spine.* St. Augustine, FL: Institute of Graduate Physical Therapy; 1991.
3. Paris SV. *S3 Course Notes.* St. Augustine, FL: Institute of Graduate Physical Therapy; 1992.
4. Paris SV, Nyberg R, Irwin M. *S2 Course Notes.* St. Augustine, FL: Institute of Physical Therapy; 1993.
5. Patla CE, Paris SV. *E1 Course Notes: Extremity Evaluation and Manipulation.* St. Augustine, FL: Institute of Physical Therapy; 1993.
6. American Physical Therapy Association. *Guide to Physical Therapist Practice, Revised 2nd ed.* Alexandria, VA: American Physical Therapy Association; 2003.
7. Kaltenborn FM. *The Spine: Basic Evaluation and Mobilization Techniques.* 2nd ed. Oslo, Norway: Olaf Norlis Bokhandel; 1993.
8. Kaltenborn FM. *Manual Mobilization of the Joints: The Kaltenborn Method of Joint Examination and Treatment. Volume I: The Extremities.* 6th ed. Oslo, Norway: Olaf Norlis Bokhandel; 2002.
9. Maitland GD. *Peripheral Manipulation.* 3rd ed. Woburn, MA: Butterworth-Heinemann; 1991.
10. Maitland GD, Hengeveld E, Banks K, English K. *Maitland's Vertebral Manipulation.* 6th ed. Woburn, MA: Butterworth-Heinemann; 2001.
11. Wyke B. Neurological aspect of low back pain. In: Jayson MIV, ed. *The Lumbar Spine and Back Pain.* 2nd ed. London: Pitman Publishing; 1976.
12. Cyriax JH, Cyriax PJ. *Cyriax's Illustrated Manual of Orthopaedic Medicine.* 2nd ed. Woburn, MA: Butterworth-Heinemann; 1993.
13. Kendall F, McCreary E, Provance P. *Muscles: Testing and Function with Posture and Pain.* 4th ed. Baltimore, MD: Lippincott Williams & Wilkins; 1993.
14. Gonella C, Paris SV. Reliability in evaluating passive intervertebral motion. *Phys Ther.* 1982;62:436-444.
15. Mahar C, Adams R. Reliability of pain and stiffness assessments in clinical manual lumbar spine examination. *Phys Ther.* 1994;74(9):801-811.
16. Chesworth BM, MacDermid JC, Roth JH, Patterson SD. Movement diagrams and "end-feel" reliability when measuring passive lateral rotation of the shoulder in patients with shoulder pathology. *Phys Ther.* 1998; 78:593-601.
17. Hayes K, Peterson C. Reliability of assessing end-feel and pain and resistance sequence in subjects with painful shoulders and knees. *J Orthop Sports Phys Ther.* 2001;31:432-445.
18. Peterson CM, Hayes W. Construct validity of Cyriax's selective tension examination: association of end-feels with pain at the knee and shoulder. *J Orthop Sports Phys Ther.* 2000;30:512-527.
19. Greenman, PE. *Principles of Manual Medicine.* 2nd ed. Baltimore, MD: Lippincott Williams Wilkins; 1996.
20. Snook SN, Campanelli RA, Ford RJ. *A Study of Back Injury at Pratt and Whitney Aircraft.* Hopkinton, MA: Boston Liberty Mutual Company; 1980.
21. Nachemson AL. The natural course of low back pain. In: White AA, Gordon S, eds. *American Academy of Orthopedic Surgeons Symposium on Low Back Pain.* St. Louis, MO: CV Mosby Co; 1982:46-51.
22. Wiesel S, Tsourmas N, Feffer HL, et al. A study of computer-assisted tomography, I: The incidence of positive CAT scans in an asymptomatic group of patients. *Spine.* 1984;9:549-551.
23. Frymoyer JW, Newberg A, Pope MH, et al. Spine radiographs in patients with low back pain: an epidemiological study in men. *J Bone Joint Surg Am.* 1984;66:1048-1055.
24. Boden SD, Davis DO, Dina TS, et al. Abnormal magnetic-resonance scans of the lumbar spine in asymptomatic individuals: a prospective investigation. *J Bone Joint Surg Am.* 1990;72:403-408.
25. Mulligan BR. *Manual Therapy NAGS, SNAGS, MWMS, etc.* 5th ed. New Zealand: Plane View Services Ltd.; 2004.
26. Paris SV. *The Spinal Lesion.* Christchurch, New Zealand: Pegasus Press; 1965.
27. Paris SV. Anatomy as related to function and pain. *Orthop Clin N Am.* 1983;14:475-489.
28. Paris SV, Nyberg R. Innervation of the posterolateral aspect of the lumbar intervertebral disc. Abstract. Presented at the International Society for the Study of the Lumbar Spine; May 1989; Kyoto, Japan.
29. Paris SV, Nyberg R, Mooney V, Gonyea W. Three level innervation of the lumbar facet joints. Presented at the International Society for the Study of the Lumbar Spine; 1980: New Orleans.
30. Selby D, Paris SV. Anatomy of facet joints and its clinical correlation with low back pain. *Contemp Orthop.* 1981;312:1097-1103.
31. Bogduk N, Tynan W, Wilson AS. The nerve su`ly of the human lumbar intervertebral discs. *J Anatomy.* 1981;132:39-56.
32. Erhard RE, Bowling R. The recognition and management of the pelvic component of low back pain and sciatica pain. *Bull Orthop Section Am Phys Ther Assoc.* 1977;2:4-15.

The Australian Approach

Christopher H. Wise, PT, DPT, OCS, FAAOMPT, MTC, ATC

[*This chapter is dedicated to the memory of Geoffrey Douglas Maitland (1924–2010)*]

Chapter Objectives

At the conclusion of this chapter, the reader will be able to:

- Identify the major influences leading to the development of the Australian approach to orthopaedic manual physical therapy (OMPT).
- Understand the value of using compartmental thinking when interacting with patients.
- Conduct an interrogation with empathy when performing a subjective examination.
- Emphasize the relationship between pain and stiffness when assessing range of motion (ROM).
- Understand the importance of the comparable sign in guiding intervention.
- Appreciate the myriad of ways in which motion may be tested within this approach and how overpressure may be implemented.

- Use the findings from the ROM examination and slump testing to reach a differential diagnosis.
- Interpret the Maitland movement diagram.
- Understand the emphasis placed on analytical assessment in leading to one of four diagnostic classification groupings.
- Understand the system used for grading of mobilization and how the therapist's choice may be guided by the diagnostic classification.
- Appreciate the differentiating characteristics of this approach and to what extent the current best evidence supports it.

HISTORICAL PERSPECTIVES

Getting Started

The development of the *Australian approach* to orthopaedic manual physical therapy (OMPT) has long been attributed to the work of Geoffrey Maitland. Geoffrey Douglas Maitland was born in Adelaide, Australia, in 1924. After serving in the Second World War in Great Britain, he trained as a physical therapist from 1946 to 1949. While working part-time at the Royal Adelaide Hospital and part-time as a private practitioner, Maitland rapidly developed a keen interest in the management of patients suffering from neuromuscular disorders. His strict attention to detail served him well as he labored over the works of James and John Mennell, Alan Stoddard, Robert Maigne, and Edgar and James Cyriax. Maitland's interest in the detailed examination and evaluation of patients with neuromuscular disorders was innovative and became the primary focus of his

teaching endeavors in manual therapy at the University of South Australia, where he began as an instructor in 1954.

Development and Collaboration

In 1961, Maitland received a grant to study overseas. During his study tour through London, Maitland had the opportunity to interact with many of the leaders of his day in the area of manual therapy. It was during this collaborative venture, that he began to further refine his approach to manual physical therapy. Gregory Grieve and James Cyriax were among those to have the greatest impact on the development of Maitland's concepts. In 1962, Maitland presented a paper to the Physiotherapy Society of Australia in which he advocated the use of gentle passive mobilization techniques as opposed to the more forceful manipulation techniques that were traditionally being used at that time. The culmination of Maitland's work was realized in 1964 with the first edition of his text entitled *Vertebral Manipulation*, with the second edition to follow in 1968. The first edition of *Peripheral Manipulation* was published in 1970 (Fig. 8-1).

The Legacy

During his long and distinguished career, Maitland established a legacy of innovation and attention to detail. Among his accomplishments, Maitland was cofounder of the International Federation of Orthopaedic Manipulative Physical Therapists (IFOMPT) in 1974, an organization that continues to be the primary voice for manual physical therapists internationally. Among his greatest accomplishments, Maitland would , no doubt, cite his extensive interaction with patients among his greatest. Maitland viewed the clinic as a laboratory that provided a means to further enhance and refine his theories. Despite a busy lecture and research agenda, Maitland continued to regularly see patients for over 40 years, eventually closing his practice in 1988.[1] Farrell and Jensen write that the "essence" of the *Australian approach* is the insistence on using a sound foundation of basic biological knowledge to reach clinical decisions, the need for clinicians to develop high

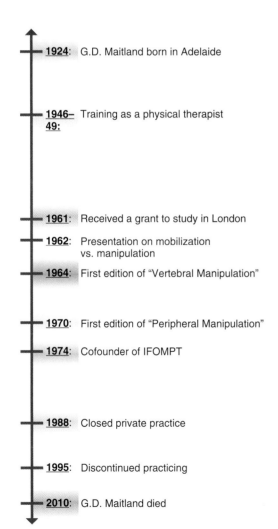

FIGURE 8-1. G.D. Maitland's biographical timeline.

- **1924**: G.D. Maitland born in Adelaide
- **1946–49**: Training as a physical therapist
- **1961**: Received a grant to study in London
- **1962**: Presentation on mobilization vs. manipulation
- **1964**: First edition of "Vertebral Manipulation"
- **1970**: First edition of "Peripheral Manipulation"
- **1974**: Cofounder of IFOMPT
- **1988**: Closed private practice
- **1995**: Discontinued practicing
- **2010**: G.D. Maitland died

levels of skill in problem-solving, the developing nature of the clinical hypothesis throughout the examination, and the necessity for a detailed examination and the need for continuous reexamination.[2] By many, Maitland is considered to be the "father of manual physical therapy." The impact that his well-articulated concepts have had on our current understanding of musculoskeletal dysfunction and the practice of manual physical therapy is profound and far-reaching.

PHILOSOPHICAL FRAMEWORK
Central Theme

It was not until 1978, during a discussion with a colleague after teaching one of his first courses in Europe, that Maitland came to realize that his ideas represented a specific concept of thought and action rather than a method of technique application. His concepts represented an entire manner of approaching the patient that guided the choice and performance of manual techniques. The specific manner of thinking and personal commitment to understanding the patient serves as the central theme of this approach. A sincere desire to understand what the patient is enduring and to engage in active listening as the patient describes the site and behavior of the symptoms lies at the core of this concept.[1,3] The requirement for an optimal outcome lies in the ability of the therapist to listen to the patient in an open, nonjudgmental fashion. Believing that what the patient is expressing is true, relevant, and of value is paramount. The therapist's ability to read and interpret both verbal and nonverbal communication is the major determinant in identifying dysfunction, choosing an intervention, and achieving optimal patient outcomes.

NOTABLE QUOTABLE

"It is open-mindedness, mental agility, and mental discipline linked with a logical and methodological process of assessing cause and effect which are the demands of this concept."

G.D. Maitland

Compartmental Thinking

The therapist's mode of thinking, interpreting, planning, and reaching conclusions related to diagnosis, intervention, and prognosis are germane to this approach. This approach requires that the therapist think and make clinical decisions within two distinctly separate, yet interdependent, compartments.

The **theoretical compartment** contains information that the therapist either knows or speculates. This information is typically obtained through formal education or research. Included in this compartment is information related to pathology, biomedical engineering, neurophysiology, and anatomy, all of which contribute to the patient's formal diagnosis.

The **clinical compartment** contains information that is obtained during the course of the examination from direct interaction with the patient. It is imperative that during the course of the examination and reexamination process the therapist disallows the theoretical compartment from obstructing the search for clinical facts.

The theoretical compartment may influence the aggressiveness and choice of technique and in so doing inform the clinical compartment. However, the therapist must not enter into a patient encounter with a preconceived bias based on theoretical knowledge. Such bias may inhibit the search and acquisition of pertinent clinical data. The choice of technique or intervention is made in relation to the patient's symptoms and signs and is not based on the predetermined diagnostic title. When a mechanical disorder that is influenced by movement or position is present, the clinical compartment takes precedence. However, when a serious disorder that requires medical management is present, the theoretical diagnosis takes precedence. It is incumbent on the manual therapist, therefore, to separate these two interdependent compartments by a *semipermeable brick wall* that divides, but allows communication, between each compartment (Fig. 8-2).[1,3]

PRINCIPLES OF EXAMINATION
General Principles

An inherent aspect of the Australian approach to OMPT is the depth and detail with which the examination is performed (Box 8-1). Most examination procedures used are standard and not unique to this approach. The emphasis on understanding the intensity, behavior, and relationship of symptoms to stiffness and movement makes this approach unique. With strict attention to detail throughout the examination, the therapist attempts to ascertain important information such as the presence of *through-range pain*, *end-range pain*, *latent pain*, and the *level of symptom irritability*. The relationship between pain and movement serve as the foundation for the implementation of passive movement techniques. This approach mandates an appreciation for fine differences in movement. A thorough examination yields pertinent data regarding symptom behavior as it relates to resistance to movement in each direction of available range.

The essence of this approach's view of the examination process is summarized by the acronym **S.I.N.S.**, which stands for severity, irritability, nature, and stage (Box 8-2). **Severity** denotes the intensity of the patient's current symptoms. This determination is based on the degree to which symptoms limit the patient's activity and normal sleeping patterns. **Irritability** is determined by the amount of activity required to produce

Box 8-1 AUSTRALIAN APPROACH EXAM PROCEDURES

Subjective Exam

1. Nature or kind of disorder
2. Area of symptoms
3. Behavior of symptoms
4. Present history
5. Past history

Objective Exam

1. Special tests, including neurological, vertebral artery, quadrant
2. Active physiologic test movements
3. Passive physiologic test movements
4. Passive accessory movements
5. Combined physiologic and accessory movements
6. Test variations

Box 8-2 FACTORS THAT DETERMINE LEVEL OF IRRITABILITY

1. **Nature of the activity:** A minimally aggressive activity that produces symptoms, suggests high irritability
2. **Degree and quality of symptoms:** The greater the severity of symptoms, the higher the level of irritability
3. **Amount of time to return to baseline:** The longer it takes for symptoms to return to baseline after an activity, the higher the level of irritability

and increase symptoms, the magnitude of symptoms, and the amount of time it takes for symptoms to return to a baseline level (Box 8-3). The **nature** of the condition includes a consideration of the suspected pathology as well as patient characteristics such as personality, pain tolerance, and cultural components. **Stage** refers to the phase of the condition. This feature takes into consideration the length of time since onset (acute, subacute, chronic) and the stability of the condition (improving, stable, unstable). Within this approach, S.I.N.S. is used to develop a working hypothesis related to the most probable origin of dysfunction.[4]

In attempting to reach a differential diagnosis, it is imperative that the therapist identifies the exact location and type of symptoms that the patient is experiencing. The therapist may employ standard test movements; however, additional procedures may be needed to provide further clarification of the patient's condition. Such procedures may include functional movements, combined movements, accessory movements, differentiating movements, countering abnormal rhythms, confirmation tests, compression tests, the use of overpressure, and the alteration of test movement sequence and position. When

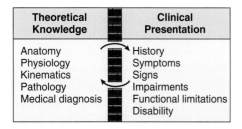

FIGURE 8-2. Two-compartment thinking separated by the semipermeable brick wall.[3]

Box 8-3 S.I.N.S.

S: *Severity* denotes the intensity of the patient's current symptoms.

I: *Irritability* is determined by the amount of activity required to produce and increase symptoms, the magnitude of symptoms, and the amount of time it takes for symptoms to return to a baseline level.

N: *Nature* of the condition includes a consideration of suspected pathology as well as patient characteristics, including personality, pain tolerance, and cultural components.

S: *Stage* refers to the phase of the condition. This feature takes into consideration the length of time since onset (acute, subacute, chronic) and the stability of the condition (improving, stable, unstable).

considering each patient's movement patterns, the overarching feature of this approach emphasizes the importance of *never thinking of range without thinking of pain and never thinking of pain without thinking of range.*[1,3]

NOTABLE QUOTABLE

"Never think of RANGE without thinking of PAIN and never think of PAIN without thinking of RANGE."

G.D. Maitland

The Subjective Examination

Hearing is passive, but listening is an acquired discipline, an art, that demands attention. This approach requires the therapist to engage in active listening for the purpose of truly understanding the plight of the patient. The subjective examination takes on the characteristics of an *interrogation with empathy*. It is an opportunity to explore a depth of questioning that enables the therapist to get an impression of the patient's experiences related to his or her disorder and to better understand the impact that the disorder is having on the patient's life. The questions used during the subjective examination are designed to explore one of three main areas of thought. The subjective examination seeks to identify the kind of structures involved, develop and provide clarification regarding the therapist's initial working hypothesis, and identify the stage, current stability, and irritability of the disorder. During this portion of the examination, the therapist begins to develop an initial hypothesis related to the origin of the patient's presenting symptoms.

NOTABLE QUOTABLE

"The patient is a person, a person needing our skills. Our duty is to the person."

G.D. Maitland

When planning the subjective examination, the initial line of questioning focuses on identifying the kind of disorder that may be present. To ascertain this information, the manual physical therapist engages in four distinct lines of questioning that eventually lead to information related to the *diagnosis, stage of the disorder,* and *stability of the disorder* (Fig. 8-3). The **site of symptoms** questions are the first step toward clarifying the depth, nature, behavior, and chronology of symptoms. The objective of this line of questioning is to provide an indication regarding the pain-sensitive structures that are likely to be involved. The next category of questioning is the **behavior of symptoms** questions. During this series of questioning, the therapist seeks to differentiate local pain from referred pain and to ascertain the patient's level of irritability. When a patient has been identified as irritable, testing procedures must only be taken to the onset of symptoms so as to avoid an exacerbation. **Special questions** are those questions that must be asked in order to detect any inherent risks to the performance of

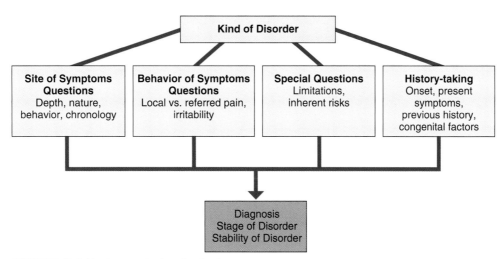

FIGURE 8-3. Subjective examination planning.[1]

manual therapy and to isolate any factors that may limit the effectiveness of intervention. During the *history-taking* aspect of the subjective exam, the therapist strives to understand the onset and development of the present symptoms and any previous history, including episodic and congenital factors.[1,3,5]

QUESTIONS *for* REFLECTION

- How would a therapist go about determining which disorder is serious in nature and requires *medical* management and which disorder is *mechanical* in nature?
- What are the *red flags* that might indicate that a medical referral is necessary?
- How does a therapist with theoretical knowledge *avoid bias* when examining patients?

By the conclusion of the subjective examination, a rapport between the patient and therapist must be established. The patient should be made to feel at ease and confident that the therapist is able to assist him or her. Based on an individual's presenting pattern of symptoms, the therapist should have several well-established clinical hypotheses regarding the origin of such symptoms that will serve to guide the remainder of the examination (Table 8-1). The challenge to the therapist, much like putting together a puzzle, is to make the features and findings of the examination fit together into a clinically recognizable pattern that can be adequately addressed through specific intervention strategies (Fig. 8-4).

The Objective Examination

In planning the objective examination, the manual physical therapist must consider which structures are the most likely contributors to the patient's presenting symptoms, what limitations to the examination exist, and what additional aspects must be considered to further refine the diagnosis. The *first goal* of the objective examination is entirely related to determining the culpable structures and movement directions. The *second goal* is to determine the antecedent factors that have resulted in the onset of symptoms. The objective examination may include a variety of standard testing procedures that are typically used in most physical examination schemes. Covered here are the objective examination procedures that are unique to the Australian approach to OMPT.

Within this approach, it is believed that joint dysfunctions are best determined by using passive movement tests and muscular dysfunctions are best determined by using isometric resistance testing, both of which seek to minimize movement

Table 8-1	Common Pain-Sensitive Structures of the Spine and Their Patterns of Pain
STRUCTURE	**PAIN PATTERN**
Intervertebral Disc	Broad, ill-defined, unilateral, bilateral symmetrical or unsymmetrical, central, more distressing than other sources, not to distal extremity, deep, difficult to change after period of prolonged positioning, location of pain varies based on speed, pain through range, latent pain after sustained positions, latent pain, provoked by stretch or compression; lumbar–across back, gluteal, thigh, abdomen; cervical–suprascapular, upper arm
Ligamentous or Capsular	Pain is local and specific, referred pain is poorly defined, distal is less severe than proximal symptoms; provoke through stretch or compression causing sharp or stretch pain locally
Zygapophyseal (Facet) Joint	Acute phase when local pain may spread and be severe; pain-free phase; chronic phase with no local pain, yet referred pain in distant localized area (i.e., abdominal pain from thoracic lesion)
Dura and Nerve Root Sleeve	Distal never greater than proximal, not referred into foot, no presence of paresthesia, depends on location: Anterior midline = central pain, lateral = vague referral similar to nerve root
Nerve Root and Nerves	Often only in distal dermatome; specific area of referral based on the nerve involved

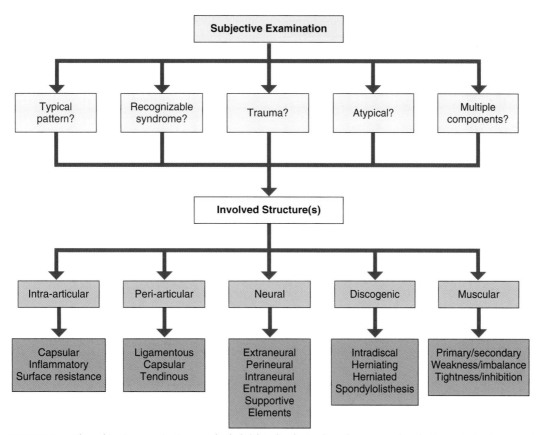

FIGURE 8–4. The subjective examination may be helpful in developing hypotheses regarding the types of structures involved.[1]

to the joint. Identification of a joint-related dysfunction, however, does not enable the examiner to implicate the exact pathoanatomical structure (i.e., disc, joint, capsule). For the manual therapist, joint-related dysfunction simply conveys a disturbance in normal movement patterns that may involve any or all of these interdependent structures (Table 8-2).[1,3,5]

As in most other approaches, the objective examination typically progresses from active movement testing to passive movement testing. A unique feature that is paramount to this approach, however, is the concept of the **comparable sign**. This term is defined as a combination of pain, stiffness, and spasm that the examiner identifies upon examination and considers to be the exact reproduction of the signs and/or symptoms with which the patient has presented. The terms used to

define a manual therapist's perception of spinal stiffness are poorly defined. Cluster analysis procedures were used to reduce 31 stiffness descriptors into 3, which consisted of limited mobility, increased mobility, and viscoelasticity.[6] These categories may be considered to be the fundamental characteristics of the clinical concept of spinal stiffness. Further clarification and development of methods to reliably measure these attributes are required.[6] Lumbar motion segment stiffness has been found to be related to the pathoanatomical structures involved.[7] A decrease in motion segment stiffness was found to occur in the initial stages of disc degeneration, with an increase in stiffness noted with severe degeneration, through comparison of magnitude of the resistance to distraction versus the range of motion via pressure-volume discography on cadaver specimens.[7]

Despite the confusion that exists related to the concept of stiffness during passive movement testing, when the exact symptom that has brought the patient to seek care is reproduced by a test movement, the significance of that movement and its contribution to the patient's current presentation becomes apparent. If, however, pain is produced without reproduction, the results are considered to be less definitive. The primary goal of the objective examination is to find one or more of the patient's comparable signs. Test movements are relevant, thus denoted by *asterisks*, only if such movements produce symptoms that are comparable to the patient's presenting complaints. Within this paradigm, such findings during the objective examination are known as "asterisk signs."

Table 8-2	Type of Dysfunction and Recommended Examination Procedures Used to Confirm	
TYPE OF DYSFUNCTION	**EXAM PROCEDURE**	
Joint Dysfunction	Passive Movements	
Muscle Dysfunction	Isometric Tests w/o movement	

For individuals whose pain complaints appear to be secondary to their motion limitations, firm **overpressure** must be applied at end range of all test movements for the purpose of identifying end-feel and to ascertain the patient's symptomatic response (Box 8-4). For those whose pain appears to be of primary significance, test movements should be performed in neutral positions that are fully supported and pain free and should only be brought minimally beyond the point of pain in order to assess how quickly the symptoms increase. It is of critical importance to note that within the Australian approach, movement is not considered to be normal unless the range is pain free both actively, passively, and in response to overpressure (Box 8-5).

Active movements are the first movements to be formally tested. The examination begins by asking the patient to perform **functional reproducing movements**. The patient is encouraged to demonstrate a particular movement that is known to reproduce symptoms. By establishing the comparable sign, the therapist has addressed the abnormal movement pattern that reproduces symptoms. This movement pattern must, therefore, be specifically addressed during intervention. This comparable sign is intermittently performed throughout the patient's care as a means of gauging improvement. A randomized single-blind clinical trial comparing facet injections with exercise to exercise only in a population of individuals with chronic, work-related spinal disorders (n = 421) found that detection of segmental rigidity using three-segment true lumbar active movement testing with inclinometry was highly reliable among experienced therapists and that segmental

Box 8-4 GOALS OF OVERPRESSURE

1. Determine the true end range of passive movement
2. Determine symptomatic response at end range
3. Determine nature of resistance at end range or end-feel

Box 8-5 NORMAL MOVEMENT

Normal movement requires the following:

1. Normal range for that patient and that joint
2. No symptoms upon active and passive movements
3. No symptoms upon overpressure at end range

rigidity does not appear to be related to the presence of confirmed facet joint involvement.[8]

Passive movements are also used for the purpose of producing the comparable sign. Along with recording the symptomatic movements, reductions in the quantity of passive movement is noted. Passive movements can be divided into two groups of tests. **Passive physiologic movements** consist of osteokinematic motions such as flexion, abduction, external rotation, etc. **Passive accessory movements** are defined as the arthrokinematic motions that accompany the osteokinematic motions (see Chapter 2). While performing these procedures, the presence and location of symptoms should be determined. The available range, nature of the limitation, and changes in pain behavior during testing must also be evaluated. A comparison between the results of active and passive movement testing is useful in identifying the culpable structure(s). The measurement of passive accessory movement, although more challenging to perform and interpret, is an invaluable component of the examination. These movements are performed in the open-packed or midrange position or at the limit of range depending on the patient's level of irritability.[1,3,5,9]

QUESTIONS for REFLECTION

- What kind of information does a *passive movement assessment* versus an *active movement assessment* provide?
- How will the results of these assessments influence your course of intervention?
- Are there occasions in which you are able to (or may wish to) not perform one or the other type of assessment?

QUESTIONS for REFLECTION

- Why do therapists routinely assess *active and passive movement* for the extremities, but rarely assess passive movement in the spine?
- Why do many therapists routinely assess *active and passive movement*, but rarely assess *accessory movement*?
- What can be gained by assessing *accessory movement* that cannot otherwise be achieved?

Some authors have reported **passive accessory intervertebral mobility (PAIVM)** testing to be unreliable for diagnosis of spinal dysfunction. Agreement among examiners on spinal level and intervertebral mobility was found to be poor.[10,11] Some suggest that increased reliability may be obtained through a consideration of abnormal motion along with an appreciation of tissue resistance and provocation of symptoms when detecting spinal dysfunction that is symptomatic.[11,12] Others have found poor association between the intervertebral segment found to be most painful upon testing and the segment with the least amount of motion.[13] The basis for accessory motion testing is generally considered to be weak. A profound need for future research that is directed toward the anatomical basis for accessory motion testing in addition to research directed toward identifying methods for improving the reliability of these procedures is needed.[14]

Once the comparable sign has been determined, the therapist moves into **differentiation testing**. These tests are designed to determine the source of the patient's symptoms by distinguishing between two or more potentially involved joints or structures. These tests are performed by facilitating active or passive movements simultaneously across at least two adjacent joints while attempting to reproduce symptoms. There are five types of differentiation tests that might be used. The *first group* of testing includes identification of the primary site of the disorder including the exact joint and location from which the symptoms emanate. **Confirmation tests** are used to assist in identifying the primary site.[3] These tests consist of a series of specific movements. Through stabilization of joints adjacent to the suspected dysfunctional joint, these tests attempt to differentiate which joint, within a multijoint movement system, is the primary source of the comparable sign. For example, in a patient with occipital headaches, the comparable sign may be elicited through performance of cervical rotation to the right actively. In a multijoint system, such as the cervical spine, it may be difficult for the manual therapist to identify the primary origin of dysfunction and, therefore, where to direct intervention. Confirmation testing may include passive accessory motion overpressure that is provided by the therapist at the C1-C2 segment during active right rotation that results in an increase in the comparable sign. Further confirmation testing may reveal that a reduction in symptoms is noted when movement at C1-C2 is inhibited through manual pressure while the adjacent segments actively move into right rotation. Furthermore, inhibition of movement at other segments fails to produce a change in the comparable sign. The results of such confirmation testing would suggest that the C1-C2 segment is

the primary site of dysfunction or a contributing factor in the patient's headache-related symptoms.

The *second group* of testing seeks to identify the contribution of adjacent regions to the comparable sign.[3] For example, in the case of the patient presenting with occipital headaches, the suboccipital spine may be implicated as the primary source of dysfunction. However, the temporomandibular joint and other plausible structures may also be examined for their potential contribution. The *third group* attempts to differentiate between joint or neurogenic causes.[3] In our patient, the question of whether the headache is caused by compression of the greater occipital nerve or whether the headache is the result of joint-related pain within the upper cervical spine is an important consideration that is determined during third group testing. The *fourth group* seeks to differentiate between intra-articular versus periarticular structures.[3] In our example, this group of tests attempts to answer questions regarding whether or not the symptoms emanating from the suboccipital spine are produced from intra-articular spondylitic changes, for example, or from the periarticular musculature such as increased tone in the muscles of the suboccipital triangle. The *fifth group* attempts to identify if referred symptoms, when present, are originating from the joint, the viscera, peripheral nerve compromise, or are radicular in nature.[3]

In addition to using the aforementioned active and passive movement tests, there is a combination of additional procedures that the manual physical therapist may also incorporate into the examination process. These additional tests are indicated when the examiner is unable to elicit a comparable sign through standard movement testing. The use of overpressure can be superimposed on any of the movement tests that have been described. As mentioned, a joint is not considered to possess normal movement unless firm overpressure can be applied without pain. If a comparable sign is identified through standard movement testing, the use of overpressure is not indicated.

Combined movement testing includes a combination of both accessory and physiologic movement. These tests may be used when neither physiologic movement testing (osteokinematic movements) nor accessory movement testing (arthrokinematic movements) reproduces the patient's symptoms individually. When using combined movements, it is important to note the sequence of recruitment, which may also be varied to assess the patient's response. Using combined movements and altering the sequence in which movements are performed may reveal an antecedent comparable sign that was previously undetected (Fig. 8-5). For example, if cardinal plane active cervical spine movements do not elicit a comparable sign, the manual therapist may have the patient perform an active physiologic motion while

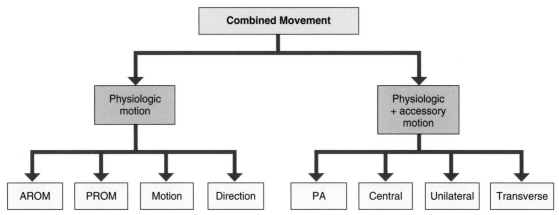

FIGURE 8–5. Types of combined movements used during examination.[1]

superimposing passive accessory movement in order to identify a comparable sign as in the cervical spine confirmation testing scenario described above.

> ### CLINICAL PILLAR
>
> Slight variations in the direction, location, duration, rhythm, and force of gliding may yield useful results in better identifying the exact location and origin of the comparable sign.

Manual therapists may also choose to use **compression tests** when seeking to identify the comparable sign. These tests involve the use of compressive forces that are placed through the joint to assess the patient's response.[1,3] In a patient with neck pain, for example, cervical right side bending may produce the comparable sign. The therapist may then attempt to compare the effect of performing this activity in extension (a position of greater facet joint compression) compared to flexion (a position of less facet joint compression). Adding compression to the comparable sign movement pattern and assessing the impact of this activity on the patient's reported symptoms may serve to refine the therapist's understanding of the condition. Another method of performing compression tests involves the testing of movement patterns in weight-bearing positions or in non-weight-bearing positions with compression provided manually by the therapist.[1,3] These findings may provide additional insight regarding the origin and behavior of the patient's symptoms.

> ### QUESTIONS *for* REFLECTION
>
> In the early stages of joint pathology, *compression* is believed by many to be contraindicated. Unique to this approach is the use of compression in performing manual techniques.
>
> - If techniques are directed toward enhancing motion and reducing symptoms in a joint, why would we consider techniques that include compression?

Abnormal rhythms of movement are common and may be a contributing factor to a patient's disorder. Abnormal rhythms are defined as movement patterns that do not follow the expected kinematics of the joint in question. A patient presenting with poor dissociation of movement between the scapula and the humerus during active arm elevation provides an example of an abnormal rhythm. If the therapist applies **counterpressure** to the abnormal rhythm that is identified at a particular joint complex during active movement using manual contacts and the symptoms are altered (reproduced, increased, or decreased) compared with active movement without manual resistance, then the abnormal rhythm represents a compensation that is directly associated with the disorder. For example, if a comparable sign is elicited or reduced when excessive scapular upward rotation is countered, or restricted, manually by the therapist during active shoulder elevation, then the abnormal rhythm of the scapulothoracic joint is considered to be directly associated with the patient's shoulder disorder. The relationship between these abnormal rhythms and the chief presenting disorder is made only when countering such rhythms directly impacts the comparable sign.

> ### CLINICAL PILLAR
>
> Consider the presence of **abnormal rhythms**:
>
> 1. *If countered rhythm reduces symptoms:* it is an *antecedent factor* predisposing the patient to dysfunction (i.e., poor scapulohumeral rhythm may lead to impingement).
>
> 2. *If countered rhythm increases symptoms:* it is a *secondary compensation* for the primary dysfunction (i.e., pain from primary impingement alters scapulohumeral rhythm).

Occasionally, the patient may be asked to perform **injuring movements**. Injuring movements are those movements that require the patient to actually reenact, if possible, the initial mechanism that led to their current symptoms. For example, a golfer who has developed back pain may perform a swing

- If you are able to successfully *counter an abnormal rhythm* that you have identified in the shoulder complex and symptoms *decrease,* what valuable information do you now possess regarding the origin of these symptoms?
- What would it tell you if symptoms *increased* from countering the abnormal rhythm?
- Reflect on patients that you have seen and construct a list of common abnormal rhythms at various locations throughout the body.

that is identical to that which precipitated the onset of his or her disorder. When a comparable sign cannot be otherwise identified, injuring movements may be a useful adjunct to other procedures. In the absence of positive findings during standard movement testing, injuring movement testing may provide valuable information regarding the origin of the patient's symptoms and serve as evidence of clinically meaningful progress (Box 8-6).[3]

The slump test is an examination procedure used within this approach that incorporates many of the aspects of the objective examination already discussed. The slump test endeavors to identify the comparable sign through use of overpressure, if needed. Its purpose is to ascertain the presence of neurological compromise. Much like the straight leg raise maneuver, the slump test is designed to identify the presence of dural root tension signs within the sciatic nerve complex. It is performed in the sitting position and involves the progressive

Box 8-6 EXPANDED LIST OF TEST MOVEMENTS

1. Active Movements
- Functional reproducing movements
- Active physiologic

2. Passive Movements
- Passive physiologic
- Passive accessory

3. Differentiation Tests
- *Group 1:* Primary site (confirmation tests)
- *Group 2:* Adjacent contributions
- *Group 3:* Joint versus neurogenic
- *Group 4:* Intra-articular versus extra-articular
- *Group 5:* Origin of referred symptoms

4. Test Variations
- Overpressure
- Combined movement
- Compression tests
- Gliding tests
- Counter abnormal rhythms
- Injuring movement

passive tensioning of the nerve through the performance of slumped posturing, knee extension, and ankle dorsiflexion. Cervical flexion and extension is used as a sensitizing maneuver designed to further differentiate between muscular restrictions, namely within the hamstrings, and nerve compromise. If positive, the slump test can be used for intervention. See Chapter 28 for a complete description of the slump test.

The literature suggests that the cervical spine sensitizing maneuvers can have an effect on knee extension indicating the presence of neurologic compromise and the ability of these procedures to differentiate between hamstring tightness and neurologic involvement. Repeated performance led to increased knee extension and decreased hamstring electromyographic activity.[15] An association between individuals with a chronic history of hamstring strains and a positive slump test was found; however, a causal relationship could not be determined.[16] When used for intervention, a modification of the slump test maneuver was found to increase sympathetic nervous system outflow in the target upper extremity (see Chapter 19).[17]

- How does the *slump test* differ from the *straight leg raise* test?
- Why would you use one as opposed to the other?
- If positive, how would you incorporate these tests into your intervention regimen?

Documentation of Findings

The Australian approach to OMPT advocates using the written record to display the therapist's clarity of thought and ability to extract pertinent information from the examination. Such a record also encourages the manual physical therapist to adopt a methodological approach to examination of the patient. In 1970, a method of diagrammatically representing the abnormalities that were observed during the passive movement examination process was proposed.[18] The **movement diagram** may serve as a dynamic map that represents the quality and quantity of a patient's passive movement test findings. The movement diagram provides a visual depiction of the amount, behavior, and relationship between pain and range of motion. Movement diagrams are essential in communicating the relationship that exists between abnormalities in movement quantity and the patient's symptoms. The attributes of passive movement testing that are included in the movement diagram include pain (indicated by **P**), protective involuntary muscle spasm (indicated by **S**), and spasm-free resistance or stiffness (indicated by **R**) (Fig. 8-6; Box 8-7).[1,3,18]

The reliability of using movement diagrams and evaluation of end-feel for external rotation in 34 patients using two physical therapist examiners revealed high levels of intrarater and interrater reliability. Both maximum pain and resistance were

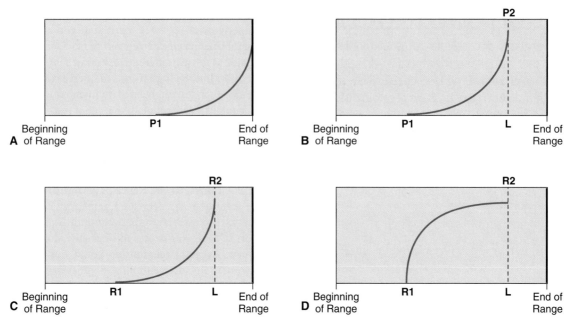

FIGURE 8–6. Examples of Maitland movement diagrams used to depict observed movement patterns. **A.** Pain in range that gradually increases but does not limit motion. **B.** Pain in range that gradually increases and limits motion referred to as pain- or symptom-dominant. **C.** Resistance in range that gradually increases and limits motion, referred to as resistance-dominant. **D.** Resistance in range with abrupt increase that limits motion. L = limitation of motion; P1 = first onset of pain; P2 = final onset of pain; R1 = first onset of resistance; R2 = final onset of resistance. (From: Hengeveld E, Banks K, eds. *Maitland's Peripheral Manipulation.* 4th ed. Edinburgh: Elsevier-Butterworth-Heinemann; 2005.)

NOTABLE QUOTABLE

"Geography would be incomprehensible without maps. They've reduced a tremendous muddle of facts into something you can read at a glance. Now I suspect (passive movement) is fundamentally no more difficult than geography. Except that it's about things in motion. If only somebody would invent a dynamic map."

C.P. Snow, 1965

strongly associated with range of motion as measured by the movement diagram. Good reliability was noted between the movement diagrams and assessment of end-feel.[19]

Analytical Evaluation

Flawless, analytical assessment, or evaluation, is the vital link of this concept. It is the foundation without which the entire approach breaks down. Developing skill in examination and intervention are important, yet not equivalent in value to becoming proficient in the detailed analytical evaluation of the data obtained through a thorough examination of the patient.[1–3]

The three types of evaluations that are used within this approach are based upon when they are performed within the patient's plan of care. They include (1) the **initial evaluation,** which is made at the time of the first visit and designed to relate examination findings to symptom behavior while

Box 8-7 COMPONENTS OF THE MAITLAND MOVEMENT DIAGRAM

AB: The range of full available motion
A: Beginning of range
B: Limit of normal passive range that lies beyond the limit of active movement
AC: The degree of the components being plotted
A: Absence of the component being plotted
C: Maximum degree of the component being plotted
L: The limit of available range (**L** before **B** = hypomobility, **L** after **B** = hypermobility)
P1: Position where pain is initially experienced
P2: Pain that restricts further movement (placed on the **CD** line above **L**)
P1-P2: A line that represent a visual image of pain during movement
P': Pain that does not limit further motion (placed at the point in the range where it is experienced)
R1: Position where pain-free resistance to movement is initially experienced
R2: Resistance that restricts further movement (placed on the **CD** line above **L**)
R1-R2: A line that represents a visual image of pain during movement
S1: Position where muscle spasm resistance to movement is initially experienced
S2: Muscle spasm resistance that restricts further movement (placed on the **CD** line above **L**)

identifying the stage and irritability of the disorder; (2) the **intervention to intervention evaluation**, which seeks to determine intervention effectiveness related to specific techniques during the course of the patient's care; and (3) the **retrospective evaluation**, which is performed at distinct times throughout intervention and at the conclusion of intervention to determine overall effectiveness and future prognosis (Box 8-8). By carefully listening to the patient, thinking through the hands during the examination, and continual reconsideration of the patient's symptomatic response to chosen interventions, the therapist will obtain valuable data that could make the difference in achieving optimal outcomes.

Continual reevaluation is required to ensure that the manual physical therapist is addressing the patient's specific needs related to his or her comparable sign. At the time of

the initial examination and throughout each patient interaction, the manual therapist must attempt to identify the specific site(s) of symptomatic origin and the relationship between movement and symptoms (Fig. 8-7). This information will lead the examiner to the process of differential diagnosis, which will dictate the most preferred course of intervention (Box 8-9).[1,3]

Within this approach, analytical evaluation results in the assignment of the patient into one of four diagnostic classification groupings. These classification groupings are as follows: (1) **Group 1: pain-dominant behavior** is present when pain is the primary origin of the movement disorder; (2) **Group 2: stiffness-dominant behavior** is present when joint restrictions are the primary origin of the movement disorder; (3) **Group 3a and 3b: pain and stiffness combined behavior** is more common and is present when both pain and stiffness are contributing to the movement disorder, with *a* denoting pain as the primary limitation and *b* denoting stiffness as the primary limitation; (4) **Group 4: momentary pain behavior** patients present with no loss of joint range, but intermittent pain associated with certain movements. Most Group 4 patients do not seek intervention because their symptoms are not significant enough to impact their normal level of function.

Early in the examination process, the therapist must determine if the patient is exhibiting either pain-dominant behavior, with pain serving as the primary limitation, or stiffness-dominant behavior, with joint restriction serving as the primary limitation. The determination of the patient's dominant behavior is integral to decisions regarding the most appropriate plan of care (Fig. 8-8, Table 8-3).[1,3,5,9]

Box 8-8 TYPES OF EVALUATION AND REASONS FOR EACH

1. Initial Evaluation
- Connection between subjective and objective
- Diagnosis and classification

2. Intervention to Intervention Evaluation
- Response to interventions
- Periodically performed throughout

3. Retrospective Evaluation
- Change over time
- Prognosis and need for further intervention

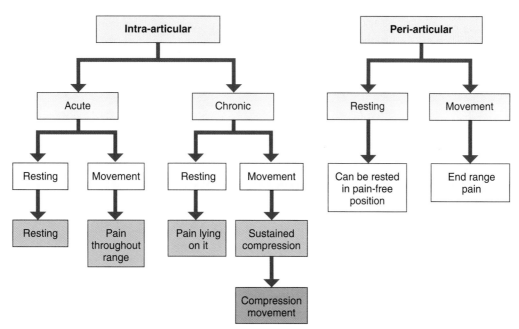

FIGURE 8–7. Differentiation between intra-articular and periarticular disorders. (From: Maitland GD. *Peripheral Manipulation.* 3rd ed. Woburn, MA: Butterworth-Heinemann; 1991, with permission.)

Box 8-9 SUMMARY OF THE EVALUATION PROCESS

1. During first evaluation, therapist collates information to understand disorder stage, stability, and makes diagnosis.

2. Relate or dissociate patient's history to physical findings.

3. Evaluate patient's personality and pain threshold

4. By end of first visit, anticipate prognosis.

5. At beginning of each session, evaluate changes in patient's status subjectively and objectively and the symptom behavior between visits.

6. During each session, effectiveness of each intervention is evaluated before, during, and after application.

7. Periodically, the overall effect of intervention, as a whole, is evaluated (every four visits).

8. At the conclusion of intervention, evaluation of long-term prognosis, including the need for prophylaxis, is determined.

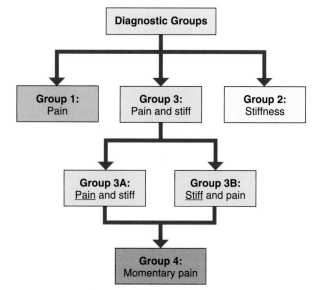

FIGURE 8–8. Australian approach diagnostic classification groupings.[3]

Table 8-3	Characteristic Variables Related to Examination and Intervention in Pain Versus Stiffness-Dominant Disorders[5]

Subjective Presentation

VARIABLE	PAIN/SYMPTOM DOMINANT	STIFFNESS/RESISTANCE DOMINANT
Location	Diffuse	Localized
Night pain	Worse	Mild/moderate
Use of analgesics	Medium/high dose	Low dose
Pain/symptom characteristics	Burning, sharp	Stiff, restricted
Pain/symptom frequency	Constant/variable	Intermittent
Response to activity	Aggravated by low levels	Aggravated by vigorous only
Pain/symptom intensity	>5/10	<5/10
Pain/symptom duration	Slow to reduce after activity	Short duration
History	Recent onset	Chronic (>6 months)
Location	Diffuse	Localized
Night pain	Worse	Mild/moderate
Use of analgesics	Medium/high dose	Low dose
Pain/symptom characteristics	Burning, sharp	Stiff, restricted
Location	Diffuse	Localized

Objective Presentation

VARIABLE	PAIN/SYMPTOM DOMINANT	STIFFNESS/RESISTANCE DOMINANT
Range	Pain or fear of pain with movement	Limited
Pain/symptoms	Resting, early and midrange	End range only
Spasm	Often present	Seldom present
Repeated movements	Aggravates, except if in preferred direction	Increases range

Table 8–3	Characteristic Variables Related to Examination and Intervention in Pain Versus Stiffness-Dominant Disorders[5] —cont'd	

Intervention

VARIABLE	PAIN/SYMPTOM DOMINANT	STIFFNESS/RESISTANCE DOMINANT
Grades of movement	Grade I and II	Grade III and IV
Goal of intervention	Eliminate pain/symptoms	Increase range (pain may be produced)
Relationship of intervention to barriers (P1, R1, S1)	Short of barriers	Progress into and through barriers
Focus of evaluation	Pain behavior	Range of motion while respecting pain
Preferred movement direction	Direction of least painful/restricted	Direction of most restriction
Potential mechanism	Active inflammation	Fibrosis/scarring
Stage of healing	Inflammatory	Proliferative, fibrotic, maturation

NOTABLE QUOTABLE

"Manual therapy depends on clarity of thought. The business of methodical, critical thinking is terribly important. Novices must expect to get fewer results more slowly than those who are experienced and they must resist the temptation to take shortcuts. For the novice, arriving at the right result more slowly, having proved the correctness of every step along the way, will pay in the future. Unless therapists sort out their knowledge into these clear-cut proven facts, they will end up with wishy-washy knowledge which is of little use in the different situations which come along."

J. Hickling

PRINCIPLES OF INTERVENTION
Principles and Definitions

Unlike other approaches to manual therapy, the Australian approach de-emphasizes technique performance and places a greater value on the development of examination and assessment skills. Within this approach, there is no definitive set of techniques that are advocated. Likewise, the suggested methods for performance of manual techniques are nonprescriptive. Therapists are encouraged to modify, reverse, enhance, and even invent new techniques to specifically meet the needs of the patient. Similar to other approaches, the most important skill that is required to achieve an effective mobilization is the development of movement perception. To better sense movement, the therapist is encouraged to use the body as opposed to using the fingers or hands as the prime movers.

The techniques espoused by Maitland all have a few basic components in common. Almost all of the techniques involve some level of oscillatory movement. Generally, a rate of two or three oscillations per second is suggested; however, variations are common. When beginning to use these techniques,

the therapist is encouraged to place the joint in a neutral position so as to require the least amount of force with the greatest effect. Within this approach, mobilization techniques focus on the use of the following passive movements: *physiologic movements, accessory movements, combined physiologic movements, combined physiologic with accessory movements,* and *combined accessory movements.*[1,3,5,9]

Techniques may be used in the case of a stiffness-dominant joint for the purpose of increasing its range. In this instance, techniques are performed in the direction of stiffness and done at the point where the resistance is encountered. Techniques may also be used in the case of a pain-dominant joint in which the objective is to relieve symptoms. In this instance, the therapist performs a large amplitude mobilization with gentle pressure that is halted before resistance or pain is encountered. In such an instance, the therapist may choose to reverse the direction of the technique or perform the technique on a nonpainful adjacent region first. Before engaging in passive manual techniques, it is of vital importance that the therapist is cognizant of the passive movements or positions that provoke or relieve the patient's symptoms.[5,9]

CLINICAL PILLAR

Two important questions must be continually asked throughout intervention:

1. What is the *site* from which symptoms originate?
2. What is the *relationship* between movement and symptoms?

Proper performance of manual techniques within this approach requires the therapist to use the examination findings to determine the rhythm at which the technique should be performed, the position in the range where the technique should be performed, and the amount of force that should be used when performing the technique. The unique characteristics of this intervention approach include freedom given to therapists to readily modify the technique based on patient response, the emphasis on the use of oscillations, and the intermittent use of joint compression. The key concept to consider is that the *"technique is the brainchild of ingenuity"*; the manual physical therapist should not be a slave to the technique, but rather the technique should be directed by the process of examination and evaluation.[3] The manual therapist should use innovation, creativity, and discipline in the selection and application of manual techniques to achieve optimal results (Box 8-10).

NOTABLE QUOTABLE

"A technique is the brainchild of ingenuity."

G.D. Maitland

Within this approach, the amplitude and rhythm used to perform techniques are placed into one of four grades (Box 8-11). These grades are widely used by manual therapists and considered by most to be the preferred method of describing and documenting the type of passive movement performed. Despite their widespread acceptance, the validity of this grading system has been challenged.[20] The grades of movement used in the application of passive movement are

Box 8-10 BASIC ASPECTS OF TECHNIQUE PERFORMANCE

1. Techniques are nonprescriptive and should be modified to meet patient needs.

2. Techniques based on therapist's ability to sense movement.

3. Requires the use of the body as prime movers, not the fingers.

4. Regular use of oscillations usually ranges between two and three cycles per second.

5. May be best to initiate techniques with the joint in neutral.

6. Use the least force possible.

Box 8-11 REASONS FOR GRADING MOVEMENTS

1. They form the basis of communication for teaching and while treating a patient.

2. They encourage the therapist to think more critically about the technique that is being performed.

3. They provide an effective method of abbreviation when recording interventions.

(1) **Grade I**: small amplitude movement near the beginning of range; (2) **Grade II**: large amplitude movement that goes well into the range, occupying any part of the range that is free of stiffness or muscle spasm; (3) **Grade III**: large amplitude movement that moves into stiffness or muscle spasm; and (4) **Grade IV**: small amplitude movement moving into stiffness or muscle spasm. Occasionally a plus (+) or minus (–) is used to provide a more specific description of mobilization amplitude and location. A *Grade II–* is a large amplitude movement at the beginning of the resistance-free range, and *Grade II+* is a mobilization taken deeply into the range, yet still short of resistance. Similar interpretation is used for *Grades III–, III+* and *Grades IV–, IV+*. The position of *Grade IV* as compared to *Grade IV+* is subjective and depends on the force used by the therapist at end range. A *Grade IV+++* is indicative, for example, of very strong pressure elicited at end range.[1,3,5,9] These grades can be depicted diagrammatically using a movement diagram that contains a line representing a range of movement from resting position (**A**) to the end of the given range of motion (**B**) (Figs. 8-9, 8-10, 8-11, 8-12).[18,19]

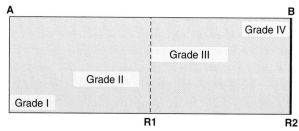

FIGURE 8–9. Grades of mobilization in a normal range of motion, where A and B represent the start and end ranges, respectively, of available movement at any given joint. R1 is the first onset of resistance to motion and R2 is the final onset of resistance. (Maitland Australian Physiotherapy Seminars. *MT-1: Basic Peripheral.* Cutchogue, NY: Maitland Australian Physiotherapy Seminars; 2005.)

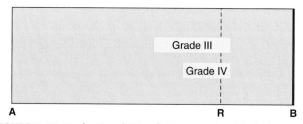

FIGURE 8–10. Grades III and IV in relation to a soft end-feel, where resistance (R) is experienced before the end range of movement (B).[1]

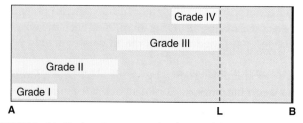

FIGURE 8–11. Grades of movement in a hypomobile joint where the pathologic end range of movement (L) precedes the normal end range of the joint (B).[1]

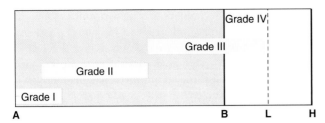

FIGURE 8–12. Grades of movement in a hypermobile joint where the typical end range of movement (B) precedes the end range of movement of the hypermobile joint (H).[1]

Movement diagrams will vary depending on the type of end-feel. If a soft, as opposed to hard, end-feel is noted, then the resistance (**R**) that is experienced precedes the end range (**B**) and the relationship of Grades III and IV will vary as compared to that noted for a hard end-feel. The location within the range at which the technique is applied and the amplitude and rhythm of the mobilization will vary depending on the nature of the identified end-feel.[1,3,18,19] A *Grade III–* mobilization indicates that movement occurs up to and slightly into resistance, whereas a *Grade III+* mobilization moves well into the resistance. Similar grading is used for *Grade IV* movements. It is important to note that *Grades I* and *II* are always, by definition, resistance-free movements.[1,3,5,9]

Although the therapist considers the specific structures that may be contributing to a particular movement restriction, the patient's symptoms and signs have the highest priority in determining the treatment technique and the manner in which the chosen technique is applied. Decisions regarding the most appropriate technique to use are based on the correlation between the patient's symptoms and the type and location of the movement restriction (Box 8-12).

Grade I and *Grade II* mobilizations are believed to primarily have a neurophysiologic effect that reduces joint-related pain. *Grade III* and *Grade IV* mobilizations are believed to have a greater influence on increasing joint range of motion through elimination of joint restrictions by engaging the tissue barrier. Grade III mobilizations that use accessory motion have also been found to alter sympathetic nervous system function that may be associated with analgesia. Grade III mobilizations to the cervical spine and to the glenohumeral joint have been found individually to alter sympathetic outflow as observed by changes in skin temperature and skin conductance.[21,22]

Box 8-12 DECISIONS REGARDING TECHNIQUE SELECTION

1. Position in range
2. Amount of force
3. Duration of technique
4. Speed of technique
5. Rhythm of technique
6. Acceptable degree of pain during technique

Application of Techniques

Application of the most appropriate treatment technique requires accurate, repeated assessment that informs the therapist's decision regarding type, direction, grade, speed, rhythm, and duration of the technique. When a particular technique is applied without producing a change, the technique is performed at least one more time with more force and then abandoned if no change is noted. If improvement is noted with a particular technique, the same technique is repeated. If symptoms increase in response to a particular technique, it should not be repeated; however, it may be attempted again more gently at a later stage. In general, it is critical for the manual physical therapist to continue the performance of a technique until it is clear that the technique is ineffective.[5,9]

QUESTIONS *for* REFLECTION

- Why would you consider using *passive mobilization* techniques instead of other, less time-consuming interventions?
- What are the indicators or predictors that are evident in the patient's examination that would suggest that the patient might benefit from passive mobilization?
- How might passive mobilization techniques be used to prevent injury?

The depth with which a particular technique is applied is determined by the relationship between pain, muscle spasm, and resistance. The severity and relative position of these factors in the range of movement are important guides. Pain upon movement is the most important guide regarding the depth to which a technique should be applied. If the disorder is pain-dominant and the pain is present early in the range, then *Grade I* techniques are used with progression to *Grade II*. As progress with these techniques plateaus, the grade of mobilization is increased for the purpose of engaging the movement barrier. Greater care is required when a technique produces referral into a distal region. When moving into the pain, assessment over the 24 hours following intervention will indicate whether or not the technique should be continued. With a stiffness-dominant disorder, engaging the resistance can be done with either large-amplitude *Grade III* or small-amplitude *Grade IV* movements. The small-amplitude *Grade IV* mobilizations are used in the treatment of end-range pain. The larger-amplitude *Grade III* mobilizations may be used for through-range pain and to relieve soreness produced from the use of *Grade IV* movements. When a mobilization produces a muscular response, or spasm, then it is critical that the technique initially be performed more slowly and at a depth that avoids spasm (Fig. 8-13).[3,5,9]

In regard to duration and frequency of intervention, it is important to note that the duration of the initial treatment is often less than subsequent interventions because of the

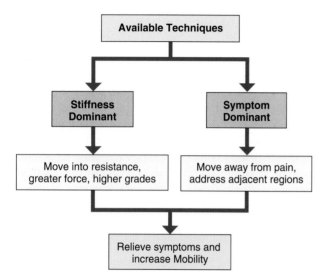

FIGURE 8–13. General concepts of technique selection based on the relationship between movement and symptoms.[1]

expected cumulative effects from the examination and first applied intervention. The duration of subsequent interventions depends on the patient's reaction to the previous sessions. As a general guideline, three or four mobilizations of a joint, each lasting approximately 30 seconds, is considered to be optimal. A highly irritable disorder requires a reduction in these parameters by half. If interventions are perpetuating soreness or failing to yield results over a number of sessions, treatment may be temporarily discontinued.

CLINICAL PILLAR

- Perform each technique at least twice before abandoning it.
- Be sure that you know the effects of a technique before attempting another.

When applying passive movement techniques, a variety of options are available. Passive movement techniques may include the use of physiologic or accessory movements. Techniques may also include **combined physiologic movements** (i.e., passive movement of the patient into combined lumbar right side bending and rotation), **combined accessory movements** (i.e., a unilateral posteroanterior pressure produces a combination of PA glide and rotation), or **combined physiologic with accessory movements** (i.e., cervical spine is passively moved into rotation while the therapist applies a unilateral posteroanterior glide). It is important to note that **distraction** and **compression** are intermittently used throughout intervention as well. When symptoms are dominant, slight distraction may be used to improve patient tolerance for the technique. Compression may be used when the patient's level of pain is a less significant factor.[3]

The next consideration in technique application is the determination regarding the direction in which passive movements

may be performed. Techniques may be performed in a biomechanical direction (in accordance with the joint's physiologic plane of movement) or in a nonbiomechanical direction (without attention to the joint's physiologic plane of movement). Within this approach, there is little regard for strict adherence to the rules of joint kinematics.[1,3] Knowledge of expected joint movement is theoretically useful but should not permeate intervention to the point that treatment options are restricted and bound by such principles (Table 8-4).

During the examination, the therapist attempts to identify the primary movement that either reduces or increases the comparable sign. If, for example, cervical flexion produces the comparable sign and other motions do not, then flexion is considered to be the primary movement. The therapist would then identify the effect of combined movements on the symptoms. For example, do the symptoms increase when side bending is added to flexion? The therapist may add side bending to flexion or flexion to side bending to determine which produces the most significant comparable sign. The last component to add to the combined movement is the accessory movement. For example, the effect of a unilateral posteroanterior pressure at C6 on the comparable sign with the patient prepositioned in flexion and side bending may be useful in guiding intervention. Depending on the symptom behavior, the therapist may choose to begin in a less provocative direction and progress toward the most provocative position.

QUESTIONS *for* REFLECTION

- To what extent should knowledge of joint kinematics guide the manner in which techniques are performed?
- Structure is said to dictate function. If this is true, should not passive mobilization techniques be bound by the kinematics of the joint?

In addition to the aforementioned principles of technique application, the rhythm with which a technique is performed must also be considered. Rhythms of mobilization consist of **stationary holding rhythms, slow rhythms,** and **staccato**

Table 8-4	The Type of Technique Is Dictated by the Nature of the Symptoms
SYMPTOMS	**TYPE OF TECHNIQUE**
End-of-range symptoms	End-of-range techniques
Through-range symptoms	Through-range techniques
Constant pain	Accessory movements in neutral physiologic positions
Mild aching in weight-bearing	Techniques under compression
Stiffness of periarticular structures with pain	Stretching into stiffness to point of pain provocation

rhythms. Slow rhythms are indicated for painful joints. With patients who have difficulty relaxing, using broken rhythms and changing the amplitude of rhythms may be effective. Stationary holding involves applying movement slowly up to the motion limitation, which is then held for a period of time. When pain or limitation subsides, further movement into the restricted range is achieved. Small oscillatory movements may then be performed short of the limit (Fig. 8-14).[3,5,9]

CLINICAL PILLAR

- The uninvolved side is your best comparison.
- Let patients help refine your skills; their comments are priceless.
- Recognize difference and dominance of pathophysiologic versus pathomechanical conditions.
- Avoid "brick" or "iron" hands; use gentle touch and "see" with your hands.
- Let features of the examination fit a presentation; do not try to fit a bias on the presentation.
- Make the first visit a success.
- Only add a second technique when you know the effect of the first.
- Do not hold too long at end range; go in and do it!
- Do not be "greedy"; treat briefly early on.
- Start active exercise once passive techniques are under control.
- Predetermine treatment outcome, not grades of movement.
- Give the patient your attention; think about theories later.
- Use the least possible force to have the greatest effect.
- Do not get paralysis from analysis.
- Avoid the diagnostic trap; treat the patient not the diagnosis, X-ray, magnetic resonance imaging, etc.
- Never pay for the same real estate twice (i.e., if you got more motion, do your best to maintain it, including getting the patient involved).

DIFFERENTIATING CHARACTERISTICS

Although most approaches within manual therapy ascribe to the performance of a comprehensive subjective examination and history, most do not ascribe to the same level of intense preoccupation with truly understanding the experience of the patient through a detailed interrogation process that is the key

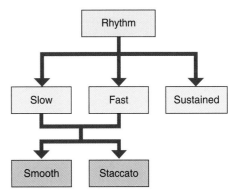

FIGURE 8–14. Choice of rhythms to use during mobilization. (From: Maitland GD: *Peripheral Manipulation.* 3rd ed. Woburn, MA: Butterworth-Heinemann; 1991, with permission.)

feature of this approach. Empathetic interrogation is accomplished through an astute listening process that requires both verbal and nonverbal communication (Fig. 8-15).

This approach, like most, attributes value to identifying the pathological tissue(s) in question. The Australian approach, however, assigns theoretical knowledge as having a secondary role compared to therapist observation during the firsthand interaction with the patient. Maitland's process of compartmental thinking is designed to avoid clinical bias in determining the origin of symptoms. Within this approach, examination of accessory movement may occur in loose-packed, end range, or painful positions. Within this approach, intervention is almost entirely guided and informed by the relationship between observed movement and reported symptoms. There is a profound de-emphasis on establishing a definitive tissue-based diagnosis in favor of a symptom-based diagnosis determined by the identification of one or more comparable signs. The Australian approach places preferential emphasis on the evaluation component of patient management and views actual technique performance as a secondary consideration. This concept is evident in the nonprescriptive manner in which techniques are applied, with therapists encouraged to use innovation and creativity when implementing techniques. Manual techniques are applied with variability in direction, type of movement, rhythm of movement, position, grade, and duration. Techniques may combine accessory movements with physiologic movements. This approach also uses compressive forces during examination and/or intervention. The techniques used for intervention are often the identical techniques used during examination. The overarching guide for technique selection and performance is identification and elimination of the observed comparable sign.

Although the manual therapy techniques used in this approach emanate from the osteopathic, chiropractic, and traditional medical literature, Maitland's emphasis on critical thinking, through a process of continual evaluation, is the distinguishing feature of this approach. These innovative concepts have contributed to our present-day clinical decision-making models within physical therapy. Maitland's attention to careful clinical examination, differential diagnosis, and

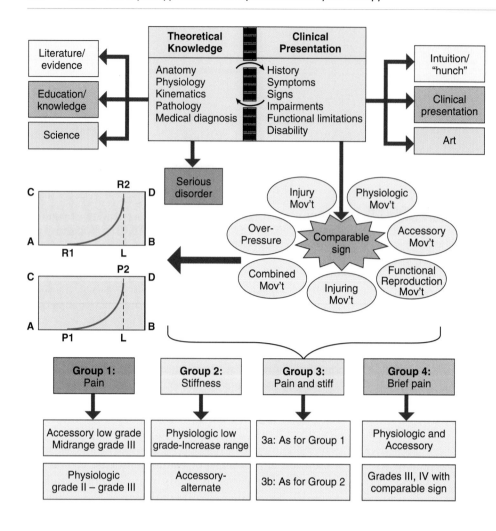

FIGURE 8–15. Australian approach to orthopaedic manual physical therapy conceptual framework displaying the primary features of this approach, including compartmental thinking that leads to examination procedures designed to identify one or more comparable signs. Ultimately, identification of a comparable sign, along with an appreciation of the relationship between resistance and pain during passive motion testing, leads to diagnostic group classification. The diagnostic classification then dictates intervention.

commitment to fully understanding what the patient is enduring has been a hallmark of this approach since its inception. Twomey expressed it best when he exclaimed, *"Maitland's emphasis on careful and comprehensive examination leading to the precise application of treatment by movement and* *followed in turn by the assessment of the effects of that movement on the patient, form the basis for the modern clinical approach . . . which is as close to the scientific method as is possible within the clinical practice of physical therapy and serves as a model for other special areas of the profession."*[23]

CLINICAL CASE

History of Present Illness (HPI)

A 45-year-old female presents with neck and right arm pain beginning 2 years ago when she experienced a whiplash-associated disorder (WAD) caused by a motor vehicle accident (MVA). Her symptoms completely resolved about 1 year ago. However, she reports that last week, while playing tennis, there was a return of symptoms secondary to forcefully serving the ball. Her symptoms progressively increased over the next several hours after the initial onset. On subsequent days, her symptoms were worse upon awakening in the morning and eased after a warm shower with stretching. Her symptoms presently consist of lower cervical pain with occasional paresthesia into the medial border of the scapula and distally into the upper extremity to the elbow on the right. Increased symptoms are noted upon performance of cervical extension, right side bending, and right rotation. Her symptoms are similar to those noted previously.

Observation: Increased muscle tone/tension noted in the right anterior scalene and sternocleidomastoid muscles. Forward head and rounded shoulder posture are also noted.

AROM: Limited by 50% in active physiologic extension and right side bending, both of which produce the comparable sign of right medial border of scapular and arm paresthesia.

PAIVM Testing: Comparable sign noted with Grade II+, unilateral PA glides at C4-C5 on the left by P2.
Strength: 4–/5 noted in right biceps, brachialis, brachioradialis; otherwise 5/5
Neurological: Intact and symmetrical deep tendon reflex (DTR) and light touch, sharp/dull sensation
Special Tests: Right lower quadrant sign = + with peripheralization of symptoms
Radiographs: Unremarkable

1. Based on this presentation, in what diagnostic group would you put this patient? Would you classify her as having a pain-dominant or stiffness-dominant disorder? Explain your rationale and the process of coming to this conclusion.
2. Given this presentation, what is the most likely origin of this patient's symptoms? What tissue-based diagnostic title might you offer? What was revealed in the patient's history and/or subjective report and/or what was revealed in the physical examination that guided you toward this conclusion?
3. Describe how your differential diagnosis as noted above would impact your selection and application of manual therapy techniques according to the Australian approach to OMPT.
4. Is there any additional information that you would like to have before initiating intervention?
5. Identify three specific manual therapy techniques that you would implement at the time of this patient's first visit to physical therapy. Describe each in detail (i.e., grade, position, direction, duration, etc.) and perform them on your partner (see Chapter 30 for details of specific techniques).
6. At the time of the patient's next visit to physical therapy, how would you assess the success of your previous intervention? If there was a negative response to the previous intervention, what would you do at this time? If there was a positive response to the previous intervention what would you do at this time?
7. Draw a movement diagram that accurately depicts your current findings.
8. What additional nonmanual interventions would you use with this patient? How would these interventions relate to and support the OMPT interventions chosen?

HANDS-ON

With a partner, perform the following activities:

1 Allow your partner to portray the patient described in the clinical case scenario above. What are the three most important questions required to determine your initial course of intervention? Describe the process of clinical compartmental thinking that you will use to reach conclusions about this patient. Describe how theoretical compartmental thinking may influence your evaluation, diagnosis, prognosis, and plan of care.

2 Grasp your partner's second MCP joint between your index finger and thumb, being sure to place your fingers as close to the joint line as possible. While using the grades of mobilization diagram, perform Grades I–IV accessory glide mobilizations on your partner. As you perform the technique, are you able to identify when R1 and R2 are engaged? Is P1, P2 or S1, S2 present? Ask your partner for feedback as you perform these techniques. Perform Grades I–IV glide mobilizations on your partner's wrist, elbow, shoulder, hip, knee, and ankle.

3 Choose one spinal technique and one extremity technique from Part III: Practice of OMPT and perform each technique on your partner using Grades I–IV in the same manner as described above.

4 Draw a movement diagram that accurately depicts your findings during performance of the mobilization techniques described above.

5 While performing the chosen techniques above, practice changing the direction of mobilization, patient and therapist position, mobilization rhythm, mobilization grade, and attempt incorporation of compression and distraction.

6 Choose a technique from Part III: Practice of OMPT that involves a combination of physiologic and accessory movements and perform this technique on your partner. Identify R1, R2, P1, P2, S1, S2 when present and document using a movement diagram.

7 Switch partners and perform these techniques on another person. Teach your chosen techniques to one other person and provide him or her with feedback regarding his or her performance.

8 If possible, video your performance of these techniques. Self-assess your performance of the chosen techniques by writing down three areas of deficiency and three areas of proficiency when using these techniques. Focus on such factors as therapist position, patient position, hand placement, force direction, instruction to the patient, etc. Critique the performance of others in a similar fashion.

REFERENCES

1. Maitland GD, Hengeveld E, Banks K, English K. *Maitland's Vertebral Manipulation*. 6th ed. Woburn, MA: Butterworth-Heinemann; 2001.
2. Farrell JP, Jensen GM. Manual therapy: a critical assessment of role in the profession of physical therapy. *Phys Ther*. 1992;72:843-852.
3. Maitland GD. *Peripheral Manipulation*. 3rd ed. Woburn, MA: Butterworth-Heinemann; 1991.
4. Koury MJ, Scarpelli E. A manual therapy approach to evaluation and treatment of a patient with a chronic lumbar nerve root irritation. *Phys Ther*. 1994;74:548-560.
5. Maitland Australian Physiotherapy Seminars. *MT-2: Basic Spinal*. Cutchogue, NY: Cayuga Professional Education; 1985.
6. Maher CG, Simmonds M, Adams R. Therapists' conceptualization and characterization of the clinical concept of spinal stiffness. *Phys Ther*. 1998;78:289-300.
7. Brown MD, Holmes DC, Heiner AD. Measurement of cadaver lumbar spine motion segment stiffness. *Spine*. 2002;27:918-922.
8. Mayer TG, Gatchel RJ, Keeley J, et al. A randomized clinical trial of treatment for lumbar segmental rigidity. *Spine*. 2004;29:2199-2205.
9. Maitland Australian Physiotherapy Seminars. *MT-3: Intermediate Spinal*. Cutchogue, NY: Cayuga Professional Education; 1999.
10. Binkley J, Stratford PW, Gill C. Interrater reliability of lumbar accessory motion mobility testing. *Phys Ther*. 1995;75:786-795.
11. Phillips DR, Twomey LT. A comparison of manual diagnosis with a diagnosis established by a uni-level lumbar spinal block procedure. *Manual Ther*. 1996;2:82-87.
12. Jull G, Treleaven, Versace G. Manual examination: is pain provocation a major cue for spinal dysfunction? *Aust J Physiother*. 1994;40:159-165.
13. Beneck GJ, Kulig K, Landel RF, Powers CM. The relationship between lumbar segmental and pain response produced by a posterior-to-anterior force in persons with nonspecific low back pain. *J Orthop Sports Phys Ther*. 2005;35:204-209.
14. Riddle DL. Measurement of accessory motion: critical issues and related concepts. *Phys Ther*. 1992;72:865-874.
15. Fidel C, Martin E, Dankaerts W, Allison G, Hall T. Cervical spine sensitizing maneuvers during the slump test. *J Man Manip Ther*. 1996;4:16-21.
16. Turl SE, George KP. Adverse neural tension: a factor in repetitive hamstring strain. *J Orthop Sports Phys Ther*. 1998;27:16-21.
17. Slater H, Vicenzino B, Wright A. "Sympathetic slump": the effects of a novel manual therapy technique on peripheral sympathetic nervous system function. *J Man Manip Ther*. 1994;2:156-162.
18. Hickling J, Maitland GD. Abnormalities in passive movement: diagrammatic representation. *Aust J Physiother*. 1970;13:105-114.
19. Chesworth BM, MacDermid JC, Roth JH, Patterson SD. Movement diagrams and "end-feel" reliability when measuring passive lateral rotation of the shoulder in patients with shoulder pathology. *Phys Ther*. 1998;78: 593-601.
20. Chester R, Swift L, Watson MJ. An evaluation of therapist's ability to perform graded mobilization on a simulated spine. *Physiother Theory Pract*. 2003;19:23-34.
21. Petersen N, Vicenzino B, Wright A. The effects of a cervical mobilization technique on sympathetic outflow to the upper limb in normal subjects. *Physiother Theory Pract*. 1993;9:149-156.
22. Simon R, Vicenzino B, Wright A. The influence of an anteroposterior accessory glide of the glenohumeral joint on measures of peripheral sympathetic nervous system function in the upper limb. *Man Ther*. 1997;2:18-23.
23. Twomey LT. A rationale for the treatment of back pain and joint pain by manual therapy. *Phys Ther*. 1992;72:885-892.

The McKenzie Method®
of Mechanical Diagnosis
and Therapy®

Kay A.R. Scanlon, PT, DPT, OCS, Dip MDT
Angela R. Tate, PT, PhD, Cert MDT
Nancy Parker Neff, PT, DPT, Cert MDT

Chapter Objectives

At the conclusion of this chapter, the reader will be able to:

- Briefly describe the confluence of factors leading to the development of the Mechanical Diagnosis and Therapy (MDT) approach.
- Discuss the philosophical underpinnings upon which the MDT approach is based.
- Describe, in detail, the three primary syndromes used to classify patients within the MDT approach.
- Discuss the concept of centralization and peripheralization and the implications of these concepts on prognosis and pathology.
- Describe the primary methods that may be used to differentially classify patients into one of the three primary syndromes.

- Understand the criteria required to determine an individual's principle of intervention.
- Identify the criteria needed to determine the presence of a lateral shift.
- Articulate the manner in which forces are progressed within this approach and when manual interventions may be applied.
- Describe and demonstrate the progression of intervention for each of the syndromes.
- Identify the key features that differentiate this approach from that of others.

HISTORICAL PERSPECTIVES
Personal Background

Robin McKenzie was born in Auckland, New Zealand, in 1931. He graduated from the School of Physiotherapy of New Zealand in 1952 and began a private practice in Wellington, where he specialized in the treatment of spinal disorders. His insight and study of mechanical spinal disorders has made Robin McKenzie a pioneer in the classification and treatment of these conditions. In addition to publishing in the *New Zealand Medical Journal*, among others, he has authored five books: *Treat Your Own Back*; *Treat Your Own Neck*; *The Lumbar Spine: Mechanical Diagnosis and Therapy*; *The*

Cervical and Thoracic Spine: Mechanical Diagnosis and Therapy; and, in collaboration with Stephen May, *Mechanical Diagnosis and Therapy of the Human Extremities*.

Among his many honors, Robin McKenzie was made an *Honorary Life Member* of the American Physical Therapy Association (APTA) for "distinguished and meritorious service to the art and science of physical therapy and to the welfare of mankind." Additionally, he was elected to membership in the *International Society for the Study of the Lumbar Spine*, and he is a *Fellow of the American Back Society*, an *Honorary Fellow of the New Zealand Society of Physiotherapists*, and an *Honorary Fellow of the Chartered Society of Physiotherapists* in the United Kingdom. In the 1990

Queen's Birthday Honours, he was made an *Officer of the Most Excellent Order* of the British Empire, and in 2000 Her Majesty the Queen appointed Robin McKenzie as a *Companion of the New Zealand Order of Merit*. McKenzie received an Honorary Doctorate from the Russian Academy of Medical Sciences in 1993. In 2004, McKenzie was named the most influential and distinguished physical therapist in the field of orthopaedic physical therapy by a random sampling of 320 physical therapists in the Orthopaedic Section of the APTA.

Development of the Mechanical Diagnosis and Therapy Approach

Like most physiotherapists in New Zealand in the 1950s, Robin McKenzie treated many patients for low back pain with variable success. McKenzie's practice was forever changed when a patient with sciatic pain inadvertently positioned himself in end-range lumbar extension. To the complete astonishment of McKenzie, this patient's constant leg pain had vanished. Over several additional visits, McKenzie continued to use this position with his patient, which culminated in complete resolution of his pain and full restoration of lumbar range of motion. At that time, the use of extension was not considered a beneficial practice in the care of lumbar spine disorders and was contrary to all that McKenzie and his colleagues had been taught.[1]

McKenzie's search for an explanation of the dramatic changes that he had witnessed in this patient led him to the writings of *James Cyriax* (see Chapter 5). McKenzie extrapolated from Cyriax's work that his patient's recovery likely occurred *"because the pressure on his sciatic nerve was removed."*[2] Operating under the premise that movement of the lumbar spine can alter pressures on painful structures, McKenzie continued to explore this intervention concept with other patients. He noticed that in some individuals, end-range extension resolved their symptoms. For others, movements such as end-range flexion or lateral movements were necessary for symptom resolution. Over time, McKenzie formalized his process of examining and treating patients based on their symptomatic response to movement and position. From this rather inauspicious beginning, the *McKenzie Method® of Mechanical Diagnosis and Therapy® (MDT)* was born.

MDT is a comprehensive approach to the conservative management of most activity-related spinal disorders. It is a system of patient examination, classification, and intervention that is based on an individual's symptomatic and mechanical response to movement and position.

This chapter presents an overview of the methodology as it applies to the lumbar spine. It is intended to familiarize the reader with the approach and basic techniques used in examination and intervention only. Expertise and interrater reliability is developed by clinical practice and postgraduate study through the *McKenzie Institute® International*, which now has a presence in 29 countries.[3]

Since 1990, the McKenzie Method® has evolved to include management of mechanical disorders of the cervical and thoracic spine, as well as the extremities. The conceptual approach is the same, but the process incorporates regional differences in movements and positions. Further discussion of these concepts as they apply to these other regions is beyond the scope of this chapter.

PHILOSOPHICAL FRAMEWORK AND FUNDAMENTAL CONCEPTS
Philosophical Underpinnings

Underlying the MDT approach is the belief that most individuals with mechanical spinal disorders have the physical capacity, intellectual wherewithal, and the self-discipline to successfully manage their condition when provided with appropriate education, guidance, and exercise. Given this, it is the responsibility of the MDT practitioner to correctly classify responders to MDT, prescribe effective interventions, create therapeutic alliances, educate patients on fundamental principles of mechanical pain, and provide strategies to control or prevent symptoms and restore function (Box 9-1).

A variety of exercises and orthopaedic manual physical therapy (OMPT) procedures may be required for a successful episode of care. Early in the intervention process, most patients are instructed in self-intervention procedures and

Box 9-1 THE PRIMARY ROLE OF THE THERAPIST WITHIN THE MDT APPROACH

The primary role of the therapist within the MDT approach is to do the following:

1. To classify responders
2. To progress the appropriate intervention correctly
3. To create a therapeutic alliance with the patient
4. To discourage patient dependency
5. To educate the patient on the fundamental principles of mechanical pain
6. To provide strategies to control and prevent the patient's symptoms
7. To provide strategies to restore function

behavior modification designed to control their symptoms and, once controlled, to prevent their return. OMPT procedures are incorporated into intervention when patients are unable to make improvements in response to self-intervention techniques. For the patients that require hands-on care to progress their rehabilitation, the goal of the practitioner is to provide that service only until individuals are able to self-manage their symptoms.

QUESTIONS *for* REFLECTION

- What is the major differentiating characteristic of the **MDT approach** compared to most other approaches covered in this text?
- What is the MDT approach's view of OMPT, and how does that view influence its use in the MDT plan of care?

The emphasis on identifying the patient's symptomatic response to movement makes it safe for nearly all patient populations. The MDT approach is invaluable when treating individuals with precautions for OMPT because the system requires gradual progression of forces and establishes the appropriate direction in which forces are most safely applied. MDT is not intended to be all inclusive and endeavors to quickly identify responders and nonresponders. Patients presenting with contraindications to the use of OMPT, including an inability to provide relevant feedback, are not appropriate for MDT, and other medical or physical therapy interventions should be considered.

CLINICAL PILLAR

The **MDT approach** is considered safe for conditions ranging from acute to chronic for the following reasons:

1. A **gradual progression** of forces is used.
2. Prior to force application, the **direction** in which forces may be safely applied is established.
3. It involves the **careful monitoring** of each individual's symptomatic response.

CLINICAL PILLAR

To appropriately use the principles and procedures of the **MDT approach** to classify and treat the patient, that individual must be able to provide **relevant verbal feedback**. The effectiveness of this approach rests on the interaction between patient and therapist.

Fundamental Concepts and Diagnostic Classification

MDT is a systematic approach to the conservative management of most activity-related spinal disorders that is "diagnostic, prognostic, therapeutic, and prophylactic."[1] Perhaps one of the greatest features of this approach is the use of a well-defined classification system (Fig. 9-1) that categorizes patients according to their symptomatic response to movement and position, rather than a system that is based on a pathoanatomical diagnosis. The value of using impairment-based classification systems to guide intervention in this population has been well established (see Chapter 17).[4–8]

MDT is consistent with the **Quebec Task Force** classification system for activity-related spinal disorders (Fig. 9-2)[9] and meets the criteria for classification schemes described in the APTA's **Guide to Physical Therapist Practice**.[10] Unless contraindicated, all patients with spine-related pain, with or without referred symptoms, are suitable for mechanical examination.

QUESTIONS *for* REFLECTION

- Why is classification of spinal syndromes so challenging?
- What are the most valuable aspects of the MDT system for classification of spinal disorders?
- What aspects of this system need to be further refined and investigated?
- What are the recommended criteria for creating a system of classification for spine-related disorders?
- Does the MDT system of classification satisfy these parameters?

Classification by MDT focuses on the use of repeated movements and positions. At the conclusion of the examination, the individual is classified as having a **derangement syndrome, dysfunction syndrome, postural syndrome,** or **"other."** Individuals classified within one of these mechanical syndromes are considered to be ideal candidates for MDT, whereas those falling into the "other" category require additional examination or referral. The hallmark features for each of the three mechanical syndromes are summarized in Table 9-1.

The Derangement Syndrome

The derangement syndrome is the most frequently observed and best studied of the mechanical syndromes.[11,12] The pathoanatomical model for the presence of a derangement is an internal displacement of the intervertebral disc, which affects the normal resting position of the joint surfaces. Displacement of intradiscal material is presumed to obstruct normal segmental spinal motion to varying degrees. Derangements typically develop as a result of sustained or repetitive loading (often into flexion and/or rotation), chronic postural stresses (often into flexion and/or rotation), or trauma.

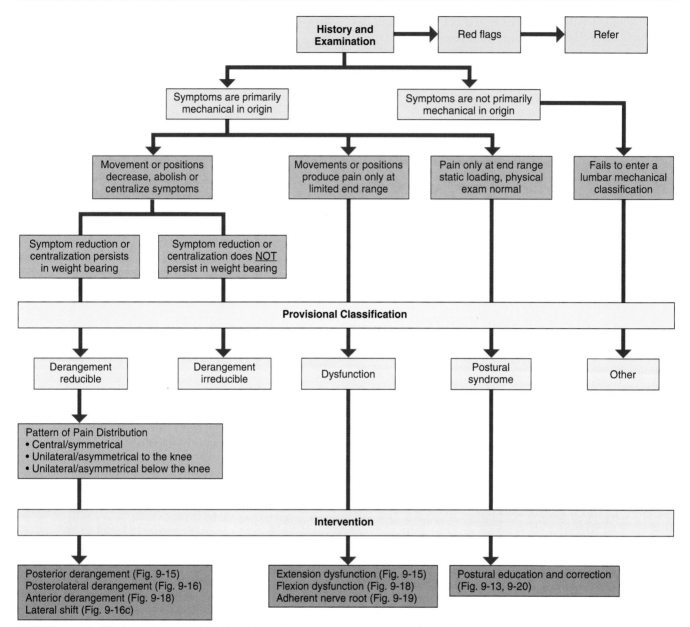

FIGURE 9–1. Classification and treatment algorithm. (Adapted from: McKenzie R, May S. *Mechanical Diagnosis & Therapy.* Waikanae, New Zealand: Spinal Publications; 2003, with permission.)

The displacement of intradiscal material may produce localized effects such as pain or paresthesia and motion loss. Large derangements may cause not only motion loss, but also an obstruction to normal posture such as an acute lateral shift (Fig. 9-3) and reduced lumbar lordosis. When the disc material compresses the nerve root, which lies in close proximity to the disc, symptoms may peripheralize into the lower extremities and symptoms such as leg pain, motor weakness and/or sensory changes may occur.

As the extent and location of the derangement changes with movement and position, the location and intensity of symptoms may change. The **centralization phenomenon** occurs when symptoms migrate from a distal location to a more proximal location. For example, symptoms are said to centralize when during the course of intervention pain that was once present in the lateral foot now resides in the posterolateral thigh only. Conversely, **peripheralization** is defined as the process by which symptoms move from a proximal to a more distal location. The ability to centralize symptoms is considered to be a favorable prognostic indicator,[2,13–18] whereas the inability to centralize symptoms has been reported as the strongest predictor of chronic pain and disability.[19]

Centralization is possible only in the case of a **competent disc** in which the annular wall remains intact. In such cases, the derangement is considered to be reducible and lasting changes are often achieved. Mechanically determined **directional preference** is the term given to the direction of movement that causes the symptoms to centralize. This movement, or positional bias, gives the practitioner and patient a powerful tool that may be used to positively affect symptom behavior

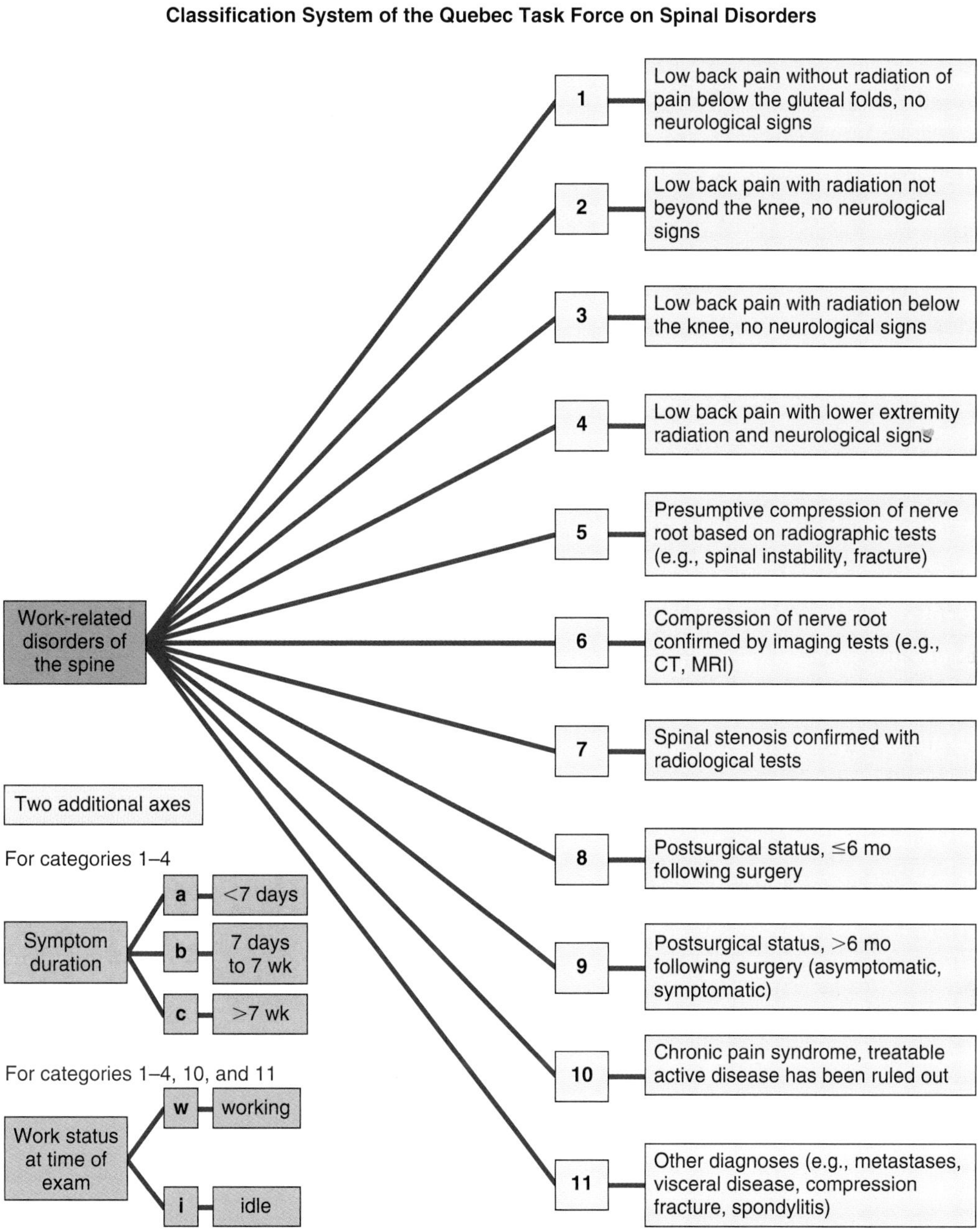

Classification System of the Quebec Task Force on Spinal Disorders

FIGURE 9–2. Quebec Task Force Classification System for activity-related spinal disorders (From: Riddle D. Classification and low back pain: a review of the literature and critical analysis of selected systems. *Phys Ther.* 1998;78:708-735, with permission).

and guide intervention. Identifying an individual's direction of preference will allow the therapist and patient to intentionally move the lumbar spine in the direction that reduces the derangement while intentionally avoiding the direction of movements or positions that worsen the condition. In the presence of an **incompetent disc**, or disc in which the annular wall is compromised, symptoms may appear to be centralized in non-weight-bearing but do not remain centralized in standing. In such cases, a derangement is deemed as *irreducible*.

An individual with a disc derangement often presents with distinctive features that are uniquely identified throughout

the patient history and mechanical examination (Table 9-1). During the interview, patients often report symptoms that are better with some activities and worse with others. During the physical examination, repeated movement testing often reveals the phenomena of centralization and/or peripheralization. Derangements are named by the direction in which the internal disc displacement is presumed to have occurred (posterior, anterior, or lateral) and the pattern of symptom distribution (Fig. 9-4).[2]

In randomized controlled trials, patients classified and treated using the McKenzie Method® demonstrated better

Table 9–1	Characteristics of MDT Mechanical Syndromes		
	DERANGEMENT	DYSFUNCTION	POSTURAL
Suspected Pathology	Disc injury or inflammation	Adaptively shortened tissues	Stressed normal tissue
Demographics Typical age range	20–55	Over 30*	Under 30
Pain Rating/Frequency			
• Intermittent	Yes/no	Yes	Yes
• Constant	Yes/no	No	No
History Pain location			
• Local (trunk)	Yes/no	Yes	Yes
• Referred (buttock, lower extremity)	Yes/no	ANR, Yes	No
Time Frame to Develop Condition			
• Acute	Yes	No	Yes
• Subacute	Yes	No	No
• Chronic	Yes	Yes	No
Mechanism of Injury			
• Gradual onset	Yes/no	Yes	Yes
• Sudden onset (trauma/injury)	Yes/no	No*	No
Examination Findings Neurological			
• (+) motor or sensory deficits	Yes/no	No	No
• (+) abnormal reflexes	Yes/no	No	No
• (+) dural signs	Yes/no	ANR Yes	No
Movement Loss			
• Range of motion loss	Yes—Obstructed	Yes—Restricted	No
Test Movements (repeated)			
• Changes in pain location	Yes	No	No
• Pain during movement	Yes	No	No
• End range pain	Yes	Yes	Yes**

ANR, adherent nerve root.
*Except ANR following trauma or derangement.
**Sustained end-range positioning.

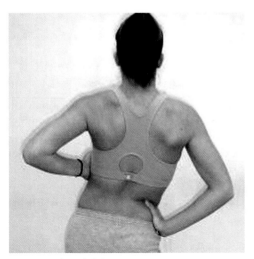

FIGURE 9–3. Acute lateral shift.

outcomes when compared to patients who were treated by other interventions including intense strength training,[20] mobilization,[21] back school,[22] or intervention based on the *Agency for Health Care Policy and Research (AHCPR)* guidelines.[23] Additionally, outcomes were significantly better in patients for whom exercises were prescribed based on their mechanically determined directional preferences.[24]

The Dysfunction Syndrome

For patients classified with a dysfunction syndrome, it is hypothesized that the periarticular soft tissues surrounding one or more of their spinal segments are contracted, adhered, or adaptively shortened. Movement or prolonged positioning becomes painful when restricted soft tissues are brought to the end of their available motion. Pain with movement may lead to the avoidance of end-range positions, which results in greater restrictions and a more profound loss of movement.

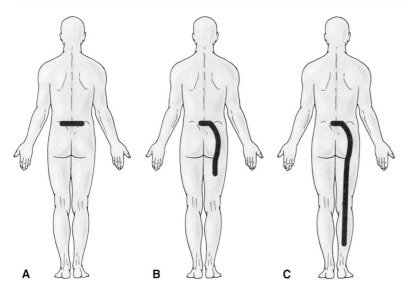

FIGURE 9–4. Patterns of symptom distribution. In derangement, the distribution is described as **A.** Central/symmetrical, **B.** unilateral/asymmetrical to the knee, or **C.** unilateral/asymmetrical below the knee.

Dysfunction may result as a secondary complication of lumbar surgery, sciatica, trauma, or disc derangement, typically emerging at a minimum of 6 weeks following the insulting event. Prolonged poor postural habits and long-term restrictions in joint mobility, as in the case of arthritis and stenosis, may also result in the development of a dysfunction. Dysfunction syndrome is the second most common syndrome; however, it only accounts for between 4% and 19% of patients with mechanical low back pain.[24,25]

Patients with dysfunction syndrome are consistent in their mechanical presentation. When restricted tissues are stressed,

pain is produced. Conversely, when stress is relieved by bringing the tissues into a more neutral position, the pain dissipates. In patients with dysfunction, motion restriction is observed in the same direction in which pain is produced. Dysfunction syndromes may appear in single or multiple planes of motion.

Dysfunction syndromes are named by the direction in which motion is restricted and symptoms are produced (Box 9-2). For example, in a **flexion dysfunction syndrome,** symptoms are produced at the end range of flexion and abate as the patient moves away from this position. The patient has local pain in the lumbar region and limited motion with

---

Box 9-2 THE MDT DIAGNOSTIC SPINAL CLASSIFICATION SYNDROMES

The Postural Syndrome

1. Pain is experienced when normal soft tissues experience abnormal stresses.

2. Structures such as joint capsules and ligaments strain in response to prolonged static loading at end range.

3. There is no reproduction of symptoms in response to single or repeated movements.

4. There are low levels of pain in response to maintenance of prolonged positions only.

5. *Prolonged sitting postures may lead to a loss of extension over time, culminating in a progression into one of the more advanced syndromes.*

The Dysfunction Syndrome

1. Pain results as abnormally restricted soft tissues are brought to the end of their available motion.

2. When stress is relieved by bringing the joint into a more neutral position, the pain is expected to dissipate.

3. Dysfunction syndrome may result as a complication secondary to lumbar surgery, sciatica, trauma, or disc derangement, typically emerging a minimum of 6 weeks following

4. Symptoms remain local and are not expected to refer into the extremities.

5. The specific dysfunction syndrome that exists is named by the direction in which motion is restricted and symptoms are reproduced.

The Derangement Syndrome

1. Internal displacement of the intervertebral disc occurs, which affects the normal resting position of the joint surfaces.

2. Lateral shift postural deformity is often present.

3. Repeated movement testing often reveals the phenomena of centralization and/or peripheralization, which is unique to patients with derangements.

4. Derangements are named according to the direction in which the internal disc displacement is presumed to have occurred.

5. Derangements are more specifically defined by the central versus peripheral location of the primary symptoms and on the degree of spinal deformity.

6. There are seven specific derangement subtypes.

flexion. However, no pain should be produced with any other lumbar motion. The opposite pattern of motion occurs with an extension dysfunction syndrome.

One special case of dysfunction is the **adherent nerve root (ANR) syndrome**. This syndrome is created by adhesions that have formed around the spinal nerve root or dura preventing normal mobility.[26] In contrast to the other types of dysfunction, which produce symptoms local to the spine, a lumbar ANR syndrome may include symptoms that radiate into the extremity. This syndrome may mimic a posterior derangement and, therefore, be confusing to the examiner. Differentiation may be accomplished through identifying the patient's symptomatic response to end-range *flexion in standing (FIS)* compared with *flexion in lying (FIL)*. In the case of a derangement, alteration of pressure gradients within the intervertebral disc through movement leads to compression of the nerve root regardless of the weight-bearing status. Therefore, in the case of a derangement, peripheralization will occur in both the flexion in standing and flexion in lying positions. With an ANR, lower extremity symptoms are only produced when adequate tension is placed through the nerve root and dural sheath. The flexion in standing movement (Fig. 9-5a), which involves the combined motions of trunk flexion, hip flexion, knee extension, and ankle dorsiflexion, is expected to be symptomatic in the presence of an ANR, whereas flexion in lying with hips and knees flexed (Fig. 9-5b) reduces tension through the sciatic nerve and is asymptomatic in the presence of an ANR.

The Postural Syndrome

In patients presenting with postural syndrome, it is theorized that lumbar pain is experienced when normal soft tissues experience abnormal stresses, typically in response to prolonged static loading at end range. The effects of a postural syndrome are most commonly experienced after prolonged slouched sitting (Fig. 9-6) in sedentary individuals such as students and deskbound workers. McKenzie states that "low back pain starts for the same reason as pain arising in the forefinger when it is bent backwards far enough to stimulate the free nerve endings of periarticular structures. No pathology needs to exist, and no chemical intervention will cure this form of mechanical pain."[27]

Individuals with postural syndromes do not often seek intervention. Patients with a postural syndrome report no reproduction of symptoms in response to single or repeated movements during the examination and will exhibit normal range of motion. These individuals typically report low levels of localized pain in response to prolonged positioning only. The postural syndrome is considered to be the least common disorder causing low back pain;[25] however, persistence of this syndrome is considered a precursor to the other, more advanced conditions and serves as a warning that demands behavior modification and postural reeducation.[28] Poor postural habits may lead to a loss of extension over time, culminating in a progression of the individual into one of the more advanced syndromes.

Other Syndromes

Individuals who fail to meet the criteria for classification into one of the mechanical diagnostic syndromes after examination

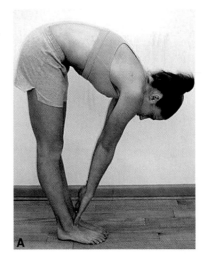
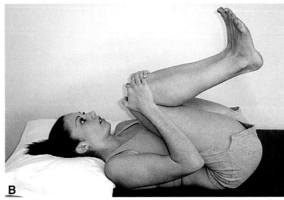

FIGURE 9-5. Differentiating ANR from derangement. In adherent nerve root, symptoms are produced when tension is placed on the nerve with **A.** flexion in standing, but not with **B.** flexion in lying. Patients with posterior derangement will have pain produced/worsened with lumbar flexion in both positions.

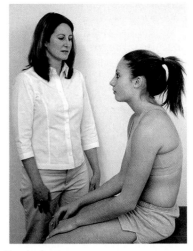

FIGURE 9-6. Slouched sitting.

and provisional intervention may be classified within the *other syndrome* category. It is important to note that individuals with other syndrome pathologies may have concomitant mechanical back pain and should be afforded an MDT examination to determine if their pain can be managed through mechanical intervention. Intervention for these conditions is outside the scope of this chapter (Box 9-3).

PRINCIPLES OF EXAMINATION

Examination begins with a thorough review of the patient's history, proceeds to a mechanical examination, and concludes in the provisional classification of the patient's condition. The classification directs the practitioner to the optimal mechanical intervention to address the patient's complaints. The McKenzie Institute® has developed examination protocols, complete with McKenzie assessment forms (Figs. 9-7 and 9-8), which may be accessed on the Institute's website at www.mckenziemdt.org/forms.cfm. The reader is also referred to McKenzie's *The Lumbar Spine: Mechanical Diagnosis & Therapy, Volume Two* for more detailed information.

QUESTIONS *for* REFLECTION

- What is the value of using an organized, sequential approach to examination?
- How might the use of examination forms serve to improve the efficiency and thoroughness of your examination?
- Using the first page of the MDT examination form, as shown in Figure 9-7, complete a full history on your role-playing partner. Then have your partner take a full history as you role-play without the use of the form. Which history was more thorough? Which was more efficient?

Throughout taking the history and performing the physical examination, the examiner should be aware of the presence of any red flags that may suggest serious spinal or systemic pathology for which medical intervention is required. Patients

Box 9-3 CRITERIA FOR INCLUSION IN THE "OTHER" SYNDROME CATEGORY

1. Fail to meet criteria for any of the other syndromes
2. Presence of *red flag* signs or symptoms
3. *Nonmechanical* symptom behavior, including suspected cauda equina syndrome, malignancy, fracture, and systemic inflammatory disorders
4. Patients meeting strict diagnostic criteria for conditions such as spinal stenosis, symptomatic hip pathology, symptomatic sacroiliac joint dysfunction, and symptomatic spondylolisthesis
5. Pregnancy-related lower back pain (LBP)
6. LBP status after lumbar surgery

with spinal pain who have undiagnosed serious pathologies, including cancer, infections, fractures, bone-weakening diseases, cauda equina syndrome, cord signs, and inflammatory arthropathies, make up less than 2% of the population of patients with back pain.[29]

The History

The first page of the *McKenzie Institute® Lumbar Spine Assessment®* (Fig. 9-7) summarizes the patient history. Within this approach, the process of history taking can be referred to as *empathetic interrogation* owing to the detailed manner in which this information is obtained. This interrogation is undertaken to denote the patient's mechanical behavior throughout the course of a typical day.

NOTABLE QUOTABLE

"The patient interview must be as an empathetic interrogation."
-Robin McKenzie

A comprehensive history is designed to efficiently gather information about the present episode of symptoms, including the *mechanism of injury*, *symptom presentation*, and *functional limitations*. During the examination, the quantity of data to be collected that relates to the impact of movement and position on the patient's symptoms is extensive. The examiner begins to formulate an idea of the patient's mechanical classification during the interview. These key characteristics related to the mechanical syndromes are summarized in Table 9-1. The reader is encouraged to refer to Figure 9-7 throughout the following discussion related to the subjective history.

CLINICAL PILLAR

Empathetic interrogation involves a series of follow-up questions that are designed to provide greater insight regarding the individual's current condition and any contributing factors. Such a series of questioning is imperative in order to fully understand the nature of the current condition.

Demographics
Date of Birth

In addition to the characteristic age ranges found in Table 9-1, other spinal conditions may be more prevalent at different stages of life. Knowledge of the patient's age and epidemiological factors increase the examiner's awareness that the patient may have a particular disorder.

Work/Leisure and Postures/Stresses

This portion of the history provides insight into the overall physical activity level of the patient and the presence of existing

The McKenzie Institute Lumbar Spine Assessment

Date _____

Name _____ Sex M/F _____

Address _____

Telephone _____

Date of birth _____ Age _____

Referral: GP/Orth/Self/Other _____

Work/Leisure _____

_____

Postures/Stresses _____

Functional disability from present episode _____

Functional disability score _____

VAS score (0–10) _____

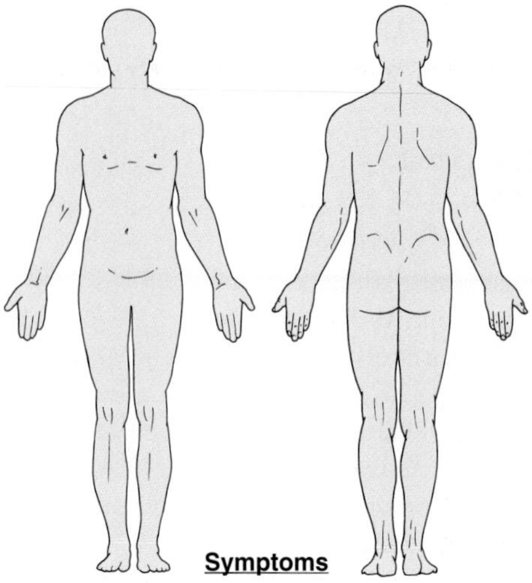

<u>Symptoms</u>

<u>History</u>

Present symptoms _____

Present since _____ Improving/Unchanging/Worsening

Commenced as a result of _____ Or no apparent reason

Symptoms at onset: Back/Thigh/Leg _____

Constant symptoms: Back/Thigh/Leg _____ Intermittent symptoms: Back/Thigh/Leg

Worse	Bending	Sitting/Rising	Standing	Walking	Lying
	AM/As the day progresses/PM			When still/On the move	
	Other_____				
Better	Bending	Sitting	Standing	Walking	Lying
	AM/As the day progresses/PM			When still/On the move	
	Other_____				

Disturbed sleep   Yes/No   Sleeping postures: Prone/Sup/Side R L   Surface: Firm/Soft/Sag

Previous episodes 0 1–5 6–10 11+   Year of first episode _____

Previous history _____

_____

Previous treatments _____

_____

Specific Questions

Cough/Sneeze/Strain/+ve/–ve   Bladder: Normal/Abnormal   Gait: Normal/Abnormal

Medications: Nil/NSAIDS/Analg/Steroids/Anticoag/Other _____

General Health: Good/Fair/Poor _____

Imaging: Yes/No _____

Recent or major surgery: Yes/No _____ Night pain: Yes/No _____

Accidents: Yes/No _____ Unexplained weight loss: Yes/No

Other: _____

FIGURE 9–7. Lumbar Spine Assessment form, page 1. (Reprinted with permission from the McKenzie Institute International.)

EXAMINATION

Posture

Sitting: Good/Fair/Poor   Standing: Good/Fair/Poor   Lordosis: Red/Acc/Normal   Lateral shift: Right/Left/Nil

Correction of posture: Better/Worse/No effect _____ Relevant: Yes/No

Other observations: _____

Neurological

Motor deficit _____   Reflexes _____

Sensory deficit _____   Dural signs _____

Movement Loss

	Maj	Mod	Min	Nil	Pain
Flexion					
Extension					
Side gliding R					
Side gliding L					

Test Movements

Describe effect on present pain–During: produces, abolishes, increases, decreases, no effect, centralising, peripheralising.
After: better, worse, no better, no worse, no effect, centralised, peripheralised.

Symptoms During Testing	Symptoms After Testing	Mechanical Response		
		↑Rom	↓Rom	No Effect
Pretest Symptoms Standing:				
FIS				
Rep FIS				
EIS				
Rep EIS				
Pretest Symptoms Lying:				
FIL				
Rep FIL				
EIL				
Rep EIL				
If Required Pretest Symptoms:				
SGIS R				
Rep SGIS R				
SGIS L				
Rep SGIS L				

Static Tests

Sitting slouched _____   Sitting erect _____

Standing slouched _____   Standing erect _____

Lying prone in extension _____   Long sitting _____

Other Tests _____
_____

Provisional Classification

Derangement   Dysfunction   Posture   Other

Subclassification _____

Principle of Management

Education _____   Equipment provided _____

Mechanical therapy _____

Extension principle _____ Lateral principle _____ Flexion principle _____

Other _____

Treatment goals _____

FIGURE 9–8. Lumbar Spine Assessment form, page 2. (Reprinted with permission from the McKenzie Institute International.)

or previous biomechanical risk factors. Biomechanical risk factors for low back pain include repeated forward bending or twisting, frequent or heavy lifting, and prolonged sitting or standing.[28]

Functional Disability

Perceived disability is documented through functional disability questionnaires, such as the *Oswestry Low Back Pain Disability Questionnaire*, the *Roland and Morris Disability Questionnaire*, or the *Quebec Back Pain Disability Scale*, among others.

Pain Rating

A baseline pain rating (verbal rating scale and/or visual analog scale) is reported for each symptomatic region. Identifying changes in baseline pain is extremely valuable throughout the mechanical examination process as the patient's symptomatic response to positions and movements will establish classification and subsequent intervention. In addition to its value during the initial examination, these baseline scores are used to assess progress upon subsequent visits.

QUESTIONS *for* REFLECTION

- How is an individual's verbal *numeric pain rating (NPR) scale* used during the typical MDT examination?
- What is the value of establishing an individual's baseline pain rating?
- How often should the individual's pain rating be obtained during the examination?
- In addition to pain intensity (1–10), what other factors related to pain (i.e., location, duration, etc.) are important to identify and why?

Body Diagram

The diagram is helpful in establishing classification. Back pain is commonly reported in all three mechanical syndromes, but the only syndromes that include the presence of lower extremity symptoms are derangement syndromes or a dysfunction with an adherent nerve root (ANR syndrome). Patients with "other" spinal disorders, such as stenosis with nerve entrapment, may exhibit leg pain as well.

Present Symptoms

This section is designed to document only those symptoms that have occurred within the last 24 to 48 hours.

Present Since

The duration of symptoms establishes if the condition is acute, subacute, or chronic and assists in classification, indicates the irritability of the patient's condition, and guides the aggressiveness of the examination. It is imperative that the examiner establishes when "this particular episode" started, even if the patient has had recurrent episodes of back pain.

Both derangement and postural syndromes may have an acute onset, but pain that is due to a dysfunction syndrome occurs only after soft tissues have become adaptively shortened, contracted, or fibrotic over time.

Improving/Unchanging/Worsening

It is important for the examiner to identify the patient's perception of the change in his or her condition since the onset of this episode of back pain by circling the appropriate description.

Commenced as a Result of

It is important to distinguish between pain with onset for *no apparent reason (NAR)* and pain associated with a specific incident.

Symptoms at Onset

The examiner circles the body part(s) where symptoms appeared at onset and describes the specific details of the symptoms at that time.

Constant Symptoms or Intermittent Symptoms

For each symptomatic body segment, the examiner circles the symptoms as being either constant or intermittent. *Constant pain* is present 100% of the time, although it may vary in intensity. *Intermittent pain* is present less than 100% of the time, even if pain-free times are brief. Unremitting, constant pain that does not abate even with recumbency may indicate serious nonmusculoskeletal pathology.[30] When pain is most intense or present only at night and causes difficulty with returning to sleep, it may be a red flag for malignancy.[31]

Worse/Better

For each activity or position, the patient is asked to describe if the symptoms become worse, meaning that symptoms are either produced, made more intense, or peripheralize; better, meaning that existing symptoms are reduced; or whether the movement has had no effect. Activities that consistently affect symptoms are circled. Those activities that sometimes affect symptoms are underlined, and those activities that have no effect are crossed through.

In order to provide greater detail, the form should be annotated to reflect conditions that may affect symptom response. For example, if a patient reports that sitting for longer than 20 minutes always provokes pain, the examiner should write "*>20 min*" next to sitting and circle it. Additionally, it is important to note if symptom location varies. For example, if a patient reports that walking for longer than 20 minutes worsens the back pain but reduces the leg pain, circle walking in the *worse* section, write in "*>20 min back*," and circle walking in the *better* section and write "*>20 min leg*." Drawing these parallels between the examination and daily functions will reinforce actions that patients will need to take to manage their condition.

Disturbed Sleep

If sleep is disturbed, the examiner must explore if this is due to the *sleeping postures*, the *sleeping surface*, or possibly a more sinister cause, as described above.

Previous History

It is well recognized that "the strongest risk factor for future back pain is history of past back pain."[2] The examiner must obtain details regarding previous history and any previous intervention that may or may not have been helpful.

Specific Questions

Cough/Sneeze/Strain

Symptoms that are worsened by coughing, sneezing, and or straining suggest the presence of an active condition that is aggravated by sudden or increased internal pressures. These characteristics often occur in the presence of a derangement syndrome.

CLINICAL PILLAR

Classic signs/symptoms of disc derangement include the following:

1. Symptoms into the leg often distal to the knee
2. Poor tolerance for flexed postures and movements
3. If advanced, neurological signs, including hyporeflexia, dermatomal hypoesthesia, and myotomal weakness
4. Symptoms worsened with coughing, sneezing, straining
5. Possible presence of dural root tension signs (i.e., positive straight leg raising, slump test)

Changes in bladder function (initiation, retention, or incontinence) and/or saddle anesthesia that occur in conjunction with low back pain may be indicative of a systemic problem such as bladder pathology or cauda equina syndrome and require immediate referral.

Gait

A new onset of gait dysfunction should be explored to expose the underlying cause(s). *Antalgia*, for example, may arise from a derangement with a lateral component or from an adherent nerve root, when the sciatic nerve is tensioned at heel strike. Other gait issues such as *drop foot or ataxia* may arise from neuropathy or myelopathy, and additional examination procedures are warranted.

Medications

It is important to review all medications that are being taken by the patient prior to examination. Strong analgesics taken prior to examination may alter the patient's pain perception during testing. Anticoagulants or long-term steroid use is considered a precaution for the use of manual techniques. Aspirin that provides disproportional relief of symptoms is a "*red flag for bone cancer.*"[32]

General Health

During this portion of the examination, the therapist identifies the patient's perception of his or her overall health, including a list of **comorbidities**. Constitutional symptoms such as fever,

chills, or night sweats occurring in concert with complaints of low back pain suggest a systemic, rather than musculoskeletal, origin. A previous history of cancer that is not being monitored warrants referral if other warning signs are present.

Imaging Studies

Imaging studies are essential for the purpose of ruling out serious pathology in individuals with a history of trauma or symptoms that suggest the presence of malignancy. A significant percentage of asymptomatic individuals have been found to have substantial abnormalities, such as a herniated nucleus pulposus, upon imaging.[33,34] Therefore, the results of the mechanical examination rather than the results of diagnostic imaging must be used to determine the course of intervention.

QUESTIONS *for* REFLECTION

- Why is it preferable to treat an individual based on the results of the mechanical examination as opposed to the results of diagnostic imaging (MRI, CT, etc.)?
- What does the evidence say concerning the prevalence of false-positive imaging results?
- How might "treating the image" lead to poor outcomes?

Recent or Major Surgery

Information regarding previous surgeries can alert the examiner to the potential for other causes of symptoms. Patients with constant, unremitting pain, especially if accompanied by fever, following a recent surgical procedure may suggest the presence of an infection.

Night Pain

As mentioned, unremitting night pain may be indicative of a more serious spinal pathology such as cancer or ankylosing spondylitis.

Accidents

The presence of fractures, instabilities, and other injuries must be ruled out following trauma. Modification of testing procedures is often indicated after trauma and in the presence of active inflammation. The examiner should restrict range of motion and repeated movement testing to remain within the pain-free limits.

Unexplained Weight Loss

While some patients lose their appetites secondary to pain or medication side effects, more gain weight because of decreased activity levels. Unintentional weight loss greater than 10% of a patient's total body weight over a 4-week period of time is indicative of malignancy.[35]

The Working Hypothesis:

After completion of the first page of the ***Lumbar Spine Assessment***®, the examiner should attempt to develop an initial working hypothesis regarding the origin and nature of the patient's condition. First and foremost, the examiner must determine whether or not there are any "red flags." Additionally, the examiner must determine if the history should influence the remainder of the physical examination and whether or not there are any psychosocial issues, such as fear avoidance or depression.[36]

The Physical Examination

The physical examination is designed to confirm or reject the working hypothesis by testing the patient's symptomatic response to loading and by observing the quality and quantity of movement. During the examination, *testing error* must be minimized. The reader should refer to Figure 9-8 throughout this discussion.

Postures

Sitting

The patient's posture is grossly assessed while the examiner is obtaining the subjective history. If pain is reported in sitting, the location of the pain is recorded. The examiner corrects any aberrant postures (Fig. 9-9a) and monitors the patient's response to postural correction. If symptoms are reduced, the patient is educated on how to reproduce this posture, including the use of a lumbar roll (Fig. 9-9b).

Standing

When the patient is standing, posture is assessed in the sagittal and frontal planes. The presence of a reduced or accentuated **lordosis** is noted. If pain is reported in standing, the location is recorded as well as any response to postural correction. Chronic deviations, such as scoliosis, may be present but have no effect on symptoms. Acute deviations, such as a **lateral shift,** also known as an acute lumbosacral or sciatic scoliosis, may also be present. This postural deviation is nonstructural and is caused by pressure on a nerve root from a disc herniation or other space-occupying lesion.[37] The lateral shift is named by the direction in which the upper torso is displaced. The criteria for confirming the presence of a lateral shift that is relevant to the current condition includes the following: (1) the deformity is clearly visible; (2) the onset is concurrent with the present episode of pain; (3) the lateral shift cannot be voluntarily corrected or maintained; (4) both flexion and extension movements are painful in weight-bearing; and (5) the pain is worse in standing or walking than it is when lying down.

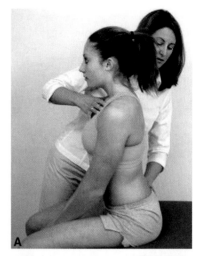

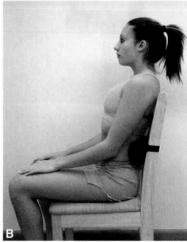

FIGURE 9–9. Postural correction. **A.** Postural correction by clinician. Slouched posture is corrected by the application of force through the lumbar spine and sternum to align the patient's shoulders over hips and head over shoulders. **B.** Correct sitting with a lumbar roll. The lumbar roll should support but not exaggerate the lumbar lordosis.

CLINICAL PILLAR

Criteria for determining the presence of a *lateral shift* that is clinically relevant includes the following:

1. Deformity must be clearly visible.
2. Onset must be concurrent with the current episode of pain.
3. It cannot be voluntarily corrected or maintained.
4. Flexion and extension movements are painful in weight-bearing.
5. Pain is worse in standing or walking than it is when lying down.

QUESTIONS *for* REFLECTION

- Briefly define what is meant by a *lateral shift*.
- How is a lateral shift named?
- What are believed to be the etiologic factors that lead to a lateral shift?
- What does the evidence reveal regarding the reliability of identifying a lateral shift and its clinical relevance?
- Briefly describe the procedures that may be used to reduce a lateral shift. Perform these maneuvers on a partner.

If a lateral shift is confirmed during the examination, lateral shift correction techniques (Fig. 9-10) should be commenced prior to initiation of repeated movement testing and intervention. Poor tolerance for repeated movements is often noted in the presence of a lateral shift.

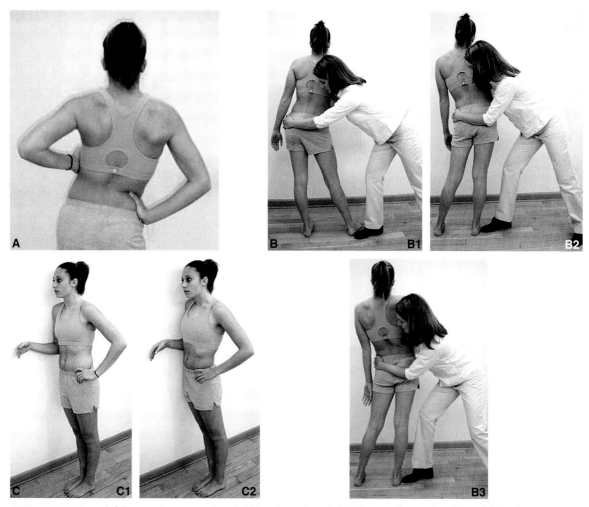

FIGURE 9–10. Lateral shift correction progression. **A.** Right relevant lateral shift. **B.** Manual correction of lateral shift (shown for correction of a right lateral shift): The patient stands with feet shoulder-width apart and weight evenly distributed. Her right elbow is flexed 90 degrees and placed against the trunk above the level of the iliac crest. The clinician stands perpendicular to the patient on her right side in a lunge position, with her right shoulder against the patient's right upper arm. The clinician's hands are clasped around the patient's left iliac crest **(B1)**. The clinician gently pulls the patient's pelvis toward her while simultaneously pushing the patient's trunk away by the pressure exerted through the clinician's right shoulder. The patient must remain weight-bearing symmetrically. Intermittent gentle pressure is applied and partially released, with more pressure given with each repetition until a slight overcorrection of the deformity is accomplished **(B2)**. The patient is then asked to perform extension while the therapist maintains a slight overcorrection of the shift **(B3)**. **C.** Self-lateral shift correction against a wall. The patient stands with feet together about shoulder's width from the wall with the side of the shift near the wall (usually the shoulder contralateral to the painful side). The patient's elbow is flexed above the level of the iliac crest, and the upper arm is placed against the wall **(C1)**. The patient then uses her other hand to apply rhythmic pressure through the pelvis toward the wall until overcorrection is achieved **(C2)**. In this position, lordosis is restored by performing extension in standing in the overcorrected position.

Neurological

If the patient reports symptoms such as weakness or gait dysfunction, paresthesia/anesthesia, or pain in the lower extremities, *motor deficits*, *sensory deficits*, *dural signs*, and *reflexes* are examined.

Movement Loss

Spinal movements are assessed in standing prior to repeated movement testing. Movement loss is visually assessed and recorded on a continuum from *nil* to *major loss* of motion. It is common for individuals with limited lumbar mobility to compensate elsewhere. It is critical that the examiner observe both

the quantity as well as the quality of motion. Observation of deformity, sufficient curve reversal, and any deviations from the normal path of movement are noted by circling the observed direction of deviation. Visual estimation is typically used, although other more reliable methods such as goniometry, inclinometry, or tape measurement (Schober method) may also be used.

Test Movements

The use of **repeated movement testing** during the examination is one of the distinguishing features of the MDT approach. The patient's symptomatic and mechanical response to loading guides the examiner to the appropriate classification and course of intervention. During and immediately following test movements, the examiner carefully records any changes in the patient's symptoms and the patient's mechanical response (Table 9-2).

The sequence of repeated movement testing is displayed in Figure 9-11. From a neutral position and after recording the baseline location and intensity of symptoms, the patient moves as far as possible through a test movement for one repetition and then repeats for 10 repetitions. During and immediately following these movements, the examiner records the effect on the patient's symptoms. Once the patient returns to the neutral position and rests for a few moments, the effect of movement on symptoms is recorded (Table 9-2). Repeated movements in the offending direction are immediately abandoned if peripheralization of the symptoms remain after testing.

If symptoms are improving or centralizing during repeated movement testing, the examiner should continue to see if the symptoms can be completely abolished. If symptoms are significantly reduced or abolished during movement testing in the prone position, it is important to have the patient rise from the table while maintaining a lordosis to determine if the symptoms

remain improved in full weight-bearing. Maintenance of improved symptoms upon assumption of a weight-bearing posture is an indicator of a **reducible derangement.**

If the patient reports no effect in response to repeated movements, additional repetitions may be performed to confirm this finding. If there is no conclusive symptomatic or mechanical response to sagittal plane movements, a **laterally displaced derangement** may be present. Repeated movement testing should then be performed with a lateral bias, such as extension in lying position with the hips displaced laterally to one side, then the other (Fig. 9-12a), or side gliding in the standing position (Fig. 9-12b).

Static Tests

Although not routinely performed, static tests may be necessary if repeated movement testing is inconclusive. Additionally, static tests may be preferable for patients with acute deformity or severe pain or when a postural syndrome is suspected. Selected positions include *sitting erect, sitting slouched, long sitting, standing slouched, standing erect,* or *lying prone in extension* (Box 9-4).

Other Tests

If testing fails to identify a mechanical disorder, other tests may be performed to ascertain the potential contribution from adjacent regions. Such procedures include *sacroiliac joint screening* and *hip joint assessment.* Within this approach, these conditions are recognized, yet strict criteria for classification is not provided.

The Provisional Classification

At the conclusion of the mechanical examination, the examiner should have sufficient information to make a provisional classification. Refer to the classification algorithm (see Fig. 9-1) and characteristics (Table 9-1) to guide the decision-making process. If the classification is a derangement, the pattern of pain presentation should be identified, as well as the directional preference, in order to select the appropriate intervention. If the classification is a dysfunction, the direction of restriction must be identified in order to select the proper intervention.

If there is insufficient evidence at the conclusion of the initial examination to make a provisional classification, patients are asked to keep a record of their symptomatic response to movement and position. At the conclusion of the examination, the therapist should have identified a *mechanical versus nonmechanical condition,* the *syndrome classification,* the *directional preference,* and the subsequent *principle of intervention.*

PRINCIPLES OF INTERVENTION
General Principles

As previously stated, mechanical classification drives the intervention. In a derangement syndrome, the primary objectives of intervention are to reduce the internal displacement,

Table 9-2	Effects on Pain During and After Test Movements

Description of symptom change that may occur *during* movement:

P	Produce: Symptoms that were not present prior to movement are now present.
I	Increase: Symptoms that were present are increased in intensity.
PE	Peripheralizes: The pain moved from a proximal to a more distal body part.
D	Decrease: Symptoms that were present are decreased in intensity.
A	Abolish : Symptoms that were present prior to movement are completely gone.
C	Centralizes: The pain moved from a distal to a more proximal body part.
NE	No effect.

Description of symptoms that occur *after* movement:

B	Better: Symptoms remain improved after completion of repeated movements.
NB	No better: Symptoms improve only temporarily with repeated movements.
C	Centralized: Distal symptoms move proximally and remain after movement testing.
W	Worse: Symptoms remain worse after completion of repeated movements.
NW	No worse: Symptoms worsen only temporarily with repeated movements.
PE	Peripheralized: Proximal symptoms move distal and remain after movement testing.
NE	No effect: Symptoms do not change following repeated movement testing.

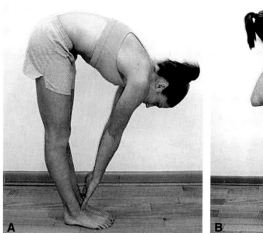
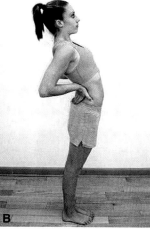
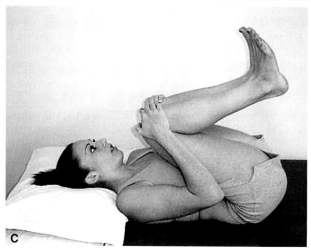
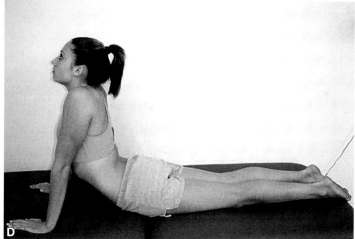

FIGURE 9–11. Sequence of repeated movement testing. **A.** Flexion in standing (FIS): Stand with feet shoulder-width apart. Bend forward from the waist and slide the hands down the legs as far as possible while keeping the knees straight. **B.** Extension in standing (EIS): Stand with feet shoulder-width apart. Place the hands in the small of the back and arch backward as far as possible while keeping the knees straight. **C.** Flexion in lying (FIL): From the hook-lying position, bring the knees toward the chest as far as possible. Clasp the hands over the knees to further flex the lumbar spine. **D.** Extension in lying (EIL): Place hands directly under the shoulders. Extend the elbows slowly to raise the upper body off the plinth. Keep the hips and thighs relaxed, and allow the abdomen to sag.

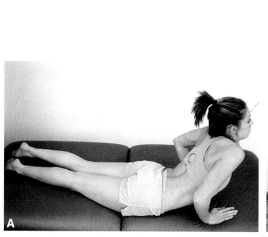
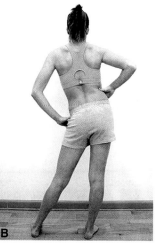

FIGURE 9–12. Repeated movement test movements with lateral bias. **A.** Extension in lying (EIL) with hips off center: In prone, translate the hips laterally, usually away from the pain. Perform EIL: Place hands directly under the shoulders. Extend the elbows slowly to raise the upper body off the plinth. Keep the hips and thighs relaxed, and allow the abdomen to sag. **B.** Side glide in standing (SGIS): Directions for right SGIS. Stand with feet shoulder-width apart. Translate the hips to the left while maintaining the trunk in neutral with shoulders parallel to the ground. The clinician may initially guide the movement at with hands at the right iliac crest and left shoulder.

Box 9-4 SPINAL MOVEMENTS AND POSITIONS TESTED DURING THE MDT EXAMINATION

Sequence of Spinal Movements

1. Flexion in standing (FIS)
2. Repeated flexion in standing (RFIS)
3. Extension in standing (EIS)
4. Repeated extension in standing (REIS)
5. Flexion in lying (FIL)
6. Repeated flexion in lying (RFIL)
7. Extension in lying (EIL)
8. Repeated extension in lying (REIL)
9. Side glide in standing right (SGIS R)
10. Repeated side glide in standing right (RSGIS R)
11. Side glide in standing left (SGIS L)
12. Repeated side glide in standing left (RSGIS L)

Static Postures

1. Sitting slouched
2. Standing slouched
3. Lying prone in extension
4. Sitting erect
5. Standing erect
6. Long sitting

maintain the reduction, and restore full movement. In a dysfunction syndrome, the primary objectives are to remodel adaptively shortened tissues and reduce movement restrictions. The objective of intervention for patients presenting with a postural syndrome is to remove abnormal stresses on normal tissues. A critical principle of intervention is the confirmation or rejection of the provisional classification. Upon subsequent visits, if the patient's symptoms are worse, or not improved, compliance and technique are checked before assuming an incorrect mechanical diagnosis has been made. Confirmation of the classification should be determined within five sessions.

CLINICAL PILLAR

Primary intervention objectives for the mechanical classifications are as follows.

Postural syndrome: Remove the abnormal stress that is being applied to normal tissue.

Dysfunction syndrome: Facilitate the remodeling of adaptively shortened tissues, thus reducing the primary and secondary movement restrictions. Intervention typically involves movement into the painful direction.

Derangement syndrome: Reduce the internal displacement, maintain the reduction, and restore full movement. Intervention typically involves movement away from the painful direction.

A key feature of this approach is the emphasis on holding the patient responsible for his or her own care, which begins on the first visit, through a substantial amount of patient education. Patients are educated on appropriate posture and body mechanics, given their classification, including proper sitting and sleeping postures, transitional movements, and postural support. The use of a lumbar roll in the region of the lumbar lordotic curve when sitting is often incorporated to improve sitting posture by preserving lumbar lordosis and reducing the effects of prolonged flexion forces (Fig. 9-13a and b).

Patients are provided with a specific prescription for exercise(s) to perform until the next appointment, usually in 1 to 2 days. Patients are informed about warning signs, such as peripheralization, and are given instructions regarding what to do if such a situation arises.

When performing exercises, force progression is considered to be a valuable concept for two reasons: (1) physiologically, mechanical pain may resolve using a range of forces, and (2) philosophically, using the least amount of force necessary to resolve the symptoms is safer. Therefore, only when individuals are unable to control their own symptoms should additional forces be introduced. The sequence of force progression begins with **patient-generated forces** that take place in midrange with eventual progression to end range and end range with *self-overpressure*. Once patient-generated forces have been exhausted, intervention may progress to **clinician-generated forces**, which involve assisting the patient with movement from midrange to end range with *therapist overpressure*. Passive nonthrust and thrust mobilization performed by the clinician are considered when patient-generated forces are inadequate to produce the desired outcome. Once the patient's directional preference has been confirmed, progression along the force continuum is dictated by symptom response. A patient who has responded well to movement into end-range extension but continues to display movement loss (Fig. 9-14a) should progress to end-range extension with self-overpressure (Fig. 9-14b). Additionally, once improvement plateaus, modifications such as altering the *starting position* (loaded or unloaded), the *direction of loading* (sagittal, frontal, or combination), and *duration of the technique* may be explored.

Lastly, this approach espouses the use of *prophylactic measures* designed to equip patients with the knowledge and activities to prevent and manage future episodes by using *"first aid"* exercises. Patients using an MDT approach demonstrate high

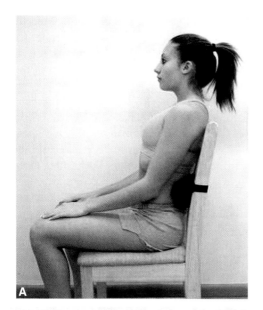

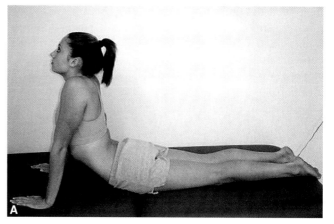

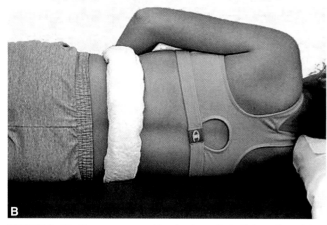

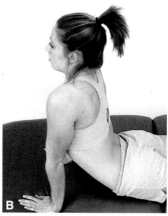

FIGURE 9–14. Progression of forces. Forces are progressed when symptoms have decreased but have reached a plateau. **A.** The force progression for extension in lying is as seen in b. **B.** Extension in lying with self-overpressure.

FIGURE 9–13. Correct posture with a lumbar roll. **A.** Sitting roll. In sitting, the lumbar roll should support but not exaggerate the lumbar lordosis. **B.** Night roll. Patients who find side lying worsens symptoms are often more comfortable with a rolled towel fastened around the waist to support the spine in neutral.

levels of satisfaction in their ability to manage their current symptoms and recurrences,[38] demonstrate lower rates of recurrence,[39,40] have less sick leave,[41] and seek less medical assistance.[41]

Intervention for Derangement Syndrome

Reduction of a derangement is achieved and maintained by consistent application of the loading strategy that centralized the patient's symptoms during the examination. Once reduced, it is important to educate the patient to consistently avoid the provocative positions and movements. Extensive patient education regarding centralization and peripheralization principles as well as postural education and correction are vital to maintaining reduction and preventing recurrence.

Ideally, exercises must be performed 10 times every 1 to 2 waking hours, or more frequently if symptoms recur. Assuming the mechanical classification given at examination is correct, patients should report a decrease in symptoms with

centralization, increased mobility, and tolerance for progression of forces. If centralization is not achieved within five sessions, it is unlikely that centralization will occur.[17] A common error is that patients may not have achieved end range and then are mistakenly believed to be noncentralizers.

When the patient's symptoms are no longer provoked or peripheralized with movements or postures, the derangement is considered to be fully reduced. During intervention, provocative motions are avoided to reduce the risk of rederangement. A return to provocative motions must be done gradually, with the goal of restoring any residual motion loss and with an awareness that any limitation in spinal motion is a risk factor for future derangement.[2] Intervention is complete when the patient reports restoration of normal activities and pain-free movement in all directions.

Empowering patients to intelligently manage their own pain by providing them with the tools needed to recognize and manage recurrences is one of the greatest virtues of the MDT approach. When warning signs are present, patients should initiate self-management measures for 48 hours, such as (1) avoiding positions and movements that provoke pain, (2) sitting with the lumbar spine unsupported for no longer than 5 to 10 minutes at a time and resting in either the prone or supine position, and (3) commencing with prior exercise 10 to 15 times every 1 to 2 waking hours. Patients are instructed to continue their exercise program for at least 6 weeks after discharge, maintain good postural habits, reduce their biomechanical risk factors, and incorporate general fitness activities into their lifestyle.

Four groups of derangements are typically seen with unique directional preferences. The intervention approach is the same for each group although the exact loading strategies may vary.

Intervention for Posterior Derangement Syndrome

The intervention for a **posterior derangement** follows the **extension principle** (Fig. 9-15). Most patients who present with a derangement fall into this subclassification.[12]

Extension in lying (EIL) is the exercise of choice for a posterior derangement because of reduced compressive forces. In some individuals, the first few repetitions may provoke pain because motion is obstructed by the posterior displacement of the disc. However, as the patient performs more repetitions, reduction occurs, pain resolves, and motion improves. **Extension in standing (EIS)** is performed throughout the day when extension in lying is not possible. Preservation of the lumbar lordosis in sitting (see Fig. 9-13) by using a lumbar roll for mechanical and tactile cueing is essential in order to maintain the reduction. Additionally, maintenance of lumbar lordosis during transfers and activities of daily living may require patient education and cueing by the therapist. To be effective, the patient must take primary responsibility for performing exercises and avoiding provocative movements and positions.

Prior to discharge, intervention for a patient with a posterior derangement must include restoration of pain-free flexion (Fig. 9-11c). Once patients can reliably manage their symptoms, movement into flexion is explored in a controlled fashion. While supervised, patients perform up to 10 repetitions of **flexion in lying (FIL)**. If pain is not worsened or

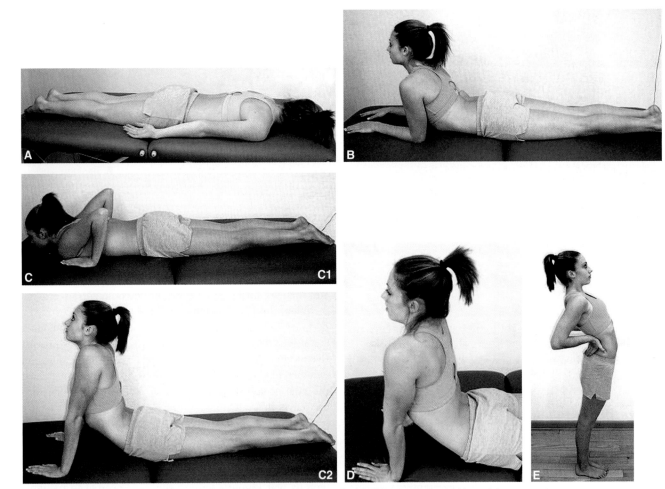

FIGURE 9–15. Extension Principle/progression of forces. **A.** Lying prone. The head is rotated to one side and the arms relaxed by the side of the trunk. The position may be modified if the patient has an acute kyphotic deformity by placing pillows under the abdomen to accommodate the deformity, then sequentially removing pillows until lying prone is attained. **B.** Lying prone in extension: Place elbows directly under the shoulders with the forearms parallel and the hips flat on the plinth. The lumbar spine should sag into lumbar lordosis. **C.** Extension in lying (EIL): Place hands directly under the shoulders **(C1)**. Extend the elbows slowly to raise the upper body off the plinth. Keep the hips and thighs relaxed and allow the abdomen to sag **(C2)**. **D.** Extension in lying with self-overpressure. Perform EIL. Apply self-overpressure: Lock the elbows at end-range extension, exhale fully, and allow the abdomen to sag prior to lowering the chest to the table. **E.** Extension in standing (EIS): Stand with feet shoulder-width apart. Place the hands in the small of the back and arch backward as far as possible while keeping the knees straight.

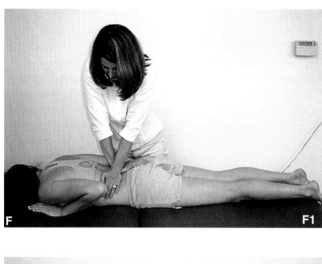
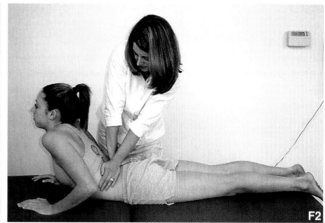
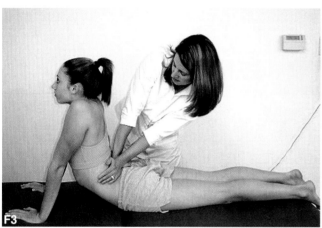
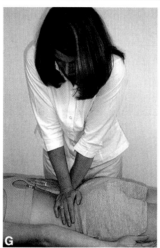

FIGURE 9–15. cont'd F. Extension in lying with clinician overpressure: The clinician places the heels of her hands on the selected transverse processes of the lumbar segment **(F1)**. The patient performs EIL. As the patient progresses into greater extension **(F2, F3)**, the clinician shifts her body backward to maintain a force "parallel to the motion segment."[42] Overpressure is maintained until the patient fully lowers to the start position. **G.** Extension mobilization. The clinician places her hands perpendicular to each other over the transverse processes of the spinal segment. The clinician's shoulders must be directly over her hands and her elbows extended. Gradual rhythmic and symmetrical pressure is applied in a posteroanterior direction to end range. Symptom response is monitored at each segment. Mobilization is provided to the same segment 10 times before progressing to the next segment.

peripheralized and extension range of motion is not reduced, then FIL is added to the intervention plan. If there is a poor response, then the derangement is unstable and repeated flexion should be delayed.

Intervention for Posterior Derangement Syndrome With Lateral Component

Some patients with a posterior derangement require the application of either frontal or transverse plane directed forces along with sagittal plane-directed forces (Fig. 9-16) in order for a complete reduction to occur. These patients are said to have a lateral component to their derangements. In this syndrome, the patient's symptoms are unilateral or asymmetrical, and during examination the symptoms do not respond to or are worsened by pure sagittal plane movements.

Intervention begins with EIL, with the hips shifted laterally (Fig. 9-16a), and progresses by adding clinician overpressure (Fig. 9-16b). To reduce or centralize symptoms, the hips are most frequently shifted *away from, but occasionally*

toward, the painful side. Other options for reduction of symptoms using lateral forces include **side gliding in standing (SGIS)** (Fig. 9-16c), rotation mobilization in extension bilaterally (Fig. 9-16d1) or unilaterally (Fig. 9-16d2), rotation in flexion (Fig. 9-16e), and rotation mobilization in flexion (Fig. 9-16f).

When symptoms have centralized or become symmetrical, EIL in the pure sagittal plane should be retested to see if it is safe to perform, after which the treatment plan is progressed to pure extension-biased exercises. If pain is worsened or peripheralized, then the derangement is not sufficiently stable to cease lateral forces.

Intervention for Lateral Shift

A lateral shift is defined as a frontal plane postural deviation in which the upper trunk is displaced laterally relative to the lower trunk and the upper trunk is unable to move past the midline. The majority of patients with a relevant lateral shift will deviate *away from the painful side*. The specific mechanisms underlying the etiology and direction in which the lateral deviation occurs has yet to be confirmed in the literature.

Correction of the lateral shift must be achieved before attempting to restore extension range of motion. Attempts to apply sagittal forces in the presence of a true lateral shift will worsen the patient's symptoms. Manual correction of a lateral shift is one of the more common manual therapy procedures used within the MDT approach (Fig. 9-10). Correction, or overcorrection, in which the patient's shifted trunk is brought to midline and then slightly beyond, may be painful and may produce *vasovagal syncope*. Once overcorrection is achieved, patients must immediately perform extension in standing while overpressure is maintained by the clinician to maintain

the correction (Fig. 9-17). Following lateral shift correction in the clinic, it is imperative that the patient maintain lordosis at all times to prevent recurrence. Additionally, patients are instructed in self-correction techniques, including SGIS (Fig. 9-10c). The patient stands with the shoulder (on the side to which the shift has occurred) against the wall and the feet together, approximately 12 inches away from the wall. The opposite hand is placed on the outside hip as the patient moves the pelvis toward the wall; the position is held for several seconds and repeated until the shift is corrected. After self-correction, the patient immediately performs EIS or EIL with hips offset. The shift correction is maintained by avoiding trunk flexion and strict adherence to good posture.

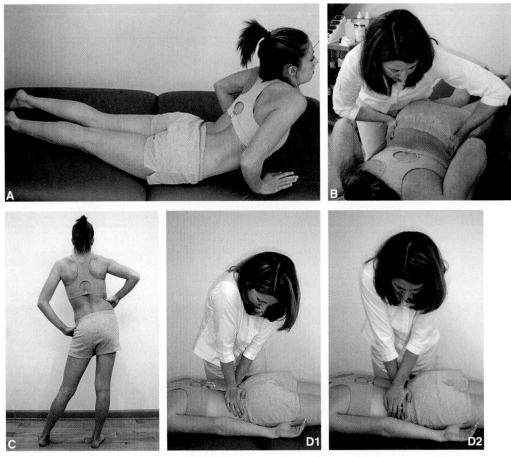

FIGURE 9–16. Treatment principle for posterior derangement with lateral component/progression of forces. When sagittal plane movements do not reduce a posterior derangement (Fig. 9-15) lateral forces may be necessary. **A.** Extension in lying (EIL) with hips off center: In prone, translate the hips laterally, usually away from the pain. Perform EIL: Place hands directly under the shoulders. Extend the elbows slowly to raise the upper body off the plinth. Keep the hips and thighs relaxed and allow the abdomen to sag. **B.** EIL with hips off center with lateral overpressure by clinician: With the patient positioned in prone with hips off center, the clinician applies and maintains overpressure at the iliac crests to further enhance lateral forces as EIL is performed. **C.** Side glide in standing (SGIS): Directions for right SGIS. Stand with feet shoulder-width apart. Translate the hips to the left while maintaining the trunk in neutral with shoulders parallel to the ground. The clinician may initially guide the movement with hands at the right iliac crest and left shoulder. **D1.** Rotation mobilization in extension: The clinician's hands are placed perpendicular to each other with hypothenar eminences over the area of the transverse processes of the spinal segment to be mobilized and shoulders over the hands. The mobilization is performed by alternating forces from one side of the spinal segment to the other. First, an anteromedially directed force is applied by shifting the shoulders forward over the extended arm. The shoulders are then shifted back to apply force through the opposite hypothenar eminence. Rhythmical application of forces is continued. If application of force on one side centralizes the symptoms, a unilateral rotation mobilization is performed **(D2)** by placing one hand on top of the other. Rotation in flexion: In hook-lying position, the patient rotates the knees to the side (usually toward the side of the pain).

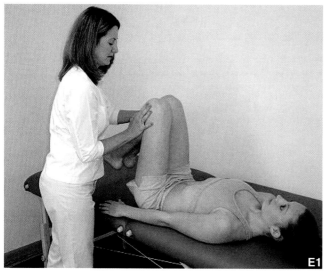
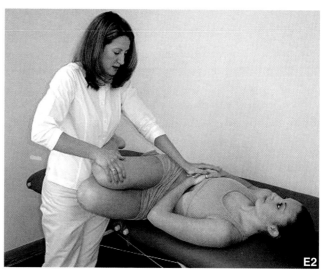
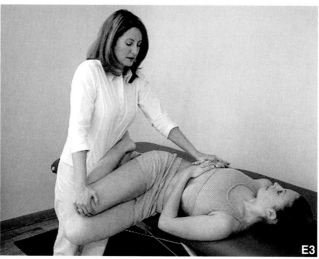

FIGURE 9–16. cont'd E1. Rotation mobilization in flexion: The patient lies supine with hips and knees extended. The clinician stands to the side of the patient, facing proximally. The clinician passively flexes the patient's hips and knees to 90 degrees and presets the pelvis by rotating it prior to bringing the knees to one side (usually toward the side of pain). **E2.** The patient's ankles rest on the clinician's hips or pelvis. The hand closest to the patient fixes either the far shoulder or rib cage through the patient's clasped hands. **E3.** The therapist's far hand pushes the knees downward, either sustaining the force or by applying intermittent pressure. Symptom response is monitored. The lower extremities are passively returned to the starting position.

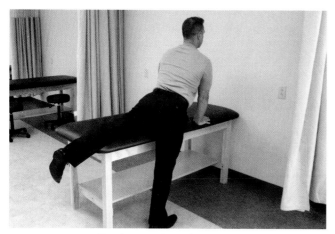

FIGURE 9–17. Transition from standing to lying prone following lateral shift correction. Every effort is made to avoid flexion, which presumably causes the lateral shift to return. Once prone, extension progressions are performed.

Once a shift is corrected, exercise proceeds as for a posterior derangement (Fig. 9-15).

Intervention for Anterior Derangement Syndrome

The intervention of an anterior derangement follows the flexion principle (Fig. 9-18), which increases compressive forces anteriorly. Ten repetitions of the selected exercise must be performed every 1 to 2 hours. A progression of force is made when the patient's symptoms have improved, but are no longer progressing with the current exercise regimen. It is important to note that less than 7% of all derangements are anterior.[2]

Intervention for Dysfunction Syndrome

There are four types of dysfunction syndromes, which are named by the restricted direction or the direction in which symptoms are reproduced. They are flexion dysfunction,

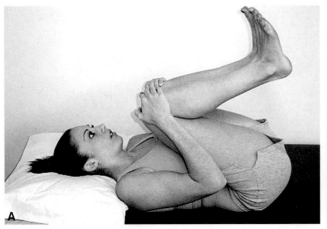
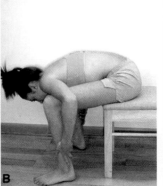
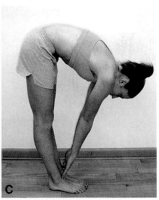
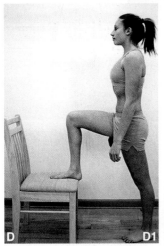
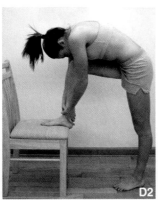
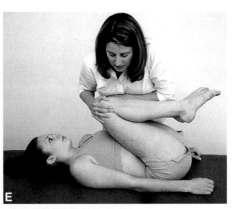

FIGURE 9–18. Flexion principle/progression of forces. **A.** Flexion in lying (FIL): From the hook-lying position, bring the knees toward the chest as far as possible. Clasp the hands over the knees to further flex the lumbar spine. **B.** Flexion in sitting (FISit): The patient sits in a straight-back chair and bends forward, bringing the head between the knees, and then returns to the full upright position. **C.** Flexion in standing (FIS): Stand with feet shoulder-width apart. Bend forward from the waist and slide the hands down the legs as far as possible while keeping the knees straight. **D.** Flexion in step standing (FISS): This procedure is used when there is a deviation in flexion. The patient stands with one leg on a chair so that the knee is flexed 90 degrees and the other leg extended **(D1)**. The leg on the chair is on the side contralateral to the side of deviation. The patient forward flexes her lumbar spine by grasping her ankle and bringing her shoulder to the raised knee **(D2)**. Between each repetition, the patient must return to standing and restore the lordosis. **E.** Flexion in lying with clinician overpressure: The patient performs FIL. The clinician evenly applies overpressure through the patient's knees.

extension dysfunction, side gliding dysfunction, and adherent nerve root dysfunction (Box 9-5).

As described, with the exception of an *adherent nerve root dysfunction syndrome*, a dysfunction produces only local symptoms without peripheralization. The progression of intervention for an ANR is displayed in Figure 9-19. Progressions are made when the prescribed exercises are no longer producing symptoms, but full range of motion has not yet been achieved. Many ANRs occur as complications of a previous posterior derangement; therefore, flexion exercises should be avoided during the first 4 hours of the day and should always be immediately followed by extension procedures.[27]

The appropriate intervention for a patient presenting with a dysfunction syndrome is progressive movement in the direction of restriction. The main goal of intervention is to improve motion by gradually eliminating the barriers to full motion. Patient education regarding the warning signs of

overstretching, such as pain lasting more than 20 minutes after the completion of exercises, as well as postural education and correction, are an integral part of the plan of care for a patient with a dysfunction syndrome.

Exercises must be performed 10 times every 2 to 3 waking hours. Patients should move into the range of motion where symptoms are reproduced; however, the increase in symptoms should only be temporary and localized to the spine, except for the case of an ANR, as mentioned above. The symptoms should abate rapidly when the position is released, and there must be no lasting or residual increase in pain.

Progressions are made when exercises no longer produce end-range pain or when additional increases in range have ceased, but full range of motion has not yet been achieved. A response to intervention is expected within 4 to 6 weeks. As in the management of the other syndromes, patients are provided with a structured home exercise program and instructed

Box 9-5 Quick Notes

The Four Subtypes of Lumbar Spinal Dysfunction Syndromes

- Named for the direction of restriction or the direction in which the symptoms are reproduced
- Posture poor, spinal deformities atypical
- Movement loss present and pain produced with some test movements, but subsides when returning to start position
- Peripheralization only with adherent nerve root

1. Flexion dysfunction
2. Extension dysfunction
3. Side gliding dysfunction
4. Adherent nerve root dysfunction

to see their physical therapist as necessary to monitor pain and range of motion and to progress their program. Manual techniques are rarely required in the case of a dysfunction; however, they may be indicated when patient-generated forces have been exhausted and progress has plateaued. The progression for intervention of an extension dysfunction is presented in Figure 9-15 and the progression for a flexion dysfunction is displayed in Figure 9-18.

Intervention for Postural Syndrome

Education is the key to the management of a postural syndrome. Spinal joint capsules, spinal ligaments, and muscles are strained at the end of their range of motion owing to prolonged static loading. It is vital to discuss how this concept translates into patients' lives and to instruct patients in good postural habits for sitting, standing, and sleeping, as well as proper body mechanics for functional activities. The

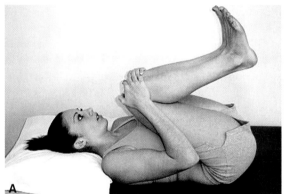
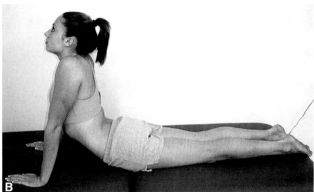
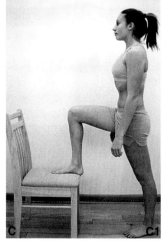
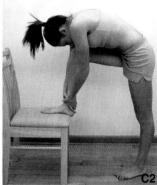
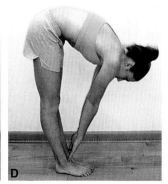

FIGURE 9–19. Adherent nerve root progression. **A.** Flexion in lying (FIL): From the hook-lying position, bring the knees toward the chest as far as possible. Clasp the hands over the knees to further flex the lumbar spine. **B.** Extension in lying (EIL): Place hands directly under the shoulders. Extend the elbows slowly to raise the upper body off the plinth. Keep the hips and thighs relaxed and allow the abdomen to sag. **C.** Flexion in step standing (FISS): In ANR, stand with the asymptomatic leg on a chair so that the knee is flexed 90 degrees and the symptomatic leg extended **(C1)**. The patient forward flexes her lumbar spine by grasping her ankle and bringing her shoulder to the raised knee **(C2)**. Between each repetition, the patient must return to standing between each repetition and restore the lordosis. **D.** Flexion in standing (FIS): Stand with feet shoulder-width apart. Flex the lumbar spine by sliding the hands down the legs as far as possible while keeping the knees straight. Between each repetition the patient must return to standing and restore the lordosis.

slouch-overcorrect exercise (Fig. 9-20) is given to teach patients how to find good posture in sitting. Intervention for postural syndrome must include a discussion of the long-term consequences of poor posture, including the increased risk for future back and neck pain.

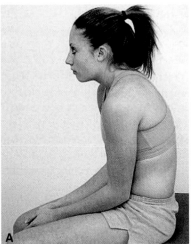

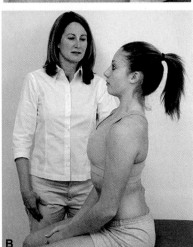

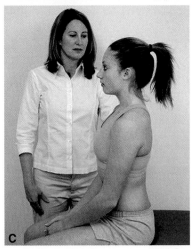

FIGURE 9–20. Slouch-overcorrect exercise. **A.** The patient is instructed to sit slouched, **B.** then sit erect in exaggerated good posture with the lumbar spine arched, chest up, and cervical spine in retraction. **C.** The patient is then instructed to relax 10% into good sitting posture.

DIFFERENTIATING CHARACTERISTICS

In summary, the ***McKenzie Method® of Mechanical Diagnosis and Therapy®*** is a systematic approach to conservative management of activity-related spinal disorders. As defined, McKenzie's system may not be considered a manual therapy approach in the truest sense. MDT encourages a more active approach that places the responsibility of care in the hands of the patient.

Considered a comprehensive approach, MDT includes a full continuum of procedures ranging from examination to intervention to prevention of recurrence. The progression through each phase of management is logical and sequential and guided by the results of the examination. This system is unique in that it clearly identifies patients who present with *mechanical versus nonmechanical* conditions and then specifically assigns individuals into one of the three *mechanical syndrome classifications.*

The use of diagnostic classification systems in the care of spinal conditions has been deemed as an important initiative.[5–8] An impairment-based system of classification is preferred over a pathoanatomical tissue-based system that attempts to identify the specific anatomical origin of an individual's reported back pain. The MDT approach uses a classification system that is based on an individual's *mechanical response to movement and position.* Aina et al[11] performed a systematic review of 14 studies and found assessment of centralization to be reliable (kappa values 0.51–1.0) on both subacute and chronic back pain patients.

Another unique feature of this approach is the manner in which active movements are tested. To classify patients, examination includes the use of repeated movements. Typically, 8 to 10 repetitions are performed as patients report their pain levels, the specific location of their symptoms, the point within the movement at which symptoms occur, and if the symptoms are provoked during the movement or at end range. Side gliding in standing, replaces the typically performed rotational and side-bending movements. Repeated movements are tested both in weight-bearing (i.e. EIS, FIS, SGIS) and non-weight-bearing positions (i.e. EIL, FIL).

The concept of *centralization* and *peripheralization* and the manner in which intervention is guided by these features are unique to this approach. Sufka et al[14] found centralization occurred less frequently among those with chronic symptoms and those with more pain; however, Werneke et al[16] found leg pain at intake (not severity) to be a significant predictor of chronic pain and disability. Centralization and peripheralization of symptoms in the presence of a derangement syndrome is used to gauge a patient's progress in response to intervention. Centralization is associated with favorable outcomes, whereas noncentralization is associated with poorer outcomes.[11,14] Using these principles to guide intervention has been shown in the literature to be effective and predictive.[12,14,18,33]

The MDT approach espouses a *criterion-based progression of forces.* The value of this approach lies in its simplicity. The examination findings of greatest relevance involve an appreciation of the patient's symptomatic and mechanical response to active movement and/or position. The movements used for *examination become the intervention.*

This approach is preoccupied with empowering patients to take personal responsibility for their own care. Significant emphasis is placed on patient education and self-care procedures. Each patient is instructed in a specific course of exercises based on his or her syndrome classification that are to be performed routinely throughout the day along with following specific guidelines related to posture and body mechanics. OMPT procedures are not enlisted until self-management measures have reached their maximal benefit.

EVIDENCE SUMMARY

Lumbar Extension in Examination and Intervention

Several authors have attempted to study the validity of lumbar extension as an examination tool and the efficacy of lumbar extension as a primary intervention strategy. Stankovic et al[43] compared the findings of computed tomography (CT) and/or magnetic resonance imaging (MRI) with the validity of various clinical tests for patients with a suspected herniated nucleus pulposus. The diagnostic sensitivity of 82.6% and specificity of 54.7% for clinical tests of disc herniation were reported. Agreement for the type and spinal level of diagnosis between radiological findings and clinical measures, which included the slump test, lumbar extension, and neurological examination, was found in 68.6% of patients.

Alexander et al[44] examined the outcome of conservative intervention based on a subject's ability to achieve lumbar extension by using repeated extension exercises. In the 33 patients examined at long-term follow-up, 94% were satisfied with the results of conservative management, 82% returned to work, 73% required no analgesics, and only 9% of the individuals required surgery or other more invasive procedures. The ability to achieve extension in the first 5 days was highly predictive of successful nonsurgical management ($P = 0.0001$).

Hahn et al[45] found that if within-session improvements were found in flexion, extension, lateral-flexion, and straight leg raising, then there was a higher likelihood that between-session improvement would be experienced. Clare et al[46] found better globally perceived effect scores in patients with a derangement who have a directional preference of extension. These studies suggest that improvement in lumbar extension is an important indicator of positive outcomes and therefore should be routinely considered.

Individuals with a posterior derangement syndrome often present with a loss of extension and reduced lumbar lordosis. Although identifying a loss of lordosis has been found to be reliable, the presence of a reduced lordosis was not related to the presence of symptoms.

Passive extension is indicated for those having a posterior derangement. Fiebert and Keller[47] attempted to determine if the extensor muscles remain passive during activities such as extension in lying, lying in prone, neutral standing, and extension in standing. Electromyographic activity was greatest for extension in lying exercises ($p < 0.05$) and least during prone lying ($p < 0.05$). Despite evidence supporting their use, the extension exercises advocated in this approach do not appear to be truly passive.

Detection and Clinical Significance of a Lateral Shift

Donahue et al[48] determined the interrater reliability of evaluating the presence of clinically relevant lateral shifts using the two-step process described by McKenzie. The first step was observational analysis for the presence of a lateral shift. The second step was the side-glide test. Interrater agreement on the identification of a clinically relevant lateral shift had a kappa value of 0.16 and percentage of agreement of 47%. However, when assessing the degree of agreement for the side-glide test, the kappa was 0.74, confirming that symptom response is superior to visual inspection.

Clare et al[49] found moderate interrater reliability for identifying lateral shifts regardless of experience. First year physical therapy students had an intrarater reliability of 0.56 and an interrater reliability of 0.53, with a kappa value of 0.36. Graduate physical therapists had an intraclass correlation coefficient (ICC) of 0.48 and 0.49 for intrarater and interrater reliability, respectively, and a kappa value of 0.26. McKenzie-trained physical therapists had an intrarater ICC of 0.59, interrater ICC of 0.64, and a kappa value of 0.38, revealing only moderate reliability even for those with the most training in this approach.[50]

Some authors have studied the clinical significance of a lateral shift. Gillian et al[51] identified resolution of a lateral shift after 90 days of MDT intervention as compared to controls. Results revealed no relationship between the presence of a lateral shift and self-reported disability. However, this study did not follow the five-step process for identification of a lateral shift. The positive side-gliding test was found to possess high reliability.[51]

In an effort to understand the differences between SGIS and lateral side bending, Mulvein and Jull[52] performed a kinematic analysis that revealed mean side bending and side gliding of 16.6 and 5.5 degrees at the L1-L4 levels, respectively, and 3.6 and 2.5 degrees at L4-S1, respectively. They concluded that SGIS may be an effective method of examining lower lumbar levels.

The Centralization and Peripheralization Phenomena

Researchers have attempted to relate the ability to centralize to a pathoanatomical source. From 61 composite pain drawings, Young and Aprill[53] concluded that pain at or above L5, obstruction to movement, change in the loss of movement, as well as peripheralization/centralization suggests a discogenic origin of symptoms.

The ability to reduce a derangement is predicated on the belief that the disc is competent. Donelson et al[54] attempted to relate the clinical findings from active movement testing to the results of a discogram. Thirty-one subjects (49.2%) centralized, 16 (25.4%) peripheralized, and 16 (25.4%) experienced no change. Twenty-three of the 31 patients who centralized (74%) had a positive discogram ($p < 0.007$), and the annulus was deemed competent in 21 (91%; $P < 0.001$). Of the 16 who peripheralized, 11 (69%) had a positive discogram ($P < 0.004$), with 6 presenting with the annular wall intact (54%) ($P = 0.093$). Those deemed as centralizers were more likely to have an intact annulus. Furthermore, this method was able to differentiate between whether the annulus was competent or not, which was superior to that reported by MRI ($P < 0.0001$).[54]

Werneke et al[36] studied the reliability of two examiners in categorizing patients using three pain pattern groups based on changes in pain location over time. Of those patients, 46% exhibited a partial reduction, 23.2% were noncentralized, and 30.8% centralized. Patients were reliably classified, and those who centralized had less frequent visits and less intense pain than did those in the other groups ($P < 0.001$).[36]

Laslett et al[55] attempted to examine the diagnostic predictive power of the centralization in 107 patients with chronic low back pain using provocation discography. Pain distribution and intensity ratings had a sensitivity of 40%, specificity of 94%, and a positive likelihood ratio of 6.9. Although centralization was highly specific to positive discography, in the presence of severe disability specificity was reduced.

Some authors have studied the use of centralization as an outcome predictor. In 53 subjects with acute low back pain, 47 were able to centralize, 98% of whom had a favorable outcome ($P < 0.001$). Eight-six percent of the individuals with symptoms for 4 to 12 weeks and 84% with symptoms for more than 12 weeks also demonstrated centralization. Of those who centralized, 77% and 81% had good to excellent results. Conversely, the noncentralized individuals had a significantly lower incidence of good or excellent outcomes (50% and 33%, respectively). These results provide support for centralization as a useful predictor of favorable outcomes.[13] Long[17] affirmed the value of using centralization as a predictor by reporting a decrease in pain and higher return-to-work rates (68.4% versus 52.2%) when compared to noncentralizers at 9-month follow-up.

Werneke and Hart[36] attempted to analyze the predicative power of centralization in determining who might develop a chronic condition. Results suggest that overt pain behavior, perceived disability upon discharge, and pain pattern classification were the most common factors affecting an individual's report of pain and disability. Pain pattern classification and leg pain were predictors of perceived disability, and those with chronic pain and noncentralizers did not return to work, continued to use health care resources, continued to report pain, and refused to participate in activities.

Werneke and Hart[19] found that if noncentralization was noted upon the initial visit, the patient was 8 times more likely to have nonorganic signs, 13 times more likely to have overt pain behavior, 3 times more likely to have fear avoidance, and 2 times more likely to have somatization of their symptoms. Centralization was reported in 46%, indicating a more favorable prognosis.

Sufka et al[14] documented the prevalence of centralization, categorized centralizers, and compared outcomes to noncentralizers on self-perceived disability. Twenty-five of 36 were centralizers and had higher score changes on the Spinal Function Sort (SFS) self-assessment disability questionnaire ($p = 0.015$).

Likewise, George et al[56] found that initial disability, the centralization phenomenon, and fear-avoidance beliefs were good predictors of disability. Karas et al[18] concurred by demonstrating that centralizers (n = 92) had a higher incidence of return to work than did noncentralizers (n = 34) ($x^2 = 4.31$, $P = 0.038$). Inability to centralize indicated decreased return to work, regardless of the Waddell score. In the Donelson[54] study, 73% of the patients were found to have centralization of symptoms. Werneke et al[57] compared first-visit to multiple-visit classification of centralization. The results revealed that many patients were reclassified after multiple visits, suggesting the value of considering changes in the patient's symptomatic response to mechanical forces over time.

The Reliability of the MDT System of Classification

In 1993, Riddle and Rothstein[58] performed a multicenter (eight clinics, n = 363), interrater reliability study on the MDT system of classification. For comparisons of therapists with at least one postgraduate course on the McKenzie system, there was 27% agreement, or kappa = 0.15. Kappa coefficients between the eight clinics ranged in values from 0.02 to 0.48, with percent agreement ranging from 22% to 60%. These results demonstrated that the MDT method of classification is unreliable when noncredentialed McKenzie therapists are used.

Razmjou et al[25] investigated the interexaminer reliability between two McKenzie-trained physical therapists in determining diagnostic syndromes and subsyndromes in patients with low back pain. Agreement between the two raters revealed kappa = 0.70, with a 93% agreement for syndrome, and kappa = 0.96, or a 97% of agreement for individuals with a derangement syndrome. Moderate interrater reliability was found for identification of a lateral shift with kappa = 0.52. Kappa values for identification of a relevant lateral shift was 0.85, for relevance of a lateral component was 0.95, and for identification of sagittal plane deformity was 1.00. Fritz et al[59] substantiated these findings. The percentage of agreement for the total sample was 87.7%, with a 95% confidence interval and a kappa coefficient of 0.777 to 0.809. Licensed physical therapists achieved 89.7% agreement (kappa = 0.823), and physical therapy students achieved 85.9% agreement (kappa = 0.763). For therapists with more than 6 years of experience, 90.2% agreement was demonstrated (kappa = 0.873). Therapists with less than 6 years of experience had a percentage of agreement of 88.8% (kappa = 0.817).

In 2004, Clare et al[60] found the percentage of agreement for assignment into syndromes by trained McKenzie therapists from patient assessment forms to be 91%, with the kappa point estimate of 0.56, with a 95% confidence interval. There was 76% percent agreement for subsyndromes (kappa = 0.68) with a 95% confidence interval ratio. In 2005, Clare et al[49] found 100% agreement in classifying lumbar syndromes (kappa = 1.0) and a 92% agreement for subsyndromes (kappa = 0.89). For cervical patients, there was 92% agreement (kappa = 0.63) and 88% (kappa = 0.84) agreement for subsyndromes.

Kilpikoski et al[61] examined the interexaminer reliability of both MDT clinical testing and eventual classification of syndromes in 39 individuals with low back pain. For the presence of lateral shift, 79% (kappa = 0.2; $P < 0.248$) agreement was reported, with 77% (kappa = 0.4; $P < 0.003$) agreement for direction of lateral shift, and 85% (kappa = 0.7; $P = 0.000$) agreement for the relevance of the lateral shift. Ninety-five percent agreement (kappa = 0.7; $P < 0.002$) was identified for using static end-range loading to define centralization during repeated movements, and 90% agreement (kappa = 0.9; $P < 0.000$) was found for defining the directional preference. For individuals who were classified into the McKenzie main syndromes and into specific subgroups, agreement was 95% (kappa = 0.6; $P < 0.000$) and 74% (kappa = 0.7; $P < 0.000$), respectively.

Efficacy of MDT for Lumbar Spine-Related Disorders

Ponte et al[42] attempted to compare the Williams regimen to the MDT approach on their effectiveness in managing low back pain. Individuals receiving the McKenzie protocol improved significantly greater in forward flexion ($P < 0.001$) and straight leg raise ($P < 0.001$) than did subjects in the Williams group and in a shorter period of time. Nwuga and Nwuga[62] attempted to compare these two approaches in patients with prolapsed intervertebral discs. The McKenzie protocol was found to be superior to the Williams protocol in postintervention total flexion and extension ($P < 0.01$), side bending ($P < 0.05$), and rotation ($P < 0.01$). In addition, the mean intervention time was significantly lower for the McKenzie group ($P < 0.001$).

Dettori et al[63] found that after 1 week of intervention, individuals with acute low back pain improved in both the flexion and extension groups, and after 8 weeks, there was no difference between the two groups. In addition, there were no differences between groups in rate of reoccurrence after 6 to 12 months.

Long[24] compared outcomes of patients receiving intervention matched to their directional preference to those receiving either exercise opposite their directional preference or midrange exercise and stretching of the hips. The group receiving exercises matched to their classification had better outcomes, suggesting the value of using directional preference to guide intervention.

ACKNOWLEDGMENT

Course information, additional reading, and assessment forms are available through the McKenzie Institute® International at www.mckenziemdt.org.

The contents of this chapter have been approved and permission has been granted for publication of these materials by the McKenzie Institute® International.

CLINICAL CASE

Patient History

JP is a 39-year-old photographer who comes to your clinic today with pain rated 8/10 in his right buttock, thigh, and calf. His history is significant for four previous episodes of low back pain with occasional radiation into the thigh, which began about 2 years ago, with a typical episode lasting a few days. Last week, after bending over to pick up his photography equipment, he felt pain in his back as he was slinging the pack over his left shoulder and straightening up. He continued to work for several hours, then went home and sat in his recliner and watched TV. When he attempted to get up from the recliner, he had difficulty straightening up and had pain going down his right leg. Since then he can only sit for 15 minutes and walk for 10 minutes because of pain. He is worse sitting and rising from sitting. He has difficulty sleeping and has been unable to work. He feels best lying on his right side. During this episode his pain is intermittent in the back, buttock, thigh, and right leg to the midcalf. His Oswestry Disability Index score is 45%.

Physical Examination

Posture: Poor in sitting with a reduced lordosis, no change in symptoms with postural correction.

Neurological: (+) Extensor hallucis weakness on the right (L5), sensory and reflexes intact, (+) straight leg raise at 40 degrees, (+) slump test

Motion Loss:
- **Flexion:** minimum
- **Extension:** moderate
- **Side-gliding right:** moderate with severe distal pain produced
- **Side-gliding left:** nil

Test Movements

Pretest symptoms standing: pain in the right buttock, leg to midcalf at 8/10 level of intensity

- **Flexion in standing (FIS):** produces right foot pain
- **Repeated FIS × 2:** peripheralized into foot, worse
- **Extension in standing (EIS):** increased right foot pain
- **Repeated EIS:** increased right foot pain, worse

  Pretest symptoms lying: pain right buttock, right posterior thigh at 6/10 level of intensity

- **Flexion in lying (FIL):** produced right foot pain
- **Repeated FIL:** increased right foot pain, worse/peripheralized
- **Extension in lying (EIL):** increased right foot pain
- **Repeated EIL:** increased right foot pain, worse

  Pretest symptoms lying: pain right buttock, posterior thigh, foot

- **EIL with hips offset left:** abolished foot, increased thigh and back pain, symptoms centralizing
- **Repeated EIL with hips offset left:** abolished foot, abolished thigh, increased back pain, centralization with increased range of motion (ROM) noted

1. What is your provisional classification, directional preference, and principle of intervention for this patient?
2. What procedures would be indicated on day 1 of intervention? Include a home exercise program and recommendations for sitting and sleeping.
3. What would your reexamination include at the following session? How will you determine and document the patient's response to your intervention?
4. Three days following the initial examination, the patient reports pain that is present in the right thigh and buttock. What procedures are indicated?
5. One week following the initial examination, the patient reports pain that is present symmetrically in the buttocks and

low back. What is your principle of intervention now, and has it changed from your initial plan? What would guide your decision to use either self-generated or clinician-generated procedures, and which would be most appropriate at this time?
6. Two weeks following the initial examination, the patient reports only intermittent lumbar discomfort rated 2/10. How would you determine if the patient is ready to begin procedures to restore full flexion mobility, and what precautions must the patient be instructed in?
7. Upon discharge from therapy, what instructions should be given to this patient?

HANDS-ON

With a partner, perform the following activities:

1   Role-play the case study provided above. Incorporate the extension principle with the lateral component that was present acutely. Practice the following:
- Perform manual lateral shift correction (see Fig. 9-10b)
- Demonstrate and instruct the patient in self-correction of lateral shift/side gliding against a wall (see Fig. 9-10c).
- Perform extension in lying with hips off center without (see Figure 9-16a) and with lateral overpressure (see Fig. 9-16b) and rotation mobilization in extension bilateral (see Fig. 9-16d1) and unilateral (see Fig. 9-16d2).

2   Practice the following procedures incorporating the extension principle, which is invariably used for central/symmetrical pain with an extension directional preference,

but may also be appropriate for unilateral/asymmetrical pain if the desired response is achieved with sagittal procedures.

Static procedures:
- Lying prone (see Fig. 9-15a)
- Lying prone in extension (see Fig. 9-15b)
- Correct sitting posture without (see Fig. 9-10b3) and with a lumbar roll (see Fig. 9-10c)

Dynamic procedures:
- Extension in lying (EIL) (see Fig. 9-15c)
- Extension in lying with self-overpressure (see Fig. 9-15d)
- Extension in lying with clinician overpressure (see Fig. 9-15f)
- Extension mobilization (see Fig. 9-15g)
- Extension in standing (see Fig. 9-15e)
- Slouch-overcorrect (see Fig. 9-21)

3 Instruct your partner in the process of recovering flexion after a posterior derangement. Remember that flexion procedures after a posterior derangement should not be performed for the first 4 hours upon awakening and should always be followed by extension movements. Demonstrate the following procedures:
- Flexion in lying (Fig. 9-17a)
- Flexion in sitting (Fig. 9-17b)
- Flexion in standing. (Fig. 9-17c)

4 Demonstrate how you would determine if a patient with back and leg pain from a motor vehicle accident 4 months ago has a derangement or an adherent nerve root.

REFERENCES

1. McKenzie Institute USA. *Intro to the McKenzie Method®: Part 4: Overview and Validation* (Video). McKenzie Institute USA. Available at: www.mckenziemdt.org/eduCourseOnline.cfm. Accessed January 16, 2006.
2. McKenzie R, May S. *The Lumbar Spine Mechanical Diagnosis and Therapy.* Vol 1. Waikanae, New Zealand: Spinal Publications; 2003.
3. McKenzie Institute USA. A History of Success. McKenzie Institute USA website. www.mckenziemdt.org/hist.cfm. Accessed January 10, 2006.
4. McClure P. The degenerative cervical spine: pathogenesis and rehabilitation concepts. *J Hand Ther.* 2000;4-6:163-174.
5. Fritz JM, George S. The use of a classification approach to identify subgroups of patients with acute low back pain: interrater reliability and short-term treatment outcomes. *Spine.* 2000;25:106-114.
6. Riddle D. Classification and low back pain: a review of the literature and critical analysis of selected systems. *Phys Ther.* 1998;78:708-735.
7. Borkan JM, Koes B, Shmuel R, Cherkin D. A report from the second international forum for primary care research on LBP: reexamining priorities. *Spine.* 1998;23:1992-1996.
8. Leboeuf-Yde C, Lauritzen JM, Lauritzen T. Why has the search for causes of LBP largely been nonconclusive. *Spine.* 1997;22:877-881.
9. Spitzer WO. Scientific Approach to the Assessment and Measurement of Activity-Related Spinal Disorders: A Monograph for Clinicians—Report of the Quebec Task Force on Spinal Disorders. *Spine.* 1987;12(7 suppl):1-59.
10. American Physical Therapy Association. *Guide to Physical Therapist Practice, Revised 2nd ed.* Alexandria, VA: APTA; 2003.
11. Aina A, May S, Clare H. The centralization phenomenon of spinal symptoms–a systematic review. *Man Ther.* 2004;9:134-143.
12. Hefford C. McKenzie classification of mechanical spinal pain; profile of syndromes and directions of preference. *Man Ther.* 2008;13:75-81.
13. Donelson R, Silva G, Murphy K. Centralization phenomenon. Its usefulness in evaluating and treating referred pain. *Spine.* 1990;3:211-213.
14. Sufka A, Hauger B, Trenary M, et al. Centralization of low back pain and perceived functional outcome. *J Orthop Sports Phys Ther.* 1998;3:205-212.
15. Donelson R, Grant W, Kamps C, Medcalf R. Pain response to sagittal end-range spinal motion. A prospective, randomized, multicentered trial. *Spine.* 1991;6 (suppl):S206-212.
16. Werneke M, Hart DL, Cook D. A descriptive study of the centralization phenomenon. A prospective analysis. *Spine.* 1999;24:676-683.
17. Long A. The centralization phenomenon: its usefulness as a predictor of outcome in conservative treatment of chronic low back pain (a pilot study). *Spine.* 1995;20:2513-2521.
18. Karas R, McIntosh G, Hall H, Wilson L, Melles T. The relationship between nonorganic signs and centralization of symptoms in the prediction of return to work for patients with low back pain. *Phys Ther.* 1997;77:354-360.
19. Werneke M, Hart DL. Centralization phenomenon as a prognostic factor for chronic low back pain and disability. *Spine.* 2001;26:758-765.
20. Petersen T, Kryger P, Ekdahl C, Olsen S, Jacobsen S. The effect of McKenzie therapy as compared with that of intensive strengthening training for the treatment of patients with subacute or chronic low back pain: a randomized controlled trial. *Spine.* 2002;27:1702-1709.
21. Schenk R, Jozefczyk, Kopf A. A randomised trial comparing interventions in patients with lumbar posterior derangement. *J Man Manip Ther.* 2003;11:95-102.
22. Stankovic R, Johnell O. Conservative treatment of acute low-back pain. A prospective randomized trial: McKenzie Method of treatment versus patient education in "mini back school." *Spine.* 1990;15(2):120-123.
23. Fritz JM, Delitto A, Erhard RE. Comparison of classification-based physical therapy with therapy based on clinical practice guidelines for patients with acute low back pain. *Spine.* 2003;28:1363-1372.
24. Long A, Donelson R, Fung T. Does it matter which exercise? A randomized control trial of exercises for low back pain. *Spine.* 2004;29: 2593-2602.
25. Razmjou H, Kramer J, Yamada R. Intertester reliability of the McKenzie evaluation in assessing patients with mechanical low-back pain. *J Orthop Sports Phys Ther.* 2000;30:368-389.
26. Cooper RG, Greemont AJ, Hoyland JA, et al. Herniated intervertebral disc-associated periradicular fibrosis and vascular abnormalities occur without inflammatory cell infiltration. *Spine.* 1995;20:591-598.
27. McKenzie RA. *The Lumbar Spine Mechanical Diagnosis and Therapy.* Waikanae, New Zealand: Spinal Publications; 1981;150.
28. Bakker EW, Verhagen AP, Lucas C, et al. Daily spinal mechanical loading as a risk factor for acute non-specific low back pain; a case-control study using the 24-hour Schedule. *Eur Spine J.* 2007;16:107-113.
29. Waddell G. *The Back Pain Revolution.* Edinburgh, Scotland: Churchill Livingstone; 1998.
30. Deyo RA, Rainville J, Kent DL. What can the history and physical examination tell us about low back pain? *JAMA.* 1992;268:760-765.
31. Boissonault WG. *Primary Care for the Physical Therapist Examination and Triage.* St. Louis, Missouri: Elsevier Saunders, 2005;70.
32. Goodman CC, Snyder TEK. *Differential Diagnosis in Physical Therapy.* 2nd ed. Philadelphia, PA: WB Saunders Company, 1995;16.
33. Boden SD, David DO, Dina TS, Patronas NJ, Wiesel SW. Abnormal magnetic-resonance scans of the lumbar spine in asymptomatic subjects. *J Bone Joint Sur.* 1990;72A:403-408.
34. Boden, S. Current concepts review: the use of radiographic imaging studies in the evaluation of patients who have degenerative disorders of the lumbar spine. *J Bone Joint Sur.* 1996;78:114-124.
35. Goodman CC, Snyder TEK. *Differential Diagnosis in Physical Therapy.* 3rd ed. Philadelphia, PA: WB Saunders Company, 2000;48.
36. Werneke M, Hart L. Centralization: association between repeated end-range pain responses and behavioral signs in patients with acute non-specific low back pain. *J Rehabil Med.* 2005;37:286-290.
37. Lorio MP, Bernstein AJ, Simmons EH. Sciatic spinal deformity-lumbosacral list: an "unusual" presentation with review of the literature. *J Spinal Disorders.* 1995;8:201-205.
38. May S, Donelson R. Evidence-informed management of chronic low back pain with the McKenzie Method. *Spine.* 2008;8:134-141.
39. Laslett M, Michaelsen DJ, Williams MM. A survey of patients suffering mechanical low back pain syndrome or sciatica treated with the "McKenzie Method." *NZ J Physiother.* 1991;8:24-32.
40. Larsen K, Weidick F, Leboeuf-Yde C. Can passive prone extensions of the back prevent back problems? A randomized, controlled intervention trial of 314 military conscripts. *Spine.* 2002;27:2747-2752.
41. Stankovic R, Johnell O. Conservative treatment of acute low back pain. A 5-year follow-up study of two methods of treatment. *Spine.* 1995;20: 469-472.
42. Ponte D, Jensen G, Kent B. A preliminary report on the use of the McKenzie protocol versus Williams protocol in the treatment of low back pain. *J Orthop Sports Phys Ther.* 1984;9-10:130-139.
43. Stankovic R, Johnell O, Maly P, Wilner S. Use of lumbar extension, slump test, physical and neurological examination in the evaluation of patients with suspected herniated nucleus pulposus. A prospective study. *Man Ther.* 1999;4:25-32.
44. Alexander H, Jones A, Rosenbaum D. Nonoperative management of herniated nucleus pulpous: patient selection by the extension sign: long term follow up. *Orthop Rev.* 1992;21:181-188.
45. Hahn A, Keating J, Wilson S. Do within-session changes in pain intensity and range of motion predict between-session changes in patients with low back pain? *Aus J Physiother.* 2004;50:17-23.

46. Clare HA, Adams R, Maher CG. Construct validity of lumbar extension measures in McKenzie's derangement syndrome. *Man Ther*. 2007;12: 328-334.

47. Fiebert, I. Keller, C. Are "passive" extension exercises really passive? *J Orthop Sports Phys Ther*. 1994;19:111-116.

48. Donahue M, Riddle D, Sullivan M. Intertester reliability of a modified version of McKenzie's lateral shift assessments obtained on patients with low back pain. *Phys Ther*. 1996;76:706-716.

49. Clare H, Adams R, Maher C. Reliability of McKenzie classification of patients with cervical or lumbar pain. *J Man Psychol Ther*. 2005;28(2): 122-127.

50. Landis JR, Koch GG. The measurement of observer agreement for categorical data. *Biometrics*. 1977;33:159-174.

51. Gillian M, Ross J, McLean I, Porter R. The natural history of trunk list, its associated disability and the ability and the influence of McKenzie management. *Eur Spine J*. 1998;7:480-483.

52. Mulvein K, Jull G. Kinematic analysis of the lumbar lateral flexion and lumbar lateral shift movement techniques. *J Man Manip Ther*. 1995;3:104-109.

53. Young S, Aprill C. Characteristics of a mechanical assessment for chronic lumbar facet joint pain. *J Man Manip Ther*. 2000;8:78-84.

54. Donelson R, April C, Medcalf R, Grant W. A prospective study of centralization of lumbar and referred pain. *Spine*. 1997;22:1115-1122.

55. Laslett M, Oberg B, April C, McDonald B. Centralization as a predictor of provocation discography results in chronic low back pain, and the influence of disability and distress on diagnostic power. *Spine J*. 2005;5: 370-380.

56. George S, Bialosky J, Donald D. The centralization phenomenon and fear-avoidance beliefs as prognostic factors for acute low back pain: a preliminary investigation involving patients classified for specific exercise. *J Orthop Sports Phys Ther*. 2005;35:580-588.

57. Werneke M, Hart D. Discriminant validity and relative precision for classifying patients with nonspecific neck and back pain by anatomic pain patterns. *Spine*. 2003;28:161-166.

58. Riddle D, Rothstein J. Intertester reliability of McKenzie's classifications of the syndrome and types present in patients with low back pain. *Spine*. 1993;18:1333-1344.

59. Fritz J, Delitto A, Vignovic M. Busse R. Interrater reliability of judgments of the centralization phenomenon and status change during movement testing in patients with low back pain. *Arch Phys Med Rehabil*. 2000;81: 57-61.

60. Clare H, Adams R, Maher C. Reliability of the McKenzie spinal pain classification using patient assessment forms. *Physiotherapy*. 2004;90: 114-119.

61. Kilpikoski S, Airakinen O, Kankaanpaa M, et al. Interexaminer reliability of low back pain assessment using the McKenzie Method. *Spine*. 2002;27:E207-E214.

62. Nwuga G, Nwuga V. Relative therapeutic efficacy of the Williams and McKenzie protocols in back pain management. *Physiother Pract*. 1985;1: 99-105.

63. Dettori J, Bullock S, Sutlive T, Franklin R, Patience T. The effects of spinal flexion and extension exercises and their associated postures in patients with acute low back pain. *Spine*. 1995;20:2303-2312.

The Mulligan Concept

Donald K. Reordan, PT, MS, OCS, MCTA
Christopher H. Wise, PT, DPT, OCS, FAAOMPT, MTC, ATC

Chapter Objectives

At the conclusion of this chapter, the reader will be able to:

- Identify the history and key contributing factors in the development of the Mulligan concept approach to orthopaedic manual physical therapy (OMPT).
- Understand the theoretical underpinnings that are believed to be responsible for the clinical effectiveness of the Mulligan concept.
- Describe the clinical features that may be used to confirm the efficacy of mobilization with movement (MWM) techniques.
- Articulate and implement the clinical practice guidelines for the use of MWM.

- Develop introductory level proficiency in the performance of spinal and peripheral MWM techniques.
- Describe how the concepts and techniques within the Mulligan concept can be integrated into a comprehensive examination and intervention scheme.
- Identify and discuss the current best evidence related to this approach.
- Discuss the characteristics that differentiate this approach from other manual and nonmanual therapy strategies.

HISTORICAL PERSPECTIVES

Personal Background

The **Mulligan concept** approach to orthopaedic manual physical therapy (OMPT) was conceived by a New Zealand physiotherapist by the name of **Brian R. Mulligan.** Mulligan qualified as a physiotherapist in 1954 and achieved his Diploma in Manipulative Therapy in 1974. In 1996 he was made an Honorary Fellow of the **New Zealand Society of Physiotherapists** for his contribution to physiotherapy. Some of Mulligan's other honors include being a life member of the **New Zealand Manipulative Physiotherapists Association** (1988); life member of the **New Zealand College of Physiotherapy** (1998); honorary teaching fellow at the University of Otago, Department of Physiotherapy (2003); fellow of the **American Academy of Orthopaedic Manual Physical Therapists** (2004); and recipient of the International Service Award from the **World Confederation of Physical Therapy** (2007).

In addition to maintaining active clinical practice, Brian Mulligan has been teaching manual therapy in New Zealand since 1970 and internationally since 1972. He first began teaching in the United States in 1979. He is the author of numerous journal articles that have appeared in the *New Zealand Journal of Physiotherapy* as well as other international publications (Fig. 10-1).

Mulligan credits **Freddy M. Kaltenborn** of Norway (see Chapter 6) as being his primary mentor in the area of practical learning. Upon this foundation, Mulligan's clinical observations, born out of inquisition and experimentation, have led to an entirely new approach to OMPT. To meet the increasing international demand from therapists wishing to learn the Mulligan concept and to ensure high standards of instruction, Mulligan established the **Mulligan Concept Teachers Association (MCTA)** in 1993. In addition to instruction, the MCTA is dedicated to the generation of funding and promotion of research related to the validity of these concepts and the clinical efficacy of these techniques. MCTA instructors are accessible at **www.bmulligan.com** and **www.na-mcta.com.**

NOTABLE QUOTABLE

"In the field of scientific discovery, chance always favors the prepared mind."

-Louis Pasteur

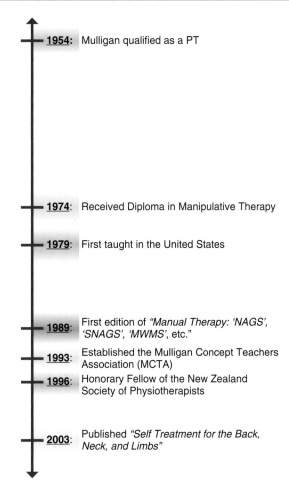

FIGURE 10–1 B.R. Mulligan's biographical timeline.

1954: Mulligan qualified as a PT

1974: Received Diploma in Manipulative Therapy

1979: First taught in the United States

1989: First edition of *"Manual Therapy: 'NAGS', 'SNAGS', 'MWMS', etc."*

1993: Established the Mulligan Concept Teachers Association (MCTA)

1996: Honorary Fellow of the New Zealand Society of Physiotherapists

2003: Published *"Self Treatment for the Back, Neck, and Limbs"*

As in most other approaches to OMPT, the Mulligan concept approach is based on a firm understanding of functional anatomy and kinematics. However, there are several components of this approach that render it unique. The first edition of Mulligan's book entitled, ***Manual Therapy: NAGS, SNAGS, MWMS, etc.***,[1] was published in 1989, and the sixth edition of this text was completed in 2010. Mulligan's second book, which was written for patients in 2006 and is currently in its second edition, is entitled, ***Self Treatment for the Back, Neck, and Limb***[2]. In 1993, Mulligan also developed a 2-hour DVD entitled ***Mobilisations with Movement***[3], which includes footage of actual patient intervention. Two 90-minute teaching DVD's) entitled, ***Spinal Techniques: The Cervical Spine***[4] and ***Spinal Techniques: The Thoracic and Lumbar Spine***[5] were produced in 1997.

Concept Development

From his clinical experiences at his thriving practice in Wellington, New Zealand, Mulligan began to appreciate the importance of assessing the immediate effectiveness of his manual interventions. His intolerance for the use of interventions that lacked timely results led him toward the pursuit of new paradigms (Box 10-1).

Box 10-1 MOBILIZATION WITH MOVEMENT

One of the foundational differentiating characteristics of these techniques is the **combination** of various forms of movement consisting primarily of performing passive **accessory movement** during active or passive **physiologic movement**.

NOTABLE QUOTABLE

"Endless perseverance with no lasting benefit to the patient cannot be justified."

–B.R. Mulligan

In the process of treating an individual who presented with pain and movement restrictions in the proximal interphalangeal joint of her second digit, Mulligan became frustrated after exhausting all of the traditional intervention options. Frustration gave way to inspiration when Mulligan attempted a technique that he had not been taught nor had previously performed. He changed the direction of joint mobilization from a traditional sagittal plane posterior-to-anterior (PA) glide of the concave joint surface (proximal end of middle phalanx) to a passive accessory glide in the frontal plane that accompanied active movement (Fig. 10-2) (Box 10-2). Both Mulligan and the patient were pleased to acknowledge that upon application of this technique, the previously restricted and painful motion was immediately restored to normal pain-free range.

NOTABLE QUOTABLE

"Expect a miracle each day."

–B.R. Mulligan

This unexpected experience led to further experimentation using similar mobilizations in other joints of both the spine and extremities. Mulligan consistently found that, when indicated, the combination of *accessory* joint mobilization with concurrent *physiologic* movement provided immediate, significant, and lasting changes in the patient's condition. The improvements that Mulligan observed in response to these new techniques occurred so quickly and were of such magnitude that they could not be explained by the gradual nature of the typical healing process.

QUESTIONS *for* REFLECTION

- Briefly define the terms *accessory* joint movement and *physiologic* joint movement.
- Why are both necessary in the production of normal movement?

- What are the clinical manifestations of accessory motion loss? Of physiologic motion loss?
- Which of these two types of motion is traditionally addressed through joint mobilization techniques?
- What are the advantages to using mobilization that combines these movements? What are the challenges?

THEORETICAL FRAMEWORK

Through empirical evidence gained by frequent and consistent trials using the strategy of combining accessory movement with physiologic movement, Mulligan further developed the theory that a joint may assume a faulty position that might restrict movement and produce pain. Such a *positional fault* may be the result of trauma, aging, muscle imbalance, or poor posture and may not be detectable through traditional diagnostic imaging procedures.

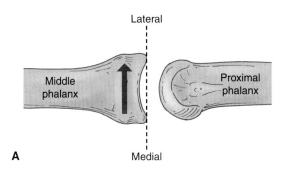

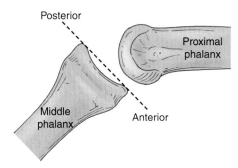

FIGURE 10–2 Mobilization with movement (MWM) of the proximal interphalangeal (PIP) joint in the frontal plane. **A.** Superior view of the PIP, with the dotted line representing the treatment plane of the joint, the red arrow indicating the laterally directed frontal plane mobilization force that is performed as the joint is actively flexed and extended. **B.** Lateral view of the PIP, with the dotted line representing the treatment plane of the joint and the yellow arrow representing the sagittal plane direction in which the joint glides during flexion and extension.

Box 10-2 TRIPLANAR MOBILIZATION

Unlike most other approaches that seek to restore joint motion through application of sagittal plane-directed forces (i.e., P-A, A-P glides), the *Mulligan concept approach* uses predominantly frontal and transverse plane glides for sagittal plane provocative movements.

This theory is in contrast to traditional approaches that use joint mobilization for the purpose of stretching or breaking adhesions or for the purpose of gaiting pain that may be associated with restrictions in joint mobility.

Mulligan's description of the **positional fault theory** is neither new nor unique to this approach (Box 10-3). The concept that articular malalignment may lead to altered kinematics and eventual dysfunction is a fundamental principle within several OMPT approaches. Hinman et al[6] discuss the concept of "tracking problems" in the management of patellofemoral syndrome, and VanDillen et al[7] describe the "displaced path of the instantaneous center of rotation" in patients with movement impairments.[6,7]

To test the positional fault theory, the manual physical therapist need only reposition the joint and have the patient undertake the previously restricted or provocative movement, while taking note of any changes in the patient's range of motion or symptoms. The immediate results often experienced in response to these techniques seem to provide face validity for the positional fault theory. This is not to say that capsular restrictions do not exist. However, their role as the primary limiting factor in full, pain-free motion may be reconsidered. Perhaps, the nonresponders to these techniques are those individuals who are truly experiencing issues with adaptive shortening and capsular adhesions. When applied as one component of the physical examination, this process of clinical exploration may assist in determining the cause of a movement restriction and in guiding subsequent intervention.

QUESTIONS *for* REFLECTION

- What are the advantages and limitations to using the patient's symptomatic response to movement as the primary guideline for directing intervention?
- Which has been found to be more valid and reliable for guiding intervention in the literature, the reproduction of symptoms or the identification of movement restrictions?

CLINICAL PILLAR

Within the *Mulligan concept approach*, the following sequence is used to determine the impact of each procedure on the patient's condition:

1. Examination

2. Trial Intervention

3. Reexamination

The patient's motion and symptomatic response to joint repositioning confirms or refutes the presence of a positional fault.

Box 10-3 THE POSITIONAL FAULT THEORY

Articular malalignment may lead to altered kinematics and eventual dysfunction. Therefore, the *Mulligan concept approach* is based on the need to identify and reduce positional faults for the purpose of improving joint kinematics

PRINCIPLES OF EXAMINATION

This approach advocates the use of a comprehensive examination. However, the primary examination procedure that is used to make clinical decisions and guide subsequent intervention lies in the concept of the **trial treatment**, or trial intervention. The specific procedures chosen for this trial intervention are based primarily on the location of symptoms and the specific movements or positions that either provoke or increase the patient's chief complaint (Box 10-4).

The impact of each trial manual intervention on the patient's chief impairment provides immediate efficacy and therefore becomes the primary indicator for intervention. As the trial mobilization is performed, the therapist queries the patient regarding the influence of the procedure on his or her symptoms. In order to ascertain the effect of each chosen technique on the patient's chief impairment, the process must involve examination and trial intervention, followed immediately by reexamination (Box 10-5).

No time is wasted as the value of these techniques will be immediately apparent. If such a response is not realized, the therapist should make slight alterations in the location, direction, and/or the amplitude of force. If the patient continues to fail to respond, the technique may be abandoned altogether in favor

Box 10-4 THE TRIAL INTERVENTION APPROACH

- This approach involves the initiation of a *low-dosage* intervention that is employed for the primary purpose of evaluating the immediate and delayed effects of such an intervention on the patient's primary presenting impairment.
- The specific procedures chosen for this trial intervention are based primarily on the *location* of symptoms and the specific joint *movements* or *positions* that either provoke or increase the patient's chief complaint.

Box 10-5 MOBILIZATION WITH MOVEMENT

Effective MWMs are PILL:

- P—pain free
- I—immediate
- L—long
- L—lasting

The majority of improvement from MWM should be retained at the next visit. If not, look for the cause.

of another. Common errors in technique performance include failure to apply force in the ideal direction of the facet joint treatment plane, reduction of the mobilizing force during the active movement, application of force over the wrong segment or joint, or mobilization with either too little or too much force.

CLINICAL PILLAR

Common errors in the performance of MWMs are as follows:

- Failure to apply force in the ideal *direction*
- Failure to *maintain* force throughout the physiologic motion
- Application of force in the wrong *location*
- Mobilization applied with *too much* or *too little* force

PRINCIPLES OF INTERVENTION

The transition from examination to intervention is immediate and lends to the overall efficiency of this approach. The specific trial procedure that was proven to be effective in altering symptoms and enhancing motion during the examination, becomes the intervention. Mulligan has chronicled a collection of techniques that have proven to be effective for a myriad of disorders. These techniques have collectively become known as **mobilization with movement (MWM)** based on the fact that active or passive physiologic movement occurs simultaneously with passive accessory mobilization.

Mobilization With Movement Clinical Practice Guidelines

The chief tenets of Mulligan's MWM approach are not entirely new to the specialty of manual therapy. Although specific manual contacts may differ, the application of articular accessory glides used during MWM follows the mobilization principles espoused by Kaltenborn (see Chapter 6)[8] and others. In particular, two fundamental principles of the *Nordic approach* are strictly followed when performing MWM. First, the manual therapist must be sure to gain contact and apply force as close to the joint as possible. Second, the mobilizing force must be applied parallel to the treatment plane, which is defined by the line that extends across the concave articular surface of the joint.

QUESTIONS *for* REFLECTION

- Briefly define the term *treatment plane*.
- How is the treatment plane used to determine the direction of mobilizing force?
- How does the manual therapist identify the treatment plane of a given joint?
- Does the treatment plane change if the position of the joint changes?

There are several important clinical practice guidelines that make the performance of MWM unique. First and foremost, MWM techniques must be performed under *pain-free conditions*. If pain is produced, then either the technique is not indicated or the technique is being performed incorrectly and the manual physical therapist must modify or discontinue the technique immediately. During performance of a technique, the manual physical therapist must be sure to use the *minimum amount of force necessary* to achieve pain-free mobilization. The mobilizing force is typically applied directly to the region from which symptoms are emanating. The manual physical therapist's hand contacts must enable the application of an accessory glide *parallel to the treatment plane*. When performed in the spine, force is applied in accordance with the anatomical features of the joint along the plane of the concave joint surface. This force is applied as the pain-producing *physiologic motion is superimposed* either actively or passively. It is paramount that the manual therapist *sustains the mobilizing force throughout the entire range* of physiologic movement until the joint returns from the provocative range. Once the end of available range is accomplished, passive **overpressure** is applied that may be assisted by the patient. Lastly, many MWM techniques are performed in *weight-bearing*, which is presumed to enhance retention. Furthermore, using the weight-bearing position is often considered to be more functional; it is the posture in which active range is often examined and, in many cases, the posture in which pain is produced. Once efficacy has been established, sufficient repetitions (usually 5–10 repetitions) for effective training are performed to sustain the corrected articular position and mobility after the force is released.

CLINICAL PILLAR

Force application during mobilization with movement should do following:

- Sustain the corrected articular position
- Be maintained to the end of the range of motion
- Include passive overpressure
- Avoid restricting movement
- Be maintained until returning from the provocative zone

CLINICAL PILLAR

- MWMs are performed in **weight-bearing** whenever indicated.
- The **physiologic motion** performed is the symptomatic and/or restricted movement.
- **Accessory glides** are applied in **combination** with active or passive physiologic motion.
- Mobilizing force is often applied directly to the **region of pain**.

- Accessory glides are performed in accordance with the **treatment plane** of the joint.
- Mobilizing force must be **maintained** with the correct amount of force and direction throughout the entire range of provocative physiologic motion.
- Passive overpressure should be applied at the end range.
- The mobilization must be entirely **pain free.**
- **Efficacy** is immediately determined through patient response.
- Once efficacy is determined, MWM is performed for **5 to 10 repetitions** and may be followed with **self-mobilization** or **taping** if function is not normalized on release of mobilization.

MWM techniques typically use patient-assisted overpressure at end range as opposed to the use of oscillations. Furthermore, the primary objective in using MWMs is to eliminate positional faults through the application of light, sustained pressure as opposed to stretching a restricted structure. Therefore, unlike traditional joint mobilization, the guiding indication for the degree of mobilizing force is not the joint's end-feel, but rather the onset of the patient's symptoms and functional restrictions.

NOTABLE QUOTABLE

"Treat with confidence, but do not over-treat."

–B.R. Mulligan

Efficacy is determined by repositioning the joint using the appropriate amount of force, then repeating the previously restricted and/or provocative motion and noting any changes in movement or symptoms. If either the range of movement or symptoms are significantly improved, MWM is indicated in the management of the patient and the presence of a positional fault is suspected. If the provocative and/or restricted joint motion is improved but not cleared in response to mobilization, the manual physical therapist may slightly modify the direction, force, or location of the mobilization to attempt to improve the response. The manual physical therapist must make every attempt to persist with minor modifications until, ideally, symptoms are eliminated and full motion has been restored.

CLINICAL PILLAR

If there is no *immediate* improvement with the application of a MWM, either the technique has not been applied correctly, or it is inappropriate for the patient.

To maintain improvement and reduce recidivism, the patient may be instructed in the performance of *self-MWM*. These techniques are designed to allow the patient to become an active participant in his or her own care and to maintain improvement between visits. If MWM is initially effective but there is a return of symptoms upon retesting the movement, then adhesive tape may be applied to sustain the articular positional corrections achieved through manual mobilization.

In this chapter, a collection of Mulligan concept techniques will be described to provide the reader with the clinical application of the principles being discussed. The reader is encouraged to obtain Mulligan's text[1] for additional information on the philosophy and practice of this approach.

Mobilization of the Spine

The use of MWMs in the management of spinal conditions has become widely practiced among the OMPT community owing to repeated claims of their clinical efficacy. A survey of 3,295 physical therapists in Britain was conducted to investigate the current use of MWM for the management of low back pain. Over 40% of the respondents reported using MWM techniques in their plan of care, and more than 50% were using MWMs on a weekly basis. Over 50% reported that the most common immediate finding was an increase in range of motion, and 27.5% reported an immediate relief in pain.[9]

Sustained Natural Apophyseal Glides

Spinal **sustained natural apophyseal glides (SNAGs)** are nonoscillatory mobilizations that may be applied throughout the entire spine. These techniques were among the first procedures described by Mulligan in his exploration into the concept of MWM.

Cervical Sustained Natural Apophyseal Glides

This technique is often effective in managing deficits in cervical rotation (Fig. 10-3). Interestingly, the process of applying accessory force that opens a joint concurrently with physiologic motion that closes it appears to be counterintuitive. It is, therefore, difficult to explain the reported clinical effectiveness of this technique on the basis of biomechanical causes alone. Hearn and Rivett[10] attempted to identify the likely biomechanical effects of a unilateral cervical SNAG, which is performed ipsilateral to the side of pain when treating cervical rotation. Presumably, an accessory glide that is applied ipsilateral to the side of pain will serve to reduce the *downglided* segment, thus allowing physiologic active movement toward that side to be improved.

To perform a cervical SNAG, the patient is seated with the therapist standing behind. The medial side of the contact thumb is placed over the articular pillar of the involved segment

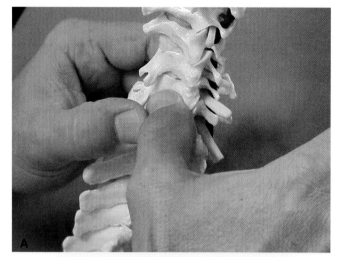
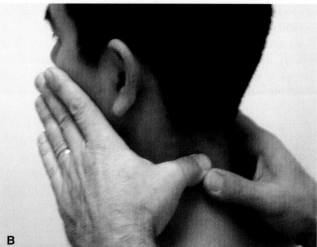

FIGURE 10–3 Cervical sustained natural apophyseal glides (SNAGs). **A.** Thumb over thumb hand contact at painful segment. **B.** With the patient seated, the therapist contacts the painful and/or restricted segment and applies thumb-over-thumb force in the direction of the treatment plane as the patient actively moves into the painful and/or restricted active movement.

for a unilateral condition or over the spinous process for a bilateral condition. For right rotation unilateral SNAGs with report of pain on the right, the right thumb is placed at the involved segment on the right. The other thumb is placed over the lateral border of the contact thumb to provide the mobilizing force. For example, pain on the right at C5-C6 during right rotation requires thumb-over-thumb pressure on the articular pillar of C5 on the right, which is applied during active right cervical rotation. Force is provided in an upward and forward direction toward the patient's eye to match the treatment plane. It is imperative that the force be maintained as the patient moves throughout the entire range of motion and be sustained with patient-assisted overpressure at end range. Overpressure is accomplished by having the patient use his or her hand at the side of the cheek while holding for 5 seconds or more. The force is sustained until the patient returns from the provocative movement. To maintain this force in the correct direction, the therapist must move as the patient moves. If there is no effect from this technique, altering the technique slightly is indicated, or pressure may be applied to the C5 articular pillar on the left or to the spinous process of C5.

The SNAG process just described may be used for cervical side bending, extension, and flexion, as well as combined movements. A foam pad may be used to improve the therapist's grasp on the segment and to decrease soreness that may be caused from thumb pressure (see Fig. 2-19). Effective intervention may be followed by encouraging the patient to use his or her newly acquired range of motion between visits.

Lumbar Sustained Natural Apophyseal Glides

As with cervical SNAGs, the patient should be treated in his or her provocative position (Fig. 10-4). If the patient is symptomatic in both sitting *and* standing, sitting is attempted first, and if indicated, improvement will typically be noted in both positions.

To perform lumbar SNAGs in sitting, the therapist stands behind the seated patient with a belt around the therapist's hips and just inferior to the patient's anterior superior iliac spine (ASIS). The belt is used to offer counterforce to the anterior pressure of the mobilizing hand. The therapist's mobilizing hand contacts the spinous process or transverse process of the superior vertebra of the segment to be mobilized, with the hypothenar border just distal to the pisiform. The mobilizing hand is supinated to hook onto the soft tissue, and force is applied in a cranial direction to match the treatment plane of the apophyseal joint as the patient moves. If SNAGs are indicated, an accessory glide will result in full, painless motion through the previously provocative range. At L5, performance of a SNAG requires mobilization using thumb over thumb contact of both thumbs.[1] Mulligan's thoracic SNAGs may be the treatment of choice when high-velocity thrust is contraindicated, as in cases of osteoporosis.

Natural Apophyseal Glides

Natural apophyseal glides (NAGs) (Fig. 10-5) depart from the MWM practice guidelines previously described. These techniques do not include the combination of accessory and physiologic movement as used when performing SNAGs, but rather they use *oscillatory mobilization* that is directed parallel to the *treatment plane* of the joint. The direction of force is critical and is dictated by the position of the therapist's mobilizing hand. These techniques are once again performed in a weight-bearing position. Cervical NAGs are performed with the therapist standing

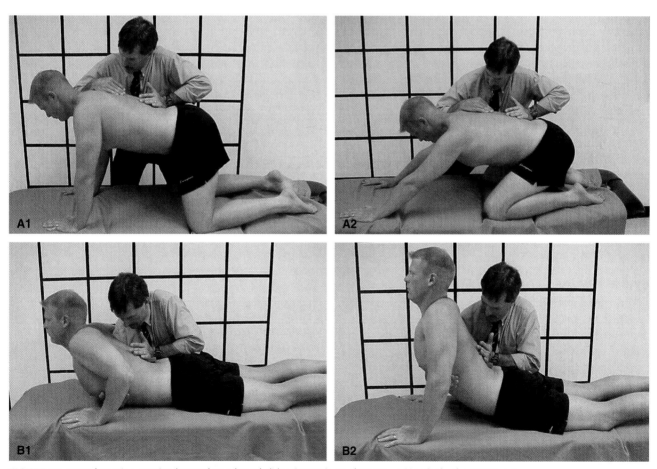

FIGURE 10–4 Lumbar spine sustained natural apophyseal glides (SNAGs). An alternate position for lumbar SNAGs is in **A1.** quadruped for flexion and **B1.** prone position for extension. **A2.** For a flexion SNAG, the patient brings the buttocks to the heels (i.e., lion exercise) while the therapist applies supero-anterior force. **B2.** For an extension SNAG, the patient performs a prone press-up while the same force is applied by the therapist. For both techniques, the therapist's stabilizing arm securely encircles the patient's upper abdomen, alternately draping an arm over the patient's shoulder for flexion.

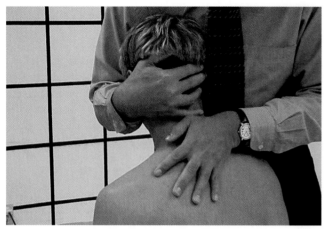

FIGURE 10–5 Cervical natural apophyseal glides (NAGs). With the patient seated, the therapist stabilizes the head and body and makes contact with the middle phalanx of the fifth digit of the stabilizing hand. Force is placed through this contact in the direction of the treatment plane. This technique may be used throughout the cervical spine. Repeat five to six times, retest; the therapist may need to do several sets and/or levels.

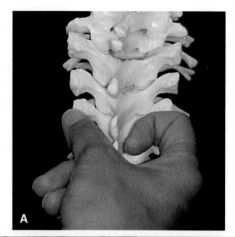

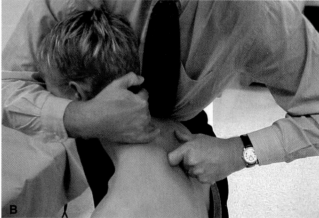

FIGURE 10–6 Reverse natural apophyseal glides. With the patient seated, the therapist stabilizes the head and body as for NAGs. The fingers of the stabilizing arm are placed around the posterior aspect of the superior vertebra of the segment to be mobilized. **A.** In the cervical spine a V is formed with thumb and flexed index finger of the opposing hand and placed over the articular pillars of the inferior vertebra of the segment to be mobilized. Force is applied up and forward along the treatment plane through the V-hand contact. **B.** Separate thumb and index finger to contact transverse processes when mobilizing the upper thoracic spine. This is most used in the thoracic spine and may be useful if NAGs prove to be unsuccessful.

using the lower trunk to block body movement through contact at the patient's anterior shoulder. The therapist cradles the patient's head using the forearm, which is angled against the side of the patient's face. The middle phalanx of the fifth digit of the contact hand gains purchase on the spinous process of the superior vertebra of the segment to be mobilized as the lateral aspect of the thenar eminence of the mobilizing hand applies force through this "dummy finger" contact. Slack is taken up in the joint until the barrier is reached, at which time oscillatory mobilization is performed.

To achieve maximum contact, the head-cradling hand may bring the cervical spine into flexion. As flexion is introduced, the direction of mobilizing force in the midcervical spine becomes more horizontal. Glides are performed rhythmically (two to three per second). If pain is experienced, gentle traction may be applied by the therapist shifting weight or standing more upright. Modifications may be incorporated that involve the application of unilateral force over the articular pillar as opposed to the spinous process.[11]

Reverse Natural Apophyseal Glides

For the manual intervention of patients with end-range cervical movement loss, the therapist may choose to use **reverse natural apophyseal glides (RNAGs)** (Fig. 10-6). These techniques are designed to produce downglide of the segment in question through application of force applied to the inferior vertebra of the segment. These techniques approximate the forces that occur during neck retraction (axial extension) exercises. For example, reverse NAGs for a restriction at C5-C6 would involve the setup and force application similar to that described for NAGs, but with the therapist positioned to the side of the patient. The fingers of the mobilizing hand are placed into the "V-hand position," a position similar to that which is used by golfers to place their tee into the ground. The V hand is placed over C6 with the apex of the V capturing the spinous process. As force is applied through this contact over C6, a downglide of C5 relative to C6

is, in effect, taking place. As with NAGs, the force direction respects the treatment plane. It is critical that the therapist take up slack in the joint before mobilizing, and oscillations must occur at the midrange to end range of segmental motion.

Sustained Natural Apophyseal Glides for Headaches

The cervical SNAG technique previously described may be adapted to specifically manage headaches. These techniques are identified as **headache SNAGs** and are performed in a nonoscillatory, sustained fashion. Identical positioning and handling as described for cervical NAGs is adopted; however, the spinous process of C2 is contacted. A minimal degree of force is applied in a posteroanterior direction and sustained for a minimum of 10 seconds. Slightly modifying the direction of horizontal force to the right or left may afford better symptom resolution in the case of less than complete relief. Mobilization through C2 moves C2, which in turn engages C1, resulting in a posteroanterior mobilization of C2 and C1 relative to the occiput. If the headache is cervicogenic in origin, this technique is often quite effective in producing a relief of the symptoms during the sustained hold. If improvement is noted, the patient may perform the **self-headache SNAG** technique, which involves performance of a chin tuck while using a towel to provide counterforce over C2 in a PA direction (Fig. 10-7).

Reverse headache SNAGs are performed by the therapist supporting the occiput with one hand and using an open lumbrical grasp to hold C2. C2 is held in position as the occiput is moved anteriorly, thus producing a posteroanterior mobilization of the occiput and C1 relative to C2, which is the opposite effect of the headache SNAG. If reverse headache SNAGs are effective, the complementary self-treatment would be *fist traction*, where the patient places his or her fist between the chin and chest and with the other hand applies a flexion moment force to the occiput (Fig. 10-8). The primary indication for use of the fist traction technique is pain or restriction with cervical flexion. Proper screening procedures must be performed prior to subcranial mobilization.

Spinal Mobilization With Extremity Movement (SMWAM and SMWLM)

When symptoms that are thought to be referred from the spine are present within the periphery, the use of mobilization at the appropriate spinal level should be considered in conjunction with extremity movement. Mobilizing force is applied to the appropriate spinal level and sustained as the patient actively performs the previously provocative extremity movement.

As with other forms of MWM, immediate improvement in symptoms and range is anticipated, thus establishing its efficacy. The terminology used to describe these techniques is either **spinal mobilization with arm movement (SMWAM)** or **spinal mobilization with leg movement (SMWLM).**

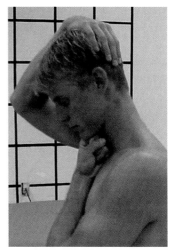

FIGURE 10–8 Fist traction. In sitting, the patient flexes the neck and places a closed fist between the sternum and chin. The patient's other hand is placed over the occiput and gently applies a traction force against the counter-resistance of the fist. This position is held for 10 seconds and repeated three times; it can be performed routinely throughout the day.

For SMWAM, dummy-thumb contact with reinforcing thumb or finger is placed alongside the spinous process of the suspected cervical level. This level is determined by the location of reported spinal pain if present, the location of the patient's reported extremity symptoms, or the findings from the neurological screen. For example, radiating paresthesia into the middle digit of the hand with diminished sensation and a reduction in the triceps deep tendon reflex (DTR) on that side all suggest the C7 nerve root as the culpable segment. This nerve root exits the spine at the C6-C7 segment. Thumb contact for this mobilization would then be made at the side of the spinous process at C6 to mobilize this segment. The force direction for this mobilization is lateral, and it is sustained as the patient actively performs the symptom-producing arm movement. The patient may perform any cardinal plane or combined plane shoulder motion that is provocative, and the elimination of symptoms is expected as the spinal mobilization force is provided and maintained throughout the motion. If the desired effect is not observed, then the therapist may attempt mobilization at another level or in a slightly different direction (Fig. 10-9).

Spinal mobilization with extremity movements can also be performed in the lumbar spine using lower extremity movement; however, assistance in their performance is often required. These techniques are advocated in the presence of a lumbar lesion that results in symptoms or signs distal to the knee, as provoked by supine side leg raising (SLR), for example, or in the presence of a femoral nerve sign. In side-lying position, the involved extremity is uppermost as the patient's hip is brought into a slight degree of abduction to tolerance. The therapist applies transverse pressure along the side of the spinous process of the superior aspect of the segment to be mobilized. For symptoms involving the sciatic nerve, the target segment would be L4 or L5. Overpressure may be applied, but care is taken not to overtreat (Fig. 10-10).[12]

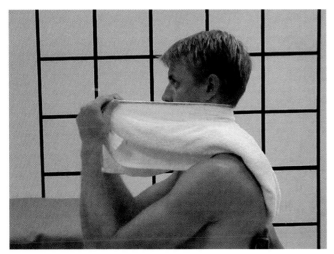

FIGURE 10–7 Self-headache SNAG. With the patient seated, a towel is placed specifically over C2. The patient then performs cervical retraction while holding the towel securely. This position is held for 10 seconds and repeated 6 to 10 times, and it can be performed routinely throughout the day.

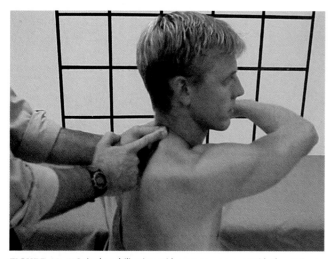

FIGURE 10–9 Spinal mobilization with arm movement. With the patient sitting, the therapist places index finger pressure over lateral side of thumb at the side of the spinous process of the superior aspect of the involved segment. A laterally directed force is applied and maintained as the patient performs the provocative arm movement. Immediate improvement in arm motion and symptoms is expected. Overpressure is applied to the arm movement by the patient if pain free.

The prone SMWLM involves the patient angled obliquely so as to allow the leg to move off the edge of the table. The therapist stands on the patient's involved side with thumb-over-thumb contact to the side of the spinous process of the superior aspect of the involved segment as an assistant provides force in the opposite direction on the inferior aspect of the involved segment. Another assistant supports the extremity as it is slowly brought to the floor within tolerance, after which the assistant returns the leg to its start position (Fig. 10-10). Several case studies have demonstrated the effectiveness of SMWLM[13] and SMWAM[14] in patients with pain of suspected spinal origin.

Mobilization of the Extremities

In the periphery, Mulligan classifies synovial joints into one of two major types, which will dictate the direction in which forces are to be applied during MWM. The *freely mobile*, or *hinge-type*, joint is used to describe such joints as the knee or interphalangeal joints. MWM for freely mobile joints requires the mobilization glide to take place in the frontal plane for a loss of sagittal plane movement; that is, the mobilizing force is

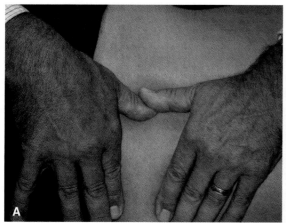
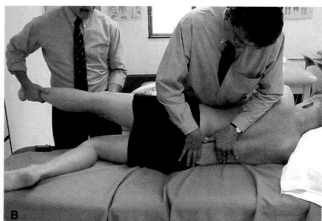
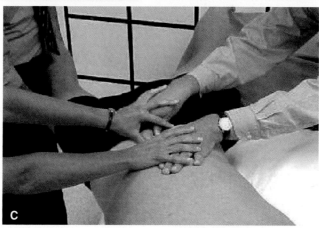

FIGURE 10–10 Spinal mobilization with leg movement. **A.** Hand contact using thumb-over-thumb placement to the side of the spinous process of the superior vertebra of the involved segment, **B.** With the patient in side-lying position with the involved side uppermost, the therapist applies a laterally directed force at the side of the spinous process at the superior aspect of the involved segment while the patient slowly brings the leg into the provocative SLR position. An assistant supports the full weight of the leg. **C.** With the patient in prone position, one therapist applies a laterally directed force to the side of the spinous process of the superior aspect while another therapist applies a laterally directed force in the opposite direction at the inferior aspect of the involved segment. An assistant fully supports the leg and provides light resistance to an active SLR from the table toward the ground into the provocative SLR position.

applied at a right angle to the plane of physiologic motion. If knee extension, for example, is either painful or restricted, force would be applied to the tibia in a frontal plane direction (either medially or laterally) during performance of active knee extension. If the joint motion is not cleared by such a glide, a transverse plane mobilization (i.e., rotation or spin) may be attempted. If the condition is recalcitrant, the manual physical therapist may attempt a *combined mobilization* that includes both transverse plane mobilization and a medial or lateral frontal plane glide.

The second type of extremity synovial joint is referred to as the *adjacent long bone* joint. This type of joint includes the intermetacarpal joints or the radioulnar joints. The primary direction of mobilizing force applied to these joints during MWM is PA with respect to the treatment plane. In the case of applying MWM to adjacent metacarpals four and five, force may be applied posteriorly (dorsally) to the fourth metacarpal while counterforce is applied to the fifth metacarpal in an anterior volar direction. Exelby[15] offered several postulates regarding the cause for the immediate improvement noted in range and symptoms in response to MWM in the periphery.

Mobilization With Movement for the Hip

MWM for the hip incorporates a mobilizing glide that is perpendicular to the direction of joint movement. MWM for the hip may be performed either in weight-bearing or non-weight-bearing. For a loss of hip internal rotation, which is commonly experienced in individuals with low back pain,[16-18] MWM may be performed with the patient supine as the therapist places a mobilizing strap around his or her hips and the patient's proximal femur. The therapist's cephalad hand is placed inside the strap contacting the patient's lateral iliac crest as the therapist's elbow is placed onto the ASIS for stabilization of the pelvis. It is imperative that this stabilization be maintained throughout the mobilization. The therapist's caudal hand encircles the patient's flexed knee. A lateral glide is provided via the mobilization strap by the therapist protruding his or her hips, during which time the patient's hip is passively moved into internal rotation (Fig. 10-11).[19] In standing, the therapist stands on the side to be mobilized with the strap placed in the same location as the patient unilaterally bears weight. As the patient rotates his or her trunk toward the weight-bearing side, hip internal rotation is produced. This is performed as a lateral glide is applied through the mobilization belt while the therapist provides counterforce at the lateral aspect of the iliac crest. MWM for hip extension and abduction may also be performed in standing. To restore *hip extension*, the uninvolved foot is placed on a chair, and the patient lunges forward on the chair as *lateral glide* is provided to the involved hip via the mobilizing strap in a lateral direction. For *hip abduction*, the uninvolved foot is placed on a chair, and the patient leans over the chair as a *posterior glide* is performed via the mobilizing strap.

Mobilization With Movement for Straight Leg Raising

Restricted hip flexion may also be treated with the *SLR with traction* technique. The patient is brought into the SLR position

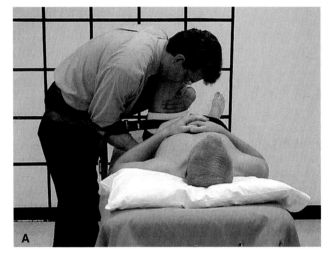

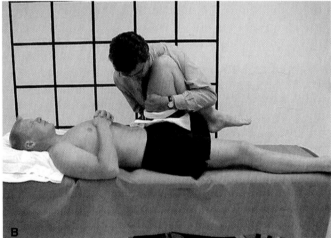

FIGURE 10–11 Hip mobilization with movement for flexion and internal rotation. **A.** To improve hip internal rotation, with the patient in supine position and the hip and knee flexed, the therapist places the mobilizing strap at the proximal femur. The therapist's arm is placed within the strap between the patient's iliac crest and the therapist's ASIS. The other arm is wrapped around patient's flexed knee. The arm inside the strap stabilizes while a lateral distraction force is applied via the strap. While maintaining this lateral glide, the therapist moves the patient's hip into internal rotation. **B.** To improve flexion, the same patient position is used and a lateral glide is imparted via the strap, the therapist moving the femur into hip flexion.

short of the point of limitation or pain. The therapist then uses a flexed elbow and opposing hand to grasp just proximal to the ankle to provide a distraction force through the long axis of the extremity. As distraction is applied, the therapist will note an increase in the available range of SLR without symptoms or report of tightness. As resistance is experienced, the therapist may choose to slightly alter the hip position to allow more abduction or rotation. As with the other MWM techniques, it is critical that the therapist maintain sustained distraction throughout the entire technique.

It is likely that distraction produces an increase in the firing frequency of the *Golgi tendon organs* of associated muscles, thus producing the desired effect of decreased tone, or relaxation, which allows the motion to proceed. Distraction in this fashion may also be considered as another form of hamstring stretching that uses distraction across the muscle to promote elongation through plastic deformation. The latter explanation, however, is less likely given the immediate results that are often appreciated.[20]

Mobilization With Movement for the Knee

MWM of the knee involves the application of a medial or lateral accessory glide for medial and lateral knee pain, respectively, while active flexion or extension is performed. The patient may either lie prone or stand with one foot on a chair, with knee flexion produced by a forward lunge, while the therapist maintains a frontal plane glide manually or with a belt at the tibia (Fig. 10-12). In addition to medial/lateral gliding, the MWM technique of choice for the knee is often the use of tibial rotation. The MWM may be progressed from the supine to a more functional position with the patient's foot on a chair. Flexion of the knee is introduced as the patient lunges, while the therapist provides a mobilizing force into tibial internal rotation through tibial and fibular contacts (Fig. 10-12). Self-mobilization may be performed in a similar fashion, and an innovative taping technique, to be discussed later, may be used to maintain improvement.

Mobilization With Movement for the Ankle

A loss of motion or pain with plantar flexion is addressed in the following manner. The patient is supine, with his or her knee flexed to 90 degrees and the calcaneus planted on the table. The therapist maintains the ankle in neutral and grasps the lower leg, providing a posterior glide of the leg that is maintained while the talus is grasped between the thumb and index finger of the other hand and rolled into plantar flexion over the fulcrum of the calcaneus.

MWM to improve dorsiflexion is most effective and includes placing the involved foot on a chair as the patient is instructed to lean forward, moving the ankle into dorsiflexion. The therapist kneels in front of the patient's chair with the

mobilizing strap fixed around his or her hips and the patient's posterior leg, with the bottom edge of the belt approximately 2 inches above the level of the malleoli. The space between the therapist's thumb and index finger contacts the talus anteriorly and is reinforced by the other hand. As the patient leans forward, an anteroposterior glide of the talus is performed while posteroanterior force is applied through the mobilizing strap (Fig. 10-13).

It is hypothesized by Mulligan that inversion sprains do not routinely involve damage to the strong *anterior talofibular (ATF) ligament* as traditionally thought. Rather, during the course of the inversion sprain, the ATF ligament moves the distal fibula into a more anteriorly displaced position, which is deemed the culprit for the symptoms associated with lateral ankle sprains.[21] Rather than management directed toward the ATF ligament, immediate repositioning of the fibula is required. This is accomplished by the therapist placing their thenar eminence over the anterior aspect of the lateral malleolus and applying a supero-posterolateral glide. This glide is maintained while the patient performs active inversion and plantar flexion with therapist-assisted overpressure at end range (Fig. 10-14). Taping, as described later in this chapter, may then be applied to maintain the reduction.

Mobilization With Movement for the Shoulder

With the patient seated and the therapist standing on the opposite side of the involved extremity, hand contact is made at the anterior aspect of the humerus, providing an posterolateral glide as the patient performs the symptomatic movement of flexion, abduction, or internal/external rotation in an elevated position (i.e., 90 degrees of abduction). The therapist may also apply a mobilizing strap through which force is delivered to the anterior humerus for larger patients (Fig. 10-15).

MWM for glenohumeral internal rotation involves the patient adopting a position of functional internal rotation, which includes extension and adduction. This can be done with a

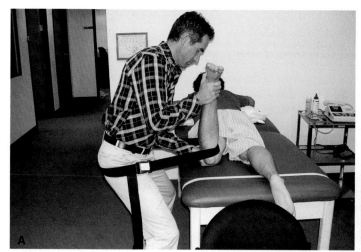
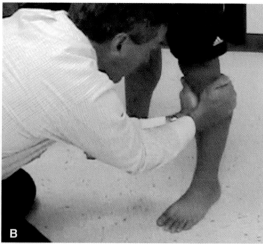

FIGURE 10–12 Knee mobilization with movement for flexion. **A.** The mobilizing strap is applied to the proximal tibia in prone so as to provide a medial glide for medial knee pain and a lateral glide for lateral knee pain as the patient actively flexes the knee. **B.** For the proximal tibiofibular joint, an internal rotation is provided via tibia and fibula contacts as the patient actively flexes the knee in weight-bearing. If improvement is noted, three sets of 10 repetitions may be performed.

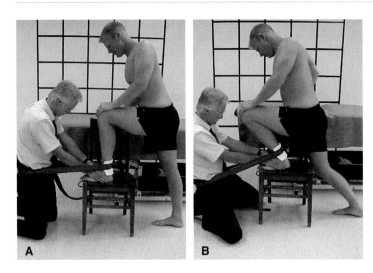

FIGURE 10–13 Ankle mobilization with movement for dorsiflexion. **A.** With the foot to be mobilized resting on a chair, the mobilization strap is applied just proximal to the talocrural joint and around the legs of the therapist. Hand-over-hand contact is made at the anterior aspect of the talus. **B.** As the patient leans over the foot to produce dorsiflexion, anteroposterior force is applied to the talus while posteroanterior force is applied to the distal tibia and fibula via the mobilization strap. If improvement is noted, repeat three sets of 10 repetitions are done.

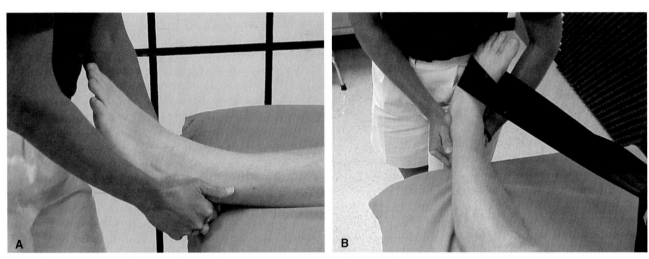

FIGURE 10–14 Distal tibiofibular mobilization following inversion sprain. **A.** With the patient in supine position, the therapist contacts the anterior aspect of the distal fibula with the thenar eminence and applies an anteroposterior and cranial force. **B.** This force is maintained while active inversion is performed, and if the patient is pain free, overpressure is added. If improvement is noted, repeat three sets of 10 repetitions. Follow with taping.

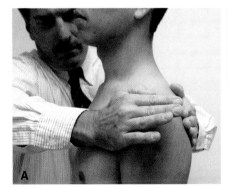
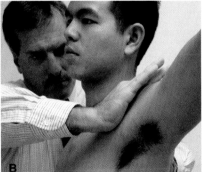
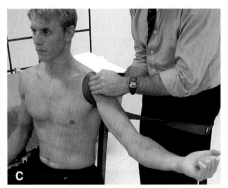

FIGURE 10–15 Shoulder mobilization with movement for elevation. **A.** The therapist stands on the side opposite the involved shoulder. One hand stabilizes at the scapula while the mobilizing hand is placed at the anterior aspect of the humeral head. **B.** As the patient actively performs the provocative movement of elevation, an anteroposterior-lateral force is applied through the humeral head contact, which is maintained throughout the movement. If improvement is noted, repeat three sets of 10 repetitions, with overpressure if the patient is pain free. **C.** A mobilization strap may be used for large patients or to free the therapist's mobilizing hand for another use.

towel held high by the uninvolved hand and draped over the shoulder and grasped behind the back by the patient's involved hand. Standing to the side of the patient, the therapist places his or her hand in the axilla for scapula stabilization and hooks the opposite thumb onto the patient's flexed elbow. While stabilizing the scapula, an inferior glide is performed with the mobilizing hand at the elbow and simultaneous pressure into adduction applied by the therapist's body against the patient's lateral/distal arm. The therapist's hand in the axilla acts as a fulcrum to provide a lateral glide of the humeral head concurrent with the inferior glide as the patient pulls the involved hand cephalad into greater degrees of functional internal rotation. A mobilizing strap may also be used to provide the inferior gliding force (Fig. 10-15).

Mobilization With Movement for the Elbow

In the elbow, a loss of flexion or extension, or pain with either, may be addressed through the use of a lateral glide. This may be applied with the patient in supine or sitting position, and a mobilizing belt or the therapist's manual contacts alone may be used. This lateral glide, like the others, is applied during the patient's active performance of the symptomatic movement, which may include elbow flexion, extension, or repeated hand gripping (Fig. 10-16). For lateral epicondylalgia, the same lateral glide may be applied with active gripping for three sets of 10 repetitions. Improved grip strength and less pain is the desired result. Self-mobilization may be performed using a doorway for stabilization of the humerus as lateral glide is performed.

Mobilization With Movement for the Wrist and Hand

To restore wrist flexion or extension, the *freely mobile joint* guidelines are in effect. With the patient seated, the therapist grasps the distal aspect of the radius with the stabilizing hand and the proximal row of carpal bones with the mobilizing hand. The patient then performs the symptomatic/restricted movement and applies overpressure at end range using his or her uninvolved hand. Slight alterations in the direction of glide should be made, or use of rotation, if the initial mobilization is not immediately effective (Fig. 10-17). Similar techniques are conducted for the metacarpophalangeal (MCP) and interphalangeal (PIP, DIP) joints as well.[22]

Loss of supination or pronation requires application of the adjacent long bone guidelines. The patient sits with his or her elbow flexed to 90 degrees. The therapist applies thumb-over-thumb pressure at the ulnar head in a dorsovolar direction as the patient moves into either supination or pronation, with self-overpressure applied with the uninvolved hand at end range (Fig. 10-17).

Ancillary and Adjunctive Procedures

Pain Release Phenomenon

Pain release phenomenon (PRP) techniques are used for individuals presenting with chronic conditions when the early stages of healing have occurred. These techniques involve reproduction of a patent's pain complaint through either an

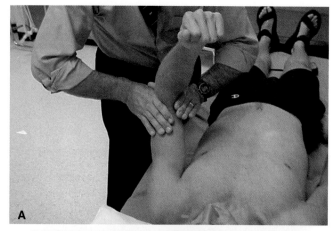

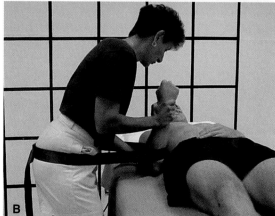

FIGURE 10–16 Elbow mobilization with movement for flexion and extension. This may be performed entirely manually or with a strap. With the patient supine, **A.** hand contact or **B.** mobilization strap is placed over the proximal radius and ulna and the therapist's legs while the distal humerus is manually stabilized. A gentle lateral glide is provided through the strap while the patient actively performs the provocative motion of elbow flexion or extension. If improvement is noted, repeat three sets of 10 repetitions. A transverse plane rotation of the ulna on the humerus may be indicated if the lateral glide is ineffective, and if so, the treatment may be followed with taping.

active contraction of the painful region or stretch of the involved structures. Typically, the painful activity is maintained for a maximum of 20 seconds, within which symptoms should resolve.[23] These techniques operate in a fashion similar to the concept of deep friction massage as espoused by Cyriax (see Chapter 5).[24]

In managing tendonopathy, active contraction or stretch of the involved tendon that produces moderate pain may be held for the recommended 20 seconds, at which time symptoms are expected to resolve. This process may be used for conditions such as medial and lateral tendonopathy and DeQuervain's syndrome, among others.

PRPs may also involve the use of joint compression, which includes physiologic movements or accessory glides. PRPs for a painful second MTP joint involves sustained compression of the proximal phalanx and metatarsal with concurrent performance of an alternating caudal-to-cranial gliding of the articulation for up to 20 seconds, during which time pain should

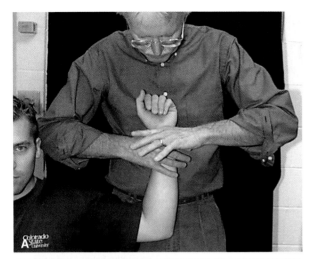

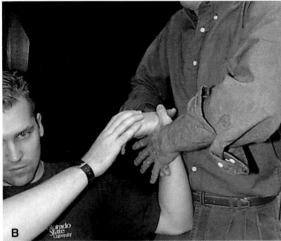

FIGURE 10-17 Wrist mobilization with movement for flexion, extension, supination, pronation. **A.** With the patient sitting and elbow flexed, the therapist provides stabilization at the distal radius and ulna with the web space of one hand while a lateral glide is applied to the proximal row of carpal bones with the other. **B.** This force is maintained while the patient actively performs the provocative flexion or extension movement with overpressure. If improvement is noted, repeat three sets of 10 repetitions. The treatment may be followed by taping.

subside. For PRPs to be effective, pain must be present and provoked. With this in mind, it is important for the manual physical therapist to remember that these techniques are effective in the management of chronic conditions only.

Principles of Self-Mobilization

A common criticism of OMPT relates to the passive role adopted by the patient during intervention. The Mulligan concept is cognizant of this limitation and appreciative of the potential for recidivism that may follow the often dramatic changes that occur in response to these manual interventions. To address these issues, patients who have responded favorably to MWM in the clinic but have some return of dysfunction are introduced to **self-mobilization** techniques, which are to be performed between sessions and possibly after discharge. These techniques serve to provide lasting improvement, increase the efficiency of intervention, allow the patient to take a more active role in his or her care, and may be used as preventative measures.

Self-SNAGs

When performing *self-SNAGs*, the patient-directed mobilizing force is provided by using a towel or self-mobilization strap (see Fig. 2-26) at the segment in which symptoms are reported while the patient actively performs the provocative symptomatic motion (Fig. 10-18). The force must follow the treatment plane and be maintained throughout the entire movement until the patient returns to neutral. As with SNAGs, the mobilization must occur completely free of symptoms.

A patient with pain upon right rotation at C5-C6 would be instructed to place the unfolded edge of a towel over C5. Using a towel that is gathered will reduce the specificity of the technique. With arms crossed, the patient grasps the edge of the towel. If the patient is rotating to the right, the right hand is placed over the left. The left hand holds the towel against the patient's chest as the right hand places the towel in line with the C5-C6 treatment plane toward the eye. The left hand holds, while the right hand pulls the towel along the midcervical treatment plane toward the eye as the patient performs rotation to the right. The mobilizing force must be maintained within the correct plane throughout the entire motion. This is accomplished by ensuring that the space between the towel and the patient's cheek does not change throughout the entire movement. In this case, the left elbow may be hooked around the back of the chair to prevent the trunk from rotating with the neck during movement. Because of the complexity of the hand positioning with this technique, it may be advisable to provide a picture of the technique with step-by-step instructions to ensure correct performance (Fig. 10-18). Self-SNAGs are also commonly performed in the lumbar spine as well (Fig. 10-19). A strap, belt, or the fist is used over the symptomatic segment while trunk movement is performed.

Self-MWMs

Following the concept of MWM for freely mobile joints, wrist medial or lateral glide or rotation may be applied to the proximal row of carpal bones during active wrist flexion or extension through the use of the other hand. Similar glides may also be easily performed over the proximal or distal interphalangeal joints (PIP, DIP) during flexion and extension.

Self-MWMs are often used to enhance movement of the knee, particularly into flexion. In keeping with the general principles of MWM, the involved foot is placed on a chair, and the patient leans forward using both hands to produce tibial internal rotation through hand contacts at the proximal tibia and fibula. As with other MWMs, the force is maintained throughout the entire motion and sustained at end range. If MWM is asymptomatic, but symptoms return upon retesting, taping to sustain tibial internal rotation relative to the femur is attempted.

Adhesive Taping Strategies

The use of adhesive tape within this approach is based on the positional fault theory, which states that articular malalignment may lead to altered kinematics and eventual dysfunction. Adhesive tape may be used between OMPT interventions and during activities of daily living (ADL) and sport participation for prophylaxis and to maintain a more optimal articular alignment. For

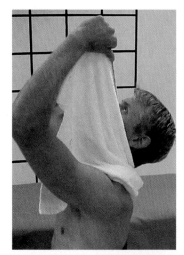

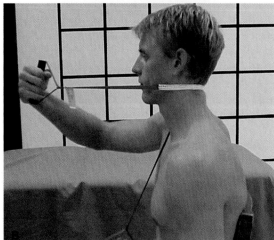

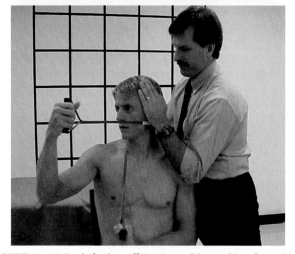

FIGURE 10–18 Cervical spine self-SNAGs. In sitting position, the patient places the very edge of a towel at the involved level to be mobilized. **A.** Mid cervical/lower cervical extension: The patient pulls antero-cranially with both hands and must move as the treatment plane moves. **B.** Mid-cervical/lower cervical rotation: One hand holds the strap in place while the other hand pulls in the direction of the cervical treatment plane. This force is maintained as the patient actively performs the provocative movement, which must now be asymptomatic. **C.** Use of a self-mobilization strap showing positioning of strap and utilization of strap for rotation with therapist overpressure.

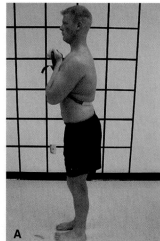

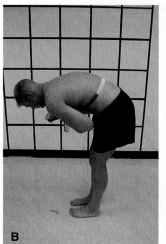

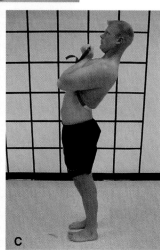

FIGURE 10–19 Lumbar spine self-SNAGs. **A.** With the patient in standing position, the lumbar self-SNAG strap or belt is placed over the involved level and force is applied in the direction of the lumbar spine treatment plane. Force is maintained as the patient actively performs the provocative movement into either **B.** flexion or **C.** extension.

most of the taping procedures described, two strips of tape are used. The first strip is the base strip, which often uses 2-inch cloth athletic tape. The 1-inch locking strip, created from tearing a strip of 2-inch tape longitudinally, is placed over the base strip. Various brands of tape are currently used for these procedures, and the success of this intervention may depend on the strength and durability of the tape that is applied. Hair removal is necessary, and the use of tape adhesive may increase the longevity of the tape.

Adhesive Taping of the Knee

The knee MWM used to improve knee flexion in closed chain, as previously described, involves the application of internal tibial rotation. Adhesive tape may subsequently be used to maintain this corrected articular position (Fig. 10-20). In standing with the knee slightly flexed, the patient's tibia is internally rotated manually. The tape is applied in a spiral fashion, beginning at the proximal posterolateral tibia, angling obliquely just inferior to the patella, and spiraling around the medial aspect of the knee and ending at the posterolateral thigh.

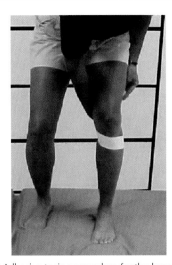

FIGURE 10–20 Adhesive taping procedure for the knee. In standing with the knee slightly flexed, the patient's foot and tibia are internally rotated and the femur externally rotated. The tape is applied in a spiral fashion beginning at the proximal posterolateral leg anteriorly crossing the knee joint just below the patella and spiraling around the medial thigh and ending at the posterior thigh.

Adhesive Taping of the Ankle

As previously described, a potential sequela of an inversion ankle sprain involves the anterior migration of the distal fibula, thus producing a positional fault of the distal tibiofibular joint. Similar to the taping procedure just described for the knee, ankle taping involves two strips of spiraled tape (Fig. 10-21). Taping for this articular malalignment includes the application of the mobilizing force to the distal fibula in the posterolateral and superior direction, which is held while tape is applied. The tape originates at the lateral malleolus and spirals posteriorly and cephalad across the posterior calf, ending at the anteromedial aspect of the tibia.

Adhesive Taping of the Wrist

One or two diagonal strips of tape from medial to lateral across the dorsal and/or ventral aspects of the wrist may be effective at maintaining a lateral glide of the carpal bones relative to the distal radius and ulna. Such a procedure may be useful at improving wrist flexion and extension and pain associated with either (Fig. 10-22).

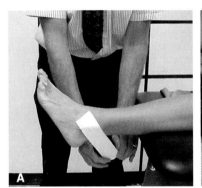 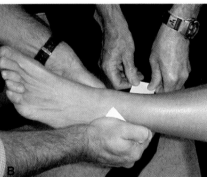 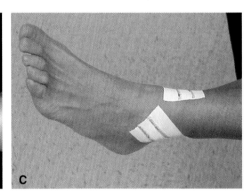

FIGURE 10-21 Adhesive taping procedure for the ankle. **A.** Beginning at the lateral malleolus, **B.** anteroposterior-cranial mobilizing force to the distal fibula is held while tape is applied spiraling posteriorly and cephalad across the posterior compartment, and **C.** ending at the medial aspect of the distal tibia.

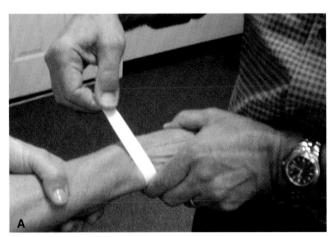 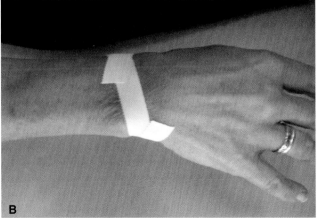

FIGURE 10–22 Adhesive taping procedure for the wrist. **A.** A diagonal strip of tape is applied from medial to lateral across the dorsal aspect of the wrist to maintain a lateral glide of the carpal bones relative to the distal radius and ulna. **B.** A second strip of tape may be necessary across the ventral wrist to counter any unwanted rotation from the first strip. Such a procedure may be useful for improving wrist flexion and extension and any pain associated with either movement.

Adhesive Taping of the Spine

After mobilization, symptoms may return if patients do not maintain proper posture. The application of adhesive tape may be a useful adjunct to OMPT by providing the patient with tactile cues for better posturing. To accomplish this, one horizontal strip may be applied from one scapula to the other at approximately the T4-T6 region. In addition, an X consisting of two diagonal strips of tape may be applied in the lumbar region. Tactile feedback occurs as the patient begins to slump or lean forward, thus cueing the patient to return to a more upright posture.

DIFFERENTIATING CHARACTERISTICS

The Mulligan concept approach to OMPT may be elevated as the quintessential endeavor into clinical experimentation that arose from a general dissatisfaction with the status quo. The MWM techniques, which have now become widely used, were created inadvertently and then further developed through careful observation. Although other approaches describe mobilization that includes a combination of both accessory and physiologic motion,[25] this approach was the first to apply these techniques to various regions of the body and to provide detailed descriptions of their performance. No other approach has articulated effective intervention in such simple terms, and few have demonstrated such immediate effects.

NOTABLE QUOTABLE

"There is still so much to discover and learn."

-B.R. Mulligan

It is well-established that a primary role of the physical therapist is in the areas of prevention and education.[26] The self-mobilization techniques espoused within this approach move beyond the emphasis of most manual paradigms that consist of passive procedures only and effectively engender patient participation. The self-mobilization techniques described within this approach are technically easy to perform and require little or no equipment.

Other approaches have discussed the concept of positional faults and the impact that such faults may have on joint kinematics.[6,7] Within the Mulligan concept, the positional fault theory is considered to be the basis upon which intervention is directed. This approach is one of the first to incorporate the use of innovative adhesive taping techniques into its plan of care. As with mobilization, the objective for the application of tape is the reduction of joint positional malalignments that may be contributing to dysfunction.

Overall, the Mulligan concept has made valuable and innovative contributions to the specialization of OMPT. It stands on a firm foundation of functional musculoskeletal anatomy and joint kinematics and espouses principles of examination and intervention that are supported through the current best evidence. The sometimes dramatic effects experienced as a result of using these techniques makes them worthy of consideration as an important

component in the toolbox of the manual physical therapist. Exelby[27] has demonstrated how these concepts can be used in the management of a variety of specific conditions and how these concepts can be integrated into other paradigms.

As manual physical therapists have become more acquainted with the basic tenets of this approach, new techniques are forever emerging. Indeed, modifications to the standard techniques originally described by Mulligan are seen clinically and in the literature. In the spirit of clinical science, the Mulligan concept approach to OMPT is an ever-evolving system of concepts and techniques designed to better meet the needs of each individual patient . . . *but of course!*

EVIDENCE SUMMARY
Evidence for Mobilization With Movement of the Extremities

The extremity mobilization techniques that are espoused within this approach have been more extensively studied than have those for the spine. Abbott et al[28] investigated the effects of MWM of the elbow in 25 subjects with lateral epicondylalgia. A laterally directed glide was performed while the patient performed the provocative motion up to 10 repetitions.[28] Vicenzino et al[29] replicated these results in 24 patients with unilateral chronic lateral epicondylalgia. Using a randomized, double-blind, repeated measures design, a 58% increase in pain-free grip strength and a 10% change in pain pressure thresholds were observed during and after application of elbow MWM compared to the placebo and control groups.[29]

Kochar and Dogra[30] studied the effect of MWM and ultrasound therapy versus ultrasound alone. Forty-six subjects were randomized into one of two treatment groups, with the remaining 20 serving as controls. Results revealed that the group receiving MWM had greater improvement than did the group with ultrasound alone and the control groups on the visual analog scale (VAS) ($p < 0.05$; $p < 0.05$), weight test ($p < 0.01$; $p < 0.001$), and grip strength (not significant; $p < 0.05$). The MWM group showed immediate improvement.[30]

Several studies have attempted to identify the mechanisms that are responsible for the effects noted in response to MWM for this condition. It appeared that tolerance for the initial hypalgesic effect did not occur, as demonstrated by a lack of reduction in the effect with repeated application between sessions. The pain-free grip strength measure, but not the pain pressure threshold measure, improved over repeated sessions. These results concur with other studies and suggest that the hypalgesia produced by these techniques possesses a nonopioid mechanism.[31,32] These findings are in agreement with similar studies performed to ascertain the mechanisms underlying hypoalgesia subsequent to spinal manual therapy procedures.[33,34] It was demonstrated that MWM for lateral epicondylalgia produced an initial hypalgesic effect with concurrent sympathoexcitation that was similar to that which is reported in response to spinal mobilization.[35,36] Sympathoexcitation was observed by changes in blood pressure, heart rate, and cutaneous sudomotor, and vasomotor function.[37]

Several case studies have also been performed that substantiate the use of MWM for this condition. Stephens[38] demonstrated similar results in a 43-year-old female with history of repetitive motion injuries, including bilateral carpal tunnel. The MWM technique included lateral glide of the forearm during active wrist extension, forearm supination, and hand grip. In addition, a dorsal glide of the hand was applied during active radial deviation, and the carpometacarpal joint of the thumb was mobilized toward the palm during thumb opposition. Adhesive tape was applied to the elbow to maintain the restoration of positional relationships. The patient's pain level reduced to 0/10 after the first visit.[38]

Vicenzino and Wright[39] showed similar results in a 39-year-old subject who was involved in manual labor. A visual analog scale and a pressure algometer were used to measure pain. A grip dynamometer, function VAS, and pain-free function questionnaire were used to measure changes in function. Four interventions revealed immediate improvements in all dependent variables in response to the MWM technique, with a greater effect noted in pain reduction versus functional improvement. Furthermore, improvements continued into the 6-week follow-up phase, with attainment of full function achieved within this period.[39]

Few researchers have considered the relationship between the level of force applied with a particular technique and the resultant hypalgesic effect. McLean et al[40] performed a randomized controlled trial involving six subjects with diagnosis of lateral epicondylalgia. Four levels of force measured with a pressure mat were applied to the subject in a lateral glide direction while the subject performed a pain-free grip test using a digital hand-grip dynamometer, with the elbow in extension and the forearm in pronation. The mean force data produced by the therapist during mobilization ranged from 36.8 N to 113.2 N. The relationship between force and pain-free grip strength revealed that there was a significantly greater change in this variable between the second (1.9 N/cm) and third (2.5 N/cm) levels of force. These results suggest that there may be a critical level of force required during mobilization in order to obtain the desired result, with the critical level being somewhere between 1.9 N/cm and 2.5 N/cm (50%–66% of the therapist's maximum force).[40] Clinically, the effectiveness of MWM techniques appear to be linked with the requirement for a sufficient quantity of force.

In 23 subjects with lateral epicondylalgia, Abbott[41] revealed significant increases in shoulder internal and external rotation of both involved and uninvolved extremities in response to MWM of the elbow. Because both the involved and uninvolved extremity improved in range, it appears more likely that the cause was neurophysiologic in nature.

In addition to the MWMs for shoulder dysfunction previously described, Mulligan[42] has published a case series in which techniques designed to address faults of other joints within the shoulder are explained and then applied to actual cases, revealing favorable results. With the patient in the seated position, the therapist stands on the uninvolved side, with one hand over the inner third of the clavicle and the thenar eminence of the other hand at the spine of the scapula. The therapist first provides compression force through both hand contacts. In addition, the scapular hand provides inferior, upward rotation and medial glide of the scapula toward the spine. While holding this scapular position, the patient actively elevates his or her arm. Slight alterations in scapular repositioning may be required as well as therapist assistance for arm

elevation.[42] The statistical significance of the results of this case series was not reported. Further evidence is required to determine the clinical efficacy of this technique.

The use of MWM for injuries of the hand, particularly for injuries to the thumb, have also been considered in the literature. Several case studies have been performed that reveal the effectiveness of MWM techniques in the management of DeQuervain's tenosynovitis.[43,44] Techniques that involve long-axis rotation were shown to be most effective.[43] Other MWM techniques described for the management of DeQuervain's tenosynovitis include a lateral glide that is applied to the proximal row of carpal bones during movement, followed by sustained ulnar glide of the trapezium and trapezoid along with the active performance of carpometacarpal (CMC) radial abduction. Radiocarpal mobilization was performed to enhance tolerance for weight-bearing through the wrist, and elastomer inserts were added to the patient's splint to maintain the corrected positional relationships. A 25% reduction in pain was noted after the first visit, and a 50% reduction was noted following the third intervention. The results suggest a relationship between tendon function and joint position.[44]

In a case study using thumb MWM, Hsieh et al[45] attempted to use magnetic resonance imaging (MRI) to measure the effect of this intervention on joint position. MRI, including stress views, revealed a healed fracture of the metacarpal head and bony irregularity at the proximal and distal phalanges of the thumb, as well as a long-axis rotational fault of the MCP joint. During the initial examination, a MWM that was described as supination of the proximal phalanx (presumed to be long-axis rotation of the proximal phalanx) with active flexion relieved the patient's pain. MRIs before, during, and after MWM revealed a long-axis rotation positional fault of the MCP joint preintervention, which was corrected when viewed during application of the MWM. Following a course of MWM intervention, although symptoms were completely resolved, a positional fault that was similar to that which was noted prior to intervention remained. This suggests that additional mechanisms are responsible for the effects often reported in response to MWM.[45]

Carson[46] examined the intervention of an 11-year-old swimmer who was repeatedly disqualified from competition owing to an asymmetrical swimming pattern. This case demonstrated the use of an eclectic intervention strategy that included MWM for the shoulder and hip. Using an eclectic approach to intervention was effective at improving function, yet further evidence is required to see the direct effect of hip MWM on athletic performance.[46]

Hall et al[20] studied the effects of the SLR with traction technique on range of movement for hip flexion. The results revealed that this technique was effective in improving pain-free range of SLR in normal subjects (an increase of 13.3 degrees from 49.9 degrees to 63.2 degrees), which involved both hip flexion (10.6% increase) and posterior pelvic rotation increases (2.7% increase), with the former being most significant.[22] This degree of improvement was greater than that found in the literature in response to standard stretching and stretching that involved Proprioceptive Neuromuscular Facilitation (PNF) techniques.[47-49]

Kavanagh[50] compared the degree of anterior-to-posterior (AP) distal fibula excursion in patients with acute or chronic ankle sprains to normal subjects. The degree of excursion of the sprained ankles was compared to the degree of excursion in the normal ankles. The results support the hypothesis that there is a significantly greater degree of movement per unit force in the AP direction in two out of six patients with acute ankle sprains, suggesting a distal tibiofibular joint positional fault of an anteriorly displaced distal fibula in cases of inversion ankle sprains.[50] A larger degree of excursion, however, does not automatically indicate that the start position was aberrant.

Collins et al[51] investigated the use of MWM in the care of subacute ankle sprains using the weight-bearing AP talar glide with dorsiflexion technique. Fourteen subjects with subacute grade II lateral ankle sprains were randomly assigned. Results revealed immediate improvement in dorsiflexion range with no effect on mechanical and thermal pain threshold measures. Based on these findings, it was determined that a mechanical, rather than a hypalgesic, effect was the most likely contributor to these improvements.[51]

Evidence for Mobilization With Movement of the Spine

Several studies have demonstrated the effectiveness of SNAGs in the management of thoracic pain. Horton[52] investigated the effects of SNAGs for acute thoracic pain and deformity in a 20-year-old male and found that a central SNAG procedure to the spinous process of T8 followed by use of two strips of adhesive tape applied diagonally across the midback region produced 95% improvement. Improved thoracic pain was noted in a 51-year-old female with 9 months of thoracic, chest, sternal, and left shoulder pain in response to mobilization with movement and spinal manipulative procedures.[53]

Exelby[54] performed a lumbar SNAG on the right articular pillar of L4 while bringing buttock to heels in quadruped (i.e., the lion stretch) in a 46-year-old female with acute onset of right low back pain, which resulted in complete symptom resolution. An adhesive tape strip was applied after mobilization over this segment, and the patient was instructed to perform these activities without the mobilization force independently at home. However, in a double blind study with 49 asymptomatic individuals, no difference in flexion range of motion was found when comparing individuals who received an L3, L4 SNAG mobilization technique for flexion with a sham intervention.[55]

In 2010, Billis described the characteristics, effectiveness, clinical indications and contraindications of lumbar SNAG techniques for the purpose of promoting their proper use. In addition, potential mechanisms of action based on recent evidence was proposed.[56]

CLINICAL CASE

CASE 1: Upper Extremity MWM   *By Ed Wilson, Great Britain (MCTA)*
Visit 1

Subjective: An 18-year-old female is referred to your clinic with diagnosis of *complex regional pain syndrome (CRPS)* of her right hand with a request for intensive physical therapy. She reports the onset of symptoms secondary to striking her right hand on her chest of drawers at home approximately 8 weeks ago. Since that time, a gradual increase in pain, swelling, and stiffness has ensued.

Radiographs: Unremarkable.

Observation: Extremely edematous and mottled right hand is noted. The majority of edema and pain was noted at the MCP joint of the second digit.

Palpation: Increased sensitivity to light touch throughout the right hand. Shooting pain is noted upon palpation or finger movement.

AROM: She has 25% of full motion at MCP, PIP, DIP of the second phalanx; 50% of full motion at MCP, PIP, and DIP of digits 3–5.

Strength: Inability to perform grip strength testing because of pain.

Intervention: The most painful and restricted motion of MCP flexion and extension was initially addressed using a trial MWM intervention to assess its efficacy. A gentle lateral glide was applied to the MCP joint with active flexion and extension. Upon performance, the elimination of symptoms and an increase in range of motion (ROM) by 75% was noted. After two sets of 10 repetitions of this technique, reexamination revealed no pain and 75% improvement in range of motion.

Visit 2

This patient returned 1 week later with no discoloration, minimal edema, reduced hypersensitivity, and 75% of full ROM with persistent complaint of pain and weakness. Based on these findings, MWM techniques were reapplied to the PIP, DIP, as well as the MCP, of the second digit and digits 3–5. The patient was instructed in how to perform self-MWM for these joints and instructed to do so regularly throughout the day. Grip strength was measured using a hand dynamometer, which revealed right = 6 kg, left = 26 kg. Adhesive tape was applied to the wrist and grip strength was retested, revealing an increase in right grip strength from 6 kg to 19 kg. The patient was shown how to self-tape for writing and to continue with self-mobilization.

Visit 3

The patient returned for one more session and was discharged the following week with full ROM, no pain, and grip strength on the right at 28 kg without the use of adhesive tape.

1. Briefly classify and describe the metacarpophalangeal (MCP) and interphalangeal (PIP, DIP) joint according to the Mulligan concept approach.
2. Based on the type of joint described in question 1, what type of glide is most appropriate according to the Mulligan concept approach? Briefly describe the theory that supports the effectiveness of these techniques. How does the use of MWM techniques increase range of motion, decrease pain, and reduce edema?
3. Briefly describe any indications in the patient's presentation that encourages the use of these techniques.
4. Briefly explain the improvement in grip strength that was noted in response to wrist taping. What is the objective of using adhesive tape as an adjunct to manual interventions?
5. Practice the techniques used in this case on your partner. Instruct your partner in self-MWM of the hand, and attempt these techniques on yourself as well.

CASE 2: C2 SNAG's for Management of Vertigo   *By Gaetano Milazzo, Australia (MCTA)*

Subjective: A 53-year-old male presents to your clinic upon referral from a neurologist for treatment of *benign paroxysmal positional vertigo (BPPV)*. The symptoms were present for 2 months and were not associated with any known incident or trauma. Various medications had not had any effect. Symptoms were worse when changing positions, especially when transferring from the lying to the sitting position.

Objective: Clinical assessment demonstrated segmental hypomobility in the upper cervical spine (C1-C2) with poor activation of deep neck stabilizing muscles. The patient was asked to perform changes in posture, first getting up toward the right side, then getting up toward the left side. The posture change with body movement to the right produced more dizziness than when performed to the left.

Intervention: The initial trial intervention was performed with the patient in sitting position and used the Mulligan concept approach technique for dizziness/vertigo, which consisted of a C2 SNAG. One set of five repetitions was performed. Upon reexamination, the dizziness experienced was reported to be less, but still present. The technique was repeated, but there was no additional change reported. The technique was then modified so as to use a sustained pressure while the patient performed the changes in posture. A C1 SNAG was performed in the lying position. This technique consisted of a unilateral PA pressure at the right lateral mass of C1 that was maintained while the patient changed positions. The technique was repeated three times, and the worker reported no dizziness with each repetition. When the patient was retested without the SNAG, there was a return of his dizziness, but the intensity was reported to be less than 50% of the original intensity. The patient was instructed in self-SNAGs and was advised to perform these self-mobilizations three times a day, five repetitions each, for the next 3 days.

Evaluation: The patient was contacted 3 days later at which time he reported that he has not had any dizziness since the day following intervention. He noted the ability to change positions even without application of a SNAG. Contact with the patient 2 weeks after the initial consultation revealed that the dizziness had not returned and that he was no longer doing the exercises.

1. How might this patient's response to the C2 and C1 SNAG techniques help in reaching a differential diagnosis regarding the etiology of his chief complaint of vertigo? Did this patient truly have BPPV? Explain your answer.
2. What is your explanation for the improvement noted in response to the SNAG? Why was the SNAG performed during the provocative change in posture, and why was this strategy effective?
3. Identify additional indications that may suggest the use of these techniques.
4. Perform a C1 SNAG on your partner. Instruct your partner in a C1 self-SNAG, and perform this technique on yourself.
5. The technique used in this case is based on those described in Mulligan's text (i.e., upper cervical SNAGs); however, the application of this technique is unique in this case. Is it appropriate to modify techniques to better meet each patient's individual needs? What are the advantages and limitations of doing this? What indicators might be used to guide the modification of your chosen technique?

HANDS-ON

With a partner, perform the following activities:

1 Your partner presents with left midcervical and trapezius pain at 50% of active cervical rotation to the left. Perform a Mulligan concept technique to help correct this. Be careful to attend to correct patient positioning, therapist positioning, hand contact, and force direction. How would you evaluate the success of this technique? Partners should provide feedback regarding technique performance, then switch places.

2 Your partner presents with weight-bearing wrist extension of 60 degrees, which causes pain. Perform a MWM in non-weight-bearing and progress to mobilization in weight-bearing. What is your rationale for treatment in weight-bearing? Teach your partner self-mobilization techniques to facilitate progress.

3 Your partner presents with right knee pain when stepping down a 6-inch step. Perform a partial weight-bearing MWM to help correct this. Progress to a MWM performed in combination with the provocative movement. Based on the results of this mobilization, apply adhesive taping to your partner to maintain this improvement.

4 Your partner presents with right low back and buttock pain during active forward bending in standing, which is also limited to 25% of normal range. Perform a MWM to help correct this presentation. Teach your partner self-mobilization techniques to facilitate progress.

5 Get in groups of three. Review one Mulligan concept approach technique described in this chapter for each body region. Perform each technique on both partners in your group. While performing the technique, solicit feedback from the individual receiving the technique and from the third partner who is watching you perform the technique. When possible, instruct your partners in self-mobilization activities for carryover of the mobilizations that you just performed.

REFERENCES

1. Mulligan BR. *Manual Therapy: NAGS, SNAGS, MWMS, etc.* 6th ed. New Zealand: Plane View Services Ltd; 2010.
2. Mulligan BR. *Self-Treatments for Back, Neck and Limbs.* 2nd ed. New Zealand: Plane View Services Ltd; 2006.
3. Mulligan BR. *Mobilisations with Movement* [DVD]. New Zealand: Mulligan Concept; 1993.
4. Mulligan BR. *Spinal Techniques: The Cervical Spine.* New Zealand: Mulligan Concept; 1997.
5. Mulligan BR. *Spinal Techniques: The Lumbar Spine and Thoracic Spine*; New Zealand: Mulligan Concept; 1997.
6. Hinman RS, Crossley KM, McConnell J, et al. Efficacy of knee tape in the management of osteoarthritis of the knee: blinded randomized controlled trial. *BMJ.* 2003;327:135-140.
7. VanDillen LR, Sahrmann SA, Norton BJ. Movement system impairment-based categories for low back pain: stage 1 validation. *J Orthop Sports Phys Ther.* 2003;33:126-42.
8. Kaltenborn FM. *Mobilization of the Extremity Joints.* Oslo, Norway: Olaf Norlis Bokhandel, 1980.
9. Konstantinous K, Foster N, Baxter D. The use and reported effects of mobilization with movement techniques in low back pain management; a cross-sectional descriptive survey of physiotherapists in Britain. *Man Ther.* 2002;7:206-214.
10. Hearn A, Rivett DA. Cervical snags: a biomechanical analysis. *Man Ther.* 2002;7:71-79.
11. Mulligan BR. NAGS–Modified mobilisation techniques for the cervical and upper thoracic spines. *NZ J Physiother.* 8:1982.
12. Mulligan BR. Spinal mobilisation with leg movement (further mobilisation with movement). *J Man Manip Ther.* 1995;3:25-27.
13. Mulligan BR. Update on spinal mobilisations with leg movement. *J Man Manip Ther.* 1997;5:184-187.
14. Mulligan BR. Spinal mobilisations with arm movement. *J Man Manip Ther.* 1994;2:75-77.
15. Exelby L. Peripheral mobilisation with movement. *Man Ther.* 1996;1: 118-126.
16. Mellin G. Correlations of hip mobility with degree of back pain and lumbar spine mobility in chronic low-back pain patients. *Spine.* 1988;13:668-670.
17. Chesworth BM, Padfield BJ, Helewa A, Stitt LW. A comparison of hip mobility in patients with low back pain and matched healthy subjects. *Physiother Can.* 1994;46:267-274.
18. Cibulka MT, Sinacore DR, Cromer GS, Delitto A. Unilateral hip rotation range of motion asymmetry in patients with sacroiliac joint regional pain. *Spine.* 1998;23:1009-1015.
19. Mulligan BR. Mobilisation with movement for the hip joint to restore internal rotation and flexion. *J Man Manip Ther.* 1996;4:35-37.
20. Hall T, Cacho A, McNee C, Riches J, Walsh J. Effects of the Mulligan traction straight leg raise techniques on range of movement. *J Man Manip Ther.* 2001;9:128-133.
21. Hubbard TJ, Hertel J, Sherbondy P. Fibular position in individuals with self-reported chronic ankle instability. *J Orthop Sports Phys Ther.* 2006;36:39.
22. Mulligan BR. Extremity joint mobilisations combined with movement. *NZ J Physiother.* 4:1992.
23. Mulligan, BR. Pain release phenomenon techniques – PRPS. *NZ J Physiother.* 4:1989.
24. Cyriax, J. *Textbook of Orthopaedic Medicine, Volume One.* 8th ed. London: Bailliere Tindall; 1982.
25. Maitland GD, Hengeveld E, Banks K, English K. *Maitland's Vertebral Manipulation.* 6th ed. Woburn, MA: Butterworth-Heinemann; 2001.
26. APTA. *Guide to Physical Therapist Practice.* Rev., 2nd ed. Alexandria, VA: American Physical Therapy Association; 2003.
27. Exelby L. Mobilization with movement: a personal view. *J Physiother.* 1995;81:724-729.
28. Abbot J, Patla C, Jensen R. The initial effects of an elbow mobilization with movement technique on grip strength in subjects with lateral epicondylagia. *Man Ther.* 2001;6:163-169.
29. Vicenzino B, Paunmail A, Buratowski S, Wright A. Specific manipulative therapy treatment for chronic lateral epicondylalgia produces uniquely characteristic hypoalgesia. *Man Ther.* 2001;6:205-212.
30. Kochar M, Dogra K. Effectiveness of a specific physiotherapy regimen on patients with tennis elbow. *Physiother.* 2002;88:333-341.

31. Paungmali A, Vicenzino B, Smith M. Hypoalgesia induced by elbow manipulation in lateral epicondylalgia does not exhibit tolerance. *J Pain*. 2003;4:448-454.
32. Paungmali A, O'Leary S, Souvlis T, Vicenzino B. Naloxone fails to antagonize initial hypoalgesic effect of a manual therapy treatment for lateral epicondylalgia. *J Manipulative Physiol Ther*. 2004;27:180-185.
33. Zusman M, Edwards B, Donaghy A. Investigation of a proposed mechanism for the relief of spinal pain with passive joint movement. *Manual Medicine*. 1989;4:58-61.
34. Vicenzino B, O'Callaghan J, Kermode F, Wright A. An investigation of the interrelationship between manipulative therapy-induced hypoalgesia and sympathoexcitation. *J Manipulative Physiol Ther*. 1998;21:448-453.
35. Sterling M, Jull G, Wright A. Cervical mobilization: concurrent effects on pain, sympathetic nervous system activity and motor activity. *Man Ther*. 2001;6:72-81.
36. Vicenzino B, Collins D, Benson H, Wright A. An investigation of the interrelationship between manipulative therapy-induced hypoalgesia and sympathoexcitation. *J Manipulative Physiol Ther*. 1998;21:448-453.
37. Paungmali A, O'Leary S, Souvlis T, Vicenzino B. Hypoalgesic and sympathoexcitatory effects of mobilization with movement of lateral epicondylalgia. *Phys Ther*. 2003;83:374-383.
38. Stephens G. Lateral epicondylitis. *J Man Manip Ther*. 1995;3:50-58.
39. Vicenzino B, Wright A. Effects of a novel manipulative physiotherapy technique on tennis elbow: a single case study. *Man Ther*. 1995;1:30-35.
40. McLean S, Naish R, Reed L, Urry S, Vicenzino B. A pilot study of the manual force levels required to produce manipulation induced hypoalgesia. *Clin Biomech*. 2002;17:394-308.
41. Abbott J. Mobilization with movement applied to the elbow affects shoulder range of movement in subjects with lateral epicondylalgia. *Man Ther*. 2001;6:170-177.
42. Mulligan BR. The painful dysfunction shoulder. A new treatment approach using 'mobilization with movement.' *NZ J Physiother*. 2003;31:140-142.
43. Folk B. Traumatic thumb injury management using mobilization with movement. *Man Ther*. 2001;6:178-182.
44. Backstrom K. Mobilization with movement as an adjunct intervention in a patient with complicated DeQuervain's tenosynovitis: a case report. *J Orthop Sports Phys Ther*. 2002;32:86-97.
45. Hsieh C, Vicenzino B, Yang C, Hu M, Yang C. Mulligan's mobilization with movement for the thumb: a single case report using magnetic resonance imaging to evaluate the positional fault hypothesis. *Man Ther*. 2002;7:44-49.
46. Carson P. The rehabilitation of a competitive swimmer with an asymmetrical breaststroke movement pattern. *Man Ther*. 1999;4:100-106.
47. Tanigawa MC. Comparison of the hold relax procedure and passive mobilization on increasing muscle length. *Phys Ther*. 1972;52:725-735.
48. Pollard H, War G. A study of two stretching techniques for improving hip flexion range of motion. *J Manipulative Physiol Ther*. 1997;20:443-447.
49. Hanten WP, Chandler SD. Effects of myofascial leg pull and sagittal plane isometric contract relax techniques on passive straight leg raise angle. *J Orthop Sports Phys Ther*. 1994;20:138-144.
50. Kavanagh J. Is there a positional fault at the inferior tibiofibular in patients with acute or chronic ankle sprains compared to normals? *Man Ther*. 1999;4:19-24.
51. Collins N, Teys P, Vicenzino B. The initial effects of a Mulligan's mobilization with movement technique on dorsiflexion and pain in subacute ankle sprains. *Man Ther*. 2004;9:77-82.
52. Horton S. Acute locked thoracic spine: treatment with a modified SNAG. *Man Ther*. 2002;7:103-107.
53. Aiken DL, Vaughn D. The use of functional and traditional mobilization interventions in a patient with chronic thoracic pain: a case report. *J Man Manip Ther*. 2013;21(3):134-138.
54. Exelby L. The locked lumbar facet joint: intervention using mobilizations with movement. *Man Ther*. 2001;6:116-121.
55. Moutzouri M, Billis E, Strimpakos N, Kottika P, Oldham JA. The effects of the Mulligan sustained natural apophyseal glide (SNAG) mobilisation in the lumbar flexion range of asymptomatic subjects as measured by the Zebris CMS20 3-D motion analysis system. *BMC Musculoskeletal Disorders*. 2008:9;1-9.
56. Billis E. Mulligan's "SNAG" Mobilization Techniques: A Clinical Approach for non-specific Low Back Pain. *Physiotherapy Issues*. 2010:6(2);73-81.

The Canadian Approach

Jim Meadows, BSc., PT, FCAMPT

Chapter Objectives

At the conclusion of this chapter, the reader will be able to:

- Briefly review the history of orthopaedic manual physical therapy in Canada.
- Identify the rationale, purpose, and techniques of the differential diagnostic examination.
- Identify the rationale, purpose, and techniques of the biomechanical examination.
- Integrate and analyze the data generated from the differential diagnostic examination either to generate a provisional examination and management plan or to determine the need for biomechanical testing.
- Integrate and analyze the data generated from the biomechanical examination to generate a diagnosis concerning the movement status of the spinal segment or peripheral joint, such as hypomobility (pathomechanical, pericapsular, or myofascial); hypermobility

(irritable or nonirritable); or instability (ligamentous or segmental).

- Identify the rationale and need for nonmanual interventions such as mechanical traction; specific exercise prescription for hypomobility, pain and instability; electrophysiological agents; ergonomic advice and modifications; and activities of daily living advice and modifications.
- Identify the rationale and need for manual interventions such as passive mobilization for pain and hypomobility, manipulative therapy, segmental and general proprioceptive neuromuscular facilitation (PNF) techniques for movement reeducation in cases of instability and hypomobility.

INTRODUCTION

Orthopaedic manual physical therapy (OMPT) may best be defined as an entire approach to musculoskeletal dysfunction rather than a series of techniques, whose purpose it is to mobilize or stabilize a particular joint or segment in order that other techniques, particularly specific exercise, may have a more optimal effect. The Canadian approach to OMPT claims its inception to date back to 1972 when the first meeting of, what would eventually become the *International Federation of Manipulative Physical Therapists (IFOMPT),* was held in the Canary Islands. Upon returning to Canada, these qualified manual therapists organized a series of manual therapy courses that became the foundation of this approach. Since its beginning, the *Canadian Physiotherapy Association,*

through its Orthopaedic Division, has sponsored courses and certification examinations in OMPT that have been standardized nationally. Canada has been a full member of IFOMPT for two decades and has established long-term residencies in OMPT. Several prominent Canadian manual physical therapists were involved in the leadership of IFOMPT and in the early development of the Canadian approach to OMPT. Among them, were the late *David Lamb*, *Cliff Fowler*, *John Oldham*, *Alun Morgan*, *Jim McGregor*, and others. The later development of this approach was credited to the work of several manual physical therapists, such as *Bob Sydenham*, past president of IFOMPT, *Erl Pettman*, *Diane Lee*, *Marilyn Atkins*, *D'Arcy Bain*, *Rick Adams*, *Wendy Aspinal*, and *Jim Meadows*, author of this chapter.

"Manual therapy is an entire approach to musculoskeletal dysfunction, not just a series of techniques, whose purpose is to mobilize or stabilize a particular joint or spinal segment so other techniques can have an optimal effect."

-J. Meadows

The eclectic nature of the Canadian approach and the organized and obsessive attention to clinical reasoning are, perhaps, its most distinguishing characteristics. Early in its development, the Canadian approach embraced such interventions as muscle energy, muscle balancing, peripheral nerve mobilization, Maitland's[1] oscillatory mobilization, Norwegian concepts of biomechanics and locking techniques,[2,3] medical exercise training concepts,[4] cranial osteopathy, craniosacral, dural release, Janda's[5] and Sahrmann's[6] concepts related to muscle tightness, MacConaill's[7] approach to biomechanics and taping procedures, and Cyriax's[8] system of examination. Organized clinical reasoning in the Canadian approach was initially in the form of applied anatomy and pathology as advocated by Cyriax.[8] The introduction of what is known as the *quadrant courses*, first by Pettman and later with Meadows, brought concepts of clinical reasoning to the performance of functional activities and biomechanics.

QUESTIONS *for* REFLECTION

The *Canadian approach* to orthopaedic manual physical therapy is eclectic in nature.

- What are the advantages of adopting an approach to OMPT that integrates concepts and techniques from a variety of different approaches?

The *Canadian approach* is founded on a body of knowledge that incorporates the current best evidence from basic science constructs. To facilitate clinical application, basic science is blended with the current best evidence from clinical research, clinical experience, expert opinion, and face validity. The overarching theme of this approach is its preoccupation with clinical reasoning and de-emphasis on the adoption of any particular cadre of manual techniques.

QUESTIONS *for* REFLECTION

- What is the difference between *criterion* and *construct* validity?
- Is one type of validity more valuable than the other?
- Most of the evidence supporting the *Canadian approach* concepts have construct validity, but lack criterion validity. How might this impact your view and use of this approach in your clinical practice?

The purpose of this chapter is to delineate the standard procedures of examination and intervention germane to this approach, as expressed by the **North American Institute of Orthopedic Manual Therapy (NAIOMT).** The concepts and principles covered in this chapter will be applied primarily to the lumbar spine for the purpose of demonstrating the clinical utility of this approach, but are applicable to all regions of the body. The concepts and content in this chapter are based on the previously published home-study course sponsored by the **Orthopaedic Section** of the **American Physical Therapy Association (APTA)** and are used with permission.[9]

PRINCIPLES OF EXAMINATION
The Subjective Examination

The Canadian approach elevates the *subjective examination* to a level that possesses greater value than the objective examination. This is especially true when it comes to identifying the presence of serious pathologies through red flags. This system espouses the adoption of the *hypothetico-deductive model* of reasoning that encourages the use of a clinical decision-making algorithm. Through meticulous inquiry, the manual physical therapist arrives at a working hypothesis that is then used to guide the remainder of the examination. The objective examination subserves this working hypothesis by either supporting or refuting its veracity by using specific testing procedures. If refuted, another hypothesis should take its place and then be tested using specific questions and physical examination procedures. Final proof for the validity of the chosen hypothesis is evidenced by a successful outcome. The information that must be obtained during the subjective portion of the examination is listed in Box 11-1.

The Objective Examination

The *objective examination* for the individual with musculoskeletal dysfunction falls into two major components. First, the manual physical therapist performs a **differential diagnostic examination** to reach a definitive diagnosis. This examination is followed by a **biomechanical examination** to determine the motion status of the involved joints (Box 11-2).

The differential diagnostic examination used within this approach is primarily based on information obtained during the detailed history and the results of **selective tissue tension (STT)** testing, as developed by James Cyriax (see Chapter 5).[8] This approach does not, for the most part, offer new testing procedures but rather sequences and assigns new meaning to tests that have been described elsewhere. The overriding principle of the systematic objective examination is based on an understanding of anatomy and pathology. The validity of selective tissue tension testing has recently been questioned.[10,11] However, the methodology, assumptions, external validity, and the conclusions drawn from this evidence still provide direction for the manual physical therapist.

Cyriax divided the neuromusculoskeletal system into **contractile tissue, inert tissue,** and **conduction tissue.** These

Box 11-1 INFORMATION OBTAINED DURING THE SUBJECTIVE EXAMINATION

- Pain:
  - Type (neuropathic or somatic)
  - Location and distribution (segmental, multisegmental, nonsegmental)
  - Onset (sudden or gradual)
  - Progression (worsening, stable, or improving)
  - Severity (mild, moderate, severe, excruciating)
  - Aggravating and relieving factors
- Paresthesia:
  - Location and distribution (segmental, multisegmental, cord, peripheral nerve)
  - Severity (mild, moderate, severe, excruciating)
  - Aggravating and relieving factors
- Central nervous system:
  - Type (visual, auditory, taste, smell, etc.)
  - Location and distribution (brainstem, cord, cerebral)
- Dizziness:
  - Type (vertigo, oscillopsia, presyncope, disequilibrium)
  - Severity (mild, moderate or profound (sit down or fall down)
  - Persistent or nonpersistent
  - Directionally consistent if vertigo
  - Onset (traumatic, nontraumatic)

- Aggravating and relieving factors (medications, head versus body movement etc.)
- Related to other symptoms (headaches, neurological symptoms)
- Pain irritability:
  - How long does the pain last after a given trigger? Mild trigger with severe long-lasting pain suggests high levels of irritability that is probably related to inflammation, whereas strong stress with mild short-duration pain is probably mechanical in nature, and of course all stops in between.
- Relationships of multiple symptoms:
  - Associate and dissociate. Are they from the same or different sources? Are they aggravated and relieved by the same triggers? Are they progressing with each other, or is one or more getting better while the others are getting worse?
- Behavior:
  - How do the symptoms respond to daily stresses? Are particular times of day worse? Is it better at work or during leisure activities? Are there trigger and relieving factors? What are the effects of drugs, etc.?

Box 11-2 Quick Notes! TWO COMPONENTS OF THE CANADIAN APPROACH EXAMINATION

1. **The differential diagnostic examination:** Designed to reach a definitive diagnosis, including identification of pathological conditions that are outside the purview of physical therapy

2. **The biomechanical examination:** Designed to determine the movement characteristics of involved joints and associated structures

tests may provide misleading results for the examiner, and the interpretation of these findings must be carefully considered. To test contractile tissues, Cyriax suggested a submaximal isometric contraction in midrange with progression to a maximal contraction as needed.[8] A more efficient method for using maximal contractions involves performance in the stretched position, which may be used in routine cases.

Inert, or noncontractile, tissues are the tissues mainly affected by passive movement and ligament stress testing. The most provocative tests for these tissues are passive movements, with concentration on end-feel and reproduction of pain.

In addition to determining the ability of neural tissues to conduct neural impulses, these structures must also be examined for irritability and mobility. The tests for the latter are provocative passive movement tests (see Chapter 19), whereas those for the former include muscle strength testing, sensation testing, and reflex testing.

The Differential Diagnostic Examination
Active Movement Testing

Active movement involves both contractile and inert tissues and requires normal neurological function. An abnormal result suggests a problem in one or more of these tissues. Specifically, these tests evaluate range of motion, patterns of restriction, quality of motion, symptom reproduction, and willingness to move.

Hypermobility, or even instability, may be present in a joint where a normal degree of active movement seems to be available. Symptoms, or fear of symptoms, may cause patients to actively limit their motion, causing them to present with movement that appears to be normal. These movement aberrations may not be identified until passive **overpressure** is applied. Overpressure will reveal less than expected resistance to further motion at end range and may produce symptoms or apprehension from the patient.

If a reduction in mobility is identified, an appreciation of the pattern of restriction (i.e., capsular versus noncapsular) is noted. There is debate in the literature regarding the concept of **capsular** and **noncapsular patterns**.[10,12–16] The capsular pattern of restriction suggests the presence of arthritis or arthrosis within the joint. A noncapsular pattern suggests the presence of an extra-articular restriction.

Movement quality is observed as the patient moves into the desired motion and as the patient returns to the neutral starting position. When testing spinal motion, the presence of an angulation, an area of increased mobility that is often particularly noticeable during extension or side bending, may suggest the presence of a segment with excessive mobility.

Passive Movement Testing

Passive movement testing includes range of motion and stress testing as well as *neuromeningeal tests*, such as the straight leg raise and prone knee bend tests (see Chapter 19). While passive movement testing predominantly tests inert tissues, these tests will also produce tension within the periarticular contractile tissues. Therefore, it is critical that the results of passive movement testing be considered in light of other test findings. Examination of passive movement includes an appreciation of the range of available motion, patterns of restriction, reproduction of symptoms, end-feel, apprehension, and intra-articular joint sounds.

Most approaches advocate the application of overpressure only when pain is not produced during passive movement testing. However, the primary reason to perform passive movement testing is to evaluate **end-feel**. When applying overpressure, the nature of the symptoms determines how aggressive forces may be applied during intervention (Table 11-1).

CLINICAL PILLAR

Unlike other approaches, application of **overpressure** at the end ranges of painful, as well as painless, movements are advocated to determine the nature of the end-feel. If overpressure is performed only during painless movement, the examiner may miss important information. Most end-feels suggesting acute or serious pathology are found within the painful ranges of motion.

Resistance Testing

Franklin[11] challenged the construct validity of resistance testing on an individual with exercise-induced muscle soreness. This subject did not have a documented contractile lesion; therefore, the generalizability of these findings to actual patient populations is dubious.

Despite Cyriax's recommendations to fully challenge the musculotendinous unit, a maximum contraction in the lengthened position must be elicited. It is important for the clinician to be aware of any reproduction of symptoms and to perform a bilateral comparison of force output as opposed to evaluating the absolute force output of each muscle individually. For this reason, it is important that the manual physical therapist performs resistance testing in the same fashion bilaterally.

CLINICAL PILLAR

During resistance testing, in addition to testing muscle performance in the neutral position, as advocated by Cyriax, the manual therapist should also test the muscle in its maximally lengthened position. Testing in both positions will provide more accurate information regarding the status of the muscle. This position may place inert structures on tension and may result in comparatively less force from the muscle. Therefore, it is important to test the muscle in the exact fashion bilaterally and to compare force output rather than consider the absolute force generated from each muscle individually.

The results of resistance testing should reflect the degree of damage to the contractile tissue. If the isometric test in the lengthened position is positive, then the test should be repeated in neutral to ascertain the degree of association between test results and the degree of damage. Because of the anatomical and functional overlap between contractile and inert tissue, differential diagnosis based on resistance testing alone is challenging (Table 11-2).

There are four primary conclusions that may be drawn from isometric resistance testing as defined by Cyriax[8] (see Chapter 5). Testing that results in a painful and weak response

Table 11-1	Pathological End-Feels With Descriptors and Potential Contributors	
END-FEEL	**DESCRIPTOR**	**POTENTIAL CONTRIBUTORS**
Hard capsular	Stiff	Ligamentous or capsular adhesions, scarring, or hypertrophy
Soft capsular	Not stiff enough	Hypermobility or ligamentous tearing if found on a stress tests
Bony	Unyielding	Bone on bone, osteophytosis, fracture angulation
Springy	Rebound	Meniscal derangement, loose body, nuclear prolapse or extrusion
Early range spasm	Abrupt sudden stop early in the range; usually associated with pain	Arthritis, grade 2 muscle tear, fracture, neoplasm
Late range spasm	Abrupt stop or muscle flicker at the end of range; may not be associated with pain.	Irritable hypermobility
Empty	The therapist stops the test because of the extreme pain being experienced by the patient.	Serious pathology

Table 11–2	Matching the Patient's Level of Acuity With Manual Intervention Based on the Relationship Between Pain and Resistance During Passive Movement		

PAIN/RESISTANCE ASSOCIATION	ACUITY	MANUAL INTERVENTION
Pain and no resistance (empty end-feel)	Possible serious pathology	None
Constant unvarying pain	Hyperacute	None
Pain before resistance	Very acute	Sub-barrier techniques (Grade I or II mobilizations)
Pain at the same time as resistance	Acute	Sub-barrier techniques (Grade I or II mobilizations)
Pain after resistance	Sub or nonacute	Barrier techniques (Grade III or IV mobilizations)
Pain and no resistance	Nonacute, stiff	Stretch barrier techniques (Grade III++ or IV++)

is suggestive of a grade two tear, hyperacute arthritis, fracture near the insertion of the contractile tissue, or possibly, bone cancer.

Spinal segmental tissues (i.e., facet joint capsule, intervertebral disc) are typically more vulnerable to damaging forces than is the paraspinal musculature. If symptoms are reproduced with active or passive movement testing, it is important to avoid isolated resistance at the end range of motion as the resulting compression may produce more damage to the segmental structures. In such cases, resistance testing should always be performed submaximally in the neutral position when examining a patient with spinal dysfunction.

CLINICAL PILLAR

When examining patients with spinal dysfunction, resistance testing should be performed submaximally in the neutral position. Performing isolated resistance testing to spinal segments at end range in joints that are painful during active and passive movement testing may produce compressive forces that lead to further damage.

Neurological Testing

Compression of the spinal nerve or nerve root is a common sequela of low back and neck pain. Clinically detectable and relevant neurological deficits may be challenging to definitively ascertain and often suggest the presence of large impingement forces. Testing of these structures does not differ substantially from those used in other approaches, the details of which are described elsewhere (Table 11-3).

Special Testing

Special tests are performed when more information is required to make a definitive diagnosis. These tests are usually the last component of the examination to be performed and are therefore used to either confirm or refute the working hypothesis. There is no particular construct advocated within this approach (Table 11-4).

The Biomechanical Examination

Movement dysfunction through an appreciation of normal and abnormal joint kinematics is the focus of this portion of the examination.[1] Within this approach, the patient's symptomatic

Table 11–3	Segmental Neurological Tests		

LEVEL	MYOTOME	DERMATOME	REFLEX
L1 and 2	Hip flexion	Upper outer groin and thigh	None
L3	Knee extension	Medial lower thigh and knee	Adductor magnus and quadriceps
L4	Ankle dorsiflexion and inversion	Medial lower anterior tibia	Tibialis anterior
L5	Great toe extension and eversion	Medial dorsum of foot	Extensor digitorum brevis and peroneus longus
S1	Ankle plantar flexion and eversion	Lateral foot and two toes	Achilles tendon and peroneus longus
S2	Knee flexion and hip extension	Lateral posterior thigh	Hamstring
S3	None	Medial upper and midthighs	None
S4	None (bladder and bowel weakness)	Saddle area	Anal wink
Spinal Cord	Extrasegmental and nonspecific	Anywhere in the legs	Babinski, clonus, hyperreflexia

Table 11–4	Examination Procedure Sequence as Determined by Patient Position to Improve Efficiency and Patient Comfort

PATIENT POSITION	EXAMINATION PROCEDURES
Standing	Observation Trunk flexion, extension, side flexion, and rotation movements overpressure Isometric tests S1 myotome (plantar flexion)
Sitting	Trunk rotation, sitting straight leg raise, and slump test
Supine	Straight leg raise and adjunct test L1, L2, L3, L4, L5, S1, S3 dermatomes L1, L2, L4, L5 myotomes Quadriceps, adductor magnus, tibialis anterior, peroneus, extensor digitorum, hamstrings, and Achilles deep tendon reflexes Cord reflexes Primary anterior sacroiliac stress test Compression, traction
Side lying	Primary posterior sacroiliac stress test L5 myotome (abduction)
Prone	Torsion, posteroanterior pressures S2 myotome (knee flexion and hip extension or gluteal tightening) S2 dermatome

response to movement is not a necessary ingredient in the diagnosis of movement dysfunction and may complicate such a diagnosis. To establish the efficacy of manual physical therapy, however, improvement in the patient's symptoms and function must be documented.

CLINICAL PILLAR

Unlike other approaches, the *Canadian Approach* de-emphasizes the use of patient symptomatic response to reach conclusions during movement testing. Patient response may confound results. The efficacy of manual interventions, however, is based on improvement in patient symptoms and function.

There are two main types of hypomobility commonly encountered by the manual physical therapist. **Articular hypomobility** leads to a decrease in range in both **passive physiologic intervertebral movement (PPIVM)** and **passive arthrokinematic (accessory) intervertebral movement (PAIVM)**. There are two potential causes of articular hypomobility. **Pericapsular restrictions**, owing to inextensibility of the periarticular tissues, may cause such restrictions, as well as a **subluxed joint**, which is independent of tissue extensibility.

The origin of articular hypomobility is determined by end-feel, with the pericapsular restriction producing a *hard capsular end-feel* and the subluxation producing a jammed or *pathomechanical end-feel*. The pathomechanical end-feel is more clearly identified when more specific segmental movement tests are used during the biomechanical examination. This end-feel is abrupt, nearly hard, with a slight springy feel.

Extra articular hypomobility is typically due to inextensibility of muscle secondary to scarring or adhesions or due to an increase in muscle tone. Extra-articular hypomobility results in a restriction during PPIVM testing without a decrease noted during PAIVM testing (Box 11-3).

Hypermobility is defined as an increase in physiologic range of motion that is beyond the joint's normal range. If pathologic, the joint is defined as possessing instability. If the observed hypermobility is *nonirritable*, then the excessive range can be appreciated along with a soft, capsular end-feel. If the condition is irritable, the excessive range of motion cannot be observed as protective spasm prevents further entry into this range. In such cases, joint hypermobility may present clinically as a hypomobile condition. Hypermobility must, therefore, be deduced by the presence of muscle spasm at the end range of normal motion (Box 11-4).

Instability may be further defined as increase in the range of the neutral zone of the joint. The neutral zone is the area within

Box 11-3 Quick Notes! TWO TYPES OF *HYPO*MOBILITY AND THEIR CLINICAL FEATURES

1. Articular hypomobility:
- Decreased range during PPIVM *and* PAIVM testing
- Caused by pericapsular restriction (hard capsular end-feel) or a subluxed joint (jammed, pathomechanical end-feel)

2. Extra articular hypomobility:
- Decrease range during PPIVM testing *only*
- Caused by inextensibility of muscle due to scarring, adhesions, increased tone

Box 11-4 Quick Notes! TWO TYPES OF *HYPER*MOBILITY AND THEIR CLINICAL FEATURES

1. Nonirritable hypermobility:
- Presents with increased physiologic range that is appreciated along with a soft, capsular end-feel

2. Irritable hypermobility:
- Patient presents with normal or reduced physiologic range as the result of protective muscle spasm preventing further entry into the range.
- Hypermobility is deduced by the presence of muscle spasm at the end range of normal motion.

a range of motion in which there is no resistance to that motion. Perhaps a more useful definition of instability would be the presence of motion where no appreciable motion should exist.

QUESTIONS *for* REFLECTION

- How is it possible for *hypermobility*, or even *instability*, to be present in a joint that demonstrates normal active range of motion (AROM)?
- What strategies might the manual therapist use to uncover the presence of any existing hypermobility?
- Why is this information so critical for the therapist when developing the plan of care?

Ligamentous instability results from rupture or laxity of the ligamentous support system. Spinal **segmental instability** occurs as a result of degeneration of the zygapophyseal joint surfaces and intervertebral discs of the spine. Ligamentous instability is typically detected during the differential diagnostic examination. However, segmental instability must be determined from the biomechanical examination and the patient's history (Box 11-5). Table 11-5 lists the various biomechanical movement dysfunctions and their principle clinical characteristics.

Box 11-5 Quick Notes! TWO TYPES OF INSTABILITY AND THEIR CLINICAL FEATURES

1. Ligamentous instability:
- The result of rupture or laxity of the ligamentous support system
- Identified through the differential diagnostic examination

2. Segmental instability:
- The result of degeneration of the zygapophyseal joint surfaces and intervertebral discs of the spine
- Identified through the biomechanical examination and the patient history

---

When applying these concepts to the spine, it has long been documented that it is possible for a patient's gross range of motion to appear normal while intervertebral motion testing reveals abnormalities. Therefore, the biomechanical examination is designed to use the concepts of normal joint kinematics to make determinations regarding joint mobility. In the spine, the biomechanical examination of the spinal segment involves testing *PPIVM*, *PAIVM*, and the stability of the segment through **segmental stability tests (SST)** (Box 11-6). The purpose of the biomechanical examination is to generate a profile of the movement characteristics of the segment or joint.

When evaluating the mobility of a spinal segment, it is most valid to compare the degree of mobility between adjacent segments as opposed to evaluating a segment's range against a normal population. Segmental comparison, although difficult, is possible for the more experienced clinician.

QUESTIONS *for* REFLECTION

- When evaluating spinal segmental mobility, what is the best gauge for determining normalcy?
- Why is comparison to a hypothetical normal range deemed to be erroneous?
- Why is it imperative that the manual therapist fully understand the etiology of the observed restriction?

In addition to the range of segmental mobility, end-feel must be evaluated. It is imperative that the manual physical therapist fully understands the etiology of the observed restriction. If hypomobility is identified, the type of hypomobility must be determined before manual interventions can be applied. For example, if flexion is limited by inextensible muscle tissue, stretching interventions that target the restricted tissue is indicated. Conversely, an articular restriction such as an adherent joint capsule requires joint glide mobilization.

PPIVMs consist of isolated segmental tests that explore the range and end-feel of various combined (multiplanar) or uncombined (uniplanar) physiologic movements. When combined

---

Table 11-5	Biomechanical Movement Dysfunctions and Their Principle Clinical Characteristics	
DYSFUNCTION	**DEFINED**	**PRINCIPLE EXAMINATION FINDINGS**
Extra-articular (myofascial) hypomobility	Inextensibility of muscle or tendon caused by hypertonicity, adhesions or scarring	Decreased PPIVMs but normal PAIVMs
Articular (pericapsular) hypomobility	Inextensibility of joint capsule or ligaments	Decreased PPIVMs and decreased PAIVMs with hard capsular (stiff) end-feel
Articular (subluxation, pathomechanical) hypomobility	All tissues are extensible, but the joint is jammed at one end of its range.	Decreased PPIVMs and PAIVMs with a pathomechanical (jammed) end-feel
Nonirritable hypermobility	Increased range of physiological motion	PPIVMs excessive with soft capsular end-feel
Irritable hypermobility	Normal range of physiological motion	PPIVMs normal range with spasm end-feel
Instability	The presence of movement where no movement should exist	Nonphysiologic movements (movements that should not exist) are present

Box 11-6 BIOMECHANICAL MOVEMENT TESTS AND THEIR CLINICAL USE

1. Passive physiological intervertebral movement testing (PPIVM):
   - Identifies the presence of physiologic movement (i.e., flexion, side bending) and/or accessory movement (i.e., glide) restrictions.
   - The movement restriction may be articular or extra-articular and does not differentiate which is present.

2. Passive arthrokinematic (accessory) intervertebral movement testing (PAIVM):
   - Identifies an accessory movement restriction.
   - Identifies the presence of an articular restriction versus an extra-articular restriction.

3. Segmental stability test (SST):
   - Identifies movements that are not expected to exist at an appreciable degree.
   - Identifies the presence of abnormal joint play in each direction.

movements are used as PPIVMs, test movements will maximize zygapophyseal joint motion. The potential movements that are used during both combined and uncombined physiologic movement testing are displayed in Table 11-6.

Table 11-7 displays the joint and specific movement that is tested during each combined movement pattern that may be used during PPIVM motion testing. Unlike the cervical spine, where good consensus regarding coupled movement exists among clinicians, lumbar spine coupling mechanics is controversial. In addition, there is little agreement between leading clinicians and radiographic[17] or cadaveric[18] evidence regarding such mechanics. During testing, the examiner may either impose a rotation or allow rotation to occur naturally in response to the primary motion. The component of the test that determines the

Table 11-6   Uncombined (Uniplanar) and Combined (Multi planar) Movements Utilized During PPIVM Testing

SYMMETRICAL (UNCOMBINED/ UNIPLANAR) MOVEMENT TESTING	ASYMMETRICAL (COMBINED/ MULTIPLANAR) MOVEMENT TESTING
Flexion	Flexion-right side bending-rotation
Extension	Flexion-left side bending-rotation
Right side bending	Extension-right side bending-rotation
Left side bending	Extension- left side bending-rotation
Right rotation	
Left rotation	

Table 11-7   Combined Movement PPIVMs and the Joint and Movement That Is Being Tested

COMBINED MOVEMENT	JOINT/MOTION TESTED
Flexion-right side bending	Left zygapophyseal flexion
Flexion-left side bending	Right zygapophyseal flexion
Extension-right side bending	Right zygapophyseal extension
Extension-left side bending	Left zygapophyseal extension

degree of flexion or extension is side bending. For example, if a segment side-bends to the right, the superior facet of the right zygapophyseal joint glides inferiorly, or extends, while the left facet glides superiorly, or flexes. If right side bending is imposed on flexion, then the left facet joint is maximally flexed while the right facet is not extended but rather moving toward neutral. If the segment was extended and right side-bent, the right facet joint would be maximally extended while the left facet would be moving toward neutral.

If hypermobility is detected from PPIVM testing, PAIVM testing, which is used to determine the type of hypomobility, is not indicated. In cases of hypermobility, the therapist endeavors to identify the presence of instability through *segmental stability testing (SST)*. Segmental stability testing uses movements that are not expected to exist, such as pure rotation of the segment, anterior, posterior, and transverse shear forces. The objective of SST is to assess the presence of abnormal joint play in each direction.

The PPIVMs, PAIVMs, and SSTs are carried out in non-weight-bearing. In side lying, lumbar PPIVM testing occurs by flexing, extending, side bending, and rotating the patient by using the legs and/or pelvis as levers while the segment being tested is palpated for motion and end-feel. If deficits in normal movement are noted during PPIVM testing, the appropriate PAIVM is tested; if excessive motion is palpated, SSTs are performed to rule out instability. Figure 11-1 displays a decision-making algorithm that uses PPIVM, PAIVM, and SST testing.

Symmetrical movement dysfunctions, tests, and interventions have been identified as *uncombined/uniplanar* while **asymmetrical movement** dysfunctions, tests, and interventions have been identified as *combined/multiplanar or triplanar* (Box 11-7). Perhaps, better terminology for these dysfunctions would be *symmetrical* for dysfunctions that are equal bilaterally and *asymmetrical* for dysfunctions that are unequal bilaterally, or unilateral, in nature. The most important reason for using such terminology is to indicate whether the dysfunction is on both sides of the segment (symmetrical) or only/to a greater extent on one side of the segment (asymmetrical). These terms are routinely used within this approach (Table 11-8).

Symmetrical (Uniplanar) Movement Tests

For examination of symmetrical movement dysfunctions, PPIVM mobility is first assessed to identify physiologic movement restrictions. Once identified, more specific PAIVM testing

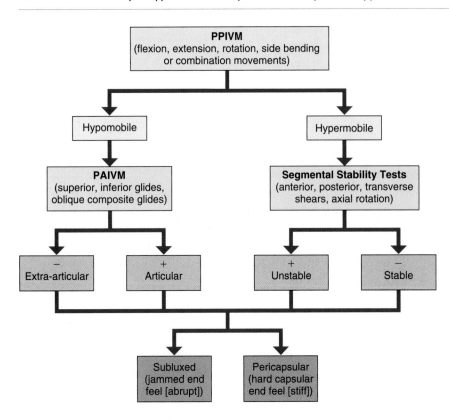

FIGURE 11-1 Decision-making algorithm for determining the movement characteristics of the joint using PPIVM, PAIVM, and SST testing.

Box 11-7 Quick Notes! PATTERNS OF MOVEMENT RESTRICTIONS

1. Symmetrical movement dysfunctions:
- Identifies the presence of physiologic movement (i.e., flexion, side bending) and/or accessory movement (i.e., glide) restrictions
- The movement restriction may be articular or extra-articular and does not differentiate which is present.

2. Asymmetrical movement dysfunctions:
- Identifies the presence of an accessory movement restriction
- Identifies the presence of an articular restriction versus an extra-articular restriction

---

is used to identify the presence of accessory movement restrictions. When using this method of examination, a more complete profile of the movement characteristics of the segment can be obtained.

Flexion

In side lying, the therapist holds the patient's thighs against his or her own thigh with the patient knees flexed. The neutral position of the spine for flexion/extension is found by palpating the L5 spinous process and alternately flexing and extending the hips until movement is felt. The therapist maintains the hold on the patient's thighs and palpates the interspinous space. The degree of interspinous separation is compared to the segment above as the test is carried out sequentially from level to level.

If reduced motion is found, the superior spinous process is stabilized while the inferior vertebra is moved and end-feel is appreciated. PAIVM is tested by stabilizing the inferior vertebra and gliding the superior segment superoanteriorly and comparing its end-feel with adjacent segments.

Extension

In the same side-lying position and with the spine in neutral, the therapist palpates the interspinous space, but this time extends the patient's hips and evaluates the closing of the two processes by comparing it with the segment above. If reduced closing is noted, the superior processes are stabilized by holding it caudally as the inferior is flexed (thereby extending the segment) until the end-feel can be appreciated. If reduced motion is present, PAIVM testing is performed by stabilizing the superior vertebra by holding it inferiorly and gliding the inferior vertebra superoanteriorly and comparing its end-feel with the segments above and below.

Rotation

Left rotation is tested with the patient in the right side-lying position and right rotation with the patient in the left side-lying position. In side lying, the neutral position of flexion/extension and rotation is found, and the underside of two adjacent spinous processes is palpated with the therapist's caudal hand. The patient's trunk is rotated by the therapist's contact at the patient's anterior shoulder with his or her forearm, which is placed under the patient's uppermost arm. The pelvis is prevented from rotating by the stabilization of the caudal-most forearm at the posterior hip. The therapist feels for the superior spinous process of the segment to move downward toward the plinth. If both spinous processes move simultaneously, hypomobility

Table 11-8	**Key Descriptors for Identification of Symmetrical Versus Asymmetrical Dysfunctions**	

DESCRIPTORS	SYMMETRICAL DYSFUNCTIONS	ASYMMETRICAL DYSFUNCTIONS
Motion Characteristics	Hypomobile, hypermobile, or unstable	Hypomobile, hypermobile, or unstable
Sagittal Symmetry/Asymmetry	Equally dysfunctional on both sides into flexion or extension	Dysfunctional into flexion or extension on one side of the segment more than the other
Transverse and Frontal Symmetry/Asymmetry	Rotation and side flexion affected equally on both sides	Rotation and side flexions are not affected equally and may be affected on one or both sides, depending on how it couples and the dysfunctions present
Positional Findings	No positional findings for those who look	Positional findings include ERSR, FRSR, ERSL, or FRSL or any combination
Etiology	Causes include fixed postural deficits, acute pain states, bilateral traumatic or systemic arthritis, acute fractures, bilateral hypermobility or instability	Causes include unilateral zygapophyseal joint arthritis, arthrosis, fibrosis, disc protrusions and herniations, unilateral myofascial restriction, unilateral hypermobility or instability

is present. Too much movement of the superior process, when compared with segments above and below, suggests hypermobility. By stabilizing the lower spinous process and rotating the superior, the segment's end-feel may be appreciated.

If reduced movement occurs, PAIVMs are tested by taking the segment into its maximum rotation and carrying out an oblique posteroanterior pressure toward the feet and toward the head to assess the glides of both facet joints. PAIVM testing during rotation involves flexion of one facet and extension of the other.

Side Bending

Right side bending is tested with the patient in the left side-lying position and left side bending is tested with the patient in the right side-lying position. In side lying with the spine in neutral, the therapist palpates the interspinous space with his or her cranial hand and places his or her caudal forearm on the patient's uppermost ilium in the region between the greater trochanter and the iliac crest. The therapist's chest is then applied to his or her forearm, and by leaning on the forearm the therapist side flexes the patient's spine by pushing the pelvis down toward the table, causing it to side bend over the greater trochanter. The therapist palpates for the spinous processes to come together as they lift up and away from the table. If excessive angulation occurs (as compared with the segment above), hypermobility is suspected, which requires stability testing. If insufficient closing occurs, the segment is deemed as hypomobile. End-feel is appreciated by stabilizing the upper vertebra downward and repeating the test. Since side bending is considered to be pure glide, no PAIVM can be tested that has not already been tested with the PPIVM, and the determination of whether an articular or extra-articular hypomobility is present must be based on integrating the findings from this test with the results of the others.

Considering the direction of the side-bending dysfunction with the flexion or extension dysfunction, integrating the appropriate PAIVM, and appreciating end-feel serves to identify the site and type of hypomobility and dictates the appropriate

intervention. The direction of the rotation hypomobility is irrelevant to determining the location of the dysfunction but may be more sensitive than the other tests for detecting motion dysfunction. If rotation is found to be abnormal, but the other tests feel normal, retesting of these motions is indicated. If hypermobility is found, then the stability test will often determine the direction of the instability.

If right side bending and flexion are both limited together with the flexion PAIVM tests, then the left facet joint is believed to be demonstrating an *opening*, or *flexion*, *restriction*. If the end-feel at the end range of these movements is pathomechanical, then the left facet joint is likely subluxed into extension with an inability to flex or open. If the end-feel is hard capsular, then the left joint is limited into flexion by inextensible periarticular tissues but is not locked into extension. If right side bending and flexion are limited, but the PAIVMs are normal, then an extra-articular restriction is suspected. If left side bending and extension and their PAIVMs are limited, then a *closing*, or *extension*, *restriction* is suspected at the left facet joint.

Asymmetrical (Multiplanar) Movement Tests

With symmetrical PPIVM testing, the segment's motion is appreciated through palpation of the interspinous spaces. During asymmetrical PPIVM testing, the segment is placed into its end range position, and the restriction is evaluated by its end-feel. By recruiting combined movement patterns that traverse multiple planes (ideally triplanar), the therapist is able to be more specific in differentially diagnosing the nature of the restriction.

Prior to performance of formal movement testing pretest screening procedures may be used to improve efficiency. **Screening tests** focus on a specific segment so that a more detailed examination can occur. These tests are not intended to be exhaustive and are inclusive rather than exclusive. The screening tests advocated by NAIOMT faculty include *position tests*, *quadrant tests* (both peripheral and spinal), and the *H and I tests*.

Asymmetrical Movement Screening Tests

Positional Screening Tests

Positional testing and *diagnosis*, as used within the osteopathic approach to determine intervention,[19] are incorporated. However, in this approach, these procedures are used as a screening tool that provides guidance regarding which segments and movements require attention (see Chapter 4).

For example, the finding of a left transverse process that was found to be posterior during position testing in flexion would suggest that one of four possibilities may be present: (1) hypomobility into flexion of the left facet joint, (2) hypermobility into flexion at the right facet joint, (3) a developmental anomaly making the vertebra appear rotated (which would be present in all positions), and (4) a compensatory response to an aberration located at a distance from the segment in question. Although passive movement testing is required to determine which of these possibilities is correct, position testing improves efficiency by leading the examiner to the appropriate segment and motion of interest.

If the PPIVM to be tested was determined from the position test, then rotation is often used to de-rotate the segment in the extended or flexed position. If this cannot be accomplished, then flexion or extension would be considered to be limited; if it can be de-rotated, then flexion or extension was not limited.

In the above scenario, the initial hypothesis is that the cause of the positional abnormality is hypomobility of the left facet joint, disallowing the joint to move into flexion to the same degree as the contralateral side of the segment. Within the osteopathic approach, such a finding denotes a positional diagnosis of what is known as **ERS Left,** for a segment that is said to be relatively *extended (E), rotated (R), and side-bent (S)* to the *left (L)*. Even without this understanding of lumbar-coupled movements (which is under debate), the putative dysfunction can be determined when it is understood that normal coupling is not occurring. The vertebra is rotating about an abnormal axis provided by the hypomobile (or in the case of hypermobility, the less mobile, yet normal, joint) and so must rotate and side flex to the same side. Based on this understanding, the **positional diagnosis (PD)** identifies a segment that is rotated and side-bent to the left when observed in a flexed position. To confirm the positional diagnosis, PPIVM and PAIVM testing must be performed. The motions used for testing, when found positive, become the intervention technique of choice.

In this case, the patient is placed on the left side (on the side of the posterior transverse process), and the hips are flexed until movement arrives into flexion at the involved segment. Further lumbar flexion and rotation are produced from above by pulling the patient's lower arm up and out. Further rotation can be obtained by partly extending the lower leg without extending the spine and rotating the pelvis toward the floor.

Once the lumbar spine is fully flexed and rotated to the right, PPIVM testing is performed to the segment of interest by specifically rotating it to the right through its spinous processes and evaluating the end-feel. If the end-feel is normal as compared with the segments above and below, then the presence of hypomobility is ruled out. If the end-feel is abnormal, PAIVM testing is performed by gliding the cephalad vertebra of the segment superoanteriorly on the stabilized caudal vertebra and evaluating the end-feel. If the end-feel is normal, the hypomobility is caused by an extra-articular (myofascial) restriction. If PAIVM testing reveals abnormal findings, then the restriction is believed to reside within the intra-articular structures.

Identification of the positional diagnosis indicated performance of PPIVM testing of the segment to verify hypomobility into flexion. If PPIVM testing reveals negative findings, then an alternate hypothesis regarding the origin of the positional diagnosis must be developed. If hypomobility into flexion is noted, the examiner must then determine if the restriction is inter- or extra-articular, which is accomplished through PAIVM testing as described. In this manner, positional screening serves to develop an initial working hypothesis that must then be tested through PPIVM and PAIVM procedures.

If PPIVM testing reveals an end-feel that is normal, then flexion of that side of the segment is deemed normal and a second hypothesis must be considered. The positional diagnosis that was identified may be the result of the right side of the segment displaying hypermobility into flexion. To test this hypothesis, the patient is placed on the side contralateral to the posteriorly positioned transverse process (the right side in this case). Flexion is again produced by the same means, but this time it is the right side of the segment that is being tested by evaluating its rotation via its end-feel. If there is a spasm end-feel or a soft capsular end-feel, then hypermobility is considered to be present (irritable with spasm, nonirritable with the soft capsular end-feel). If the end-feel is normal, then flexion of the right facet joint is considered to be normal. This normal finding, coupled with a normal finding for flexion during PPIVM testing on the left, suggests that overall flexion at this segment is considered to be normal. The only other possibilities then remaining for the positional diagnosis are congenital or developmental structural abnormalities or compensations. Neither of these can be directly tested in the clinical setting and therefore become a diagnosis of exclusion based on the negative findings from movement testing.

If the positional screening test demonstrated a posterior left transverse process in extension, then an **FRS Left** is deemed to be the positional diagnosis. In this case, the hypomobility is considered to be on the right side causing relative flexion *(F), rotation (R), side bending (S)* to the *left (L)* as the vertebra rotates around the left side of the segment.

The major limitation with position testing is that these tests are carried out in non-weight-bearing and are inadequate for identifying the presence of symmetrical dysfunctions. The therapist is cautioned to use positional screening only as a guide and to base the differential diagnosis upon formal movement testing.

Quadrant Screening Tests

During *quadrant testing* the patient is asked to actively move into each of the four quadrants: (1) flexion, right side bending, right rotation; (2) flexion, left side bending, left rotation; (3) extension, right side bending, right rotation; (4) extension, left side bending, left rotation. As the individual does so, the therapist listens for complaints of pain or other symptoms; looks for abnormal movement in the spine such as angulations, restrictions, or excessive movements; and then feels for abnormal motion barriers by providing overpressure and evaluating the end-feel. If, for example, flexion, left side bending, and left rotation is determined to be restricted, then the patient is assessed for a left flexion hypomobility as he or she was in the case described above of the ERS Left found in position testing.

The limitations in using this method are that symmetrical restrictions reduce its sensitivity. Furthermore, a painful hypermobility may present in a fashion very similar to a painful hypomobility. The strength of using quadrant testing is that it is carried out in weight-bearing and may therefore demonstrate unstable fixations (subluxations) more easily than do the positional tests.

H and I Screening Tests

The patient is asked to move into the quadrant test positions, as described above, but this time in a strictly ordered sequence. Where quadrant tests allow the patient to move into all three planes in a combined manner, *H and I tests* do not. During H and I testing, the patient is asked to perform motions in the following specific sequence: (1) flexion, right side bending followed by right side bending, flexion; (2) flexion, left side bending followed by left side bending, flexion; (3) extension, right side bending followed by right side bending, extension; (4) extension, left side bending followed by left side bending, extension. The H and I patterns of movement that are performed by the patient give these tests their name (Fig. 11-2).

This test is designed to differentiate between a **stable hypomobility** and an **unstable hypomobility**. A stable hypomobility will limit the quadrant range of motion regardless of the manner in which the patient achieves this position. Conversely, an unstable hypomobility will present with restrictions in only one of the sequences for accessing end range of the quadrant position. This finding indicates an instability that fixates (subluxes) in response to compressive forces from weight-bearing.

There are four permutations of the right flexion quadrant position (flexion, right side bending and right side bending, flexion) (Fig. 11-3). If the quadrant has full range in both sequences,

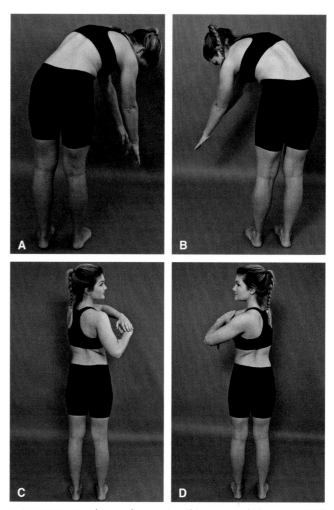

FIGURE 11–3 Lumbar quadrant testing. This testing includes testing of all four quadrants. Overpressure is applied at the end range of all quadrants. **A**. Flexion, right side bending, right rotation. **B**. Flexion, left side bending, left rotation. **C**. Extension, right side bending, right rotation. **D**. Extension, left side bending, left rotation.

then it is presumed to indicate normal range. If the quadrant has reduced motion in both sequences, then a stable hypomobility is indicated. If the quadrant has full flexion but limited side flexion, then an instability, possibly in the flexion range, is indicated. Lastly, if the quadrant has full side flexion but limited flexion, then an instability, possibly in the side flexion range, is suggested.

The limitation with this screening test is the presence of symmetrical restrictions or an instability that is not currently fixating (subluxing), causing a false negative as well as the effect of pain in restricting motion. The strength of this test is that it is performed in weight-bearing and thus shares the same characteristics as the quadrant test.

Direct Asymmetrical Movement Tests

Without the use of positional testing as a screen, all PPIVMs must be tested. Within this approach, side bending is used to determine which side is flexing and which is extending. Right side bending involves the superior articular process of the right zygapophyseal joint gliding inferiorly (extension) while the superior articular process of the left zygapophyseal joint glides

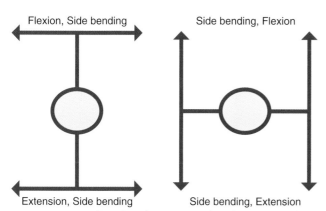

FIGURE 11–2 H and I testing. This testing involves the use of quadrant test positions that are performed in a strictly ordered sequence as indicated by the pattern of an H and an I. This test is useful in differentiating between a stable and an unstable hypomobility.

superiorly (flexion). If side bending is combined with flexion or extension, one joint will maximally flex or extend while the other moves back toward the neutral position. The end-feel is appreciated by stabilizing one vertebra and applying overpressure into further side bending. PAIVM testing for flexion is appreciated by stabilizing the inferior vertebra of the segment and gliding the superior vertebra of the segment superoanteriorly. PAIVM testing for extension is performed by stabilizing the superior vertebra and gliding the inferior vertebra superoanteriorly.

To move the segment into flexion and right side bending, the patient is positioned in right side lying with the hips flexed and the uppermost arm lying across the chest, this will help maintain flexion of the trunk during positioning (Fig. 11-4). The lowermost arm is pulled parallel to the floor (flexing the trunk) but toward the feet (producing right side flexion). Left rotation is produced, but it should be minimal so as not to detract from the flexed position. This same flexed position can be obtained in left side lying and flexion obtained by pulling the inferior arm cranially while maintaining the position of all other segments. These positions will be delineated more specifically within the intervention section of this chapter.

To position the patient in extension and right side bending, the patient is placed in right side-lying position with the uppermost arm hanging behind the patient to maintain extension (Fig. 11-5). The lower arm is pulled perpendicular to the floor (extending the trunk) and toward the feet (side flexing the trunk to the right). The rotation is a minor consideration, and the therapist may choose to forego this component. Alternately, the patient may be positioned in left side lying with the lowermost arm pulled cranially to attain the same position while keeping all other components the same.

For the novice, symmetrical testing is less challenging to perform and interpret. For the experienced manual physical therapist, asymmetrical testing integrates osteopathic positional testing

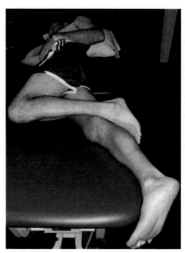

FIGURE 11–5 Trunk extension pre-position. Prior to extension mobilization, the patient is pre-positioned into lumbar extension to the level of the target segment by extending the lower hip and allowing the uppermost arm to lie behind the patient. This position will maintain extension of the trunk during mobilization. The lower arm and pelvis may be used to provide additional specificity to the mobilization.

techniques and is therefore considered to be a more efficient testing procedure while at the same time providing more complete testing of the extreme ranges of motion, including end-feels.

Segmental Stability Tests

The diagnosis of *segmental instability* is best made through performance of stability tests that are carried out on the hypermobile segment that was previously identified. Therefore, if hypermobility is appreciated upon either symmetrical or asymmetrical movement testing, the manual physical therapist should consider differentially determining the presence of instability by using SSTs.

Examination of Anterior Shear/Stability

The examination of anterior shear/stability is carried out indirectly by stabilizing the superior vertebra of the suspected segment and shearing the inferior vertebra posteriorly through the legs (Fig. 11-6). The patient is positioned in side-lying position and neutral flexion/extension. The therapist stabilizes the spinous process of the superior vertebra of the segment while palpating the inferior vertebra. The patient's hips are flexed to 45 degrees for testing of the lumbosacral junction and to 80 degrees for the remaining segments. The patient's knees are placed between the therapist's thighs, which are then used to generate a posterior shear. The inferior vertebra's spinous process is palpated for any shifting or excessive movement or joint sounds, which suggests the presence of anterior instability.

Examination of Posterior Shear/Stability

To test posterior shear (Fig. 11-7), the patient assumes a seated position with the legs over the side of the table and the therapist standing in front. The patient then places his or her forearms on the therapist's chest as the therapist reaches around and stabilizes the lower vertebra of the segment being tested

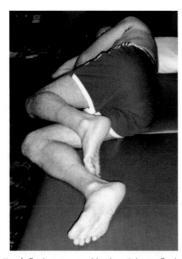

FIGURE 11–4 Trunk flexion pre-positioning. Prior to flexion mobilization, the patient is pre-positioned into lumbar flexion to the level of the target segment by flexing the hips and allowing the uppermost arm to lie across the chest. This position will maintain flexion of the trunk during mobilization. The lower arm and pelvis may be used to provide additional specificity to the mobilization.

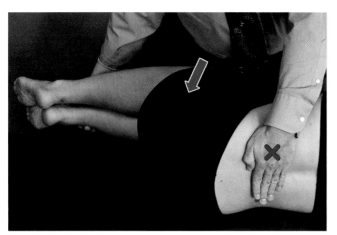

FIGURE 11–6 Segmental stability test for anterior shear/stability. (*Bob Wellmon Photography, BobWellmon.com*)

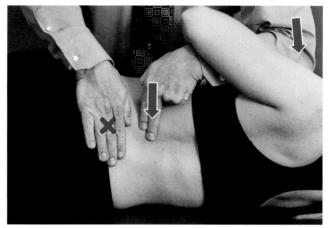

FIGURE 11–8 Segmental stability test for torsional stability. (*Bob Wellmon Photography, BobWellmon.com*)

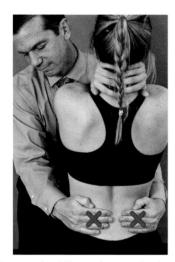

FIGURE 11–7 Segmental stability test for posterior shear/stability. (*Bob Wellmon Photography, BobWellmon.com*)

and palpates the spinous process of the superior vertebra for excessive movement. The patient is then asked to gently push into the therapist's chest using scapular protraction. In the presence of a posterior instability, the superior vertebra will be felt to slip backward on the stabilized segment.

Examination of Torsional Stability

For testing of segmental torsional stability (Fig. 11-8), the patient is positioned in side lying on the side opposite to the direction that is to be tested. The spine is positioned in neutral flexion/extension, but gently rotated until rotation is recruited among all of the segments. Segmental locking may occur if excessive rotation is recruited; therefore, the examiner must use caution in order to prevent bringing rotation to end range. Once rotation is recruited, the therapist pushes the spinous process of the superior vertebra of the segment toward the floor while lifting the inferior spinous process away from the floor to produce pure segmental rotation.

The specificity and sensitivity of these tests have yet to be established. Although these tests may demonstrate signs of clinical segmental instability, the history, along with other aspects

of the examination, must be considered to determine the presence of *functional instability* (see Chapter 18).[20–22] In order to be classified as functional instability, the disability must be functionally restrictive in some capacity.

PRINCIPLES OF EVALUATION

The patient's presenting diagnosis is often a medical diagnosis that falls into a general category, waiting to be confirmed by imaging or laboratory findings. These more general diagnoses are often based on the presence of red or yellow flags indicating that an immediate medical referral may be warranted (Table 11-9).

Clinical reasoning is the application of knowledge to information gained from the patient during the examination. There is good evidence that an algorithmic approach to clinical reasoning that is based on pattern recognition is adopted by most experts.[23]

Evaluation of Findings From the Differential Diagnosis Examination

An abnormal end-feel is determined by an end-feel that is different from that which is expected or an end-feel that occurs at a point in the range other than what is deemed as normal end range. As pain is generally not the limiter of movement in passive tests (unless an empty end-feel is present), these tests are based on determining a limitation using tissue resistance rather than patient willingness to move. Table 11-10 provides the manual intervention that is recommended for each abnormal end-feel that may be experienced. Therefore, passive movement tests and end-feels are deemed as being better at determining the pattern of restriction when compared with active movement tests.

If pain is reproduced during movement testing, it is important to correlate the onset of pain with the onset of tissue resistance. Apprehension that limits movement suggests instability. Apprehension in the early part of the range is often the result of anxiety owing to pain (Table 11-2). A consistent click or shifting of the bone during movement is suggestive of instability during ligamentous stress testing, as is excessive movement or joint play.

Table 11-9	Common Clinical Presentations That Suggest the Possibility of Medical Pathology for Which OMPT Is Not Indicated*	

CLINICAL PRESENTATION	PATHOLOGICAL CONDITION TO BE RULED OUT
Severe bilateral root pain in the elderly patient	Neoplasm
Vertebral wedging	Fracture (traumatic, osteoporotic, neoplastic
Onset/offset unrelated to specific lumbar stress or to general physical activity	Visceral
Severe pain with relatively good movements	Neoplasm
Bilateral capsular pattern (extension loss, symmetrical side flexion and rotation loss, and least loss of flexion)	Arthritis (traumatic or systemic)
Three levels involved	Neoplasm, early cauda equina pressure
Back pain with bladder dysfunction	Prostatitis
Back and leg pain with bladder dysfunction	Cauda equina compression
Back and leg pain with hyperreflexia and Babinski	Multiple sclerosis
L1 or L2 palsy	Neoplasm
Paralysis or anesthesia	Neurological disease, peripheral neuropathy or neoplasm

*These conditions must be ruled out through extensive medical management prior to initiating intervention.

Table 11-10	Matching of the Most Appropriate Manual Intervention to the Identified Pathological End-Feel		

END-FEEL	TYPE OF RESTRICTION	MANUAL INTERVENTION
Empty	Pain	None
Spasm	Pain and reflex	None
Hard capsular	Pain and articular	Arthrokinematic oscillations
Hard capsular	Joint adhesions	Arthrokinematic stretch
Elastic-capsular	Muscle adhesions	Physiological stretch
Light elastic-severely abrupt	Hypertonicity	Hold-relax, belly release, prolonged stretch, traction oscillations
Abrupt and slight springy	Pathomechanical	High-velocity thrust or Grade III+
Abrupt and unyielding	Bone	None

Evaluation of Findings From the Biomechanical Examination

For the purposes of determining whether identified dysfunctions are causal or contributive to the patient's primary condition, the lower quadrant is divided into functional units. The *lumbo-pelvic* *region* includes the lumbar spine, sacroiliac joint, and the hip joints. The *knee* includes the tibiofemoral and patellofemoral joints. The *foot* includes the intertarsal, talocrural, and superior and inferior tibiofibular joints.

The influence of identified dysfunction may be mechanical, neurological, neurophysiological, or a combination of two or more influences. These influences may be *ascending* (that is lying distal to the symptomatic area) or *descending* (that is lying proximal to symptomatic area). While mechanical influences may be most destructive within a given unit, influences external to the unit may be equally damaging. External influences may include hypertonicity caused by segmental facilitation, axoplasmic flow interruption caused by minor compression of a spinal or peripheral nerve, and mechanical stresses caused by leg length discrepancies and postural deficits.

The majority of acute patients will respond to local interventions consisting of manual techniques and exercise. The patient who is experiencing a more chronic condition, however, may require the therapist to search for remote impairments. Acuity is based on the relationship between the onset of pain and resistance and not on the amount of time since onset (Table 11-2).

Operant Definitions

While the basic language used by therapists is fairly standard, some terms have grown to possess different meanings. **Axoplasmic transportation (AXT)** is a non-impulse-based condition along the core of the nerve fiber of trophic nutrients to the tissues innervated by the nerve, neurotransmitter substances to the synapses of the nerve, and metabolites back to the central nervous system.

A **trigger** is considered to be the immediate provoking agent and not the cause. For a trigger to cause symptoms for the first time, a predisposition in the form of an asymptomatic pathology must already be present. This word typically lacks usefulness when describing the aggravating factor of an already symptomatic condition.

The *body tilt test* is an examination procedure that involves holding the head, neck, and trunk together so that they are moved as a single entity through tilting the seated trunk forward/backward and side to side. This maneuver is designed to stimulate the labyrinth, but not the cervical proprioceptors or the vertebral artery. Any dizziness produced, therefore, is likely to be generated by the vestibular system.

The *de Kleyn test* is an occlusive test for the neurovascular system of the neck and head. The full test is to position the neck in rotation and extension with the head overlying the edge of the plinth. A *minimized de Kleyn (MdeK)* consists of maintaining the same position on the bed, and a *progressive minimized de Kleyn (PMdeK)* consists of arriving at the minimized de Kleyn in stages, taking care that each stage is either symptom free or any symptoms that are provoked are investigated and cleared before progressing on to the next, more aggressive, position. Generally, the positive response for this test is dizziness, but it is rarely a true positive for *vertebral basilar insufficiency (VBI)*.

Intervertebral disc herniations may be defined in many ways, and confusion often exists when using the term. For the purposes of this discussion, the term "disc herniation" will be used to describe the migration of the nucleus pulposus through the annulus fibrosis. An incomplete migration is termed a *prolapse*, a herniation that escapes the annulus is an *extrusion*, and a fragmentation of the herniated nuclear material is known as a *sequestration*.

The **initial working hypothesis (H1)** is the provisional diagnosis that is subject to change as the hypothesis is tested against new information generated by the subjective and objective examination. **Neuropathic pain** is the pain produced by most neurological tissues when they are damaged or seriously inflamed. It is described as lancinating or causalgic, and both are felt through the areas subserved by the injured nerve tissue. **Lancinating pain** is a short, sharp flash of pain that is intense and electrical in nature, which runs along the involved dermatome and is narrow banded, spanning only an inch or two in width. Such pain would be described as intolerable if it lasted more than a brief moment. This type of pain is typical of true nerve root pain. **Causalgia** is a prolonged dry, burning, itching type of pain that is usually recalcitrant even to narcotics, only yielding to antiscizure medications. Causalgia is rarely caused by nerve root damage but rather usually by central lesions, particularly those involving the thalamus and peripheral nerves. It is important to note that neither type of pain can be generated by nonneurological tissue; therefore, their presence most certainly signifies neurological involvement. **Segmental facilitation** is a state of heightened excitation of the spinal cord segment resulting in a decreased response threshold caused by prolonged nociceptive input. The effect of segmental facilitation is segmentally distributed hypertonicity, increased deep tendon reflex briskness, vasoconstriction, and nonfatigable weakness due to neuromuscular incoordination. Somatic tissues are incapable of producing neuropathic pain and most neurological tissues, including the nerve root, are incapable

of producing somatic pain. As a point of interest, the somatic pain that is felt down the back of the leg in disc herniations is not directly from the nerve, but more likely from the dura mater or even the disc itself.

To demonstrate the application of clinical reasoning within this approach, the reader is encouraged to refer to the algorithms presented in Figures 11-9, 11-10, 11-11, and 11-12.

PRINCIPLES OF INTERVENTION
General Guidelines

As with other interventions, manual physical therapy should seek to use the least amount of force possible to achieve the desired effect. The *grade* of the mobilization will, in part, determine the intervention dosage. Movement diagrams may be used to plot the relationship between pain and resistance relative to range of motion (Table 11-2) (see Chapter 8). Other aspects of dosage that must be considered are the duration of the mobilization and, to a lesser extent, the *frequency* with which mobilization is performed. Table 11-11 contains the common contraindications and potential complications for high-velocity thrust and nonthrust mobilization of the spine according to the *Canadian approach*.

Technique Selection

Within the Canadian approach, knowledge of the pathoanatomical structure at fault is considered to be important. If hypermobility is noted during the examination, manual techniques can be used to reeducate more normal movement patterns.

Muscular restrictions are often the first barrier to be treated with light *hold-relax techniques*. The use of *Grade III or IV oscillations* may be used to control the patient's symptoms. As pain is reduced, the primary barrier to movement is approached. If periarticular tissue is at fault, then *Grade IV+ rhythmical oscillations* are used to stretch the tissue, and if the joint is subluxed, *Grade III+ mobilizations* may be applied to restore normal positional relationships.

Reeducation is imperative immediately following nonthrust or high-velocity thrust mobilizations. While the joint is positioned in the newly acquired range, gentle isometric contractions are performed alternately between the agonists and antagonists. Such techniques assist in reducing postintervention soreness and aid in reducing recidivism. In order to avoid injury to adjacent regions, *locking techniques* are used over the areas that serve as levers.

Intervention for Myofascial Restrictions

Restrictions in periarticular myofascia of the spine is identified by a reduction in PPIVM in the presence of normal accessory or PAIVM. When myofascial restrictions are present, the endfeel may be characterized as *elastic* in cases of hypertonicity or *hard capsular* when scarring is present.

Clinically, it may be observed that muscles causing hypomobility are often hypertonic as opposed to being structurally shortened. Structural shortening is the result of posttraumatic scarring or adaptive shortening that occurs from prolonged

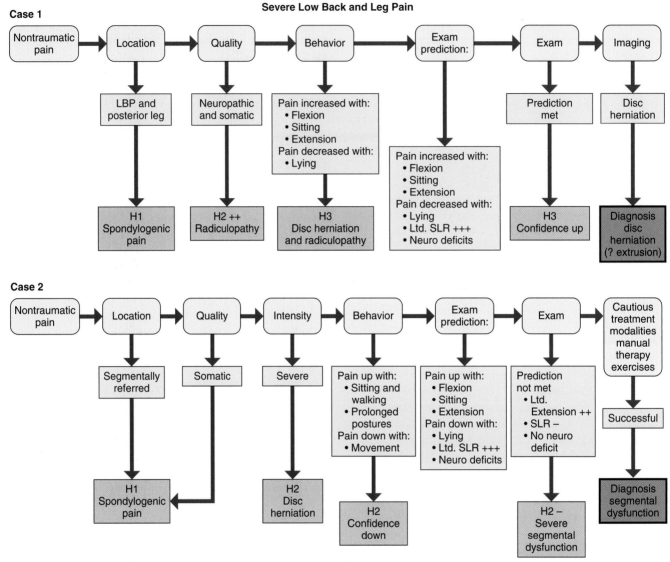

FIGURE 11–9 Algorithmic approach to two cases of severe low back pain and leg pain.

periods of immobility. Janda[5] advocates the use of techniques that involve stretch that occurs in a nonrepetitive fashion. Sahrmann[6] advocates strengthening of the antagonist in an attempt to reduce tone. Activities such as phasic eye exercises, hold-relax techniques, muscle belly pressure techniques, and brief oscillatory spinal traction are all believed to reduce tone. If techniques designed to selectively reduce muscle tone do not yield favorable results, then adaptive structural shortening is suspected and stretching techniques are implemented. Stretching is designed to gradually stretch the scar or adhesion, whereas high-velocity thrust techniques aim to rupture the restriction.

Hypertonicity may result from segmental facilitation where nociceptive input into the spinal segment produces a number of responses into structures that share the same segmental distribution.[24] One of the responses caused by segmental facilitation is muscle hypertonicity that is the result of an increased stretch response that modifies muscle tone.

Another source of nonneurological hypertonicity may be a dysfunction in the vestibular system.[24,25] Such a dysfunction

may produce hypertonicity in the muscles of the neck to reduce head movement in an effort to diminish the intensity and frequency of dizziness. Increased tone in the trunk and limbs may be due to an uninhibited vestibulospinal response. This response appears to be most marked in the limbs for which there is increased tone of the flexor muscle group in the upper extremities and of the extensor muscle group in the lower extremities.

Whatever the cause of the hypertonicity, decreasing tone is the object of the intervention as opposed to techniques designed to change the length of shortened structures. *Hold-relax* (or *contract-relax*) techniques are frequently all that are necessary.

Intervention for Capsular Restrictions

Inextensibility of the joint's *capsuloligamentous complex* are known within this approach as *articular restrictions*. The intervention for a joint that displays a spasm end-feel must address the cause of

Post Motor Vehicle Accident Dizziness: Case 1

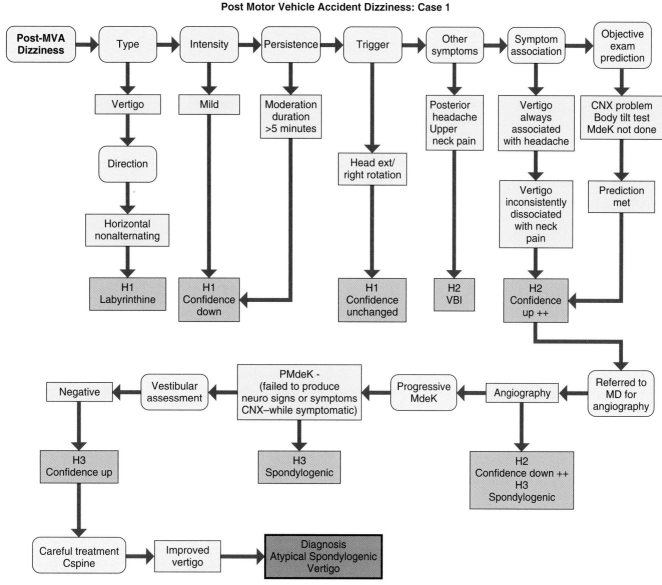

FIGURE 11–10 Algorithmic approach to a case of dizziness following a motor vehicle accident. Clinical case one.

the spasm to be effective. For the most part, intervention consists of rest and anti-inflammatory modalities. Stretching the muscle or aggressive treatment of the joint will usually increase the inflammatory response and increase the degree of spasm.

Adhesions, or scarring, of the periarticular structures require stretching. In the larger peripheral joints, this stretching may be nonspecific and is often more effective than more specific mobilization. However, in the spine, generalized stretching may damage adjacent structures and produce hypermobility if the stiff joint does not mobilize easily. It is difficult to attribute a specific mechanism to the often effective results achieved through joint mobilization. Perhaps, short duration, segmental mobilization exerts its greatest effect through neurophysiologic as opposed to mechanical effects.

The term "specific" may refer to preintervention *locking* of segments adjacent to those being mobilized, despite the fact that most OMPT interventions have a regional, as well as a local effect. Nevertheless, attempts to lock adjacent segments

prior to performance of manual interventions may serve a useful purpose.

Whereas locking is used to provide leverage, *barriering* moves the target joint to its abnormal barrier, thereby allowing the barrier to be engaged immediately by the therapist and, therefore, minimizing the amount of force required to mobilize the restriction. In the case of an acutely painful segment, the segment to be treated is placed in a neutral position, and Grade 1 or 2 techniques that do not reach the barrier are used.

The techniques described in this section pre-position the segment in side bending to flex or extend the target joint rather than rotation. Likewise, the mobilizing force that is used in these techniques will be a side-bending force. Although more challenging to perform, side-bending mobilizations are believed to be less likely to produce postintervention soreness by limiting the amount of torque experienced by the segment.

Within this approach, a common technique used to flex the right facet joint of the hypomobile segment begins with the

Post Motor Vehicle Accident Dizziness: Case 2

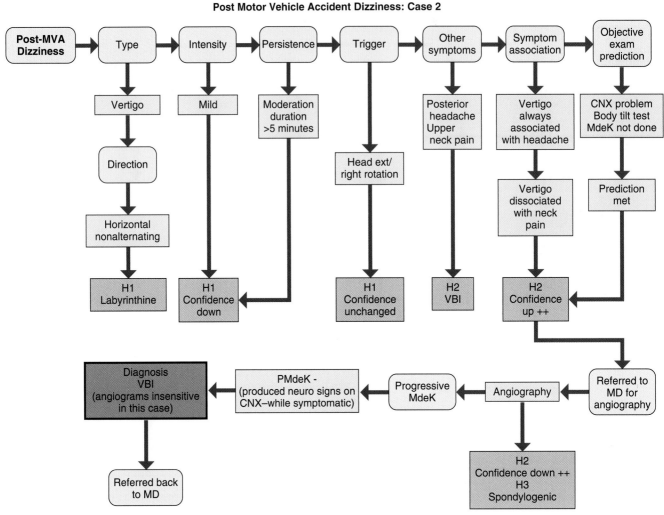

FIGURE 11–11 Algorithmic approach to a case of dizziness following a motor vehicle accident. Clinical case two.

patient positioned in right side-lying position. The patient's hips are flexed and pelvis posteriorly rotated until the target segment is flexed. The patient's upper arm (left) is positioned anteriorly over the side of the bed. This position will bias the trunk into flexion when the segments above the target segment are side-bent by pulling the lower arm (right) cranially and parallel to the bed (see Figs. 11-13 and 11-14). The therapist then undoes the flexion of the segments below the target segment (L5-S1 in this case) by extending the patient's lower leg and rotating the pelvis in the opposite direction until very slight movement of the inferior vertebra of the target segment (L5) is palpated. In addition, the segments below the target segment (L5-S1) are now rotated to the left by pulling the pelvis forwards towards the therapist until L5 is felt to move slightly. This will undo the flexion at L5-S1 and so limit the ability of the corrective force from mobilizing flexion at that level. The L4-5 segment is now positioned in flexion and left side bending so that the right zygapophyseal joint is at its flexion barrier as the left joint is moved away from the barrier. The patient is log-rolled (pelvis, lumbar spine, and thoracic spine as a unit) into the therapist, bringing both patient and therapist into a better position for effective intervention. The therapist places the flexor aspect

of his or her forearm on the patient's pelvis between the trochanter and the iliac crest and slightly posterior (Fig. 11-14).

The therapist then rocks the pelvis cranially by adducting the patient's shoulder until the pelvis and spine are side-bent to the left. The therapist remains above the pelvis as force is delivered (thrust or nonthrust), which moves the pelvis into further side bending and farther into the abnormal end-feel (Fig. 11-15).

This approach also advocates the use of a technique to flex the right joint of the hypomobile segment in left side-lying position. To begin, the patient is positioned in left side-lying position with the hips flexed and the upper (right) arm positioned anteriorly over the side of the bed, with flexion recruited through posterior rotation of the pelvis to the target segment. The lower arm (left) is pulled caudally and parallel with the bed so as to side-bend the trunk to the left (Fig. 11-16).

The lower leg is extended, ensuring the upper leg accompanies it so that the pelvis rotates anteriorly until the sacrum is felt to move; this serves to bring the L5-S1 segment out of flexion for locking. The patient is log-rolled until the therapist's arm is positioned on the pelvis and the segments below the target segment are locked with right rotation by

Nontraumatic Headache

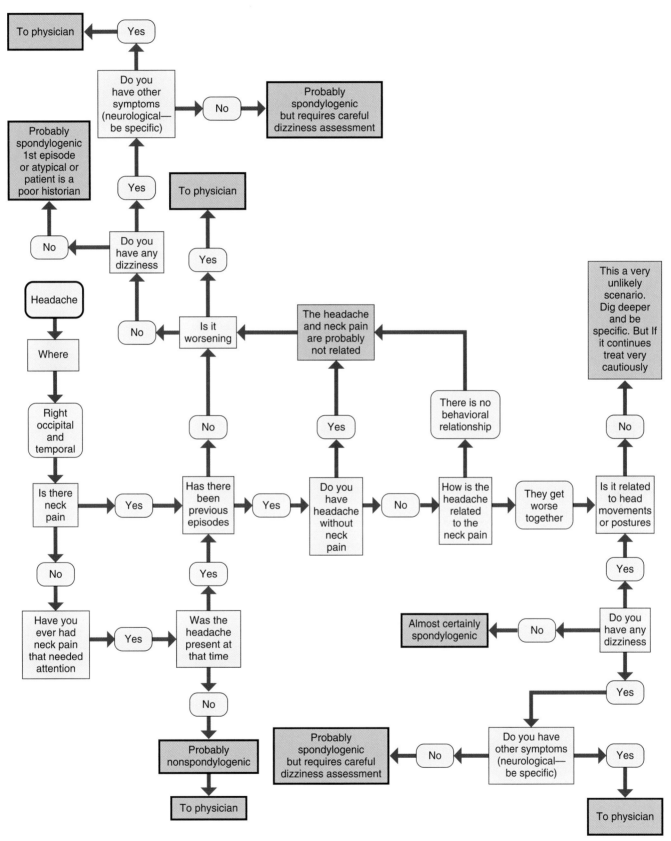

FIGURE 11–12 Algorithmic approach to a case of nontraumatic headache.

Table 11–11   Contraindications and Precautions for Thrust and Nonthrust Mobilization of the Spine and Potential Complications That May Occur as a Result of Inappropriate Use

CONTRAINDICATIONS	CHARACTERISTICS AND POTENTIAL PROBLEMS
Neoplastic disease	Medical diagnosis—possibility of fracture
Cauda equina signs and symptoms	Bilateral multisegmental lower motor neuron signs and symptoms, including bladder dysfunction—possibility of serious compression damage and permanent palsy
Spinal cord signs and symptoms	Multisegmental upper motor neuron signs and symptoms—possibility of serious compression damage and permanent deficit
Nonmechanical causes	Minimal musculoskeletal signs and symptoms—waste of effort and delay in getting appropriate care
First and second lumbar nerve root palsies	Hip flexor weakness. Levels often affected by neoplastic disease—delay in getting appropriate care and possibility of fracture
Trilevel segmental signs	Disc compression can impact a maximum of two levels of nerve root—possibility of neoplastic disease or spondylolisthesis or cauda equina compression
Sign of the buttock	Empty end-feel on hip flexion Painful weakness of hip extension Limited SLR, trunk flexion, and hip flexion Noncapsular pattern of restriction of the hip Swollen buttock Possible serious disease such as sacral fracture, neoplasm, infections, etc.
Various serious pathologies	Empty end-feel and severe multidirectional spasm
Adverse joint environment	Spasm—acute inflammation, fracture
Acute fracture or dislocation	Immediate onset of posttraumatic pain and function loss
Bone disease	Deep pain and relatively minimal musculoskeletal signs—wasted effort and the possibility of fracture
Acute rheumatoid arthritis episode	Medical diagnosis—possibility of increased tissue damage and severe exacerbation
Infective arthritis	Severe inflammation and reddening—delay in getting appropriate medical care
Emotionally dependent patients	Desires manipulation—long-term dependency without much hope of benefit
Chronic pain/fibromyalgia type syndromes	Inadequate signs to explain the patient's widespread symptoms—long-term dependency without much hope of benefit
Precautions	
Rheumatoid arthritis	Medical diagnosis—possibility of increased tissue damage and severe exacerbation
Osteoporosis	Medical diagnosis—fracture
Spinal Nerve (Root) Compression	Segmental neurological signs—probable wasted effort and possibility of increasing the compression
Spondylolisthesis	Radiographic evidence—exacerbation of signs and symptoms
Hypermobility	Clinical finding—increased hypermobility and pain
Acute pain states	Pain onset before or simultaneous with tissue resistance—possibility of severe exacerbation
Pregnancy	Risk of ligamentous damage as a result of the relaxin hormone effect and risk of coinciding with a miscarriage
Repeated steroid injections	Tearing of collagen tissue
Long-term systemic steroid use	Tearing of collagen tissue and fracture
History of neoplastic disease	Risk of recurrence
Distal pain on movement	Acute root compression or severe joint inflammation
Nuclear prolapse or meniscoid entrapment	Springy end-feel
Central or lateral stenosis	Paresthesia dominating pain

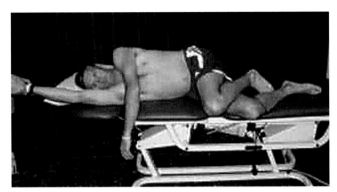

FIGURE 11-13 Trunk flexion, side bend left in right side-lying pre-positioning.

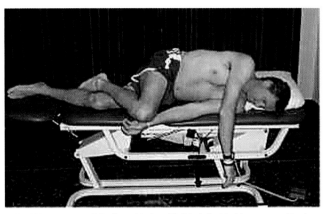

FIGURE 11-16 Trunk flexion, side bend left in left side lying pre-positioning.

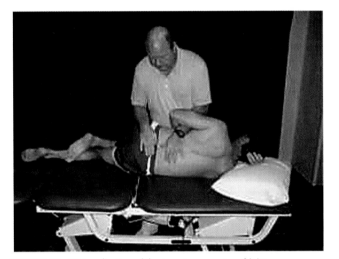

FIGURE 11-14 Localization of the target segment and joint.

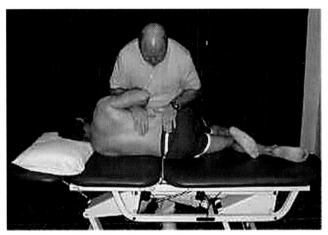

FIGURE 11-17 Localization of the target segment and joint.

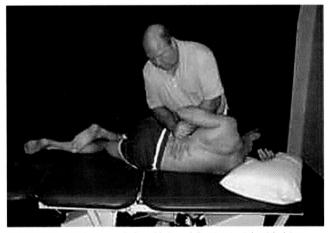

FIGURE 11-15 Flexion, side bend left mobilization in right side lying.

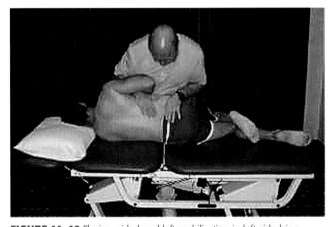

FIGURE 11-18 Flexion, side bend left mobilization in left side lying.

pulling the pelvis forward toward the therapist until the lower vertebra of the segment (L5) is felt to move slightly (Fig. 11-17).

The therapist then applies his body weight through the patient's pelvis while using the arm to produce side bending of the trunk to the left by rocking the patient's pelvis onto the caudal side of the lower trochanter, and the force (thrust or nonthrust) is applied into the abnormal end-feel (Fig. 11-18). Pure side bending is difficult to achieve; therefore, a small

amount of rotation is provided by applying force roughly through the long axis of the femur.

Extension of the target joint is achieved in a similar fashion. This time, however, the legs are extended, and the upper arm is positioned behind the patient's trunk. The arm is pulled either caudally or cranially depending on which side the patient is lying, but it is angled obliquely rather than parallel (Figs. 11-5, 11-19). Figure 11-20 displays the technique for extension of the left joint in right side lying.

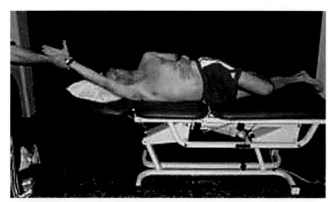

FIGURE 11–19 Trunk extension, side bend left in right side lying pre-positioning.

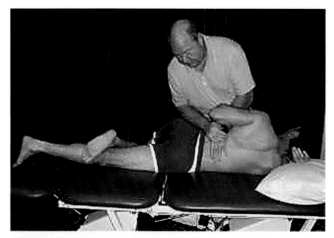

FIGURE 11–20 Extension, side bend left mobilization in right side lying.

If it is not possible to barrier from the top with side bending and flexion or extension, then the vertebrae superior to the target segment may be locked using rotation combined with either flexion or extension. To flex and rotate left, the legs are flexed and the upper arm is positioned in front of the patient. The lower arm is pulled away from the patient parallel to the bed so that the trunk rotates to the left (Fig. 11-21). It is essential for the therapist to carefully palpate for the first movement at the superior vertebra of the target segment (L4)

so that rotation does not enter the segment and confound the results.

To extend and rotate left, the legs are extended and the upper arm lies behind the patient. The arm is pulled away from the patient, but now at an oblique angle to the bed so that left rotation and flexion occur (Fig. 11-22). As previously, careful monitoring to avoid rotation into the target segment is critical. In these techniques, the rotation component is simply used as a locking strategy for the adjacent segments.

Intervention for Subluxation Hypomobility

A term preferable to "subluxation" may be *pathomechanical hypomobility*. Regardless of the terminology, the manual physical therapist must appreciate that the joint is restricted at one end of its range. Some theorize that the joint has lost alignment as a result of instability. Some believe that this condition is due to a joint whose surfaces are caught up on the secondary contours of the joint or on articular surface deficiencies. Others attribute this condition to muscular hypertonicity. The lumbar pathomechanical hypomobility is recognized by a loss of flexion or extension, a loss of its associated arthrokinematics, and an abrupt, hard end-feel. The most effective technique is *high-velocity thrust*, which consists of a low-amplitude high-velocity thrust, or traction technique whose intention is to "unlock" or "unjam" the joint.

The grading of mobilization is a means of applying a graduated and, if required, progressive force to the articulation. Within the *Canadian approach* to OMPT, Maitland's general model of graded mobilization based on the amplitude of motion is followed.[1] The range of motion is the available range, not the full range, and is usually in one direction only (see Chapter 8).

Intervention for Hypermobility and Segmental Instability

The underlying principle behind intervention for hypermobility or instability, as identified by positive findings upon segmental stability testing, is the removal of the causal stress. The cause may be due to repetitive motion, a single traumatic event,

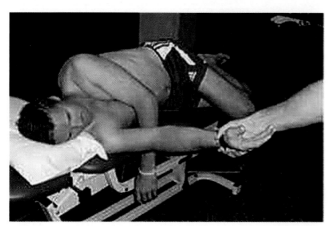

FIGURE 11–21 Flexion with left rotation locking.

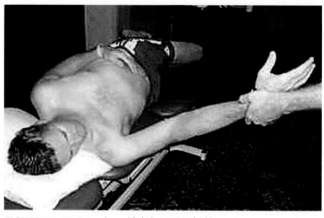

FIGURE 11–22 Extension with left rotation locking.

or may occur as a compensation for adjacent hypomobility. In such cases, it is imperative to reduce compensatory movement. If necessary, temporary support of the segment with an orthosis may be indicated. If hypomobility is present, mobilization designed to increase the segment's contribution to the movement pattern must be performed in a manner that does not impact the already hypermobile segment.

The care of segmental instability involves using interventions designed to manage, as opposed to correct, the culpable structural deficiencies observed. Within this approach, intervention for instability uses three intervention routes: *global*, *regional*, and *segmental*.

Global Intervention for Instability

Within this phase, the patient is asked to avoid or minimize the activities that are contributing to the instability. Alternative strategies for the performance of daily activities must be identified. External support using lumbar orthoses, trunk taping techniques for proprioceptive cues, and correction of leg length discrepancies may also prove to be effective strategies.

Regional Intervention for Instability

If the patient is unable to avoid the insulting activity, and adaptations in the environment are not feasible, then the patient must be taught strategies for protection, including correct lifting techniques. During performance of material handling tasks, it is often useful to instruct the patient in dynamic stabilization activities for trunk support. This regimen typically involves maintenance of neutral lumbar spine postures through abdominal and deep spinal musculature cocontraction.[24] (See Chapter 17 for details related to dynamic spinal stabilization.)

Segmental Intervention for Instability

An attempt should be made to reeducate the muscles to ensure that those controlling the segment are active during trunk movement. The therapist's job is to reeducate optimal movement patterns that involve recruitment of both segmental muscles, such as the transverse abdominis and multifidus, as well as the larger multisegmental muscles, such as the rectus abdominis and erector spinae.

Within this approach, reeducation often begins in side-lying position to avoid the need to stabilize against gravity. Segments do not move in isolation, and therefore no attempt is made to train the deep stabilizers alone. During this process, diagonal patterns that display signs of instability and combinations of patterns must be used (see Chapter 13).

This process typically consists of slow contractions performed throughout the affected range. The first type of contraction used is typically *eccentric*. Once the patient exhibits good control in this activity, the speed of movement is increased, followed by implementation of another contraction type. Finally, new diagonal patterns are added until the patient is able to perform eccentric, concentric, and isometric contractions at varying speeds in any direction. Once this is accomplished, the patient is trained to switch from a fast eccentric contraction moving toward the instability to a slow concentric contraction into the instability and all of the variations in between. Once these diagonals are performed in side-lying position, the patient is progressed to a seated position, then standing. In addition, the patient is instructed in a home exercise regimen designed to simulate the exercises performed in the clinic. Manual interventions may be used in conjunction with these exercises to optimize the dynamic process of segmental stabilization.

DIFFERENTIATING CHARACTERISTICS

The *Canadian approach* to OMPT is an eclectic approach that integrates principles and techniques from various schools of thought. Clinical problem-solving and differential diagnosis that integrates information generated throughout the examination to ascertain causal and contributive factors from remote regions is another key feature of this approach.

A substantial portion of the examination process is based on the principles of differential diagnosis as espoused by *James Cyriax*. Such concepts include examination of end-feel, selective tissue tension testing, and identification of capsular patterns. Refinement of the diagnosis and subsequent intervention is based on concepts related to the clinical application of biomechanical principles as developed by *MacConaill* and *Kaltenborn*. The concept of positional diagnosis, which is borrowed from *osteopathy*, serves to improve the efficiency of reaching a differential diagnosis by narrowing the number of tests needed to determine the dysfunction. As in many approaches, the grading of mobilization according to *Maitland* is commonly used to gauge and document the aggressiveness of the intervention techniques. Along with appreciating the value of OMPT in mobilizing joints, various techniques designed to improve stabilization are also routinely incorporated.

In summary, the *Canadian approach* to OMPT is somewhat of a misnomer in that there is no one school of thought or one method of doing things. Rather, the approach encourages individual variation in the intellectualization and the practical aspects of manual physical therapy. The principles are much the same as those espoused within other approaches, namely rational, scientific thought. If a single maxim can summarize this approach it is: "*be scientific, be creative, look beyond the obvious, and be iconoclastic.*"

NOTABLE QUOTABLE

"*If a single maxim can summarize this approach it is, 'be scientific, be creative, look beyond the obvious, and be iconoclastic'.*"

-J. Meadows

CLINICAL CASE

History of Present Illness (HPI)

A 35-year-old right-hand dominant male in evident good health and reasonable fitness level with no history of significant medical conditions complains of right elbow pain. Pain is present along lateral side of the right elbow from an area 1 inch above the lateral epicondyle to 4 inches below it on the dorsum of the forearm. Occasionally, when severe, the pain can spread to just above the posterior aspect of the wrist. Patient reports onset of symptoms 2 weeks earlier that began with an aching while he was painting a fence at his home for 4 hours. The pain worsened over that evening, reaching its peak the next morning when he found that almost any use of his hand caused severe pain at an 8/10 level of intensity. There was no previous history of similar pain or other pains, except for mild aching after prolonged, heavy, or unusual activity levels.

He was seen by his physician on the third day when there was no improvement, and he was unable to work at his occupation, as an electrician. The physician diagnosed him with lateral epicondylitis, gave him NSAIDs, and told him to buy a tennis elbow support and return in 10 days. He was instructed to try to work. The patient stated that the NSAIDs provided some relief for an hour or so after taking them but did not allow him to use the hand for anything without moderate to severe pain. Recently, the pain had subsided a little but was easily exacerbated, and he was still unable to work. Upon seeing his physician for follow-up, he was referred for physical therapy.

Aggravating and Relieving Factors

Anything involving the use of the right hand aggravates the pain. Strong gripping attempts cause severe pain and provoke severe-moderate aching for up to 2 hours afterward. Gentle prolonged use such as holding a book or the steering wheel of the car provoke immediate mild pain that worsens as time goes on and causes mild aching for about an hour afterward. The tennis elbow support allows him to function with fewer consequences. Ice and NSAIDs eased the postactivity pain, but only nonuse allows him to be pain free. He also complains of tenderness over the lateral elbow region. He had no complaints of neck, thoracic, shoulder, or hand pain, and using these areas did not reproduce the elbow symptoms.

Initial Hypothesis (H1): The most likely cause of local lateral elbow pain is tennis elbow, which is also known as lateral epicondylitis or tendonitis (H1). The term lateral epicondylitis is a misnomer because it is not the epicondyle but rather the common extensor tendon that is potentially inflamed. Without additional information, it is hypothesized that it is a tendonopathy because there is no evidence indicating whether the tendon is inflamed (tendinitis, H1) or degenerative (tendinosis, H2).

Hypothesis Two (H2): The lack of unfamiliar overuse would suggest that playing tennis was a trigger rather than a cause and that there is a potential predisposition specific to the patient. That predisposition is likely to be, at least in part, degeneration of the tendon from cumulative stress or vascular insufficiency.

Hypothesis Three (H3): In addition to the presence of either H1 or H2, this patient must be cleared for potential contributors that have predisposed this patient to this condition. These contributors may be located at some distance from the site of symptoms. All contributors must be addressed if this patient is to achieve full recovery.

Diagnostic and Biomechanical Examination

Confirmation of H1/H2 would both reveal the following upon physical examination:

Wrist:
- *Active ROM*
  - Extension painful but probably full range (contraction of the muscle)
  - Flexion painful and limited range (stretching of the muscle)
  - Radial deviation painful but less so and full range
  - Ulnar deviation possibly painless and full range
- *Passive ROM*
  - Extension pain free and full range
  - Flexion very painful and limited possibly by spasm
  - Radial deviation painless
  - Ulnar deviation painless or mild pain with full range
- *Isometric Resistance*
  - Extension very painful and weak
  - Painless and strong

- Painful and strong
- Ulnar deviation painless and strong

Elbow:

- *Active ROM*
  - Flexion pain free full range
  - Extension slightly painful and limited
  - Supination pain free and full range
  - Pronation pain free and full range
- *Passive ROM*
  - Flexion pain free full range
  - Extension painful and limited possibly with spasm end-feel
  - Supination pain free and full range
  - Pronation pain free and full range
- *Isometric Resistance*
  - Flexion pain free and full range
  - Extension slightly painful and limited
  - Supination pain free and full range
  - Pronation pain free and full range
- *Palpation*
  - Very tender somewhere along the lateral elbow between the epicondylar ridge, the epicondyle, the tendon body or the musculotendinous junction. The area of tenderness extends over more than one of the structures, but will be focused on the epicondyle.
    Confirmation of potential contributors (H3) would reveal the following upon upper quadrant examination:
- Abduction fixation at the ulnohumeral joint
- Right extension C5-C6 hypermobility. The effect of the C5-C6 extension hypermobility is to produce a dynamic lateral stenosis that may cause changes in the structure of the common extensor tendon by neurotrophic malnutrition resulting from reduced *axoplasmic transportation* or *segmental facilitation*. Another possibility is a C5-C6 asymptomatic palsy. However, the lack of segmental weakness or sensory loss during the cervical scan examination would argue against the possibility of segmental dysfunction.
- C2-C3 and T2-T3 right extension hypomobilities were discovered, both of which may stress C5-C6 in greater amounts of extension to compensate for the regional loss of motion.

Conclusion/Confirmation

If this is a common extensor tendonopathy, regardless of whether it is a tendinosis or tendonitis, it will be provoked by characteristic tests. First, isometric wrist extension, and less certainly, radial deviation, will be painful. Second, there will be tenderness over the pathology, usually the epicondylar part of the common tendon. If there is inflammation, the pain upon palpation and isometric testing will be considerably higher, and there may be painful weakness with isometric testing. In this case, there was no painful weakness, and the pain caused by the isometric test was moderate at maximum contraction. H2 is, therefore, strengthened.

The moderate to severe pain with gripping noted as a provoking activity is consistent with both tendinosis and tendinitis and thus do not favor either H1 or H2. However, the lack of irritability is strongly indicative of the absence of inflammatory processes and thus suggests H2, or tendinosis. Tendinosis is confirmed throughout the course of the examination; however, additional information from the examination provides a more complete statement concerning diagnosis and etiology. Although H2 seems to be the most definitive diagnosis, its etiology is unknown. If good and lasting results are to be expected, then the examiner must look deeper. The search for etiology is guided by the results of examination findings that direct the therapist toward potential contributors. This condition is an *epicondylar tendinosis* resulting from a predisposition of an *ulnohumeral abduction fixation* and a *C5-C6 dynamic stenosis* owing to an extension hypomobility. These primary etiologies were in turn caused by *C2-C3* and *T2-T3 hypomobilities*. For complete resolution of this condition and prevention of recidivism, the manual therapist must address all of the identified contributing factors. Therefore, a common straightforward presentation such as lateral elbow pain, if not responding to standard care, may require a deeper investigation of potential contributors that may be located at some distance from the locus of discomfort (see Fig. 11-23).

Lateral Elbow Pain

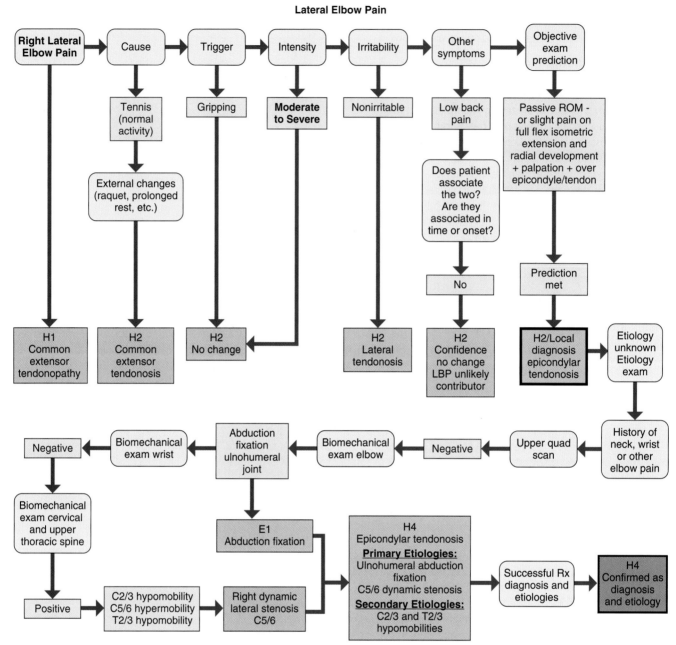

FIGURE 11-23 Algorithmic approach to a case of lateral elbow pain.

1. What were the indicators in this case that caused you to look deeper and consider the possibility of additional etiologic factors or predispositions contributing to the initial and secondary hypotheses?

2. Prior to viewing Figure 11-22, attempt to construct an algorithm that may be used to guide the manual physical therapist's examination that will ultimately lead to differential diagnosis. Compare your algorithm with Figure 11-22.

3. To which of the following tissues do you attribute this patient's primary symptoms? Secondary symptoms? Is it contractile, inert, or conduction tissue? How would you proceed in your differentiation of one from the other?

4. Is determining end-feel important in this case? If so, how is it important, and what type of end-feel would you expect to find at this patient's elbow, wrist?

5. According to the Canadian approach, how would you classify the type of dysfunction that is present at this patient's elbow? At C5-C6? At C2-C3 and T2-T3? What examination procedures might you use to confirm or refute your hypothesis? Consider Table 11-5 when answering.

6. How would you determine if spinal instability was present in this patient? Perform each of the SSTs on your partner. See Figures 11-5, 11-6, and 11-7.

7. In regard to this patient's contributing factors at the cervical and thoracic spine, how would you identify the presence of a symmetrical versus an asymmetrical dysfunction? Would you use screening tests to improve the efficiency of your examination? If so, which ones? Perform symmetrical and asymmetrical movement testing and any screening tests that you may choose to use on your partner.

HANDS-ON

With a partner, perform the following activities:

1 Perform selective tissue tension testing on your partner's elbow as your partner simulates either a contractile, inert, or conduction tissue disorder. Consider the key features of each presentation when attempting to make your diagnosis. Review these factors with your partner. Discuss the variables that may confound your diagnosis.

2 Perform passive range of motion (PROM) with application of overpressure at end range for each of the following motions. Be sure to identify differences in end-feel for each motion.
- Cervical rotation
- Shoulder external rotation
- Elbow extension
- Hip abduction
- Knee flexion
- Ankle eversion

3 Perform positional screen testing on your partner's thoracic spine. Attempt to identify the presence of either ERS (extension, rotation, side bending) or FRS (flexion, rotation, side bending) positional diagnoses. How does positional screening improve the efficiency of the examination?

4 Perform the following symmetrical movement tests on your partner:
- Flexion symmetrical movement tests
- Extension symmetrical movement tests
- Rotation symmetrical movement tests
- Side-bending symmetrical movement tests

5 Perform the following segmental stability tests on your partner. Discuss with your partner what constitutes a positive test and how these findings may guide your intervention.
- Anterior shear
- Posterior shear
- Torsion

6 Engage in role-play by having your partner portray one of the clinical cases described within the evaluation portion of this chapter (low back pain/leg pain, dizziness following motor vehicle accident, nontraumatic headache). As your partner acts out each of the cases, attempt to differentiate between each of the probable hypotheses. Use the decision-making algorithms to guide your conclusions.

7 Review with your partner the specific techniques that you may use for the following dysfunctions, then practice performing each on your partner:
- Myofascial restrictions
- Pericapsular restrictions
- Hypermobility and segmental Instability

8 Pre-position your partner in a triplanar fashion to facilitate maximal opening and maximal closing of the following facet joints prior to mobilization:
- Right C4-C5
- Left T9-T10
- Right L2-L3

9 During spinal mobilization, why is side bending preferred over rotation for pre-positioning and mobilization? After careful triplanar pre-positioning, mobilize each of the joints listed in number 8 using a side-bending force.

10 Within this approach, why is the use of overpressure advocated even for movements that are already painful? After careful pre-positioning, perform overpressure for each of the joints listed in number 8.

11 Construct an algorithm to help guide your use of PPIVM and PAIVM testing and SSTs for reaching a conclusion regarding the nature of an individual's dysfunction according to the Canadian approach. Compare your algorithm with Figure 11-1.

12 Using the table below, list your expected examination findings for each type of dysfunction. Identify which of the examination procedures would be of greatest value for differentially diagnosing and classifying each condition.

EXAMINATION PROCEDURE	EXTRA-ARTICULAR (MYOFASCIAL) HYPOMOBILITY	ARTICULAR (PERICAPSULAR) HYPOMOBILITY	ARTICULAR (SUBLUXATION, PATHOMECHANICAL) HYPOMOBILITY	NONIRRITABLE HYPERMOBILITY	IRRITABLE HYPERMOBILITY	INSTABILITY
AROM						
PROM						
Resistance Testing						
Neurological Testing						
Symmetrical Movement Testing						
Asymmetrical Movement Testing						
PPIVM						
PAIVM						
Segmental Stability Testing (SST)						
Positional Screening						
Quadrant Screening						
H and I Screening						

REFERENCES

1. Maitland GD. *Vertebral Manipulation*. 4th ed. Sydney, Australia: Butterworths; 1977.
2. Kaltenborn FM. *The Spine: Basic Evaluation and Mobilization Techniques*. 2nd ed. Oslo, Norway: Olaf Norlis Bokhandel; 1993.
3. Kaltenborn FM. *Manual Mobilization of the Joints: The Kaltenborn Method of Joint Examination and Treatment, Volume I: The Extremities*. 6th ed. Oslo, Norway: Olaf Norlis Bokhandel; 2002.
4. Gustavsen R. *Training Therapy Prophylaxis and Rehabilitation*. New York: Thieme Inc.; 1985.
5. Janda V. Muscles and back pain: assessment and intervention, movement patterns, motor recruitment. Course notes, 2nd ed.; 1994.
6. Sahrmann SA. *Diagnosis and Treatment of Movement Impairment Syndromes*. St. Louis, MO: Mosby; 2002.
7. MacConaill M, Basmajian J. *Muscles and Movement: A Basis for Human Kinesiology*. Baltimore, MD: Williams & Wilkins; 1969.
8. Cyriax J. *Textbook of Orthopedic Medicine, Volume 1*. 8th ed. Philadelphia, PA: WB Saunders; 1982.
9. Meadows J. *The Principles of the Canadian Approach to the Lumbar Dysfunction Patient* in *Management of Lumbar Spine Dysfunction*. 9.3.6. Alexandria, VA: Orthopaedic Section, APTA Inc.; 1999.
10. Hayes KW. An examination of Cyriax's passive motion tests with patients having osteoarthritis of the knee. *Phys Ther*. 1994;74:697.
11. Franklin ME. Assessment of exercise induced minor muscle lesions: the accuracy of Cyriax's diagnosis by selective tissue tension paradigm. *J Orthop Sports Phys Ther*. 1996;24:122.
12. Browder DA, Erhard RE. Decision-making for a painful hip: a case requiring referral. *J Orthop Sports Phys Ther*. 2005;35:738-744.
13. Fritz JM, Delitto A, Erhard RE, Roman M. An examination of the selective tissue tension scheme, with evidence for the concept of a capsular pattern. *Phys Ther*. 1998;78:1046-1061.
14. Greenwood MJ, Erhard RE, Jones DL. Differential diagnosis of the hip vs. lumbar spine: five case reports. *J Orthop Sports Phys Ther*. 1998;27: 308-315.
15. Winters JC, Groenier KH, Sobel JS, Arendzen HH, Jongh BM. Classification of shoulder complaints in general practice by means of cluster analysis. *Arch Phys Med Rehabil*. 1997;78:1369-1374.

16. Zimny NJ. Clinical reasoning in the evaluation and management of undiagnosed chronic hip pain in a young adult. *Phys Ther*. 1998;78:62-73.

17. Pearcy M, Treadwell SB. Axial rotation and lateral bending in the normal lumbar spine measured by three dimensional radiography. *Spine*. 1984;9:294.

18. Oxland TR. The effect of injury on rotational coupling at the lumbosacral joint. A biomechanical investigation. *Spine*. 1992;17:74.

19. Mitchell F, Moran PS, Pruzzo NA. *An Evaluation and Treatment Manual of Osteopathic Muscle Energy Procedures*. Valley Park, MO: Mitchell Moran and Pruzzo Associates; 1979.

20. Meadows JTS. *Differential Diagnosis in Orthopedic Physical Therapy: A Case Study Approach*. New York: McGraw-Hill; 1999.

21. Grieve G. Lumbar instability. *Physiother*. 1982;68:2.

22. Schneider G. Lumber instability. In: Boyling JD, Palastanga N, eds. *Grieve's Modern Manual Therapy*. 2nd ed. Edinburgh; Churchill Livingstone; 1994.

23. Jensen GM, Gwyer JM, Hack LM, Shepard KF. *Expertise in Physical Therapy Practice*, 2nd ed. Philadelphia, PA: Saunders/Elsevier; 2006.

24. Patterson MM. A model mechanism for segmental facilitation. *J Am Osteopath Assoc*. 1976;78:62.

25. Chester JB, Jr. Whiplash, postural control, and the inner ear. *Spine*. 1991;16:716.

RECOMMENDED READING

Herdman S, ed. *Vestibular Rehabilitation*. Philadelphia, PA: FA Davis; 1994.

Richardson CA, Jull GA. Concepts of assessment and rehabilitation for active lumbar stability. In: Boyling JD, Palastanga N, eds. *Grieve's Modern Manual Therapy*. 2nd ed. Edinburgh: Churchill Livingstone; 1994.

The Functional Mobilization Approach

Gregory S. Johnson, PT, FFCFMT, FAAOMPT

Vicky Saliba Johnson, PT, FFCFMT, FAAOMPT

Rachel A. Miller, PT, MS, WCS, CFMT

Leslie Davis Rudzinski, PT, OCS, CFMT and

Kristina M. Welsome, MSPT, DPT, OCS, CFMT, MTC

Chapter Objectives

At the conclusion of this chapter, the reader will be able to:

- Identify the major influences leading to the development of the Functional Mobilization approach to orthopaedic manual physical therapy (OMPT).
- Understand the examination and treatment philosophy of The Institute of Physical Art and Functional Mobilization.
- Conduct a functional examination, including assessment of rolling and gait.
- Understand the use of functional movement patterns and proprioceptive neuromuscular facilitation patterns to identify biomechanical dysfunctions.

- Understand the importance of the impact test.
- Use Functional Mobilization to identify, localize, mobilize or stabilize, and reeducate dysfunctional movement segments.
- Appreciate how the Functional Mobilization approach to OMPT can combine treatment of structural dysfunctions, neuromuscular dysfunctions, and motor learning into one treatment.
- Understand how to involve the patient in treatment through movement education, active release, and neuromuscular control and reeducation.

INTRODUCTION

Functional Mobilization (FM) is an inherent component of *Functional Manual Therapy (FMT)*, a systematic approach to patient care designed to identify the mechanical, neuromuscular, and motor control factors inhibiting and preventing efficient function. Differing from traditional passive approaches, FM couples active and resisted movements with specific, directional pressures to restore functional mobility. FM offers a seamless progression from assessment of mobility to a three-dimensional approach to intervention.

NOTABLE QUOTABLE

"The Functional Manual Therapy Approach offers concepts and tools for examination and intervention. . . . Examination is performed through the use of observation of form and motion,

palpation to determine condition, and resistance to explore neuromuscular control. Through intervention, we improve the interplay of motor control, structure, and functional capacity. . . ."

-G. Johnson

Functional Mobilization, developed by *Gregory S. Johnson* in 1980, represents a synergy of eclectic study and clinical experience. Following graduation from the University of Southern California in 1971, Johnson attended a yearlong **proprioceptive neuromuscular facilitation (PNF)** residency under *Margaret "Maggie" Knott* at Kaiser Rehabilitation Hospital in Vallejo, California (Fig. 12-1). Continuing at Kaiser as senior faculty in the residency program until 1978, Johnson's experiences reinforced his understanding of the importance of evaluating function, applying manual resistance,

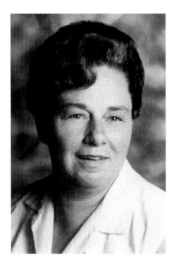

FIGURE 12–1 Margaret "Maggie" Knott, developer of proprioceptive neuromuscular facilitation.

and using developmental postures and motions for movement reeducation.

From 1972 to 1978, Johnson augmented his training in PNF with extensive study in joint mobilization approaches and alternative therapies. In 1978, together with his wife and co-founder of the *Institute of Physical Art*, *Vicky Saliba Johnson*, Johnson began teaching continuing education directed at the enhancement of function. The principles of PNF, joint mobilization, and soft tissue mobilization laid the foundation for the development of FM as a dynamic three-dimensional approach.[1–5]

The FM approach has been influenced by a variety of orthopaedic manual physical therapy (OMPT) approaches, including the Nordic (Chapter 6), Australian (Chapter 8), Paris (Chapter 7), Osteopathic (Chapter 4), Cyriax (Chapter 5), and Canadian (Chapter 11) schools of thought, in addition to a variety of soft tissue and alternative approaches.[6–14] Although many neuromuscular reeducation philosophies influenced the development of the FM approach, PNF provided the philosophical framework.[15–21]

PHILOSOPHICAL FRAMEWORK

FMT seeks to promote optimal function while addressing the patient's subjective complaints. A functional manual therapist seeks to facilitate each patient's existing potential by addressing the following: (1) the *mechanical* system, which determines optimal alignment and functional capacity[1–5]; (2) the *neuromuscular* system, which provides muscular initiation, strength, and endurance, creating both stability and mobility[21,22]; and (3) *motor control*, which integrates both centrally mediated and automatic patterns to produce coordinated, purposeful, and automatic activities.[21,22]

The FMT approach alleviates symptoms and improves performance by facilitating three-dimensional function to the joints, soft tissues, and neuromuscular system. FM, an inherent component of FMT, offers strategies for facilitating a mechanical system that normalizes the distribution of forces through the body and restores neuromuscular control.

PRINCIPLES OF EXAMINATION
Function-Based Examination Tools
Functional Tests

Functional tests provide an objective measure of postural and structural integrity coupled with assessment of motor control capacity (Box 12-1). These tests provide proprioceptive feedback that may be assessed before and after FM intervention. Shifting the focus from pain to function, functional tests encourage the therapist to assume a global rather than segmental approach to the patient.

Vertical Compression Test

The **vertical compression test (VCT)** is performed through application of a slow and progressively applied vertical force to the patient's shoulders to assess the integrity of the structural system, which is measured by the attenuation of force through the segments to the base of support (Fig. 12-2). An efficient system allows for force attenuation without any buckling or shear. For a more detailed description of the VCT, see Chapter 13.[5,22]

Elbow Flexion Test

The **elbow flexion test (EFT)** is performed through application of a slow and progressively applied vertical force through the forearms to assess the neuromuscular and motor control response to forearm loading (Fig. 12-3). In an efficient state,

> **Box 12-1 Quick Notes! FUNCTIONAL TESTS**
>
> *Functional tests* provide an objective measure of postural and structural integrity coupled with assessment of motor control capacity, and they include the following:
> - Vertical compression test (VCT)
> - Elbow flexion test (EFT)
> - Lumbar protective mechanism (LPM)
> - Functional squat (FS) test

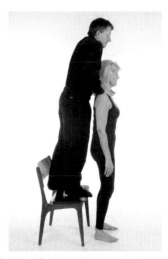

FIGURE 12–2 The vertical compression Test (VCT).

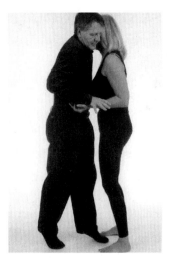

FIGURE 12–3 The elbow flexion test (EFT)

the patient responds with primary initiation of the trunk core muscles supplemented by global muscles to produce an appropriate balance and strength response. For a more detailed description of the EFT, see Chapter 13.[5,22]

Lumbar Protective Mechanism Test

In 1983, Johnson developed the term **lumbar protective mechanism (LPM)** to refer to the trunk's ability to automatically stabilize against external force in the efficient state. To perform this test, the patient is positioned against a stable surface with the trunk unsupported or in a stride stance. A slow and progressive force is applied to the shoulders in anterior-posterior and posterior-anterior diagonal directions to reveal the patient's stabilizing response (Fig. 12-4). For a more detailed description of the LPM, see Chapter 13.[5,22]

Functional Squat Test

The **functional squat (FS) test** is an excellent method to examine common functional movement patterns that involve the entire body. The patient stands with a normal base of support and squats as far as possible without pain while keeping the

heels on the ground. During the squat, the patient's balance and sequence of motion are noted (Fig. 12-5). This test is progressed to the step and step-down test. For a more detailed description of the functional squat test, see Chapter 13.[2,3,5]

Functional Palpation Examination

Skilled **functional palpation** should identify the exact condition of the underlying joint, soft tissue, nerve, and organ during normal motions. Functional palpation uses passive, active, and resisted PNF patterns and normal functional motions to effectively examine the quantity and quality of the three-dimensional motions of joints and soft tissues. Based on function, these tissues are examined during various postures and movements (Figs. 12-6, 12-7, 12-8).[1–5,16–18,21] The quality of end-feel, accessory motion, and tissue extensibility are the *pillars* of the functional palpation examination.

QUESTIONS *for* REFLECTION

- Functional palpation uses which motions during examination?
- What are considered to be the pillars of functional palpation?
- What are the three dimensions in which end-feel should be assessed?
- Define "muscle play" and how this might be used to determine the presence of soft tissue restrictions.

End-Feel

End-feel is defined as "the quality of resistance felt in a tissue or joint at the end of physiologic or accessory range."[1–5] A springy end-feel is indicative of the efficient state. Dysfunctional tissues have varying degrees of hard end-feel and motion loss. The goal is to assess end-feel and localize restrictions in three dimensions (*location*, *direction*, and *depth*).

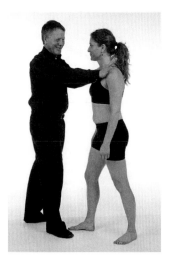

FIGURE 12–4 The lumbar protective mechanism (LPM).

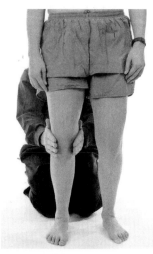

FIGURE 12–5 Observation of balance and the sequence of motion during the functional squat (FS) test.

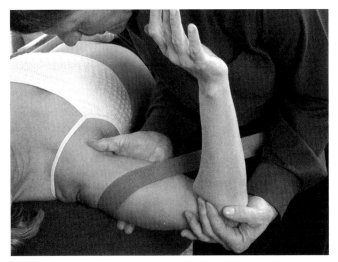

FIGURE 12–6 Functional palpation examination of the shoulder to assess end-feel, accessory motion, and tissue extensibility.

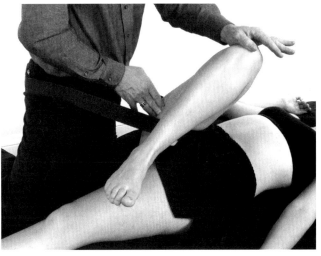

FIGURE 12–7 Functional palpation examination of the hip to assess end-feel, accessory motion, and tissue extensibility.

FIGURE 12–8 Characteristics of neuro-muscular control.

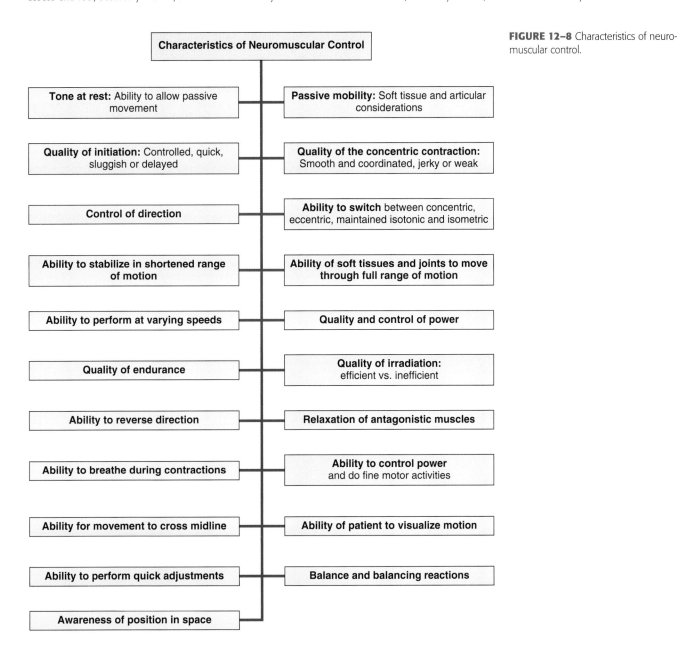

Accessory Motion

Accessory motion is a term generally used in reference to joint mobility. Mennell[23] adopted the term *joint play* to describe accessory joint motion. Unique to the FM approach is the consideration of the motion that normally occurs between all soft tissue structures. The interfaces between soft tissue structures are separated by fascia (extracellular matrix), and lubricated by the ground substance, and may be termed **functional joints.**[24] In the FM approach, motion occurring between muscles is termed **muscle play**, which highlights the ability of muscles to move freely in relationship to each other.[1,5] Refer to Chapter 13 for a complete discussion.[2,3,5]

CLINICAL PILLAR

Assessment of soft tissues, such as joints, should include the following:

- Examination using both active and passive motion
- Examination using three-dimensional motions
- Examination using both WB and NWB postures
- Examination using end-feel in three dimensions
- Examination of accessory motion

Tissue Extensibility

Tissue extensibility is defined as the ability of tissues to optimally elongate and fold (shorten) while maintaining a springy end-feel.[1,5] Evaluation of true soft tissue extensibility and flexibility is achieved by palpating the tissues through their full passive, active, and resisted ranges of motion.

Neurovascular Mobility and Neural Dynamic Examination and Intervention

Patients with chronic pain often exhibit underlying dysfunction within the peripheral and central nervous systems.[25–31] The FM strategy for neurovascular examination and intervention expands upon the work of others (see Chapter 19). FM incorporates the use of specific **tracing and isolating procedures**, which use passive and active movement with functional palpation to assist in localizing the specific peripheral and central adherences.

Upper Limb Tension Testing

The *upper limb tension tests (ULTT)*, developed by Elvey[27] provide the foundation for the FM neurovascular examination and intervention. FM uses active and resisted motions in addition to passive positioning to trace and isolate neurovascular restrictions. The patient is guided through motions to reproduce repeated slack and tension, as traditionally described, while the therapist palpates the nerve from the neural foramen to the hand. Often, several locations of impeded mobility are identified (i.e., double crush injury).[28] Once an adherence is identified, the therapist treats the localized restriction(s) with sustained pressure at the barrier,

coupled with mobilization through repeated upper extremity motion (Fig. 12-9).

The FM protocol proceeds from the periphery to evaluation of each associated cervical vertebra. In the case of a median nerve restriction, for example, it is critical to enhance the mobility of C5-T1. Next, the therapist places pressure at the lateral aspect of each cervical vertebra while performing the median nerve ULTT. Dysfunction is identified by (1) a change in end-feel, (2) increased pressure against the palpating finger, or (3) a positional change in the vertebra. Dysfunction is treated by blocking the vertebra while tension is produced through upper extremity motion until the vertebra no longer moves in response to neural tensile forces (Fig. 12-10).[3]

QUESTIONS *for* REFLECTION

What is unique about the manner in which *upper and lower limb tension tests* for the examination of neural mobility are performed within the **FM approach** to OMPT compared with typical methods as described in Chapter 19?

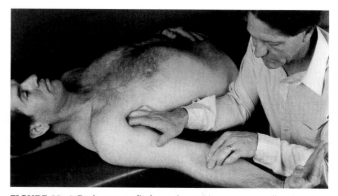

FIGURE 12–9 During upper limb tension testing, once an adherence is identified, the therapist treats the localized restriction(s) with sustained pressure at the barrier, coupled with mobilization through repeated upper extremity motions.

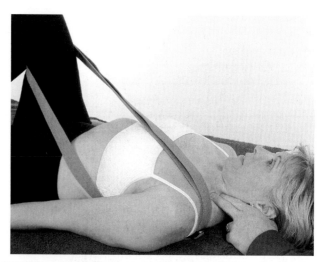

FIGURE 12–10 Blocking the involved vertebra while intermittent tension is produced from passive, active, or resisted upper extremity motion.

Lower Limb Tension Testing

Utilization of tracing and isolation, as described for ULTT, may also be performed in the lower extremity.[4]

Dural Mobility Testing

To assess upper quadrant dural mobility, the therapist performs the **turtle neck test** by positioning the patient in hook-lying position and cradling the head with gentle traction.[3] The patient performs lower trunk rotation while the therapist palpates for any caudal pull.

Examination of dural mobility can be combined with lower limb tension testing using the *slump-sitting test* developed by Maitland[25] and the **extension sitting test** developed by Johnson[4] (Figs. 12-11, 12-12). The extension sitting test is conducted on a table with the patient facing the therapist and feet suspended using a mobilization belt between the therapist's pelvis and patient's spine. The therapist segmentally moves the belt cephalad to maximize the anterior translation of each individual vertebra. While sustaining anterior pressure through the strap, increased neural tension is elicited through knee extension, dorsiflexion, and neck

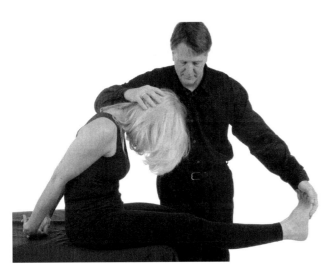

FIGURE 12–11 Slump-sitting test developed by Maitland.

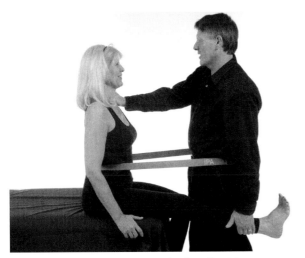

FIGURE 12–12 Extension sitting test developed by Johnson.

flexion/extension. If tension exists, tracing and isolating is performed (Fig. 12-13).[3,4]

Describe the specific methods used within the **FM approach** to OMPT to assess *dural mobility*.

Functional Movement Patterns

The use of **functional movement patterns (FMP)**[2,5] provides a mechanism to efficiently identify mechanical, neuromuscular, and motor control dysfunctions (Box 12-2). FMPs are based on the **awareness through movement (ATM)** approach, developed by *Moshe Feldenkrais*[7] (see Chapter 20), and PNF diagonal patterns. FMPs include the pelvic clock, arm circles, trunk side bending, hip rotations, and shoulder girdle clocks. The presence of a dysfunctional active motion directs the therapist to assess the FMP through palpation of the soft tissues, joints, and neuromuscular recruitment patterns. Once the specific source of the dysfunctional motion is identified, the FMP becomes the intervention (Fig. 12-14).[2]

Examination of Rolling and Gait

Similar to the use of FMPs, observation and palpation during the performance of normal functional activities reveals soft

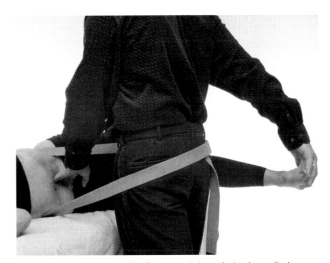

FIGURE 12–13 Tracing and isolating restrictions during lower limb tension testing.

Box 12-2 Quick Notes! FUNCTIONAL MOVEMENT PATTERNS

Functional movement patterns consist of the following:
- Pelvic clock
- Arm circles
- Trunk side bending
- Hip rotations
- Shoulder girdle clocks

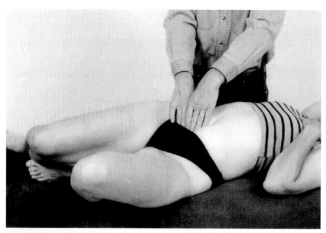

FIGURE 12–14 Assessment of the functional movement pattern (FMP) through functional palpation of the soft tissues, joints, and neuromuscular recruitment pattern.

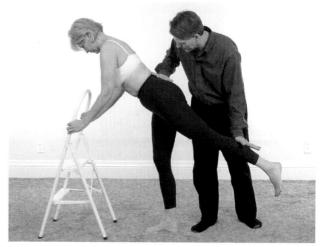

FIGURE 12–15 Observation and palpation during the performance of standing hip extension reveals soft tissue, articular dysfunctions, and any associated inefficient movement patterns.

tissue and articular dysfunctions and any associated inefficient movement patterns (Fig. 12-15).[22] Typically, examination includes activities such as *rolling, supine to sitting, sitting, sitting to standing, walking, bending, reaching, pushing, pulling,* and *lifting.* During these activities, the patient's ability to maintain a neutral posture and base of support, move efficiently, and demonstrate graceful motions is observed.[1–4,22]

CLINICAL PILLAR

Functional palpation during activities of daily living seeks to assess the following:

● The patient's mechanical and neuromuscular ability to attain and maintain a neutral posture

● The patient's ability to move about efficient axes of motion

● The patient's ability to establish and function within an effective base of support

● The patient's ability to demonstrate graceful motions

● The specific mechanical restriction or inefficient neuromuscular pattern contributing to the movement dysfunction

---

Examination of Rolling Patterns

There is often a direct relationship between the strategies used in rolling and those performed during gait.[32,33] During normal growth and development, the extremity phasic muscles (global muscles) dominate early movement.[32,34] A child ambulates most efficiently after mastering the motor planning of rolling and crawling. In adulthood, efficient performance can be lost because of trauma, misuse, and inhibition of the core musculature. Evaluation of rolling is performed, specifically noting the method of initiation and integrated use of the head, trunk, and extremities. Efficient rolling from supine to prone uses a **mass**

flexion pattern. Appropriate mass flexion is initiated with pelvic anterior/elevation progressing to lower extremity flexion/adduction, scapular anterior depression, followed by upper extremity extension/adduction. A common dysfunction involves pushing into hip extension. Through functional palpation, the therapist localizes the dysfunction by assessing passive, active, and resisted pelvic and lumbar motions during the activity. Once identified, the dysfunction is treated using the same motions coupled with joint and soft tissue mobilization and neuromuscular facilitation. The transition from mechanical treatment to motor control occurs by using repeated movement and prolonged holds to "*reset*" the motor control system.

Examination of Gait

The primary focus of the gait evaluation is observation and palpation of the pelvis and trunk. An *optimal gait cycle* can be broken down into four pelvic girdle motions based on PNF diagonals.[4,15–18,21,22,33] The four PNF diagonals are as follows. (1) **Anterior elevation (AE)** is most efficient when the iliopsoas and abdominals contract synergistically to promote trunk stabilization during the initial swing phase. (2) **Anterior depression (AD)** occurs as the pelvis assists the leg to elongate down and forward for initial contact with the ground. The ability for the right quadratus lumborum to elongate with good eccentric control is critical for proper deceleration of the limb. (3) **Posterior depression (PD)** is necessary for effective midstance and push off. The therapist should be able to palpate the gluteal muscles or observe plantar flexors firing in an efficient recruitment pattern during this phase. (4) **Posterior elevation (PE)** promotes trunk stability in conjunction with contralateral anterior elevation. Dysfunctional pelvic motions noted during gait are further assessed by evaluating the pelvic patterns in the side-lying position.

The FM approach considers the *iliosacral (IS)* joint movement of the ilium on the sacrum to be an extension of lower extremity motion and the *sacroilial* joint movement of the sacrum on the ilium to be an extension of axial skeleton spinal motion. The therapist evaluates innominate motion using a standing **leg swing mobility test** (Fig. 12-16).[4] As the patient swings the leg from flexion to extension, the therapist palpates the posterior superior iliac spine and anterior superior iliac spine. If there is an abrupt stop, the restriction correlates to the direction in which hip motion is limited. Additional localization of the restriction occurs through adding hip internal and external rotation.

The Impact Test

The **impact test** is adapted from the work of *Herman Kabat, MD*.[35] This test identifies aggravating activities or movement patterns that inhibit central and peripheral muscles.[3,4] These findings assist the therapist in training the patient in more efficient body mechanics.

Patients with back pain have reflexive inhibition of spinal stabilizing muscles at the segment and side of pain.[36–42] These patients lack the ability to control segmental function through the local muscles and instead attempt to stabilize with the global phasic muscles. The impact test specifically correlates peripheral weakness to central inhibition.

Progression of the Impact Test

Muscle Tests

Lower or upper extremity muscle tests are used to identify muscular response and endurance.[3,4,22,43] It is important to note the presence or absence of proper trunk stabilization, irradiation of the contraction, and the presence of any movement compensations. If any dysfunctions exist, treatment progresses to segmental facilitation.

Segmental Facilitation Procedure

The purpose of this procedure is to discover if central segmental facilitation can enhance central stabilization and improve the peripheral response. The facilitation procedure consists of a prolonged (hold) contraction (cervical axial elongation or lumbar abdominal series) to facilitate the inhibited tonic components.[3,4,44] Following the identification of upper extremity muscle weakness, the therapist performs a resisted prolonged hold to *cervical axial elongation* (retraction) in supine.[3,44–47] There are two types of resisted axial elongation. **General resistance** is applied to the cervical spine and chin to facilitate the short neck flexors. **Specific segmental resistance** is applied to the articular pillars of the inhibited level (Fig. 12-17). In a dysfunctional state, the patient is unable to effectively maintain the position. The therapist uses a very slowly applied resistance (the **tonic spread**) to facilitate the core muscles. If the patient attempts to produce the stabilizing contraction with a phasic response, an oscillating contraction (**phasic shake**) will occur secondary to fatigue. With continued appropriate resistance, this phasic contraction transitions into a stabilizing or tonic contraction (Box 12-3).

In the lumbar spine, the **abdominal series** is performed to test if there is central inhibition related to weakness of the lower extremities.[4] There are four separate components to the supine abdominal series: (1) resistance of bilateral hip flexion, emphasizing traction (Fig. 12-18); (2) resistance of crossed hip flexion (hands on opposite thighs) (Fig. 12-19); (3) resistance of hip

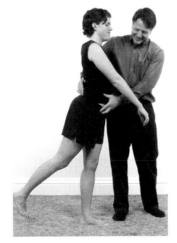

FIGURE 12–16 The leg swing mobility test.

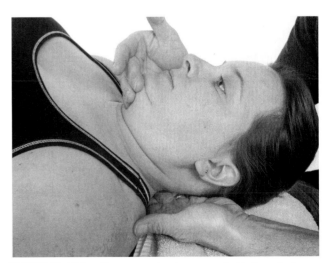

FIGURE 12–17 Specific segmental resistance applied to the articular pillars of the inhibited level.

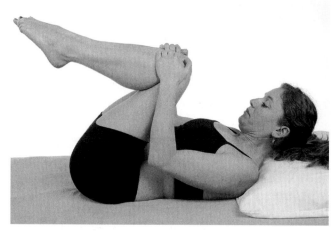

FIGURE 12–20 Resistance of hip extension, emphasizing traction.

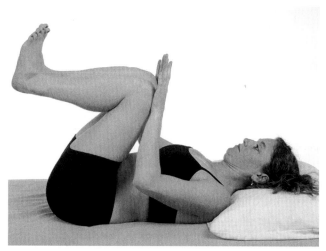

FIGURE 12–18 Resistance of bilateral hip flexion, emphasizing traction.

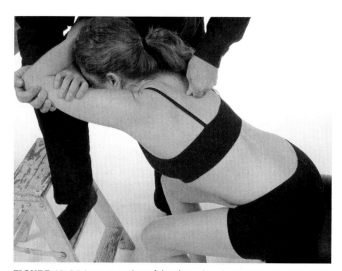

FIGURE 12-21 Impact testing of the thoracic spine.

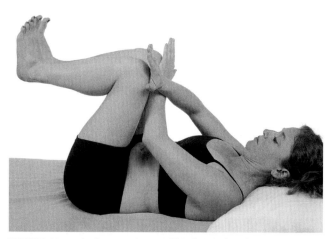

FIGURE 12–19 Resistance of crossed hip flexion (hands on opposite thighs).

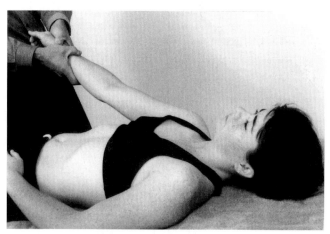

FIGURE 12–22 Impact testing involving traction of the upper extremity.

extension, emphasizing traction (Fig. 12-20); and (4) resisted bilateral hip flexion, emphasizing traction. It is important to perform each component of the series, using a tonic spread. If segmental facilitation does not produce any changes, the patient's prognosis is not optimal for successful conservative care.

Examples of cervical and lumbar impact testing include prolonged flexion, rotation, or extension; axial compression; traction of an extremity; or any functional movement identified as a possible aggravating factor (Figs. 12-21, 12-22). The patient's peripheral response is tested after each position, movement, or stress.

The findings of the impact test direct the therapist in selecting specific FM techniques. For example, the cervical patient is instructed to perform resisted axial elongation in supine or sitting by self-resistance or by using exercise tubing at the level of inhibition (Figs. 12-23, 12-24). While the lumbar patient is instructed in the abdominal series, the goal is to progress them into a functional stabilization program.

PRINCIPLES OF INTERVENTION
Components of Functional Mobilization
Soft Tissue Mobilization

The FM approach emphasizes the enhancement of soft tissue mobility prior to mobilizing restricted joints and developing motor control. **Functional soft tissue mobilization (FSTM)** seeks to identify the accessory mobility (muscle play), intrinsic tone, and functional excursion (ability of the muscle to lengthen and fold) of the myofascial structures.[1,5] Evaluation begins with skin and superficial fascia and proceeds to soft tissue attachments along bony contours and assessment of the myofascial complex function. Treatment intervention follows the cascade of techniques detailed in Chapter 13 of this text.

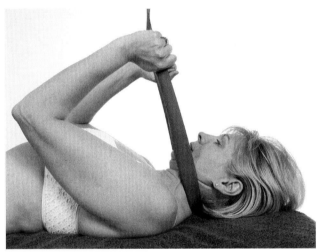

FIGURE 12–23 Resisted axial elongation in the supine position by using exercise tubing at the level of inhibition.

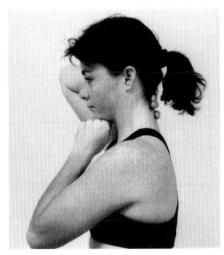

FIGURE 12–24 Resisted axial elongation in the sitting position using self-resistance to the neck and chin.

Joint Mobilization

The FM approach integrates traditional joint mobilization with passive, active, and resisted PNF or FMPs. For those patients who require thrust manipulation, functional manipulation couples thrust with a graded resisted contraction.

Neuromuscular Reeducation and Motor Control

Proper timing and initiation of core (local) muscles is a critical component of neuromuscular control. In an efficient state, local muscles perform a preparatory contraction prior to the initiation of the action (feed forward) to prepare and protect the surrounding structures.[1-4,16,21] Evaluation of inherent movement patterns and sequencing of motor recruitment becomes an important aspect of intervention. Dysfunction may produce repetitive trauma to both the articular and myofascial systems, which lead to structural dysfunction and symptoms.[36,48-52] Intervention facilitates improved mobility, automatic core stabilization (tonic contractions), and efficient patterns of movement (phasic contractions). The use of neuromuscular facilitation in newly acquired ranges enhances the patient's proprioceptive awareness and promotes retention of the new range of motion (ROM).

Once mechanical and neuromuscular function is improved, FM progresses to segmental motor control. Movement patterns perpetuated by mechanical dysfunctions, ineffective neuromuscular function, and inefficient body mechanics lead to loss of coordination, balance, and options for advanced motor planning and degenerative changes.[46,50-61] Effective motor learning progresses from reflexive or volitional (cognitive) motor responses toward associative and automatic motor control.[2-4,16-18,21,23] FM uses the principles and procedures of PNF to seamlessly progress from the mobilization aspect to progressive motor control training. The training begins at the local level where mobilization facilitates an improvement in mechanics. Once local control is established, the patient is progressed into functional movements to incorporate the new mobility and control into larger, more complex activities.[3,21,22,33,35]

Proprioceptive Neuromuscular Facilitation

The use of PNF to augment traditional mobilization techniques evolved from the need to place a more functional demand on the body and to engender patient participation. The PNF treatment strategy of considering normal development as a foundation for rehabilitation led to the incorporation of these procedures when managing the orthopaedic population.

QUESTIONS *for* REFLECTION

- Why is PNF deemed to be an important component within the **FM approach**?
- How are the principles and procedures of PNF incorporated into this approach?
- Briefly describe both upper- and lower-extremity diagonal 1 (D1) and diagonal 2 (D2) patterns.

General Principles of PNF

Body Position

The therapist's body position determines the direction in which the force is applied, facilitating the desired motor response. A three-point or diagonal stance allows the therapist to use his or her entire body to create resistance as opposed to using only the arms and legs.

Manual Contacts

Motor responses are influenced by the stimulation of skin receptors. Pressure is applied either in the direction of the desired motion or over the muscle group being facilitated.

Appropriate Resistance

Johnson and Johnson changed the original PNF term, *maximal resistance*, to *appropriate resistance* in 1982. This shift in terminology emphasizes the use of an appropriate response to facilitate fiber-specific motor recruitment.[15]

Traction and Approximation

The use of separate force vectors, coupled with appropriate resistance, enhances the efficiency of the body's motor response. Traction is especially important for facilitation of the core muscles.

Patterns of Facilitation

Inherent within the body's mechanical and neuromuscular systems exists specific patterns of movement that allow for optimum motor function of synergistic muscle groups. The spiral and diagonal PNF patterns of facilitation represent efficient patterns of movement that exist in functional activities.[15–21] Within the FM approach, these diagonal patterns are used to identify specific motion loss and subsequent intervention options.

Identification and Facilitation of Appropriate Contractions

The use of resistance provides a vehicle to selectively evaluate the ability to perform and integrate stabilizing (isometric) and movement (isotonic) contractions. PNF defines a contraction by the *intended purpose* of the contraction.[15–21, 62–76]

Isometric Contractions

Traditionally, an **isometric contraction** is characterized by a state in which the external force is equal to the internal force, thus preventing external movement.[76,77] In contrast, PNF defines an isometric contraction by the patient's *intention to maintain* a consistent position in space. The use of slowly building and matching resistance, coupled with the verbal command, *"keep it there,"* allows for specific isolation of a motor contraction while avoiding any compensations.[15–21]

Movement Contractions

Traditionally, an **isotonic contraction** is characterized by a state in which motion occurs when the internal force of the contraction overcomes the external force.[76,77] Within PNF, an isotonic contraction is one in which the *intention is to move*.[16–18,22] The term **concentric** means an active shortening of a muscle group; **eccentric** means a controlled active lengthening of a muscle group. **Maintained contraction**

refers to a dynamic contraction in which the patient's intention to produce movement is limited by a greater external force. This type of contraction is facilitated by asking the patient to push or pull into resistance while preventing any motion through increased resistance. This procedure is applied to promote an active contraction when a patient demonstrates diminished awareness of a desired movement. This contraction can also be used to increase motor output through appropriate irradiation following the specific activation of a muscle group with isometric resistance.[3,4,21]

PNF Techniques

PNF techniques are selected secondary to the identification of a specific dysfunction manifested by inefficient mechanics or poor neuromuscular control.

QUESTIONS *for* REFLECTION

- Describe each of the following PNF techniques, including purpose and clinical performance:
  - Combination of isotonics
  - Reversal of antagonists
  - Contract/hold-relax

Combination of Isotonics

Combination of isotonics (COI)[15,21] facilitates the ability to perform controlled and purposeful movements and enhances mobility of joint and soft tissues. COI identifies the patient's capacity to transition between the three types of isotonic contractions. To ensure an appropriate response, the therapist should initiate the motor contraction with an isometric hold and transition into COI. For enhancing mobility of joint and soft tissue restrictions, the therapist places the segment in a loose-packed position and proceeds to alternate between the various contractions, progressively moving into the eccentric range.

Reversal of Antagonists

Most activities depend on coordinated control of antagonistic muscle groups.[76,77] When an agonist fails to work in accordance with the demand of the activity, function is impaired. The reversal of the antagonist technique, based upon Sherrington's principle of successive induction, provides a mechanism to facilitate improved motor control.[78,79] There are two techniques: **isotonic reversals**, to restore reciprocation,[15,21] and **stabilizing reversals**, to promote core control.

Contract and Hold-Relax

The techniques of **contract and hold-relax**[15,21,63–75] are designed to stretch the intrinsic muscular connective tissue elements. The contract-relax technique uses either a concentric or a maintained isotonic contraction, whereas the hold-relax uses an isometric contraction.

To perform these techniques, place the segment at the point of limitation within the movement pattern. Resistance is applied either to the restricted agonist **(autogenic inhibition)** or to the antagonist (**reciprocal inhibition**). With contract-relax, a few degrees of motion occur (Fig. 12-25). Upon full relaxation, the segment is passively or actively moved into the new available range. Provide resistance in the new range of motion for reinforcement of that range. For treatment of pain, use hold-relax in a pain-free range of motion. Slowly build and release the isometric contraction.

Functional Mobilization Intervention Progression

The FM intervention progression can be broken down into the following phases (Box 12-4).[3,4] **Identification** is discovering three-dimensional joint or soft tissue dysfunction in static and dynamic postures and movements. **Localization** is determining

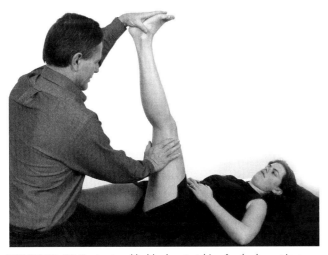

FIGURE 12–25 Contract and hold-relax stretching for the hamstrings.

Box 12-4 FUNCTIONAL MOBILIZATION TREATMENT PROGRESSION

- *Identification phase*: Discovering three-dimensional joint or soft tissue dysfunction in static and dynamic postures and movements
- *Localization phase*: Determining the exact depth and direction of the barrier's hardest end-feel, accompanied by passive or active movements of the specific body part
- *Mobilization phase:* Maintaining pressure on the dysfunctional structure while performing passive techniques, patient active movements, and resisted patterns
- *Neuromuscular reeducation (NMR) (stabilization) phase:* Using prolonged holds at the end of the newly gained range to assist in maintaining the new range and to protect the joint by stabilizing the segment
- *Motor control phase*: Using a combination of isotonics and isotonic reversal techniques to enhance local and global coordinated movement

---

the exact depth and direction of the barrier's hardest end-feel accompanied by passive or active movements of the specific body part. The **mobilization phase** includes the performance of FM by maintaining pressure on the dysfunctional structure while performing passive techniques, patient active movements, and resisted patterns. *Passive techniques* include traditional sustained, oscillatory, percussion, and thrust techniques to enhance mobility. *Patient active movements* can be simple, unidirectional movements of a single joint, or they can be more complicated functional motions. During the active movement, the therapist applies maintained pressure on the dysfunction as the patient moves, creating tension on the restriction.[3,4,78–86] During *resisted movements*, the therapist applies sustained pressure to the restriction while maintained resistance is applied to a regional body part that mitigates pressure specifically on the restriction. An alternative method uses isometric resistance to facilitate the specific motor contraction that engages the muscles directly connected to the soft tissue or joint structures being mobilized. When the restriction begins to release, progression from the sustained contraction to the eccentric phase of a COI procedure is initiated. The technique continues with alternating eccentric, concentric, and holding contractions as the therapist evaluates the response of the restriction.

When performing techniques, it is essential to address dysfunction of adjacent segments to avoid treating through a *"dirty lever arm."*[82] For example, prior to treating the pelvic girdle, it is essential to address a dysfunction of the hip.

Following achievement of improved motion, this approach progresses immediately to the **neuromuscular reeducation (NMR) (stabilization) phase**. This phase uses prolonged holds at the end of the newly gained range to maintain the new range and protect the joint. Once the stabilizing contraction is facilitated and the mechanical and neuromuscular control components are addressed, the **motor control phase** begins. This phase involves utilization of a combination of isotonic reversal techniques to enhance local and global coordinated movement. When using COI, initially the focus is on those contractions that are performed well with progression to those that are more challenging. The addition of stabilizing reversals encourages coordinated, alternating movement.

The intervention strategy progresses to the development of motor control and automatic functional training using the tools of ***Back Education and Training (BET)***.[22] Patients must gain a kinesthetic awareness of the more efficient postures and movements through training and repetition. The key to this learning process is using a combination of manual resistance, appropriate verbal commands, and manual interventions. Home programs are designed in accordance with the patient's functional deficits to produce automatic use of more efficient movement patterns.

Principles of Functional Stabilization

The strategy for managing a hypermobile segment includes mobilization of the regional hypomobile segments and facilitation of motor control of hypermobile or unstable segments.[48,83,84,87–98] It is important to establish local stability prior to encouraging global movement.[35,82–105] To begin, the segment is placed in a midrange, weight-bearing position by using *prolonged holds* and *stabilizing reversals.* Manual resistance is applied directly to the unstable segment to facilitate the stabilizing muscles. Once a stabilizing contraction is achieved, treatment progresses to controlled movement through *combinations of isotonics.* As neuromuscular control is achieved, training is progressed through the segment's full range, followed by the inclusion of functional activities (Fig 12-26).

CLINICAL PILLAR

Principles of Functional stabilization include the following:

- Mobilize hypomobile segments and facilitate motor control of hypermobile or unstable segments.

- Establish local stability prior to encouraging global movement.

- Begin with the segment placed in a midrange, weight-bearing position.

- Use *prolonged holds* and *stabilizing reversals.*

- Apply manual resistance directly to the unstable segment to facilitate the stabilizing muscles.

- Treatment progresses to controlled movement through *combinations of isotonics.*

- Once neuromuscular control in midrange is accomplished, training is progressed throughout the full range.

- Stabilization training is then progressed to include functional training.

MANAGEMENT OF THE UPPER QUADRANT

Management of the Thoracic Girdle

The restoration of upper thoracic mobility prior to focusing on cervical spine or upper extremity symptoms is a primary emphasis of the FM approach. The thoracic girdle's primary structures are the first thoracic vertebra, first ribs, and the manubrium. Additional structures include the second thoracic vertebrae, second ribs, and the sternoclavicular joints.[3]

The *manubrium* is the first bony structure treated after addressing the soft tissues. Assessment begins by *spring testing* the right/left and superior/inferior aspects (i.e., four quadrants) of the manubrium to identify the location and direction of greatest restriction. With the patient's hand placed behind the neck (an FMP termed **lazy Cobra**); the therapist uses assisted diagonal cervical flexion and extension to localize the restriction to the hardest end-feel and then applies directed resistance to the elbow to enhance the speed and effectiveness of the mobilization.

For example, during left cervical flexion the left inferior pole of the manubrium is restricted in the posterior and inferior direction. The treatment hand provides sustained pressure to the restriction while the assisting hand resists cervical flexion/left diagonal through the elbow (Fig. 12-27). Once the restriction begins to soften, the procedure transitions into a COI and progresses into the new ROM, which is followed by a prolonged hold for training. This procedure is a **direct technique** because the resistance is in the same direction as the restriction. **Indirect techniques** (resistance applied in the opposite direction of the restriction) are appropriate when direct techniques produce pain or are ineffective.

If the cervical spine is flexion sensitive, use the upper extremity to assist in the mobilization of the manubrium.

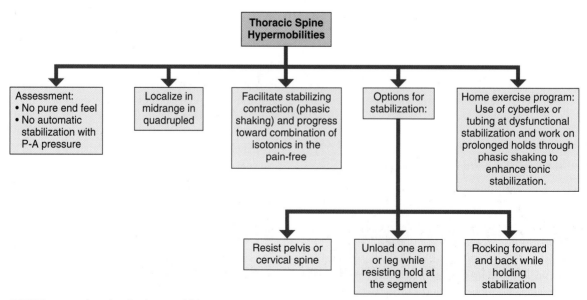

FIGURE 12–26 Thoracic spine hypermobilities.

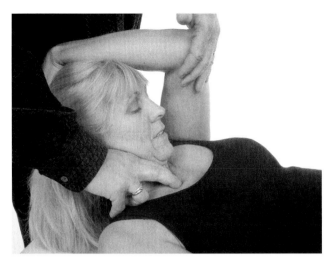

FIGURE 12–27 The lazy cobra position.

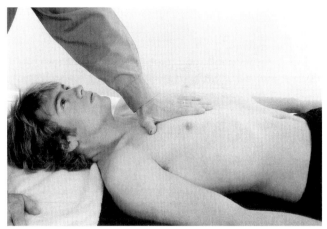

FIGURE 12–29 Resisted sternal breathing is performed by placing the heel of the hand on the manubrial body to evaluate motion during full inhalation and exhalation. If the manubrium is limited in exhalation, with full exhalation the therapist blocks inhalation to mobilize, then takes up the slack during exhalation. For limited inhalation, the therapist facilitates full sternal elevation through resisting a full inhalation, then applies a hold followed by an attempt at further inhalation.

For example, if the restriction is on the left, use the right upper extremity. Place the patient's right hand on the left shoulder, the **cover position**, and apply resistance through the elbow into the upper extremity extension-adduction pattern (Fig. 12-28). Directed breathing is used to enhance the mobilization process.

Resisted sternal breathing is performed once normal mobility of the manubrium is achieved. Place the heel of the hand on the manubrial body to evaluate motion during full inhalation and exhalation. If the manubrium is limited in exhalation, then with full exhalation the therapist blocks inhalation to mobilize and takes up the slack during exhalation (Fig. 12-29). For limited inhalation, the therapist facilitates full sternal elevation through resisting a full inhalation then a hold followed by an attempt at further inhalation.

The second structures evaluated and treated in the supine progression of the thoracic girdle are the *first ribs*. Initially, the therapist examines the posterior-anterior and anterior-posterior mobility of the first ribs, which are coupled with cervical rotation. The direction of greatest limitation (the

hardest end-feel) is identified and mobilized through one or a combination of the following: active cervical rotation, lower trunk rotation, resisted lazy cobra, axial elongation, the cover position (Fig. 12-30).

The second phase, first rib *distraction and depression* (inferior glide) (Fig. 12-31) are examined in supine or sitting position through palpation of the first rib, which migrates inferiorly during ipsilateral cervical side bending. If it is restricted, then intervention is localized to the hardest end-feel and mobilization using breathing, cervical rotation/lateral flexion, lower trunk rotation, or the cover position is performed, the latter of which is most effective.

The final phase of first rib mobilization is **scalene elongation.** To perform scalene elongation, the first rib is stabilized with one hand as the cervical spine is passively side-bent contralaterally, and the specific region of tightness is localized

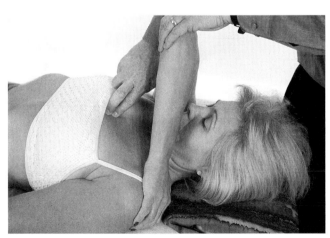

FIGURE 12–28 The cover position with resistance applied through the elbow into the upper extremity extension-adduction pattern.

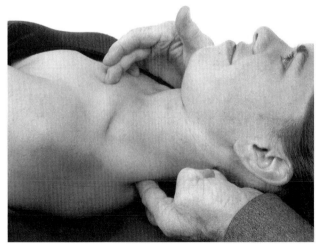

FIGURE 12–30 Examination of anterior-to-posterior and posterior-to-anterior first rib mobility.

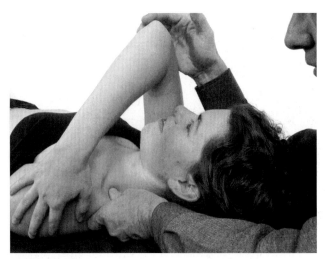

FIGURE 12–31 First rib distraction and depression (inferior glide) mobilization in the cover position.

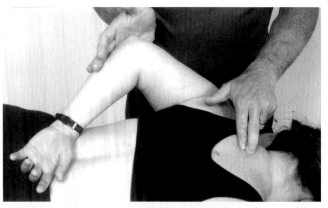

FIGURE 12–33 Position 1 of the mobility examination for T1-T2 includes placing the back of the patient's hand on the buttocks or lumbar spine while examining the ability of the vertebrae to rotate superiorly.

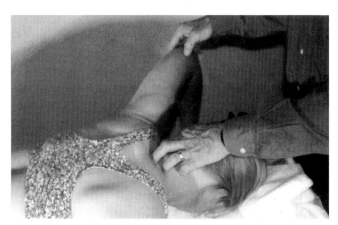

FIGURE 12–34 Position 2 of the mobility examination for T1-T2 includes placing the hand flat on the table above the shoulder to test pure rotation.

through cervical rotation. Once localized, the structures are treated with contract-relax stretching and STM.[3–5,16,21,82–84] Self-mobilization of the first rib between sessions is performed using a towel or strap (Fig. 12-32).

Improvement in *T1-T2* mobility is critical for enhancing cervical rotation and the alignment of the head over the thoracic cage. In the standing position, the relationship of the lower cervical to the upper thoracic spine is observed. Motion palpation in the sitting position, with the patient's hands interlaced behind his or her neck, is the most effective evaluation position. However, the prone position is used for the initial mobilization by placing the upper extremities in four distinct positions. **Position one,** with the back of the patient's hand on the buttocks or lumbar spine, examines the ability of the vertebrae to rotate superiorly (Fig. 12-33). **Position two,** with the hand placed flat on the table above the shoulder, tests vertebral movement into pure rotation (Fig. 12-34). **Position three,** with the hand on the back of the head, tests the ability of the vertebrae to rotate inferiorly (Fig. 12-35). **Position four** includes the addition of anterior to posterior motion. The

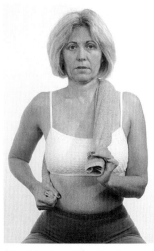

FIGURE 12–32 Self-mobilization of the first rib.

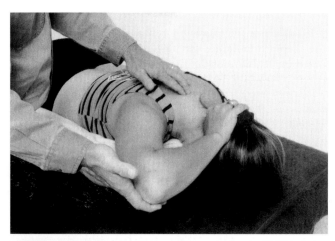

FIGURE 12–35 Position 3 of the mobility examination for T1-T2 includes placing the hand on the back of the head to test the ability of the vertebrae to rotate inferiorly.

patient is positioned in prone on the elbows with his or her hand on the opposite shoulder (cover position) and the forehead resting on the elbow with the face in the bend of the arm to prevent upper cervical extension (Fig. 12-36). Localization of restrictions is accomplished through thoracic extension

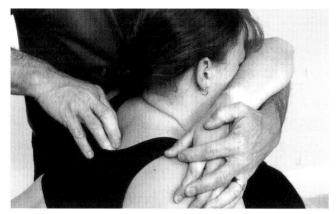

FIGURE 12–36 Position 4 of the mobility examination for T1-T2 includes the addition of anterior-to-posterior motion. The patient is in the cover position with the forehead resting on the elbow and the face in the bend of the arm to prevent upper cervical extension.

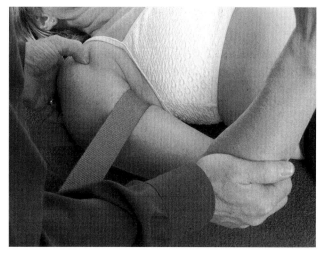

FIGURE 12–37 Lateral gapping or scaption distraction mobilization.

diagonals. For the mobilization phase, resistance is applied to trunk flexion, and as always, the procedure is completed with NMR and progressed into weight-bearing positions, such as sitting (Fig. 12-21).

Management of the Glenohumeral Joint

Treatment of the glenohumeral (GH) joint occurs subsequent to managing the thoracic girdle and scapula.[3] The scapula's position and mobility, which dictate GH mechanics, are determined by the structure and function of the underlying thoracic cage.[106–123]

The first components of the treatment progression seek to address *accessory motions* of the GH joint. These motions are lateral gapping, inferior translation, inferior glide, and posterior translation/internal rotation.

Lateral Gapping or Scaption Distraction Mobilization

During normal function, the humerus has the ability to distract an average of 0.5 mm from the glenoid fossa and is controlled by the rotator cuff.[120] Using a mobilization strap, end-feel assessment is performed by manually moving the head of the humerus away from the glenoid fossa (Fig. 12-37). The free hand palpates the anterior/medial joint line to monitor the distraction. At the point of restriction, mobilization is performed by resisting shoulder abduction at the elbow.

Neuromuscular reeducation follows the mobilization phase to enhance the ability of the rotator cuff to set the humeral head within the glenoid fossa. Initially, isotonic resistance for abduction is used while setting is evaluated. Once the therapist is aware of the setting procedure, facilitation by using the rotator cuff only (without resisted abduction) is performed. NMR with prolonged holds and COI continues until stability is achieved. Training automatic setting of the humeral head during functional activities is then pursued (Fig. 12-38).[117–123] By using a strap or towel roll for a fulcrum in sitting position, GH gapping may also be performed (Fig. 12-39).

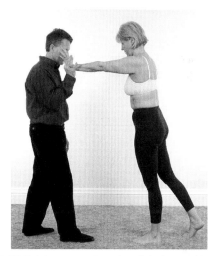

FIGURE 12–38 Training automatic setting of the humeral head during functional activities.

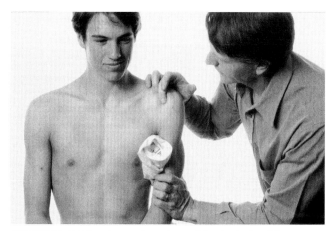

FIGURE 12–39 Glenohumeral gapping mobilization in the sitting position using a towel roll as a fulcrum.

Inferior Translation Mobilization

Assessment is performed in supine position with the arm placed at the side, elbow flexed. With a strap placed around the elbow, the therapist assesses *inferior translation* of the humerus and separation of the head from the acromion process. Following normalization of inferior translation, a prolonged hold to facilitate the tonic fibers of the supraspinatus then progressing to COI for motor reeducation is pursued (Fig. 12-40).

Inferior Glide Mobilization

To mobilize the inferior capsule, the patient is sitting next to the treatment table with the affected arm resting on the table at 80 to 90 degrees of abduction. The therapist is at the patient's side with the heel of the hand assessing the ability of the humeral head to glide inferiorly. Restrictions are localized and *inferior glide* mobilization through upper extremity adduction into the table is performed (Fig. 12-41). To conclude, NMR is pursued through manual resistance to humeral head depression, beginning with prolonged holds and progressing to COI to facilitate the infraspinatus, teres minor, and subscapularis (Fig. 12-42).

Internal Rotation Mobilization

The goal of intervention is to improve the ability of the humeral head to remain stable within the glenoid and accomplish pure

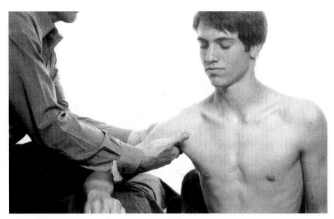

FIGURE 12–42 Neuromuscular reeducation through manual resistance to humeral head depression.

rotation. With the patient in the supine position, the therapist is seated at the side of the table with the strap over the proximal humerus and under the therapist's foot (Fig. 12-43). The elbow rests on the therapist's knee as close to 90 degrees of abduction as possible. An anterior-posterior pressure to the humerus is applied by placing force on the strap while taking the GH joint to full available internal rotation. Mobilization is performed through resisted external rotation followed by NMR into the new range of internal rotation. With the patient in the prone position, the same technique may be used for mobilization into *external rotation* (Fig. 12-44).

After accessory motions are addressed, evaluation and treatment of the joint through the range of PNF patterns is implemented. To evaluate the condition of the soft tissues, acromioclavicular, sternoclavicular, and GH joints, position the shoulder at the end range of each diagonal (Fig 12-45).

Flexion, Abduction, and External Rotation Pattern Mobilization

In the hook-lying position, the shoulder is passively moved to end range while the GH joint is localized by using a strap to

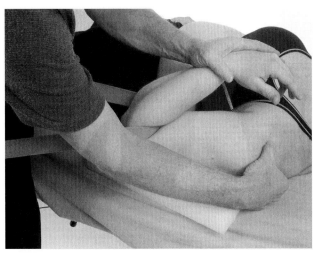

FIGURE 12–40 Glenohumeral inferior translation mobilization with mobilization belt.

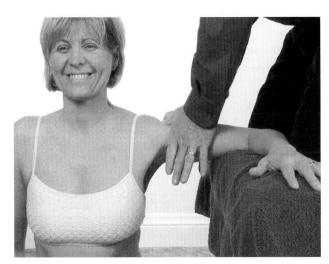

FIGURE 12–41 Glenohumeral inferior glide mobilization with shoulder in abduction.

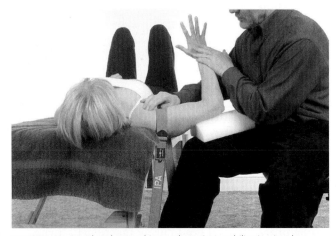

FIGURE 12–43 Glenohumeral internal rotation mobilization involves anterior-posterior pressure to the humerus applied by placing force on the strap while taking the GH joint to full available internal rotation with patient in supine position.

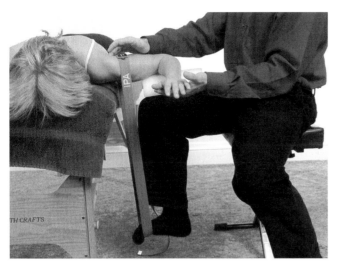

FIGURE 12–44 Glenohumeral external rotation mobilization involves posterior-anterior pressure to the humerus applied by placing force on the strap while taking the GH joint to full available external rotation with patient in prone position.

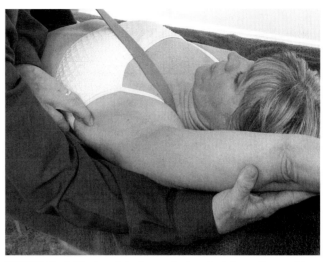

FIGURE 12–46 Flexion, abduction, and external rotation pattern mobilization, which includes localizing the GH joint by using a strap to stabilize the scapula.

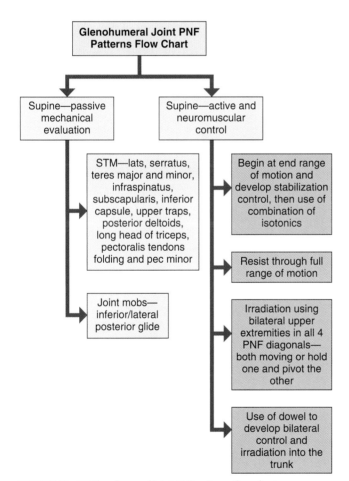

Glenohumeral Joint PNF Patterns Flow Chart

Supine—passive mechanical evaluation

Supine—active and neuromuscular control

STM—lats, serratus, teres major and minor, infraspinatus, subscapularis, inferior capsule, upper traps, posterior deltoids, long head of triceps, pectoralis tendons folding and pec minor

Joint mobs—inferior/lateral posterior glide

Begin at end range of motion and develop stabilization control, then use of combination of isotonics

Resist through full range of motion

Irradiation using bilateral upper extremities in all 4 PNF diagonals—both moving or hold one and pivot the other

Use of dowel to develop bilateral control and irradiation into the trunk

FIGURE 12–45 Glenohumeral joint PNF patterns flow chart.

stabilize the scapula as the following components are assessed and treated (Fig. 12-46).[3,16,17]

- *Myofascia:* Evaluate individually the latissimus dorsi, teres major and minor, infraspinatus, subscapularis, triceps,

pectoralis major and minor, the inferior capsule, and neurovascular structures.

- *Acromioclavicular joint:* Evaluate the distal end of the clavicle for anterior motion in relationship to the acromion process.
- *Sternoclavicular joint:* Evaluate the proximal end of the clavicle for distraction and downward glide relative to the manubrium.
- *Glenohumeral joint:* Evaluate and perform joint mobilization within this pattern with an anterior/inferior glide using a strap around the posterior aspect of the humerus and the therapist's shoulder applying posterior-anterior pressure (Fig. 12-47).
- *Neuromuscular reeducation:* NMR begins with prolonged holds at the end of the range until a stabilizing

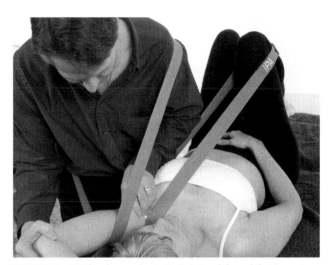

FIGURE 12–47 Glenohumeral anterior/inferior glide mobilization using a strap looped around the posterior aspect of the humerus with the therapist's shoulder applying the posterior-anterior pressure.

contraction is established. Once stabilization is established, perform COI through the range.

Extension, Adduction, Internal Rotation Pattern Mobilization

The end range of this pattern is with the arm across midline.[3,16,17]

- *Myofascia:* Individually evaluate the upper trapezius, levator scapulae, deep cervical fascia, serratus posterior superior, supraspinatus, deltoids, pectoralis tendon, bicipital groove, infraspinatus, and teres major and minor.
- *Acromioclavicular joint:* Evaluate the distal end of the clavicle for posterior motion in relationship to the acromion process.
- *Sternoclavicular joint:* Evaluate the proximal end of the clavicle for compression, hinging, and upward glide relative to the manubrium.
- *Glenohumeral joint:* Perform evaluation and joint mobilization using a mobilization strap, the therapist's forearm, or a small foam roll as a fulcrum for gapping, and superior motion of the GH joint (Fig. 12-48).
- *Neuromuscular reeducation:* NMR includes resistance of the PNF pattern into the new range of motion (Fig. 12-49).

Flexion, Adduction, and External Rotation Pattern Mobilization

The pattern crosses midline with the elbow bent.[3,16,17]

- *Myofascia:* Evaluate the same soft tissues as those evaluated with the flexion, abduction pattern.
- *Acromioclavicular joint:* Evaluate the distal end of the clavicle for posterior motion in relationship to the acromion process.
- *Sternoclavicular joint:* Evaluate the proximal end of the clavicle for compression, hinging, and inferior motion.
- *Glenohumeral joint:* Perform evaluation and joint mobilization for distraction, inferior, and lateral motion (Fig. 12-50).
- *Neuromuscular reeducation:* NMR includes resistance of the pattern to develop control in the new range of motion.

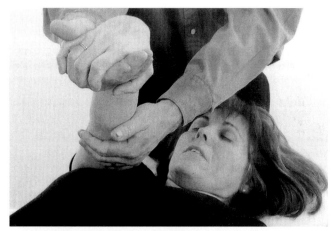

FIGURE 12–49 Neuromuscular reeducation includes resistance of the PNF pattern into the new range of motion.

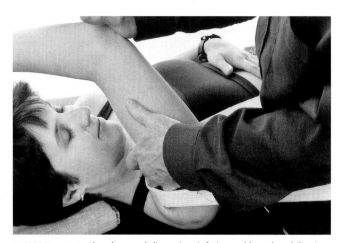

FIGURE 12–50 Glenohumeral distraction, inferior and lateral mobilization.

Extension, Abduction, and Internal Rotation Pattern Mobilization

The pattern moves in extension off the edge of the table.[3,16,17]

- *Myofascia:* Evaluate the same soft tissues as those evaluated with the flexion, abduction pattern.
- *Acromioclavicular joint:* Evaluate the distal end of the clavicle for anterior motion in relationship to the acromion process.
- *Sternoclavicular joint:* Evaluate the proximal end of the clavicle for distraction and superior motion.
- *Glenohumeral joint:* Perform evaluation and joint mobilization for distraction and posterior motion (Fig. 12-51).
- *Neuromuscular reeducation:* NMR includes resistance of the pattern to develop control in the new range of motion.

MANAGEMENT OF THE LOWER QUADRANT
Management of the Coccyx

Within the FM approach, the coccyx is the key structure of the lumbopelvic girdle region. Clinical experience has demonstrated that normalization of a dysfunctional coccyx enhances

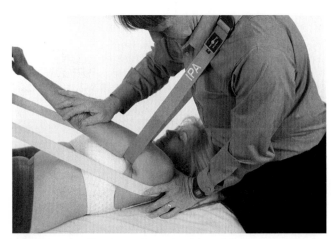

FIGURE 12–48 Glenohumeral superior glide mobilization using the therapist's forearm or a small foam roll as a fulcrum for gapping.

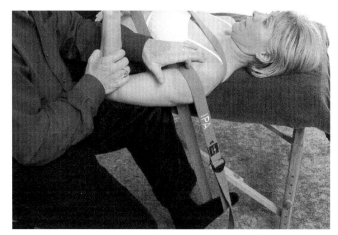

FIGURE 12-51 Glenohumeral distraction, posterior mobilization

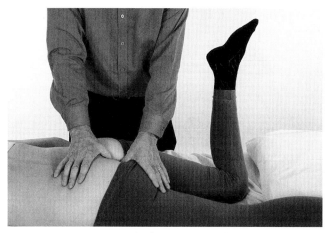

FIGURE 12-52 Intervention for the sacrococcygeal junction rotation involving pressure applied to the restriction with active or resisted hip rotation ipsilaterally.

objective signs in other lumbopelvic girdle structures.[4,124–132] Conversely, when related structures (sacrum, innominate, lumbar spine, and hips) are treated, coccygeal dysfunctions rarely improve. The impact of coccygeal mobilization on other structures may be attributed to the attachment of the terminalis of the dura to the second coccygeal segment, the attachment of the pelvic floor muscles, and/or the extensive anterior and posterior fascial and ligamentous insertions.

In the efficient coccyx, the transition from the sacrum to the coccyx is smooth, with a springy end-feel, and the body possesses a normal curve without deviation. Possible dysfunctions at the *sacrococcygeal junction* include compression, rotation, lateral translation, and posterior and anterior shear. Possible dysfunctions at the *body of the coccyx* include deviation (side bending), extension, and flexion.

Intervention for the Sacrococcygeal Junction

Compression

In the efficient state, caudal pressure placed against the coccyx will identify a springy separation of the joint surfaces. When a dysfunction is identified, force is applied directly into the restriction with active or resisted bilateral hip rotation.

Rotation

Rotation is identified through a unilateral hard end-feel and lipping of the coccyx above the sacral component of the joint. Lipping and a hard end-feel on the right is indicative of a right rotation. Treatment consists of pressure applied to the restriction with active or resisted hip rotation ipsilaterally (Fig. 12-52).

Posterior Shear

Posterior shear is identified through bilateral lipping of the coccyx with a palpable hard end-feel. This condition is often seen after childbirth and is treated with bilateral hip rotation or upper quadrant press-ups.

Anterior Shear

Anterior shear is often the result of a direct fall and is most effectively treated with an internal mobilization.

Lateral Translation

This condition involves shifting of the coccyx to the right or left of the joint line. The most effective treatment position is in the side-lying position using unilateral hip rotation.

Intervention for the Body of the Coccyx

Deviation

This condition is present when there is less space and a hard end-feel between one side of the coccyx and the lateral structures. A deviated coccyx is not functioning along its normal axis and should be treated prior to treating a flexion/extension dysfunction. The patient is positioned in the side-lying position with the deviated side up, and localization is accomplished through hip flexion/extension, abduction/adduction, and rotation. Mobilization occurs through active or resisted hip flexion/extension or rotation of the superior leg (Fig. 12-53).

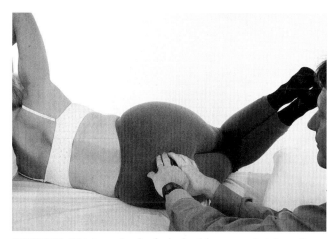

FIGURE 12-53 Intervention for the body of the coccyx deviation with the patient positioned in side-lying position with the deviated side up and localization accomplished through hip flexion/extension, abduction/adduction, and rotation. Mobilization occurs through active or resisted hip flexion/extension or rotation of the superior leg.

Extension

This condition is characterized by a restriction of the body in a posterior-to-anterior direction. Treatment occurs in prone with knees flexed while resisting knee extension. Mobilization may also occur during active upper quadrant press-ups.

Flexion

A flexed coccyx is often difficult to contact directly; therefore, internal treatment is often necessary. An effective external option is in the quadruped position, which provides easier access to the tip. Apply pressure toward extension with traction as the patient sits back toward his or her heels (Fig. 12-55). Additional precautions are implemented for individuals with osteoporosis.

Following management in non-weight-bearing positions, conduct assessment of the coccyx, sacrum, innominates, and lumbar spine in sitting. The lumbar spine should be cleared first, followed by intervention that progresses caudally to the coccyx (Fig. 12-56). Once a dysfunction is identified, accomplish localization through trunk flexion/extension and diagonal motions. Perform FM with either direct or indirect techniques followed by NMR (Figs. 12-57, 12-58).

Lower Quadrant Strategies

Because the pelvic girdle is central to the function of the lower quadrant, early management of mechanical and motor control dysfunctions are a primary focus. The emphasis of sacral management is the assessment of the sacrum's ability to nutate and attain a form closure position in relationship to the innominates. There are eight innominate motions that are evaluated and treated, and they are named according to their associated hip motions: flexion, extension, internal and external rotation, abduction and adduction, elevation and depression. An essential aspect of pelvic girdle management is the enhancement of hip mobility and development of optimal motor control.

The efficient function of the knee depends upon the mobility of the innominate-hip complex and the foot-ankle complex.

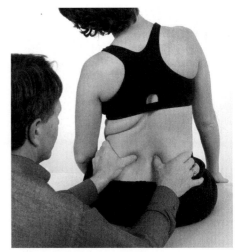

FIGURE 12–55 Clearing the lumbar spine through palpation of the transverse processes during the combined position of extension, side bending, and rotation.

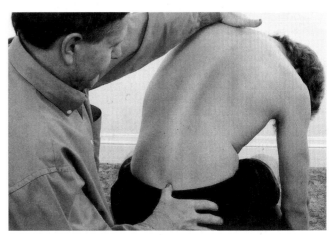

FIGURE 12–56 Intervention for the body of the coccyx involves clearing the lumbar spine first followed by intervention that progresses caudally to the coccyx. Localization is accomplished through trunk flexion and diagonal motions.

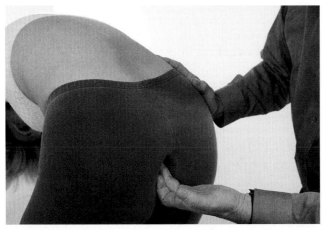

FIGURE 12–54 An effective external option for palpation of a flexed coccyx is in the quadruped position, which provides easier access to the tip. Apply pressure toward extension with traction as the patient sits back toward his or her heels.

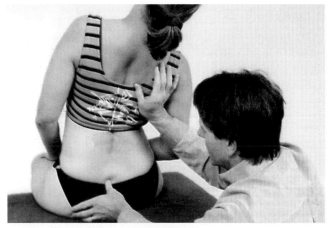

FIGURE 12–57 Intervention for the body of the coccyx involves clearing the lumbar spine first followed by intervention that progresses caudally to the coccyx. Localization is accomplished through trunk extension and diagonal motions.

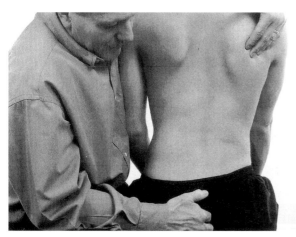

FIGURE 12–58 Intervention for the body of the coccyx involves clearing the lumbar spine first followed by intervention that progresses caudally to the coccyx. Localization is accomplished through trunk rotation.

The FM approach provides tools to manage the surrounding soft tissues and patella, the fibula head, the intrinsic mobility between the tibia and femur, and a unique approach for treating meniscal tears.

Management of foot and ankle impairment involves a step-by-step systematic management system. In both non-weight-bearing and weight-bearing positions, the therapist seeks to enhance foot and ankle mechanics and neuromuscular control. Treatment begins by first assessing calcaneal motion in all directions for mechanical restrictions. To restore calcaneal motion, it is essential that treatment be performed in full dorsiflexion. The progression proceeds to the Achilles tendon and posterior soft tissues and then to the talus for medial, lateral, anterior, and posterior directions. Weight-bearing treatment of the talus is an essential component for attaining efficient function. Evaluation and treatment is progressed to address the anterior soft tissues, interosseous membrane, and fibular head. Clinical observations indicate that the midfoot is the location of primary dysfunction in most patients. It has been noted that the cuneiforms (primarily the first and second) are immobile in most infants and adults. A variety of foot conditions, such as supinated feet, compensated supinated feet, and hallux valgus deformity, may originate from this region of immobility. Once the midfoot and forefoot are managed, general conditioning of the foot intrinsic musculature is addressed. See Figure 12-59 for an outline of the FM lower extremity treatment progression.

ACTIVITIES OF DAILY LIVING: INTERVENTION AND PROGRESSION STRATEGIES
Motor Control Development Through Resisted Rolling

Evaluation of rolling patterns identifies underlying motor planning and neuromuscular control issues. The initial goal is to facilitate the core muscles through prolonged holds to mass trunk flexion and extension patterns emphasizing pelvic,

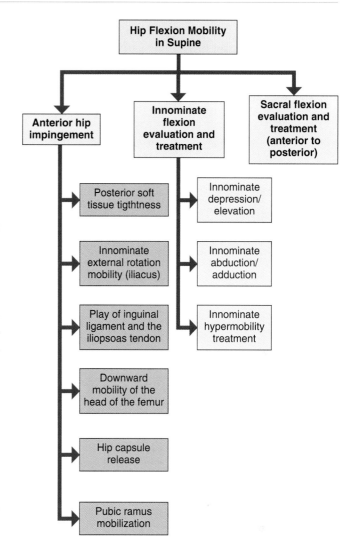

FIGURE 12–59 Hip flexion mobility in supine.

foot, head, and neck components. For example, if a patient ambulates with an accentuated lumbar lordosis, then the tonic stabilizers of mass trunk flexion need facilitation to decrease the need for the overactive erector spinae. To accomplish this, the patient is positioned in mass flexion in the side-lying position with the dysfunctional side up, and facilitation through resisted prolonged holds (as previously described) of scapular anterior depression and pelvic anterior elevation is performed. Using resistance and traction assists in the learning process (Fig. 12-60).[30] Treatment progresses to motor control training, which uses a COI and isotonic reversals in the new range of motion through repeated rolling. As the patient masters rolling, the motion can be added to the home program by adding resistance through a band or SportCord.

Gait Training

Initially, the emphasis is placed on assessing the motion and stability of the lumbo-pelvic-hip complex. Once the mechanical dysfunctions are addressed, PNF resisted gait techniques are used to train more efficient patterns of ambulation.[4]

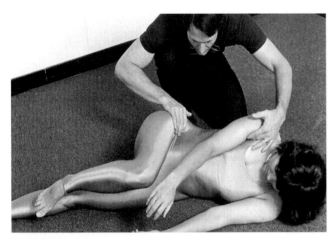

FIGURE 12–60 Motor control development through resisted rolling. The patient is in mass flexion in side-lying position with the dysfunctional side up, and facilitation occurs through resisted prolonged holds of scapular anterior depression and pelvic anterior elevation.

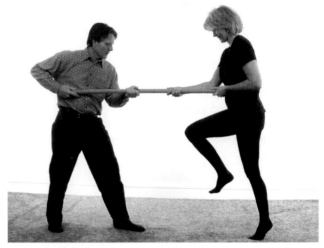

FIGURE 12–62 With the use of dowels held in the upper extremities, core, stabilization is enhanced through pushing and pulling techniques at waist height, which are later progressed to stepping activities.

There are several options for the management of gait dysfunctions. The first option is to regress the patient to non-weight-bearing and resist rolling then crawling to engage the pelvis. Once more efficient use of the pelvis is restored, gait can be facilitated through applied resistance in several directions, including forward, backward, and lateral directions, as well as braiding and resisted hopping and skipping (Fig. 12-61). With dowels held in the upper extremities, core stabilization is enhanced through pushing and pulling techniques, which are later progressed to stepping activities (Fig. 12-62, 12-63).

The home program uses five phases. **Rockette walking** emphasizes pelvic anterior elevation with the verbal cues of using a "long leg" walk from the thoracolumbar junction. **Prancing** is used to emphasize the initiation of hip flexion and involves taking high steps while walking. The last technique, **rollerblading**, is used to emphasize push-off and propulsion. It involves initiating motion in the trunk through a subtle lean forward and then propelling the body forward

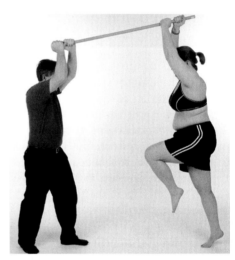

FIGURE 12–63 With the use of dowels held in the upper extremities, core stabilization is enhanced through pushing and pulling techniques overhead, which are later progressed to stepping activities.

through the lengthening of the hip and push-off through the foot. For cool down, the patient combines the rockette and rollerblade walking to create more pelvic mobility.

DIFFERENTIATING CHARACTERISTICS

The FM approach offers a variety of unique examination and intervention strategies not found in other OMPT paradigms (Box 12-5). At the core of this approach is the predominant *focus on function*. Unlike many other forms of manual therapy, FM endeavors to examine the patient as a whole and seeks to reestablish efficient function throughout the entire system. Although management is not directed specifically toward an individual's presenting pain complaints, restoration of efficient structure and function is believed to not only provide pain reduction, but also to reduce the likelihood of symptomatic reoccurrence through improved mechanics and neuromuscular control.

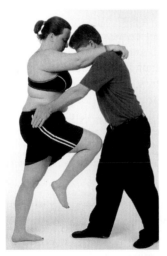

FIGURE 12–61 Gait can be facilitated through applied resistance in several directions, including forward, backward, and lateral directions, as well as braiding and resisted hopping and skipping.

Box 12-5 DIFFERENTIATING CHARACTERISTICS OF THE FUNCTIONAL MOBILIZATION APPROACH TO OMPT

- Focus on function
- Eclectic
- Integration of neuromuscular reeducation, soft tissue mobilization, and joint mobilization
- Systematic
- Patients participate
- Creative

The *eclectic* nature of the FM approach is another distinguishing feature that renders it unique. This approach seeks to incorporate the best philosophies and practices from several OMPT schools of thought. The ability to integrate a combination of philosophies into the one system provides the therapist with a flexible framework from which to manage patients.

The integration of NMR, STM, and joint mobilization differentiates FM from other forms of OMPT that may focus on only one of these components. Improved efficiency and effectiveness is enhanced by integrating various schools of thought into one congruent regimen.

FM provides a *systematic approach* to the management of each articulation without depending on preconceived protocols. Appropriate intervention requires each therapist to use his or her own scientific and clinical knowledge to reach effective solutions to solve complex problems.

Unlike some approaches, the FM approach requires *patient participation*. Individuals who play a major role in their own recovery are less likely to become dependent. Within this approach, the manual physical therapist's primary role is to facilitate function and teach patients to take responsibility on their road toward recovery.

Lastly, FM is an extremely *creative* form of OMPT. FM encourages each therapist to modify and adapt his or her technique to meet the needs of each unique individual. Alterations in technique performance are encouraged in pursuit of optimal outcomes. The techniques that compose the FM approach are limited only by the creativity and ingenuity of the clinicians who continually seek to discover alternate solutions to restoration of efficient function.

CLINICAL CASE

History of Present Illness (HPI)

A 40-year-old male presents with low back and buttock pain beginning 20 years ago when he sustained a fall while skiing. His symptoms completely resolved after the initial incident, but he has suffered from episodic returns throughout the years. Six months ago, he caught himself in a flexed over position during a hard landing when he slipped and fell down a short flight of stairs. His symptoms returned and worsened over the next several days until he was unable to resume an upright position. His symptoms were worse upon upright standing and walking and eased by supine lying with knees bent and his back flat. Increased symptoms are noted with extension, right side bending, and right rotation.

Observation: Increased lumbar spine lordosis with bilateral genu recurvatum is noted. Right pelvis is anteriorly rotated. Right hip is in external rotation.

Active Range of Motion (AROM): Limited by 50% in active physiological forward bending, backward bending, right side bending, right rotation.

Palpation: Left rotation at L4 and L5 noted via palpation of transverse processes. Right (R) > left (L) psoas decreased play, extensibility.

Accessory: Hard end-feel noted left L4 and L5 transverse process spring testing in left extension quadrant.

FMP: (+) Armadillo R > L; (+) corkscrew to L > R; (+) leg swing right flexion

Functional Examination Findings: Deficits in gait and rolling

Neurological: Intact and symmetrical deep tendon reflex (DTR) and light touch, sharp/dull sensation

Special Tests: Impact test (+) lower quadrant (LQ) facilitation after right hip extension

LPM = 2/5   EFT = 2/5   VCT = 2/5

Radiographs: (+) L5 spondylolisthesis present, (+) L4-L5 and L5-S1 disk protrusion and encroachment of right L5 nerve root

1. Given this presentation, what is the most likely origin of this patient's symptoms? What was revealed in the patient's history and/or subjective report that may influence your choice of examination/intervention positioning or vigor? What positions, movements, ROM, or intensity would you select?

2. Based on this presentation, with what dysfunction(s) would you diagnose this patient? Would you treat the patient to address symptoms or correct biomechanical dysfunction? Explain your rationale and the process of coming to this conclusion.

3. Describe how your differential diagnosis as noted above would influence your selection and application of manual physical therapy techniques according to the Functional Mobilization approach to OMPT.

4. Is there any additional information that you would like to have before initiating intervention?

5. Identify three specific manual physical therapy techniques that you would implement at the time of this patient's first visit to physical therapy. Describe each in detail (i.e., position, direction, duration, vigor, etc.). In addition, perform them on your partner.

6. At the time of the patient's next visit to physical therapy, how would you evaluate the success of your previous intervention? If there was a negative response to the previous intervention, what would you do at this time? If there was a positive response to the previous intervention, what would you do at this time?

7. Document your current findings.

8. What additional interventions would you use with this patient? How would these interventions relate to and support the OMPT interventions chosen?

HANDS-ON

With a partner, perform the following activities:

1 Allow your partner to portray the patient described in the clinical case scenario above. According to the FM approach philosophy, identify the possible structural, neuromuscular, and motor control dysfunctions that may be present.

2 Conduct a functional evaluation and identify any movement dysfunctions in rolling and gait.

3 Perform the impact test to identify central inhibition of extremity strength.

4 At the L5 motion segment, use the FM approach to OMPT to identify a dysfunctional end-feel, localize it to the depth and direction of maximal end-feel, and perform an FM mobilization technique. Ask your partner for feedback as you perform these techniques.

5 Perform an FM stabilization technique at the L5 motion segment in quadruped using fiber-specific isometric recruitment in the mid-range of motion, progressing to combination of isotonics to reeducate the neuromuscular control of the segment. Ask your partner for feedback as you perform these techniques.

6 Choose an extremity technique you are currently familiar with and adapt it to a FM technique that combines into one intervention the treatment of structural dysfunctions, neuromuscular dysfunctions, and motor learning.

7 Document your evaluation findings. Perform and document the techniques that you have chosen.

8 Practice involving the patient in the treatment by increasing awareness during performance of a technique through movement education, active release during passive movement, or movement, and patient awareness. Switch partners and perform these techniques on one another. Provide each other with feedback regarding performance.

9 If possible, video your performance of Functional Mobilization. Self-evaluate your performance of the chosen techniques by writing down three areas of deficiency and three areas of proficiency when using these techniques. Focus on such factors as therapist position, patient position, hand placement, force direction, instruction to the patient, etc. Analyze the performance of others in a similar fashion.

REFERENCES

1. Johnson GS. *FO I: Functional Orthopaedics I*. Steamboat Springs, CO: The Institute of Physical Art; 2010.

2. Johnson GS. *FO II: Functional Orthopaedics II*. Steamboat Springs, CO: The Institute of Physical Art; 2010.

3. Johnson GS. *FMUQ: Functional Mobilization for the Upper Quadrant*. Steamboat Springs, CO: The Institute of Physical Art; 2010.

4. Johnson GS. *FMLQ: Functional Mobilization for the Lower Quadrant*. Steamboat Springs, CO: The Institute of Physical Art; 2010.

5. Johnson GS, Saliba VL. Soft tissue mobilization. In: Donatelli RA, Wooden MJ, eds. *Orthopaedic Physical Therapy*. 3rd ed. New York: Churchill Livingston; 2002.

6. Rolf I. *Rolfing: Reestablishing the Natural Alignment and Structural Integration of the Human Body*. Rochester, VT: Healing Arts Press; 1989.

7. Feldenkrais M. *Awareness Through Movement: Health Exercises for Personal Growth*. New York: Harper & Row; 1972.

8. Aston Judith. *Aston Postural Assessment Workbook: Skills for Observing and Evaluating Body Patterns*. San Antonio, TX: Therapy Skill Builders; 1998.

9. Liskin J. *Moving Medicine: The Life and Work of Milton Trager, MD*. Barrytown, NY: Barrytown/Station Hill Press; 1996.

10. Dicke E, Shliack H, Wolff A. *A Manual of Reflexive Therapy of Connective Tissue (Connective Tissue Massage) "Bindegewebsmassage."* Scarsdale, NY: Sidney S. Simone; 1978.

11. Ebner M. *Connective Tissue Massage: Theory and Therapeutic Application*. Malabar, FL: R.E. Krieger Publishing; 1975.

12. Todd ME. *The Thinking Body*. Gouldsboro, ME: Gestalt Journal Press; 1997.

13. Heller J. *Bodywise*. New York: St. Martin's Press; 1986.

14. Jones F. *Body Awareness the Alexander Technique*. New York: Schocken Books; 1979.

15. Saliba V, Johnson G, Wardlaw C. Proprioceptive neuromuscular facilitation. In: Basmajian J, Nyberg R, eds. *Rational Manual Therapies*. Baltimore: Williams & Wilkins; 1993:243-284.

16. Knott M, Voss DE. *Proprioceptive Neuromuscular Facilitation*. 2nd ed. New York: Harper & Row; 1968.

17. Adler S, Becker D, Buck M. *PNF in Practice*. 3rd ed. Berlin: Springer; 2007.

18. Knott M. In the groove. *Phys Ther*. 1973;53:365-372.

19. Voss DE. Proprioceptive neuromuscular facilitation. *Phys Ther*. 1967;46: 838-899.

20. Kabat H. Proprioceptive facilitation in the therapeutic exercise. In: Licht E, ed. *Therapeutic Exercise*. 2nd ed. New Haven, CT: E Licht Publisher;1961.

21. Johnson GS, Saliba-Johnson VL. *PNFI: The Functional Approach to Movement Reeducation*. Steamboat Springs, CO: Institute of Physical Art; 2010.

22. Saliba-Johnson VL. *Back Education and Training: Course Outline*. Steamboat Springs, CO: Institute of Physical Art; 2010.

23. Mennell J. *Joint Pain*. Boston: Little, Brown; 1964.

24. Gratz C. Fascial adhesions in pain in the low back and arthritis. *JAMA*. 1938;3:1813-1818.

25. Maitland GD, Hengeveld E, Banks K, English K. *Maitland's Vertebral Manipulation*. 6th ed. Woburn, MA: Butterworth-Heinemann; 2001.

26. Scott W, Stevens J, Binder-Macleod SA. Human skeletal muscle fiber type classifications. *Phys Ther*. 2001;81:1810-1816.

27. Elvey RL. Intervention of arm pain associated with abnormal brachial plexus tension. *Austral J Physiother*. 1986;32:224.

28. Shacklock M. *Clinical Neurodynamics*. Edinburgh, Scotland: Elsevier; 2005.

29. Butler D. *The Sensitive Nervous System*. Adelaide, Australia: NoiGroup Publications; 2001.

30. Edgelow P. *The Edgelow Neuro/Vascular Entrapment Self-Treatment Program – Patient Booklet*. Available at: www.vascularweb.org/educationandmeetings/2013-Vascular-Annual-Meeting/Documents/P2-Wed-755_Physical_Therapy_for_nTOS_Edgelow.pdf%3FMobile%3D1+&cd=1&hl=en&ct=clnk&gl=us.

31. Edgelow P. Neurovascular Consequences of Cumulative Trauma Disorders Affecting the Thoracic Outlet: A Patient-Centered Treatment Approach. In: Donatelli, R., ed. *Physical Therapy of the Shoulder*. 4th ed. New York: Churchill Livingstone; 2003: 205–238.

32. Bly L. The components of normal movement during the first year of life and abnormal motor development. Therapy Skill Builders; 1994.

33. Johnson GS, Saliba-Johnson VL. *Functional Gait*. Steamboat Springs, CO: Institute of Physical Art; 2010.

34. Goddard S. *Reflexes, Learning and Behavior*. Eugene, OR: Fern Ridge Press; 2002.

35. Kabat H. *Low Back and Leg Pain from Slipped Disc in the Neck: Instruction Manual for Patients*. St. Louis, MO: Warren H. Green; 1983.

36. Richardson C, Hodges P, Hides J. *Therapeutic Exercise for Lumbopelvic Stabilization*. 2nd ed. New York: Churchill Livingstone; 2004.

37. Hides JA, Stokes MJ, Saide M, Jull GA, Cooper DH. Evidence of lumbar multifidus muscle wasting ipsilateral to symptoms in patients with acute/subacute low back pain. *Spine*. 1994;19:165-172.

38. Hides J, Richardson C, Jull G. Multifidus muscle recovery is not automatic after resolution of acute, first-episode low back pain. *Spine*. 1996;21: 2763-2769.

39. Kay AG. An extensive literature review of the lumbar multifidus: anatomy. *J Man Manip Ther*. 2000;8:102-114.

40. Yoshihara K, Nakayama Y, Fujii N, Aoki T, Hiromoto I. Atrophy of the multifidus muscle in patients with lumbar disk herniation: histochemical and electromyographic study [abstract]. *Orthobluejournal*. 2001;493-495.

41. Yoshihara K, Shirai Y, Nakayama Y, Uesaka S. Histochemical changes in the multifidus muscle in patients with lumbar intervertebral disc herniation [abstract]. *Spine*. 2001;26:622-626.

42. Hodges PW, Richardson A. Inefficient muscular stabilization of the lumbar spine associated with lower back pain. *Spine*. 1996;21:2640-2650.

43. Kendall F, McCreary E, Provance P. *Muscles Testing and Function with Posture and Pain*. 4th ed. New York: Williams & Wilkins; 1993.

44. Friberg R, Thurmond S. Facilitation of the lumbar multifidi and erector spinae using prolonged isometric contraction; Construct validity of lumbar spine classification system. Poster presentations. AAOMPT Conference; Salt Lake City, UT; October 14-16, 2005.

45. Abdulwahab S, Sabbahi M. Neck retractions, cervical root decompression, and radicular pain. *J Orthop Sports Phys Ther*. 2000:31:4-12.

46. O'Leary S, Jull G, Kim M, Vicenzino, B. Specificity in retraining craniocervical flexor muscle performance. *J Orthop Sports Phys Ther*. 2007:37:3-9.

47. Falla DL, Jull GA, Hodges PW. Patients with neck pain demonstrate diminished electromyographic activity of the deep cervical flexor muscles during performance of the craniocervical flexion test. *Spine*. 2004:29: 2108:2114.

48. Lee HWM. Progressive muscle synergy and synchronization in movement patterns: an approach to the treatment of dynamic lumbar instability. *J Man Manip Ther*. 1994:2:133-142.

49. Ylinen J, Salo P, Nykanen M, Kautiainen H, Hakkinen A. Decreased isometric neck strength in women with chronic neck pain and the repeatability of neck strength measurements. *Arch Phys Med Rehabil*. 2004;85:1303-1308.

50. Kong WZ, Goel VK, Gilbertson LG, Weinstein JN. Effects of muscle dysfunction on lumbar spine mechanics: a finite element study based on a two-motion segments model. *Spine*. 1996;21:2197-2207.

51. O'Sullivan PB, Twomey L, Allison GT. Dysfunction of the neuro-muscular system in the presence of low back pain: implications for physical therapy management. *J Man Manip Ther*. 1997;5:20-26.

52. Stevans, J, Hall KG. Motor skill acquisition strategies for rehabilitation of low back pain. *J Orthop Sports Phys Ther*. 1998;3:165-167.

53. Van Dieen JH, Cholewicki J, Radebold A. Trunk muscle recruitment patterns with low back pain enhance the stability of the lumbar spine. *Spine*. 2003;28:834-841.

54. Beattie P. Current understanding of lumbar intervertebral disc degeneration: a review with emphasis upon etiology, pathophysiology, and lumbar magnetic resonance imaging findings. *J Orthop Sports Phys Ther*. 2008;38: 329-340.

55. Buckwalter JA. Aging and degeneration of the human intervertebral disc. *Spine*. 1995;20:1307-1314.

56. Dolan KJ, Green A. Lumbar spine reposition sense: the effect of a "slouched" posture. *Man Ther*. 2006;11:202-207.

57. Lundon K, Bolton K. Structure and function of the lumbar intervertebral disk in health, aging, and pathologic conditions. *J Orthop Sports Phys Ther*. 2001;31:291-306.

58. O'Sullivan P, Mitchell T, Bulich P, Waller R, Holte J. The relationship between posture and back muscle endurance in industrial workers with flexion-related low back pain. *Man Ther*. 2006;11:264-271.

59. Pettman, E. What is a typical posteriolateral disc protrusion and how is it so successfully managed by the passive extension protocol innovated by Robin McKenzie, an evidence based review. Excerpt from Level I NAIOMT course at Andrews University, Eugene, OR. Date unknown.

60. Ames DL. Overuse syndrome. *J Fla Med Assoc*. 1986;73:607.

61. Farfan HF. Mechanical factors in the genesis of low back pain. In: Bonica JJ, ed. *Advances in Pain Research and Therapy*. Vol 3. New York: Raven Press; 1979.

62. Cholewicki J, Silfies SP, Shah RA, et al. Delayed trunk muscle reflex responses increase the risk of low back injuries. *Spine*. 2005;30: 2614-2620.

63. Davis DS, Ashby PE, McCale KL, McQuain JA, Wine M. The effectiveness of 3 stretching techniques on hamstring flexibility using consistent stretching parameters. *J Strength Con Res*. 2005;19:27-32.

64. Ferber R, Osternig LR, Gravelle DC. Effect of PNF stretch techniques on knee flexor muscle EMG activity older adults. *J Electromyogr Kinesiol*. 2002;12:391-397.

65. Godges JJ, Mattson-Bell M, Thorpe D, Shah D. The immediate effects of soft tissue mobilization with proprioceptive neuromuscular facilitation on glenohumeral external rotation and overhead reach. *J Orthop Sports Phys Ther*. 2003;33:713-718.

66. Grzebellus M, Hering G. The Effect of contralateral PNF Patterns on Patients After Knee Surgery. IPNFA Meeting Vallejo, 1998.

67. Hight AB, Duncan PW, Nelson SG. Electromyographic Activity of Two Contralateral Lower Extremity Muscles During a PNF Pattern.

68. Kofotolis N, Vrabas IS, Vamvakoudis E, Papanikolaou A, Mandroukas K. Proprioceptive neuromuscular facilitation training induced alterations in muscle fibre type and cross sectional area. *Br J Sports Med*. 2005;39:e11.

69. Kotoftolis N, Kellis E. Effects of two 4-week proprioceptive neuromuscular facilitation programs on muscle endurance, flexibility, and functional performance in women with chronic low back pain. *Phys Ther*. 2006;86: 1001-1012.

70. Marek SM, Cramer JT, Fincher AL, et al. Acute effects of static and proprioceptive neuromuscular facilitation stretching on muscle strength and power output. *J Athl Train*. 2005;40:94-103.

71. Moor MA, Kukulka CG. Depression of Hoffman reflexes following voluntary contraction and implications for proprioceptive neuromuscular facilitation therapy. *Phys Ther*. 1991;71:321-333.

72. Nakamura R, Kosaka K. Effect of proprioceptive neuromuscular facilitation on EEG activation induced by facilitating position in patients with spinocerebellar degeneration. *Tohoku J Exp Med*. 1986;148:159-161.

73. Spernoga SG, Uhl TL, Arnold BL, Gansneder BM. Duration of maintained hamstring flexibility after a one-time, modified hold-relax stretching protocol. *J Athl Train*. 2001;36:44-48.

74. Stevenson J, Maitland M, Anemaet W, Beckstead J. Body weight support treadmill training compared with PNF training in persons with chronic spine. *J Neuro Phys Ther*. 2004;12.

75. Wang R. Effect of proprioceptive neuromuscular facilitation on the gait of patients with hemiplegia of long and short duration. *Phys Ther*. 1994;74:1108-1115.

76. Gowitzke BA, Milner M. *Scientific Basis of Human Movement*. Baltimore: Williams & Wilkins; 1988.

77. Basmajian JV. *Muscles Alive. Their Functions Revealed by Electromyography*. Baltimore: Williams & Wilkins; 1978.

78. Sherrington CS. *The Integrative Action of the Nervous System*. New Haven, CT: Yale University Press; 1961:340.

79. Sherrington CS. *Selected Writings of Sir Charles Sherrington: A Testimonial Presented by the Neurologists Forming the Guarantors of the Journal Brain*. D Denny-Brown, ed. Oxford, UK: Oxford University Press, 1979.

80. Vicenzino B, Branjerdporn M, Teys P, Jordan K. Initial changes in posterior talar glide and dorsiflexion of the ankle after mobilization with movement in individuals with recurrent ankle sprain. *J Orthop Sports Phys Ther*. 2006;36:464-470.

81. Vicenzino B, Cleland JA, Bisset L. Joint manipulation in the management of lateral epicondylalgia: a clinical commentary. *J Man Manip Ther*. 2007;15:50-56.

82. Flynn T. *The Thoracic Spine and Rib Cage: Musculoskeletal Evaluation and Treatment*. Boston, MA: Butterworth-Heinemann; 1996.

83. Riemann B, Lephart S. The sensorimotor system, part I: the physiologic basis of functional joint stability. *J Athl Train*. 2002;37:71-79.

84. Riemann B, Lephart S. The sensorimotor system, part II: the role of proprioception in motor control and functional joint stability. *J Athl Train*. 2002;37:80-84.

85. Evjenth O, Hamberg J. *Muscle Stretching in Manual Therapy, Vol. 1 & 2*. Alfta, Sweden: Alfta Rehab; 1984.

86. Nouwen A, Van Akkerveeken PF, Versloot JM. Patterns of muscular activity during movement in patients with chronic low-back pain. *Spine*. 1987;12: 777-782.

87. Kirkaldy-Willis WH. *Managing Low Back Pain*. 2nd ed. New York: Churchill Livingstone; 1988.

88. White A, Panjabi M. *Clinical Biomechanics of the Spine*. New York: Lippincott; 1978.

89. Johnson GS, Johnson SV. The application of the principles and procedures of PNF for the care of lumbar spinal instabilities. *J Man Manipul Ther*. 2002:10:83-105.

90. Paris SV. Physical signs of instability. *Spine*. 1985;10:277-279.

91. Fritz JM, Erhard RE, Hagen BF. Segmental instability of the lumbar spine. *Phys Ther* 1998:8:889-896.

92. Morgan FP, King T. Primary instability of the lumbar vertebrae as a common cause of low back pain. *J Bone Joint Surg Br*. 1957;39:6-21.

93. Pope MH, Panjabi MM. Biomechanical definitions of spinal instability. *Spine*. 1985;10:255-256.

94. Frymoyer JW, Selby DK. Segmental instability: Rationale for treatment. *Spine*. 1985;10:280-286.

95. Panjabi MM. The stabilizing system of the spine: part II. Neutral zone and instability hypothesis. *J Spinal Disord*. 1992;5:390-396.

96. Panjabi MM, Abumi K, Duranceau J, et al. Spinal stability and intersegmental muscle forces: a biomechanical model. *Spine*. 1989:14: 194-200.

97. Pope MH, Panjabi MM. Biomechanical definitions of spinal instability. *Spine*. 1985;10:255-256.

98. Frymoyer JW, Selby DK. Segmental instability: Rationale for intervention. *Spine*. 1985;10:280-286.

99. Radebold A, Cholewicki J, Panjabi MM, Patel TC. Muscle response pattern to sudden trunk loading in healthy individuals and in patients with chronic low back pain. *Spine*. 2000;25:947-954.

100. Hodges P, Cresswell A. Altered trunk muscle recruitment in people with low back pain with upper limb movement at different speeds. *Arch Phys Med Rehabil*. 1999;80:1005-1011.

101. Hodges P, Cresswell A, Thorstensson A. Preparatory trunk motion accompanies rapid upper limb movement. *Exp Brain Res*. 1999;124: 69-79.

102. Hodges P, Richardson C. Contraction of the abdominal muscle associated with movement of the lower limb. *Phys Ther*. 1997;77:132-143.

103. Hodges P, Richardson C. Inefficient muscular stabilization of the lumbar spine associated with low back pain. A motor control evaluation of transversus abdominis. *Spine*. 1996;21:2640-2650.

104. Janda V. Introduction to functional pathology of the motor system. In: Janda Compendium: Minneapolis, MN: OPTP; 1994;25-29.

105. Nouwen A, Van Akkerveeken PF, Versloot JM. Patterns of muscular activity during movement in patients with chronic low-back pain. *Spine*. 1987;12:777-782.

106. Cleland JA, Childs JD, Fritz JM, Whitman JM, Eberhart SL. Development of a clinical prediction rule for guiding treatment of a subgroup of patients with neck pain: use of thoracic spine manipulation, exercise, and patient education. *Phys Ther*. 2007;87:9-22.

107. Cleland JA, Glynn P, Whitman JM, et al. Short-term effects of thrust versus nonthrust mobilization/manipulation directed at the thoracic spine in patients with neck pain: a randomized clinical trial. *Phys Ther*. 2007;87:431-440.

108. Do DT. Resolution of chronic non-cervicogenic dizziness following manual physical therapy directed at the ribcage: a case report. AAOMPT Conference, Charlotte, NC, October 20-22, 2006.

109. Lee D. Biomechanics of the thorax: a clinical model of in vivo function. *J Man Manip Ther*. 1993;1:13-21.

110. Liebler E, Tufanao-Coors L, Douris P, et al. The effect of thoracic spine mobilization on lower trapezius strength testing. *J Man Manip Ther*. 2001;9:207-212.

111. McGuckin N. Modern manual therpay of the vertebral column. In: *The T4 Syndrome*. Grieve GP, ed. New York: Churchill Livingstone; 1986: 238.

112. Viti James, Paris S. The use of upper thoracic manipulation in a patient with headaches. *J Man Manip Ther*. 2000;8:25-28.

113. Burkhart SS, Morgan CD, Kibler WB. The disabled throwing shoulder: spectrum of pathology part III: the SICK scapula, scapular dyskinesis, the kinetic chain, and rehabilitation. *Arthroscopy*. 2003;19: 641-661.

114. Cools AM, Witvrouw EE, Declercq GA, et al. Scapular muscle recruitment patterns: trapezius muscle latency with and without impingement symptoms [abstracted by Hoops J, *IAOM Quarterly Review*. 2005;]. *Am J Sports Med*. 2003;31:542-549.

115. Laudner K, Myers J, Pasquale M, Bradley J, Lephart S. Scapular dysfunction in throwers with pathological internal impingement [abstracted by Harris PM, *IAOM-US Quarterly Review*. 2006;56:2-3]. *J Orthop Sports Phys Ther*. 2006;36:485-494.

116. Levangie PK, Cook HE. The shoulder girdle: kinesiology review. *PT Magazine*. 2000;12:48-62.
117. McClure P, Michener L, Karduna A. Shoulder function and 3-Dimensional scapular kinematics in people with and without shoulder impingement syndrome. *Phys Ther*. 2006;86:1075-1090.
118. Rundquist P. Alterations in scapular kinematics in subject with idiopathic loss of shoulder range of motion. *J Orthop Sports Phys Ther*. 2007;37:19-25.
119. Tate AR, Mcclure P, Kareha S, Irwin D. Effects of the scapula reposition test on shoulder impingement symptoms and elevation strength in overhead athletes. *J Ortho Sports Phys Ther*. 2008;38:4-111.
120. Thigpen CA, Padua DA, Morgan N, Krops C, Karas SG. Scapular kinematics during supraspinatus rehabilitation exercise: a comparison of full-can versus empty-can techniques. *Am J Sports Med*. 2006;34: 644-652.
121. Senbursa G, Baltaci G, Atay A. Comparison of conservative treatment with and without manual physical therapy for patients with shoulder impingement syndrome: a prospective, randomized clinical trial. *Knee Surg Sports Traumatol Arthorosc*. 2007;7:915-921.
122. Flatow EL, Soslowski LJ, Ticker JB, et al. Excursion of the rotator cuff under the acromion. patterns of subacromial contact. *Am J Sports Med*. 1994;22:779-788.
123. Donatelli, R., *Physical Therapy of the Shoulder*. 3rd ed. New York: Churchill Livingstone; 1997.
124. Maigne JY, Doursounian L, Chatellier G. Causes and mechanisms of common coccydynia. *Spine*. 2000;25:3072-3079.
125. Maigne JY, Guedj S, Straus C. Idiopathic coccygodynia. Lateral roentgenograms in the sitting position and coccygeal discography. *Spine*. 1994;19:930-934.
126. Maigne JY. Management of Common Coccydynia. 2002;1-10 Available at www.sofmmoo.com/english_section/7_coccyx/coccyx.htm.
127. Thiele GH. Coccygodynia, the mechanism of its production and its relationship to anorectal disease. *Am J Surg*. 1950;110-116.
128. Heinrich S. Treatment of sacro-coccygeal dysfunction: dealing with a delicate issue in therapy. *Phys Ther Forum*. 1992;22:5.
129. Maigne JY, Chatellier G. Comparison of three manual coccydynia treatments. *Spine*. 2001;26:479-484.
130. Maigne JY, Chatellier G, Faou ML, Arachambeau M. The treatment f chronic coccydynia with intrarectal manipulation: a RCT. *Spine*. 2006;31:E621-7.
131. Schapiro S. Low back and rectal pain from an orthopedic and proctologic viewpoint. *Am J Surg*. 1950;117-128.
132. Barral J, Mercier P. The coccyx. *Visceral Manipulation*. 2nd ed. Seattle, WA: Eastland Press; 2006:259-263.

CHAPTER

13

Soft Tissue Mobilization in Orthopaedic Manual Physical Therapy

Leslie Davis Rudzinski, PT, OCS, CFMT

Gregory S. Johnson, PT, FFCFMT, FAAOMPT

Chapter Objectives

At the conclusion of this chapter, the reader will be able to:

- Identify the major influences that led to the development of the functional orthopaedics approach to soft tissue mobilization.
- Understand the relationship between structure and function and how it relates to the application of soft tissue mobilization.
- Conduct an examination including structural evaluation and functional testing consisting of the vertical compression test, elbow flexion test, and lumbar protective mechanism.

- Understand the importance of muscle play.
- Understand and apply the concept of three-dimensional identification of soft tissue restrictions.
- Understand and apply the cascade of techniques for soft tissue mobilization.
- Demonstrate entry-level performance of soft tissue mobilization of superficial fascia, bony contours, and myofascial dysfunctions on all regions of the body.

HISTORY AND DEVELOPMENT

Massage may be the oldest form of medical care. The history of massage dates back to ancient times. In China, as early as 2700 BC, massage was recommended for a variety of ailments in *The Yellow Emperor's Classic of Internal Medicine*.[1] In the 5th century BC, *Hippocrates*, the father of Western medicine, stated that "the physician must be experienced in many things, but assuredly in rubbing . . . for rubbing can bind a joint that is too loose and loosen a joint that is too rigid."[2] The physician *Galen*, in the late first century AD, also advocated the use of massage for a variety of maladies.[2]

In the late 19th and early 20th centuries, clinical interest in the cause and treatment of pain of muscular origin continued in the medical community.[3,4] St. George's Hospital in London had a department of massage until 1934.[1] It was in 1894 that

physical therapists began using massage techniques based on the work done by the Swedish physician, *Per Henrik Ling*.[1] In the mid-1930s, a German physical therapist, *Elizabeth Dicke*,[5] developed a more specific manipulative technique for connective tissue called *Bindegewebemasssage*. This form of connective tissue massage (CTM) later spread to the English-speaking world through the work of another physical therapist, *Maria Ebner*.[6] With the advent of clinical modalities, however, massage fell out of favor within the medical community.[7]

Today, many forms of sophisticated soft tissue intervention techniques have emerged, bringing us back to a more hands-on approach to the treatment of myofascial pain and dysfunction. *Travell and Simons's*[3] trigger point therapy (see Chapter 16), *Cyriax's*[8,9] deep friction massage (see Chapter 5), Dicke and Ebner's[5,6] connective tissue massage, and osteopathic myofascial release (see Chapters 4 and 14), as well as alternative approaches including *Rolfing*,[10,11]*Feldenkrais*[12] (see Chapter 20), *Hellerwork, Aston patterning*,[13] and *Trager*[7,14] have emerged to promote the use of myofascial manipulation for the enhancement of structure and function.

The **soft tissue mobilization (STM)** principles and procedures described in this chapter represent an eclectic approach (Box 13-1). This approach was developed by the co-author, *Gregory S. Johnson*, together with his wife, *Vicky Saliba Johnson*. Johnson developed *Functional Orthopedics I (FOI)* in 1980 as a way to present an integrated, systematic approach to soft tissue mobilization. FOI became the foundational course in a series of eight courses identified collectively as *Functional Mobilization* (see Chapter 12). This approach presents STM as an adjunct to other manual physical therapy techniques, neuromuscular reeducation, exercise, and body mechanics training for the purpose of restoring efficient function.

NOTABLE QUOTABLE

"The key to optimal function is to balance the system by addressing planes both vertically and horizontally. The body is like a model of blocks or segments that, when misaligned, are unstable . . ."

-*Ida Rolf*

NOTABLE QUOTABLE

"Habitual patterns of inefficient movement ultimately lead to inefficient posture. By learning efficient movement patterns, dysfunctional postures can be changed."

-*Moshe Feldenkrais*

In the Functional Orthopedics approach, efficient movement patterns are used to reinforce the changes made through STM. Teaching patients efficient movement patterns following STM will reduce recidivism. In addition, the benefits of STM will be greatly enhanced by retraining patients' postures and breaking habitual patterns of movement.[15] A complete description of the *Functional Mobilization Approach* is provided in Chapter 12 of this text.

Box 13-1 The Functional Orthopedics Approach to STM

The Functional Orthopedics approach includes concepts from the following:

1. Cyriax's deep friction massage
2. Travell's trigger point therapy
3. Dicke's connective tissue massage
4. Myofascial release
5. Trager's oscillations
6. Rolf's concepts of postural efficiency
7. Feldenkrais's awareness through movement

NOTABLE QUOTABLE

"In the Functional Orthopedic Approach, efficient movement patterns are used not as much to change structure, but to reinforce the changes made through STM."

-*G.S. Johnson and V.L. Saliba-Johnson*

CLINICAL PILLAR

The benefits of STM will be greatly enhanced by retraining patients' postures and breaking habitual patterns of movement through the use of a combination of *education*, *neuromuscular reeducation*, and *exercise*. Teaching patients efficient movement patterns following STM will increase the longevity of the results.

ANATOMY AND PATHOANATOMY OF SOFT TISSUE
The Anatomy of Connective Tissue

The properties of connective tissue (CT) are dependent on the **extracellular matrix (ECM)**, which consists primarily of fibers (elastin and collagen), proteoglycans (PGs), and glycoproteins. Proteoglycans are characterized by a core protein covalently bonded to **glycosaminoglycans (GAGs).** There are six major GAGs, of which chondroitin sulfate 4 and 6 and hyaluronic acid (HA) are the most widely recognized. All GAGs are negatively charged, creating an osmotic imbalance that results in the absorption of water that hydrates the matrix. The proportions of the various ECM components determine the mechanical properties of the CT, which depend on the nature and extent of the loads placed upon them.[16–22]

The ECM is regulated by the balance between stimulatory *cytokines* and growth factors and the degradation and inhibition of *metalloproteinases*. Any alteration of this balance changes the properties of the CT matrix. Connective tissue disease and injury may result in a disruption of this balance.[23,24] Refer to Chapter 14 for more details on CT structure and function (Box 13-2).

Box 13-2 Quick Notes! CONNECTIVE TISSUE FUNCTIONS

1. Mechanical support
2. Movement facilitation
3. Tissue fluid transport
4. Cell migration
5. Wound healing
6. Control of metabolic processes

The Anatomy of Fascia

Fascia is comprised of both dense and loose CT and, along with muscle, is the primary focus of STM. Fascia is composed of irregular sheaths of collagen and elastin fibers and a high degree of HA (Fig. 13-1). These fascial sheaths are continuous with one another, creating an interweaving network that extends from the basement membrane of the dermis to the periosteum of the bone.[18,22]

The fascia allows for a relationship between the superficial and deep layers of muscle,[11] as well as a relationship between muscles and other structures such as nerves and bones (Fig. 13-2; Box 13-3).[25] The superficial fascia is thinner and more delicate, and the deeper sheaths are thick and tough. Fascia serves to compartmentalize structures into functional units.[11,22] The space that is created between structures acts as a functional joint or *"space built for motion."*[26] These functional joints require movement, without which the fascia will thicken and harden (Box 13-4).[11]

CLINICAL PILLAR

The space created by the compartmentalization of fascia forms a functional joint *"built for motion."* As movement specialists, the manual therapist must facilitate movement between the layers of fascia so as to avoid reductions in fascial elasticity, mobility, and adaptability.

Cross-sectional dissections show that fascia may exhibit spiral patterns of orientation. In a neutral standing position, the pattern of fascial orientation in the spine is primarily vertical. As active movement increases, a spiraling occurs around the vertebrae and muscles. The elastic recoil that is created greatly influences the subsequent smooth diagonal and spiral movement.[11] If fibers become densely packed or aligned in a fashion that resists motion, the elastic potential may be lost.[11,27] Fascia also absorbs shock, assists in the exchange of metabolites, stores energy, protects from infection,[11,18,22] and enhances active contraction.[28]

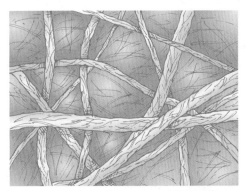

FIGURE 13-1 Dense irregular connective tissue. (Adapted from: Gray H, *Anatomy of the Human Body*. Philadelphia: Lea & Febiger, 1966, with permission.)

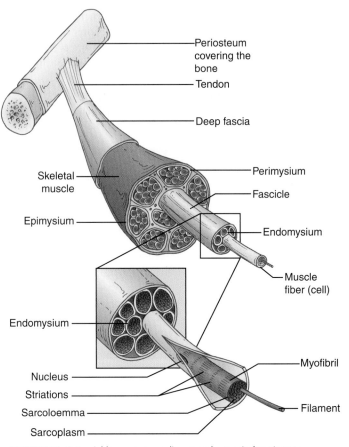

Periosteum covering the bone
Tendon
Deep fascia
Skeletal muscle
Perimysium
Fascicle
Epimysium
Endomysium
Muscle fiber (cell)
Endomysium
Myofibril
Nucleus
Striations
Sarcolemma
Filament
Sarcoplasm

FIGURE 13-2 Fascial layers surrounding muscle. Fascia functions to compartmentalize structures into functional units.

Box 13-3 Quick Notes! MECHANICAL PROPERTIES OF CONNECTIVE TISSUE

1. Properties are determined by the proportions of components in the *extracellular matrix (ECM)*.

2. Properties are determined by the nature and extent of loading.

3. **Tendons** are parallel to the muscle secondary to the line of pull.

4. **Ligaments** are primarily parallel, with some multidirectional fibers.

5. **Bone** is in orthogonal arrays in alternating sheets.

6. **Fascia and skin** are irregular and multidirectional.

The fascia between two muscles allows each muscle to function independently and glide freely alongside one another during movement. The ability of muscle to move in this fashion is termed **muscle play** (Fig. 13-3).

Connective Tissue and Healing

The synthesis of collagen begins with the alignment of amino acids followed by the assembly of three alpha chains that

Box 13-4 FASCIA IMPACTS MOVEMENT

1. As active movement increases, a *spiraling* and *narrowing* of the fascia occurs, creating *elastic recoil*, which becomes a factor in regular movement.

2. *Stretch* and *recoil* of the fascia supports the continuity of movement and creates smooth diagonal and spiral movement.

3. If fascia becomes densely packed or aligned against a typical direction of motion, as might occur with poor posture or holding patterns, then the elastic potential may be lost.

4. Fascia provides *separation* between structures that allows independent movement between adjacent structures such as muscle.

5. Fascia also *absorbs shock*, assists in the *exchange of metabolites*, *stores energy*, and provides *protection* against the spread of infection.

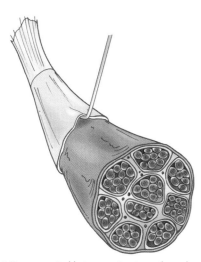

FIGURE 13–3 Space created between structures through compartmentalization of fascia acts as a functional joint, or *"space built for motion."*

combine to form *tropocollogen*. As the process continues, cross-links are formed and more bonding occurs, ultimately resulting in the formation of collagen fibers.[22]

QUESTIONS *for* REFLECTION

- What type of collagen is typically addressed through the use of STM?
- Where is this type of collagen most abundantly found?
- What are the primary structural features of this type of tissue and how are these features influenced through the application of STM?

The *maturation phase* of healing (Box 13-5) begins once levels of collagen reach their maximum at 2 to 3 weeks

Box 13-5 PHASES OF CONNECTIVE TISSUE HEALING

1. **Reaction phase:** This phase is stimulated by physical disruption of the soft tissue, which causes damage to the blood and lymph vessels and results in a transient vasoconstriction in an attempt to slow blood flow as the hemostatic process is activated.

2. **Inflammatory phase:** Vasodilation along with chemotaxis is regulated by humoral factors that follow a cascade effect where each successive factor is activated by its predecessor. Neutrophils are the cells to initially migrate to the site, followed by macrophages.

3. **Proliferative phase:** This phase is marked by fibroplasia and the development of a vascular network of granulation tissue. There is a concurrent process of angiogenesis that reestablishes the circulatory network. This new vascular system allows delivery of oxygen, amino acids, glucose, vitamins, and minerals necessary for the complete formation of collagen.

4. **Maturation phase:** This phase begins once levels of collagen reach their maximum at about 2 to 3 weeks. Initially, type III collagen, or scar tissue, is laid down. This type of collagen is poorly organized and has inadequate tensile strength. As maturation continues, type I collagen replaces type III, producing an increase in the strength of the wound. The maturation process has been shown to be stimulated by stress.

following injury. Initially, type III collagen, or scar tissue, is laid down. This type of collagen is poorly organized and has inadequate tensile strength. As maturation continues, type I collagen replaces type III, producing an increase in the strength of the injured tissue. Because stress stimulates the maturation process,[29] appropriate STM techniques can facilitate healing after connective tissue injury.[8,9] The tensile strength of connective tissue will continue to increase for up to 1 year following injury, and these tissues may return to between 80% and 100% of their original strength.[30–33]

As collagen synthesis proceeds, collagen lysis also takes place. The rate of turnover and the balance between lysis and synthesis determines the nature of the scar. Collagen lysis is stimulated by the enzyme *collagenase*, which is brought to the site of healing by granulocytes and macrophages. In the event of extreme oxygen deprivation or severe deficiency of protein or vitamins, lysis will continue and synthesis will cease, resulting in incomplete healing of the wound.[34] Clinically, this balance is important for the formation of strong, but mobile, scars. In the case of synthesis-dominant healing, the potential for hypertrophic and immobile scar tissue exists, often resulting in decreased mobility.[35,36] Immobile scar tissue, in the skin or in the deeper connective tissue, will limit mobility of soft tissue structures.

Fibrosis is defined as the laying down of fibrous tissue and is normally considered pathological. Fibrosis, however, occurs as part of the normal wound-healing process. Fibrosis follows a similar pathway to normal wound healing except there is a chronic progression of the fibrotic process characterized by continuous insult or stimulus that is either chemical or mechanical in nature.

SOFT TISSUE IMPAIRMENT

Mechanisms and Cellular Processes of Soft Tissue Injury

A detailed manual physical therapy clinical examination provides evidence that myofascial restrictions exist.[3,37–41] Various etiologic hypotheses leading to soft tissue dysfunction are often identified.[7] Among these are (1) *mechanical restrictions* in the form of cross-linking of collagen fibers or scar tissue adhesions, (2) ground substance *dehydration*, (3) *interstitial fluid changes* such as lymphatic stasis and/or interstitial swelling,(4) *neuroreflexive* causes, and (5) *electrochemical* or *biochemical* causes.[7,29,42–44]

QUESTIONS *for* REFLECTION

- How does collagen fiber direction influence motion in the presence of restrictions?
- How does the collagen fiber direction influence the application of STM techniques?

The most widely accepted etiology of connective tissue pathology is the presence of mechanical restrictions that prevent mobility between fascial layers.[35,36,44–47] Postural stresses or continued use of the injured tissue may act as a continuous mechanical insult causing excessive synthesis of collagen and extracellular matrix components resulting in hypertrophic scar tissue.[42,49,50]

Ida Rolf[10] believed that habitual tension leads to an increase in fibroblastic activity and deposition of collagen. Continued mechanical injury results in disruption of sarcomeres with leakage of the cellular components into the ECM, which stimulates tissue scarring.[44,47]

Connective tissue adhesions are a common by-product of the reparative process following surgery.[44–47,50] This suggests that mechanical stimuli can lead to adhesion formation.[50] Early passive mobilization using STM may improve the healing process through the initiation of gliding motions that disrupt adhesions and produce a change in the cellular response by alternating between stress and relaxation.[51]

QUESTIONS *for* REFLECTION

- What is the primary role of *proteoglycans (PG)* and *glycosaminoglycans (GAG)*?
- Where do these molecules primarily reside?
- How would you describe the structure of these molecules?
- Against what forces are they effective in resisting?
- How does restoring normal mobility to a structure help to maintain the health of this structure?

After a 9-week immobilization period, Akeson et al[52,53] found an increase in *periarticular connective tissue (PCT)* cross-links. In addition, a reduction in water content, hyaluronic acid, and chondroitin suggests a loss of lubrication at the fiber-to-fiber interfaces.

CLINICAL PILLAR

Physical forces produced through motion are able to *modulate the synthesis* of proteoglycans and collagen in connective tissue. Furthermore, regular movement *reduces the formation of collagen cross-linking*.

These findings suggest that motion is able to modulate the synthesis of proteoglycans and collagen in connective tissue. Regular movement reduces the formation of collagen cross-linking due to frequent changes in the location of intercept points between fibers, with the converse being true in the presence of immobility (Fig. 13-4). In vivo, animal arthrographic measurements showed significant contracture formation following just 2 weeks of immobilization. The amount of tension increased 10 times, and the area of hysteresis increased by as much as 23 times that of the control group.[52–55] In addition to the mechanical causes of soft tissue restrictions, *dehydration* has also been identified as a factor in cross-linking.[52–55]

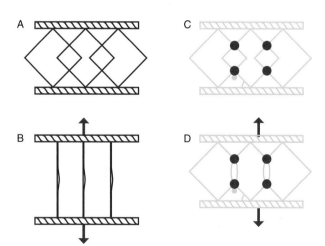

FIGURE 13–4 Cross-linking between collagen fibers limits extensibility. When movement is restricted, cross-links form where collagen fibers intercept, ultimately resulting in adhesions and decreased flexibility. Regular movement reduces the formation of collagen cross links. **A.** In normal muscle that is in a relaxed state, there is no crosslinking present. **B.** As the fibers are elongated during motion, a normal amount of excursion takes place. **C.** As a result of immobility and/or injury, cross-linking at intercept points may occur in the relaxed/shortened state. **D.** This limits the ability of the muscle to elongate leading to deficits in ROM. (From: Akeson WH, Amiel D, Woo S. Immobility effects on synovial joint: the pathomechanics of joint contracture. *Biorheology.* 1980;17:95-110, with permission.)

QUESTIONS *for* REFLECTION

- What are the current hypotheses regarding the etiologic mechanisms underlying soft tissue dysfunction?
- How do our STM techniques address these factors?
- Are there specific techniques that are designed to address specific etiologies?
- How does poor posture and habitual patterns of activity contribute to soft tissue dysfunction?

The association between HA and scar production has been demonstrated in mouse fetal limb wound repair. Scarless repair occurs in the 14-day fetal mouse limb; however, later in the gestational period, repair with scarring occurs. These results provide support for the notion that hyaluronic acid plays a key role in limiting scar tissue formation.[24,52,56]

Miller et al[57] studied the effect of injecting gel compositions of HA, calcium, and NSAIDs on adhesion formation in chickens. Because water binds to HA, the presence of HA may have allowed for better hydration and fewer adhesions. The addition of NSAIDs and calcium resulted in "*less dense*" scars. This suggests that *inflammation* may also affect interstitial flow, which facilitates fibrosis.[29]

In a study by Ng et al,[29] it was suggested that the biophysical environment that precedes fibrosis, such as swelling, increased microvascular permeability, and increased lymphatic drainage plays a role in fibrogenesis. Muscle biopsies of the upper trapezius in assembly line workers with chronic localized myalgia as a result of postural stress demonstrated cellular pathology consistent with localized hypoxia.[58] This suggests that localized hypoxia resulting from postural stress could contribute to the production of a fibrotic state.[48,49,58]

Additional animal studies have shown that HA-treated groups demonstrated higher GAG content and up to 50% decrease in stiffness. HA injections to reduce pain and stiffness in arthritic knees are becoming commonplace. Is the mechanism whereby such positive effects are exerted due to a reduction in the formation of adhesions, or does HA provide the needed lubrication and spacing that enables freer movement? Evidence also suggests that HA may exert a positive feedback on its own production.[59]

The ECM protein, TN-C, has been shown to be present in regions where high mechanical forces are transmitted, such as the myotendinous and osteotendinous junctions. It is likely that TN-C plays an important role in providing elasticity to the myofascial system, and a reduction in the quantity of this protein may contribute to stiffness.[60]

Despite the fact that most studies have been performed on animal subjects, collectively they suggest that mechanical, as well as biochemical, processes are involved. Such processes, which affect hydration and interstitial fluid interaction, including swelling and lymphatic stasis, are all involved in the formation of soft tissue restriction. Furthermore, *neuroreflexive processes* may also play an additional role in the development of soft tissue dysfunction.[61,62]

CLINICAL PILLAR

Trigger points are myofascial aberrations that present as hyperirritable nodules or bands of myofascial tissue that represent a **neuroreflexive dysfunction**. Trigger points are thought to occur secondary to sensitization of muscle afferent nerve endings or a convergence of afferent fibers from the TrP and those from the referred pain zone onto a common **spinothalamic tract neuron**. Intervention must address the neuroreflexive nature of trigger points.

Myofascial Impairment

Janda[63–65] states that muscle imbalances are *reflexive* in nature and can be considered a systemic deviation in the quality of muscle function that results from an adaptation to lifestyle. This results in various patterns of muscle tightness and weakness through a region or even throughout the entire body. Janda outlined three specific muscle imbalance syndromes, which are described in Table 13-1. As the manual physical therapist evaluates muscle dysfunction, therefore, it is important to examine the body as a whole, keeping in mind the effect that weakness, posture, and coordination have on a given muscle group. Muscular pain syndromes reflect dysfunction of the entire system and must not be considered in isolation.[66]

NOTABLE QUOTABLE

*"Muscle imbalances are **reflexive** in nature and can be considered to be a systemic deviation in the quality of muscle function that results from an adaptation to lifestyle. This results in various patterns of muscle tightness and weakness through a region or even throughout the entire body."*

–Vladimir Janda

CLINICAL PILLAR

As the manual therapist evaluates muscle dysfunction, it is important to examine the body as a whole, keeping in mind the effect that weakness, posture, and coordination have on a given muscle group. Muscular pain syndromes reflect dysfunction of the whole system and must not be considered simply as a localized affliction.

Muscle tightness, as described by Janda,[63,65,66] is the result of chronic overuse or poor posture. Tight muscles are painful when palpated but are not spontaneously painful. Tight muscles have a lower threshold, making them more

Table 13–1	Janda's Classification of Common Muscular Imbalance Syndromes Noted During Structural Observation That Require Closer Examination

MUSCLE IMBALANCE SYNDROMES	MUSCLES INVOLVED
Crossed Pelvic Syndrome	**Tight:** Hip flexors, paraspinals **Weak:** Gluteals, abdominals
Proximal Crossed Syndrome	**Tight:** Upper trapezii, levator scaulae **Weak:** Scapular stabilizers
Layer Syndrome	**Tight:** Hamstrings, thoracolumbar paraspinals, neck, upper trapezii, levator scapulae **Weak:** Gluteals, L4-S1 paraspinals, scapular stabilizers

easily activated, which contributes to their overuse and cycle of pain and tightness.[66–68] Over time, strength diminishes in the shortened muscle as active fibers are replaced by non-contractile tissue.[63]

Muscle adapts to increased length by increasing sarcomeres, and the weight of the muscle increases secondary to changes in protein content. No deleterious biochemical changes have been reported in lengthened muscle.[27] Muscles immobilized in a shortened position undergo a decrease in the number of sarcomeres of up to 40%. *Biochemical* changes also occur in the shortened muscle, which favor catabolism. Shortened muscles show a steep passive tension curve compared to controls, which may indicate that connective tissue loss occurs at a slower rate than does muscle loss. Endomysium and perimysium also become thicker, with immobilization in a shortened range further contributing to the reduction in extensibility.[27] Tardieu et al[69] found a similar increase in the passive tension curve slope when the triceps surae muscles of humans were immobilized in a shortened position.

Clinically, patients often present with muscle imbalances and postural dysfunctions that leave certain muscle groups shortened for prolonged periods of time. Clinically, it is important to understand that these muscles may have reduced protein content, increased infiltration of connective tissue, and a thickened endomysium and perimysium, all of which may contribute to the clinical presentation of "*tightness.*"

NOTABLE QUOTABLE

"Muscle spasm is an involuntary and inappropriate, reversible, prolonged bracing of a muscle or group of muscles, attributable to overactivity of motor units or changes of excitability of muscle fibers."

—M. Emre

Janda[65] describes muscle tightness as a result of overuse creating physiologic shortening (Box 13-6). Based on this premise, he suggests the use of stretching techniques that are based on the work of Knott[70] and to include timing for the contraction and relaxation phases of the stretch.[65,70,71]

CLINICAL PILLAR

- "*Tight*" muscles are not just in a shortened state. In addition, these muscles may have **reduced protein** content, relatively **increased connective tissue**, and a **thickened endomysium and perimysium**, all of which contribute to the clinical representation of "*tightness.*"

- Muscle dysfunction can present in many forms; therefore, intervention should be directed at the specific cause of the dysfunction.

- Treating shortened muscles with stretching techniques that include **specific timing** for the contraction and relaxation phases of the stretch is recommended.

The accessory motion of muscle, as previously described, is termed muscle play,[43,72] that is, the ability of each muscle to move freely in all directions in relation to the surrounding muscles and fascia. Normal gliding motion is possible through adequate hydration of the ground substance provided by water binding to proteoglycans. The mobility of the fascia allows one muscle to move past another as muscles are stretched or contracted. In the dysfunctional state, however, the independent movement between muscle groups is limited or even lost.

Any intervention directed toward increasing muscle length must take muscle play into account. Simply stretching the muscles will not necessarily restore muscle play, and without restoring muscle play, the efficiency of muscle elongation cannot be achieved. Clinically, restoring muscle play through STM can often restore normal length without the need for stretching.[43,72] The STM techniques described throughout the remainder of this chapter, are classified as either *muscle play techniques*, *muscle tone techniques*, or *muscle excursion* techniques.

Box 13-6 JANDA'S TYPES OF MUSCLE DYSFUNCTION

1. Muscle imbalance
2. Muscle and joint correlation and associated muscle patterns
3. Muscle coordination, movement patterns, movement programming
4. Muscle contraction speed
5. Increased muscle tone or hypertonicity

- In the same way that the physiologic motion of a joint is determined in part by its *accessory motion*, the length and function of a muscle is also determined in part by its accessory motion.

- The accessory motion of muscle is termed *muscle play* and defined as the ability of each muscle to move freely in relation to the surrounding muscles and fascia.

- Simply stretching muscles will not restore muscle play. Without restoring muscle play, efficiency of muscle elongation cannot be obtained.

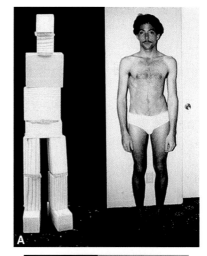

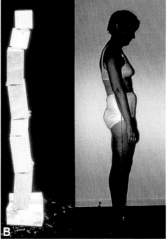

FIGURE 13–6 The frontal **(A)** and sagittal plane **(B)** postural alignment deviations are identified during the structural examination. If even one block or segment is out of alignment, the structure becomes less stable and therefore less efficient. Intervention is directed toward facilitating functional efficiency through restoring normal alignment. (From: Johnson GS, Saliba-Johnson VL. *Functional Orthopaedics I,* course lecture material. Steamboat Springs, CO: The Institute of Physical Art, 2003, with permission.)

PRINCIPLES OF EXAMINATION

The Objective Examination

The Structural Examination

The functional orthopedics approach bases its examination on identifying inefficiencies in both structure and function. The objective examination begins with a **structural examination.** The goal of this examination is to determine inefficiencies in the patient's structure that may lead to inefficiencies in function. Rolf[10] described the body as a model of blocks or segments that, when misaligned, are unstable and therefore inefficient. Rolf contended that many postural dysfunctions and inefficiencies are produced from abnormal tension in the soft tissue.[10] These structural inefficiencies present as compensatory postures and can be altered through soft tissue intervention (Figs. 13-5, 13-6).[10]

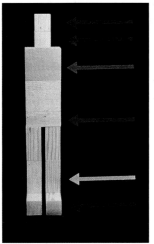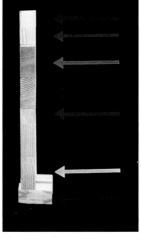

FIGURE 13–5 The frontal and sagittal alignment of segments are much like the stacking of building blocks. If the blocks are in good vertical alignment, the structure is stable and can support superincumbent weight. (From: Johnson GS, Saliba-Johnson VL. *Functional Orthopaedics I,* course lecture material. Steamboat Springs, CO: The Institute of Physical Art; 2003, with permission.)

When examining the structure for vertical and horizontal alignment, the therapist should initially focus only on the bony structure. Using Rolf's analogy of blocks, the examiner can evaluate whether any of the segments are misaligned. Visually, the therapist gets an idea of the efficiency of the structure and estimates where the structure might buckle under pressure.

Once the osseous examination has been completed, the therapist seeks to identify the presence of soft tissue restrictions. During this process, it is important for the therapist to appreciate the three-dimensional components of length, depth, and width of each segment and to evaluate whether each segment is proportional to adjacent segments. For example, in the case of a protruding abdomen, increased anterior length creates excessive lordosis, resulting in compression of the lower lumbar facet joints.

CLINICAL PILLAR

When conducting the **structural examination**:

1. Begin observation in a *natural setting* with the patient unaware that he or she is being observed.

2. Observe the efficiency of *transitional movements.*

3. *Look "through"* the patient, initially, without focusing on any one specific region.

4. Observe the *pattern of weight-bearing and base of support.*

5. Appreciate the *three-dimensional position* of each segment.

6. Focus first on the *osseous structures* that serve as the structural framework.

7. Progress to observation of the *symmetry, proportions, and contours of the soft tissues.*

8. Visualize how the soft tissue structures may *function during movement.*

9. Note any *mechanical stress points* and patterns of structural dysfunction.

10. Note any areas of potential *compensation*.

Examination of the soft tissues includes evaluation of symmetry, proportions, and contours. It is important to observe from caudal to cephalad looking for soft tissue torsions, muscle atrophy or hypertrophy, and any other asymmetries. Posteriorly, the therapist examines the verticality of the Achilles tendons, the position of the calves, and the relationship between the calves and the hamstrings. The contour of the hamstrings and the gluteals, including the presence of any holding patterns or atrophy, should also be determined. Throughout the soft tissue portion of the examination, observation of creases, folds, bands, constrictions, holding patterns, and asymmetries in the soft tissue should be noted. Regions where the skin looks shiny may indicate areas of constant tension or possible autonomic changes. During observation, the therapist should continually visualize how the structure might function during movement.

The two most common postural dysfunctions are the **anteriorly rotated pelvis** and the **anteriorly sheared pelvis**.[73] An anteriorly rotated pelvis is typically accompanied by hyperextension of the knees, increased lumbar lordosis, a backward bent costal cage, an elevated sternum, and forward head. An anteriorly sheared pelvis causes the sway back posture with the knees flexed, costal cage posterior, a depressed sternum, and forward head.[38] The depressed sternum is usually associated with scapular depression and downward rotation, whereas the elevated sternum is more likely to be associated with an elevated or anteriorly tipped scapula.[74] The clinician must determine, not only the primary dysfunction, but also any secondary compensations (Table 13-2). The anteriorly tilted pelvis is most often associated with tightness of the iliacus and hip internal rotators. The anteriorly sheared pelvis is associated with tightness of the psoas and the hip external rotators.[75]

STM endeavors to address soft tissue dysfunction for the purpose of returning structures to their most efficient neutral state. In neutral, minimal muscle activity is required for erect standing or sitting postures. The key to determining the quality of a particular posture lies in whether the structure functions efficiently.

Table 13-2	Common Postural Dysfunctions Identified During the Structural Examination and Their Associated Joint and Muscular Involvement	
POSTURAL DYSFUNCTION	**JOINT POSITIONS**	**ASSOCIATED MUSCLE IMBALANCES**
Anteriorly Rotated Pelvis	**Pelvis:** Anteriorly rotated **Knees:** Hyperextended **Lumbar:** Increased lordosis **Ribs:** Posterior to pelvis **Scapulae:** Elevated, anteriorly tilted **Sternum:** Elevated **Head:** Forward	**Tight:** Iliacus, hip internal rotators, paraspinals **Weak:** Gluteals, abdominals
Anteriorly Sheared Pelvis	**Pelvis:** Anteriorly sheared **Knees:** Flexed **Lumbar:** Swayback **Ribs:** Posterior to pelvis **Scapulae:** Depressed, downwardly rotated **Sternum:** Depressed **Head:** Forward	**Tight:** Psoas, hip external rotators **Weak:** Gluteals, paraspinals

Movement Testing

In the context of examining soft tissue dysfunction, movement tests are performed to identify how these structures *fold* and *elongate* during movement.[76,77] When examining trunk mobility, *pelvic shear* or *side gliding* is a valuable examination tool[78] as it involves the use of a complex movement pattern that requires efficient hip, pelvic, lumbar, and thoracic function. Any movement that is limited, inefficient, or painful can be performed following intervention to assess treatment efficacy.

The Vertical Compression Test

The **vertical compression test (VCT)** (Fig. 13-7) is a useful method of examining the alignment and efficiency of a patient's structure to allow optimal weight transfer.[43,72] Vertical compression is applied through the patient's structure in a caudal direction to evaluate how well the inherent structure is aligned. To perform the VCT, the therapist places his or her hands between the patient's first ribs and the acromion process and applies a gentle vertical pressure caudally. To ensure pure caudally directed force, the therapist's forearms should be positioned as vertically as possible. The patient should remain relaxed while the therapist carefully evaluates for the presence of movement within the system or the production of pain. In an efficient posture, force is transmitted to the feet with a springy and stable response without unwanted movement. A hard end-feel may indicate active resistance to pressure (Fig. 13-7a). In an inefficient posture, the patient will buckle or shift, most commonly into lumbar extension, anterior or lateral shear, or rotation (Fig. 13-7b). The test is graded on a 1 to 5 scale using a method found to have 80% interrater reliability by Johnson, anecdotally. *Grade 1* indicates no buckling with the amount of pressure

needed to contact bony structures. Each subsequent grade requires the addition of the same amount of force used for grade 1. An immediate improvement in the VCT is often realized through subtle modifications in the patient's posture or following minimal cueing. A positive response may suggest the presence of instability.[79]

The Lumbar Protective Mechanism (LPM)

The **lumbar protective mechanism (LPM)** (Fig. 13-8) examines the efficient timing of the core and global muscle systems' response to an outside force.[80] The patient stands in a diagonal stance with the therapist facing the patient in the same diagonal. To allow initiation of the abdominals to prevent trunk movement, pressure is slowly applied and gradually progressed through the infraclavicular region in a posterior diagonal. The command is *"hold, don't let me move you."* In the efficient state, the patient should be able to maintain an erect vertical alignment without buckling, shifting, rotating, or developing pain. The therapist continues to provide more force until maximum force is applied without compensation or until movement or pain occurs as initiation, strength, and endurance of the stabilizing contraction is evaluated. LPM should be tested both in anteroposterior and posteroanterior directions and in both diagonals, and graded on a 1 to 5 scale.

The Elbow Flexion Test (EFT)

For the **elbow flexion test (EFT)** (Fig. 13-9), the patient stands with elbows flexed to 90 degrees with palms up as vertical force is applied through the patient's forearms. The therapist evaluates the patient's ability to maintain an erect posture with scapulae correctly positioned on the rib cage. Compensations may include movement of the thoracic cage

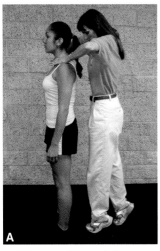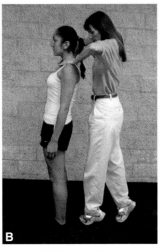

FIGURE 13–7 The vertical compression test (VCT) is a useful method for examining the alignment and efficiency of a patient's posture. **A.** In an *efficient posture*, the clinician will sense the force transmitted through the feet and into the floor with a solid, but not hard, end-feel during the application of vertically directed force. **B.** In an *inefficient posture*, the patient will buckle or shift somewhere along the kinetic chain upon application of vertically directed force. Most commonly when inefficient, the patient will shift into lumbar extension.

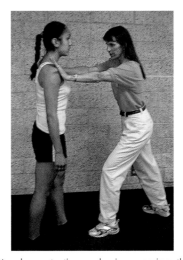

FIGURE 13–8 Lumbar protective mechanism examines the efficiency of the trunk to stabilize against an outside force. It is a dynamic test of the efficiency of the structure and of the neuromuscular response of the stabilizing musculature. The patient stands in a diagonal stance, and the clinician stands facing the patient in the same diagonal. Pressure is applied by the clinician through the patient's infraclavicular region in a posterior diagonal direction. The command is *"hold, don't let me move you."* The clinician slowly applies force, evaluating the patient's ability to initiate the abdominals and prevent movement of the trunk.

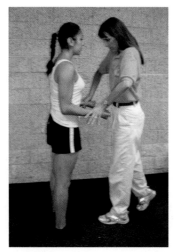

FIGURE 13–9 The elbow flexion test is a dynamic test of structural efficiency. The patient stands with elbows bent to 90 degrees and palms facing up. Vertical force is applied down through the patient's forearms. The assessment is of the patient's ability to maintain an erect vertical posture with scapulae correctly positioned on the rib cage. Compensations from an inefficient posture may include movement of the thoracic cage behind the pelvis, shoulder girdle movement into elevation, protraction or anterior tipping (winging), or overuse of the upper trapezius.

behind the pelvis; shoulder girdle movement into elevation, protraction, or anterior tipping; or overuse of the upper trapezius. Like the other tests, the EFT is graded on a scale from 1 to 5.

The Functional Squat

The **functional squat (FS)** is an excellent method to examine movement patterns that involve the entire body. The patient stands with a wide base of support and is asked to squat as far as possible without pain while keeping the heels on the ground. The therapist makes an overall evaluation of the coordination and efficiency of the movement. The efficiency of the lower extremity is often determined by the alignment of the patellae in relationship to the foot. The effort required to keep the patellae tracking correctly is helpful in determining whether the dysfunction is more structural or more functional in nature. In the efficient state, there should be a natural weight transfer. Inefficient movement results in either flexion at the spine or an attempt to keep the spine vertical, causing a loss of balance. General inefficiency during the FS may indicate that this is not the patient's preferred method for bending (Table 13-3).

Table 13–3	**Special Tests Designed to Examine Postural and Structural Efficiency and Alignment**			
TEST	**PURPOSE**	**PATIENT/THERAPIST POSITION**	**PERFORMANCE**	**INTERPRETATION OF FINDINGS**
Vertical Compression Test (VCT)	• To determine alignment and efficiency of weight transference	• Behind patient, hands on shoulder between first rib and acromion process • Forearms vertical	• Apply downward force with patient in relaxed posture. • Instruct patient to relax everything but the knees. • Monitor for pain and movement.	• **Positive:** Patient buckles or shifts (lumbar extension, anterior or lateral shear, rotation) • **Negative:** Force transmitted to floor with solid and springy, not hard, end-feel • **Grade 1:** Weight of hands produces buckling • **Grade 2:** Minimum force without buckling • **Grade 3:** Minimum-moderate force without buckling • **Grade 4:** moderate-maximum force without buckling • **Grade 5:** Maximum force without buckling
Lumbar Protective Mechanism (LPM)	• To determine the efficiency of trunk to stabilize against outside force and timing of muscle responses	• Patient and therapist in opposing diagonal stance	• Pressure applied through the infraclavicular region in an anterior-posterior, posterior-anterior diagonal • Monitor initiation of muscle response and trunk movement	• **Positive:** Poor timing and initiation of the core versus global muscle systems and decreased strength and endurance resulting in loss of erect alignment • **Negative:** Efficient initiation, strength and endurance of core muscles maintaining an erect position

Table 13–3	Special Tests Designed to Examine Postural and Structural Efficiency and Alignment—cont'd			
TEST	**PURPOSE**	**PATIENT/THERAPIST POSITION**	**PERFORMANCE**	**INTERPRETATION OF FINDINGS**

				• **Grading:**
				• **Initiation:** Absent
				  Sluggish
				  Efficient
				• **Strength and Endurance:** 1–5 with 1 being poor and 5 being good or efficient

Elbow Flexion Test (EFT)	• To determine efficiency of core and global muscle systems', position and balance control, and ability to maintain an erect posture with scapulae on rib cage	• Patient standing with elbows flexed to 90 degrees and palms facing up	• Downward force through patient's forearms without forward or backward force	• **Positive:** Decreased strength of the upper extremity, decreased strength and stability of the shoulder girdle allowing for protraction, firing of global versus core muscles, backward bending of thoracic spine, loss of balance • **Negative:** Maintain an erect vertical posture with scapulae correctly positioned on the rib cage and efficient balance
Functional Squat (FS)	• To examine movement patterns that involve the entire body • To evaluate the interrelationships of most segments of the body	• Patient stands with a wide base of support	• Patient squats as far as possible without pain while keeping heels on the ground.	• **Positive:** Suggests that this is not the preferred method of bending. Excessive pronation, external rotation, or decreased ROM at the ankles. Patellar tracking medial to the great toe with increased effort. Flexion at spine or attempt to keep spine vertical. • **Negative:** Patellae track in line with the second metatarsal. Natural weight transfer. As knees flex, hips flex, allowing trunk to become horizontal. Spine in neutral, pelvis drops back and down.

Palpation Examination and Localization of Soft Tissue Dysfunction

Once these areas have been identified, the palpation examination allows the therapist to localize the specific dysfunction. Just as joints are evaluated for end-feel, so should soft tissues be evaluated for mobility and end-feel.[81–83] Normal soft tissue end-feel is expected to be *"springy."*

The key to successful STM, within this approach, is three-dimensional localization of the restriction, which includes *location*, *depth*, and *direction.* Cyriax advocates the concept that (1) all pain arises from a lesion; (2) to be effective, the technique must reach the lesion; and (3) intervention must exert a beneficial effect on the lesion.

Dividing the body into four layers helps to isolate restrictions. The *first layer* consists of the skin and superficial fascia.

Layers two and *three* are myofascial layers deep under the skin but short of the underlying bony structures. The *fourth layer* consists of the deepest myofascial structures that lie against the underlying bone.[84,85] Although the layers are not distinct, they aid in the specificity of the examination and intervention.

Superficial restrictions should always be cleared before moving to the deeper layers. The depth at which STM is applied is determined by the angle of the therapist's fingers to the target tissue and does not require an increase in pressure. To address the superficial layer, the treatment hand is nearly parallel to the surface. Deeper layers are reached by increasing the angle of the treatment hand to gradually become more perpendicular to the surface. This method disallows the need to increase force required to exert the desired effect.

A convenient method of indicating the specific direction of a soft tissue restriction is to use the image of a clock as a visual tool for the therapist to determine the specific restricted direction. This method of examination has been identified as **tracing** and **isolating**.[43] Once specific localization of the dysfunction with regard to depth and direction has been determined, specific intervention may commence.

CLINICAL PILLAR

When addressing soft tissue lesions, the following concepts must be followed:

1. Be *specific* in localizing the *depth* and *direction* of any given lesion.

2. Clear the more *superficial restrictions* before addressing lesions in the deeper layers.

3. The depth of a technique is determined by the *angle of the therapist's fingers*, with deeper layers impacted as the angle becomes more perpendicular.

4. *Tracing and isolating* involves visualizing the face of a clock and checking soft tissue mobility in all directions.

PRINCIPLES OF INTERVENTION
The Effects of Soft Tissue Mobilization

Improvement in palpatory findings, increased range of motion (ROM), postural changes, and functional improvements can be identified as a result of STM.[5,35,72,86–88] Maitland and others[89,90] profess that joint mobilization permanently elongates the soft tissues that restrain joint mobility through the use of external force and may also explain the effects of STM on myofascial structures. In the case of postsurgical scars, STM can improve scar mobility and consequently lead to improvement in joint ROM and function.[35,36] In the same way, adhesions within the fascial sheaths may also be altered by direct force.

Mechanical stress, in the form of tension or pressure, is thought to facilitate the process of healing by speeding the fibroblastic secretion of collagen.[11] In addition, Ng et al[29] found that when granular tissue fibroblasts were subjected to tension, in vivo, differentiation into myofibroblasts was increased indicating that mechanical forces facilitate myofibroblastic differentiation. Myofibroblasts in turn secrete hyaluronic acid.

Other effects of STM may be circulatory or neuroreflexive. STM causes mast cells to release a histamine-like substance that leads to vasodilation.[63] Because vasodilation is a normal part of the healing process, techniques that facilitate vasodilation could promote healing in tissues that were previously not amenable to such processes.

When treating trigger points (TrPs) or muscle hypertonicity, neuroreflexive changes are thought to play a role in the reduction of pain and hypersensitivity (Box 13-7).[3] Some have used dry needling to decrease the hyperirritability that is associated with active TrPs through mechanical disruption of the sensory nerve endings that mediate TrP activity (see Chapter 16).[3]

Lastly, electrochemical influences may also play a role in the effect that STM plays in reducing pain and restriction. The interaction between biological tissues and electromagnetic fields may prove to relate to myofascial dysfunction. In addition, such phenomena as the piezoelectric effect may exist not only in the physical sciences, but also may present in a similar way in biological tissues.

Preparing for Intervention

Beginning the intervention with the patient in the neutral position places tissues on slack, reduces muscle guarding due to pain, and allows the therapist to evaluate without the influence of external forces. As intervention progresses, STM can be performed in more functional positions (see Chapter 12).

Box 13-7 JANDA'S ETIOLOGIES OF MUSCLE HYPERTONICITY

1. **Limbic dysfunction:** Not spontaneously painful and presents as a gradual change between the normal and the hypertonic muscle

2. **Interneuronal dysfunction:** Rare and exists as an altered balance of antagonistic muscles similar to that found in neural infections

3. **Incoordinated contraction:** Causes increased tone in a specific part of the muscle and is commonly referred to as trigger points

4. **Pain irritation:** Presents as a guarding or protective action by the muscle and is most often seen following acute injury. Under these circumstances, it is possible to record spontaneous EMG activity, which indicates that the whole reflex arc is activated, making it comparable to a voluntary muscle contraction.

5. **Muscle tightness:** Usually a result of chronic overuse or poor posture. Tight muscles are painful to palpation but are not spontaneously painful. Tight muscles present with a lowered threshold, making them more easily activated. This contributes to their overuse, keeping the cycle of tightness going. Initially, strength increases in the shortened muscle; however, in time, strength decreases as the active fibers are replaced by noncontractile tissue.

CLINICAL PILLAR

TIPS FOR PROPER PERFORMANCE OF STM

1. Place the patent in *neutral alignment* with adequate support to facilitate comfort and ease of application and progress toward end-range positions.

2. The therapist's *body generates the pressure* and creates movement, which is accomplished by placing the therapist's shoulders and hips in the direction of movement, with the feet positioned in a *diagonal stance* so that movement is produced by *weight shifting* from one foot to the other.

3. Identify specific parameters to evaluate the success of STM, keeping in mind specific goals that are commensurate with the stage of the condition.
   - *Acute stage*: Reduce pain, muscle tone, spasm
   - *Subacute stage*: Reduce tone, improve mobility
   - *Chronic stage*: Address soft tissues and associated compensations in more *lengthened ranges* and during functional motions

4. Maintain *constant communication* with the patient regarding his or her comfort and response to intervention.

5. The patient must take responsibility and become an *active participant* in his or her own care. The primary role of the manual therapist is to *facilitate* an efficient postural state and to *teach* patients how to maintain and care for themselves.

The Soft Tissue Mobilization Cascade of Techniques

Intervention should proceed in a methodical fashion, continuously searching for specificity while focusing on function. Most of the cascade of techniques that follow require both hands; therefore, descriptions consist of details regarding the *treatment hand* and the *assisting hand* (Box 13-8).

Soft Tissue Mobilization for the Skin and Superficial Fascia

Collagen fibers within the integument run in all directions. However, there is usually a predominate fiber direction that runs parallel to the direction that the skin is folded (shortened) and becomes stretched during normal movements. The skin is loosely attached and moves easily in relation to the underlying *tela subcutanea* or *superficial fascia*.[22,91]

Scar tissue is the extreme example of skin/superficial fascial immobility. More commonly, minor adhesions form between these layers, resulting in limitations in movement. To examine the skin and superficial fascia, the clinician places one or both open hands with palms down on the area to be examined with enough pressure to "*tack*" down the skin. As the hands are moved, the skin slides along the underlying tissues. This form

Box 13-8 CASCADE OF STM TECHNIQUES

1. Sustained pressure
2. Sustained pressure with assisting hand either *shortening* or *lengthening* the surrounding tissues
3. Unlocking spiral performed by treatment hand
4. Sustained pressure with shortening or lengthening of a body part
5. Sustained pressure with associated oscillations
6. Direct oscillations with the treatment hand
7. Functional Mobilization

of examination is called **skin sliding** and is typically performed around the image of a clockface.[43]

Because tissues in various regions move differently, the focus of the examination is on identification of end-feel rather than excursion. Once the slack is taken up, overpressure is applied to assess end-feel. Dysfunctional tissues are identified as having a hard end-feel. By moving into all directions of the imaginary clock, the direction of hardest end-feel and greatest restriction can be identified. **Finger gliding** of one finger along the skin normally reveals that the finger glides easily, creating a wave of skin in front of it (Fig. 13-10).[43] Dysfunctional tissues will cause a slowing down of the finger glide or resistance. The therapist then moves along the surface in parallel, adjacent rows as though mowing a lawn, while ensuring that the finger remains on layer one by remaining parallel to the surface of the skin.

The manual physical therapist must be careful to maintain contact with the patient at all times in order to instill in him or her a feeling of confidence and security. Intervention begins with sustained pressure from the treatment finger, making sure the restriction remains isolated and is taken to its end range. Pressure is applied gently and follows the direction of greatest restriction, which may change as the restriction releases. With the assisting hand, the tissues around the restriction can be shortened, creating slack around the restriction, or lengthened, producing traction on the restriction. *Shortening* of the tissues can be applied in any direction around the restriction, whereas *lengthening* is usually performed along the direction of the restriction (Fig. 13-11).

If sustained pressure combined with shortening or lengthening of tissues fails to provide a release, then a *rotational* force from the treatment hand may be used. This technique is called the **unlocking spiral**. This is performed by maintaining pressure on the restriction and superimposing a clockwise or counterclockwise motion through the treatment hand. The rotation is produced by the therapist's forearm moving toward pronation or supination. The tissue's resistance to the rotation is evaluated in both directions, and the spiral is performed in the direction of greatest ease until the restriction releases.

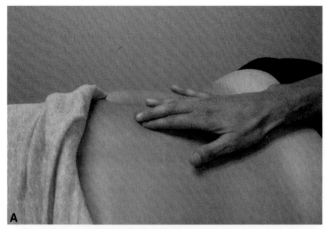

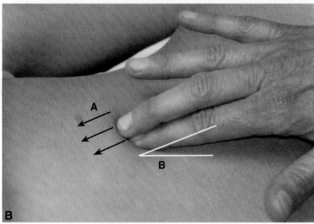

FIGURE 13–10 Finger gliding in order to *trace* and *isolate* a single dysfunctional region. **A.** In normal tissue, the finger glides easily. **B.** In dysfunctional tissue, resistance is noted under the finger. The therapist then moves along the surface in parallel, adjacent rows (A). Remaining on the proper layer is accomplished through attention to the angle of the finger and arm (B).

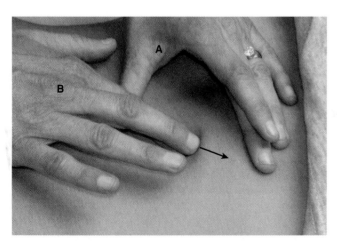

FIGURE 13–11 *Shortening* or *lengthening* of superficial fascia, may be applied with A. the assisting hand, as B. the treatment hand releases the restriction. Tissues around the restriction can be shortened, creating slack around the restriction, or lengthened, producing traction on the restriction. Shortening of the tissues can be applied in any direction, whereas lengthening is performed along the direction of the restriction.

The more aggressive techniques are typically reserved for the deeper layers. The only exception to this is scar tissue, which is more resistant to intervention and may require more aggressive techniques to gain mobility. Following intervention of the superficial fascia, reexamination is required. Releasing the skin and superficial fascia may have profound effects on deeper structures as well. Not only will ROM improve, but these techniques may also produce changes in the aforementioned functional tests.

Soft Tissue Mobilization for Bony Contours

Because soft tissues attach to bone, clearing restrictions at the site of attachment is a good starting point. By improving mobility along these bony contours, release of tissue tension in the muscles that attach to the same site is facilitated (Fig. 13-12).[64] For example, clearing restrictions along the iliac crest can impact the thoracolumbar fascia, paraspinals, quadratus lumborum, latissimus dorsi, and oblique abdominals.[7] In addition, clearing bony contours is necessary since fascial sheaths may become "*snagged*" on bony hooks such

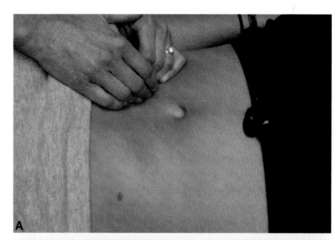

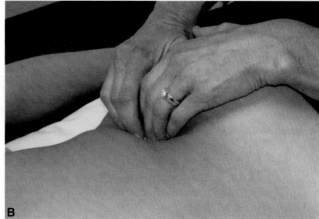

FIGURE 13–12 By improving mobility along *bony contours*, release of tissue tension can occur in all of the muscles that attach there. For example, clearing restrictions along the **A.** lower border of the rib cage or **B.** iliac crest can affect muscles throughout the trunk. Once a restriction is identified, further localization is accomplished by angling the finger toward or away from the bone. The assisting hand can then shorten or lengthen the surrounding tissues.

as the coracoid process, resulting in a modified flow of the fascia from the neck to the hand. The coccyx may also interrupt the continuity of fascial tissue both inside and outside the pelvis.

The bony contours that frame the lumbar spine consist of the iliac crest, 12th rib, sacral sulcus, coccyx, and spinal groove. Once the superficial fascia is cleared, the therapist evaluates the deeper layers by changing the angle of the treatment hand. For example, when treating along the iliac crest, progression from layer one to layer two is accomplished by angling the hand and forearm about 30 degrees from the horizontal. Depth can also be accomplished by curling the hand so that the fingers themselves become more perpendicular to the structures that are being addressed. Once a restriction is identified, further localization of the restriction is accomplished by angling the finger toward or away from the crest as the assisting hand shortens or lengthens the surrounding tissues. In order for intervention to be successful at deeper layers, the assisting hand must be kept at the same layer as the treating hand.

Releasing recalcitrant restrictions may require more aggressive techniques, which may not necessarily require more force. If unsuccessful with shortening or lengthening, the clinician moves down the cascade of techniques, which leads to *shortening* or *lengthening of a body part*. In the example of the iliac crest, the obvious option is to shorten by pushing up on the ischial tuberosity or lengthening by pulling down on the iliac crest while maintaining the direction and depth of the restriction with the treating hand. Active movement such as hip rotation, for example, can be effective in facilitating tissue tension changes.

With progression, the patient advances from basic to more complex movements.[12,92] Feldenkrais[12] used repeated coordinated movements, which resulted in the development of efficient movement patterns that ultimately improve structure (see Chapter 20). By adding STM to these functional movement patterns, the process of releasing soft tissue restrictions is accelerated while simultaneously teaching the patient to move efficiently within the newly acquired ROM.[92]

The next intervention technique that uses the concept of shortening and lengthening of a body part in conjunction with gentle oscillations is called **associated oscillations.** The oscillations used within the FO approach derive their origin from the ***Trager method.***[14] In this form of *"body work,"* oscillatory movements are incorporated at various locations throughout the body. The use of repetitive movement induces relaxation of the muscles. Although no direct manual contact to the muscle occurs, these oscillations are effective in reducing tightness.

The key to performing associated oscillations is *rhythm.* Using the previous example, the clinician's hand is placed on the ischial tuberosity, and pressure is applied cranially. Once the pelvis reaches its end range cranially, the pressure is released, allowing the pelvis to return to its initial position. The therapist's hand must remain in contact with the ischial tuberosity both during the shortening (or lengthening) and the relaxation phase of the oscillation. The oscillatory force

is produced through movement of the therapist's body, which moves with the patient, creating a smooth, rhythmic motion. Associated oscillations can be performed in any region of the body and can be done either along the *longitudinal axis* of the body or the *transverse axis*, which creates a greater rotational force.

The most aggressive technique, reserved solely for unyielding restrictions, is the **direct oscillation**. Once the restriction has been isolated, direct oscillations are performed through the treatment hand directly into the restriction. Although the technique is considered to be direct, the force is produced through the body and is simply transmitted through the hand. This technique is similar to a grade III or IV joint mobilization and, as with associated oscillations, the patient's body should move along with the oscillation.

Soft Tissue Mobilization for Myofascial Restrictions

Muscle Play Techniques

When addressing *muscle play restrictions*, the treatment hand performs (1) *perpendicular deformation*, (2) *strumming*, and (3) *parallel mobilization*. Examination of muscle play is typically performed by **perpendicular**, or **transverse, deformation** of the muscle (Fig. 13-13). In the lumbar spine, for example, the therapist should place the heels of his or her hands on one side of the spine with the fingers in a relaxed and slightly flexed posture, allowing the fingertips to rest on the opposite side of the spine. In this way, both hands come together to produce a single *"tool"* consisting of a row of fingertips that engages the border of the muscle. Other options include using the heel of the hand or thumbs, which is a more general technique. Movement of the spinalis muscle away from the spine allows the clinician to evaluate its capacity for deformation, the extent of its excursion, and most importantly,

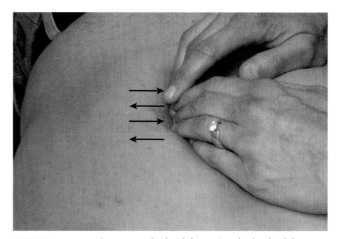

FIGURE 13–13 During *perpendicular deformation*, the heels of the hands are placed on one side of the spine, with the fingertips resting on the opposite side of the spine. Both hands come together to produce a single "tool," consisting of a row of fingertips that engages the border of the muscle. The set up for *strumming* is similar; however, once the perpendicular deformation is performed, the therapist allows his or her fingers to slide over the muscle belly. Muscle deformation is generated by the therapist's body, not his or her hands.

its end-feel. As with the intervention of bony contours, the process of examining myofascial structures must proceed from superficial to deep.

A progression of the perpendicular mobilization is a technique called **strumming**. Strumming can be used both as an examination and mobilization technique for muscle play dysfunctions. The setup for strumming is the same as that for perpendicular mobilization. However, once the perpendicular deformation is performed, the therapist allows the fingers to slide over the muscle belly and then back to the starting position. The therapist may strum repeatedly at a given location to assess the mobility and end-feel of the muscle and then repeat the process along the entire length of the muscle. As with all techniques, the muscle deformation is generated by the therapist's body, producing an oscillatory effect on the patient's body. Strumming takes time to master, but it can be an excellent method for treating muscle play dysfunctions and identifying areas of increased tone.

The third examination and intervention option is the **parallel technique.** This technique is performed by applying finger pressure parallel to the muscle, either between the bone and the muscle or between two adjacent muscles. The therapist slides his or her finger along the muscle, attempting to separate it from the surrounding tissues. Dysfunctions will present as a "*stitch*" in the tissues that makes continued gliding of the finger difficult. The therapist will trace and isolate to the specific depth and direction and treat accordingly.

Muscle Tone Techniques

Muscle tone dysfunctions present as tight nodules or bands of sensitivity within a muscle belly. Because of their neuroreflexive nature, these dysfunctions are often more resistant to lasting improvement[72,73,92]; therefore, intervention requires patient participation and retraining of posture and movement.[15] The patient's feedback is helpful in localizing the exact "*epicenter*" of the dysfunction.

Intervention is applied with sustained pressure at the exact point and direction of the dysfunction. As relaxation occurs, the therapist takes up the slack by moving farther into the tissue. The emphasis of intervention is to allow the patient to recognize the increased tone and reduce it by using various "*self-relaxation*" techniques such as (1) *breathing into the pressure*, (2) *breathing through the pressure*, (3) attempting to "*let go*," (4) using *visualization or imagery*, and (5) *contracting the isolated point followed by relaxation*. Muscle belly dysfunction can also be treated by localized strumming or general *ironing* techniques that broaden the muscle.

Muscle Excursion Techniques

Muscle tightness may exist in isolation[65,93] or in conjunction with muscle play/tone dysfunctions. Stretching in conjunction with soft tissue techniques are more effective than stretching alone.[10] To examine muscle length passively, the segment is brought to end range along its primary plane of movement followed by moving diagonally to isolate the direction of maximal restriction. For example, when testing hamstring length, the patient is asked to perform passive straight leg raising. Further isolation may be accomplished by slightly abducting and adducting, then medially and laterally rotating the leg in order to identify maximal three-dimensional tension.[94,95] STM during passive stretching and in conjunction with proprioceptive neuromuscular facilitation (PNF) may also be performed (Table 13-4).

General Myofascial Techniques

General techniques are performed using a broader contact. They are still performed specific to the location, depth, and direction of the restriction. They are effective when large

Table 13–4	Soft Tissues Typically Targeted for Mobilization Techniques Including a Description of Their Mechanical Properties and Recommended Principles of Examination and Intervention to Be Implemented for Each Tissue		
TARGET TISSUE	**TISSUE PROPERTIES**	**PRINCIPLES OF EXAMINATION**	**PRINCIPLES OF INTERVENTION**
Skin and Superficial Fascia	• Collagen run in all directions. Primary fiber direction is parallel to direction that skin is folded and stretched. • Easy gliding between skin and fascia and stretching of the skin occurs during normal movement. • Large amount of elastin allows stretching, deformation.	• Place one or both open hands with palms down. "*Tack*" down the skin so that the skin slides along the underlying tissues. This form of examination is called *skin sliding*. • Excursion of the tissues varies in different regions and directions. • Identify end-feel rather than excursion. Once the slack has been taken up, apply gentle overpressure. • Slowly move the hand in all directions, looking for the	• Sustained pressure from the assessing finger isolates the restriction and takes it to end range. • Pressure applied gently and follows direction of greatest restriction • With assisting hand, tissues around the restriction are shortened or lengthened, producing traction on the restriction. • Unlocking spiral is performed by maintaining pressure on the restriction and superimposing a clockwise or counterclockwise motion through the treating hand. Rotation produced by the therapist's forearm moving

Table 13–4	Soft Tissues Typically Targeted for Mobilization Techniques Including a Description of Their Mechanical Properties and Recommended Principles of Examination and Intervention to Be Implemented for Each Tissue—cont'd		
TARGET TISSUE	**TISSUE PROPERTIES**	**PRINCIPLES OF EXAMINATION**	**PRINCIPLES OF INTERVENTION**
		hour on the clock with the hardest end-feel. • Take one finger and slide along the skin in the established direction, a technique called *finger gliding*. • Move along the surface in parallel adjacent rows with the finger in layer one.	toward pronation or supination. Spiral performed in the direction of ease until the restriction releases. • Scar tissue is more resistant to intervention and may require more force and more aggressive techniques.
Bony Contours	• *Type I* fibers that present in orthogonal arrays in alternating sheets to resist multidirectional forces, including shear. • Clearing restrictions along the iliac crest can affect the thoracolumbar fascia, paraspinals, quadratus lumborum, latissimus dorsi, and oblique abdominals. • Fascial sheaths may become *"snagged"* on bony hooks like the coracoid process. • The coccyx may also interrupt the continuity of fascial tissue. • The tissue-layering concept is important because multiple layers of muscle and fascia attach to these bony contours.	• A quick screen of the superficial fascia along the bony contours progresses to deeper layers by angling the hand and forearm to 30 degrees.	• *Isolation* occurs by angling the finger toward or away from the crest to further localize the restriction. The assisting hand shortens or lengthens the surrounding tissues. • Keep the assisting hand at the same layer as the treating hand. • *Shorten* the region by pushing up on the ischial tuberosity or *lengthening* it by pulling down on the iliac crest while maintaining specific direction and depth with the treating hand. • Simple active movements are performed, including hip internal and external rotation progressing to more complex movements, including functional movements. • *Associated oscillations* are performed with treating hand on the ischial tuberosity with pressure applied cranially, followed by a release of the pressure without removing the hand. The oscillation is produced by movement through the clinician's whole body, not just the hands. Oscillations into hip or shoulder rotation are used to create rotational forces. • Once the restriction has been isolated, *direct oscillations* are performed through the treating hand.
Myofascia	• Includes both dense and loose connective tissue • Composed of irregular sheaths of collagen and elastin and a high degree of HA • Fascial sheaths are continuous, creating a network that extends from the dermis to the periosteum. • Muscles are covered by **endomysium**, **perimysium**, and **epimysium,** which are considered fascial sheaths	• Examine the body as a whole, keeping in mind the effect that weakness, posture, and coordination have on a given muscle group. • Examination of muscle play is performed by *perpendicular* or *transverse deformation* of the muscle. • In the lumbar spine, therapist places heels of hands on one side of the spine with fingers in a relaxed posture, allowing fingertips to rest on the opposite	• **Muscle play techniques** include the following: • Maintain *sustained deformation* pressure with the intervention hand with the assisting hand *shortening* or *lengthening* tissues or lengthening the body part by pulling down on the iliac crest. • *Direct oscillation* in combination with assisting hand techniques to rhythmically deform the muscle in the direction of the restriction. • *Strumming* can be set up the same as that for perpendicular mobilization.

Continued

Table 13-4 Soft Tissues Typically Targeted for Mobilization Techniques Including a Description of Their Mechanical Properties and Recommended Principles of Examination and Intervention to Be Implemented for Each Tissue—cont'd

TARGET TISSUE	TISSUE PROPERTIES	PRINCIPLES OF EXAMINATION	PRINCIPLES OF INTERVENTION
	and allow for independent movement between each structure. • Intervention for muscle play dysfunction will usually be maintained once treated; the muscle tone dysfunctions are more resistant to lasting intervention.	side of the spine; this allows both hands to produce a single *"tool"* that engages the border of the muscle. • Examining myofascial structures proceeds from superficial to deep. Once a restriction is identified, angle fingers slightly caudally and then cranially to further trace and isolate to establish the three-dimensional location of the restriction. • Examination then progresses between any two muscle bellies. • To examine muscle length, passively stretch the muscle to the end of its range. Then isolate the direction of maximal restriction by moving diagonally.	Once the perpendicular deformation is performed, the therapist allows fingers to slide over the muscle belly, strumming repeatedly at a given location, then repeating along the entire length of the muscle. • *Parallel technique* is performed by applying finger pressure parallel to the muscle, either between the bone and muscle or between two adjacent muscles. The therapist slides finger along the muscle, attempting to separate it from the surrounding tissues. • **Muscle tone techniques** include the following: • Intervention must include patient participation, which includes the retraining of posture and movement. • Intervention is applied with sustained pressure at the exact point and direction of the dysfunction. The pressure should begin at a level that does not cause the surrounding muscles to contract. As relaxation occurs, the therapist takes up the slack by moving further into the tissue. The emphasis of intervention is to allow the patient to recognize the increase of tone and learn to reduce it by using various *"self-relaxation"* techniques. While sustained pressure is maintained by the therapist, several techniques can be applied by the patient. These include (1) breathing into the pressure, (2) breathing through the pressure, (3) attempting to "let go," (4) using visualization or imagery and (5) specifically contracting that isolated point of muscle followed by relaxation. Muscle belly dysfunction can also be treated by localized strumming or by general ironing techniques that attempt to broaden the muscle. These techniques should also be performed with patient involvement. **Muscle excursion techniques** include the following: • *Stretching* of muscle in conjunction with STM involves applying STM principles during the passive stretch to increase its effectiveness and applying STM in conjunction with PNF techniques.

muscle groups are involved and can effectively *"iron out"* the muscle. In the lumbar spine, general techniques can be performed along the paraspinals, using the heel of the hand, knuckles, or proximal ulna. The stroke should be applied cranial to caudal and medial to lateral to facilitate lymph drainage and is most effective with a posterior tilt of the pelvis. Using the elbow or knuckles on the piriformis with hip rotation is often effective.

Circumferential techniques are typically performed on the extremities for the purpose of restoring muscle play so that soft tissue is able to move circumferentially around long bones. Hands are placed posteriorly and anteriorly and enough pressure is provided to take up slack and prevent hands from sliding over the skin. The soft tissues are then rotated clockwise and counterclockwise around the bone until full excursion is accomplished. End-feel is assessed, and the most restricted direction is established. The therapist then angles the pressure proximally and distally to isolate the exact angle of the restriction. To progress, the patient attempts to rotate the extremity against the therapist's pressure. Following relaxation, the therapist takes up the slack and the process is repeated.

Soft Tissue Mobilization Techniques for Selected Regions

Soft Tissue Mobilization for the Abdominal Region

In the abdominal region, examination of the superficial fascia should be performed first along with assessment of the umbilicus mobility through a 360 degree range. Specific attention should be given to surgical scars, which are common in the abdomen and can significantly affect the mobility of the spine and create locomotor dysfunction and associated pain syndromes.[35] The bony contours of the abdomen consist of the lower border of the rib cage and the anterior aspect of the ilium. Both of these bony contours lead directly to examination and intervention of the diaphragm and iliacus muscles. The diaphragm is mobilized by placing both hands on the upper abdomen with the fingers resting laterally on the rib cage (Fig. 13-14). As the patient inhales, the therapist's hands move cranially and into ulnar deviation to spread the rib cage. During exhalation, the therapist maintains the spread of the rib cage, providing a stretch to the diaphragm.[96] The iliacus can be palpated by sliding the fingers posteriorly along the iliac fossa.

After the diaphragm and iliacus have been treated, the rectus abdominis should be evaluated for muscle play. Its lateral borders, indicated by the lineae semilunares on each side of the linea alba, should be palpated. The therapist then slides the fingers medially to slide under the rectus, which is then lifted and glided from right to left.

Before progressing to the psoas, the abdominal contents are assessed. The viscera is surrounded by fascia and can therefore develop restrictions. With hands on either side of the abdomen, the entire abdomen is moved to the left and right. Isolation of the restricted direction through angling the pressure is critical. Intervention is most easily performed by having the

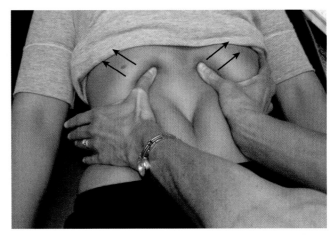

FIGURE 13–14 The *diaphragm release* is performed by placing both hands on the upper abdomen with the fingers resting laterally on the rib cage. As the patient inhales, the therapist's hands move into ulnar deviation to spread the rib cage. During exhalation, the therapist attempts to maintain the spread of the rib cage.

patient shorten or lengthen the region by rotating the spine through the lower extremities. Lastly, the therapist should treat the psoas. Soft tissue restrictions of the psoas can refer pain to the back and impact movement.[97-99] The psoas is palpated by moving deeply into the abdomen approximately midway between the umbilicus and the anterior superior iliac spine. The therapist verifies position by flexing the hip. Any of the previously mentioned techniques can be used to treat the psoas. Lengthening or shortening a body part can be performed by changing the hip angle, moving the pelvis into rotation, or rotating the spine through the legs, all of which can be performed passively or actively (Fig. 13-15).

Soft Tissue Mobilization for the Anterior Chest Region

Addressing soft tissue restrictions of the anterior chest is vital to the outcome of most neck and shoulder dysfunctions.

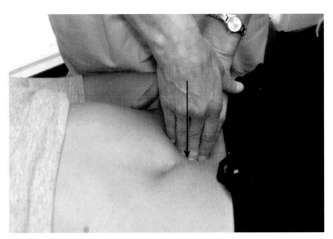

FIGURE 13–15 The *psoas release* is performed by moving deeply into the abdomen midway between the umbilicus and the anterior superior iliac spine. Gentle strumming of the psoas allows for assessment of both muscle play and tone. Once the muscle is palpated, the therapist can move more cranially and caudally to isolate restrictions.

Treating soft tissues in the anterior chest can be beneficial at improving posture and the efficiency of the cervical and thoracic spine and shoulders. In supine position, the manual physical therapist should evaluate the position of the scapulae and the breathing pattern. Intervention begins with intervention of superficial fascia. Bony contours include the manubrium, sternum, costosternal junctions, clavicle, and anterior/lateral ribs. The deep and superficial cervical fascia attaches to the clavicle, and shoulder movement into rotation is an effective way of altering fascial tension. The lateral border of the scapula should also be assessed because many of the involved muscles attach to this region. The myofascial structures treated in this region may include the *pectoralis major/minor, subscapularis, teres major/minor, serratus anterior, latissimus dorsi, infraspinatus, intercostals, sternocleidomastoid, scalenes, upper trapezii, levator scapulae, platysma*, and the *longus colli*.

CONCLUSIONS

Soft tissue mobilization as a means of addressing myofascial pain has been in existence since the beginning of time, and through the years, many clinicians and researchers from a variety of disciplines have contributed to the existing body of knowledge. The approach to STM delineated in this chapter represents a unique system developed by Gregory S. Johnson. This approach uses STM as an integrated component of Functional Manual Therapy for the reduction of pain, the enhancement of efficient function, and the restoration of myofascial mobility in preparation for the application of joint mobilization, neuromuscular reeducation, and motor control training.

To effectively implement STM, it is vital that the manual physical therapist has an appreciation for normal soft tissue anatomy and healing, as well as a complete understanding of the mechanisms that may contribute to soft tissue impairment. Effective use of STM requires the manual physical therapist to localize the soft tissue dysfunction three-dimensionally, that is, by location, direction, and depth. Localization is best accomplished through a method called tracing and isolating. Once localization of the dysfunctional lesion has occurred, a cascade of STM techniques may be implemented. These techniques should be used to address soft tissue dysfunctions, first of the skin and superficial fascia, followed by clearing of bony contours, and ultimately they should address myofascial dysfunction, more specifically, limitations in muscle play.

Soft tissue restrictions may need to be addressed in order to allow other interventions to have a more profound effect. The prevalence of soft tissue lesions requires the manual physical therapist to possess a thorough understanding of soft tissue anatomy and potential mechanisms, along with examination and intervention strategies designed to restore structural efficiency and symptom-free function.

CLINICAL CASE

CASE 1

History of Present Illness (HPI): The patient is a 29-year-old male with a history of degenerative disc disease at L4-L5 and L5-S1 and multiple episodes of low back pain and bilateral buttock and posterior thigh pain. This current episode began a couple of days ago for no apparent reason and has progressively worsened. Currently, he complains of nearly constant pain, difficulty walking, and the inability to forward bend.

Past Medical History (PMH): The original onset of symptoms was approximately 5 years ago during a ski trip. Since that time he has had five episodes of low back pain, with each resolving in response to physical therapy.

Observation: The patient presents with a 50% right lateral shift, reduced lumbar lordosis, positive pelvic anterior shear, and pelvic asymmetry with the left ilium postured superiorly.

Active Range of Motion (AROM): Backward bending = 10%; left shear = 80%; right shear = −40%.

VCT: 3/5

1. Based upon observation and the AROM findings, within what muscle groups would you expect to find myofascial impairment? Be specific and explain your rationale. Where would you expect this patient to buckle upon performance of the VCT? Explain your rationale. What other examination procedures would you perform to confirm your suspicions?

2. Describe in detail how you would examine the lumbar spine to determine the most appropriate soft tissue mobilization techniques. Assuming you identified the presence of muscle spasm, what soft tissue techniques might be most beneficial? Include direct and indirect techniques and explain your rationale. What would you monitor to determine the success of your intervention, both during the intervention and immediately after?

3. After two visits, the patient no longer presents with a lateral shift; however, the rest of the observational assessment remains the same. He now presents with left shear 80% and right shear 60%. At this time, he is not complaining of

difficulty walking and complains of a general ache in the lumbar region. What tests would you now perform to determine function?

4. During soft tissue palpation, you discover decreased muscle play on the left at L4, level 3, in the direction of 10 o'clock. Explain how this restriction might limit his right shear. Describe two myofascial techniques you could use to treat this restriction. Be specific and include the position of both the treatment hand and the assisting hand. What could you have the patient do to assist you in releasing the restriction?

5. What other interventions would you use to complement the STM techniques described above?

CASE 2

HPI: The patient is a 35-year-old female complaining of an insidious onset of right shoulder and arm pain. She complains of pain with lowering of the arm from an elevated position. In addition, she reports an episode of right neck pain about 2 months ago, with pain into the right lateral brachial region. She reports awakening with pain, with a worsening of symptoms throughout the day. She reports resolution of symptoms in response to medication.

PMH: The patient reports similar symptoms in the left shoulder approximately 2 years ago. At that time, she was diagnosed with calcific tendonitis of the supraspinatus tendon. Symptoms resolved completely in response to physical therapy.

Observation: The patient presents with forward head and rounded shoulders, increased upper thoracic kyphosis, depressed sternum, and increased internal rotation of both upper extremities. In the supine position, the right scapula rests 4 inches above the table, the left 3 inches. The patient is a chest breather.

AROM: Cervical rotation right = 60%; left = 50%. Shoulder abduction in internal rotation right = 120 degrees; left = 160 degrees.

VCT: 3/5

EFT: Elbow flexion is positive with anterior tilting of the scapulae and excessive anterior cervical muscle activity.

1. Based on the above presentation, how might you explain the development of this patient's widespread symptoms over time? Where would you begin your palpation of the soft tissues, keeping in mind restoration of function rather than reduction of pain? Provide your rationale. Explain in detail how you would progress your examination.

2. List several soft tissue groups that you would expect to find dysfunctional in this patient. Explain your rationale. What specific areas would you examine and treat with soft tissue mobilization to improve respiration?

3. During further examination, you discover that the first rib on the right is elevated. What soft tissues could you treat that may help to resolve this dysfunction? In examining the upper thoracic spine, what specific bony contours would you clear?

4. Soft tissue palpation reveals decreased muscle play of the right upper trapezius from anterior to posterior. Describe how you might use shortening and lengthening of at least two body parts to assist in improving muscle play. What might the patient do to assist during this process? If muscle play techniques are not successful in improving ROM of the cervical spine, what other myofascial dysfunction may be present that could be preventing full cervical ROM? Describe how you might treat this dysfunction.

5. What other interventions would you use with this patient to complement the soft tissue mobilization techniques described above?

HANDS-ON

With a partner, perform the following activities:

1 Perform a structural examination of your partner and note any dysfunctions in structure as well as soft tissue contours. Then perform the three functional tests, VCT, EFT, and LPM, on your partner and grade each test using the 1 to 5 scale. Use any other movement examination techniques with which you are familiar to further identify dysfunctional areas.

2 Identify three superficial restrictions within your partner's thoracolumbar spine based on where you would suspect to find dysfunction. Identify the specific location, direction, and depth of each restriction. Treat the dysfunctions using direct pressure, direct pressure with shortening or lengthening of tissues, and/or unlocking spiral. Once you have cleared the restrictions, retest VCT, EFT, and LPM and note any changes.

3 Identify a restriction along the iliac crest of your partner. Apply direct pressure with your "treatment hand." Use your assisting hand on your partner's ischial tuberosity to apply associated oscillations. It may be helpful to practice the associated oscillation prior to attempting to use it in conjunction with intervention. Continue to locate restrictions on other bony contours and use the cascade of techniques for intervention. Be sure to solicit feedback from your partner while treating. Pay particular attention to the specificity of pressure and your body mechanics. Following this intervention, retest your partner for changes in structure, movement, and the results of functional testing (VCT, EFT, LPM).

4 Use the technique of strumming to evaluate soft tissue dysfunctions along the thoracic and lumbar paraspinal musculature. Identify the location of a muscle play restriction three-dimensionally (direction, depth, and angle). Continue to use strumming to treat the dysfunction. Have the patient perform active movements of lower trunk rotation (or any other movement pattern you choose) to assist in clearing the dysfunction. If the dysfunction is not responding to intervention, try another muscle play technique, or evaluate for the presence of tone and apply techniques as needed. Retest following intervention.

5 Locate your partner's psoas muscle and compare bilaterally. Treat the most dysfunctional side using the cascade of techniques.

6 Choose another body part, preferably one not outlined in the chapter, and attempt to examine and treat the most significant superficial fascia, bony contour, and myofascial dysfunctions.

REFERENCES

1. Carlson S. History of massage. 2006. Available at https://suite101.com/a/historyofmassage-a36. Accessed March 31, 2014.
2. Calvert R. Historic descriptions of massage. *Massage Magazine*. 2005;111.
3. Travell JG, Simons DG. *Myofascial Pain and Dysfunction: The Trigger Point Manual*. Vols. I and II. Baltimore, MD: Williams & Wilkins; 1992.
4. Kellgren JH. Observations on referred pain arising from muscle. *Clin Sci*. 1938;3:175-190.
5. Dicke E, Shliack H, Wolff A. *A Manual of Reflexive Therapy of Connective Tissue (Connective Tissue Massage) "Bindegewebsmassage."* Scarsdale, NY: Sidney S. Simone; 1978.
6. Palastange N. Connective tissue massage. In: Grieve G, *Modern Manual Therapy of the Vertebral Column*. London: Churchill Livingston; 1986.
7. Miller B. Manual therapy for myofascial pain and dysfunction. In: Rachlin ES, ed. *Myofascial Pain and Fibromyalgia*. St. Louis, MO: Mosby; 2002.
8. Cyriax J. *Textbook of Orthopaedic Medicine: Diagnosis of Soft Tissue Lesions*. 8th ed. Baltimore: Williams & Wilkins;1984.
9. Cyriax J, Cyriax P. *Illustrated Manual of Orthopaedic Medicine*. Bourough Green, UK: Butterworths; 1983.
10. Rolf R. *Rolfing*. Santa Monica, CA: Dennis-Landman; 1977.
11. Schultz RL, Feitis R. *The Endless Web–Fascial Anatomy and Physical Reality*. Berkeley, CA: North Atlantic Books; 1996.
12. Feldenkrais M. *Awareness Through Movement*. New York: Harper & Row; 1977.
13. Aston J. *Aston Patterning*. Incline Valley, NV: Aston Training Center; 1989.
14. Trager M. *Trager Mentastics: Movement as a Way to Agelessness*. Barrytown, NY: Station Hill; 1987.
15. Tsao H, Hodges PW. Persistence of improvements in postural strategies following motor control training in people with recurrent low back pain. *J Electromyogr Kinesiol*. 2008;18(4):559-567.
16. Culav EM, Clark CH, Merrilees MJ. Connective tissues: matrix composition and its relevance to physical therapy. *Phys Ther*. 1999;79:308-319.
17. Frankel VH, Nordin M. *Basic Biomechanics of the Skeletal System*. Philadelphia: Lea & Febiger; 1980.
18. Currier D, Nelson R. *The Dynamics of Human Biolgic Tissue*. Philadelphia, F.A. Davis; 1992.
19. Downey PA, Siegel MI. Bone biology and the clinical implications of osteoporosis. *Phys Ther*. 2006;86:1.
20. Akeson W. Wolff's law of connective tissue: The effects of stress deprivation on synovial joints. *Arthritis Rheum*. 1989;18(suppl 2):1.
21. Mueller MJ, Maluf KS. Tissue adaptation to physical stress: A proposed "physical stress theory" to guide physical therapy practice, education and research. *Phys Ther*. 2002;82:383-403.
22. Gray H. *Anatomy of the Human Body*. Philadelphia: Lea & Febiger; 1966.
23. Akeson WH, Amiel D, Woo S. Immobility effects on synovial joint: the pathomechanics of joint contracture. *Biorheology*. 1980;17:95.
24. Amiel D, Akeson W, Woo S. Effects of nine weeks immobilization of the types of collagen synthesized in periarticular connective tissue from rabbit knees. *Trans Orth Res Soc*. 1980;5:162.
25. Butler D. *Mobilization the Nervous System*. New York: Churchill Livingstone; 1991.
26. Gratz CM. Air injection of the fascial spaces. *Am J Roentgenol*. 1936;35:750.
27. Grossman MR, Sahrmann SA, Rose SJ. Review of length-associated changes in muscle. *Phys Ther*. 1982;62:1799.
28. Schleip R, Klingler W, Lehmann-Horn F. Active fascial contractility: fascia may be able to contract in a smooth muscle-like manner and thereby influence musculoskeletal dynamics. *Med Hypothesis*. 2005;65:273-277.
29. Ng CP, Hinz B, Swartz MA. Interstitial fluid flow induces myofibroblast differentiation and collagen alignment in vitro. *J of Cell Sci*. 2005;118: 4731-4739.
30. McCullough J. The integumentary system–repair and management: an overview. *PT Magazine*. 2004. Available at: http://web.missouri.edu/~danneckere/pt316/case/wound/integumentary.pdf .
31. Engles M. A tissue response. In: Donatalli R, and Wooden M. *Orthopaedic Physical Therapy*. Philadelphia: Elsevier; 2001.
32. Woo S, Buckwalter JA. *Injury and Repair of the Musculoskeletal Soft Tissues*. Park Ridge, IL: American Academy of Orthopaedic Surgeons; 1988.
33. Arem JA, Madden JW. Effects of stress on healing wounds. Intermittent noncyclical tension. *J Surg Res*. 1976;20:93.
34. Van der Muelen JCH. Present state of knowledge on processes of healing in collagen structures. *Int J Sports Med*. 1982;3:4.
35. Kobesova A, Morris CE, Lewit K, Safarova M. Twenty-year old pathogenic active postsurgical scar: a case study of a patient with persistent right lower quadrant pain. *J Manipulative Physiol Ther*. 2007;20:234-237.
36. Lewit K, Olsanska S. Clinical significance of active scars: abnormal scars as a cause of myofascial pain. *J Manipulative Physiol Ther*. 2004;27: 399-402.
37. Cummings GS, Crutchfield CA, Barnes MR. *Orthopedic Physical Therapy Series: Vol 1: Tissue Changes in Contractures*. Atlanta: Strokesville; 1983.
38. Kendall HO, Kendall FP, Boynton DA. *Posture and Pain*. Huntington, NY: Krieger Publishing; 1977.
39. Woo SL-Y, Buckwalter JA. *Injury and Repair of the Musculoskeletal Soft Tissues*. Park Ridge, IL: American Academy of Orthopedic Surgeons; 1988.
40. Calliet R. *Soft Tissue Pain and Disability*. Philadelphia: FA Davis; 1977.
41. Farfan HF. Mechanical factors in the genesis of low back pain. In: Bonica JJ, Liebeskind JC, Albe-Fessard D, eds. *Advances in Pain and Research and Therapy*. Vol 3. New York: Raven Press; 1979.
42. Hunt TK, Banda MJ, Silver IA. Cell interaction in post-traumatic fibrosis. *Clin Symp*. 114;1985:128-149.

43. Johnson GS, Saliba-Johnson VL. *Functional Orthopaedics I. Course Outline.* Steamboat Springs, CO: Institute of Physical Art; 2003.
44. Caprini JA, Arcelus JA, Swanson J, et al. The ultrasonic localization of abdominal wall adhesions. *Surg Endos.* 1995;9:283-285.
45. Isla A, Alvarez F. Spinal epidural fibrosis following lumbar diskectomy and antiadhesion barrier. *Neurocirugia (Astur).* 2001;12:439-446.
46. Brill AI, Nezhat F, Nezhat CH, Nezhat C. The incidence of adhesions after prior laparotomy: a laparoscopic appraisal. *Obstet Gynecol.* 1998;85:269-272.
47. Ahcan U, Amez ZM, Bajrovic F, Zoman P. Surgical technique to reduce scar discomfort after carpal tunnel surgery. *J Hand Surg (Am)* 2002;27:821-827.
48. Stauber WT, Knack KK, Miller GR, Grimmett JG. Fibrosis and intercellular collagen connections from 4 weeks of muscle strains. *Muscle Nerve.* 1996;19:423-430.
49. McNeil PL, Khakee R. Disruptions of muscle fiber plasmamembrane: role in exercise-induced damage. *Am J Pathol.* 1992;140:1097-1099.
50. Matthews P, Richards H. Factors in the adherence of flexor tendon after repair. *J Bone Joint Surg.* 1976;58B:230.
51. Gelberman RH, Vandebert JS, Lundberg GN, Akeson WH. Flexor tendon healing and restoration of the gliding surface. *J Bone Joint Surg.* 1983;65A:70.
52. Akeson WH, Amiel D, Mechanic GL, et al. Collagen cross-linking alterations in periarticular connective tissue collagen after nine weeks of immobilization. *Connect Tissue Res.* 1977;5:15-19.
53. Akeson WH, Woo SL-Y, Amiel D, Matthews JV. Biomechanical and biochemical changes in the periarticular connective tissue during contracture development in the immobilized rabbit knee. *Connect Tissue Res.* 1974;l2:4.
54. Woo S, Matthew JV, Akeson WH, et al. Connective tissue response to immobility: correlative study of biomechanical and biochemical measurements of normal and immobilized rabbit knees. *Arthritis Rheum.* 1975;18:257.
55. Woo S, Gomex MA, Woo YK, et al. The relationship of immobilization and exercise on tissue remodeling. *Biorheology.* 1982;19:397.
56. Iocono JA, Ehlich HP, Keefer KA, Krummel TM. Hyalurion induces scarless repair in mouse limb organ culture. *J Ped Surg.* 1998;33:4.
57. Miller JA, Ferguson RL, Powers DL, Burns JW, Shalaby SW. Efficacy of hyaluronic acid/ anti-inflammatory systems in preventing postsurgical tendon adhesions. *J Biomed Mater Res.* 1997;38:25-33.
58. Larsson SE, Bodegard L, Henriksson KG, Obery PA. Chronic trapezius myalgia: morphology and blood flow studied in 17 patients. *Act Orthop Scand.* 1990;61:394-398.
59. Amiel D, Frey C, Woo S, et al. Value of hyaluronic acid in the prevention of contracture formation. *Clin Orthop* 1985;196:306.
60. Jarvinen TA, Kannua P, Jarvinen TI, et al. Tenascin-C in the pathobiology and healing process of musculoskeletal tissue injury. *Scand J Med Sci Sports* 2000;10:376-382.
61. Selye H. *The Stress of Human Life.* New York: McGraw-Hill; 1978.
62. Wyke B. The neurology of joints. *Ann R Coll Sur* 1967;41:25.
63. Janda V. Muscle weakness and inhibition (pseudoparesis) in back pain syndromes. In: Grieve G, ed. *Modern Manual Therapy of the Vertebral Column.* New York: Churchill Livingstone; 1986:198.
64. Janda V. Pain in the locomotor system, a broad approach. In: Glasgow EF, ed. *Aspects of Manipulative Therapy,* Melbourne, Australia: Churchill Livingstone; 1984.
65. Janda V. *Muscles and Back Pain: Assessment and Intervention, Movement Patterns, Motor Recruitment.* Course notes. 2nd ed. 1994;4.
66. Janda V. Muscle spasm–a proposed procedure for differential diagnosis. *J Manual Med* 1991;6:136-139.
67. Emre M. Symptomatology of muscle spasm. In: Emre M, Mathies H, eds. *Muscle Spasm and Back Pain.* Carnforth, UK: Parthenon; 1988.
68. Lewit K. Management of muscular pain associated with articular dysfunction. In: Fricton JR, Awad EA. *Advances in Pain Research and Therapy. Vol 28. Myofascial Pain and Fibromyalgia.* New York: Raven; 1990.
69. Tardieu C, Tarbary J, Tardieu G, et al. Adaptation of sarcomere numbers to the length imposed on muscle. In: Gubba F, Marecahl G, Takacs O, eds. *Mechanism of Muscle Adaptation to Functional Requirements.* Elmsford, NY: Pergamon Press; 1981:103.

70. Knott M, Voss DE. *Proprioceptive Neuromuscular Facilitation.* 2nd ed. New York: Harper & Row; 1968.
71. Saliba V, Johnson G, Wardlaw C. Proprioceptive neuromuscular facilitation. In: Basmajian J, Nyberg R, eds. *Rational Manual Therapies.* Baltimore: Williams & Wilkins; 1993:243.
72. Johnson GS, Saliba VL. Soft tissue mobilization. In: Donatelli RA, Wooden MJ, eds. *Orthopaedic Physical Therapy.* 2nd ed. New York: Churchill Livingston; 1994.
73. Johnson GS, Saliba-Johnson VL. *Back Education and Training: Course Outline.* Steamboat Springs, CO: Institute of Physical Art; 1997.
74. Sahrman S. *Diagnosis and Intervention of Shoulder Movement System Impairment Syndromes.* Course notes. St. Louis, MO: Washington University; 2004.
75. Godges J. *Manual Therapy and Movement.* Course notes. 1992.
76. Kurz T. *Stretching Scientifically: A Guide to Flexibility Training.* Island Pond, VT: Stadion; 1994.
77. Rywerant Y. *The Feldenkrais Method.* San Francisco: Harper & Row; 1974.
78. McKenzie RA. *The Lumbar Spine: Mechanical Diagnosis and Therapy.* Lower Hutt, New Zealand: Spinal Publications; 1981.
79. Paris S. Physical signs of instability. *Spine.* 1985;3:277-279.
80. Saliba V, Johnson G. Lumbar protective mechanism. In: White AH, Anderson R, eds. *The Conservative Care of Low Back Pain.* Baltimore: Williams & Wilkins; 1991;112.
81. Christensen H, et al. Palpation of the upper thoracic spine: An observer reliability study. *J Manipulative Physiol Ther.* 2002;25:285-292.
82. Huijbregts P. Spinal motion palpation: a review of reliability studies. *J Man Manip Ther.* 2002;10:24-39.
83. Wainner RS, et al. Reliability and diagnostic accuracy of the clinical examination and patient self-report measures for cervical radiculopathy. *Spine.* 2003;28:52-62.
84. Hunter G. Specific soft tissue mobilization in the management of soft tissue dysfunction. *Man Ther.* 1998;3:2-11.
85. Sutton GS, Bartel MR. Soft Tissue Mobilization Techniques for the Hand Therapist. *J Hand Ther.* 1994;7:185-192.
86. Cottingham JT, Porges SW, Richmonk K. Shifts in pelvic inclination angle and parasympathetic tone produced by rolfing soft tissue manipulation. *Phys Ther.* 1988;68.
87. Godges J, Mattson-Bell M, Thorpe D, Shah D. The immediate effects of soft tissue mobilization with proprioceptive neuromuscular facilitation on glenohumeral external rotation and overhead reach. *J Orthop Sports Phys Ther.* 2008;33:713-718.
88. Senbursa G, Baltic G, Atay A. Comparison of conservative treatment with and without manual physical therapy for patients with shoulder impingement syndrome: a prospective, randomized clinical trial. *Knee Surg Sports Traumatol Arthrosc.* 2007;15:915-921.
89. Maitland GD. *Vertebral Manipulation.* 5th ed. London: Butterworths; 1986.
90. Threlkeld AJ. The effects of manual therapy on connective tissue. *Phys Ther.* 1992;72.
91. Hollinshead, WH. *Textbook of Anatomy.* 3rd ed. New York: Harper and Row; 1974.
92. Johnson GS, Saliba-Johnson VL. *Functional Orthopaedics II.* Course outline. Steamboat Springs, CO: The Institute of Physical Art; 2004.
93. Evjenth O, Hamberg J. *Muscle Stretching in Manual Therapy: A Clinical Manual.* Alfta, Sweden: Alfta Rehab Forlag; 1985.
94. Johnson GS, Saliba-Johnson VL. *PNFI: The Functional Approach to Movement Reeducation.* Steamboat Springs, CO: Institute of Physical Art; 1997.
95. Lewit K. *Manipulative Therapy in Rehabilitation of the Locomotor System.* 2nd ed. Boston: Butterworths; 1992.
96. Stoddard A. *Manual of Osteopathic Practice.* London: Hutchinson & Co; 1959.
97. Ellis J. *Lumbopelvic Integration.* Course notes; 1999.
98. Aspinall W. Clinical implications of iliopsoas dysfunction. *J Man Manip Ther.* 1993;1:41-46.
99. Ingber RS. Ilipsoas myofascial dysfunction: a treatable cause of LBP. *Arch Phys Med.* 1989;70:382-386.

Myofascial Release in Orthopaedic Manual Physical Therapy

Jay B. Kain, PhD, PT, ATC, IMT,C

Chapter Objectives

At the conclusion of this chapter, the reader will be able to:

- Delineate the history and the major contributors to present-day soft tissue approaches in orthopaedic manual physical therapy (OMPT).
- Describe the structure and function of connective tissue, including both the cellular and fibrillar components that establish the primary characteristics of connective tissue.
- Describe the effects of immobilization on connective tissue.
- Understand the differences between direct and indirect OMPT approaches to mobilization.

- Define the theory of tensegrity and the integrated systems approach to myofascial release (MFR).
- Perform a basic triplanar examination of connective tissue mobility.
- Define the primary indications and differences between soft tissue MFR and articular MFR.
- Identify and maintain a triplanar fulcrum.
- Perform several basic MFR techniques for soft tissue and articulations.

HISTORICAL PERSPECTIVES

Attempts to mobilize the myriad of connective tissues of the body have led to the development of a variety of approaches that are considered to be "*fascial*" in nature (Box 14-1). This chapter is devoted to the description of one such approach, known as **myofascial release (MFR).** The philosophical underpinnings of one form of *MFR* and its clinical application are provided.

As already delineated in Chapter 13 of this text, approaches designed to address soft tissue dysfunction may be classified in accordance with the methods used or the structures targeted.[1] ***Bindegewebsmasssage*** is considered to be an *autonomic/reflexive* approach to fascial manipulation that was developed in the 1920s by a German physiotherapist, ***Elizabeth Dicke***. This approach relies on reflexive pathways mediated through the autonomic nervous system to facilitate a therapeutic effect. Bindegewebsmasssage is performed in a very systematic fashion. Dicke's purely "*mechanical*" approach was one of the first to articulate specific clinical parameters.

Another "*reflexive*" approach, called **Hoffa massage**, requires minimal force and is designed to avoid pain.[2] Other truly

reflexive approaches include **foot reflexology, auriculotherapy, acupressure, zero balancing, and polarity therapy.**[1] Many reflexive pathways are poorly understood within the realm of traditional physiology and are better explained by concepts related to energy from within the field of applied quantum physics. A full description of these concepts is outside the scope of this chapter.

Two fascial approaches considered by Cantu and Grodin[1] to be mechanical in nature are ***Rolfing***[3] and ***Trager. Ida Rolf*** introduced Rolfing with the intent to improve the body's balance in relation to gravity. These techniques are not based on a patient's current physical status but rather on a *10-session protocol* that addresses various body quadrants. Additionally, Rolf noted that the integration of body and mind are inseparable, and both need to be addressed.[3]

Focusing on the subconscious mind, ***Milton Trager*** developed an approach that combines passive and active motions into a technique termed *mentastics*. Trager felt that the combination of relaxation and neuromuscular reeducation created a powerful tool for changing poor postural habits. Trager's approach employs movement as a mechanical tool

Box 14-1 APPROACHES TO SOFT TISSUE DYSFUNCTION AND THEIR PRIMARY METHOD TO ENACT CHANGE

- **Bindegewebsmasssage**: autonomic/reflexive approach to fascial manipulation
- **Hoffa Massage**: use of minimal force that is designed to elicit as little pain as possible
- **Rolfing**: improve the body's balance in relation to gravity through the integration of body and mind
- **Trager**: combination of tissue relaxation and neuromuscular reeducation, which focuses on the subconscious mind
- **Hellerwork**: incorporates movement reeducation through exercises that mimic everyday movement, reinforce stress-free methods of performance, and connect mental patterns to the patient's own somatic expression
- **Alexander Techniques**: supplemented by mechanical approaches that prepares a person for movement

reeducation by superimposing normal movement patterns to eliminate poor postural habits
- **Feldenkrais Awareness Through Movement**: focuses on changing old habits and patterns using a hands-on approach to slowly change inadequate movement into efficient movement
- **Aston-Patterning**: negotiating a balance of the body's tissue through touching, sensing, and hearing. Each body maintains and expresses patterns that can help or hurt an individual.
- **Functional Orthopedics Approach**: incorporates proprioceptive neuromuscular facilitation (PNF) patterns of movement with direct connective tissue manipulation

and is therefore classified as a movement approach.[1] Other mechanical fascial approaches include **shiatsu, myotherapy, and chua ka.**

In 1970, *Joseph Heller* introduced an approach that combined both mechanical and movement components.[4] *Hellerwork* emerged after years of practicing the Rolfing approach. Heller attempted to decrease fascial tension through body realignment. He observed that more upright postures require less energy. Hellerwork incorporates movement reeducation through exercises that mimic everyday movement and reinforce stress-free performance. Another component includes a dialoguing technique designed to connect mental patterns to their own somatic expression.

Movement approaches illustrate how function influences structure. *F.M. Alexander*[5] saw the head and neck as being not only representative of other dysfunctional patterns elsewhere in the body, but also the key to their correction. He found that if he superimposed normal movement patterns on existing patterns, and supplemented these patterns by mechanical approaches, then poor postural habits would be eliminated.

Moshe Feldenkrais published his classic text, *Awareness Through Movement*,[6] in 1971. He considered all individuals to be disabled in one manner or another, as demonstrated by his twofold approach. He focused on changing old patterns, then used a hands-on approach to improve movement efficiency (see Chapter 20). Both Alexander and Feldenkrais believed that all new patterns of movement are mediated through the cerebrum and transferred to the cerebellum. Permanent postural changes were best achieved if the pattern became reflexive and not processed at the cerebral level only.

Judith Aston introduced an approach called *Aston-Patterning* in 1977.[7] She believed that both mental and physical history is expressed through the body. Through three-dimensional evaluation, areas of connective tissue tension are identified. The practitioner facilitates an individual's journey in negotiating a balance of the body's tissues through touching, sensing, and hearing.

CONNECTIVE TISSUE STRUCTURE AND FUNCTION

Understanding the concept of fascial release begins with a familiarity of the basic components of connective tissue (Box 14-2). These tissues can be somewhat arbitrarily divided into two basic elements: *cells* and *extracellular matrix*. The ratio of cells to extracellular matrix varies widely among different types of connective tissues,

Box 14-2 CONNECTIVE TISSUE

- Connective tissue composes approximately 16% of our total body weight and stores 23% of the body's total water content.
- It is involved directly and indirectly in every system in the body. In essence, connective tissue represents the one system that interconnects all other systems.
- Metabolic and physiologic functions of connective tissues include protection from foreign pathogens, infection, and inflammation; transportation and storage of vital nutrients for other tissues; elimination of waste products and toxins; and provision of an avenue of communication between and among various tissues.
- Consists of hard joints (bone on bone, including *fibro-* and *hyaline cartilage articulations* in the body); soft joint (muscle to muscle, muscle to ligament, ligament to tendon, *bursa* to tendon, organ to organ); and partial soft joints (tendon to tuberosity, muscle to bone, organ to bone)
- Muscle tissue accounts for approximately 50% of the total volume of the body, connective tissue composes approximately 45%, and neural and epithelial tissues compose the remaining 5%.

The connective tissue system is comprised of components derived from the *embryological mesoderm*. This system is contiguous throughout the expanse of our body. Connective tissues comprise approximately 16% of our total body weight and store 23% of the body's total water content.

Connective tissue within the body may be subdivided into *connective tissue proper, fluid connective tissue*, and *supportive connective tissue* (Box 14-3). Connective tissues are involved directly and indirectly in every system of the body. The synchronization of motion between all types of joints is directly related to the biomechanical, intrasystem properties of connective tissue. Exemplifying intersystem relationships, loose connective tissue provides a pathway for the *reticuloendothelial system* to interact with blood, lymph, and organs in order to fight infection. Connective tissue represents a system that interconnects with all other body systems.[8-15]

The Cellular Components of Connective Tissue

All connective tissues have three primary components: cells, fibers, and ground substance. The *fibroblast* synthesizes all of the major fibrillar components of connective tissue, including *collagen, elastin,* and *reticulin*, as well as the *ground substance*. As the fibroblast matures, it transforms into the most prominent cellular element. Once mature, differentiation ceases and the fibroblast becomes a *fibrocyte*. Undifferentiated cells in mature connective tissue retain the ability to transform into other specialized cells, which is dictated by local needs (Box 14-4) (Fig. 14-1).

The Fibrillar Elements of Connective Tissue

The fibrillar elements of connective tissue include collagen, elastin, and reticulin. Depending on the type of connective tissue, there are significant differences in the ratio of cells to extracellular material. For example, in bone and muscle, there are high numbers of cells in relation to the extracellular material. In tendons and ligaments, however, the ratio of cells to matrix is low.

Collagen

Collagen is the fiber best suited to resist tensile forces, in contrast to elastin and reticulin, which both have more resiliency and elasticity.[8-15] Collagen is an adaptable material that can be as rigid as bone or as pliable as the integument.[16] Recent evidence has identified as many as twelve different types of collagen.[8-15] *Types I to IV* are the most abundant forms of collagen and appear to have the most relevance for manual physical therapy.

Accounting for 40% of all protein and comprising 70% to 90% of the dry weight of tendons and ligaments, collagen is the most abundant protein in the body. The half-life of collagen is 300 to 500 days under normal conditions, with faster and slower turnover rates in bone and cartilage, respectively.[8-15]

Box 14-3 CONNECTIVE TISSUE DIFFERENTIATION

CONNECTIVE TISSUE PROPER

Loose connective tissue differentiates into:

1. Areolar connective tissue

2. Adipose tissue

3. Reticular tissue

Dense connective tissue differentiates into:

1. Dense regular connective tissue

   a. Tendons

   b. Ligaments

   c. Aponeuroses

   d. Fascia

   e. Elastic tissue

2. Dense irregular connective tissue

   a. Capsule

   b. Skin

Ground substance of connective tissue proper: Syrupy sticky consistency. Proteoglycans made up of glycoproteins and glycosaminoglycans attach to hyaluronic acid.

FLUID CONNECTIVE TISSUE

Blood differentiates into:

1. Red blood cells (erythrocytes)

2. White blood cells (leukocytes)

Lymph: Lymphocytes

Ground substance of fluid connective tissues: Plasma, more watery and fluid than ground substance of connective tissue proper

SUPPORTIVE CONNECTIVE TISSUE:

Cartilage differentiates into:

1. Hyaline cartilage

2. Fibrocartilage

3. Elasto-cartilage

Bone

Ground substance of supportive connective tissue: Referred to as the matrix. Can range from a firm gel in cartilage to a solid matrix in bone, secondary to the combinations of calcium, salts, and collagen fibers.

Box 14-4 HISTOLOGICAL MAKE-UP OF THE CONNECTIVE TISSUE

CELLULAR COMPONENTS

1. **Fibroblasts:** Fixed stellate-shaped cells that produce all the fibrous components of connective tissue proper, as well as the ground substance

2. **Macrophages:** First line of defense for tissues against infection, inflammation, trauma, burns, etc.

   A. **Fixed macrophages:** These are scattered throughout the connective tissues, and when stimulated, they can mobilize themselves and become free macrophages.

   B. **Free macrophages:** These are highly mobile versions of fixed macrophages, but apparently performing the same functions.

3. **Monocytes:** These are actually precursors or immature macrophages and are found in the blood. Once stimulated by the immune system, they are drawn to a needed site (chemotaxis) and migrate through the endothelial lining of the capillary by a process called "diapedesis."

4. **Fibrocyte:** Fully differential mature version of a fibroblast

5. **Adipocyte:** A fixed fat cell (adipose)

6. **Melanocyte:** Stores a brown pigment (melanin)

7. **Mesenchymal cells**: Stem cells that produce fibroblasts and other connective tissue cells

8. **Mast cells:** Large cells found mainly near blood vessels. Mast cells have a dual function: secrete histamine (vasodilatation) and secrete heparin (prevents clotting). They also release serotonin and bradykinin during inflammation. Mast cells work in conjunction with basophils during allergic reactions.

9. **Plasma cells:** Develop from lymphocytes and are responsible for antibody production

10. **Lymphocytes:** Derived from lymph tissue, bone marrow, and gut and circulate in blood temporarily before entering lymph system. Eventually go back into the blood and repeat the process.

11. **White blood cells (leukocytes):** Help remove pathogen toxins, waste, and damaged cells.

    A. Granular leukocytes, which include polymorphonuclear neutrophils, polymorphonuclear eosinophils, polymorphonuclear basophils

    B. Agranular leukocytes, which include monocytes, lymphocytes

12. **Microphages:** A special phagocytizing cell that works closely with the lymphocyte

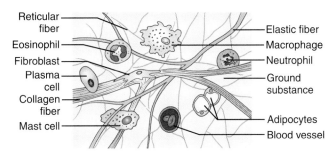

FIGURE 14–1 Cellular and fibrillar elements of connective tissue.

Elastin

Elastin is found in the skin, tendons, lungs, and the linings of arteries. It is found in varying degrees within ligaments, most predominantly in the *ligamentum nuchae*, *ligamentum flavum*, and *intervertebral discs* (Fig. 14-2). These fibers elongate in the direction of force and return to their original shape when released. Elastin is comprised of a smaller microfibrillar network compared to collagen. Elastin is more extensible in warmer temperatures and becomes brittle at 20 degrees centigrade.

Reticulin

Reticulin fibers are glycoprotein, but less tensile than collagen or elastin. There is a slight variation in the combination of protein sequences within this tissue that allows it to form networks of durable, yet pliable, meshing (Fig. 14-3). A delicate tissue distributed around organs and glands, reticulin contains type II collagen and fibronectin.

Fibronectin

One of the more recent molecular discoveries is the identification of **fibronectin** within connective tissue. It was first

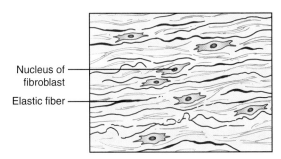

FIGURE 14–2 Elastic connective tissue.

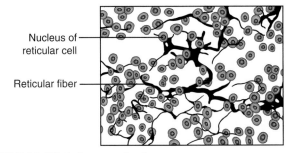

FIGURE 14–3 Reticular connective tissue.

recognized on the cell surface, then as a tissue adhesive, and most recently as a constituent of blood plasma. It is a network-forming glycoprotein that functions to allow for intracellular and extracellular communication in order to achieve homeostasis.

Ground Substance

The **ground substance** is the environment in which all connective tissue components exist (Box 14-5, Fig. 14-1). The fibroblast produces most of the elements within the ground substance. It provides a barrier against invading bacteria, allows for diffusion of waste and nutrients, and maintains fiber distance between the collagen fibers.

Box 14-5 EXTRACELLULAR MATRIX COMPONENTS

FIBERS—GLYCOPROTEINS

1. **Collagen:** Stiff but pliable molecules with high tensile strength and poor stretch capability. Type I is found in loose and dense connective tissue proper; Type II is found in cartilage; Type III is found in arteries and fetal dermas; Type IV is found at the level of the basement membrane.

2. **Elastin:** Elastin is a protein that affords extensive flexibility. It can be stretched up to 130% of its initial length. **Fibronectin:** An important constituent of blood plasma that is synthesized by many cell types, including red blood cells, lymphocytes, fibrocytes, basophils, neutrophils, eosinophils, and macrophages.

3. **Reticulin:** Composed of reticular fibers that form a meshwork that is flexible yet durable. This tissue is found predominantly in the viscera, that is, spleen and liver.

4. **Laminin:** A network-forming glycoprotein that is connected with basement membrane and adhesion to the epithelial layers (type IV collagen).

5. **Chondronectin:** A network-forming glycoprotein is associated with adhesion factors for chondrocytes and type II collagen in cartilage.

GROUND SUBSTANCE

Ground substance is a saline gel that permeates and surrounds cells throughout the entire organism. It is composed of several macromolecules.

1. **Proteoglycan:** A sugar protein complex with an electrocharge suitable for extensive water-binding capabilities.

2. **Glycosaminoglycans (GAGs):** Composed of sulfated and nonsulfated disaccharide units, including chondroitin sulfate, dermatan sulfate, hyaluronic acid, heparin sulfate, and keratin sulfate. They maintain the critical fiber distance, thus inhibiting dysfunctional cross-linking among some fibers.

The primary components of ground substance are **glycosaminoglycans (GAGs)** (Box 14-5) and water (70% of total weight), which have a lubricating effect on tissues. Large polysaccharides, called **proteoglycans** (Fig. 14-4), bind with water and become linked with the function of *hyaluronic acid* contributing to the viscoelastic properties of cartilage.[17]

GAGs are separated into sulfated groups that include *chondroitin sulfate, dermatan sulfate, heparin sulfate, keratan sulfate,* and nonsulfated groups inclusive of hyaluronic acid. Chondroitin sulfate contributes to the rigidity of the ground substance within cartilage, and hyaluronic acid binds with water.

Ground substance is in a constant state of flux as a result of metabolic changes. Within the tissues of tendon, ligament, and bone, the ground substance is referred to as the *matrix*. It serves as a facilitator as well as a barrier between cellular substances and blood.[18] In other words, the ground substance is not the inert substance it was once thought to be.

Structure and Function on a Tissue Level

Muscle tissue accounts for approximately 50% of the total volume of the body, connective tissue comprises approximately 45%, and neural and epithelial tissues comprise the remaining 5%. Despite the large volume of connective tissue, only recently has adequate attention been given to these structures, as evidenced by the frequency of diagnoses such as *fibrositis, myofibrositis,* and *fibromyalgia.*

Muscle Tissue Structure and Function

Muscle's connective tissue has similar properties to both connective tissue proper and bone. The connective tissue of the muscle's functional unit, the *myofibril*, plays an important role in structural organization (Fig. 14-5). Muscle fibers range in thickness from 10 to 100 nm and 1 to 3 cm in length.[13] Connective tissue helps compartmentalize and separate, yet also allows for communication and transport. The deepest layer of muscle's connective tissue, the **endomysium**, is loose connective tissue that encompasses each muscle fiber, while

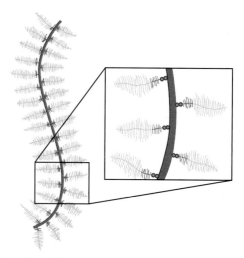

FIGURE 14–4 Proteoglycan arrangement.

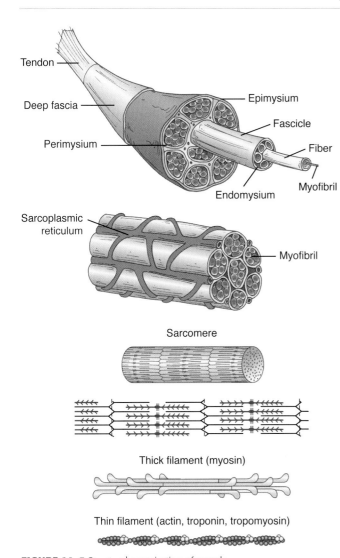

FIGURE 14–5 Structural organization of muscle.

also forming connections with adjacent fibers. These bundles of fibers, called **fascicles,** are enclosed in a dense connective tissue sheath called the **perimysium.** The **epimysium** surrounds the muscle and has additional fibers that connect to surrounding structures.[18] These structures also surround the nerves and vasculature[19] and continue beyond the muscle to form the tendon that blends with the periosteum of the bone.

Connective Tissue Structure and Function

The composition of connective tissue has already been described. It can be categorized into several groups and subgroups based on its structure and subsequent function. The first group is *connective tissue proper*, which in turn is divided into *loose* and *dense connective tissue.* These subgroups may be further subdivided into *dense regular* or *irregular* arrangements.[20] The second group of connective tissue is *supportive connective tissue*, which includes *bone* and *cartilage.* The third group of connective tissue is *fluid connective tissue*, which includes *blood* and *lymph.* Some collagen arrangements of fibers appear more parallel (i.e., ligaments and tendons), whereas

scar tissue and dermis exhibit a fibrous irregular arrangement. *Elastic tissues* have a predominance of elastin fibers and *adipose tissue* is infiltrated by fat cells (Box 14-3).

Connective Tissue Proper

Loose Connective Tissue

Loose connective tissue, or **areolar tissue,** exists as a padding that fills the interstices between the organs. It is also found between the dermis and its underlying structures (i.e., muscle or bone) and over body parts that are devoid of subcutaneous fat (i.e., the dorsum of the hand). The loose connective tissue underlying the skin and infiltrated with adipose tissue is referred to as **superficial fascia.** This tissue helps conserve body heat and is responsible for body contours. Because the fibers are loosely arranged, this tissue is able to deform without significant damage.[8–15]

Dense Regular and Irregular Connective Tissue

The multidirectional capability of this tissue to provide support, protection, and strength makes it a unique structure and difficult to replace once it is injured. Examples of dense regular connective tissue include aponeuroses and elastic tissue. Aponeuroses help attach muscle to other structures, whereas elastic tissue provides resiliency to a structure, allowing it to stretch. Dense irregular connective tissue is found in the larynx and respiratory pathways as well as in blood vessels (Figs. 14-6 and 14-7).

Areolar Tissue

Loose connective tissue, or areolar tissue, has a lower ratio of collagen (Fig. 14-8). This tissue is suited to absorb force. This resilient tissue creates a functional space between the subdermis and underlying muscle. This tissue is also found in the superficial and deep fascial layers, and sheaths of the nerves.

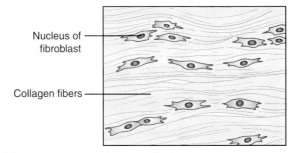

FIGURE 14–6 Dense regular connective tissue.

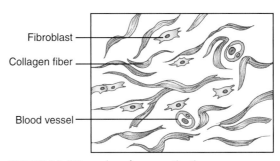

FIGURE 14–7 Dense irregular connective tissue.

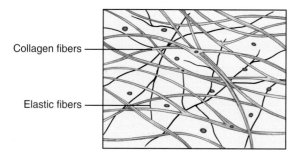

FIGURE 14–8 Areolar connective tissue.

Fascia

Microscopically, **fascia** is more organized and has a greater amount of collagen than does loose connective tissue. Macroscopically, there are two distinct fascial systems. The internal fascia, which lines the thoracic and abdominal cavity, is referred to as *endothoracic* and *endoabdominal* fascia. This barely discernible lining affixes the parietal layer of the *serous sacs*, the *pleura* in the thorax, and the *peritoneum* in the abdomen to the inner aspect of the body wall.[21] Specializations exist within these layers, such as the *suprapleural membrane*, which is a thickening of the endothoracic fascia over the dome of the lung. Unlike these specifications, the internal fascia has regional identifications based on the muscles it contacts.[22] The psoas fascia, on the right side of the body, is merely a continuation, in part, from *Toldts' fascia*, which anchors the ascending colon.

Considering the deep cervical fascia may help illustrate a portion of this tissue's adaptability. In the neck and limbs, the deep fascia is a tough fibrous connective tissue layer that surrounds each particular body part. In the back of the arm, the deep fascia is fused to the surface of the muscle, whereas in the front of the arm it forms a loosely fitting envelope around the muscle. Where greater function and separation of structure is needed, such as the cervical spine, the fascial layers become more refined, definitive, and intricate (Fig. 14-9).[23]

Ligaments and Tendons

Regional demands on connective tissue, including stress and strain, are exemplified by those made by ligaments and tendons. Skeletal ligaments are distinct kinds of connective tissue that traverse joints and, at times, blend into fibrous walls of the joint capsule. *Visceral ligaments*, which are not routinely considered by manual therapists, vary in tensile strength based on the

motility and mobility of the respective organ.[24] The stomach, for example, has a strong attachment to the diaphragm by the *gastrophrenic ligament*. Other ligaments that connect to the stomach, such as the *lesser omentum*, are actually part of the **mesentery**, a thin sheet of connective tissue with mesothelial surfaces that conduct blood and lymph vessels and nerves to other structures. The left and right *triangular ligaments* and the two portions of the *coronary ligament* that anchor the liver, are modified mesenteries that have a supportive function.[18] An increased regional thickening is noticeable the farther one moves from the diaphragm, suggesting that more passive support is required for the lower organs of the inferior abdominal region.[25,26]

Some ligaments are actually remnants from our fetal development. The *medial umbilical ligaments* are formed from the *umbilical arteries*. There are ligaments that contain smooth muscle or that are formed largely from them, such as the *ligament of Trietz*, which is also referred to as the *suspensory muscle of the duodenal jejunal junction*.[24]

The external surface is the *visceral layer*, whereas the internal layer surrounding the cavity is the *parietal layer*. The two layers are continuous through a *mesotendon*, which is separated by a thin film of fluid. In some areas, cartilage or bones (i.e., *sesamoids*) develop within tendons where excessive friction is too great for the bursa or sheathing to handle. Bursae usually develop before birth, but they can develop in adulthood in response to friction.[18]

Supportive Connective Tissue

Classified as a supportive connective tissue, cartilage and bone provide static and dynamic support for the rest of the body's systems. A significant feature of cartilage is its avascular nature. The proteoglycan chondroitin sulfate composes the gel that is the hallmark feature of cartilage. Cartilage is divided into three types: *fibrocartilage* (Fig. 14-10), *hyaline cartilage* (Fig. 14-11), and *elastic cartilage* (Fig. 14-12).[18,22,27]

Bones remain one of the body's highest metabolically active structures *Osteogenic* cells differentiate into *osteoblasts*. These bone building cells eventually form *osteocytes*, the resident cells of bone. Bone is constantly being remodeled through the work of *osteoclasts*, which engage in bone resorption through the release of enzymes along its ruffled border (Fig 14-13).[28] Mature bone may be classified as either **trabecular bone** (Fig. 14-14) (also known as cancellous or spongy) or **cortical bone** (also known as compact). The long bones throughout the body are composed of both trabecular and cortical bone (Fig. 14-15).

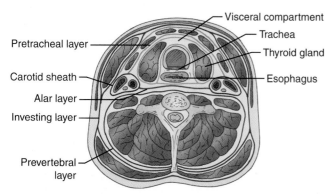

FIGURE 14–9 Transverse cross-section of deep cervical fascia.

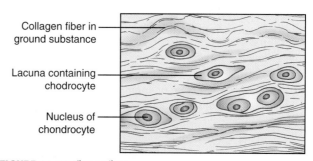

FIGURE 14–10 Fibrocartilage.

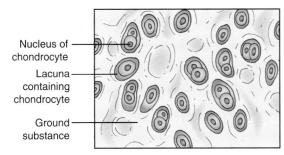

FIGURE 14–11 Hyaline cartilage.

Nucleus of chondrocyte

Lacuna containing chondrocyte

Ground substance

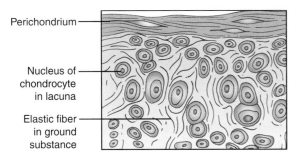

FIGURE 14–12 Elastic cartilage.

Perichondrium

Nucleus of chondrocyte in lacuna

Elastic fiber in ground substance

Connective Tissue and Immobilization

The macroscopic and microscopic impact of immobilization on the structure and function of connective tissues is far-reaching (Box 14-6). The current best evidence related to the structural and functional impact of immobilization on connective tissue is provided in Chapter 13 of this text. The reader is encouraged to review this information prior to embarking on the philosophy and practice of myofascial release.

QUESTIONS *for* REFLECTION

- Given the ubiquitous nature of connective tissue within the body and its integral role in multiple body systems, why has its role in dysfunction and strategies designed to reduce impairment of these structures not been extensively considered?
- In what ways might impairment of connective tissue influence muscle function, articular mobility, visceral organ function, etc.?
- How might a manual physical therapist begin to differentiate which structure may be contributing to impairments in mobility?

PHILOSOPHICAL FRAMEWORK OF MYOFASCIAL RELEASE

The Pathogenesis of Myofascial Impairment

Neuromusculoskeletal impairment may lead to postural dysfunction that produces fascial tension and often causes pain. The development of palpation skills is essential for accurate diagnosis of fascial dysfunction. An educated tactile sense can determine if tissue is tense, relaxed, or altered as a result of an imbalance of tissue chemistry.

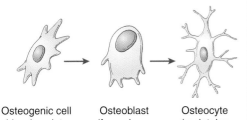
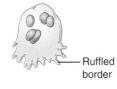

Osteogenic cell (develops into an osteoblast)

Osteoblast (forms bone tissue)

Osteocyte (maintains bone tissue)

Osteoclast (functions in resorption, the destruction of bone matrix)

Ruffled border

FIGURE 14–13 The cellular composition of bone. *Osteogenic* cells differentiate to become *osteoblasts*, which are responsible for the building of bone. *Osteocytes* are the resident mature cells that maintain the characteristic features of bone. *Osteoclasts* serve to resorb bone, a process that is useful during remodeling of bone following fracture. The balance between osteoblastic and osteoclastic activity is critical in maintaining the normal rigidity of bone. This balance will vary substantially throughout life.

FIGURE 14–14 Trabecular (cancellous, spongy) bone.

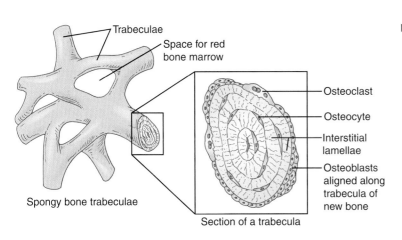

Trabeculae

Space for red bone marrow

Osteoclast

Osteocyte

Interstitial lamellae

Osteoblasts aligned along trabecula of new bone

Spongy bone trabeculae

Section of a trabecula

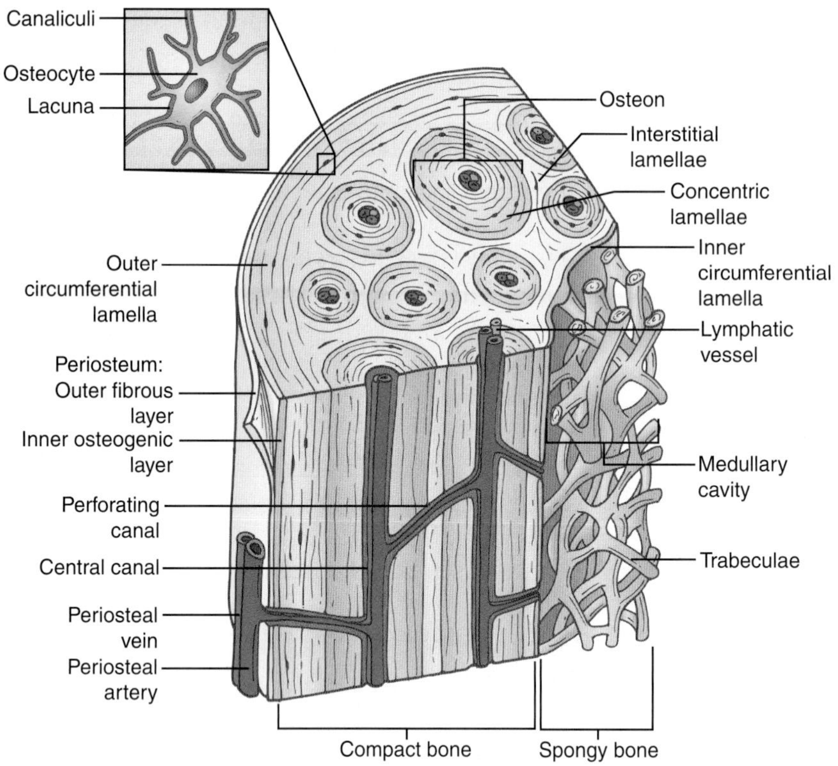

Canaliculi

Osteocyte

Lacuna

Osteon

Interstitial lamellae

Concentric lamellae

Inner circumferential lamella

Lymphatic vessel

Outer circumferential lamella

Periosteum: Outer fibrous layer

Inner osteogenic layer

Perforating canal

Central canal

Periosteal vein

Periosteal artery

Medullary cavity

Trabeculae

Compact bone   Spongy bone

FIGURE 14–15 Arrangement of trabecular and cortical bone.

Box 14-6 EFFECTS OF IMMOBILITY

- *Wolff's law* states that tissues adapt to the stresses applied or not applied to them.
- Proliferation of fibro-fatty connective tissue within articulating surfaces in addition to a thinning of articular cartilage, fibrillation, and loss of matrix staining, and distortion and shrinking of chondrocytes.
- Pressure necrosis, ulceration of cartilage with erosion to *subchondral bone*, as well as fibrillation, necrosis, and cellular distortion
- Muscle atrophy occurs rapidly, with 50% of the total loss occurring within the first week of immobilization, which is attributed to a decrease in protein synthesis that leads to a significant loss of muscle protein.
- Microscopically, water content loss ranges from 65% to 70% in the extracellular fluid. A loss of GAGs (from 30% to 40%) is the most prominent effect, specifically *chondroitin-4, chondroitin sulfate-6, hyaluronic acid*, and to a lesser degree, *dermatan sulfate*. This loss leads to a reduction in critical fiber distance between collagen fibers, which results in excessive cross-linking, adhesions, and fixation.

As described in the literature and elsewhere in this text, immobilization may result in fascial dysfunction. Long periods of immobilization produce muscle atrophy, joint stiffness, ulceration of joint cartilage, osteoarthritis, skin necrosis, infection, tendocutaneous adhesion, thrombophlebitis, and varying degrees of contracture.[29–37] Current evidence reveals that following periods of immobilization, synovial fluid develops excessive connective tissue deposition in the joint and joint recesses (e.g., heterotrophic ossification). Chronic and excessive deposition of fibrous connective tissue forms mature scars and creates intra-articular adhesions.[29–37]

The Theory of Tensegrity

An underacknowledged concept presented by Ingber[38] and Juhan[23] may add a broader base to our understanding of connective tissue. The term **tensegrity,** or **tensional integrity**, was first adopted by *Buckminster Fuller* to describe a natural phenomenon whereby a "system stabilizes itself mechanically via an intricate balance and distribution of compressional and tensional forces on the skeleton."[38]

Ingber[38] identified a consistent organizational pattern of tissues with a well-defined hierarchy in every level of body

CLINICAL PILLAR

It is incumbent upon the manual physical therapist to attain a specialized sense of touch necessary for the diagnosis of tissue disorders. An educated tactile sense can determine if tissue is tense, relaxed, or altered because of an imbalance of tissue chemistry.

NOTABLE QUOTABLE

"A system stabilizes itself mechanically via an intricate balance and distribution of compressional and tensional forces on the skeleton."

—*Buckminster Fuller*

tissue. The existence of tensional and compressive balance exists at not only the level of the muscles, fascia, tendons, and ligaments, but more importantly, it also exists at the molecular level. Specifically, Ingber showed that cells contain an internal framework of protein polymers that he referred to as the *cytoskeleton*. He was able to simulate how a finite network of contractile microfilaments actually extends through the cell, pulling the contents toward the cell nucleus. Adhesion receptors on the cell surface, known as *integrins*, help transmit these forces from the external to internal milieu of the cell. Ingber cited that "the existence of a force balance was a way to provide a means to integrate mechanics and biochemistry at the molecular level."[38] He found it possible to change the cell cytoskeleton by altering the balance of physical forces transmitted across the cell surface. Changing cytoskeletal geometry and mechanics could affect biochemical reactions and even alter the genes that are activated and thus the proteins that are created. Ingber also found that, depending on the type of stress induced at the cell surface, reactions were stimulated at the cellular level.[38]

The profound clinical implications for tensegrity can best be appreciated when examining the **fascial fulcrum concept.** By introducing stress in specific patterns, we can introduce forces down to the level of the cell and affect its functional capacity, thus moving us beyond a *pathomechanical* model to a *pathophysiological/pathochemical* model.[38]

The Integrated Systems Approach to Myofascial Release

It is most effective and efficient to use a *system-specific approach* for intervention. If the impairment has manifested itself within the connective tissue, *MFR* should be considered. Because of the predominance of connective tissue throughout the body, *MFR* may be considered even when connective tissue is not the primary component.

The 3-Planar Fascial Fulcrum Approach to MFR

MFR may produce a direct effect on collagen, elastin, ground substance, and more. As mentioned, fascial dysfunction may be the result of physical trauma, inflammation, infection, postural dysfunction, articular restriction, and any external or internal body torsion, which contributes to fascial strain. *MFR* techniques affect the continuous, contiguous, connective tissue system, which envelops every cell and fiber in the body. The goal is to relieve fascial restrictions and normalize the health of this system. At the cellular level, *MFR* affects the *elastocollagenous complex* (integrated collagen and elastin fibers), as well as the consistency of the ground substance. In response to *MFR*, it is presumed that the density and viscosity of the matrix (ground substance) decreases and the metabolic rate increases, resulting in improved metabolism and health.

MFR can be performed in a *direct* or *indirect* fashion based on the direction in which forces are delivered. The **3-planar fascial fulcrum approach,** which is the model that is

advocated and described in this chapter, is always indirect (Box 14-7). Based on its indirect nature, this form of *MFR* is considered to be more comfortable compared to direct methods, and resistance is less when the barriers are not engaged.

QUESTIONS *for* REFLECTION

- What is the difference between the direct and the indirect approach to *MFR*?
- What are the advantages to one form of *MFR* compared to the other?
- Which form of *MFR* is more comfortable for the patient?
- By what mechanism does the indirect approach to *MFR* exert its effect?
- Which form of *MFR* is adopted during performance of the **3-planar fascial fulcrum approach** that is described in this chapter?

The concept of the *fulcrum* used in this approach can best defined as a *fixed point* around which the tissues engage in a process of *pressure unwinding*, which leads to an increase in soft tissue flexibility. A fulcrum also creates a mechanoenergetic interface where energy is (hypothetically) transduced or transformed.

During *MFR*, the manual physical therapist continuously monitors tissue tension throughout the duration of the technique (Box 14-8). When tissue tension changes, softens, and relaxes, a *tissue tension release* has presumably occurred. The decrease in tissue tension that occurs in response to *MFR* has been attributed to several factors. One factor is the decrease in *efferent neuron activity* (gamma and alpha impulses), resulting in decreased resistance of the *muscle spindle* and relaxation and elongation of the sarcomere. Another factor is the change of elastic resistance to viscous compliance of the soft tissue as a result of morphological changes. During performance of these techniques, it is not uncommon for the therapist

---

Box 14-7 Quick Notes! THE FASCIAL FULCRUM MODEL OF MFR

- This model is based upon the concept of **tensegrity.**
- Introduction of minimally maintained stresses in specific patterns, impacts structures at the cellular level.
- By changing cytoskeleton configurations through force transmission from an external fascial fulcrum, we have an increased potential for affecting a multitude of pathological conditions.
- This model steps beyond a **pathomechanical** model to a **pathophysiologic** or **pathochemical** model.

Box 14-8 Quick Notes! EFFECTS OF MFR

- *MFR* techniques affect the continuous, contiguous, connective tissue system, which envelops every cell and fiber in the body.
- The goal is to relieve fascial restrictions and to normalize the health and tension of this body system.
- At the cellular level, *MFR* affects the **elastacollagenous complex** as well as the consistency of the ground substance.
- *MFR* increases soft-tissue flexibility and relieves tissue tension while decreasing the density and viscosity of the ground substance, thus increasing the metabolic rate and improved metabolism and health.

CLINICAL PILLAR

Indications for MFR:

- Primary intervention for **neuromusculoskeletal-fascial** impairments
- Secondary intervention for joint dysfunction, muscle fiber dysfunction, fascial dysfunction, neuronal dysfunction, periosteal and bone dysfunction, and circulatory dysfunction
- Positive findings with myofascial mapping
- Decreased fascial glide or compromised mobility
- Joint hypomobility
- Soft tissue tension
- Postural deviations
- Dynamic limitations in range of motion

Precautions for MFR:

- Systemic disorder
- Malignancy
- Nonunion fracture
- Cardiopulmonary impairment, such as congestive heart failure

to identify an increase in temperature emanating from the treated body tissue. In addition, the astute manual physical therapist may perceive a sensation of movement, filling of space, and a pulsation, which is defined as a **therapeutic pulse**. The amplitude of this therapeutic pulse increases during the technique and subsides as the tissue tension release occurs.

THE CLINICAL PRACTICE OF MYOFASCIAL RELEASE

Indications, Precautions, and Contraindications for Myofascial Release

Primary *neuromusculoskeletal-fascial dysfunction* is the chief indication for *MFR*. It is important to note that the use of *MFR* is not reserved for soft tissue lesions alone. *MFR* may also be indicated, and has been found to be clinically effective, in the management of such conditions as joint dysfunction, muscle fiber dysfunction, fascial dysfunction, neuronal dysfunction, periosteal and bone dysfunction, and circulatory dysfunction.

In the presence of a systemic disorder, although unlikely, *MFR* may aggravate the symptoms. In the presence of malignancy, there is no clinical evidence to suggest that *MFR* is contraindicated. In the presence of a nonunion fracture, *MFR* has been anecdotally found to promote union, and no evidence exists to suggest harm. Nevertheless, further evidence is needed to confirm its use in the presence of such conditions, and the prudent practitioner may choose to forego *MFR* in the presence of such conditions.

As described, there are two primary forms of *MFR* that may be implemented, *MFR* for soft tissue and *MFR* for joints. The protocols for these techniques differ in detail. Regardless of which form is used, *MFR* should be performed from proximal to distal, from static postural dysfunction to dynamic postural dysfunction, from most severe postural dysfunction to least severe postural dysfunction, from soft tissue *MFR* to articular *MFR*, and from superficial fascial layers to deep fascial layers.

Examination of Myofascial Dysfunction

Examination of fascial glide is necessary in order to determine the mobility of the connective tissue system. Under normal circumstances, soft tissues remain mobile and friction-free during movement. The manual physical therapist's hands are gently but firmly placed on the body. The practitioner can begin by standing at the patient's feet, with a hand on each leg, and the patient in the supine position. The practitioner can assess the fascial glide throughout the anterior surface of the body. Upon completion, the fascial glide evaluation process is

CLINICAL PILLAR

Myofascial examination:

- Three layers of fascial glide are assessed, including (1) skin on superficial fascia, (2) deeper layers of fascia, and (3) mobility of soft tissue on bone.
- Tissues are palpated for mobility, flexibility, and freedom of tissue glide.
- Mobility is assessed in three planes: (1) superiorly-inferiorly, (2) medially-laterally, and (3) clockwise-counterclockwise.
- If fascial glide is tight, hypomobile, or inflexible, document findings on the body diagram; *MFR* is indicated.

repeated with the patient in the prone position. Three layers of fascial glide are assessed, including (1) skin on superficial fascia, (2) deeper layers of fascia, and (3) mobility of soft tissue on bone. The therapist palpates tissue mobility, flexibility, and the freedom of glide in three planes: superiorly-inferiorly, medially-laterally, and clockwise-counterclockwise. If the fascial glide appears compromised, tight, hypomobile, or inflexible, then the therapist documents these findings on the body diagram and *MFR* is indicated.

Myofascial Release Technique for Soft Tissues

Indications for Soft Tissue Myofascial Release

The soft tissue *MFR* technique is best implemented when the following positive findings, indicating dysfunction, have been noted: (1) positive myofascial mapping, (2) decreased fascial glide or compromised fascial mobility, (3) joint hypomobility, (4) soft tissue tension, (5) positive deviations, (6) dynamic limitations in ranges of motion.

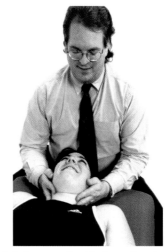

FIGURE 14–16 Soft tissue myofascial release: lateral neck hold displaying right and left hand placement over the region to be released.

CLINICAL PILLAR

MFR procedure:

- "Sandwich" body part between hands (right and left side, anterior and posterior, medial and lateral surfaces).

- Compress body part through hand contacts using 5 grams of force.

- Maintain force as hands move in opposite directions.

- Determine in which direction the tissues are most mobile and move the tissues in that direction.

- Intend to move underlying versus superficial tissues.

- Patiently hold the static fulcrum position and avoid any quick, repetitive, or forceful physiologic movements.

- Follow subtle motion of soft tissue by not allowing the hands to move.

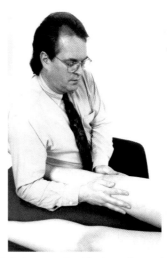

FIGURE 14–17 Soft tissue myofascial release: knee release displaying medial and lateral hand placement over the region to be released.

Procedure for Soft Tissue Myofascial Release

Prior to imparting force, the body part to be treated is "sandwiched" between the hands of the therapist on the right and left side (Fig. 14-16), laterally and medially (Fig. 14-17), or anteriorly and posteriorly (Fig. 14-18). The therapist then provides and maintains compression with a force no greater than 5 grams. The underlying tissues are then displaced as the hands move in opposite directions in three planes.

Distortion of Tissues in the Sagittal Plane

To distort soft tissues within the sagittal plane, the anterior hand moves the tissue in a superior direction while the posterior hand moves in an inferior direction. The tissues are then returned to neutral and the direction is reversed.

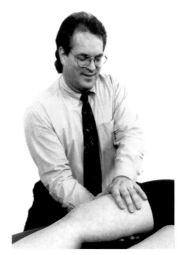

FIGURE 14–18 Soft tissue myofascial release: knee release displaying anterior and posterior hand placement over the region to be released. This technique will access the medial and lateral ligaments as well as the menisci.

While applying force in each direction, the manual physical therapist determines in which direction the tissues are most and least mobile within the sagittal plane. As noted, the type of *MFR* described in this chapter is indirect; therefore, force is elicited in the direction of least restriction.

Distortion of Tissues in the Transverse Plane

To distort the underlying soft tissues within the transverse plane, the anterior hand is moved in a medial direction while the posterior hand moves the tissue in a lateral direction. The tissues are returned to neutral, and the force direction is reversed. As for the sagittal plane, tissue mobility is assessed, and the tissues are moved into the direction of greatest ease.

Distortion of Tissues in the Frontal Plane

For distortion in the frontal plane, the anterior hand moves the tissues in a clockwise direction, while the posterior hand moves in a counterclockwise direction. As in the other planes, the tissues are returned to neutral and the force direction is reversed. The technique is then performed in the direction of least restriction.

It is important to note that the therapist's hands do not move on the skin. Rather, the hand contacts are firmly maintained throughout the technique. The hands and skin impart force and produce a distortion of the tissues that lie beneath. To impart the necessary force and avoid slippage, the use of massage cream or ointment is undesirable; therefore, *MFR* may best be performed before other interventions that require ointment.

Once the hand contacts and distortion of tissues is provided, there are now four directions in which forces are being provided and maintained from each hand onto the involved soft tissues. They include (1) slight compression, (2) sagittal plane—superior or inferior, (3) transverse plane—medial or lateral, and (4) frontal plane—clockwise or counterclockwise. The intersection of these seven forces produces a "fixed point." This fixed point is the *fulcrum* around which the fascial tissue will *unwind*, *release*, or experience a *decrease in tension*. This fulcrum is the specific point around which the three-planar myofascial fulcrum technique is performed and exerts its maximal effect.

Tissue Tension Release

It is critical that the manual physical therapist maintains the fulcrum, once the triplanar fulcrum has been established. Although there is temptation to move the hands and follow the subtle motion of the soft tissues, it is imperative to disallow the hands from moving. The objective is not a physiologic unwinding of a body part, but rather the creation of an internal "unraveling or release" of the fascial tissue. The forces generated by maintenance of the static fulcrum will produce changes in the internal environment of the connective tissue, resulting in release. This process of fascial unwinding is slow and gentle, thus making it important for the manual physical therapist to patiently hold the static fulcrum position and avoid any quick, repetitive, or forceful physiologic movements.

The therapist must also closely monitor the patient's movement patterns during performance of the technique to prevent the patient from moving quickly, without repetition, or with force. If the body part changes position in space slowly and gently in order to facilitate the internal tissue unwinding, this movement is acceptable and encouraged. At the end of the release, the hands will be in different positions compared to where they began because of the changes that have taken place within the internal body tissues.

Shoulder Girdle and Clavipectoral Fascia Soft Tissue Fulcrum MFR Technique

Indication

The primary indication for the use of this technique is the observation of a protracted shoulder girdle upon performance of a static postural examination. In addition, shoulder horizontal abduction may be limited dynamically.

Patient and Therapist Position

The patient is placed into either a supine or sitting position. The manual physical therapist places one hand on the *posterior aspect of the scapula*. The fingers are spread in an attempt to contact as many different tissues and structures as possible. The hypothenar eminences contact the *humeral head*, while the anterior hand rests on the *clavipectoral region*. The fingers are spread and contact the *supraclavicular tissue*, *clavicle*, *infraclavicular tissue*, and ribs.

Technique

Once these contacts have been achieved, the manual physical therapist compresses the clavipectoral region with both hands, squeezing gently, using the image of a soap bubble between his or her hands. The therapist must attempt to maintain gentle compression without bursting the bubble.

The *first plane* is engaged by moving the anterior hand cephalad while the posterior hand moves caudad, thus distorting the soap bubble. The hands return to neutral and reverse direction. The hands move the tissues in the direction of greatest ease, or the most mobile direction.

Once movement into the first plane has been achieved, the second plane is now added, or "stacked," on it. When engaging the second plane, it is important to maintain the first plane. It is often challenging to maintain the fulcrum in the process of stacking planes, and it is a common error to "lose" a plane as subsequent planes are engaged. The third plane is then stacked on the first two. The manual physical therapist must avoid returning the tissues to neutral.

Once this sequence of events has been achieved, the fulcrum has been established. Each hand is exerting four different directions of forces mechanically in an attempt to distort the tissue between the hands. The directions of forces are compression, superior/inferior, medial/lateral, and clockwise/counterclockwise (medial rotation or lateral rotation). Each hand will maintain the fulcrum, which is designed to facilitate a decrease in tissue tension tone throughout the duration of the technique.

As the tissue unwinds and movement occurs within the tissues, the therapist must resist the temptation to move the hands and release the fulcrum. The therapist and patient may perceive heat, paresthesia, anesthesia, vibration, fatigue, electric impulses, cold, perspiration, pain, circulatory changes, breathing changes, sympathetic skin erythema or blanching, and other phenomena. At the conclusion of the technique, the signs and symptoms will typically subside along with the desired effect of improved postural symmetry (decreased protraction) and increased horizontal abduction.

Myofascial Release Technique for Articulations

Indications for Articular Myofascial Release

Articular *MFR* is typically most effective when it follows soft tissue *MFR*. After the soft tissues have been released, residual joint dysfunction may be noted. Upon observation, static postural asymmetries may be observed within the joint. Dynamic posture evaluation may indicate positive findings of joint dysfunction and lack of articular balance. Mobility testing will often reveal joint hypomobility. Articular *MFR* is designed to address restrictions within the joint capsule and ligaments.

Procedure for Articular Myofascial Release

To begin, the manual physical therapist places his or her hands to contact the bones on either side of the articulation. Occasionally, a longer lever may be more favorable. The therapist must grip only as hard as is necessary to maintain control of the position of both joint surfaces while being careful to avoid any distraction or approximation of the joint surfaces. The therapist's hands move in opposite directions on all three planes. In the sagittal plane, one joint surface is moved superior while the other is moved inferior (superior/inferior). In the transverse plane, one joint surface is moved into internal rotation while the other is moved into external rotation (internal/external). In the frontal plane, one joint surface is moved into abduction, while the other is moved in adduction. The direction of movement is reversed within each plane in order to determine the direction of greatest mobility as performed during the soft tissue technique. Once determined, the tissues are moved in the direction of greatest ease, as each accessory joint movement is stacked upon the previous motion.

The therapist's grip on the body part is maintained in all three planes, which becomes the fulcrum around which the soft tissues (ligaments, capsule) surrounding the joint will release. The therapist must avoid hand movement throughout the technique but allow for repositioning of joint surfaces during the technique for improved articular balance. Fascial release will be slow and gentle. At the completion of the intervention, there may be joint sounds as a result of the rebalancing of joint surfaces. At the conclusion of the release, the therapist's hands will be in a neutral position, and articular balance will be improved, along with normalization of articular balance and improved joint mobility.

Glenohumeral Joint Articular Fulcrum MFR Technique

Indication

This technique is most effective for cases of static postural dysfunction that involves anterior shear of the humeral head in the glenoid fossa. This technique may also be effective for dynamic postural dysfunction, including a limitation in end ranges of shoulder motion with hypomobility of accessory movement, as noted on mobility testing.

Patient and Therapist Position

The patient is positioned either in supine or sitting position. One hand grasps the scapula to control the position of the glenoid fossa. The other hand grasps the upper arm to control the position of the humeral head. It is important to avoid approximation of joint surfaces.

Technique

The first plane is engaged by the therapist placing his or her superior hand on the shoulder girdle and lifting the glenoid fossa cephalad, while the inferior hand on the upper arm pulls the humeral head caudad. The directions are then reversed as the therapist determines which direction (cephalad/caudad or caudad/cephalad) is most mobile. The joint surfaces are returned to the position of greatest mobility and maintained. To stack the second plane, the superior hand holding the shoulder girdle moves the glenoid fossa anteriorly, while the inferior hand holding the upper arm moves the humeral head posteriorly. The superior hand then moves the glenoid fossa posteriorly, while the inferior hand pushes the humeral head anteriorly. The therapist compares the degree of mobility in each direction, then moves the joint in the direction of greatest ease. The joint is maintained in this new position. The third plane is stacked in the same fashion. The superior hand grasps the shoulder girdle and rotates the glenoid fossa externally, while the inferior hand grasps the upper arm and rotates the humeral head internally. The joint is returned to neutral, and the direction is reversed. The directions are compared, and the joint is moved in the direction of greatest mobility. (Fig. 14-19.)

Each hand has now exerted forces to mechanically position the articular surfaces in opposite directions on three planes. Each hand maintains all three directions of force, which facilitates tissue unwinding of the joint capsule and ligaments. The fulcrum is maintained as the tissue unwinds and extracellular and intracellular movements are perceived.

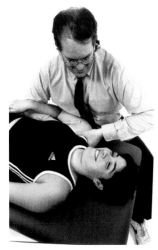

FIGURE 14–19 Articular myofascial release of the glenohumeral joint. Hand contacts at the scapula and humeral head assess, then maintain, the position in which motion is least restricted in all three planes.

The therapist maintains the fulcrum until all signs and symptoms have ceased and improved articular balance of the humeral head within the glenoid fossa has been achieved.

Myofascial Release Technique for Chronic Neurological Dysfunction

Examination of the neurologically impaired patient typically includes observation of motor behavior as well as assessment of passive and active range of motion. Intervention techniques designed to improve joint mobility are commonly integrated into the therapeutic program. These procedures affect the intra- as well as extra-articular tissues, along with the periarticular soft tissues. Individuals with neurological impairment commonly present with a synergistic pattern of spasticity that inhibits movement and contributes to decreased joint mobility. Because of the widespread nature of motion restrictions in this population, an approach that provides beneficial effects for multiple body regions may be more efficient and cost effective than other traditional approaches. Because *MFR* is a manual therapy approach that is designed to affect connective tissue that envelopes every cell and fiber in the body, it may be deemed to be a more efficient method for enhancing mobility, even in a population in which the primary impairment is not musculoskeletal in origin.

Individuals with neurologic-related synergies often exhibit typical patterns of limitation in range of motion. Certain joints present with a typical gross limitation of motion in one specific direction. This differs from motion loss related to musculoskeletal dysfunction, which often involves motion loss in more than one direction.

In a study of 10 neurologically impaired patients with severe, post-traumatic brain injury (greater than 2 years post injury), *MFR* was used to improve mobility.[39] The purpose of the study was to describe *MFR* as a process used to normalize range of motion for the neurological patient. The dependent variables were reductions in postural deviations and deformity.

The three-planar myofascial fulcrum approach, including both the soft tissue *MFR* and the articular *MFR* techniques as previously described, were used. Joints treated with *MFR* included the hip, knee, and wrist joints. Movement was measured at both the treated and untreated joints before and after *MFR* techniques were performed.

The results of this study revealed that of the treated joints, 64% of the measured directions of movement changed to more normal and 24% demonstrated no change. Interestingly, of the untreated joints, 57% demonstrated improvement. When a patient with neurological compromise is treated with passive range of motion and joint mobilization, the local tissues and structures directly addressed through intervention are affected. The techniques ordinarily applied to achieve these changes are direct approaches that include stretching or mobilizing against the tissue-resistant barrier. Conversely, the three-planar fascial fulcrum approach is an indirect approach, which does not force the tissue, requires minimal energy exertion of the therapist, and causes minimal discomfort. The results of this study suggest that both soft tissue and articular *MFR* techniques are effective in increasing ranges of motion in the severe and chronic neurological patient with gross postural deviation and deformity. The results of this study also suggest that *MFR* may affect regions of the body that have not been directly treated. These far-reaching effects may be attributed to the influence of *MFR* on the contiguous nature of the fascial system. The use of these techniques may result in a more efficient method of attaining and maintaining ranges of motion in severely impaired populations.

DIFFERENTIATING CHARACTERISTICS

MFR is an OMPT procedure that attempts to address restrictions within soft tissues, more specifically, restrictions of connective tissue. The manual physical therapist is cognizant of the fact that a combination of both articular and soft tissue restrictions may contribute to reductions in motion and altered movement patterns.

There are various methods of performing *MFR* for the reduction of tension within the fascial system. The traditional method of employing these techniques involves the use of direct forces (i.e., direct approach). The three-planar fascial fulcrum approach to MFR described in this chapter is considered to be an indirect approach that uses forces that move structures into the direction of least restriction. The indirect nature of this approach, which is philosophically similar to strain-counterstrain (see Chapter 15), departs from the more traditional methods used to enhance soft tissue mobility. Most approaches that are designed to improve flexibility of the myofascia include moving and statically holding the involved tissues into positions of elongation.

The approach to *MFR* delineated in this chapter can be adapted to impact not only the fascial system in general (i.e., soft tissue *MFR* approach), but also the periarticular fascial system (i.e., articular *MFR* approach). This adaptation alludes to the important role of the fascial system in facilitating normal joint movement.

CLINICAL CASE

Introduction

A *three-planar fascial fulcrum approach* that included both *soft tissue MFR* and *articular MFR* was used for management of a late post-acute pediatric patient. Unique to this case, a multiple hands intervention session was used.

History

An 11-year-old girl who has been receiving long-term functional rehabilitation for a stable spondylolisthesis at L5-S1 for 2 months presents to the clinic today. Following examination, the manual physical therapist establishes the goal of improving posture mobility, tone, and function.

Treatment Session

Figure 14-20 displays multiple hands performing soft tissue *MFR* and defacilitation of the spine to decrease hypertonicity, followed by a decompression technique for L5/S1. Figure 14-21 shows soft tissue *MFR* of the neck, articular *MFR* of the right shoulder, and neurofascial release on the sagittal plane.

Figure 14-22 displays transverse MFR of the respiratory abdominal diaphragm and the thoracic inlet with neurofascial release on the sagittal plane, as well as articular MFR of the right glenohumeral joint. Figures 14-23, 14-24, 14-25, 14-26 display postural and movement changes in response to MFR compared with preintervention.

1. What mechanism is responsible for the effects of MFR in a neurologically impaired population such as the individual described in this case?

2. Are there any precautions or contraindications for using MFR in this population?

3. What interventions may be used to maintain improvement and reduce recidivism from the use of MFR?

4. In addition to the postural impact from the use of MFR in this population, do you believe active muscle function may also result? If so, explain how such improvement may be facilitated.

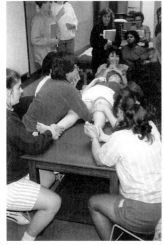

FIGURE 14–20 Mutiple hands performing soft tissue myofasical release and defacilitation of the spine technique.

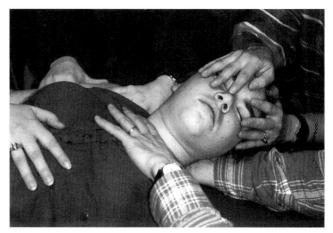

FIGURE 14–22 Myofascial release performed at multiple regions, including abdominal respiratory diaphragm release, thoracic inlet diaphragm release, neurofascial release on sagittal plan, articular myofascial release of the right shoulder.

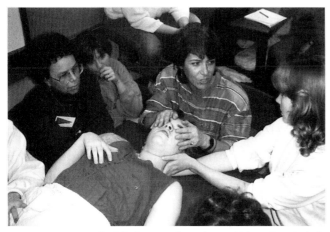

FIGURE 14–21 Myofascial release performed at multiple regions, including soft tissue myofascial release of the neck and neurofascial release on a sagittal plane.

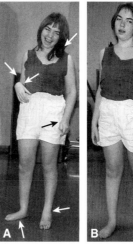

FIGURE 14–23 A. Before treatment with MFR. Arrows point to areas of significant postural deviations. **B.** After treatment with myofascial release.

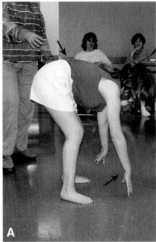

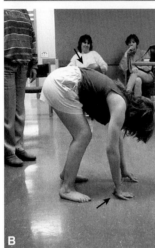

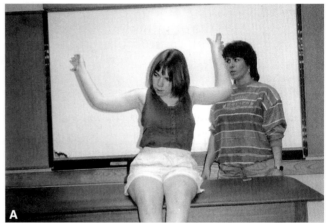

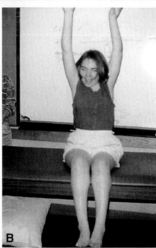

FIGURE 14–25 A. Before treatment with MFR. **B.** After treatment with myofascial release.

FIGURE 14–24 A. Before treatment with MFR. Arrows point to areas of significant postural deviations. **B.** After treatment with myofascial release.

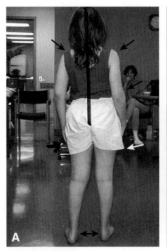

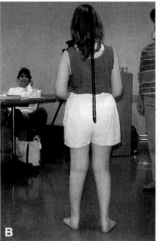

FIGURE 14–26 A. Before treatment with MFR. Arrows point to areas of significant postural deviations. **B.** After treatment with myofascial release.

HANDS-ON

With a partner, perform the following activities:

1 List the primary effects of immobilization on connective tissue. In what way might the manual physical therapist decrease or reverse these effects?

2 Discuss the primary differences between direct and indirect approaches to mobilization. Describe both the philosophical and clinical practice differences.

3 Briefly define and describe both *soft tissue MFR* and *articular MFR*. What are the primary indications for each?

4 Briefly define and describe the unique aspects of the *three-planar fulcrum approach to MFR* as delineated in this chapter. What makes this approach to *MFR* different from other approaches?

5 On the anterior aspect of your partner's thigh, assess the mobility of (1) the skin on the superficial fascia, (2) the deeper layers of fascia, (3) soft tissue on the bone. Be sure to assess mobility in all three planes of motion. Compare your findings with the other side and with another partner. Perform the same assessment on the anterior aspect of your partner's forearm, then on the paravertebral region of the lumbar spine.

6 Once you have assessed the degree of fascial mobility as described in number 5, attempt to identify and maintain a triplanar fulcrum on each region (thigh, forearm, spine) by distorting the tissues in a triplanar fashion. Be sure to provide force that moves in the direction of least restriction. Maintain the fulcrum once it has been achieved, and observe any connective tissue changes that may occur. Document the amount of time needed to produce such changes.

7 Perform the *shoulder girdle and clavipectoral soft tissue MFR* and *glenohumeral articular MFR* technique as described. Note any changes in posture or movement following each technique.

REFERENCES

1. Cantu R, Grodin A. *Myofasical Manipulation: Theory and Clinical Application.* Gaithersburg, MD: Aspen Publishers; 1992.
2. Hoffa AJ. *Technik der Massage.* Stuttgart, Germany: Ferdinand Enke; 1900.
3. Rolf IP. *Rolfing: The Integration of Human Structures.* Rochester, VT: Healing Arts Press; 1977.
4. Heller J, Hanson J. *The Client's Handbook.* Mt. Shasta, CA: Heller and Hellerwork; 1985.
5. Alexander FM. *The Alexander Technique.* New York: First Carol Publishing Group; 1989.
6. Feldenkrais M. *Awareness Through Movement.* San Francisco: Harper Collins; 1972.
7. Aston J. *Aston Patterning.* Course notes. Hartford, CT: Upledger Institute; 1993.
8. Clemente C. *A Regional Atlas of the Human Body.* Baltimore: Urban and Schwarzenberg; 1987.
9. Fitton-Jackson S. Antecedent phases of matrix formation. In: *Structure and Function of Connective Tissue and Skeletal Tissue.* London: Butterworth; 1965.
10. Frankel VH, Nordin M. *Basic Biomechanics of the Musculoskeletal System.* Philadelphia: Lea & Febiger; 1980.
11. Gray H. *Gray's Anatomy.* New York: Grammercy Books, Crown Publishers; 1977.
12. Hollinshead H, Rosse C. *Textbook of Anatomy.* 4th ed. Philadelphia: Harper Row; 1985.
13. Hukins DWL. Tissue components. In: Hukins DWL, *Connective Tissue Matrix.* Vol. I. London: McMillan Publishing; 1984.
14. Martini F. *Fundamentals of Anatomy and Physiology.* Englewood Cliffs, NJ: Prentice Hall; 1989.
15. Now VC, Holmes MH, Law WM. Fluid transport and mechanical properties of articular cartilage: a review. *J Biomech.* 1984;17:377-394.
16. Zohar D. *The Quantum Self.* New York: Quill/William Morrow; 1990.
17. Rich A, Crick FHC. The molecular structure of collagen. *J Mol Biol.* 1961;3:483.
18. Lowen F. *Visceral Manipulation.* Hartford, CT: Upledger Institute; 1990.
19. Boone E. *Origin and Development of the Fascial Structure.* Amsterdam, Holland: Upledger Institute's Europe's Fourth Biannual Congress; 1996.
20. Weiss J. Collagens and collagenolytic enzymes. In: Hukins DWL. *Connective Tissue Matrix.* Vol I. London: McMillan Publishing; 1984.
21. Barral JP. *The Thorax.* Seattle: Eastland Press; 1991.
22. Calliet R. *Soft Tissue Pain and Disability.* Philadelphia: F.A. Davis; 1988.
23. Juhan D. *Job's Body.* Barrytown, NY: Station Hill; 1987.
24. Barral JP. *Urogential Manipulation.* Seattle: Eastland Press; 1993.
25. Weiselfish S. *A Systems Approach for Treatment of TMJ Dysfunction.* Connecticut State American Physical Therapy Association Conference, 1981.
26. Bergquist R, Shaw S. *Advanced Therapeutics.* Springfield, MA: Springfield College; 1978.
27. Kain JB. *Clinical Aspects of Fascia.* Amsterdam, Holland: Upledger Institute Europe; 1996.
28. Proctor DJ, Guzman NA. Collagen disease and the biosynthesis of collagen. *Hosp Pract.* 1977:61-68.
29. Akeson WH, Woo SL, Amiel D, et al. The connective tissue response to immobility: biochemical changes in periarticular connective tissue of the immobilized rabbit knee. *Clin Orthop.* 1973;93:356-362.
30. Donatelli R, Owens-Burkhardt W. Effects on immobilization on extensibility of periarticular connective tissue. *J Orthop Sports Phys Ther.* 1981;3:67-72.
31. Noyes FR. Functional properties of knee ligaments and alterations induced by immobilization. *Clin Orthop.* 1977;123:210.
32. Woo SL, Matthews JV, et al. Connective tissue response to immobility: correlative study of biomechanical and biochemical measurement of normal and immobilized rabbit knee. *Arthritis Rheumatol.* 1975;18(3):257-266.

33. Evans E, Eggers G, et al. Experimental immobilization and mobilization of rat knee joints. *J Bone Joint Surg.* 1960;42:737-758.

34. McDonough A. Effect of immobilization and exercise on articular cartilage: a review of literature. *J Orthop Sports Phys Ther.* 1981;3:2-5.

35. Akeson WH, Amiel D. The connective tissue response to immobility: a study of the chondroitin 4 and 6 sulfate changes in periarticular connective tissue control and immobilized knees of dogs. *Clin Orthop Res.* 1967;51: 190-197.

36. Enneking W, Horowtiz M. The inter-articular effects of immobilization of the human knee. *J Bone Joint Surg.* 1972;14:198-212.

37. Hall MC. Cartilage changes after experimental immobilization of the knee joint for the young rat. *J Bone Joint Surg.* 1963;45:36-52.

38. Ingber D. The architecture of life. *Scientific American.* January 1998:48-57.

39. Weiselfish SH. *Developmental Manual Therapy for Physical Rehabilitation for the Neurologic Patient.* Vol. I, II. Ann Arbor, MI: UMI Dissertation Series; 1993.

Strain-Counterstrain in Orthopaedic Manual Physical Therapy

Sharon Giammatteo, PhD, PT, IMT,C

Chapter Objectives

At the conclusion of this chapter, the reader will be able to:

- Identify the origins of strain-counterstrain (SCS).
- Discuss the anatomical underpinnings believed to be responsible for protective muscle spasms and the mechanisms by which SCS may address these issues.
- Define protective muscle spasm, facilitated segment, myotatic reflex arc, release phenomenon, position of comfort, and tender point.

- Discuss how muscle hypertonicity/spasm may lead to tender points, postural aberrations, and restrictions in motion.
- Discuss the difference between direct and indirect techniques.
- Discuss how SCS differs from other soft tissue approaches to orthopaedic manual physical therapy.

HISTORICAL PERSPECTIVES
Eclectic Origins

The foundational origins of *strain-counterstrain (SCS),* or what is sometimes termed *positional release therapy,* have similarities to other intervention paradigms that are currently in use.[1] The practice of SCS involves an appreciation of postural deviations that may result from hypertonic muscle(s). Approaches such as yoga (see Chapter 21), Feldenkrais's awareness through movement (see Chapter 20), and tai chi, among others, focus on the practice of optimizing body position for the purpose of enhancing function.[1] These approaches each share the belief that optimal function flows from optimal positioning of body parts relative to one another. These positions are designed to stretch some regions while placing others in a position of relaxation.[2]

The concept of the **tender point** is not germane to SCS. Acupuncture points, which closely relate to the location of tender points used in SCS, have been used in the management of musculoskeletal pain syndromes for over 5,000 years.[1] Perhaps, the most widely used exposition of the existence of such tender points comes from the work of Travell and Simons,[3] who have systematically mapped the location of such tender points, along with various strategies designed to reduce their presence (see Chapter 16).

Concept Development

In 1954, *Dr. Lawrence H. Jones* was treating a patient suffering from a 4-month episode of severe low back pain who was not responding to conservative management. The patient experienced psoas spasms with a resultant analgesic posture and was having difficulty sleeping. Jones attempted to find a position that would allow the patient the ability to sleep more comfortably. Trial and error led to the discovery of a position in which the patient experienced maximal comfort, after which Jones allowed his patient to rest for 20 minutes. The patient was slowly released from this position and was able to attain an erect standing posture that was uninhibited by pain.[4–7]

Since that time, the art and science of this approach has culminated in the development of a myriad of remarkable techniques, some of which are presented in this chapter. Jones's initial discovery that precise positioning eliminated pain and disability has led to the persistent search for additional applications of these concepts. Jones also identified the presence of *tender points*, which were exquisitely painful upon palpation. He determined that these postural deviations were caused by protective muscle spasm and determined that the shortened muscles in spasm were pulling on osteoarticular structures, thus contributing to joint dysfunction. He appreciated that precise positioning, which resulted in improved movement patterns and decreased discomfort, also dissipated the pain that was emanating from the tender point. These tender points identified in the extremities were not found in the muscle being strained or stretched, but in its antagonist. The mechanism by which these tender points were present was believed to be related to a sudden stretch placed on the muscle following insult that occurred immediately following maximal shortening. This muscle is believed to continue this behavior as if it were strained despite the fact that the underlying joint was in neutral. Attempts at continued stretch would only serve to increase the symptoms emanating from this already overstretched structure.

QUESTIONS *for* REFLECTION

- What is the difference between the manner in which tender points are considered within the SCS approach compared to other approaches?
- According to the SCS approach, where are tender points typically found and what is their etiology?
- In SCS, how are tender points used to gauge progress and outcomes?
- What is the difference between tender points and trigger points?

Subsequent to these correlations, Jones began his search for painful tender points in the musculature of all of his patients. He attempted to ascertain which muscle in spasm was reflected by which tender point. During his pursuits, Jones learned that these positions of maximal comfort required maintenance of the position for exactly *90 seconds.*[7]

NOTABLE QUOTABLE

"If you listen to the body it will tell you all you need to know!"

—*Lawrence Jones*

At the time of his initial discoveries, Jones was unaware of the neuroscience underlying these observed clinical phenomena. Fifty years of investigation has led to the development of a comprehensive approach to the management of somatic dysfunction and pain. Approximately 175 tender points and their correlating precise positions of comfort have been documented by Jones (Fig. 15-1). The art of SCS has been described in several texts by many authors, and the science of SCS continues to develop.

Direct Versus Indirect Techniques

Orthopaedic manual physical therapy (OMPT) approaches may be classified as either **direct techniques,** in which force is applied in the direction of the resistance barrier, or **indirect techniques,** in which force is applied away from the resistance barrier. The majority of techniques that we typically employ to reduce soft tissue and joint limitations and, indeed, the majority of approaches covered within this text, fall under the auspices of direct techniques. Interventions such as stretching and joint mobilization would be considered direct techniques. Direct techniques load, or bind, the tissues and structures. The tissue is moved toward a barrier on one or more planes in the direction of the least mobile, most restricted, or most limited movement. At the barrier to further movement, a technique is performed, and the anticipated result is a repositioning of the barrier closer to the end of normal range of motion (Box 15-1).

Conversely, indirect techniques, such as SCS, seek to unload the involved structures. When implementing these techniques, the tissue is moved away from the barrier on one or more planes toward the most mobile or least restricted movement. The observed postural deviation is thereby exaggerated. The anticipated result is a **release phenomenon.** The hypertonic soft tissues relax, allowing an increase in the range of motion that is beyond the original barrier. In the example of an elbow flexion contracture with limited elbow extension, the elbow is moved into flexion primarily with attempts to find the path of least resistance within the other two planes of motion, which may include pronation/supination or abduction/adduction. After 90 seconds, a *"release"* is expected to occur, resulting in decreased hypertonicity and elongation of the biceps with increased range of motion into extension. The analogy of opening a drawer that is stuck closed is often used to illustrate this process. Instead of pulling the drawer open (direct technique), the drawer may be pushed in the direction of ease first until it releases, which then allows the drawer to open without restriction (indirect technique).

ANATOMICAL RATIONALE FOR STRAIN-COUNTERSTRAIN
Impairment of the Myofascial System

The intrinsic properties of musculoskeletal structures often manifest themselves as biomechanical aberrations.[8] Myofascial structures are at the juncture of both efferent and afferent stimuli that serve to regulate their function.[1] The fascial system is a collagenous network of connective tissue that is constantly adapting to mechanical influences. In response to injury, a muscle typically responds by developing a protective spasm and adhesive fibrosis. In response to injury, inflammation leads to cross-bridge formation between the collagen fibers of the matrix, rendering the fascial system in a state of reduced elasticity and therefore less able to adapt to mechanical influences (see Chapter 13).[9]

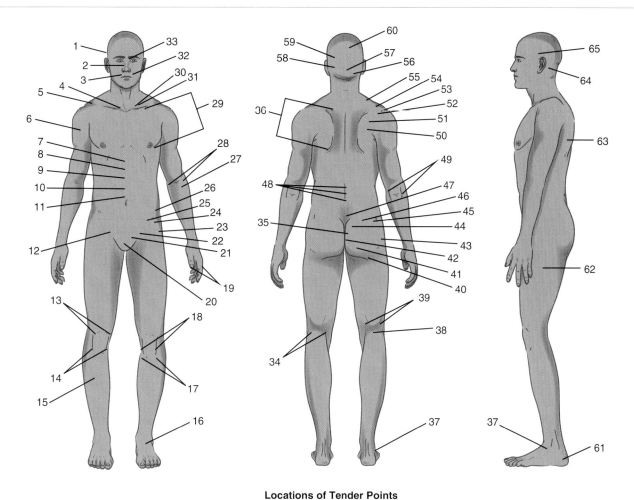

Locations of Tender Points

1. Squamosal
2. Nasal
3. Masseter-temporomandibular
4. Anterior first thoracic
5. Anterior acromioclavicular
6. Latissimus dorsi
7. Anterior seventh thoracic
8. Anterior eighth thoracic
9. Anterior ninth thoracic
10. Anterior tenth thoracic
11. Anterior eleventh thoracic
12. Anterior second lumbar
13. Medial and lateral meniscus
14. Medial and lateral extension meniscus
15. Tibialis anticus medial ankle
16. Flexion ankle
17. Medial and lateral hamstrings
18. Medial and lateral patella
19. Thumb and fingers
20. Low-ilium flare-out
21. Anterior fifth lumbar
22. Low ilium
23. Anterior lateral trochanter

24. Anterior first lumbar
25. Iliacus
26. Anterior twelfth thoracic
27. Radial head
28. Medial and lateral coronoid
29. Depressed upper ribs
30. Anterior eighth cervical
31. Anterior seventh cervical
32. Infraorbital nerve
33. Supraorbital nerve
34. Extension ankle (on gastrocnemius)
35. High flare-out sacroiliac
36. Elevated upper ribs (on rib angles)
37. Lateral ankle
38. Posterior cruciate ligament
39. Anterior cruciate ligament
40. Posterior medial trochanter
41. Also posterior medial trochanter
42. Coccyx (for high flare-out sacroiliac)
43. Posterior lateral trochanter

44. Lower-pole fifth lumbar
45. Fourth lumbar
46. Third lumbar
47. Upper-pole fifth lumbar
48. Upper lumbars
49. Medial and lateral olecranon
50. Third thoracic shoulder
51. Lateral second thoracic shoulder
52. Medial second thoracic shoulder
53. Posterior acromioclavicular
54. Supraspinatus
55. Elevated first rib
56. Posterior first cervical
57. Inion
58. Left occipitomastoid
59. Sphenobasilar
60. Right lambdoid
61. Lateral calcaneus
62. Lateral trochanter
63. Subscapularis
64. Posteroauricular
65. Squamosal

FIGURE 15–1 Location of Jones's tender points. (Adapted from Schwartz HR. *The use of counterstrain in an acutely ill in-hospital population. JAOA.* 1986;86:433-442.)

Box 15-1 Quick Notes! DIRECT VS. INDIRECT TECHNIQUES

DIRECT TECHNIQUES

- Force is applied in the direction of the resistance barrier.
- Movement is in direction that is least mobile, most restricted.
- Goal is to reposition the barrier closer to the end of normal range.

INDIRECT TECHNIQUES

- Force is applied away from the resistance barrier.
- Involved tissues and structures are unloaded.
- Movement is toward the most mobile or least restricted movement with the observed postural deviation exaggerated.
- Anticipated result is a *release phenomenon.* The hypertonic soft tissues relax allowing an increase in the range of motion that is beyond the original barrier.

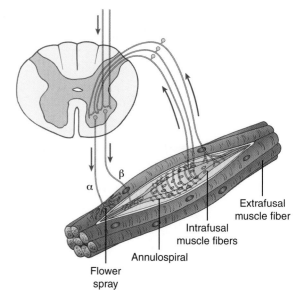

FIGURE 15–2 Control of muscle length and tension through the muscle spindle apparatus and the myotatic reflex arc. (Adapted from D'Ambrogio KJ, Roth GB. *Positional Release Therapy: Assessment and Treatment of Musculoskeletal Dysfunction.* St. Louis, MO: Mosby, 1997)

The SCS approach to OMPT places an emphasis on reducing biomechanical aberrations that may manifest themselves within the myofascial system in cases of musculoskeletal impairment. The current best evidence supports the frequency with which the myofascial system is involved in the etiology of musculoskeletal dysfunction.[1,9] In the case of injury, inflammatory processes are initiated within the myofascial structures, which result in an acute pain response.[9] The typical response of the myofascial system to injury sets into motion a cascade of events that engages not just musculoskeletal structures but neuromuscular structures as well. The myofascial impairment that results from either direct or indirect trauma engages what is known as the **myotatic reflex arc**, which is believed to be responsible for the development and perpetuation of protective muscle spasms, deficits in muscle recruitment, and limitations in joint range of motion.[1,7,10]

The Myotatic Reflex Arc as the Basis of Protective Muscle Spasm

The *myotatic reflex arc* (stretch reflex arc, the monosynaptic reflex arc, or gamma motor neuron loop) is considered to be the basis of normal resting tone within muscle (Fig. 15-2). The components of this reflex arc include the *extrafusal muscle fiber*, which has the ability to contract, relax, and elongate. The *muscle spindle*, with its *intrafusal muscle fibers*, is responsive to the length and velocity of stretch. The *afferent neuron* transmits the information regarding stretch from the spindle to the spinal cord. The *alpha motor neuron* transmits the impulse from the spinal cord to the muscle fiber leading to the elicitation of a muscle contraction. When rapid changes in length are perceived, a protective reflex engages the alpha motor neurons, resulting in increased muscle tone.

The *gamma motor neuron* innervates the intrafusal muscle fibers of the muscle spindle, allowing them to contract. These neurons are critical in creating the threshold by which the spindle is stimulated through regulating the length of the intrafusal fibers. In order to respond to changing demands, the gamma motor neurons produce a steady resting tone within the muscle spindle. This steady state of resting tone is known as **gamma bias**. In the case of myofascial dysfunction, there is an increase in gamma bias known as **gamma gain**. This process will result in changes within the extrafusal muscle fibers, namely hypertonicity and spasm, that may be challenging to address through standard soft tissue stretching regimens.[7]

QUESTIONS *for* REFLECTION

- Briefly describe the anatomical components that form the *muscle spindle.*
- What is the primary function of this nerve receptor?
- How is this receptor involved in myofascial impairment?
- How might SCS alter the function of this receptor?

When the joint is in a neutral position under normal conditions, there is an equal degree of tone in the muscles on either side of the joint. When an articulation is moved (Fig. 15-3), muscles on one side of the joint are stretched (a) while the opposing muscles are shortened (b). A stretch on the muscle (a) produces gamma gain within this muscle (a) and a reduction in neural input to the gamma system of the opposing muscle (b). This stretch results in a reflex that enacts the alpha motor neurons that innervate the extrafusal fibers of that muscle (a), resulting in a rapid attempt to reduce this stretch. This

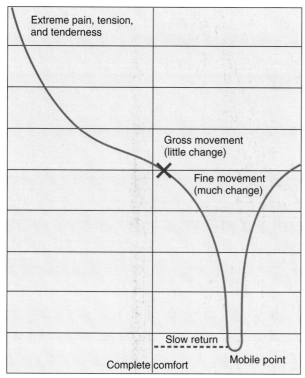

FIGURE 15–3 Ideal positioning for comfort. (Adapted from Jones LH, Kusunose R, Goering E. *Jones Strain-Counterstrain.* Boise, ID: Jones Strain-CounterStrain, Inc, 1995)

process ultimately results in increased gamma input and subsequent increased muscle tension within the previously shortened muscle (b). Following injury, the joint is malpositioned and demonstrates motion loss due to increased muscle tone resulting from increased gamma input. In order to restore normal positional relationships and motion within the joint, the degree of tension within this muscle must be normalized.

CLINICAL PILLAR

In a neutral position, there is an equal degree of tone in the muscles on either side of the joint. When an articulation is moved, muscles on one side of the joint are stretched while the opposing muscles are shortened. A stretch on the muscle produces gamma gain within this muscle and a reduction in neural input to the gamma system of the opposing muscle. This stretch results in a reflex that enacts the alpha motor neurons that innervate the extrafusal fibers of the muscle, resulting in a rapid attempt to reduce this stretch. Following injury, the joint is malpositioned and demonstrates motion loss owing to increased muscle tone that results from increased gamma input. In order to restore normal positional relationships and motion within the joint, the degree of tension within this muscle must be normalized.

Irvin Korr[11,12] is often credited with providing greater understanding of the manner in which the muscle spindle is involved in myofascial dysfunction. Korr[11,12] hypothesized that there is an increase in gamma outflow from the muscle that is hypershortened (muscle b in the example above) that leads to gamma gain in its muscle spindle. When the joint is then stretched, it experiences strain prematurely. Jones then concluded that the myofascial impairment was not a distinct lesion, but rather an ongoing process of noxious stimuli. To reduce the impairment, the shortened muscle must be maximally shortened followed by slow return to neutral. Therefore, SCS does not cure the impairment, rather these techniques seek to eliminate the irritation and inflammation produced from premature strain to the muscle, thus allowing the body to then cure itself.[7]

It is also important to consider that the resting tone of a muscle is influenced by a confluence of factors that exist from both within, as described above, as well as outside of the target muscle. For example, the supraspinatus muscle may be found to be in protective muscle spasm that may be the result of injury to itself or injury to extrinsic structures.[13] Any dysfunction within the C5 *dermatome*, *myotome*, or *scleratome* may produce a protective muscle spasm of the supraspinatus muscle. Furthermore, a glenohumeral joint dislocation, fracture of the humeral head, and subdeltoid bursitis may produce a protective muscle spasm in any or all of the muscles innervated by C5. Determining whether or not an injury has occurred directly to the supraspinatus muscle or to other structures that are also innervated by C5 is important when deciding where intervention is to be directed. Afferent information that is emanating from the supraspinatus tendon is transmitted to the C5 spinal segment. Owing to the receipt of information from this dysfunctional tissue, the C5 segment is in a state of facilitation or is said to be a **facilitated spinal segment** (Fig. 15-4) (Box 15-2). In essence, the central nervous system becomes overloaded with sensory input and becomes unable to selectively differentiate the specific origin of each individual stimulus. When C5 becomes facilitated, all muscles innervated by the C5 segment may develop an increase in tone, resulting in protective spasm. Therefore, addressing the dysfunctional structure is necessary for the elimination of the protective muscle spasm of the target structure, as well as the other muscles innervated by that same spinal segment (C5). SCS may reduce the threshold of the facilitated segment and provide an opportunity for normalization of hyperneural input.[14]

Protective muscle spasm is defined as the involuntary sustained contraction and shortening of muscle fibers at the level of the sarcomere. In this state, the sarcomere becomes hyperinnervated, owing to an increase in nerve impulses that are carried along the alpha motor nerve from the anterior horn of C5 to the supraspinatus muscle fibers. In this state, the reflex arc is said to possess **alpha gain**. If alpha gain is reduced through correction of a supraspinatus tendinitis, elimination of the protective spasm in all muscles innervated by C5 results. Improvement in voluntary motor control and increased mobility may also be experienced by the supraspinatus muscle in the absence of protective spasm.

If the neuromusculoskeletal dysfunction within the structures innervated by C5 is more diffuse, resolution of the

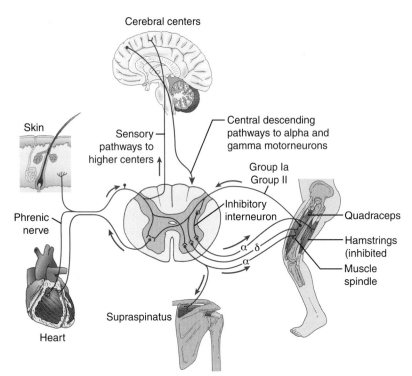

FIGURE 15–4 A facilitated segment at the C5-C7 spinal level. (Adapted from D'Ambrogio KJ, Roth GB. *Positional Release Therapy: Assessment and Treatment of Musculoskeletal Dysfunction.* St. Louis, MO: Mosby, 1997)

Box 15-2 THE FACILITATED SEGMENT

The central nervous system becomes overloaded with sensory input and becomes unable to selectively differentiate the specific origin of each individual stimulus, which leads to a misinterpretation of afferent information. When C5, for example, becomes facilitated, other regions of the body innervated by this same spinal segment may receive increased stimuli. All muscles innervated by the C5 segment may develop an increase in tone, resulting in some degree of protective muscle spasm.

supraspinatus tendinitis will not suffice. For example, along with supraspinatus tendinitis, there may also be a concomitant deltoid bursitis, anterior capsulitis, or C5 radiculopathy. When multiple conditions exist, elimination of the supraspinatus tendinitis alone will not result in complete resolution.

SCS techniques, if effective, may result in a general decrease in the level of central nervous system hyperactivity, resulting in a decrease in protective spasm in muscles that are innervated by spinal segments above and below C5. In addition, evidence exists that demonstrates a general decrease in hyperactivity of the somatic and autonomic nervous systems in response to these techniques as well.

PHILOSOPHICAL FRAMEWORK
General Description

Classically, SCS is defined as a therapeutic intervention that places the involved body part into a **position of comfort**

(POC). The POC is defined as the triplanar position, which is passively achieved for the purpose of reducing tender point irritability and achieving normalization of tissues associated with the presenting myofascial impairment (Box 15-3).[1] The manual physical therapist must exercise precision when attaining the POC because malpositioning may lead to reactivation of the facilitated segment.[1] As the POC is attained, the patient reports a reduction in tenderness as the manual physical therapist identifies a palpable reduction in the tone of the tender point, which is referred to as the **comfort zone (CZ).** When approaching the CZ, additional clinical observations including temperature changes, vibration, and breathing changes may be noted.[1]

Tender points have been described as small areas of intense, tender, edematous muscle and fascial tissue that are approximately 1 cm in diameter.[15] Tender points that reside in anterior regions of the body are usually treated using POCs that involve flexion, while posterior points are relieved by POC's that use extension. When a therapist performs SCS, the involved tissues are placed into the most shortened position

Box 15-3 POSITION OF COMFORT (POC)

The triplanar position is passively achieved for the purpose of reducing tender point irritability and achieving normalization of tissues associated with the presenting myofascial impairment. In response to achieving the ideal POC, relaxation of spastic muscles, reduction of edema, enhanced muscular recruitment, and neuromuscular reorganization ensues.

while the therapist's finger is positioned on the specific tender point. As noted, this position must be maintained for *90 seconds* when treating general musculoskeletal conditions. The author of this chapter has identified that when treating neurological conditions using SCS, as will be described later, the POC must be maintained for a minimum of *3 minutes*. Once the POC is held for the optimal amount of time, the manual physical therapist must slowly release the involved tissues to their neutral position, taking special care not to induce a quick stretch that might cause a return of increased tone in the target tissue. Once the structures have been returned to neutral, it is critical that the manual therapist reexamine the sensitivity of each tender point to determine effectiveness.[16]

Since Jones developed the foundations for this approach over 50 years ago, many clinicians and researchers have modified the techniques, enhanced our knowledge of underlying mechanisms of action, and have adopted alternative terminology. The original techniques documented by Jones are still used and found to be effective by those who regularly use this intervention approach. The author of this chapter has adopted the positions originally described by Jones. Her work in using SCS with the neurologically impaired population has led to several modifications. Individuals with neurological impairment do not have normal sensory function and thus do not feel similar pain upon pressure at the tender point. The pediatric patient, the chronic pain patient, and the geriatric patient are also unable to provide accurate feedback to the manual therapist. Typically, a baby responds to pressure on the tender point as if being tickled. The geriatric patient and the chronic pain patient often get an autonomic nervous system stimulation similar to *sympathetic dysautonomia* when the tender point is stimulated. Based on this response, this author hypothesizes that the autonomic nervous system plays a role in the development of these tender points.

The Objectives of Strain-Counterstrain

In order to normalize muscle tone and achieve improved joint mobility, SCS techniques are designed to shorten the muscle fiber of the agonist (hypertonic muscle) and strain the Golgi tendon organ (GTO) of the antagonist (the muscle on the opposite side of the joint from the hypertonic muscle). In essence, the patient's observed postural deviations are exaggerated. By exaggerating the faulty posture, the involved muscle and associated joints are moved into the direction of hypertonic muscle pull, thus placing the hypertonic muscle in a shortened state. The expected result is elongation of the muscle fiber, with a subsequent increase in joint mobility and range of motion without the need for stretching. The effect of accomplishing this objective will be a decrease in the gamma gain to the muscle spindle of the hypertonic muscle and a subsequent decrease in the hyperactivity of the myotatic reflex arc to that muscle.

Stretching activities that endeavor to elongate the involved muscle by moving the insertions of the muscle in opposite directions may lead to increased hypertonicity through the firing of the muscle spindles that serve to increase tone. Furthermore,

discomfort is often experienced by the patient upon stretching of hypertonic muscle. Discomfort may produce voluntary muscle guarding secondary to pain or fear of pain from movement.

The Kinesiological Effects of Strain-Counterstrain

During examination, the manual physical therapist may observe multiplanar postural deviations. Within this approach, the role of myofascial elements that lead to poor postures is emphasized. Postural deviations may be a reflection of the hypertonicity of the muscles in that region. The manual physical therapist may evaluate static posture and dynamic movement in order to determine the culpable hypertonic muscle(s). The postural examination that is described in this chapter is used to identify muscles that are in shortened or contracted states. For example, observation of shoulder girdle protraction during the postural examination may be the result of tightness within the pectoralis minor muscle.

Of primary importance is the impact of hypertonic muscles on normal movement patterns. Schiowitz[17] alludes to the impact of SCS on joint mobility by describing two different modifications of SCS that may be used to address tissue texture changes and restrictions in motion. SCS techniques designed to address increased tissue texture are first performed by placing superficial tissues in a position of ease. If mobility issues persist, it is recommended to place the spinal vertebra in its position of greatest ease in all three planes. Although both modifications attempt to influence spinal mobility through reduction of myofascial tone, the latter technique is believed to more specifically address the deep muscles that cross the joint.

CLINICAL PILLAR

- The most profound impairment precipitated by altered joint position secondary to hypertonic muscles is the impact on normal movement patterns.

- SCS techniques designed to address increased tissue texture are first performed by placing superficial tissues in a position of ease.

- If mobility issues persist, place the spinal vertebra in its position of greatest ease in all three planes relative to the adjacent vertebra.

One method of correcting a postural deviation that leads to improved movement patterns is the adoption of what has been termed, the *corrective kinesiologic approach* to SCS. Such an approach considers the impact of hypertonic muscles on movement. For example, if the shoulder girdle is observed to be protracted during postural observation, then there is likely to be a limitation of retraction and horizontal abduction. To address this condition with SCS, the *depressed second rib* technique may be used. The corrective kinesiologic approach to

SCS requires the reduction and elimination of the muscle spasm within the pectoralis minor, thereby reducing the protracted shoulder girdle posture and subsequently increasing the range of horizontal abduction.

The result of comprehensively eliminating hyperactivity within the facilitated segment is an elongation of the muscle fiber to its true resting length. When the muscle fiber is in a healthy, relaxed state, it does not exert abnormal tension through its bony insertions. Through elimination of protective spasm, SCS will result in normalization of joint position and improved mobility. Despite the emphasis on normalization of muscle tone, SCS may also have a profound effect on joint mobility and might be considered as an alternate means of mobilizing joints and associated structures.

PRINCIPLES OF EXAMINATION
Tenderness as an Indication for Strain-Counterstrain

As previously defined, tender points are considered to be an outward manifestation of an underlying soft tissue lesion and not the lesion itself.[1] These tender points may have tenderness in adjacent tissues, as well, with an overall increase in sensitivity that is four times greater than normal tissue.[7] Tender points are similar in nature and location to trigger points as defined by Travell and Simons[3] and are found within muscle bellies, tendons, musculotendinous junctions, fascia, and bone.[1] In a sample of 283 chronic pain patients with a minimum duration of symptoms greater than 6 months, Rosomoff et al[9] found the presence of tender points to be the most common physical finding, with 79.4% of chronic neck patients and 96.7% of chronic low back patients having more than one tender point.

As originally advocated by Jones, the application of light pressure over an identified tender point serves as the primary indicator for use of these techniques. When palpating for the identification of tender points, it is critical that the manual therapist is firm, yet gentle, when entering the tissue.[18] A quick twitch of muscle activity, known as a **jump sign**, is often used to confirm the presence of a tender point.[3,18]

Tender points are found in very specific locations within the hypertonic muscle. In addition to the specific tender points originally documented by Jones, other authors have endeavored to identify additional tender points that may be used in the application of these techniques.[19] In our previous example of pectoralis minor muscle spasm, a tender point would be found within the pectoralis minor at the midpoint of an imaginary line between the sternoclavicular joint and the axilla. A 70% to 75% reduction in tender point tenderness is typically used as the standard measure of position accuracy. Less than that amount of reduction suggests that the POC must be altered.[7,19-21]

Tender points that are associated with myofascial and visceral pain may lie within the areas of referred pain or may be located at some distance from the location of actual symptoms. The location of these tender points throughout the body and the manner in which contact reduces the degree of tenderness

associated with these points resembles acupuncture points. Melzack et al[22] demonstrated a high degree of correspondence (71%) between the spatial distribution and associated pain patterns of tender points and acupuncture points. Although a subject of debate, this relationship suggests a similarity in their underlying neural mechanisms.

Posture as an Indication for Strain-Counterstrain

Along with palpable tenderness, postural deviations may also suggest the use of SCS. As mentioned, observation of posture allows the manual physical therapist to gain an understanding of the forces acting on the patient and the movement potential of the joint in question. As mentioned, pectoralis minor hypertonicity may lead to scapular protraction, a limitation of horizontal abduction, and tenderness. The extent of postural deviations that exist are commensurate with the degree of limitation that is present in a given range of motion and the nature of positional imbalance present within the associated articular surfaces.

NOTABLE QUOTABLE

"Posture reflects the movement potential of associated articulations."

—*Sharon Giammatteo*

Identification of tender points and postural deviations are the prime indicators for the implementation of the SCS approach. The physical examination should include posture that uses a wide-angle view in all three cardinal planes. Joint mobility as well as muscle function should also be assessed before and after SCS to identify any changes in response to intervention. As increases in joint mobility are experienced during the repositioning of the articular surfaces, the patient may sense the movement through the kinesthetic receptors of the joints. Once the ideal position has been achieved, it is important that the therapist does not alter the position of the body part in any way.

As long as the patient is experiencing, or the therapist is palpating, any movement or tissue tension change, the body position should be maintained. It is only when the patient and therapist no longer experience any tissue changes or movement that the body part be returned to its neutral position, slowly and gently.

PRINCIPLES OF INTERVENTION
The Fundamentals of Strain-Counterstrain

When developing SCS, Jones established several basic principles to help guide intervention (Box 15-4). It is important when treating more than one region to address the most tender point first and to treat from a proximal to distal direction.[7]

Box 15-4 FUNDAMENTALS OF SCS

- Address the most tender point first and treat from a proximal to distal direction. Movement is in direction that is least mobile and most restricted.
- The middle tender point is treated first and used as a gauge for progress.
- Tender points that are present anteriorly are treated with flexion-biased positions. Conversely, tender points located posteriorly on the body are treated using positions of extension.
- If the tender point is lateral to midline, it is best treated using the addition of either side bending, rotation, or both, along with flexion or extension.
- Movements required to specifically achieve the POC requires skill, awareness, and patience on the part of the manual physical therapist.

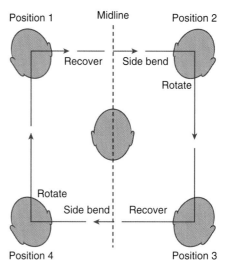

FIGURE 15–5 The *range-of-motion box* is a tool that provides a visual depiction of the manner and direction in which the cervical spine may be smoothly transitioned from one quadrant to another in pursuit of the POC. (From Woolbright JL. An alternative method of teaching strain/counterstrain manipulation. *JAOA.* 1991;4:370-376, with permission).

In addition, if there is a region that includes several active tender points, then the middle tender point is treated first and used as a gauge for progress. When attempting to identify the presence of tender points, the manual physical therapist must be aware that those that are present anteriorly are treated with flexion-biased positions. Conversely, tender points located posteriorly on the body are treated using positions of extension. If the tender point is lateral to midline, it is best treated using the addition of either side bending, rotation, or both, along with flexion or extension. The tender points described by Jones, when present, are generally located in the same exact locations throughout the body. Each tender point suggests the presence of a muscle in spasm often resulting in joint compression.

The relatively fine movements required to specifically achieve the POC requires skill, awareness, and patience on the part of the manual physical therapist. Woolbright[23] provides a method for improving the manual physical therapist's ability to specifically identify the POC through the use of what is termed the **range-of-motion box** (Fig. 15-5). Originally designed to assist the therapist in visualizing changes in direction of the patient's head and neck during SCS of the cervical spine, this tool provides a visual depiction of the manner and direction in which the cervical spine may be smoothly transitioned from one quadrant to another in pursuit of the POC.[23]

While passively moving the involved structures toward their optimal POC, the manual physical therapist maintains gentle contact on the tender point. As the POC is achieved a reduction in tenderness and palpable tone in the region of the tender point is often experienced. Once the POC has been achieved, contact on the tender point is maintained to monitor progress, but no additional pressure is added. During intervention, slight alterations to the POC may be required. The manual physical therapist must think hard through the hands to appreciate when minor adjustments are needed. Unlike other approaches, the primary effects of SCS are achieved through the attainment of the POC and not secondary to intervention directed toward the tender point.

The first phase of release involves length-tension changes within the muscle itself, 90 seconds of these changes is sufficient in most patients presenting with musculoskeletal dysfunction.[1] These effects have been found to take twice as long in the neurologically impaired patient.[1,12] The second phase of release involves the fascia, which often takes 20 to 30 minutes to achieve.[1]

It is important to remember that the POC must be entirely pain free. Secondary tender points may limit the ability to achieve these pain-free postures and occasionally require intervention first before the POC can be achieved. Occasionally, pain may be experienced initially upon achievement of the POC that soon dissipates. Allowing the patient to breathe deeply and application of gentle traction or compression may assist in diminishing symptoms and achieving the POC.

Once the release has been achieved, it is of vital importance that the involved joint slowly and passively be returned to neutral, during which time the therapist continues to monitor the status of the tender point through contact. Occasionally, slight symptoms return in the region that was treated. The manual physical therapist may experience a slight wobble, or shift, in the joint followed by a point of smooth motion, known as the **still point.**

SCS is appropriate for a wide range of presentations. Anyone who is experiencing an episode of myofascial hypertonicity, or spasticity, regardless of its origin, may be an appropriate candidate for SCS. Although outside of the purview of the physical therapist, Schwartz[20] advocates the use of SCS as an adjunctive intervention for myocardial infarction, congestive heart failure, respiratory failure, pneumonia, asthma, bronchitis, postoperative ileus, and hospital-acquired positional pain. Furthermore, SCS may be used to differentiate between disease and musculoskeletal dysfunction. For example, an anterior T11 tender point that does not respond to SCS may suggest an appendicitis.[20] Although this approach addresses soft tissue dysfunction, its effects are far-reaching and may be used to enhance movement and reduce pain and disability that results from musculoskeletal and nonmusculoskeletal origins. However, evidence supporting the latter is needed. As with other forms of manual intervention, malignancy, open wounds, healing fractures, infection, active inflammation, and rheumatoid arthritis serve as relative contraindications to SCS. Serious pathology must be ruled out before intervention is initiated.[1]

Strain-Counterstrain for Impairments of the Upper Quarter

The following SCS techniques are designed to be used in the management of cervical and upper extremity pain, postural dysfunction, and limitations in motion and are presented here as a supplement to another text written entirely on this topic by the author of this chapter.[10] In supine, sitting, and standing, observation of postural deviations within all three planes is performed, and articular postural deviations of the neck, shoulder girdle, elbow, forearm, wrist, hand, thumb, and fingers are documented.

Lateral Cervicals–Focus on C5 Strain-Counterstrain Technique (Fig. 15-6 A, B)

The tender point for this technique is on the lateral tip of the transverse process of C5. The results of the examination that indicate the need for this technique reveal postural deviations of cervical side bending to the ipsilateral side and limitations of motion for cervical side bending to the contralateral side. The position for performance of the technique is supine with the cervical spine side-bent and rotated toward the side of the tender point. Side gliding with overpressure is performed at the involved segment. Side gliding is produced by placing the hand on the side of the tender point on the lower lateral face/mandible with the contralateral hand on the opposite parietal bone. Compression of the hands bilaterally will achieve the desired side glide/side bending effect.

The objective of this technique is to reduce the protective muscle spasm of the middle scalenes. *Thoracic outlet syndrome (TOS)* is improved when scalene muscle spasm is reduced because of less compression on the brachial plexus. The scalenes insert on the first rib. This technique can reduce the pain and dysfunction associated with an elevated first rib.

Anterior Fifth Cervical Strain-Counterstrain Technique (Fig. 15-7 A, B)

The tender point for this technique is at the anterior surface of the tip of the transverse process of C5. Examination results reveal a forward head and neck posture with limitation of motion into cervical extension. The technique is performed with the patient in supine, with approximately 40 degrees of cervical flexion, approximately 25 degrees of contralateral cervical rotation, and approximately 25 degrees of contralateral side bending. This technique is designed to address C5-6 joint mobility, cervical discopathy, and referred shoulder pain.

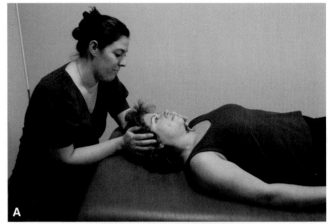
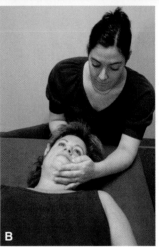

FIGURE 15–6 (A, B) Lateral cervicals strain-counterstrain technique.

First Elevated Rib (Rib Cage Dysfunction) Strain-Counterstrain Technique (Fig. 15-8)

The tender point for this technique is located beneath the margin of the trapezius muscle at the lateral aspect of the cervical spine. Findings from the examination reveal shoulder girdle elevation and limitations in cervicothoracic side bending and rotation, along with limitations for upper costal mobility during breathing. In sitting, the ipsilateral shoulder is supported by placing the patient's arm over the therapist's knee. The patient is then positioned in slight cranial extension of less than 10 degrees with a chin tuck. The therapist then moves the patient into slight cervical side bending of less than 10 degrees to the ipsilateral side and rotation to the contralateral side. An elevated first rib may cause pain at the lateral base of the neck. Cervical rotation is especially limited. Often symptoms will dissipate within a few minutes of performing this technique.

Subscapularis (SUB) Strain-Counterstrain Technique (Fig. 15-9 A, B)

The tender point is located deep within the axilla on the anterior aspect of the humerus. Postural deviations of shoulder adduction and anterior shear of the humeral head are often observed. Shoulder external rotation and abduction are consequently limited, along with posterior glide of the humeral head. The patient is placed supine with the arm off of the table.

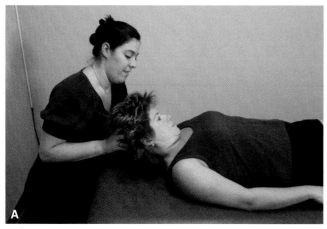

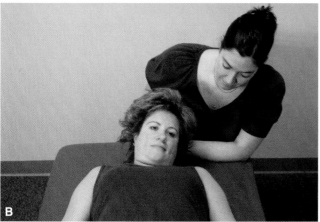

FIGURE 15–7 (A, B) Anterior fifth cervical strain-counterstrain technique.

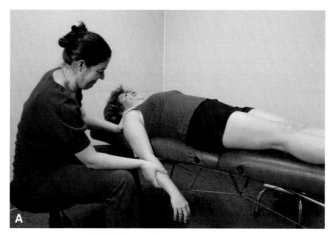

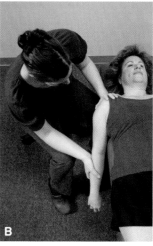

FIGURE 15–9 (A, B) Subscapularis (SUB) Strain-counterstrain technique.

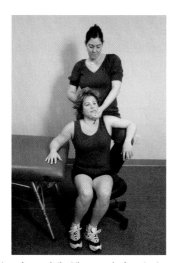

FIGURE 15–8 First elevated rib (rib cage dysfunction) strain-counterstrain technique.

The shoulder is placed into extension, internal rotation, and adduction with overpressure. This technique will decrease the adducted and internally rotated component of the spastic synergic pattern. The most problematic impact of subscapularis hypertonicity is anterior subluxation of the humeral head, which, along with inferior subluxation caused by latissimus dorsi involvement, leads to shoulder dysfunction.

Supraspinatus (SP1) Strain-Counterstrain Technique (Fig.15-10 A, B)

The tender point is found within the supraspinous fossa, 1 inch medial to the acromioclavicular joint line. Shoulder joint elevation and superior compression of the humeral head is noted during the structural examination with limitation of inferior glide of the humeral head and shoulder adduction. The patient is placed in supine with 45 degrees of flexion, 45 degrees of abduction, and 45 degrees of external rotation. Hypertonicity of the supraspinatus will compress the humeral head within the glenoid fossa. Therefore, this technique restores intra-articular joint mobility to the shoulder joint through reducing the degree of compressive forces experienced by the joint. Supraspinatus hypertonicity leads to the elevated shoulder girdle component of the synergic pattern. Jacobson et al[13] provide a comprehensive exposition of an intervention regimen that incorporates SCS for the management of supraspinatus tendonopathy.

Latissimus Dorsi (LD) Strain-Counterstrain Technique (Fig. 15-11 A, B)

The tender point is deep within the axilla on the medial (posterior) aspect of the humerus. The humeral head is stuck into inferior glide, and shoulder flexion is limited. The position for intervention is supine with the arm off of the table. The

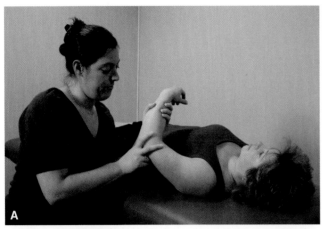

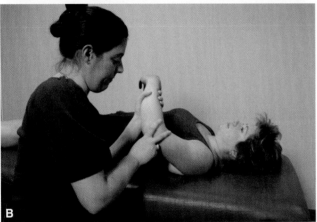

FIGURE 15–10 (A, B) Supraspinatus (SP1) strain-counterstrain technique.

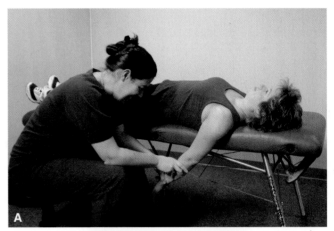

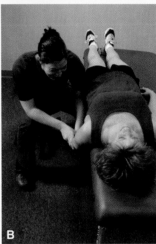

FIGURE 15–11 (A, B) Latissimus dorsi (LD) strain-counterstrain technique.

arm is brought to the end range of shoulder extension without overpressure, followed by adduction and internal rotation to end range. The extremity is then pulled inferiorly with 5 pounds of longitudinal traction force. The latissimus dorsi, besides performing shoulder joint extension, depresses the humeral head within the glenoid fossa. This technique is viewed as being among the most valuable SCS techniques for the shoulder girdle. This technique can correct an inferior subluxation/dislocation of the shoulder joint; however, the correct sequence of techniques is required. Intervention must proceed from the second depressed rib technique for the pectoralis minor, which will reduce the protracted shoulder, followed by SCS for the subscapularis, which will reduce the anterior subluxation of the humeral head, and end with SCS to the latissimus dorsi muscle. It is important for the subscapularis SCS technique, which requires only 20 degrees of shoulder extension, to be performed first so as to allow the necessary 40 degrees of extension that is required for performance of the latissimus dorsi SCS technique. The neutral position is required to obtain optimal results with this technique.

Biceps (Long Head) Strain-Counterstrain Technique (Fig.15-12 A, B)

The tender point is present at the anterior surface of the glenohumeral joint, approximately 1 inch superior to the axilla. Posturally, the patient may present with a flexed elbow joint and limited motion into extension. To treat, the patient is placed in supine with 90 degrees of shoulder flexion. The patient's forearm is supported while the elbow is flexed to 90 degrees with forearm pronation. This technique is important in addressing the elbow flexion component of the typical synergic pattern of spasticity. Biceps hypertonicity and tendinitis is a common finding. In order to obtain optimal results, SCS techniques must be performed from a proximal to distal direction, starting with the shoulder girdle techniques and progressing to the elbow region techniques. Once these regions have been addressed, the manual therapist may proceed to the wrist and hand techniques.

Medial Epicondyle (MEP) Strain-Counterstrain Technique (Fig.15-13 A, B)

The tender point is present proximally on the medial epicondyle. Postural deviation consists of forearm pronation and ulnar deviation and limitation elbow supination and radial deviation. The position for intervention is supine or sitting elbow flexion with forearm pronation and wrist flexion. This technique serves to improve supination and radial deviation. It affects the pronation component of the typical synergic pattern of spasticity.

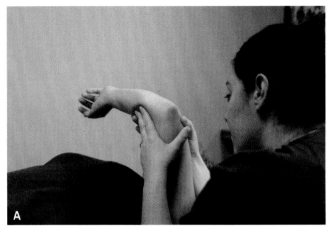

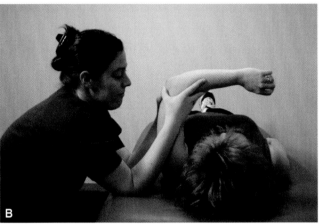

FIGURE 15–12 (A, B) Biceps (long head) strain-counterstrain technique.

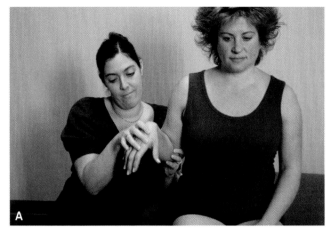

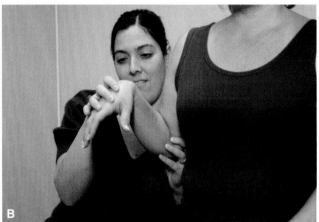

FIGURE 15–13 (A, B) Medial epicondyle (MEP) strain-counterstrain technique.

Strain-Counterstrain for Impairments of the Lower Quarter

Iliacus Strain-Counterstrain Technique (Fig.15-14 A, B)

The tender point for this muscle is found 1 inch medial and 0.5 inches caudal to the anterior superior iliac spine (ASIS) deep within the iliac fossa. Limitations in hip extension and lumbar extension are observed during examination. In supine, bilateral hips are flexed to approximately 100 degrees, and knees are flexed to 130 degrees. While ankles are crossed, both hips are externally rotated. While maintaining hip external rotation, both knees are brought toward the side of the tender point. This muscle is an important flexor of the hip, and hypertonicity of the iliacus may contribute not only to positional faults of the pelvic girdle but also, because of its relationship to lower extremity vasculature, may involve issues of claudication.

Medial Hamstrings Strain-Counterstrain Technique (Fig.15-15)

The tender point for medial hamstrings is located just proximal to the knee joint line on the medial aspect at the attachment of the medial hamstrings to the posteromedial tibia. In the presence of hypertonicity, hip flexion and lumbar flexion may exhibit restrictions. With the patient supine, the hip is flexed to 90 degrees and the knee is flexed to 100 degrees. The tibia

is externally rotated on the femur with overpressure (2 to 5 pounds of force). The medial hamstrings are among the most commonly injured muscles in the body. Hypertonicity of these muscles may predispose them to injury ranging from muscle strains, to neurological involvement of the sciatic nerve, to knee injuries caused from placing torque on the medial meniscus. This technique may be used in the prophylaxis and management of such conditions.

Piriformis Strain-Counterstrain Technique (Fig.15-16)

The tender point for the piriformis is located by first identifying the sacroiliac joint and drawing an imaginary line from this joint to the greater trochanter. At the midpoint on this line lies the tender point. Piriformis hypertonicity will lead to the primary limitation of internal rotation that is often most vividly appreciated when the hip is flexed as compared to neutral. The patient is positioned prone with the leg over the edge of the table, with the hip flexed to 120 degrees and knee flexed to 90 degrees. The hip is then brought into approximately 20 degrees of external rotation and 10 degrees of hip abduction. The piriformis muscle is commonly involved in disorders of the lumbo-pelvic-hip complex. Its insertion into the anterior aspect of the sacrum at the level of S2-S3 makes it a significant factor to consider in cases of sacroiliac joint dysfunction.

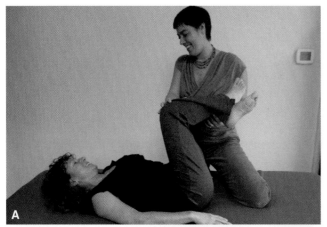

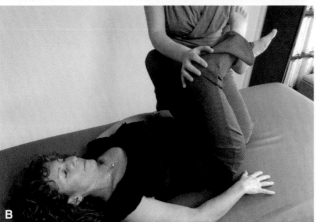

FIGURE 15–14 (A, B) Iliacus strain-counterstrain technique.

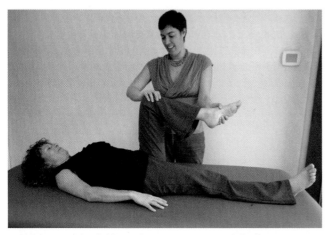

FIGURE 15–15 Medial hamstrings strain-counterstrain technique.

Hypertonicity of this muscle may limit internal rotation of the hip, which is commonly seen in individuals with low back pain, but spasm in this muscle may also produce a positional fault of the sacrum relative to the innominate bones (i.e., sacroilial fault). In most cases, the sciatic nerve exits below this muscle, and hypertonicity of this muscle may lead to a peripheral nerve entrapment syndrome known as piriformis syndrome. Therefore, by virtue of its anatomical location, hypertonicity of the piriformis may lead to impairments of the hip, sacroiliac joint, and sciatic nerve.

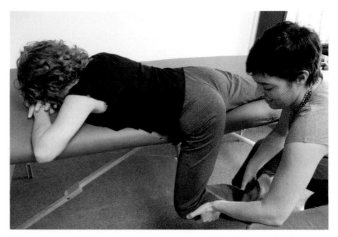

FIGURE 15–16 Piriformis strain-counterstrain technique.

Gluteus Medius Strain-Counterstrain Technique

The midaxillary line, 1 centimeter below the iliac crest, is the location for the tender point. Motion limitations typically consist of hip adduction and contralateral lumbar side bending. The treatment position consists of the patient lying prone with the hip in 10 degrees of extension, 10 degrees of abduction, and internal rotation with overpressure. The knee is kept in a relatively extended position. The gluteus medius is an important muscle for frontal plane pelvic control and stability during gait. Along with producing motion limitations, hypertonicity of this muscle may lead to less than optimal motor recruitment patterns.

Quadratus Lumborum Strain-Counterstrain Technique (Fig. 15-17)

The tender point for this muscle is found at the midaxillary line along the superior inner aspect of the iliac crest directly over the bone. Limitations are often noted in contralateral lumbar side bending when this muscle is in a state of hypertonicity. The treatment position is in side-lying on the side contralateral to the tender point with bilateral hips flexed to 45 degrees and knees flexed to 90 degrees. The feet are elevated away from the table to produce ipsilateral side bending of the trunk. This

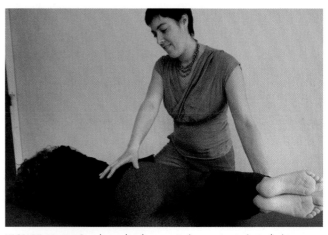

FIGURE 15–17 Quadratus lumborum strain-counterstrain technique.

muscle's anatomical location between the 12th rib and the iliac crest provides a substantial line of pull to impact both the costal cage and the pelvic girdle in cases of hypertonicity. When in spasm, the quadratus lumborum may pull the 12th rib in an anterior and caudal direction. These forces may impact the mobility of the rib cage during breathing and may produce an increase in shear at T12. In addition, the diaphragm, abdominal aorta, and esophagus may also be impacted. Hypertonicity of this muscle may also produce or occur subsequent to iliosacral positional faults such as an upslip or downslip.

Medial Gastrocnemius (EXA) Strain-Counterstrain Technique (Fig. 15-18)

The tender point for this muscle is present along the medial third of the posterior aspect of the knee joint line, approximately 1 inch in a caudal direction. Limitations in ankle dorsiflexion, which are particularly noteworthy when the knee is extended, are commonly seen when this muscle is hypertonic. The patient is placed in prone lying position with the knee flexed to 90 degrees and internal rotation of the tibia on the femur, with slight foot inversion since the gastrocnemius inserts onto the medial aspect of the calcaneus. Compression is imposed into the knee joint through the tibia, and plantar flexion is achieved with overpressure. Particularly in neurological conditions, such as in the case of an individual with hemiplegia, prolonged and premature firing of the gastrocnemius muscle may impact heel loading and weight bearing during the stance phase of gait. Hypertonicity of the gastrocnemius and loss of full dorsiflexion is also a common finding in individuals with musculoskeletal dysfunction. Ankle dorsiflexion of 10 to 15 degrees is required for normal gait, and even more range is necessary for running. If this degree of dorsiflexion is not available, then compensations will occur. Compensations such as foot abduction, overpronation, and knee flexion may lead to a reduction in movement precision and eventual impairment. This technique may be useful for individuals who are experiencing foot, ankle, or knee dysfunction related to gastrocnemius hypertonicity. Jones has carefully described a variety of techniques that may be used in the management of ankle and foot dysfunction.[7]

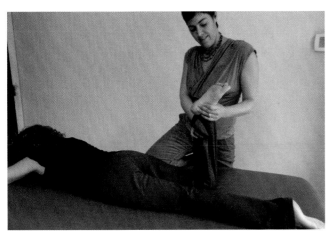

FIGURE 15–18 Medial gastrocnemius strain-counterstrain technique.

STRAIN-COUNTERSTRAIN FOR NEUROMUSCULAR IMPAIRMENT

Synergic Pattern Release and Strain-Counterstrain

Although not originally intended by Jones to address impairment in individuals with neurological conditions, the author of this chapter, with Jones's blessing, has successfully applied these concepts and techniques to this population. Each individual is believed to possess what is known as a **synergic pattern imprint**. Consider the posturing of an individual suffering from hemiplegia after a cerebrovascular accident (CVA). Immediately after the CVA, there is often a period of hypotonia, or *flaccidity*, without posturing. Within several weeks of the CVA, however, flaccidity often gives way to *spasticity*. The onset of hypertonicity, or muscle spasm, often occurs in a very characteristic pattern, which has become known as the synergic pattern.

The synergic pattern of the upper extremity most typically includes an elevated and protracted scapula, flexed, adducted, and internally rotated glenohumeral joint, flexed elbow joint, pronated forearm, flexed and ulnarly deviated wrist joint, finger flexion, and thumb flexion and adduction. The mechanisms by which SCS is able to impact both musculoskeletal, as in the case of supraspinatus tendonitis, as well as neurological conditions, such as in the case of a CVA, are not well understood. This author considers whether the internal capsule could be the home of the synergic pattern imprint. This author also hypothesizes whether the lateral reticular formation could be the site of alpha nervous system facilitation and whether the medial reticular formation could be the site of gamma nervous system inhibition. Further consideration includes whether or not the internuncial neurons in the intermediate horn of the spinal cord, between the anterior horn and the posterior horn in cross-sectional anatomy, could coordinate the alpha and gamma activity that seems to be affected by SCS. It is difficult to identify from the current best evidence if SCS exerts its influence at the spinal cord or at the supraspinal level or whether its effects are contained within the voluntary versus the autonomic nervous system. Perhaps the reason why SCS is so effective is due to the fact that a majority of individuals have some degree of protective muscle spasm and in the presence of pain begin to display some degree of synergic pattern response. Regardless of the mechanism, SCS seems to affect both the protective muscle spasm of musculoskeletal origin, as well as the synergic pattern of spasm and spasticity.

Synergic Pattern Imprint and Synergic Pattern Release: A Model for Management of Protective Muscle Spasm With SCS

When an individual experiences an upper motor neuron lesion, resting muscle tone goes unchecked by higher centers leading to **disinhibition** and hypertonicity. This process of disinhibition forms the basis for the typical spastic synergic pattern present in individuals with hemiplegia. The individual who sustains a closed head injury, with some minor exceptions, will often present with a similar pattern of spasticity. This author has observed through many years of clinical research that patterns of hypertonicity found in the mildly neurologically impaired patient are almost identical to patterns of hypertonicity present in the individual who is experiencing chronic pain. Through further investigation, it was presumed that typical synergic patterns of hypertonicity are present in all individuals, but inhibited until there is an impetus that releases this inhibition. Therefore, individuals may benefit from intervention that is designed to release the synergic pattern of hypertonicity, even in cases where symptoms have not yet emerged. The SCS techniques designed to achieve this goal are collectively known as **synergic pattern release.** Although these techniques were not originally conceived by Jones, they represent an innovative application of the principles that form the basis of SCS.

Specific synergic patterns have been identified for the upper and lower extremities, as well as the face, that result from protective spasms. The *upper extremity synergic pattern* is produced by protective spasms in the pectoralis minor, supraspinatus, subscapularis, latissimus dorsi, biceps brachii, brachioradialis, and flexors of the forearm and wrist. The *lower extremity synergic pattern* results from muscle spasms in the quadratus lumborum, piriformis, adductors, quadriceps, hamstrings, gastrocnemius, and tibialis anterior. The *face synergic pattern* is produced through spasms of the frontalis, orbicularis oculi, nasalis, masseter, temporalis, orbicularis oris, and mentalis.

DIFFERENTIATING CHARACTERISTICS

Strain-counterstrain is considered to be an OMPT approach that primarily targets impairment of soft tissue, namely muscular hypertonicity. However, as presented throughout this chapter, the existence of protective spasms within a muscle, regardless of its origin, will have a profound effect on the positional relationships of underlying joint articulations and the degree to which these associated articulations are able to move. A thorough understanding of SCS provides the manual physical therapist with an acute awareness of the relationship between soft tissue impairment and the resultant influence on joint position and movement.

SCS is performed using an indirect technique. Once muscular hypertonicity is identified, the muscle is moved away from the barrier into a position of greatest mobility and least restriction. Unlike other approaches that seek to barge through the barrier, SCS attempts to gently reduce neurological input to the hypertonic muscle by resetting the muscle spindles and therefore resetting the resting tone of the muscle. SCS is considered to be a more gentle and efficient alternative to standard stretching regimens. Placing a muscle on slack is often better tolerated by the patient with acute pain, and significantly less force is required from the therapist to achieve optimal results.

SCS differentiates itself from other OMPT approaches in its emphasis on the neuroanatomical origins of musculoskeletal impairment. All too often manual physical therapists fail to acknowledge the important role that neuroanatomical structures play in the pathogenesis of musculoskeletal dysfunction. Rather than addressing the resultant impairment (i.e., protective muscle spasm) directly, SCS seeks to eliminate the antecedent cause. In so doing, the effects of manual intervention is presumed to be longer lasting, and the potential for recidivism is therefore greatly reduced.

Similar to other approaches, the identification of active tender points serves as an important aspect of diagnosis and useful indicator of progress, and it is often the focus of intervention. However, use of the term *tender point* within this approach differs from the use of this term elsewhere. Within the SCS paradigm, tender points are considered to be present in every muscle, yet are latent and nonpathologic in the normal state. In response to dysfunction that occurs either within the hypertrophic muscle itself or within another structure that is innervated by the same neurological level, these existing tender points become symptomatic. In other approaches, tender points are the result and not the primary cause of dysfunction. They are not preexisting but rather occur in response to pathology and are absent in muscles that are in a normal state of existence.

Although manual physical therapists routinely attempt to address the issue of posture in patients with musculoskeletal dysfunction, SCS views posture as the result of underlying impairment as opposed to the cause. Within this approach, posture is used as an objective indicator of the presence of protective muscle spasm, which is presumed to have influenced normal positional relationships of the articulations over which the involved muscles lie. Posture is therefore not directly addressed but rather is expected to improve in response to the normalization of resting muscle tone. Posture is used as an indicator of impairment and as a gauge for improvement of underlying neuroanatomical influences. The frustration often experienced by manual physical therapists in correcting aberrant posture may be owing to their failure to acknowledge the neuroanatomical influences of the resultant poor postural deviations that are observed.

The emphasis on neurophysiologic origins of musculoskeletal impairment and the mandate to enact techniques that move the involved structures into positions of reduced tension are unique to this approach. When embarking on this mode of intervention, the manual physical therapist is reminded of the confluence of factors that may contribute to the emergence of muscular hypertonicity. SCS may be viewed as an effective alternative to standard interventions designed to address movement disorders that result from muscular restrictions.

CLINICAL CASE

History of Present Illness

A.W. began skiing lessons at 10 years old. After three skiing sessions, she began to complain of heel pain. She had pain at rest for more than 1 year. Her heel pain increased during standing and ambulation. She was unable to run, and she no longer was able to ski. During the year, A.W. was assessed by an orthopaedist, a physical therapist, and a podiatrist. She received mobilization techniques, after which her talocrural and subtalar joint mobility increased. She was initially issued flexible orthotics and later was fitted with a more rigid pair. In response to this course of intervention, A.W. had complete resolution of her resting pain. However, she was still unable to run, and she could not ski. After 1 year, an osteopathic physician examined and performed the gastrocnemius extended ankle (EXA) SCS technique on this patient.

When the ankle is stuck in plantar flexion, or extension, the gastrocnemius is in muscle spasm. The muscle spasm of the gastrocnemius could be the cause of heel pain, pulling on the Achilles tendon and the calcaneus. A gastrocnemius muscle spasm will cause a plantar flexion postural deviation in an orthopaedic patient. In a neurological patient, this dysfunction is referred to as an equinus posture. On standing, the tibia should be perpendicular to the floor. When there is a gastrocnemius muscle spasm, the distal tibia is in a posterior shear on the talus. During ambulation, the tibia will not glide anterior on the talus, but will be posterior on it. Furthermore, heel strike may not occur. Because of the gastrocnemius muscle spasm, the stance phase may begin with forefoot strike rather than heel strike. When forefoot strike occurs, extensor forces are transcribed up the kinetic chain. Often shin splints, chondromalacia patella, quadriceps spasm, cocontraction of the quadriceps and hamstrings, and low back pain can result. The sacrum is extended by these continual forces. L5 flexes because it moves reciprocally with S1. When L5 is flexed for long periods of time during standing and ambulation, the L5 disc may be posterior, causing discopathy.

A.W. was treated for 90 seconds on each foot with the EXA technique. The gastrocnemius muscle spasm was eliminated, as was her heel pain. Full dorsiflexion was attained with resolution of gait deviations and return of heel strike. Most importantly for the patient, she was able to return to running and skiing. Long-term follow-up has revealed no return of her symptoms.

HANDS-ON

With a partner, perform the following activities and note your findings in the table below:

1 Using the range-of-motion box in Figure 15-5, practice gently bringing your partner through each quadrant of cervical spine motion in sitting. Next, attempt to find your partner's position of comfort, the position in which the greatest degree of ease is experienced. Finally, find a tender point and gently monitor the tenderness and tone of this region while moving the patient through each quadrant of motion and while moving into the position of comfort. Are you able to perceive changes in tone and does your partner report a change in irritability as you move from one quadrant to the next? Once the position of comfort is achieved, hold that position and note any changes in the tender point.

2 Observe your partner's posture in standing and sitting and document any postural deviations. Consider what muscles may either be contributors or the result of these deviations. Discuss with your partner the insertions of these muscles and the joints over which these muscles lie. Given these postural deviations and the suspected muscles involved, consider what motions might be limited. Document your findings on the table below.

3 Confirm whether or not the suspected muscles noted above are involved in the postural deviations that you observed through palpation. Identify the location of the tender point for the involved muscle and attempt to gently identify if this tender point is active and tender. Practice palpating this tender point as you passively move the involved region and note any changes in tenderness. Attempt to palpate the tender points of other muscles that you also believe are involved

4 Perform standard stretching activities with this muscle and observe any changes in length and/or tone.

5 Based on your findings, now choose the most appropriate strain-counterstrain technique. Perform this technique on your partner. Begin by first palpating the tender point. Then passively move the body part in a triplanar fashion as needed into the maximal position of comfort. Continue to monitor the tender point for any changes in response to this technique.

6 Following performance of the technique, observe any changes in posture, tender point irritability, muscle tone, or range of motion of the involved regions.

POSTURAL DEVIATION	LENGTHENED MUSCLES	SHORTENED MUSCLES	RESTRICTED MOVEMENTS	LOCATION OF TENDER POINTS	RECOMMENDED SCS TECHNIQUE

REFERENCES

1. D'Ambrogio KJ, Roth GB. *Positional Release Therapy: Assessment and Treatment of Musculoskeletal Dysfunction.* St. Louis, MO: Mosby; 1997.
2. Hewitt J. *The Complete Yoga Book.* New York: Random House; 1977.
3. Travell JG, Simons DG. *Myofascial Pain and Dysfunction: The Trigger Point Manual.* Baltimore: Williams & Wilkins; 1983.
4. McCloskey E, Lawrence Jones DO. *Int J Applied Kinesiol Kinesiolog Med.* 2002; 13
5. Roth GB. Positional release therapy. *The Roth Institute.* http://www.rothinstitute.com/pro/SubPages/Positional-Release-Ther.html
6. Hammer W. Strain and counterstrain. *Dynamic Chiropractic.* 1994;12.
7. Jones LH, Kusunose R, Goering E. *Jones Strain-Counterstrain.* Boise, ID: Jones Strain-CounterStrain, Inc; 1995.
8. Paris SV. Manual therapy: treat function not pain. In: Michel TH, ed. *Pain.* New York: Churchill Livingstone; 1985.
9. Rosomoff HL, Fishbain DA, Goldberg M, Santana R, Steele-Rosomoff R. Physical findings in patients with chronic intractable benign pain of the neck and/or back. *Pain.* 1989;37:279.
10. Weiselfish-Giammatteo, S. *Integrative Manual Therapy for the Upper and Lower Extremities.* Vol. 2. Berkeley, CA: North Atlantic Books, 2001.
11. Korr IM. Proprioceptors and the behavior of lesioned segments. *Osteopathic Ann.* 1974;2:12.
12. Korr IM. Proprioceptors and somatic dysfunction. *J Am Osteopathic Assoc.* 1975;74:638.
13. Jacobson EC, Lockwood MD, Hoefner VC, Dickey JL, Kuchera WL. Shoulder pain and repetition strain injury to the supraspinatus muscle: etiology and manipulative treatment. *J Am Osteopath Assoc.* 1989;89:1037-1045.
14. VanBuskirk RL. Nociceptive reflexes and the somatic dysfunction: a model. *J Am Osteopath Assoc.* 1990;9:792.
15. Lewis C, Flynn T. The use of strain-counterstrain in the treatment of patients with low back pain. *J Man Manip Ther.* 2001;9:92.
16. Kam M. *Strain/Counterstrain.* Portland, OR: Sports Physical Therapy Group; 2002. http://sportstherapy.com/strain.htm.
17. Schiowitz S. Facilitated positional release. *J Am Osteopath Assoc.* 1990; 90:145-155.
18. Yunus M, Masi AT, Calabro JJ, Miller KA, Feigenbaum SL. Primary fibromyalgia (fibrositis): clinical study of 50 patients with matched normal controls. *Sem Arth Rheum.* 1981;11:151-171.
19. Cislo S, Ramirez MA, Schwartz HR. Low back pain: treatment of forward and backward sacral torsions using counterstrain technique. *J Am Osteopath Assoc.* 1991;91:255-259.
20. Schwartz HR. The use of counterstrain in an acutely ill in-hospital population. *J Am Osteopath Assoc.* 1986;86:433-442.
21. Ramirez MA, Haman J, Worth L. Low back pain: diagnosis using six newly discovered sacral tender points and treatment with counterstrain. *J Am Osteopath Assoc.* 1989;89:905-913.
22. Melzack R, Stillwell DM, Fox EJ. Trigger points and acupuncture points for pain: correlations and implications. *Pain.* 1977;3:3-23.
23. Woolbright JL. An alternative method of teaching strain/counterstrain manipulation. *J Am Osteopath Assoc.* 1991;4:370-376.

Myofascial Trigger Point Approach in Orthopaedic Manual Physical Therapy

Jan Dommerholt, PT, MPS, DPT, DAAPM and
Johnson McEvoy, PT, BSc, MSc, DPT, MISCP, MCSP

[This chapter is dedicated to the memory of David G. Simons, MD (1922–2010)]

Chapter Objectives

At the conclusion of this chapter, the reader will be able to:

- Identify the main historical events in the development of the myofascial trigger point construct and recognize the primary influences.
- Understand the main principles of muscle physiology and the motor endplate that are important in the understanding of myofascial trigger points.
- Understand the expanded integrated trigger point hypothesis.
- Understand the motor, sensory, and autonomic phenomena associated with myofascial trigger points.
- Recognize the importance of palpation and the recommended criteria for identification of myofascial trigger points with reference to current palpation reliability studies.

- Recognize the importance of the taut band, tender nodule, and referred pain pattern.
- Recognize and understand the main noninvasive interventions used to treat myofascial trigger points and the evidence available to support their use.
- Recognize and understand the invasive interventions available, with special reference to trigger point dry needling, and understand the rationale and evidence for its application.
- Recognize common perpetuating factors and formulate current management strategies.
- Learn the specific technique for palpation of myofascial trigger points.

HISTORY AND DEVELOPMENT

Drs. *Janet G. Travell* (1901–1997) and *David G. Simons* (1922–2010) brought **myofascial trigger points (MTrPs)** to the attention of clinicians and researchers worldwide,[1–3] despite the fact that MTrPs had been described as early as the 16th century[4] (Box 16-1). As a cardiologist, Travell was strongly influenced by Kellgren, who from 1938 to 1949 described, for the first time, pain referral patterns of muscles and ligaments following injection of hypertonic saline.[5–8] In 1940, Steindler introduced the term *trigger point*.[9] Travell was drawn to the potential benefits of muscular trigger point

injections and subsequently adopted the term in 1942.[10,11] In the early 1950s, Travell and Rinzler described biopsied tissues of hyperirritable trigger points in which no pathological changes were identified and concluded that these must be pathophysiological in nature.[10] They also observed that fascia referred pain in a similar fashion, leading Travell to adopt the term *myofascial pain*. In 1952, a seminal manuscript, which unknowingly mirrored the work of researchers in other continents, was published that described the pain referral patterns of 32 individual muscles.[12,13] After hearing Travell lecture on the topic, Simons became involved in

Box 16-1 EVIDENCE FOR MTrP

Many different clinicians have recognized MTrPs under different terminologies, and this has led to significant confusion in the literature. Although the earliest reference to MTrPs dates back to the 16th century, Travell and Simons are best known for developing the modern MTrP construct.

1963. Together, they coauthored several articles and book chapters, in addition to the popular and authoritative texts on this approach.[1-3] Evidence supporting the existence and management of MTrPs has grown over the past three decades, with more evidence emerging within the last decade than in the previous two combined (Table 16-1).

PHILOSOPHICAL FRAMEWORK

Although skeletal muscle comprises nearly half of the human body, there is no medical specialty that has adopted muscle as its focus organ, which prompted Simons to consider muscle as an *orphan organ*.[14] Manual physical therapy education often emphasizes joint dysfunction without careful consideration of muscle dysfunction.[13] For example, the presence of MTrPs in the extensor carpi radialis longus and brevis muscles of patients with epicondylalgia has been confirmed in randomized controlled studies, illustrating the value of addressing MTrPs as part of the standard of care in the management of musculoskeletal conditions (Fig. 16-1).[15,16]

NOTABLE QUOTABLE

"Muscle is an orphan organ."

—*David G. Simons, MD*

MTrPs may be operationally defined as *"hyperirritable spots in skeletal muscle associated with a hypersensitive palpable nodule in a taut band."*[3] MTrPs are painful upon manual compression. Based on their degree of sensitivity, they are divided into active and latent trigger points. An **active MTrP** produces symptoms, including local tenderness and pain, referral of pain or other paresthesias to a distant site, with peripheral

Table 16-1	Results of Medline Citations Search for Myofascial AND Trigger AND Point in the Last Three Decades	
DECADE	**PAPER NUMBERS**	
1997 to 2006	91	
1987 to 1996	56	
1977 to 1986	26	
Total	173	

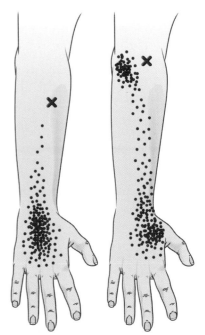

FIGURE 16–1 Referred pain patterns of MTrPs in the extensor carpi radialis brevis (left) and longus (right) muscles. (Reproduced with permission from MEDICLIP, Manual Medicine 1 & 2, Version 1.0a, 1997, Williams & Wilkins.)

and central sensitization. A **latent MTrP** produces pain only when stimulated, even though recent research has confirmed that latent MTrPs feature nociceptive qualities.[17-20] In addition to pain, MTrPs feature motor and autonomic components. Motor phenomena associated with MTrPs include disturbed motor function, muscle weakness as a result of motor inhibition, muscle stiffness, and restricted range of motion.[13] Autonomic sequelae may include, among others, vasoconstriction, vasodilatation, lacrimation, and piloerection.[21] By definition, MTrPs are located within a taut band of contractured muscle. Therefore, identification of an MTrP begins by identifying the taut band, which is best accomplished by palpating perpendicular to the muscle's fiber direction (Fig. 16-2).

Manual strumming or needling of the taut band may result in what has been termed a **local twitch response (LTR)**, which is a spinal cord reflex, leading to involuntary sudden contractions of muscle fibers within a taut band.[22-24] Identification of a taut band, MTrP, and LTR do not require a verbal response from the patient. MTrPs are present in most individuals, with the exception of infants.[3,25-28]

A survey of physician members of the ***American Pain Society*** showed overwhelming agreement that myofascial pain is a distinct clinical entity.[29] Current evidence supports the notion that active MTrPs are associated with a number of musculoskeletal pain syndromes, including migraines, tension-type headaches, craniomandibular dysfunction, epicondylalgia, low back pain, post-laminectomy syndrome, neck pain, disc pathology, carpal tunnel syndrome, osteoarthritis, radiculopathies, whiplash-associated disorders, fibromyalgia, postherpetic neuralgia, and complex regional pain syndrome, among others.[13] The integrated trigger point hypothesis as will be explained later in this chapter, is the best evidence–informed hypothesis to explain MTrP phenomena.

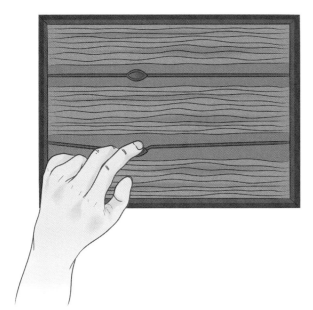

FIGURE 16–2 Palpation of a trigger point within a taut band. (Adapted from Weisskircher H-W. Head Pains Due to Myofascial Trigger Points, 1997. (CD-ROM available at www.trigger-point.com.)

MTrPs may also be associated with visceral dysfunction including endometriosis, interstitial cystitis, irritable bowel syndrome, urinary/renal and gall bladder calculosis, dysmenorrhea, prostatitis, among others.[13] Although MTrPs have been reported in the presence of acute injury,[30] they are a common and often overlooked contributor to chronic pain.[31]

MUSCLE PHYSIOLOGY
The Contractile Unit

By definition, a MTrP is located within a taut band, defined as an endogenous, localized contracture within the muscle without activation of the motor endplate.[32] In a relaxed state, there is some overlap of the actin and myosin filaments, which slide toward one another during a contraction. This process is called molecular cross-bridging (Fig. 16-3).

The efficient functioning of muscles is dependent upon the proper alignment and coordinated activity of several cytoskeletal networks, including myofibrils, the *transverse tubular (T-tubular)* system, the microtubules, and intermediate

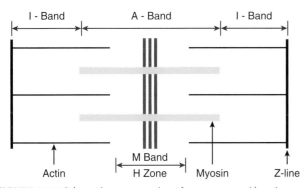

FIGURE 16–3 Schematic representation of a sarcomere with actin and myosin filaments.

filaments. The T-tubule membrane is coupled to the sarcoplasmic reticulum via the so-called *dihydropyridine* and *ryanodine receptors* (Fig. 16-4). In addition to actin and myosin, there are several other important proteins, such as titin, nebulin, and desmin, among others, which together maintain the architecture and stability of the sarcomere (Fig. 16-5).[33]

Titin is the largest known vertebrate protein, which was discovered three decades ago.[33] Titin filaments are responsible for passive tension generation when sarcomeres are stretched and provide muscle stiffness by virtue of its spring mechanism in the Iband. During sarcomere contractions, titin filaments are folded into a gel-like structure at the Z line.[34] The fourth filament system is made up by another giant protein referred to as **nebulin**, which spans the length of the actin filaments and acts as a stabilizing structure.[35] Nebulin regulates muscle contractions by inhibiting cross-bridge formation until actin is activated by Ca^{2+}.[36]

The Motor Endplate

A **motor unit** consists of all the muscle fibers innervated by the terminal branches of a single motor neuron.[37] Each branch

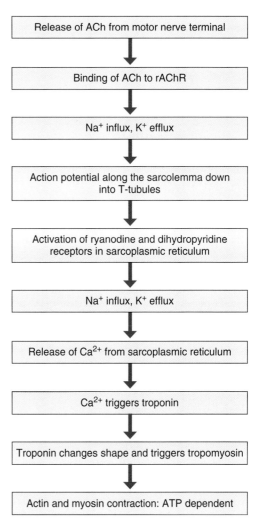

FIGURE 16–4 Sequence of events in excitation–contraction coupling.

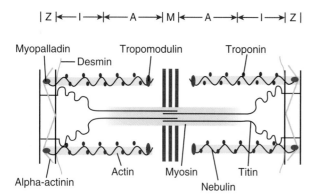

FIGURE 16–5 Expanded model of a sarcomere. (Adapted from McElhinny AS, Kazmierski ST, Labeit S, and Gregorio CC. Nebulin: the nebulous, multifunctional giant of striated muscle. *Trends in Cardiovasc Med.* 2003; 13: 195-201, with permission from Elsevier.)

terminates in multiple presynaptic boutons, each containing numerous *acetylcholine (ACh)* vesicles. The motor endplate is the polarized receptor site on the muscle fiber that synapses with the motor neuron (Fig. 16-6). The motor endplate plays a crucial role in the etiology of MTrPs.

When nerve impulses from an alpha-motor neuron reach the motor nerve terminal, voltage-gated sodium (Na^+) channels are opened. This results in depolarization of the terminal membrane. In addition, there is an influx of calcium, ACh,

and *adenosine triphosphate (ATP)* from the nerve terminal into the synaptic cleft. When ACh molecules bind to ACh receptors (nAChR) across the synaptic cleft, a Na^+ influx and potassium (K^+) efflux occurs across the muscle cell membrane. This depolarizes the postsynaptic cell and triggers a miniature endplate potential (MEPP). If sufficient MEPPs occur, they will summate to produce an action potential, which causes a release of Ca^{2+} from the sarcoplasmic reticulum. The release of Ca^{2+} triggers tropomyosin to shift its position and nebulin to allow cross-bridges to form, resulting in a muscle contraction. ACh is immediately hydrolyzed by the enzyme acetylcholinesterase (AChE) into acetate and choline. ACh release is activated by motor nerve stimulation and modulated by the concentration of AChE.

THE ETIOLOGY OF MYOFASCIAL TRIGGER POINTS

There are several possible causes of MTrPs, including eccentric contractions in unconditioned muscle, unaccustomed eccentric contractions, (sub)maximal concentric contractions, low-level contractions, uneven intramuscular pressure distributions, and direct trauma.[13,38] Eccentric training is often accompanied by cytoskeletal muscle damage. Studies have shown A band disorganization, Z line streaming, and a disruption of several cytoskeletal proteins following short bouts of eccentric exercise.[39–41] Itoh et al[42] demonstrated that eccentric exercise facilitated the formation of taut bands and MTrPs.[42] Both eccentric exercise and MTrPs have been associated with local hypoxia and impaired local circulation as evidenced by reduced oxygen saturation levels in the presence of MTrPs.[43]

Low-level contractions also result in the formation of MTrPs.[13] Treaster et al[44] found that office workers developed MTrPs after as little as 30 minutes of continuous typing.[44] In another study, piano students exhibited decreased pressure thresholds over latent MTrPs after only 20 minutes of continuous piano playing.[45] In low-level contractions, muscle fiber recruitment follows stereotypical patterns in most subjects.[46] Smaller motor units are recruited before and derecruited after larger motor units, which means that smaller type 1 fibers may be continuously activated during prolonged low-level contractions.[47,48] Several studies have suggested that such low-level contractions can lead to muscle fiber degeneration, an increase in Ca^2 release, energy depletion, and the release of various cytokines, all of which have been associated with the formation of MTrPs.[49–53] Simons and Travell considered direct trauma as an important factor in the etiology of MTrPs.[54] Several studies have explored a possible correlation between trauma, such as whiplash, and MTrPs.[55–60]

MTrPs may also occur as a result of underlying visceral disease or dysfunction. One of the first symptoms of visceral disease is hyperalgesia referred to muscle.[61,62] As early as 1952, Travell and Rinzler described MTrPs in the left pectoralis major muscle in response to an acute myocardial infarction.[12] MTrPs have also been found to be associated with prostatitis,

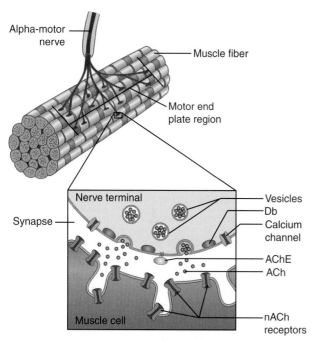

FIGURE 16–6 The motor endplate—proposed site of MTrP dysfunction. Top: The junction between an alpha-motor neuron and the muscle fiber. Bottom: Presynaptic boutons are separated from the postsynaptic muscle cell by the synaptic cleft. Within each bouton are many vesicles containing ACh, clustered around dense bars (Db). Also clustered around the Db are calcium channels. The Db is the site of ACh release into the synaptic cleft. Across the synaptic cleft, across the Db, the postsynaptic muscle cell membrane forms junctional folds that are lined with nicotinic ACh receptors (nACh). ACh released into the synaptic cleft activates nACh receptors, then is inactivated by the acetylcholinesterase enzyme (AChE).

endometriosis, and irritable bowel disease, among other diseases and dysfunctions.[61–64]

THE INTEGRATED TRIGGER POINT HYPOTHESIS

Considering the available evidence at the time, Simons and Travell proposed the **integrated trigger point hypothesis (IH)** in 1999 to explain the observed MTrP phenomena and to provide a model that could serve as the basis for future research.[3] The IH is a work in progress and has been reviewed and modified several times since its inception.[13,38,65–67]

The initial hypothesis was formulated in 1981 and became known as the **energy crisis hypothesis.**[54] This concept was based on the notion that direct trauma and subsequent damage to the sarcoplasmic reticulum or the muscle cell membrane would lead to an increase in Ca^{2+} concentration, an activation of actin and myosin, a relative shortage of ATP, and an impaired calcium pump. Under normal physiologic conditions, the calcium pump is responsible for returning intracellular Ca^{2+} to the sarcoplasmic reticulum against a concentration gradient, which requires a functional energy supply.

A 1993 study reported spontaneous electrical activity in MTrPs, which sparked a renewed consideration of the motor endplate in the etiology of MTrPs.[68] Simons realized that the observed electrical activity was in fact endplate noise, related to an excess of ACh at the motor endplate.[69] Numerous studies have now supported this new hypothesis in rabbit, human, and equine models.[67–83]

There are several mechanisms that can lead to excessive ACh, including AChE insufficiency, an acidic pH, hypoxia, a lack of ATP, certain genetic mutations, and a variety of chemicals, and increased sensitivity of the nAChRs.[38,66,84] Hypoxia leads to an acidic milieu, muscle damage, and an excessive local release of multiple nociceptive substances, including calcitonin gene-related peptide, bradykinin, and substance P.[85]

Motor Phenomena

MTrPs possess motor, sensory, and autonomic phenomena. From the motor perspective, excessive ACh will affect voltage-gated sodium channels of the sarcoplasmic reticulum and continuously increase intracellular Ca^2 levels, resulting in persistent contractures. In MTrPs, the myosin filaments may be limited by titins at the Z line, which prevent myosin from detaching, thereby maintaining the contractures and compromising local blood flow and oxygen supply.[86] Hypoxia may also trigger ACh release at the motor endplate, as has been observed in rodents.[84] There is evidence that muscle hypertonicity, as seen in MTrPs, may facilitate the excessive release of ACh.[87,88] The sequence of events leading to the formation and maintenance of MTrPs is summarized in Figure 16-7.

McPartland and Simons[66] emphasized that reduced oxygen levels combined with an increased metabolic demand result in a shortage of ATP. A decrease in ATP leads to increased ACh

and Ca^{2+} release which reinforces contractures.[66] Persistent contractures have been confirmed in several studies.[89–91]

In a study of muscle activation patterns, Lucas et al[92] demonstrated that subjects with latent MTrPs had altered shoulder abduction patterns when compared to healthy subjects.[92] Headley[93] showed that MTrPs in one muscle may actually inhibit other muscles, especially those within the area of referred pain (Figs. 16-8, 16-9).[93] It is noteworthy, that Hsieh et al[94] were able to inactivate an MTrP in the anterior deltoid by treating the MTrP in the infraspinatus.[94] Carlson eliminated pain of the masseter by treating MTrPs in the trapezius (Fig. 16-10).[95]

Sensory Phenomena

A reduction in pain threshold over active MTrPs occur within the muscle as well as the overlying cutaneous and subcutaneous tissues. In contrast, latent MTrPs do not involve cutaneous tissues.[96–98] Shah et al[99,100] found increased concentrations of bradykinin, calcitonin gene-related peptide, substance P, tumor necrosis factor-α , interleukin-1β, serotonin, and norepinephrine in the immediate milieu of active MTrPs.[99,100]

Many of these substances are well-known stimulants for various muscle nociceptive nerve endings, especially when they are present in combination.[99–102] There are numerous feedback cycles between these chemicals,[103] resulting in a poorly defined aching-type pain, which is so characteristic of MTrPs. The release of allogeneic substances may lower the tissue pH. Shah et al[99,100,104] confirmed that active MTrPs consistently have a lower pH, which may decrease the effectiveness of AChE and initiate muscle pain, allodynia, and hyperalgesia through activation of acid-sensing ion channels.[99,100,104]

Pain of muscular origin activates unique cortical structures.[105] Recent studies by Niddam et al[106,107] demonstrated that pain from MTrPs is at least partially processed at a supraspinal level, particularly in the periaqueductal gray.[106,107] Another unique feature of muscle pain is that activation of muscle nociceptors induce neuroplastic changes in the dorsal horn neurons, which has implications for referred pain from MTrPs.[108] The afferent input can engage inactive neurons in the dorsal horn in as many as 10 spinal levels, suggesting that MTrPs may refer pain extrasegmentally.[109,110,111]

In chronic myofascial pain, individuals often experience a measurable alteration in their perception of pain.[112] Although there is evidence that ongoing peripheral input is required to maintain a state of central hypersensitivity,[113] mechanical hyperalgesia may persist even after the peripheral nociceptive input has been discontinued.[114] Vecchiet and Giamberadino[115] encountered peripheral changes in the viscera that were able to maintain the state of hyperexcitability.[115]

MTrPs may trigger central sensitization as seen in a variety of conditions. Several studies have shown that patients presenting with such conditions as tension-type headaches, migraines, or osteoarthritis have more clinically relevant MTrPs than healthy controls.[116–119] Latent MTrPs also feature nociceptive qualities and can contribute to sensitization.[17–20] Differentiation between active and latent MTrPs depend on the degree

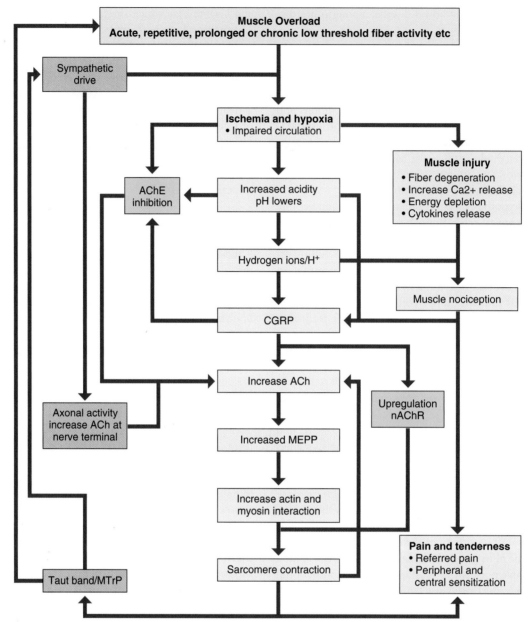

FIGURE 16-7 Muscle overload leading to the formation and maintenance of MTrPs. MEPP, miniature endplate potential; MTrP, myofascial trigger point.

of sensitization. These concepts were recently applied to an updated pain model for tension-type headache, but may be applied to other pain conditions as well.[120,121]

Autonomic Phenomena

Few researchers have focused on the autonomic features of MTrPs. Ge et al[21] provided experimental evidence of sympathetic facilitation from mechanical sensitization of MTrPs.[21] Noradrenaline was shown to increase the amplitude and duration of miniature endplate potentials of frog leg motor endplates, which may be relevant for the MTrP.[122] After exposing subjects with MTrPs in the upper trapezius muscle to stressful tasks, EMG activity increased in the MTrPs, but not in adjacent control points in the same

muscle. The effects were reversible by autogenic relaxation and by the administration of the sympathetic blocking agent, phentolamine.[76,123–125] Gerwin et al[38] speculated that the presence of alpha and beta adrenergic receptors at the motor endplate may provide a possible mechanism for autonomic interactions.[38] Stimulation of these receptors increased the release of ACh in the phrenic nerve of a rodent.[126] McPartland and Simons[66] suggested that visceral autonomic afferent input may also trigger MTrPs by viscerosomatic reflexes.[66]

PRINCIPLES OF EXAMINATION

Currently, there is no diagnostic gold standard for the identification of MTrPs (Box 16-2). Examination of MTrPs relies

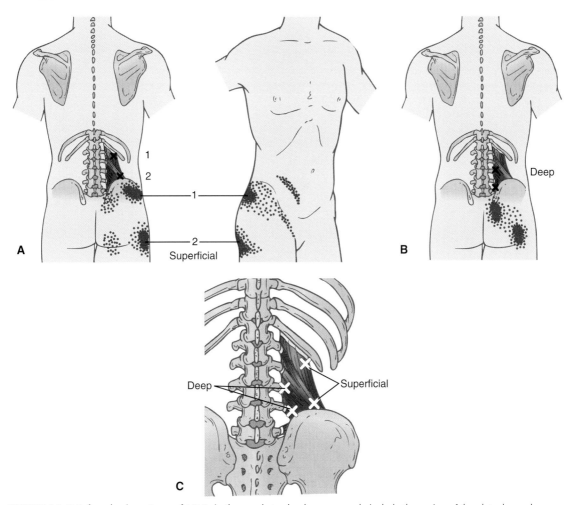

FIGURE 16–8 Referred pain patterns of MTrPs in the quadratus lumborum muscle include the region of the gluteal muscles. **A.** Referred pain patterns from superficial MTrPs. **B.** Referred pain patterns from deep MTrPs. **C.** Location of superficial and deep MTrPs within the quadratus lumborum muscle. (Reproduced with permission from MEDICLIP, Manual Medicine 1 & 2, Version 1.0a, 1997, Williams & Wilkins.)

on palpation of those muscles suspected of harboring clinically relevant MTrPs. An older pilot study found diagnostic ultrasound to be unreliable in identifying MTrPs,[127] although it was possible to visualize LTRs with needle penetration.[128] More recently, investigators were able to visualize both the taut band and the actual MTrP using high-resolution ultrasound equipment.[126] The taut band can also be visualized with magnetic resonance imaging elastography.[130,131] Pressure algometry using a pressure threshold meter is valid and reproducible for testing muscle tenderness against standard values.[132] Although tenderness is sine qua non of MTrPs, tenderness alone is not diagnostic. A piezoelectric and an electro-hydraulic shockwave emitter were tested on 114 subjects with chronic sciatic-type pain, with reproduction of pain in all cases.[133] In a prospective, randomized study of athletes with shoulder pain, electrocorporeal shockwave therapy improved isokinetic force, reduced pain, and improved overall performance.[134]

Palpation is the primary clinical tool for examination of MTrPs (Box 16-3). Criteria have been recommended based upon research and clinical expertise.[3,135] The first interrater

reliability palpation studies did not appear until 1992, with few studies presented since that time.[136] Only one study has been published on intrarater reliability.[137] Several studies have supported reliability of the combined features of spot tenderness and a taut band, which has been considered the minimum criterion for identification of an MTrP (active or latent).[13] Identification of a taut band upon physical examination is commonly used to distinguish an MTrP from other causes of muscle pain such as fibromyalgia and drug-induced myalgia.

The LTR reproduced by snapping palpation of the muscle can be difficult to elicit and has been shown to be generally unreliable. It is considered more confirmatory to the clinical assessment.[135] It is evident that the ability to accurately agree dichotomously on the presence or absence of MTrPs is directly linked to the expertise and training of the testing clinicians (Table 16-2, Box 16-4). Accurate diagnosis requires knowledge of muscle referral patterns and a comprehensive clinical history and movement analysis.[138]

As the primary tool used in the assessment of MTrPs, an astute and thorough process of palpation is critical.[3,13]

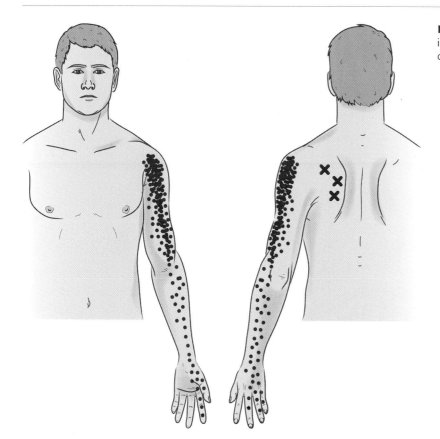

FIGURE 16–9 Referred pain patterns of MTrPs in the infraspinatus muscle include the region of the anterior deltoid muscle.

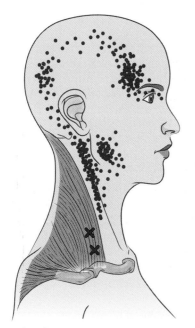

FIGURE 16–10 Referred pain patterns of MTrPs in the upper trapezius muscle include the region of the masseter muscle. (Adapted from MEDICLIP, Manual Medicine 1 & 2, Version 1.0a, 1997, Williams & Wilkins.)

Box 16-2 Quick Notes! CHARACTERISTICS OF MTrPs

- MTrPs have motor, sensory, and autonomic features.
- Latent MTrPs can alter normal movement activation patterns.
- The chemical milieu of active MTrPs is distinctly different from normal muscle tissue.
- MTrPs can contribute to local pain, referred pain, and trigger peripheral and central sensitization.

Box 16-3 IDENTIFYING AN MTrP

At minimum, the criterion for identification of an MTrP is a tender nodule on a taut band. When patient-recognized pain is produced, this is considered the criterion for an active MTrP.

Flat palpation consists of placing finger or thumb pressure perpendicular to the muscle fibers while compressing them against underlying tissue or bone (Fig. 16-11). **Pincer palpation** includes use of a pincer grip where muscle fibers are placed between the clinician's fingers and thumb and rolled in a direction that is perpendicular to the muscle fibers (Fig. 16-12).

Contracting the muscle initially to locate the muscle's fiber direction may be helpful. In cases of restricted muscle, it may need to be placed in a relaxed position prior to palpation. In overstretched muscle, a prestretch may help identify taut bands. Once the taut band is identified, the clinician feels along the taut band to identify a specific area of discrete tenderness, nodular hardening, and exquisite pain, which is

Table 16–2 Conclusions of MTrP Palpation Interrater Reliability Studies Based on Expertise and Pretraining

STUDY	EXPERT / NON-EXPERT	HANDS ON PRE-TRAINING	RELIABILITY CONCLUSIONS
Wolfe et al 1992[1]	Expert	None	Unsupported
Nice et al 1992[2]	Expert—various	None	Unsupported
Njoo and Van der Does 1994[3]	Expert/nonexpert	Yes	Good for localized tenderness with patient's recognition and jump sign
Gerwin et al 1997[4]	Expert	Yes	Supported
Lew and Story 1997[5]	Expert	None	Unsupported
Hsieh et al 2000[6]	Nonexpert	Yes	Unsupported
Sciotti 2002[7]	Expert	Yes	Supported
Bron et al 2007[8]	Expert	Yes	Supported
Donnelly and Leigh	Nonexpert	Yes	Supported

1. Wolfe F, et al. The fibromyalgia and myofascial pain syndromes: a preliminary study of tender points and trigger points in persons with fibromyalgia, myofascial pain syndrome and no disease. *J. Rheumatol.* 1992;(19): 944–951.
2. Nice DA, Riddle DL, Lamb RL, Mayhew TP, Rucker K. Intertester reliability of judgments of the presence of trigger points in patients with low back pain. *Arch Phys Med Rehabil.* 1992;73 (10):893-8.
3. Njoo, K and Van der Does E. The occurrence and inter-rater reliability of myofascial trigger points in the quadratus lumborum and gluteus medius: a prospective study in non-specific low back pain patients and controls in general practice. *Pain.* 1994; (58) 317–323.
4. Gerwin RD, et al. Interrater reliability in myofascial trigger point examination. *Pain.* 1997;69:65-73.
5. Lew PC, Lewis J, Story I. Inter-therapist reliability in locating latent myofascial trigger points using palpation. *Manual Ther.* 1997;2(2):87-90.
6. Hsieh CJ, Hong C, Adams AH, Platt KJ, Danielson CD, Hoehler FK, Tobis JS. Interexaminer reliability of the palpation of trigger points in the trunk and lower limb muscles. *Arch Phys Med Rehabil.* 2000;81(3):258-64.
7. Sciotti VM Audio lectures. Myofascial pain syndrome and trigger points: a clinical and scientific overview. DC Tracts. 2002;14(4):2,17-8.
8. Bron C; Franssen J; Wensing M; Oostendorp RAB. Interrater reliability of palpation of myofascial trigger points in three shoulder muscles. *J Manual Manipulative Ther.* 2007;15(4): 203-15.

Box 16-4 Quick Notes! CONSIDERATIONS FOR MTrP

- Interrater reliability studies suggest that clinicians should be both expert and trained in order to reliably identify MTrPs, and this has implications for physical therapy undergraduate and postgraduate education programs.
- Consider the integrated trigger point hypothesis for clinical reasoning purposes when choosing treatments for MTrPs.

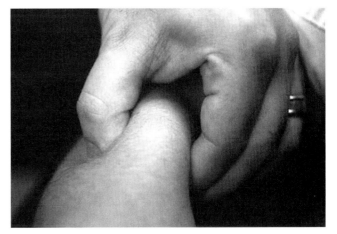

FIGURE 16–12 Pincher palpation.

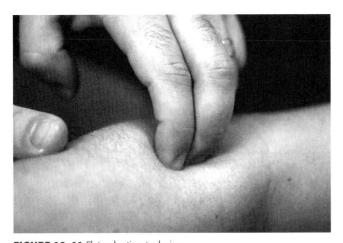

FIGURE 16–11 Flat palpation technique.

considered to be the MTrP. Confirmation of an active MTrP is achieved by placing adequate pressure upon the MTrP for 10 to 15 seconds, at which time referred pain is elicited. If the patient does not recognize the evoked pain, the MTrP would be considered a latent MTrP. It is important for the clinician to palpate the full extent of the muscle and avoid preconceived expectations based on referral diagrams. Most MTrPs are located near motor endplates within the muscle belly. *The minimum criterion for identification of an active trigger point is the presence of a taut band with exquisite point tenderness that is recognized by the patient.*

PRINCIPLES OF INTERVENTION

Traditionally, intervention options for MTrPs have been divided into noninvasive manually based, and modality-based techniques, and invasive injection and dry needling techniques (Fig. 16-13). Other intervention strategies include medical, pharmacological, or psychological therapies, which are outside of the purview of this chapter. Orthopaedic manual physical therapy (OMPT) techniques may be considered relatively invasive or noninvasive.[13,139] Invasive OMPT is referred to as **intramuscular manual therapy** when performed by physical therapists.

Noninvasive OMPT for Myofascial Trigger Points

Several reviews were published in 2005 and 2006, including a Cochrane review of acupuncture and dry needling for low back pain.[140–148] Rickards's[143,149] systematic reviews are the most complete and up-to-date reviews of noninvasive interventions.[143,149] Rickards identified five categories of noninvasive treatments, including manual therapy, laser therapy, electrotherapy, ultrasound, and magnet therapy.[143] Several manual therapies have been suggested in the literature, including massage trigger point therapy release (TPTR), formerly known as ischemic compression (IC) myofascial release, spray and stretch, postisometric relaxation, muscle energy techniques, neuromuscular therapy, manual medicine, occipital release, active head retraction and retraction extension, strain-counterstrain, trigger point dry needling, and body flexibility and stretching techniques performed by the patient.[149] Trigger point therapy release, or ischemic compression, has been considered the cornerstone of manual therapy for MTrPs.[1,3] Although unvalidated, this intervention

is believed to exert its effect by compressing the sarcomeres by direct pressure in a vertical, perpendicular manner, which leads to an elongation of the sarcomeres in a horizontal direction.[150] It is conceivable that there may also be a neural reflex component.

Massage and exercise reduced the number and intensity of MTrPs, but the overall effect on neck and shoulder pain was weak.[151] Hong and colleagues[152] reported that deep tissue massage was more effective on the immediate effects of PPT than spray and stretch and other therapies.[152] A hot pack, active range-of-motion exercises, interferential therapy, and myofascial release were most effective immediately after treatment.[153] Transverse friction massage, as described by Cyriax, was shown to be as effective as TPTR.[154] Traditional Thai massage and stretching had effects on MTrP low back pain similar to Swedish massage and stretching.[155] A recent pilot study showed that manual MTrP therapy administered by experienced massage therapists not only reduced pain, but also had a positive effect on psychological stress levels.[156]

Spray and stretch was originally used by Travell to release MTrPs. The technique includes use of a vapocoolant spray, such as ethyl chloride or fluorimethane, which is used over the muscle and into the referral zone of the MTrP. The skin cooling acts as a distraction for the stretch.[3] Because of its detrimental environmental effects, fluorimethane has been replaced.[157,158] The new spray-and-stretch product contains hydrofluorocarbons with a carbon dioxide equivalent of 1,300 or a 1,300 times greater greenhouse effect than carbon dioxide.

As an alternative, clinicians may use an ice cup and apply a few quick strokes directly over the muscle and area of referred pain. During the 1980s, Swiss physician Dejung[159] developed a comprehensive treatment strategy, which includes a combination of four effective manual therapy techniques.[159] The effectiveness of Dejung's treatment protocol was established in a nonblinded study of 83 subjects.[160] Fernández-de-las-Peñas et al[154] concluded that different compression techniques were equally effective in releasing MTrPs.[154]

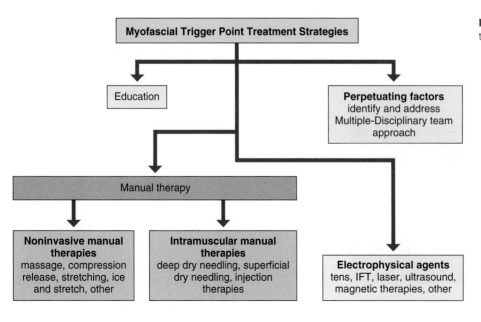

FIGURE 16–13 Myofascial trigger point treatment strategies.

Intramuscular Manual Therapy (Trigger Point Dry Needling)

Intramuscular manual therapy (IMT), or trigger point dry needling, is a relatively new form of manual therapy, which has more recently begun to gain recognition in the United States.[139,161,162] In 2009, the ***American Physical Therapy Association (APTA)*** and the ***American Academy of Orthopaedic Manual Physical Therapists (AAOMPT)*** concluded that trigger point dry needling is within the scope of physical therapist practice. Physical therapy associations in Australia, Norway, the Netherlands, South Africa, and Ireland, among others, have preceded America in reaching this same conclusion. The APTA prefers the term *intramuscular manual therapy* as used in this chapter. Despite considerable opposition by some state boards and professional organizations, an increasing number of state boards have confirmed that IMT is an integral part of modern physical therapy practice.[161,162]

Trigger point injections are generally outside the scope of physical therapy practice; therefore, this review is limited to IMT (Figs. 16-14, 16-15). Maryland was the first U.S. jurisdiction in which a board of physical therapy examiners ruled that physical therapists are permitted to perform trigger point injections.[161] The evidence suggests that there are no significant advantages of trigger point injections over IMT.[163,164] Other needling approaches, such as acupuncture, are outside the scope of physical therapy practice. These approaches are often based on different philosophical principles and generally do not target MTrPs, specifically.[139]

IMT can be divided into superficial and deep IMT. Superficial IMT was developed by Baldry,[4] who recommends inserting the needle into the tissues overlying a MTrP to a depth of 5 to 10 mm for 30 seconds.[4] If there is any residual pain, the needle is once more placed in the same region for another 2 to 3 minutes. The effects of superficial IMT are often attributed to stimulation of A-delta nerve fibers, which would activate enkephalinergic, serotonergic, and noradrenergic inhibitory systems.[4] It is, however, unlikely that superficial IMT stimulates A-delta

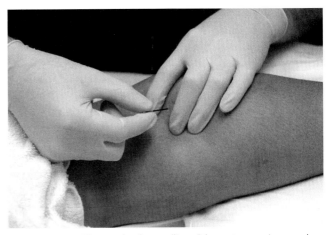

FIGURE 16–15 Trigger point dry needling of the gastrocnemius muscle.

fibers. Type I A-delta fibers respond only to noxious mechanical stimuli and Type II fibers respond to thermal stimuli.[165] Superficial IMT is a painless procedure, and there is neither noxious mechanical or thermal stimulation.[139] It is more likely that the needle causes mechanical signaling of connective tissue fibroblasts, which can lead to mechanoreceptor and nociceptor stimulation, changes in the cytoskeleton, cell contraction, variations in gene expression and extracellular matrix composition, and eventually to neuromodulation and reduction of pain.[166,167] Research on rodents suggested that the reduction of pain with superficial IMT may be due to a release of oxytocin.[168] Despite positive outcomes, the exact mechanisms of superficial IMT are unknown.[139]

With deep IMT, the needle is placed directly into the MTrP with the objective of eliciting LTRs. These involuntary spinal reflex contractions are unique to MTrP and their taut bands.[3,169] When LTRs are elicited with a monopolar Teflon-coated electromyography needle, they appear as high-amplitude polyphasic electromyographic discharges.[22] While eliciting LTRs manually can be quite difficult, when using deep IMT it is essential.[169] The evocation of a local twitch response during dry needling is linked to the effectiveness of the technique.

Shah et al[99,100] demonstrated that the concentration of nociceptive chemicals in the direct milieu of active MTrPs immediately decreased when LTRs were elicited, which illustrates that LTRs may reduce pain by normalizing the chemical environment of active MTrPs.[99,100] Chen et al[170] found that LTRs diminished the degree of endplate noise associated with MTrPs.[170] Deep IMT can easily be combined with electrotherapy, which eliminates any complications related to overcoming skin resistance and is also more effective than other applications of electrotherapy, such as N-C protein transcutaneous electrical nerve stimulation (TENS).

Deep IMT commonly triggers patients' referred pain patterns and therefore their primary pain complaint. For example, deep IMT of MTrPs in the upper trapezius or sternocleidomastoid muscles may trigger the patient's migraine or tension-type headache.[116] Deep IMT of MTrPs in the

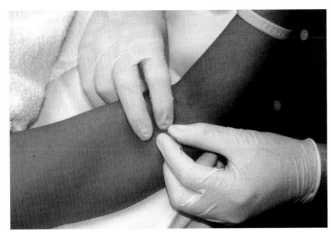

FIGURE 16–14 Trigger point dry needling of the brachialis muscle.

teres minor muscle or gluteus minimus muscle may trigger pain resembling a C8 or L5 radiculopathy, respectively.[171,172] In this fashion, IMT can assist in the differential diagnostic process. If referred pain is provoked with deep IMT, it is likely that the symptoms are primarily myofascial in nature and not neurogenic or arthrogenic.

IMT requires training and excellent palpation skills. Clinicians need to develop not only a high degree of kinesthetic perception, which allows the needle to be used as a palpation tool, but also be able to create a three-dimensional image of the pathway the needle takes within the patient's body. In many instances, patients feel an immediate relaxation of tight and contracted muscle fibers. Needling does cause some temporary postneedling soreness, which is usually an aching and poorly localized pain sensation. There are several studies and case reports that have shown that deep IMT is an effective treatment approach.[139]

Modality-Based Interventions

Several studies have shown a positive effect of laser on MTrPs.[149] TENS is the most commonly tested electrotherapy modality and is more effective in pain reduction than other forms of electrotherapy.[173,174] High-frequency/high-intensity TENS of 100 Hz with 250 µs stimulation was the most effective of four tested TENS combinations in reducing myofascial pain, but TENS had no effect on MTrP sensitivity.[175] Based on the available evidence, it is difficult to draw any conclusions on the use of TENS for MTrPs beyond the immediate short-term effects.

The potential mechanism of therapeutic ultrasound (US) is unknown. To treat MTrPs, Majlesi and Unalan[176] proposed a high-power pain threshold (HPPT) static US technique using continuous US, ramped gradually to the patient's maximum pain level, held for 4 to 5 seconds, and reduced by 50% for 15 seconds.[176] This was repeated three times at each treatment, and the HPPT technique was tested against conventional US (1.5 w/cm², continuous, 5 minutes) and results suggested that HPPT resolved active MTrPs more rapidly than did conventional treatment.[176] Trials investigating US for trapezius MTrPs yielded conflicting results. Some high-quality studies showed no effect on pain reduction,[151] while other very poor quality papers reported significantly improved pain intensity, MTrP pressure threshold, and cervical range of motion.[177] US can produce a short-term effect on MTrPs in a particular neurological segment, but not in other segments.[178] Based on current evidence, conventional US is not recommended for the management of MTrPs.

PREDISPOSING, PRECIPITATING, AND PERPETUATING FACTORS

There are five different categories of predisposing, precipitating, and perpetuating factors, which include mechanical, physiologic, medical, metabolic, and psychological categories. Any division is somewhat arbitrary as many perpetuating factors have overlapping features (Fig. 16-16).

Mechanical Precipitating Factors

Physical therapists are generally familiar with mechanical perpetuating factors. For example, patients with persistent migraine or tension-type headaches may have contributing forward head postures, which when uncorrected, are likely to

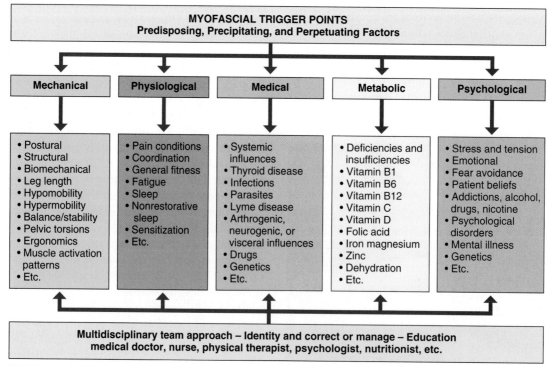

FIGURE 16–16 Overview of common predisposing, precipitating, and perpetuating factors.

trigger both the headaches and MTrPs.[179-181] Correction of postural faults is critical in the treatment of individuals with MTrPs. The initial physical therapy examination may reveal that a patient has cervical spine dysfunction with hypomobile segments in addition to MTrPs in the neck and shoulder muscles. The treatment plan should include treatment strategies to correct the mechanical spine dysfunction and to release the MTrPs. Other patients may have structural misalignments, such as a scoliosis with a leg-length discrepancy, pelvic torsion, and a loss of lumbar lordosis, which may predispose them to muscle imbalances and the recurrent development of active MTrPs.[182] Some patients with either local or systemic hypermobility may pose significant challenges.

The combination of prolonged static postures, awkward postures, excessive force, and repetitive activity are common risk factors for the development of MTrPs. Musicians are especially predisposed to developing MTrPs because of the need to assume constrained positions for prolonged periods of time while performing highly repetitive motions.[183,184] Office workers[185] and computer operators with bifocal glasses are likely to develop MTrPs in the posterior neck muscles from maintaining a posteriorly rotated position for prolonged periods. After as little as 30 minutes of continuous typing, the first signs of MTrPs appear.[44] Many health-care providers are prone to develop myalgia and MTrPs owing to prolonged static postures, overuse, poor lifting mechanics, and other stressors. Nurses, dentists, dental hygienists, and physical therapists are also at risk, and workplace and habit modification is often needed.[186-188]

Physiological Precipitating Factors

A common perpetuating factor in the etiology of musculoskeletal pain is poor sleep hygiene, irrespective of whether the sleep disturbance is caused by pain or by other factors.[189] Physical therapists should consider modifications to their standard sleeping postures for those with disturbed sleep patterns.[182]

Medical Precipitating Factors

MTrPs can be secondary to other medical diagnoses of which the patient may not always be aware. Conditions such as hypothyroidism, systemic lupus erythematosus, Lyme disease, babesiosis, ehrlichiosis, *Candida albicans* infections, myoadenylate deaminase deficiency, herpes zoster, complex regional pain syndrome, hypoglycemia, fascioliasis, amebiasis, and giardia, and most visceral diseases may produce and maintain MTrPs.[138] Samuel et al[189] confirmed that MTrPs are common with lumbar disc lesions.[189] Crotti et al[190] emphasized the role of MTrPs in thoracic outlet syndrome.[190] A more recent study confirmed that active MTrPs are nearly always present in patients diagnosed with fibromyalgia.[191]

Any of the so-called statin drugs, which lower cholesterol levels, can cause myalgia. Pain symptoms typically occur within a few weeks after starting the medication, or after increasing the dose. In a recent study, Arendt-Nielsen et al[192] observed

that glucosamine can actually induce muscle pain.[192] As physical therapy continues to move toward autonomous practice, therapists must be part of the diagnostic process and routinely screen for the presence of medical pathology.[13]

Metabolic/Nutritional Precipitating Factors

Metabolic or nutritional deficiencies are commonly linked to MTrPs. Relevant metabolic deficiencies include vitamin B_1, B_6, B_{12}, folic acid, vitamin C, vitamin D, iron, magnesium, and zinc, among others. Nutritional or metabolic insufficiencies are frequently overlooked and not necessarily considered clinically relevant by physicians unfamiliar with MTrPs and chronic pain conditions. Consistent with the integrated trigger point hypothesis, any inadequacy that interferes with the energy supply of muscle is likely to aggravate MTrPs. Although a detailed description of pertinent metabolic deficiencies is beyond the scope of this chapter, physical therapists should be familiar with the literature on the subject.[193]

Vitamin B_{12} deficiencies are very common and are thought to affect as many as 15% to 20% of the elderly and individuals with chronic MTrPs.[194,195] Patients with serum levels of vitamin B_{12} as high as 350 pg/mL may be clinically symptomatic. B_{12} deficiencies can result in cognitive dysfunction, degeneration of the spinal cord, peripheral neuropathy, and widespread myalgia, which may be misdiagnosed as fibromyalgia. A vitamin B_{12} metabolic deficiency may or may not be manifested by elevated serum or urine methylmalonic acid or homocysteine.[196,197] Close to 90% of patients with chronic musculoskeletal pain may have vitamin D deficienc.[193] Vitamin D levels are identified by measuring 25-OH vitamin D levels. Although levels above 20 ng/mL are generally considered normal, Dommerholt and Gerwin[193] have suggested that levels below 34 ng/mL may represent insufficiencies.[193]

Psychological Precipitating Factors

Many patients with persistent pain complaints, including MTrP pain, suffer from depression, anxiety, anger, feelings of hopelessness, fear, and avoidance, which can trigger and maintain pain.[198-200] Psychological stress has been shown to activate MTrPs with objective electromyographic verification, while autogenic relaxation reduces the electromyographic activity.[146,147]

SUMMARY AND CONCLUSIONS

Evidence now exists to support the acknowledgment of MTrPs as a viable contributor to pain and disability. Pioneering physicians such as Janet Travell and David Simons learned much about MTrPs through empirical research. Current evidence has almost unanimously concluded that MTrPs are a pathological condition, which may perpetuate chronic pain conditions, alter muscle activation patterns, change movement sequences, and interfere with progress. Learning how to identify MTrPs is an acquired skill and takes considerable practice through astute observation and palpation. Manual physical therapy is a critical component in the management of MTrPs and may be either invasive or noninvasive. Trigger point dry needling, or intramuscular manual therapy, is a very effective manual physical therapy technique, and a greater consideration of these procedures is warranted.

The integrated trigger point hypothesis presented in this chapter forms the foundation for basic research, clinical studies, and management. While several unexplored areas still exist, there is substantial evidence for the incorporation of MTrP management into the practice of OMPT. As the field is moving from art to evidence, the time has come to recognize the approach presented in this chapter and to expand the art of evidence-informed orthopaedic manual physical therapy.

CLINICAL CASE

Present Chief Complaint

MC is a 28-year-old male rugby player who presents with pain over the right hamstring on the posterior aspect of the thigh. In addition, he reports a feeling of tension in the hamstring. He denies pain or problems elsewhere. The complaint is intermittent and mild now, but was moderate to severe initially. The complaint is aggravated with speed, running at greater than 75% of his maximum speed, and most notable when changing direction. Jogging is generally well tolerated, but if he jogs longer than 20 minutes he feels some soreness. Improvement is noted in response to a hot bath and if he does not train. He feels better if he uses a stationary bike. The use of toe clips on the bike makes no impact. Sometimes he can feel a mild ache if he sits or drives for periods of time longer than 1.5 hours. Initially, he responded well to nonsteroidal anti-inflammatory medications (NSAIDs) that were prescribed by the team medical doctor, but now he gets no relief and they upset his stomach. If he aggravates the complaint with running, then his symptoms remain elevated for approximately 24 hours. Overall, he reports improvement, however, his symptoms still affect his ability to return to full sport participation. He has been training and can manage at a modified pace. He tried to play a match 1 week ago but retired after 15 minutes due to pain.

History of Present Illness

The patient reports that 60 minutes into a rugby match 12 weeks ago he felt a sudden onset of pain and spasm in the back of his right thigh. This was in open play and happened suddenly, with no warning. He went to the ground and was taken off the pitch with a two-person assist. He found it hard to walk, but within 1 hour he could manage to limp unaided, with pain in the posterior thigh. He was diagnosed with a hamstring tear (grade II) by the team doctor and given NSAIDs. For the next 2 days he felt very sore, but he then started to feel significantly better; within 3 days the limp was almost gone. He was seen by a physical therapist who treated him with heat, massage to the hamstring, Cyriax frictions, electrotherapies, and stretching/strengthening. He was able to go back to modified training 2 weeks after the injury, but he has struggled to get back to full training. He then rested for a month, but when he resumed activity, the problem returned.

Past Medical History

A grade II lateral ligament ankle sprain was diagnosed 6 months ago from an inversion injury. He was able to resume full sport participation in 6 weeks.

Physical Examination

Observation: In stance, symmetry is observed with structural palpation of the iliac crests, posterior superior iliac spine, anterior superior iliac spine, and greater trochanters. There is a mild increase in lumbar lordosis with an anterior pelvic rotation, and the presence of a mild Janda's double-crossed syndrome. Mild pes planus is noted but no genu varum or valgum is present.

Active Range of Motion: Lumbar spine is within normal limits for flexion and extension—without pain provocation. Repeated movements for flexion and extension are negative. Extension and rotation testing is negative. Laslett's sacroiliac joint screening tests are negative. Hips, knees, and ankles are within normal limits.

Accessory Joint Mobility: Mild tenderness and stiffness noted upon L4/L5 unilateral posteroanterior mobility testing, right equals left.

Muscle Length Testing: Thomas's test indicates mild tightness of the iliopsoas and rectus femoris, bilaterally. Hamstring flexibility reveals a straight leg raise of 85 degrees, bilaterally.

Strength: Hamstrings=4+/5, bilaterally —with no report of pain; gluteus medius and minimus Right=4/5, Left=4+/5; Repeated testing of the right gluteals=4/5; hip flexion and adduction=4+/5, bilaterally.

Neurological: Straight leg raise with tension tests and slump test are negative bilaterally. Prone knee bend is negative bilaterally. Deep tendon reflexes are intact and symmetrical.

Special Tests: Beighton hyperflexibility scale is 0/9; prone instability test is—negative; Double leg lower test—meets criteria, but when repeated become less proficient. Modified 3 point Star excursion—reveals deficits on the right with transfer of the trunk laterally to the right—with less proficiency. The anterior drawer test of the right ankle is slightly positive but without pain; mild tenderness is noted upon palpation of the anterior talofibular ligament, bilaterally, right greater than left.

Palpation: The hamstring is somewhat tender right greater than left at the biceps femoris. Exquisite tenderness of the gluteus minimus with a taut band and tender nodule and referral to the right hamstring is acknowledged by the patient as his recognized pain.

Based on the presented information answer or discuss the following:

1. What would be the main differential diagnosis for posterior hamstring pain in this patient? Discuss what parts of the assessment help to support or refute the various diagnostic possibilities.
2. Given the available information, what would be your working diagnostic impression? What particular test(s) supports your conclusion?
3. What occurs in response to muscle ischemia? Can you briefly discuss the role of fatigue in muscle performance?
4. In the initial stage of injury what role would diagnostic imaging play? What would be the role of imaging at this stage of this patient plan of care? Is it indicated presently?
5. What is the function of the individual gluteal muscles? What are their antagonists and synergists?

6. What is the significance of the noted poorer proficiency of the modified Star excursion test? What is the importance of proprioception? Would the ankle be relevant to the right limb stability?
7. The gluteus minimus palpation test identified an active MTrP that referred pain to the right hamstring. What treatment would you suggest for this gluteal muscle?
8. After deactivation of the gluteus minimus, what would be your approach to correcting perpetuating factors in this patient?
9. Is rest strongly indicated for this patient? What would be your approach to resuming training in this patient? What would your advice be in relation to graded progressive activity?

HANDS-ON

Perform the following activities in lab with a partner or partners:

1 Palpation of a muscle is the cornerstone of identifying MTrPs. This exercise is important to introduce the skill of MTrP palpation. Locate the extensor carpi radialis brevis muscle (ECRB) at the posterior lateral aspect of the forearm of your partner, who should be positioned in crook half-lying position. The forearm should be propped up on the subject's abdomen so that the elbow is significantly flexed to take the slack off of the extensor carpi radialis longus (ECRL) and the forearm pronated with the wrist in approximately neutral. In this position you have a full view of your partner's face for visual feedback of the discomfort experienced. Locate the attachments of the ECRB by palpating the lateral epicondyle of the humerus and the common extensor tendon (proximal attachment) and the base of the dorsal aspect of the third metacarpal (distal attachment). This is approximately the line of the ECRB. Place some tension on the forearm extensors by flexing the wrist slightly. Starting at the lateral epicondyle, palpate using flat palpation with two or three fingers across the line of the ECRB and move along the muscle from proximal to distal to appreciate the thin pencil-like structure of the muscle belly. Palpate in a slow, firm manner across the muscle. To improve palpation perception, instruct the subject to resist middle finger extension against your resistance. This will increase tension of the ECRB and confirm location of the muscle. When you are confident that you are in position over the ECRB, have the subject relax and flex the wrist to selectively tense the muscle. Palpate for the taut band and most tender spot on the ECRB. Try to perceive and confirm by palpation a nodular area along the taut band. This should coincide with the subject's report of exquisite tenderness. This is the minimum criteria for identifying a MTrP. Press firmly onto the tender nodule, and at this stage the subject may feel referral along the posterior forearm and into the middle digit, which is the potential referral pattern for ECRB. If this is not familiar to the subject, then this confirms a latent MTrP, and if recognized (patient's pain provoked), it is considered an active MTrP. Mark the MTrP in the ECRB with a pen and move on to exercise two.

2 With the patient in the above position, relocate the taut band and tender nodule again to confirm its position, which should coincide with the pen mark (if the subject has not moved). Using a pressure threshold meter (PPT), place the rubber disc of the PPT onto the MTrP at 90 degrees to the muscle and increase your pressure by 1 kg/sec until the subject reports the onset of pain. Record the reading from the PPT and repeat once or twice to average two to three trails. Find the mean of the readings, which is, for example, likely to be 3.0 kg in a subject with a latent MTrP.

3 To test the effect of trigger point therapy release, place firm pressure onto the MTrP in the ECRB at an approximate 5/10 on the subject's verbal analog scale. Hold the pressure steady and ask the subject to report when the pain/discomfort has fallen to 1/10. This will probably take approximately 30 to 90 seconds. At this stage, remove the pressure and retest the PPT, which should demonstrate an increase in value to, for example, 3.5 to 4.0 kg. Switch with your partner as technique development is more profound when you both palpate and are palpated. These three exercises underpin the palpation technique, the location and criteria for the identification of a latent and active MTrP, use of the PPT meter, and the effects of trigger point therapy release. Be reminded that the pincer grip palpation will be more suitable for other muscles, such as brachioradialis, upper trapezius, and pectoralis major (sternal division). Repeat this exercise with these muscles using the principles as outlined above.

4 To palpate a local twitch response, have your partner stand in a relaxed position with arms by the side. Locate the belly of the two heads of the biceps on the anterior arm. Pincer-grip the biceps by placing your index and ring fingers on the medial aspect of the biceps and the opposing thumb on the lateral aspect. The belly of the muscle should be situated in the horseshoe shape of your grasp. Do not pinch too hard and avoid compressing the medial brachial neurovascular bundle. In a slow manner, grip and slide your fingers off of the muscle anteriorly in what has been described as a snapping palpation. Avoid an overzealous grip. While motioning through this technique, observe the subject's forearm activity. The local twitch response will present as a reflex-like action at the elbow with mild transient elbow flexion and supination. Try this several times along the belly of the muscle to attempt to locate the LTR. In comparison, perform an examination for the biceps tendon reflex (BTR); the consistency of movement from the LTR and BTR will be somewhat similar.

5 Fiber direction is an important factor in determining the muscle you are palpating. To appreciate this concept, have your colleague lie prone on an adjustable plinth (set to meet your stature and reach), draped with the upper back exposed. Have a graphic muscle anatomy text open to refer to the fiber direction of the myology of the interscapular area. The three main muscles of interest for this exercise are the lower trapezius, rhomboids (major and minor), and the thoracic erector spinae (collectively). The fiber direction is approximately medial inferior to superior lateral (trapezius), superior to inferior with mild lateral superior obliqueness (erector spinae), and medial to lateral with some mild medial superior obliqueness (rhomboids). Massage some light oil over the interscapular area and massage along the fiber direction of the three muscles. Note the palpation perception of each muscle as you move with the fiber direction. Now, move transverse to the muscle fiber direction of each muscle and note the significant difference in texture as you move across the muscle. Alter your pressure to move deeper to appreciate the depth of palpation. Note the subtle and superficial flat lower trapezius in contrast to the tube like perception of the erector spinae and the subtlety of the rhomboids lying under the trapezius. Place passive tension on the rhomboids by abducting and protracting the scapula.

6 Consider other areas where muscles overlap. Repeat this exercise for the gluteal area. What are the main challenges to palpation for fiber direction in this region?

7 Discuss in a group what the likely palpation difficulties would be encountered with other muscles such as levator scapula, quadratus lumborum, multifidus, piriformis, and tibialis posterior. What effect would body type have on your ability to palpate for MTrPs? It is suggested that you repeat the palpation exercises with other subjects to appreciate the differences in the ectomorphic, endomorphic, and mesomorphic body types.

8 Consider and discuss the potential relative and absolute contraindications for trigger point therapy release and massage.

9 In the identification of MTrPs in certain muscles, the evidence suggests that clinicians should be both trained and experienced. Discuss how physical therapy students would attain both attributes. Compare MTrP palpation with passive intervertebral motion palpation of the spinal segments and discuss. What are the similar challenges to performance of both techniques? What do you think is the value of patient-recognized pain provocation?

10 Dry needling of trigger points is a growing area of physical therapy practice both in the United States and internationally. Discuss what you think would be the importance of palpation technique and practical anatomy knowledge on your ability to learn and carry out dry needling safely and efficiently.

REFERENCES

1. Travell JG, Simons DG. Myofascial Pain and Dysfunction; The Trigger Point Manual. Vol. 1. Baltimore, MD: Williams & Wilkins; 1983.
2. Travell JG, Simons DG. Myofascial Pain and Dysfunction: The Trigger Point Manual. Vol. 2. Baltimore, MD: Williams & Wilkins; 1992.
3. Simons DG, Travell JG, Simons LS. Travell and Simons' Myofascial Pain and Dysfunction; The Trigger Point Manual. Vol. 1, 2nd ed. Baltimore, MD: Williams & Wilkins; 1999.
4. Baldry PE. Acupuncture, Trigger Points and Musculoskeletal Pain. Edinburgh: Churchill Livingstone; 2005.
5. Kellgren JH. Observations on referred pain arising from muscle. Clin Sci. 1938;3:175-190.
6. Kellgren JH. A preliminary account of referred pains arising from muscle. Br Med J. 1938;1:325-327.
7. Kellgren JH. Deep pain sensibility. Lancet. 1949;1:943-949.
8. Wilson VP. Janet G. Travell, MD; a daughter's recollection. Tex Heart Inst J. 2003;30:8-12.
9. Steindler A. The interpretation of sciatic radiation and the syndrome of low-back pain. J Bone Joint Surg Am. 1940;22:28-34.
10. Travell J. Office Hours: Day and Night. The Autobiography of Janet Travell, M.D. New York, NY: World Publishing; 1968.
11. Travell JG, Rinzler S, Herman M. Pain and disability of the shoulder and arm: treatment by intramuscular infiltration with procaine hydrochloride. JAMA. 1942;120:417-422.
12. Travell JG, Rinzler SH. The myofascial genesis of pain. Postgrad Med. 1952;11:452-434.
13. Dommerholt J, Bron C, Franssen JLM. Myofascial trigger points; an evidence-informed review. J Manual Manipulative Ther. 2006;14:203-221.
14. Simons DG. Orphan organ. J Musculoskeletal Pain. 2007;15:7-9.
15. Fernández-Carnero J, et al. Prevalence of and referred pain from myofascial trigger points in the forearm muscles in patients with lateral epicondylalgia. Clin J Pain. 2007;23:353-360.
16. Fernández-Carnero J, et al. Bilateral myofascial trigger points in the forearm muscles in patients with chronic unilateral lateral epicondylalgia: a blinded, controlled study. Clin J Pain. 2008;24:802-807.
17. Ge HY, et al. Induction of muscle cramps by nociceptive stimulation of latent myofascial trigger points. Exp Brain Res. 2008;187:623-629.
18. Kimura Y, et al. Evaluation of sympathetic vasoconstrictor response following nociceptive stimulation of latent myofascial trigger points in humans. Acta Physiol (Oxf). 2009;196:411-417.
19. Li LT, et al. Nociceptive and non-nociceptive hypersensitivity at latent myofascial trigger points. Clin J Pain. 2009;25:132-137.
20. Zhang Y, et al. Attenuated skin blood flow response to nociceptive stimulation of latent myofascial trigger points. Arch Phys Med Rehabil. 2009;90:325-332.
21. Ge HY, Fernández de las Peñas C, Arendt-Nielsen L. Sympathetic facilitation of hyperalgesia evoked from myofascial tender and trigger points in patients with unilateral shoulder pain. Clin Neurophysiol. 2006;117:1545-1550.
22. Hong CZ, Torigoe Y. Electrophysiological characteristics of localized twitch responses in responsive taut bands of rabbit skeletal muscle. J Musculoskeletal Pain. 1994;2:17-43.
23. Hong CZ. Persistence of local twitch response with loss of conduction to and from the spinal cord. Arch Phys Med Rehabil. 1994;75:12-16.
24. Hong CZ, Torigoe Y, Yu J. The localized twitch responses in responsive bands of rabbit skeletal muscle are related to the reflexes at spinal cord level. J Musculoskeletal Pain. 1995;3:15-33.
25. Alfven G. The pressure pain threshold (PPT) of certain muscles in children suffering from recurrent abdominal pain of non-organic origin. An algometric study. Acta Paediatr. 1993;82:481-483.
26. Zapata AL, et al. Pain and musculoskeletal pain syndromes in adolescents. J Adolesc Health. 2006;38:769-771.
27. Kao MJ, et al. Myofascial trigger points in early life. Arch Phys Med Rehabil. 2007;88:251-254.
28. Cimbiz A, Beydemir F, Manisaligil U. Evaluation of trigger points in young subjects. J Musculoskeletal Pain. 2006;14:27-35.
29. Harden RN, et al. Signs and symptoms of the myofascial pain syndrome: a national survey of pain management providers. Clin J Pain. 2000;16:64-72.
30. Vecchiet L, et al. Muscle pain from physical exercise. J Musculoskeletal Pain. 1999;7:43-53.
31. Hendler NH, Kozikowski, JG. Overlooked physical diagnoses in chronic pain patients involved in litigation. Psychosomatics. 1993;34:494-501.
32. Mense S. Pathophysiologic basis of muscle pain syndromes. In: Fischer AA, ed. Myofascial Pain; Update in Diagnosis and Treatment. Philadelphia, PA: WB Saunders; 1997:23-53.

33. Wang K, McClure, Tu, A. Titin: major myofibrillar components of striated muscle. Proc Natl Acad Sci U S A. 1979;76:3698-3702.
34. Wang K. Titin/connectin and nebulin: giant protein rulers of muscle structure and function. Adv Biophys. 1996;33:123-134.
35. Wang K, Williamson CL. Identification of an N2 line protein of striated muscle. Proc Natl Acad Sci U S A. 1980;77:3254-3258.
36. McElhinny AS, et al. Nebulin: the nebulous, multifunctional giant of striated muscle. Trends Cardiovasc Med. 2003;13:195-201.
37. Arrowsmith JE. The neuromuscular junction. Surgery (Oxf). 2007;25:105-111.
38. Gerwin RD, Dommerholt J, Shah, J. An expansion of Simons' integrated hypothesis of trigger point formation. Curr Pain Headache Rep. 2004;8:468-475.
39. Fridén J, Lieber RL. Segmental muscle fiber lesions after repetitive eccentric contractions. Cell Tissue Res. 1998;293:165-171.
40. Lieber RL, Shah S, Fridén J. Cytoskeletal disruption after eccentric contraction-induced muscle injury. Clin Orthop Relat Res. 2002;403(Suppl):S90-S99.
41. Stauber WT, et al. Extracellular matrix disruption and pain after eccentric muscle action. J Appl Physiol. 1990;69:868-874.
42. Itoh K, Okada K, Kawakita K. A proposed experimental model of myofascial trigger points in human muscle after slow eccentric exercise. Acupunct Med. 2004;22:2-12; discussion 12-13.
43. Brückle W, et al. Gewebe-pO2-Messung in der verspannten Rückenmuskulatur (m. erector spinae). Z Rheumatol. 1990;49:208-216.
44. Treaster D, et al. Myofascial trigger point development from visual and postural stressors during computer work. J Electromyogr Kinesiol. 2006;16:115-124.
45. Chen S-M, et al. Decrease in pressure pain thresholds of latent myofascial trigger points in the middle finger extensors immediately after continuous piano practice. J Musculoskeletal Pain. 2000;8:83-92.
46. Hägg GM. The cinderella hypothesis. In: Johansson H, et al., eds. Chronic Work-Related Myalgia. Gävle, Sweden: Gävle University Press; 2003:127-132.
47. Forsman M, et al. Motor-unit recruitment during long-term isometric and wrist motion contractions: a study concerning muscular pain development in computer operators. Int J Ind Ergon. 2002;30:237-250.
48. Zennaro D, et al. Trapezius muscle motor unit activity in symptomatic participants during finger tapping using properly and improperly adjusted desks. Hum Factors. 2004;46:252-266.
49. Febbraio MA, Pedersen BK. Contraction-induced myokine production and release: is skeletal muscle an endocrine organ? Exerc Sport Sci Rev. 2005;33:114-119.
50. Gissel H. Ca2+ accumulation and cell damage in skeletal muscle during low frequency stimulation. Eur J Appl Physiol. 2000;83:175-180.
51. Gissel H, Clausen T. Excitation-induced Ca(2+) influx in rat soleus and EDL muscle: mechanisms and effects on cellular integrity. Am J Physiol Regul Integr Comp Physiol. 2000;279:R917-R924.
52. Lexell J, et al. Stimulation-induced damage in rabbit fast-twitch skeletal muscles: a quantitative morphological study of the influence of pattern and frequency. Cell Tissue Res. 1993;273:357-362.
53. Pedersen BK, Febbraio M. Muscle-derived interleukin-6–a possible link between skeletal muscle, adipose tissue, liver, and brain. Brain Behav Immun. 2005;19:371-376.
54. Simons DG , Travell J. Myofascial trigger points, a possible explanation. Pain. 198;10:106-109.
55. Dommerholt J. Persistent myalgia following whiplash. Curr Pain Headache Rep. 2005;9:326-330.
56. Baker BA. The muscle trigger: evidence of overload injury. J Neurol Orthop Med Surg. 1986;7:35-44.
57. Gerwin RD, Dommerholt J. Myofascial trigger points in chronic cervical whiplash syndrome. J Musculoskeletal Pain. 1998;6(Suppl 2):28.
58. Schuller E, Eisenmenger W, Beier G. Whiplash injury in low speed car accidents. J Musculoskeletal Pain. 2000;8:55-67.
59. Freeman MD, Nystrom A, Centeno C. Chronic whiplash and central sensitization; an evaluation of the role of a myofascial trigger points in pain modulation. J Brachial Plex Peripher Nerve Inj. 2009;4:2.
60. Ettlin T, et al. A distinct pattern of myofascial findings in patients after whiplash injury. Arch Phys Med Rehabil. 2008;89:1290-1293.
61. Gerwin RD. Myofascial and visceral pain syndromes: visceral-somatic pain representations. In: Bennett RM, ed. The Clinical Neurobiology of Fibromyalgia and Myofascial Pain. Binghampton, England: Haworth Press; 2002:165-175.
62. Giamberardino MA, et al. Referred muscle pain and hyperalgesia from viscera. J Musculoskeletal Pain. 1999;7:61-69.
63. Doggweiler-Wiygul R, Wiygul JP. Interstitial cystitis, pelvic pain, and the relationship to myofascial pain and dysfunction: a report on four patients. World J Urol. 2002;20:310-314.

64. Jarrell J. Myofascial dysfunction in the pelvis. Curr Pain Headache Rep. 2004;8:452-456.

65. McPartland JM. Travell trigger points–molecular and osteopathic perspectives. J Am Osteopath Assoc. 2004;104:244-249.

66. McPartland JM, Simons, DG. Myofascial trigger points: translating molecular theory into manual therapy. J Man Manipulative Ther. 2006; 14:232-239.

67. Simons DG. Review of enigmatic MTrPs as a common cause of enigmatic musculoskeletal pain and dysfunction. J Electromyogr Kinesiol. 2004; 14:95-107.

68. Hubbard DR, Berkoff GM. Myofascial trigger points show spontaneous needle EMG activity. Spine. 1993;18:1803-1807.

69. Simons DG, Hong C-Z, Simons LS. Endplate potentials are common to midfiber myofascial trigger points. Am J Phys Med Rehabil. 200;81:212-222.

70. Hong C-Z, Yu J. Spontaneous electrical activity of rabbit trigger spot after transection of spinal cord and peripheral nerve. J Musculoskeletal Pain. 1998;6:45-58.

71. Simons DG. Clinical and etiological update of myofascial pain from trigger points. J Musculoskeletal Pain. 1996;4:93-121.

72. Simons DG. Do endplate noise and spikes arise from normal motor endplates? Am J Phys Med Rehabil. 2001;80:134-140.

73. Simons DG, Hong C-Z, Simons L. Prevalence of spontaneous electrical activity at trigger spots and control sites in rabbit muscle. J Musculoskeletal Pain. 1995;3:35-48.

74. Chen JT, et al. Phentolamine effect on the spontaneous electrical activity of active loci in a myofascial trigger spot of rabbit skeletal muscle. Arch Phys Med Rehabil. 1998;79:790-794.

75. Chen JT, et al. Inhibitory effect of calcium channel blocker on the spontaneous electrical activity of myofascial trigger point. J Musculoskeletal Pain. 1998;6(Suppl 2):24.

76. Chen SM, et al. Effect of neuromuscular blocking agent on the spontaneous activity of active loci in a myofascial trigger spot of rabbit skeletal muscle. J Musculoskeletal Pain. 1998;6(Suppl 2):25.

77. Kuan TS, et al. Effect of botulinum toxin on endplate noise in myofascial trigger spots of rabbit skeletal muscle. Am J Phys Med Rehabil. 2002; 81:512-520; quiz 521-523.

78. Kuan TS, et al. The myofascial trigger point region: correlation between the degree of irritability and the prevalence of endplate noise. Am J Phys Med Rehabil. 2007;86:183-189.

79. Mense S, et al. Lesions of rat skeletal muscle after local block of acetylcholinesterase and neuromuscular stimulation. J Appl Physiol. 2003;94: 2494-2501.

80. Couppé C, et al. Spontaneous needle electromyographic activity in myofascial trigger points in the infraspinatus muscle: A blinded assessment. J Musculoskeletal Pain. 2001;9:7-17.

81. Macgregor J, Graf von Schweinitz D. Needle electromyographic activity of myofascial trigger points and control sites in equine cleidobrachialis muscle—an observational study. Acupunct Med. 2006;24:61-70.

82. Kuan TS. The spinal cord connections of the myofascial trigger spots. Eur J Pain. 2007;11:624-634.

83. Simons DG, Hong C-Z, Simons, LS. Spike activity in trigger points. J Musculoskeletal Pain. 1995;3(Suppl 1):125.

84. Bukharaeva EA, et al. Spontaneous quantal and non-quantal release of acetylcholine at mouse endplate during onset of hypoxia. Physiol Res. 2005;54:251-255.

85. Graven-Nielsen T, Arendt-Nielsen L. Induction and assessment of muscle pain, referred pain, and muscular hyperalgesia. Curr Pain Headache Rep. 2003;7:443-451.

86. Wang K, Yu L. Emerging concepts of muscle contraction and clinical implications for myofascial pain syndrome (abstract). In: Focus on Pain. Travell JG, ed. Mesa, AZ: MD Seminar Series; 2000.

87. Chen BM, Grinnell AD. Kinetics, Ca2+ dependence, and biophysical properties of integrin-mediated mechanical modulation of transmitter release from frog motor nerve terminals. J Neurosci. 1997;17:904-916.

88. Grinnell AD, et al. The role of integrins in the modulation of neurotransmitter release from motor nerve terminals by stretch and hypertonicity. J Neurocytol. 2003;32:489-503.

89. Reitinger A, et al. Morphologische Untersuchung an Triggerpunkten. Manuelle Medizin. 1996;34:256-262.

90. Simons DG, Stolov WC. Microscopic features and transient contraction of palpable bands in canine muscle. Am J Phys Med. 1976;55:65-88.

91. Windisch A, et al. Morphology and histochemistry of myogelosis. Clin Anat. 1999;12:266-271.

92. Lucas KR, Polus BI, Rich PS . Latent myofascial trigger points: their effect on muscle activation and movement efficiency. J Bodyw Mov Ther. 2004;8:160-166.

93. Headley BJ. The use of biofeedback in pain management. Phys Ther Pract. 1993;2:29-40.

94. Hsieh YL, et al. Dry needling to a key myofascial trigger point may reduce the irritability of satellite MTrPs. Am J Phys Med Rehabil. 2007;86: 397-403.

95. Carlson CR, et al. Reduction of pain and EMG activity in the masseter region by trapezius trigger point injection. Pain. 1993;55:397-400.

96. Vecchiet J, et al. Relationship between musculoskeletal symptoms and blood markers of oxidative stress in patients with chronic fatigue syndrome. Neurosci Lett. 2003;335:151-154.

97. Vecchiet L, Giamberardino MA, de Bigontina, P. Comparative sensory evaluation of parietal tissues in painful and nonpainful areas in fibromyalgia and myofascial pain syndrome. In: Gebhart GF, Hammond, DL, Jensen TS, eds. Proceedings of the 7th World Congres on Pain (Progress in Pain Research and Management). Seattle, WA: IASP Press: 1994:177-185.

98. Vecchiet L, Giamberardino MA, Dragani L. Latent myofascial trigger points: changes in muscular and subcutaneous pain thresholds at trigger point and target level. J Manual Medicine. 1990;5:151-154.

99. Shah JP, et al. An in-vivo microanalytical technique for measuring the local biochemical milieu of human skeletal muscle. J Appl Physiol. 2005;99:1977-1984.

100. Shah JP, et al. Biochemicals associated with pain and inflammation are elevated in sites near to and remote from active myofascial trigger points. Arch Phys Med Rehabil. 2008;89:16-23.

101. Babenko V, et al. Experimental human muscle pain and muscular hyperalgesia induced by combinations of serotonin and bradykinin. Pain. 1999;82:1-8.

102. Hoheisel U, Sander B, Mense S. Myositis-induced functional reorganisation of the rat dorsal horn: effects of spinal superfusion with antagonists to neurokinin and glutamate receptors. Pain. 1997;69: 219-230.

103. Dommerholt J, Shah J. Myofascial pain syndrome. In: Ballantyne, JC, Rathmell JP, Fishman, SM, eds. Bonica's Management of Pain. Baltimore, MD: Lippincott, Williams & Wilkins; 2010:450-471.

104. Sluka KA, Kalra A, Moore SA. Unilateral intramuscular injections of acidic saline produce a bilateral, long-lasting hyperalgesia. Muscle Nerve. 2001;24:37-46.

105. Svensson P, et al. Cerebral processing of acute skin and muscle pain in humans. J Neurophysiol 1997;78:450-460.

106. Niddam DM, et al. Central modulation of pain evoked from myofascial trigger point. Clin J Pain. 2007;23:440-448.

107. Niddam DM, et al. Central representation of hyperalgesia from myofascial trigger point. Neuroimage. 2008;39:1299-1306.

108. Wall PD, Woolf CJ. Muscle but not cutaneous C-afferent input produces prolonged increases in the excitability of the flexion reflex in the rat. J Physiol. 1984;356:443-458.

109. Hoheisel U, et al. Appearance of new receptive fields in rat dorsal horn neurons following noxious stimulation of skeletal muscle: a model for referral of muscle pain? Neurosci Lett. 1993;153:9-12.

110. Mense S. Nociception from skeletal muscle in relation to clinical muscle pain. Pain. 1993;54:241-289.

111. Hoheisel U, Koch K, Mense S. Functional reorganization in the rat dorsal horn during an experimental myositis. Pain. 1994;59:111-118.

112. Bendtsen L, Jensen R, Olesen J. Qualitatively altered nociception in chronic myofascial pain. Pain. 1996;65:259-264.

113. Herren-Gerber R, et al. Modulation of central hypersensitivity by nociceptive input in chronic pain after whiplash injury. Pain Med. 2004; 5:366-376.

114. Sluka KA, et al. Chronic muscle pain induced by repeated acid Injection is reversed by spinally administered mu- and delta-, but not kappa-, opioid receptor agonists. J Pharmacol Exp Ther. 2002;302: 1146-1150.

115. Vecchiet L, Giamberardino MA. Pain, referred. In: Aminoff MJ, Daroff RB, eds. Encyclopedia of the Neurological Sciences. Burlington, VT: Academic Press; 2003:770-773.

116. Bajaj P, Graven-Nielsen T, Arendt-Nielsen L. Osteoarthritis and its association with muscle hyperalgesia: an experimental controlled study. Pain. 2001;93:107-114.

117. Calandre EP, et al. Trigger point evaluation in migraine patients: an indication of peripheral sensitization linked to migraine predisposition? Eur J Neurol. 2006;13:244-249.

118. Giamberardino MA, et al. Contribution of myofascial trigger points to migraine symptoms. J Pain. 2007.

119. Marcus DA, et al. Musculoskeletal abnormalities in chronic headache: a controlled comparison of headache diagnostic groups. Headache. 1999; 39:21-27.

120. Fernández de las Peñas C, et al. Myofascial trigger points and sensitization: an updated pain model for tension-type headache. Cephalalgia. 2007;27:383-393.
121. Fernández de las Peñas C, et al. Bilateral widespread mechanical pain sensitivity in women with myofascial temporomandibular disorder: evidence of impairment in central nociceptive processing. J Pain. 2009;10:1170-1178.
122. Bukharaeva EA, Gainulov R, Nikol'skii EE. The effects of noradrenaline on the amplitude-time characteristics of multiquantum endplate currents and the kinetics of induced secretion of transmitter quanta. Neurosci Behav Physiol. 2002;32:549-554.
123. Banks SL, et al. Effects of autogenic relaxation training on electromyographic activity in active myofascial trigger points. J Musculoskeletal Pain. 1998;6:23-32.
124. Lewis C, et al. Needle trigger point and surface frontal EMG measurements of psychophysiological responses in tension-type headache patients. Biofeedback & Self-Regulation. 1994;3:274-275.
125. McNulty WH, et al. Needle electromyographic evaluation of trigger point response to a psychological stressor. Psychophysiology. 1994;31:313-316.
126. Bowman, WC, et al. Feedback control of transmitter release at the neuromuscular junction. Trends Pharmacol Sci. 1988;9:16-20.
127. Lewis J, Tehan P. A blinded pilot study investigating the use of diagnostic ultrasound for detecting active myofascial trigger points. Pain. 1999;79:39-44.
128. Gerwin RD, Duranleau D. Ultrasound identification of the myofascial trigger point. Muscle Nerve. 1997;20:767-768.
129. Sikdar S, et al. Novel applications of ultrasound technology to visualize and characterize myofascial trigger points and surrounding soft tissue. Arch Phys Med Rehabil. 2009;90:1829-1838.
130. Chen Q, Basford J, An KN. Ability of magnetic resonance elastography to assess taut bands. Clin Biomech (Bristol, Avon). 2008;23:623-629.
131. Chen Q, et al. Identification and quantification of myofascial taut bands with magnetic resonance elastography. Arch Phys Med Rehabil. 2007;88:1658-1661.
132. Fischer AA. Pressure algometry over normal muscles. Standard values, validity and reproducibility of pressure threshold. Pain. 1987;30:115-126.
133. Bauermeister W. Diagnose und Therapie des Myofaszialen Triggerpunkt Syndroms durch Lokalisierung und Stimulation sensibilisierter Nozizeptoren mit fokussierten elektrohydraulische Stosswellen. Medizinisch-Orthopädische Technik. 2005;5:65-74.
134. Müller-Ehrenberg H, Thorwesten L. Improvement of sports-related shoulder pain after treatment of trigger points using focused extracorporeal shock wave therapy regarding static and dynamic force development, pain relief and sensomotoric performance. J Musculoskeletal Pain. 2007;15(Suppl 13):33.
135. Gerwin RD, et al. Interrater reliability in myofascial trigger point examination. Pain. 1997;69:65-73.
136. McEvoy J, Huijbregts PA. Reliability of myofascial trigger point palpation: a systematic review. In: Dommerholt J, Huijbregts PA, eds. Myofascial Trigger Points: Pathophysiology and Evidence-informed Diagnosis and Management. Boston, MA: Jones & Bartlett; 2011.
137. Al-Shenqiti AM, Oldham, JA. Test-retest reliability of myofascial trigger point detection in patients with rotator cuff tendonitis. Clin Rehabil. 2005;19:482-487.
138. Dommerholt J, Issa T. Differential diagnosis: myofascial pain. In: Chaitow L, ed. Fibromyalgia Syndrome; A Practitioner's Guide to Treatment. Edinburgh, UK: Churchill Livingstone; 2009:179-213.
139. Dommerholt J, Mayoral O, Gröbli C. Trigger point dry needling. J Manual Manipulative Ther. 2006;14:E70-E87.
140. Beckerman H, et al. The efficacy of laser therapy for musculoskeletal and skin disorders: a criteria-based meta-analysis of randomized clinical trials. Phys Ther. 1992;72:483-491.
141. Fernández-de-las-Peñas C, et al. Manual therapies in myofascial trigger point treatment: a systematic review. J Bodywork Movement Ther. 2005;9:27-34.
142. Hey LR, Helewa A. Myofascial pain syndrome: a critical review of the literature. Physiother Can. 1994;46:28-36.
143. Rickards LD. The effectiveness of non-invasive treatments for active myofascial trigger point pain: A systematic review of the literature. Int J Osteopathic Med. 2006;9:120-136.
144. Gam AN, Thorsen H, Lonnberg F. The effect of low-level laser therapy on musculoskeletal pain: a meta-analysis. Pain. 1993;52:63-66.
145. Cummings TM, White AR. Needling therapies in the management of myofascial trigger point pain: a systematic review. Arch Phys Med Rehabil. 2001;82:986-992.
146. Furlan A, et al. Acupuncture and dry-needling for low back pain: an updated systematic review within the framework of the Cochrane Collaboration. Spine. 2005;30:944-963.
147. Gröbli C, Dejung B. Nichtmedikamentöse Therapie myofaszialer Schmerzen. Schmerz. 2003;17:475-480.
148. Gröbli C, Dommerholt J. Myofasziale Triggerpunkte; Pathologie und Behandlungsmöglichkeiten. Manuelle Medizin. 1997;35:295-303.
149. Rickards LD. Effectiveness of noninvasive treatments for active myofascial trigger point pain: a systematic review. In: Dommerholt J, Huijbregts PA, ed. Myofascial Trigger Points; Pathophysiology and Evidence-Informed Diagnosis and Management. Sudbury, MA: Jones & Bartlett; 2011:129-158.
150. Simons DG. Understanding effective treatments of myofascial trigger points. J Bodyw Mov Ther. 2002;6:81-88.
151. Gam AN, et al. Treatment of myofascial trigger-points with ultrasound combined with massage and exercise—a randomised controlled trial. Pain. 1998;77:73-79.
152. Hong C-Z, et al. Immediate effects of various physical medicine modalities on pain threshold of the active myofascial trigger points. J Musculoskeletal Pain. 1993;1:37-53.
153. Hou CR, et al. Immediate effects of various physical therapeutic modalities on cervical myofascial pain and trigger-point sensitivity. Arch Phys Med Rehabil. 2002;83:1406-1414.
154. Fernández-de-las-Peñas C, et al. The immediate effect of ischemic compression technique and transverse friction massage on tenderness of active and latent myofascial trigger points: a pilot study. J Bodyw Mov Ther. 2006;10:3-9.
155. Chatchawan U, et al. Effectiveness of traditional Thai massage versus Swedish massage among patients with back pain associated with myofascial trigger points. J Body Movement Ther. 2005;9:298-309.
156. Moraska A, Chandler C. Changes in psychological parameters in patients with tension-type headache following massage therapy: a pilot study. J Man Manip Ther. 2009;17:86-94.
157. U.S. Department of Energy. Emissions of Greenhouse Gases in the United States 2005. Washington, DC: Energy Information Administration, Office of Integrated Analysis and Forecasting, U.S. Department of Energy; 2006.
158. European Environment Agency. EEA Signals 2004. Copenhagen, Denmark: European Environment Agency; 2004.
159. Dejung B, Triggerpunkt - und Bindegewebebehandlung - neue Wege in Physiotherapie und Rehabilitationsmedizin. Physiotherapeut. 1988;24:3-12.
160. Dejung B. Die Behandlung unspezifisher chronischer Rückenschmerzen mit manueller Triggerpunkt-Therapie. Manuelle Medizin. 1999;37:124-131.
161. Dommerholt J. Dry needling in orthopedic physical therapy practice. Orthop Phys Ther Practice. 2004;16:15-20.
162. Resteghini P. Myofascial trigger points: pathophsyiology and treatment with dry needling. J Orthop Med. 2006;28:60-68.
163. Ay S, Evcik D, Tur BS. Comparison of injection methods in myofascial pain syndrome: a randomized controlled trial. Clin Rheumatol. 2010;29:19-23.
164. Ga H, et al. Intramuscular and nerve root stimulation vs lidocaine injection to trigger points in myofascial pain syndrome. J Rehabil Med. 2007;39:374-378.
165. Millan MJ. The induction of pain: an integrative review. Prog Neurobiol. 1999;57:1-164.
166. Langevin HM, et al. Subcutaneous tissue fibroblast cytoskeletal remodeling induced by acupuncture: evidence for a mechanotransduction-based mechanism. J Cell Physiol. 2006;207:767-774.
167. Langevin HM, et al. Fibroblast spreading induced by connective tissue stretch involves intracellular redistribution of alpha- and beta-actin. Histochem Cell Biol. 2006;125:487-495.
168. Uvnas-Moberg K, et al. The antinociceptive effect of non-noxious sensory stimulation is mediated partly through oxytocinergic mechanisms. Acta Physiol Scand. 1993;149:199-204.
169. Hong CZ. Lidocaine injection versus dry needling to myofascial trigger point. The importance of the local twitch response. Am J Phys Med Rehabil. 1994;73:256-263.
170. Chen JT, et al. Inhibitory effect of dry needling on the spontaneous electrical activity recorded from myofascial trigger spots of rabbit skeletal muscle. Am J Phys Med Rehabil. 2001;80:729-735.
171. Escobar PL, Ballesteros J. Teres minor. Source of symptoms resembling ulnar neuropathy or C8 radiculopathy. Am J Phys Med Rehabil. 1988;67:120-122.
172. Facco E, Ceccherelli F. Myofascial pain mimicking radicular syndromes. Acta Neurochir Suppl. 2005;92:147-150.

173. Hsueh TC, et al. The immediate effectiveness of electrical nerve stimulation and electrical muscle stimulation on myofascial trigger points. Am J Phys Med Rehabil. 1997;76:471-476.

174. Ardiç F, Sarhus M, Topuz O. Comparison of two different techniques of electrotherapy on myofascial pain. J Back Musculoskeletal Rehabil. 2002;16:11-16.

175. Graff-Radford SB, et al. Effects of transcutaneous electrical nerve stimulation on myofascial pain and trigger point sensitivity. Pain. 1989;37:1-5.

176. Majlesi J, Unalan H. High-power pain threshold ultrasound technique in the treatment of active myofascial trigger points: a randomized, double-blind, case-control study. Arch Phys Med Rehabil. 2004;85:833-836.

177. Esenyel M, Caglar N, Aldemir T. Treatment of myofascial pain. Am J Phys Med Rehabil. 2000;79:48-52.

178. Srbely JZ, et al. Stimulation of myofascial trigger points with ultrasound induces segmental antinociceptive effects: a randomized controlled study. Pain. 2008;139:260-266.

179. Fernández-de-las-Peñas C, et al. Trigger points in the suboccipital muscles and forward head posture in tension-type headache. Headache. 2006;46:454-460.

180. Fernandez-de-Las-Penas C, Cuadrado ML, Pareja JA. Myofascial trigger points, neck mobility, and forward head posture in episodic tension-type headache. Headache. 2007;47:662-672.

181. Fricton JR. Myofascial pain syndrome: characteristics and epidemiology. Adv Pain Res. 1990;17:107-128.

182. Gerwin RD, Dommerholt J. Treatment of myofascial pain syndromes. In: Boswell MV, Cole BE, eds. Weiner's Pain Management; A Practical Guide for Clinicians. Boca Raton: CRC Press; 2006:477-492.

183. Dommerholt J. Posture. In: Tubiana R, Amadio P, eds. Medical Problems of the Instrumentalist Musician. London: Martin Dunitz; 2000:399-419.

184. Dommerholt J. Performing arts medicine–instrumentalist musicians Part II: the examination. J Bodyw Mov Ther. 2010;14:65-72.

185. Sim J, Lacey RJ, Lewis M. The impact of workplace risk factors on the occurrence of neck and upper limb pain: a general population study. BMC Public Health. 2006;6:234.

186. Yamalik N. Musculoskeletal disorders (MSDs) and dental practice Part 2. Risk factors for dentistry, magnitude of the problem, prevention, and dental ergonomics. Int Dent J. 2007;57:45-54.

187. Morse T, et al. Musculoskeletal disorders of the neck and shoulder in dental hygienists and dental hygiene students. J Dent Hyg. 2007;81:10.

188. Bork BE, et al. Work-related musculoskeletal disorders among physical therapists. Phys Ther. 1996;76:827-835.

189. Samuel AS, Peter AA, Ramanathan, K. The association of active trigger points with lumbar disc lesions. J Musculoskeletal Pain. 2007;15:11-18.

190. Crotti FM, et al. Post-traumatic thoracic outlet syndrome (TOS). Acta Neurochir Suppl. 2005;92:13-15.

191. Ge HY, et al. Contribution of the local and referred pain from active myofascial trigger points in fibromyalgia syndrome. Pain. 2009;147:233-240.

192. Arendt-Nielsen L, et al. A double-blind randomizded placebo controlled parallel group study evaluating the effects of ibuprofen and glucosamine sulfate on exercise induced muscle soreness. J Musculoskeletal Pain. 2007;15:21-28.

193. Dommerholt J, Gerwin RD. Nutritional and metabolic perpetuating factors in myofascial pain. In: Dommerholt J, Huijbregts, PA, eds. Myofascial Trigger Points: Pathophysiology and Evidence-informed Diagnosis and Management. Boston, MA: Jones & Bartlett; 2011.

194. Andres E, et al. Vitamin B12 (cobalamin) deficiency in elderly patients. CMAJ. 2004;171:251-259.

195. Gerwin R. A study of 96 subjects examined both for fibromyalgia and myofascial pain (abstract). J Musculoskeletal Pain. 1995;3(Suppl 1):121.

196. Pruthi RK, Tefferi A. Pernicious anemia revisited. Mayo Clin Proc. 1994;69:144-150.

197. Gerwin RD. A review of myofascial pain and fibromyalgia—factors that promote their persistence. Acupunct Med. 2005;23:121-134.

198. Lidbeck J. Central hyperexcitability in chronic musculoskeletal pain: a conceptual breakthrough with multiple clinical implications. Pain Res Manag. 2002;7:81-92.

199. Linton SJ. A review of psychological risk factors in back and neck pain. Spine. 2000;25:1148-1156.

200. Vlaeyen JW, Linton SJ. Fear-avoidance and its consequences in chronic musculoskeletal pain: a state of the art. Pain. 2000;85:317-332.

Therapeutic Exercise Strategies for Disorders of the Spine

Christopher H. Wise, PT, DPT, OCS, FAAOMPT, MTC, ATC
Ronald J. Schenk, PT, PhD, OCS, FAAOMPT, Dip MDT

Chapter Objectives

At the conclusion of this chapter, the reader will be able to:

- Discuss the primary indications for the use of therapeutic exercise (TE) in the management of spinal disorders and how such interventions may be integrated with orthopaedic manual physical therapy into a comprehensive physical therapy regimen.
- Be aware of the current best evidence related to the use of TE in treating disorders of the spine.
- Discuss concepts related to classification and differential diagnosis, including primary reasons for classification, types of classification systems, and common systems for classification in the management of low back pain and neck pain.

- Identify the theoretical underpinnings, principles of examination/classification, and principles of intervention for three common approaches to exercise for the management of spinal disorders.
- Understand the myriad of ways in which spinal movement aberrations may be present and subsequently managed.
- Analyze exercise approaches based on the results of testing repeated end-range spinal movements, intervertebral motion testing, muscle balance testing, muscle function testing, and evaluation of kinesthesia.
- Apply appropriate exercise recommendations to decrease symptoms and improve spinal mobility and stability.

INTRODUCTION

Therapeutic exercise (TE) is routinely considered to be among the myriad of interventions deemed to be effective for the remediation of spinal dysfunction. The use of exercise to relieve symptoms, improve range of motion and muscle function, and enhance the effects of other interventions is considered to be a primary feature in the standard of care for the management of spinal dysfunction within physical therapy. Exercise is routinely used as an adjunct to prepare, support, correct, prevent, and maintain the effects before, during, or after the utilization of orthopaedic manual physical therapy (OMPT) (Fig. 17-1).

CLINICAL PILLAR

When developing a comprehensive intervention plan for individuals with spine-related disorders, therapeutic exercise may be used to

- Prepare
- Support
- Correct
- Prevent
- Maintain

the effects before, during, or after OMPT.

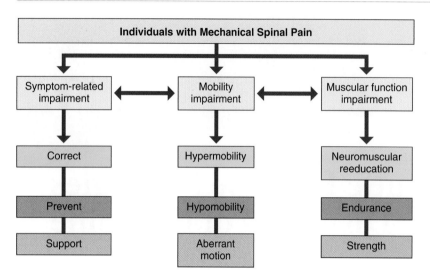

FIGURE 17–1 Primary indications for therapeutic exercise in patients with mechanical disorders of the spine.

Few studies have attempted to identify patient characteristics that warrant a specific exercise approach. A systematic review by the ***Philadelphia Panel***[1] suggests that there is "good evidence to include stretching, strengthening, and mobility exercises" in intervention programs directed toward the management of chronic low back pain (LBP).[1] While these findings are similar to other meta-analyses investigating the management of chronic LBP,[2,3] the information provided in these reviews offer little guidance regarding the efficacy of specific therapeutic exercise approaches.

This chapter will introduce three TE approaches that are commonly used in the management of spinal disorders, with an emphasis on clinical decision-making. The theoretical underpinnings, principles of examination and classification, and principles of intervention for each approach will be provided in light of the current best evidence. Based on its paramount importance in the management of spinal disorders, this chapter will begin with a discussion related to the classification of spinal disorders.

CLASSIFICATION OF SPINAL DISORDERS

Clinicians and researchers alike have advocated the role of the physical therapist in establishing a differential diagnosis.[4] The ***Guide to Physical Therapist Practice (GPTP)*** emphasizes the importance of diagnosis as a major component of the PT's role in the management of individuals with movement disorders.[5]

The Case for Classification

In 1995, and again in 1997, ***The International Forum for Primary Care Research on LBP***, an international panel spanning multiple disciplines, determined that of all research initiatives related to disorders of the spine, the item that must be given highest priority is diagnostic classification.[4] Eighty-eight investigators and clinicians from 12 countries agreed that the most important research priority related to the management of LBP should be the process of identifying homogeneous subgroups within the larger heterogeneous entity of LBP (Fig. 17-2).[6]

QUESTIONS for REFLECTION

- Why has the use of classification systems in the management of spinal disorders been given such a high priority among researchers and clinicians?
- How does classification assist the therapist in providing more efficacious care?
- Why have much of our interventions and research initiatives related to spine-related disorders resulted in equivocal outcomes, and how would classification improve this dilemma?

Not all neck and back pain is created equal. The challenge for the PT is to recognize through the utilization of valid examination procedures, astute critical thinking, and self-reflection the objective and measurable clinical patterns of presentation that serve to differentiate one individual from another.[7] In addition to directing intervention, classification systems may also demonstrate usefulness in determining prognosis, establishing a common language to facilitate communication, as well as guiding and improving the quality of research initiatives.[4] Leboeuf-Yde et al[8] concluded that classification of LBP patients into subgroups yielded better conclusions.

CLINICAL PILLAR

The four primary reasons for classifying patients with spine-related disorders include the following:

- Determining the most efficacious intervention option
- Determining prognosis
- Establishing a common language
- Guiding research initiatives

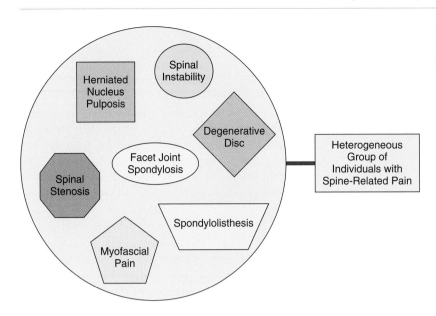

FIGURE 17–2 The heterogeneous nature of spine-related disorders, which consists of smaller pathoanatomic homogeneous subgroups.

There are two views that may be adopted when considering the concept of diagnosis and classification in the literature.[9] The **essentialist view** ascribes to the belief that disease exists fully formed and is waiting to be identified. The **nominalist view,** which now predominates, does not require the cause to be known in order for intervention to be initiated.[9]

The *International Classification of Diseases (ICD-9 and -10)*, a system in common use, includes 66 codes related specifically to the entity of LBP. The GPTP[5] uses a nominalistic, impairment-based classification system that places patients in preferred practice patterns based on the impairment without complete knowledge of the impairment's etiology. The challenges to differential diagnosis include subjectivity within the classification process, lack of mutually exclusive categories, and difficulty in deciding the level of diagnostic specificity.[9]

Fritz et al[7] compared the effectiveness and cost of a treatment-based classification approach to an approach based on the *Agency for Health Care Policy and Research* clinical practice guidelines in 78 subjects with acute, work-related LBP. Those assigned to the classification group showed a greater change in their Oswestry and SF-36 physical component score, showed greater satisfaction, were more likely to return to regular duty, and had substantially lower median total medical costs. This study, among others, demonstrated that subjects respond better when their intervention was guided by diagnostic classification.[10–14]

Types of Classification Systems

Riddle[4] defines four types of classification systems that are commonly used in health care today. The **status index** is a type of classification that defines the patient problem and is the most prevalent type used for patients with LBP. The ICD-10 classification system is a type of status index. The **prognostic index**, as its name implies, serves to predict the future status of the individual patient. The **clinical guideline index**, which is commonly used in classification systems for spinal disorders, attempts to guide intervention that flows from the assigned diagnostic classification. The popular systems of McKenzie[15] and Delitto et al[16] are both considered to be clinical guideline indices. The **mixed index** is a hybrid system that incorporates several, or all, of the other types. The Quebec Task Force[17] system is considered to be a mixed index.

Buchbinder et al,[18] in their critical appraisal of classification systems for soft tissue disorders of the neck and upper limb, identify seven major methodological criteria that can be used to judge the quality of any classification system. The seven criteria for grading methodological quality are *appropriateness of purpose, content validity, face validity, feasibility, construct validity, reliability,* and *generalizability.*

Common Classification Systems for Spinal Disorders

Newton et al[19] attempted to describe the prevalence of pathoanatomical subtypes in a population of LBP patients. Two-hundred thirteen patients were examined by PTs trained in the identification of a specific set of subtypes determined to be valid by a multidisciplinary cohort. Prevalence of the following subtypes was noted: 32% acute strain, 28% radicular syndromes, 14% chronic strain, 10% sacroiliac syndrome, 6% posterior facet syndrome, and the remaining 10% a of different syndromes.[19]

The interdependent nature of spinal structures makes the identification of a specific pathoanatomical source challenging.[4] It has therefore been suggested that spinal diagnostic classification systems focus on identifiable impairments. McClure[20] states that "basing treatment on a diagnostic label associated with pathologic anatomy, such as a herniated disc or facet joint arthrosis, may not be sound practice. Rather, new systems of classification based on symptomatic response to mechanical stress have been proposed to guide treatment, particularly physical rehabilitation."

QUESTIONS *for* **REFLECTION**

- Why is it challenging to identify the specific anatomical structure that is responsible for an individual's spine-related pain?
- Based on the challenge of using classification systems that are pathoanatomical in nature, what is the more preferred method of classifying patients with spine-related disorders?
- What is the potential role of physical examination measures and self-assessment questionnaires in classifying patients with these disorders?

NOTABLE QUOTABLE

"Basing treatment on a diagnostic label associated with pathologic anatomy, such as a herniated disc or facet joint arthrosis, may not be sound practice. Rather, new systems of classification based on symptomatic response to mechanical stress have been proposed to guide treatment, particularly physical rehabilitation."

-P. McClure

Binkley et al[21] surveyed 24 expert orthopaedic PTs to measure the levels of agreement on labels and accompanying constellations of signs and symptoms for subgroups of patients with LBP. Six of the 25 diagnostic classes did not meet the minimum criteria for agreement. The results suggest that expert opinion supports the notion that classification schemes avoid the use of pathoanatomical labels.

In an attempt to study the interrater reliability of the results of examination procedures used in the classification of patients with LBP, Van Dillen et al[22] used five trained PTs in the examination of 95 subjects with LBP and 43 asymptomatic subjects. Examination items were based on either symptomatic response to movement or judgments of alignment and movement in different positions. Percentage of agreement and kappa coefficients revealed that experienced trained examiners demonstrated better reliability for all 28 items that were related to the reproduction of symptoms (greater than or equal to 0.75) compared to those related to alignment and movement (greater than or equal to 0.40).

The aforementioned review by Riddle[4] critically analyzed four classification systems in common use (Bernard and Kirkaldy-Willis system, Delitto and colleagues system, McKenzie system, and the Quebec Task Force system) using the criteria described by Buchbinder et al.[18] The systems analyzed did not meet the majority of measurement standards. It was determined that future research should focus on analyzing the construct validity and reliability of current systems, and new systems that fulfill measurement standards should be developed.[16]

Petersen et al[23] studied eight classification systems that were selected based on their utility in guiding intervention based on symptoms and the results of clinical tests. In addition to the four systems analyzed by Riddle,[4] this study also evaluated the classification systems of Sikorski, Katz, Newton et al, and Kilsgaard et al. None of the systems fulfilled all of the criteria, and there was lack of evidence related to the reliability and validity of these systems.[23]

McCarthy et al[24] searched electronic databases for systems used to classify LBP. A review of 32 studies revealed that higher ratings were found in those systems that used a statistical cluster analysis approach as opposed to a judgment approach. The authors highlight the need for an integrated classification system that uses biomedical, psychological, and social constructs.

Systems of Classification for Low Back Pain

Mechanical Diagnosis and Therapy

This classification system (Table 17-1), espoused by Robin McKenzie,[15] is covered in detail in Chapter 9 of this text and is reviewed briefly in the Direction of Preference Model section that follows. Riddle[4] classifies this system as a *clinical guideline index* that was developed through a *judgment approach* whose purpose is to determine the most appropriate intervention option.

This system, which is based on reported pain patterns and centralization of symptoms in response to repeated movements, was shown to be highly specific to positive discography indicating disc pathology.[25] Others have confirmed the ability of this system to differentiate a discogenic from nondiscogenic origin as well as competent from incompetent annulus in symptomatic subjects.[26] This system was also found to be reliable for showing a change in patient status.[27] Several studies have demonstrated that classification, based on centralization of symptoms and pattern of pain response to end-range movement, has excellent interrater reliability.[28-32] Despite these findings, a multicenter study of 363 patients with LBP demonstrated poor reliability (kappa = 0.26) of this system for classification.[33] In this study, postgraduate training in this method of classification did not improve reliability.

The McKenzie system has been found to have significant predictive value. Patients who had an increase in radicular pain upon passive extension that abolishes within 5 days of admission was found to have an excellent chance (100%) of avoiding surgical intervention.[34] The centralization of symptoms was found to have predictive validity for determining 1 year work status, and an inability to centralize was found to correlate with a decreased ability for return to work.[34,35] The inability to centralize and an increased score on the *Fear-Avoidance Belief Questionnaire (FABQ)* was found to predict increased levels of disability.[36] Classification systems that used evaluation of specific pain patterns across multiple visits discriminated categories for change in pain and disability.[37] Among nine independent variables, classification based on pain patterns, specifically noncentralization and leg pain, were found to be the strongest predictive variables of chronicity in 223 consecutive patients with acute LBP.[38]

Activity-Related Spinal Disorders by the Quebec Task Force

This model, developed by the *Quebec Task Force on Spinal Disorders (QTFSD)*,[17] is considered to be a *mixed index* developed through a *judgment approach* whose purpose is to assist in clinical

Table 17-1	A Comparison of Common Systems of Classification for Low Back Pain			
	MECHANICAL DIAGNOSIS AND THERAPY (MCKENZIE, 1981)	**ACTIVITY-RELATED SPINAL DISORDERS MODEL (QTFSD, 1987)**	**PHYSICAL THERAPY MODEL (DEROSA, PORTERFIELD, 1992)**	**TREATMENT-BASED CLASSIFICATION APPROACH (DELITTO, 1995)**
Type	Clinical guideline index	Mixed index	Clinical guideline index	Clinical guideline index
Method of development	Judgment approach	Judgment approach	Judgment approach	Judgment approach
Purpose	Determine intervention	Clinical decision-making, establish prognosis, research	Determine intervention	Determine intervention
Classification categories	13 categories: Postural syndrome (4), dysfunction syndromes (7), derangement syndromes, hip or sacroiliac joint syndrome	11 categories with 2 axes: related to location of symptoms (4), based on imaging (3), related to time since surgery (2), related to chronicity, other (1)	3 categories: acute, reinjury, chronic	3 stages of classification: Stage I—extension, flexion, lateral shift (2), immobilization (4), traction (5), mobilization (5) Stage II—flexibility deficit, strength deficit, cardiovascular deficit, coordination deficit, body mechanics deficit Stage III—activity intolerance, work intolerance

McKenzie RA. *The Lumbar Spine. Mechanical Diagnosis and Therapy.* Wellington, New Zealand: Spinal Publications Limited; 1981.
Quebec Task Force on Spinal Disorders. Scientific approach to the assessment and management of activity-related spinal disorders. A monograph for clinicians. Spine. 1987;12:51-59.
DeRosa CP, Porterfield JA. A physical therapy model for the treatment of low back pain. *Phys Ther.* 1992;72:261-272.
Delitto A, Cibulka MT, Erhard RE, Bowling RW, Tenhula JA. Evidence for use of an extension-mobilization category in acute low back syndrome: a prescriptive validation pilot study. *Phys Ther.* 1993;73:216-228. Delitto A, Cibulka MT, Erhard RE, Bowling RW, Tenhula JA. Evidence for use of an extension-mobilization category in acute low back syndrome: a prescriptive validation pilot study. *Phys Ther.* 1993;73:216-228.

decision-making, establishing a prognosis, quality control, and to guide research initiatives.[4] This approach is comprised of 11 categories with two axes. The two axes are superimposed on the initial classification for the purpose of assisting with prognosis. These two axes include symptom duration (less than 7 days, 7 days to 7 weeks, and greater than 7 weeks) and work status at the time of the examination (working or idle) (Fig. 17-3).

A prospective study of 526 patients assessed the QTFSD system's ability to stratify patients according to severity and intervention and to assess change over time. Most patients with sciatica were classified into categories 3 to 6, and 15 patients were assigned to category 1. There were no differences in duration of pain or percentage of those working across categories 1 to 6. The results provide validation of this classification system in stratifying patients according to the severity of symptoms.[39]

Physical Therapy Model

The physical therapy model was developed by DeRosa and Porterfield[40] in an attempt to match the objectives of intervention to the classification of the patient. This system is a *clinical guideline index* developed using the *judgment approach* for the purpose of determining the best intervention option.[4] The primary feature of this approach is its simplicity; employing three categories that utilize commonly used terms (acute, reinjury, chronic). Principles of intervention are recommended that consider the stage of healing based on the assigned classification category. There is no

current evidence supporting the use of this system in clinical practice, however, this model highlights the value of employing interventions that respect the process of healing.

Treatment-Based Classification (TBC)

The classification system that has gained most favor in recent years and has undergone a substantial amount of critical analysis is the system proposed by Delitto et al.[16] This system is also a *clinical guideline index* developed using the *judgment approach* whose purpose is to determine appropriate intervention.[4] Within this approach, the first level of classification requires a determination of which individuals are appropriate for physical therapy, consultation, or referral.[16]

The second level of classification is divided into three stages. An individual classified in *stage I* is characterized by an inability to perform basic mechanical functions such as standing, walking, and sitting. In this stage, intervention is designed to relieve symptoms.[16] *Stage II* patients are able to perform basic mechanical functions but lack the ability to perform basic functional activities of daily living (ADL). Intervention strategies include pain modulation as well as interventions to eliminate signs of physical impairment.[16] *Stage III* is for the individual who is planning to return to an activity that requires a high degree of physical demand. These individuals are often asymptomatic, but are generally deconditioned from a period of inactivity.[16]

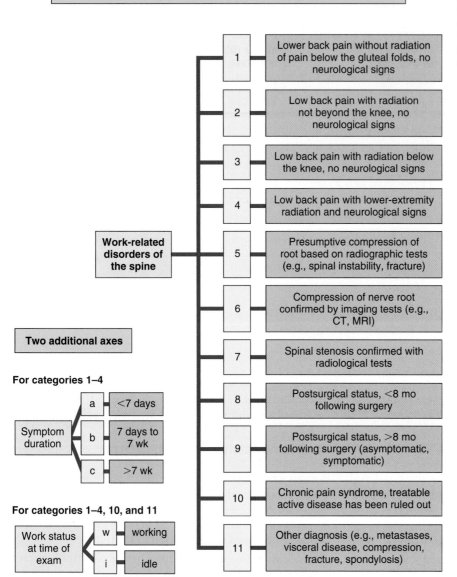

FIGURE 17-3 Description of classification categories for the activity-related spinal disorders model as developed by the Quebec Task Force on Spinal Disorders (QTFSD). (Adapted from Riddle, D. Classification and low back pain: a review of the literature and critical analysis of selected systems. *Phys Ther.* 1998;78:708-735.)

Stage I has been most extensively studied in the literature. Within stage I there are seven syndromes. The *extension, flexion,* and *lateral shift syndromes* are based on the movement direction that brings relief. If the patient fails to improve or symptoms worsen with movement, the patient is classified as having a *traction syndrome.* In the case where symptoms remain unchanged, patients are placed into the mobilization syndrome category, which consists of *lumbar* or *sacroiliac mobilization syndromes.* The *immobilization syndrome* category is for patients that present with segmental hypermobility and are classified best through the patient's history. Stage II consists of deficits in *flexibility, strength, cardiovascular, coordination, and body mechanics.* Stage III consists of activity *intolerance and work intolerance syndromes.*[16]

The TBC model has been found to demonstrate moderate interrater reliability (kappa = 0.56) when 43 LBP patients were assigned to one of the seven syndromes within stage I of this system. When the authors collapsed the seven syndromes into four based on similarities in intervention, kappa value decreased to 0.49. The percentage of patients in this study assigned to each classification was as follows: sacroiliac mobilization (27%); immobilization, extension, and flexion syndromes (18% each); lateral shift (9%); lumbar mobilization (7%); and traction syndrome (3%). It was also determined that those assigned to the immobilization category may have a less optimistic prognosis compared to those assigned to either the mobilization or specific exercise groups.[41]

Use of the TBC approach has also demonstrated more favorable outcomes when used to classify seventy-eight subjects with work-related LBP compared to a group that was treated using clinical practice guidelines. Improved disability and return to work status after 4 weeks was demonstrated in the patients treated using the TBC approach.[7] Delitto et al[42] studied the extension-mobilization syndrome category and discovered that 24 of the 39 subjects in the study were assigned to this group. Subjects were treated using extension and mobilization or a flexion exercise regimen based on classification. Subjects assigned and subsequently treated using extension and mobilization responded to intervention at a faster rate than did controls.[42]

The purpose of the TBC system is to match subgroups of patients with LBP to specific interventions based on clinical findings. George and Delitto[36] studied the discriminate validity of the TBC approach by determining whether commonly used clinical procedures were able to discriminate between TBC subgroups. One hundred thirty-one subjects were classified into the following subgroups: 38.9% specific exercise, 32,1% mobilization, 21.4% immobilization, and 7.6% traction. Evidence supporting the ability of the TBC classification system to discriminate between patients with LBP was provided.[36]

Systems of Classification for Neck Pain

Systems of classification for neck pain (NP) have not been extensively examined in the literature (Table 17-2). McClure[20] has proposed a theoretical model for classification of cervical spine disorders based on the patient's symptomatic response to mechanical stress that guides intervention (Fig. 17-4). The patient is first classified as having either *high irritability* or *low irritability*. Individuals are then classified as a *tension syndrome* or *compression syndrome* based on the movements that reproduce symptoms. This model will be covered in detail in the Direction of Preference section of this chapter.

Piva et al[43] proposed a clinical decision-making algorithm based on movement loss and the presence of radicular symptoms to classify patients and provide subsequent intervention that initially focuses on the use of cervical traction techniques (Fig. 17-5). They recommended that a patient presenting with limited flexion and upper extremity symptoms should receive traction, after which, reexamination of flexion was to be performed. If flexion remained limited, traction was to be continued. If flexion was restored to full range, then the therapist attempted to determine the presence of an opening restriction or a closing restriction for which the appropriate manual technique would be implemented.[43] Their definition of an **opening restriction** was similar to the McClure[20] tension syndrome label for which

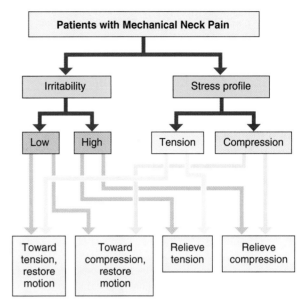

FIGURE 17–4 Clinical decision-making algorithm used to guide intervention for cervical disorders as espoused by McClure. (Adapted from McClure P. The degenerative cervical spine: pathogenesis and rehabilitation concepts. *J Hand Ther.* 2000;April-June:163-174.)

symptoms and limited motion were identified with movement away from the painful side. A **closing restriction**, similar to the McClure[20] compression syndrome label, was identified by pain and restricted motion with movement toward the painful side.[43]

A similar model was developed by Wang et al[44] to determine the effectiveness of treating NP using a clinical decision-making algorithm. An eclectic intervention regimen based on the proposed algorithm was used, including outcome measures such as cervical range of motion and numeric pain rating, among others. After 4 weeks, the experimental group showed improvement in four of the five measures compared with the control group who did not improve in any of the outcome measures. The authors concluded that an algorithmic approach to treating neck disorders may assist therapists in classifying patients into clinical patterns that provide guidelines for intervention.[44]

Table 17-2	A Comparison of Common Systems of Classification for Neck Pain			
	PIVA ET AL, 2000	**MCCLURE, 2000**	**WANG ET AL, 2003**	**CHILDS ET AL, 2004**
Type	Clinical guideline index	Clinical guideline index	Clinical guideline index	Clinical guideline index
Method of development	Judgment approach	Judgment approach	Judgment approach	Judgment approach
Purpose	Determine intervention	Determine intervention	Determine intervention	Determine intervention, establish prognosis
Classification categories	**3 stages of classification:** full/limited flexion, opening/closing restriction, presence of radicular signs, and rule out thoracic outlet syndrome	**3 categories:** compression profile, tension profile, mixed profile	**4 levels with 18 categories:** radicular pain (RAD 1-3), referred pain (REF 1-6), headache (HA 1-4), neck pain (NP 1-5)	**5 categories:** mobility, centralization, conditioning and increase exercise tolerance, pain control, reduce headache

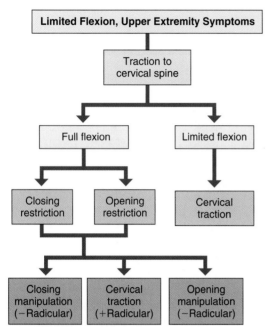

FIGURE 17–5 Clinical decision-making algorithm used to guide intervention for cervical disorders as espoused by Piva et al. (Adapted from Piva SR, Erhard RE, Al-Hugail M. Cervical radiculopathy: a case problem using a decision-making algorithm. *J Orthop Sports Phys Ther.* 2000:30(12):745-754.)

More recently, Childs et al[45] examined the literature related to classification of NP and offered a classification system based on the integration of data from the history and physical examination (Fig. 17-6). In addition to identifying the *red flags* suggestive of serious pathology, the authors identified *yellow flags*, which indicated heightened fear-avoidance behavior. Within this approach, five subgroups of NP were proposed. The *mobility category* is characterized by recent onset and

restricted range without peripheralization of symptoms. The *centralization category* includes peripheralization of symptoms with suspected cervical radiculopathy. The *exercise and conditioning category* is characterized by lower pain and disability scores and longer duration of symptoms without peripheralization. Conversely, the *pain control category* reveals high pain and disability scores, recent onset of symptoms, and poor tolerance for examination and intervention procedures. The *headache category* patient presents with unilateral headaches that are associated with NP and elicited through neck movement and manual pressure over the cervical spine. This system of classification has yet to be subjected to critical scrutiny in determining its utility for accurately and reliably classifying individuals with NP.[45]

In summary, the current best evidence suggests that the physical therapy diagnosis is best identified through a classification approach that relates the patient's relevant signs and symptoms to his or her movement behavior, with consideration given to the duration and severity of the symptoms. TE regimens should be selected based on clinically relevant, impairment-based classification that guides intervention through identification of homogeneous subgroups and not based on pathoanatomical labels. An alternative algorithm for determining exercise prescription that integrates several physical therapy approaches is presented in Figure 17-7.

THE DIRECTION OF PREFERENCE MODEL
Principles of Examination and Classification

Examination procedures intended to find the direction of preference, or the most tolerated direction of movement, requires testing of repeated end range spinal movements. This

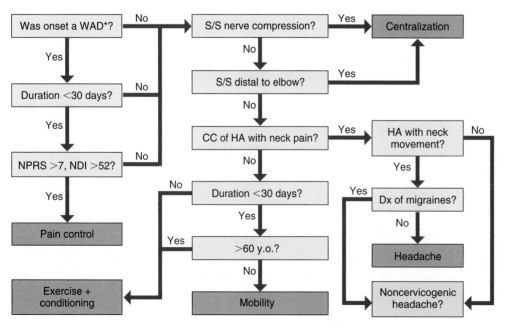

FIGURE 17–6 Modified clinical decision-making algorithm used to guide intervention for cervical disorders as espoused by Childs et al. WAD = whiplash associated disorder; SS = signs and symptoms; NPRS = numeric pain rating scale; NDI = neck disability index; CC = chief complaint; HA = headache; Dx = diagnosis; y.o. = years old. (Adapted from Childs JD, Fritz JM, Piva SR, Whitman JM. Proposal of a classification system for patients with neck pain. *J Orthop Sports Phys Ther.* 2004;34:686-700.)

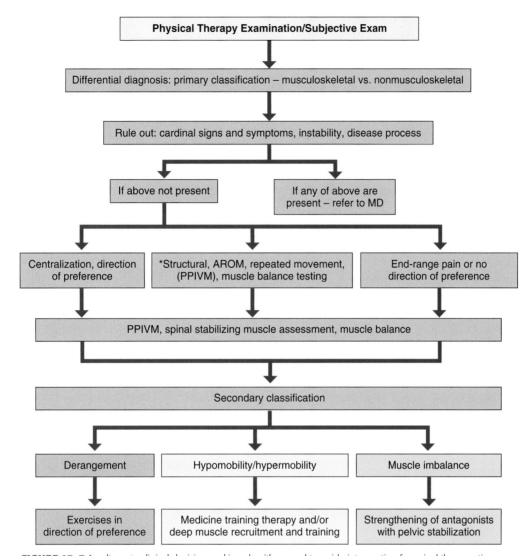

FIGURE 17–7 An alternate clinical decision-making algorithm used to guide intervention for spinal therapeutic exercise regimens, which features the integration of stability and mobility exercises for recovery of function and prevention of recurrence. AROM, active range of motion; PPIVM, passive intervertebral motion; MD, medical doctor.

concept is often attributed to the work of Robin McKenzie (see Chapter 9).[15,46]

The McKenzie approach is based on an examination scheme that is designed to identify the patient's tolerance for specific directions of movement. Intervention is then guided by what is determined as the patient's most tolerated, least provocative, most symptom-alleviating direction of movement. The direction of movement which decreases, centralizes, or abolishes symptoms constitutes the principle movement direction in which intervention will be initiated. This model is fully discussed in Chapter 9.

Prior to the advent of extension-biased regimens for spinal conditions in the early 1980s, individuals suffering from LBP were encouraged to preferentially engage in flexion. In the 1950s, *Paul C. Williams* developed a regimen of flexion-biased exercises that were believed to be indicated for most individuals with LBP.[47] This flexion-biased exercise regimen has become known as the ***Williams flexion*** regimen. Williams believed that an increase in pressure was exerted on the posterior aspect of

the vertebra and disc during typical activities that leads to rupture of the disc at L5.[47] He further postulated that extension of the spine would add further stress to this region and lead to nerve impingement.[47] Based on this theory, Williams concluded that the solution to this dilemma was to engage in postures and exercises that limited the degree of lordosis through encouraging flexion of the lumbar spine.[47]

Ponte et al[47] performed a preliminary study to determine whether the Williams flexion-biased or the McKenzie extension-biased protocol was more effective in treating 22 subjects with LBP. Changes in six distinct parameters were used to gauge each subject's response. The results indicated that those receiving the McKenzie protocol had greater improvement in a shorter period of time than those following the Williams protocol. A study by Nwuga and Nwuga[48] on 62 subjects diagnosed with a prolapsed disc showed similar findings. The McKenzie protocol was found to be superior to the Williams protocol based on changes in range of movement of straight leg raising, average time spent in treatment, decreased pain, and increased comfortable sitting time. In addition, recidivism was more common in the Williams flexion group.[48]

Although not as extensively studied as in the lumbar spine, recent research supports the use of repeated movements in classifying patients with cervical spine complaints as well.[27,28] As aforementioned, McClure[20] proposed a system for classifying mechanical NP that was based on the effects of combined movements (Table 17-3). As in the McKenzie approach, a system of classification based on the patient's symptomatic response to mechanical stress was proposed as a means to guide intervention in addition to determining the level of irritability.[20]

When symptoms are elicited prior to achieving end range, the condition is considered to be of *high irritability*. If passive overpressure is required to elicit the symptoms, the condition is deemed to be of *low irritability*. In addition to examining cardinal plane motions, combined movements are used to clarify the effect of mechanical stress on symptoms.[20] If irritability is classified as low, then the direction of preference is toward the symptom producing motion. If the level of irritability is classified as high, however, the direction of preference is away from the motion that brought on the symptoms.

McClure classifies patients into one of three symptom profiles based on their direction of preference. In the cervical spine, the *compression stress profile* would be suggested if symptoms were initially produced with extension, ipsilateral side bending, or ipsilateral rotation in reference to the painful region. Symptoms would increase and range might decrease if these motions were performed in combination, and symptoms would decrease and range might increase if

flexion, contralateral side bending, or contralateral rotation were added. Conversely, the *tension stress profile* would reveal the initial onset of symptoms with flexion, contralateral side bending, or contralateral rotation. Symptoms would increase and range might decrease if these motions were performed in combination, and symptoms would decrease and range might increase if extension, ipsilateral side bending, or ipsilateral rotation were added. In the *mixed stress profile*, elements of both the compression stress profile and the tension stress profile coexist.[20]

Principles of Intervention

Within this model of diagnostic classification, the direction of movement that alleviates symptoms, or is best tolerated, is considered to be the direction of preference and deemed as the initial movement bias in which exercise is to occur. It is important to note, that although this model directs the initial directional preference, prior to discharge, it is important for the manual therapist to consider addressing the patient's

---

CLINICAL PILLAR

When operating within the direction of preference model, be sure to begin with encouraging movement into the least provocative, most tolerated direction. Intervention, however, should eventually address movement deficits in all directions.

Table 17-3   Cervical Classification Categories and Matched Intervention Strategies as Espoused by McClure

	COMPRESSION PROFILE	TENSION PROFILE	MIXED PROFILE
Symptoms produced or increased by:	Extension, ipsilateral side bending and rotation	Flexion, contralateral side bending and rotation	Variable and Combined
Symptoms reduced by:	Flexion, contralateral side bending and rotation	Extension, ipsilateral side bending and rotation	Variable and Combined
Irritability level and matched intervention:	**High:** relieve compression through rest, modalities, meds, pain-free ROM away from compression, avoid end range, traction **Low:** restore motion through stretching into pain (compression), mobilization/ROM to improve restricted motion	**High:** relieve tension through rest, modalities, meds, pain-free ROM away from tension, avoid end range **Low:** restore motion through stretching into pain (tension), mobilization/ROM to improve restricted motion, neural tension	Variable and Combined

Piva SR, Erhard RE, Al-Hugail M. Cervical radiculopathy: a case problem using a decision-making algorithm. *J Orthop Sports Phys Ther.* 2000:30:745-754.
McClure
Wang WTJ, Olson SL, Campbell AH, Hanten WP, Gleeson PB. Effectiveness of physical therapy for patients with neck pain: an individualized approach using a clinical decision-making algorithm. *Am J Phys Med Rehabil.* 2003;82:203-218.
Childs JD, Fritz JM, Piva SR, Whitman JM. Proposal of a classification system for patients with neck pain. *J Orthop Sports Phys Ther.* 2004;34:686-700.

movement impairments in all directions to maximize function and prevent reoccurrence. Chapter 9 fully describes principles of intervention specific to the McKenzie[15] model. Like McKenzie, the Delitto[7,16] model also includes a centralization category based on testing repeated movements.

A study by Schenk et al[49] found that patients classified with a diagnosis of posterior derangement had more favorable outcomes when treated according to an exercise regimen performed in a direction of preference compared to a group treated with lumbar mobilization.[49] The importance of classifying patients was later analyzed by Cook et al,[50] who in their review of studies pertaining to exercise and patient classification, reported that there appears to be a trend toward positive outcomes with exercise intervention in trials restricted to the patient response method of classification.[50]

THE MOBILITY IMPAIRMENT/JOINT DYSFUNCTION MODEL

Principles of Examination

The *mobility impairment model* or *joint dysfunction model* attributes impairments in mobility primarily to joint dysfunction while being cognizant of the role that periarticular structures, such as muscle and the capsuloligamentous complex, play in influencing the characteristics of movement. Paris defines joint dysfunction as "a state of altered mechanics, either an increase or decrease from the expected normal, or the presence of an aberrant motion."[51] (See Chapter 7.) This approach to exercise mandates a consideration of the quantity (Q) and quality (Q) of motion along with the reproduction (R) of any symptoms that may occur as a result of movement testing (known as the QQR exam).[52]

NOTABLE QUOTABLE

"Joint dysfunction is a state of altered mechanics, either an increase or decrease from the expected normal, or the presence of an aberrant motion."

S.V. Paris

QUESTIONS *for* REFLECTION

- What structures may be responsible for the presence of mobility impairments in the spine?
- How might the manual therapist go about identifying the primary and secondary origins of such impairments during the examination?
- Why is it important to determine whether a restriction in the *joint, muscle,* or *nerve* is the most likely cause of a cervical spine mobility impairment?

CLINICAL PILLAR

When attempting to identify the origin of a cervical spine mobility impairment, consider differentiating between *joint, muscle,* and *nerve* restrictions in the following ways:

- **Joint:** Side bending is limited and does not improve with passive elevation of the shoulders. Presence of a capsular pattern (i.e., restriction on right: FB with right deviation, SB left, ROT left most limited). PPIVM, PAIVM reveals restrictions.

- **Muscle:** Side bending is limited, yet improves when the muscles are placed on slack with passive elevation of the shoulders. Side bending is more limited than rotation. There is noncapsular motion loss and palpable stiffness and trigger points.

- **Nerve:** Upper limb tension tests (i.e., ULTT, ULNT) are positive; symptoms peripheralize and are neurological in nature. Arm position affects cervical range of motion. Shoulder/scapular depression reduces cervical motion. Headaches are present.

Examination of Movement Quantity

Within this approach, the ability of the manual physical therapist to determine the extent of available motion at any given joint is paramount in determining the optimal course of intervention. During the examination, the manual therapist uses active and passive motion testing to determine the presence of either hypomobility or hypermobility. The testing of active and repeated end range spinal movements may indicate that pain is experienced at end range and that range of motion is either restricted or greater than expected.

Due to the multisegmental nature of the spine, hypomobility and hypermobility often coexist. Hypomobility in one segment is presumed to lead to adjacent compensatory hypermobility. The region of hypermobility is often found to be the symptom-producing segment. Passive accessory intervertebral mobility (PAIVM) testing and passive physiologic intervertebral mobility (PPIVM) testing will help to identify the movement characteristics of each segment relative to one another.

During the examination, the PT must differentiate between hypermobility and *instability*. In the absence of clinical symptoms and an abnormal end-feel, the former is considered to be nonpathological, whereas the latter requires stabilization of the involved segments. In a study of 172 PTs, Cook et al[53] found the following signs and symptoms to be indicators of cervical spine instability (Box 17-1): intolerance to static postures, fatigue and inability to hold head erect, improvement in response to external support including hands or collar, the frequent need for self-manipulation, the feeling of instability, shaking or lack of control during movement, frequent episodes of acute attacks, and sharp pain with sudden movements.[53]

Clinical instability has been formally defined by Panjabi[54] as "a significant decrease in the capacity of the *stabilizing system* of the spine to maintain the intervertebral *neutral zones* within physiologic limits which results in pain and disability."[54] Fritz et al[55] have summarized the work of Panjabi in describing the stabilizing system of the spine. Conceptually, the stabilizing system of the spine is composed of three subsystems (Fig. 17-8).

The **passive subsystem** is comprised of spinal osteology, facet joint capsules, ligaments, and the passive tension of the musculotendinous unit. The passive subsystem is most involved in contributing to spinal stability at or near the end ranges of movement. Mathematical models, finite element models, and serial cutting experiments have all yielded useful data related to the function of the passive subsystem.[55] These studies have identified the *direction-specific* role of spinal ligaments, facet

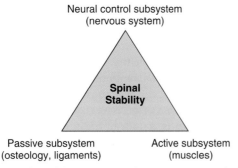

FIGURE 17–8 The stabilizing system of the spine is comprised of three subsystems: the passive subsystem, the active subsystem, and the neural control subsystem. (Adapted from Richardson C, Jull G, Hodges P, Hides J. *Therapeutic Exercise for Spinal Segmental Stabilization in Low Back Pain. A Scientific Basis and Clinical Approach*. London, UK: Churchill Livingston, 1999.)

joint capsules, and disc structures in providing stabilization at end ranges of motion.[56-59] Damage to this subsystem may have a profound effect on spinal stability and motion by increasing the size of the neutral zone and effectively placing a greater demand on the other subsystems.[55]

Vleeming et al[60] studied the role of the posterior layer of the thoracolumbar fascia during load transfer between the spine, pelvis, legs, and arms. Visual inspection and raster photography was used on 10 human cadaveric specimens to assess the response of the thoracolumbar fascia to traction forces designed to simulate a muscle contraction. In vitro, the superficial and deep laminae of the posterior layer of the thoracolumbar fascia undergoes tension from the inserting musculature, which provides effective load transmission and stabilization of the lumbar spine.[60]

The **active subsystem** is comprised of contractile skeletal muscle and is most involved in contributing to stability within the neutral zone. The **neural control subsystem** receives input from structures in the other two subsystems for the purpose of determining the requirements for stability and coordinated movement in any given task. By regulating the active subsystem through paraspinal musculature, it serves to prepare and respond to impending perturbation. For example, the neurons of the *vestibulospinal tract* originate in the lateral vestibular nucleus and carry excitatory fibers from the ipsilateral semicircular canal to influence contraction of the extensor muscles of the trunk and extremities.[61]

Regulation of spinal stability and motion quality is provided by the active subsystem through the preferential recruitment of deep/unisegmental and superficial/multisegmental spinal musculature. The deep/unisegmental spinal musculature functions as a force transducer which provides feedback on spinal position and motion to the neural control subsystem. Conversely, the larger, more superficial/multisegmental spinal musculature is best suited for producing and controlling lumbar spine motion.[55]

Cholewicki et al[62] studied the muscular activation patterns of 10 healthy subjects in the execution of slow trunk flexion-extension tasks around the neutral zone while surface electromyography (EMG) data were recorded from six abdominal and paraspinal muscles. The results demonstrated that trunk flexor-extensor muscle coactivation occurred when the spine was in the neutral zone, thus contributing to spinal stability, in the healthy population.[62] Granata and Marras[63] investigated the influence of muscle coactivation on spinal loads. They collected EMG data from five trunk muscle pairs, three-dimensional motion data, and force plate data to measure lifting kinetics in 10 healthy subjects. Results showed that healthy subjects displayed significant trunk muscle coactivity that was dramatically influenced by the compressive and anterior shear forces on the lumbar spine during lifting.[63] These studies confirm our previous assertions that the active and neural control subsystems are most involved in regulating stability and kinesthesia in the neutral zone and that this is best accomplished through muscle coactivation.

The presence of spinal instability, particularly in the cervical spine, is a serious condition. Paris[64] has identified clinical signs of spinal instability, which include a band of hypertrophy in the region of instability, failure to perform coordinated active movements, increased mobility upon PPIVM testing, and a palpable step deformity when the spine is unsupported that reduces when supported, among other signs.[64] Screening procedures may also prove useful in identifying the presence of spinal instability.[65] A complete exposition on the principles and practices of examining spinal mobility and identifying the presence of segmental instability is included in Chapters 28 to 30.

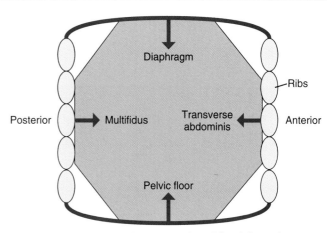

FIGURE 17–9 Diagrammatic representation of the abdominal cavity as a closed cylinder where dynamic spinal stabilization is produced by cocontraction of the transverse abdominis, multifidus, diaphragm, and pelvic floor musculature. Cocontraction reduces the volume of the abdominal cavity which increases intra-abdominal pressure. (Adapted from Richardson C, Jull G, Hodges P, Hides J. *Therapeutic Exercise for Spinal Segmental Stabilization in low Back Pain. A Scientific Basis and Clinical Approach.* London, UK: Churchill Livingston, 1999.)

> ## CLINICAL PILLAR
>
> When quantifying spinal mobility, be sure to consider the spinal *region*, spinal *segment*, and the *direction* in which motion is to occur. The degree of mobility will change based on these three variables. The manual therapist must also consider normal coupling patterns of motion and how they vary from region to region.

> ## QUESTIONS *for* REFLECTION
>
> - What is the difference between *hypermobility* and *instability*?
> - How would a manual therapist differentiate between hypermobility and instability during the examination?

Examination of Muscle Function

Examination of the Deep Stabilizers of the Trunk

When considering lumbopelvic muscle function, the *transverse abdominis* muscle appears to have a unique and specialized function.[65] This muscle is controlled independent of other trunk muscles in providing nondirectional spinal stiffness and segmental control.[65] The mechanism by which this muscle provides such control is believed to be related to the production of increased intra-abdominal pressure or an increased tension of the thoracolumbar fascia during recruitment. Evidence suggests a specialized relationship between the transverse abdominis and the deep multifidus muscle.[65] Contraction of either muscle has been observed to produce a cocontraction of the other. This cocontraction is likened to a muscular corset and is required in order to achieve optimal segmental stabilization. Along with the diaphragm and muscles of the pelvic floor, these muscles, functioning as a closed cylinder, collectively increase intra-abdominal pressure and contribute to stability through cocontraction (Fig. 17-9).[65]

The concept of global and local muscle function challenges the standard of care for spinal exercise regimens that have traditionally focused on improving performance of the global muscles as a means toward improving spinal stability. Exercises such as prone trunk extensions, posterior pelvic tilts, and sit-ups all focus, primarily, on function of the global muscles. The global muscle system is vital to trunk support, yet has limited capability in contributing to segmental stability.[66-68] These

muscles have a reduced capacity to control shear forces, may contribute to increased compression and loading, and when acting in isolation, may actually pose a challenge to spinal segmental stability.[67,68] In the presence of spinal dysfunction, the preferential use of the global system, and poor motor control of the local system is believed to be a potential contributor and/or sequela to spinal pain.[67,68]

For normal, pain-free function, the local system is required to contract at continual, low levels of tension during functional activities. The timing and coordination of local muscle recruitment is, perhaps, more important than the magnitude of force that is elicited by these muscles. In light of the evidence, examination procedures and subsequent intervention for individuals suffering from spinal instability should be reconsidered, and methods for testing the function of the local stabilizing muscles should be included during routine examination.

The clinical examination of local trunk muscle function for the lumbo-pelvic region includes the abdominal ***drawing-in maneuver*** (Fig. 17-10), the segmental multifidus test (Fig. 17-11), and the leg-loading test (Fig. 17-12).[65] Of the three, the drawing-in maneuver, which seeks to isolate recruitment of the transverse abdominis, is used most extensively. This maneuver is typically performed with the patient in prone or supine and requires an isolated contraction that is held for 10 seconds.[65] The patient is asked to draw in the abdominal wall without moving the spine or pelvis while breathing normally. The patient is advised not to hold his or her breath or to elicit activation of the global muscles. Performance of this unfamiliar task can be enhanced by focusing the patient on his or her lower abdomen and by providing verbal cues, such as "pull your belly button up and under your ribs." Proper activation of the transverse abdominis can be assessed by palpating the region just medial to the anterior superior iliac spine. If difficulty is noted in performance of this maneuver, patients may attempt to initially perform this maneuver in quadruped.[65]

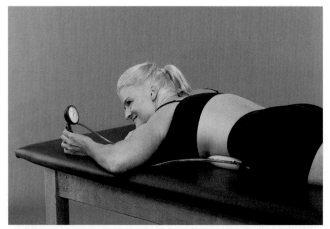

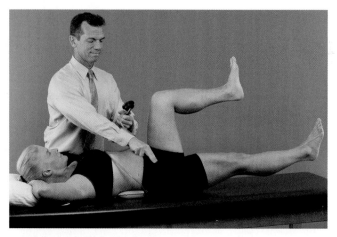

FIGURE 17–12 The leg loading test.

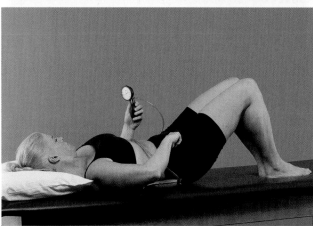

FIGURE 17–10 Examination of transverse abdominis and multifidus cocontraction using the drawing-in maneuver in **A.** prone and **B.** supine through performance of the drawing-in maneuver using the Stabilizer biofeedback unit.

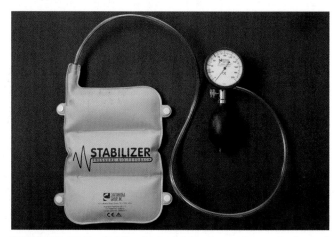

FIGURE 17–13 The Stabilizer biofeedback unit used for examination and training of deep, local muscles during segmental stabilization exercises.

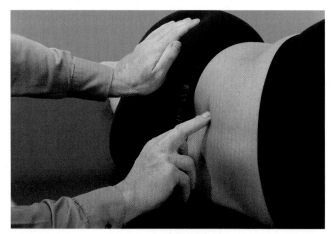

FIGURE 17–11 The segmental multifidus test.

To assist in the facilitation of the contraction and document performance, a pressure biofeedback unit, known as the *Stabilizer* (Chattanooga Pacific Pty. Ltd., Brisbane, Australia), may be used (Fig. 17-13).[65] The Stabilizer is placed with the distal edge in line with the anterior superior iliac spines. Initially, the unit is inflated to 70 mm Hg.[65] As the patient performs the maneuver, the pressure should decrease. A decrease of 6 to 10 mm Hg is considered normal.[65] If the patient is unable to achieve a reduction of this magnitude, the test is positive and poor transverse abdominis muscle function is suspected. After demonstrating the ability to isolate this muscle, the patient is asked to hold the contraction for 10 seconds as a means of testing muscle endurance. During testing, it is critical that the patient understands the emphasis on isolation as opposed to degree of force. This is facilitated through appropriate tactile feedback and verbal cues from the therapist. In a study by Haggins et al,[69] the Stabilizer was found to be effective in the instruction of asymptomatic patients in a specific stabilizing exercise regimen over a 4-week period.[69]

The association between the transverse abdominis and multifidus can be confirmed by palpating the multifidus immediately adjacent to the interspinous space at any given level during performance of the drawing-in maneuver in prone. Multifidus function is further analyzed through the segmental multifidus test, which uses tactile cues from the therapist at specific spinal segments with the instructions to "swell the muscle under my fingers," without moving the spine or pelvis.[65] This test requires astute palpatory skills and is often challenging for the novice practitioner to monitor and difficult for the patient to perform. Enhanced facilitation of multifidus recruitment may be achieved by placing the patient in side-lying position. One of the examiner's hands is placed over the pelvis to elicit resistance to rotation while the other palpates for multifidus recruitment (Fig. 17-11).

The final stage of testing for local muscle function in this region is designed to examine control of lumbo-pelvic posture through the leg-loading test.[65] This test is performed in the hook-lying position where monitoring of lumbo-pelvic position can occur as a precontraction of the deep muscles prior to limb movement. With the pressure biofeedback unit positioned under the lumbar spine and inflated to *40 mm Hg*, the patient is asked to perform various leg movements while maintaining constant pressure.[65]

Examination of the Deep Stabilizers of the Neck

In the detection of cervical spine segmental instability, a survey conducted by Cook et al[53] indicated that most PTs felt the identifiers of instability involved intricate palpation and visual assessment skills, poor tolerance to certain postures, and movement-related similarities, but added that "appropriate clinical reasoning is required for distinctive assessment."[53]

In the cervical region, the deep neck flexors and extensors such as the longus colli, longus capitus, semispinalis cervicis, and muscles of the suboccipital triangle are targeted. The goals of this examination and exercise regimen are to target the deep cervical and shoulder girdle muscles, retrain the tonic endurance capacity of these muscles, retrain patterns of activation between deep and superficial muscles, facilitate cocontraction of deep cervical flexor and extensor muscles, and reeducate the function of these muscles during posture and function.

The clinical examination of deep, local muscle function is performed using the ***craniocervical flexion test***. This procedure involves the use of the pressure biofeedback unit and/or tactile and verbal cueing from the therapist (Fig. 17-14). Prior to testing, the patient is positioned in hook-lying with the hands on the abdomen and the head in neutral, which may require adjustment using towel rolls. The biofeedback unit is placed beneath the patient's neck and inflated to *20 mm Hg* as the patient is instructed to nod his or her head so as to produce

pure rotation of head on neck. Pure rotation without retraction is monitored as the patient incrementally attempts to increase pressure from *20 to 30 mm Hg*. Through palpation, the examiner ensures that the patient is recruiting the deep stabilizing muscles as opposed to the more superficial scaleni and sternocleidomastoid muscles. If the patient is experiencing difficulty performing this maneuver, eye movement and verbal cues, including asking the patient to slide his or her head toward the shoulders then back again, may be used. The two phases of testing include testing the correct pattern of activation of local muscles followed by assessment of holding capacity, which must occur sequentially. Once the test is properly performed, the patient may hold the contraction for up to 10 seconds for 10 repetitions at *30 mm Hg* to test endurance.

QUESTIONS *for* REFLECTION

- Which muscles comprise the *deep, local muscle system* of the spine, and which muscles comprise the *superficial, global system*?
- What is the primary function of the local muscles, and how does it differ from the function of the global muscles?
- How does the anatomical arrangement of these muscles allow them to each function in their respective fashion?

Testing endurance of these muscles may also involve the graduated head lift in supine in which the patient lifts their head 1 inch above the plinth and holds the position for 10 seconds. The manual therapist may draw a line across one of the neck folds to ensure that the patient is able to maintain this position, thereby obscuring the line. An inability to maintain the contraction for 10 seconds is indicative of poor function of these muscles and suggests the need for subsequent training[70,71]

Examination of Movement Quality and Kinesthesia

Normal spine function is dependent on the seamless integration of the aforementioned subsystems, not just to provide necessary stabilization, but also to facilitate precise movement patterns.[56] Effective dynamic stability requires a balance of agonistic and antagonistic influences, controlled by the neural control subsystem, that enables precise motion to occur. Our ability to control and balance these forces requires normal *proprioception*.[57] Some consider proprioception, also known as *kinesthesia*, to be the most important sensory modality participating in the control of human movement (Box 17-2 and 17-3).[58]

Receptors and afferent nerves, capable of conveying proprioception, are located in many structures within the spine. Evidence suggests that we rely most heavily on the action of the **muscle spindle** and **Golgi tendon organ** to provide accurate information about joint position (Fig. 17-15). From these

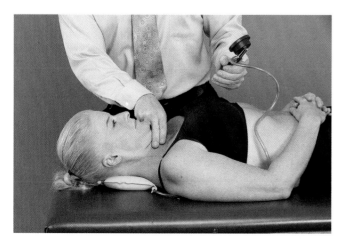

FIGURE 17-14 Examination of deep cervical muscle function through performance of the craniocervical flexion test (CCFT) using the Stabilizer biofeedback unit.

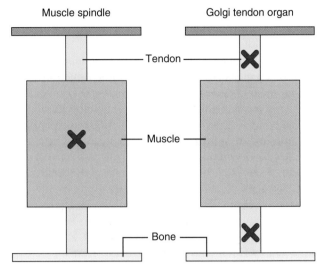

FIGURE 17–15 Diagram identifying the location of muscle spindle and Golgi tendon organ receptors relative to inert structures (tendon, bone) and contractile structures (muscle), suggesting the mechanisms by which each receptor is facilitated and thus dictating each receptor's primary function.

Table 17–4   Facilitation or Inhibition of Specialized Muscle Mechanoreceptors Relative to Mechanical Force

	MUSCLE SPINDLE	GOLGI TENDON ORGAN
Passive stretch	+	+
Active contraction	-	+
Slow, Passive Stretch	Min +	+
Long duration passive stretch	-	+
Quick, passive stretch	++	+

+ indicates facilitation of the receptor, ++ indicates increased facilitation, and - indicates inhibition of the receptor.

sensory receptors, information is projected to the brain via the dorsal column-medial lemniscal system. All afferent pathways projecting to the cerebral cortex do so through a relay nucleus in the thalamus. The lateral thalamus contains nuclei that mediate specific sensory and motor function (Table 17-4).[59]

Several authors have identified the presence of mechanoreceptors within spinal facet joints, intervertebral discs, and spinal ligaments.[72-78] Altered kinesthesia may be a predisposing factor or may occur as a result of LBP, and it may be an antecedent cause for the recurrence of LBP.

Evidence exists that reveals the impact of LBP on neuromuscular control of the spine. Newcomer et al[79] attempted to measure trunk repositioning error as a method of measuring proprioception in patients with LBP (n = 20) as compared to healthy controls (n = 20). Repositioning error was significantly higher in the LBP population during flexion, which was deemed as the more complex motion, and lower during extension, which was attributed to engagement of facet mechanoreceptors.[79]

Gill and Callaghan[56] performed a similar study to examine repositioning error in standing and four-point kneeling. Greater accuracy was noted in standing versus kneeling, however, the LBP group had greater repositioning error in both positions.[56]

Parkhurst and Burnett[57] performed a study on 88 cross-trained firefighter/EMS personnel for the purpose of investigating the relationship between low back injury and proprioception. The primary findings of this study revealed that age and years of experience were best correlated with proprioceptive deficits in the sagittal plane; injury to the lumbar spine was correlated with proprioceptive deficits in the frontal, sagittal, and in multiple planes; and proprioceptive asymmetries were associated with lumbar injury. The authors concluded that impaired proprioception from injury may predispose an individual to reinjury and restoration of normal proprioception should be a goal of intervention.[57]

Nies-Byl and Sinnott[61] compared 20 LBP patients with 26 healthy subjects in eight different positions of static balance. Compared with healthy controls, the LBP group demonstrated significantly greater postural sway in all positions, kept their center of force significantly more posterior, were less able to balance on one foot with eyes closed, and were more likely to use a hip strategy to maintain stability. The authors note that using such a strategy may limit opportunities to perform fine, controlled movements and may place undue stress on the lumbar spine.[61]

Luoto et al[80] attempted to evaluate the effects of rehabilitation on postural control parameters in individuals with LBP. In corroboration with previous work,[72] these findings suggest that impairment in postural control may be caused by LBP.[80]

Radebold et al[81] investigated the association between poor postural control and longer muscle response times to quick force. The LBP group demonstrated increased postural sway compared to healthy controls, particularly at the more challenging levels, as well as delayed muscle response times to quick force. Impaired postural control may influence dynamic stability and predispose an individual to spine-related injury.[81]

Nouwen et al[82] found that subjects with LBP displayed altered activation patterns during trunk flexion. Hodges and Richardson[83] found that in a healthy population the transverse abdominis was invariably the first muscle activated when performing extremity motions, presumably to provide spinal stiffness that precedes limb movement. The LBP population, however, demonstrated a delay in the recruitment of trunk muscles, making them subject to reactive forces.[83] Paquet et al[84] studied the interaction between the hip and the spine and muscle activation patterns during movement. The LBP group performed at a slower cadence, used their erector spinae musculature until end range of flexion, and used an alternate strategy of hip and spine motion.[84] Radebold et al[85] found that patients with LBP had a longer reaction time for muscle activation and deactivation, greater variability in their reaction times, and exhibited a pattern of cocontraction between agonists and antagonists.

The impact of muscle fatigue on spine kinesthesia in the presence of LBP has also been studied by several authors. Parnianpour et al[86] cite previous studies that have shown trunk extensors to be more fatigue resistant than trunk flexors and that the fatigability of these muscles was greater in the LBP population.[86] They further note that the most deleterious components of neuromuscular adaptation to fatigue were the reduction in accuracy, speed of contraction, and control, thus predisposing individuals to potential injury.[86]

Taimela et al[87] compared 57 LBP subjects to 49 healthy controls in their ability to sense lumbar position changes while being passively moved into rotation at a speed of 1 degree/second, which was performed before and after a fatiguing activity. The authors concluded that lumbar fatigue impairs the ability to sense position in all subjects, but particularly, in the LBP group.[87]

Brumagne et al[88] investigated the role of muscle spindles in lumbar position sense in subjects with and without LBP using paraspinal muscle vibration. Position sense was estimated by calculating the mean error in reproduction of sacral tilt angles. The decrease in position sense accuracy noted in the LBP population may be attributed to altered paraspinal muscle spindle afferents and/or central processing of this sensory input.[88]

When considering neuromuscular control, the passive subsystem should also be considered, particularly at end ranges of motion. Solomonow et al[89] performed both human and animal experiments involving electrical and mechanical stimulation of the supraspinous ligament while obtaining EMG recordings from the multifidi. Deformation of the supraspinous ligament produced multifidi activity that increased in force when greater loads were applied to the ligament.[89] Indahl et al[90] performed a similar study using 15 adult porcine specimens. The EMG response of the multifidus was measured in response to electrical stimulation of the lateral disc annulus and facet joint capsule. Stimulation of the disc produced reactions in the multifidi at multiple levels and on the contralateral side. Stimulation of the facet capsule induced multifidus activity ipsilaterally at the same segmental level. Reflexive activation is maximized when the stress in the ligament approaches injury.[90] These studies suggest that there are interactive responses between structures of the passive subsystem and paraspinal musculature.

Principles of Intervention

Intervention for Spinal Hypomobility

One method for implementation of TE within the mobility impairment or joint dysfunction model is the **medicine training therapy (MTT)** approach (Fig. 17-16), sometimes referred to as *medical exercise therapy*. This exercise approach is

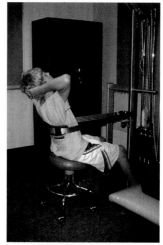

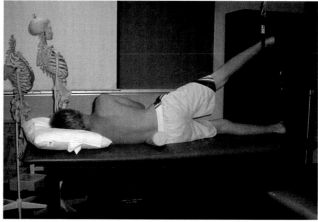

FIGURE 17–16 Medicine training therapy (MTT) exercise progression. **A.** MTT for improving hypomobility into lumbar extension at L1-2. **B.** MTT for hypomobility in side-bending right at L4-5.

based on the work of *Advar Holten*, a Norwegian physiotherapist. This approach uses belts, stabilization benches, and pulley weights to stabilize spinal segments.[91] In this approach, neighboring segments above and below the lesion are "locked out," while manual resistance and TE is used to stabilize hypermobile or hypomobile spinal segments. High repetitions (25-30) and low intensity (less than 60% of the one repetition maximum) resistive exercises are performed from the beginning to middle ranges of motion to provide stabilization to hypermobile joint segments. The parameters for hypomobile joints include 30 or more repetitions performed at a slow frequency at less than 50% of the one repetition maximum. Exercises that foster joint mobilization are performed from the middle to outer ranges of motion.

Training principles for MTT should be halted when the patient feels physically or psychologically fatigued so as to prevent incorrect motor patterns. The training program is intended to match the patient's level of motivation, with the understanding that progress is often slow in addressing improper motor patterns. Training in this manner is recommended on a daily basis or at least three times per week. Training may take place in prone, supine, side-lying, standing, and sitting positions, and resistance is individually assessed according to the patient's capacity to allow for optimal loading.

Intervention for Spinal Segmental Instability

Studies have provided evidence for the efficacy of cervical and lumbar spine stabilization exercise regimens.[92-94] The evidence suggests that for individuals with spinal pain, underlying neuromuscular impairment may not be adequately addressed through simple strength and high-load endurance training.[95] As described, stabilization approaches emphasize the retraining of specific deep or local stabilizing muscles of the spine while maintaining the region in a neutral position.[65] Deep muscle function is tested using the abdominal drawing-in maneuver and the cranio-cervical flexion test as previously described. When patients are able to effectively activate the deep muscles, they are progressed to more dynamic exercises in an effort to simultaneously train the larger, more superficial, or global, stabilizing muscles.[96]

There are three distinct phases of rehabilitation that are proposed that allow the integration of local muscle recruitment into other aspects of intervention and full function: *formal motor skill training, integration of skill into light functional tasks, and progression of skill into heavy functional tasks* (Fig. 17-17). The initial emphasis is on the ability to develop isolated recruitment of the deep muscles in a variety of positions. This motor skill is then integrated into dynamic functional tasks in which the global muscles are producing movement while the local muscles are providing stability through continual isometric recruitment. The final phase of rehabilitation must focus on the performance of heavy functional tasks that ideally simulate the individual's critical functional demands. Care must be taken with the performance of stabilization exercises in a manner that achieves functional stability without increasing spinal loads.[97] At each phase, it is critical for the manual therapist to closely monitor the exercise and use palpation to ensure proper motor recruitment.

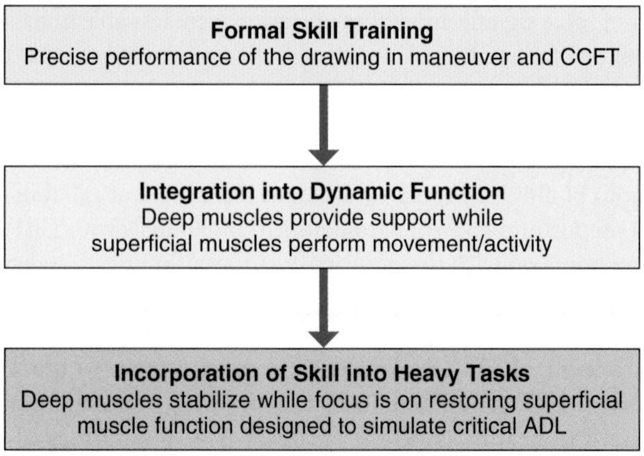

Formal Skill Training
Precise performance of the drawing in maneuver and CCFT

↓

Integration into Dynamic Function
Deep muscles provide support while superficial muscles perform movement/activity

↓

Incorporation of Skill into Heavy Tasks
Deep muscles stabilize while focus is on restoring superficial muscle function designed to simulate critical ADL

FIGURE 17-17 Phases of dynamic stabilization exercise regimen. CCFT = craniocervical flexion test; ADL = activities of daily living.

A typical exercise progression may consist of the following: single leg slide with contralateral leg support (Fig. 17-18); single knee extension with contralateral leg support (Fig. 17-19); single hip flexion with contralateral leg support (Fig. 17-20); hip adductor ball squeeze (Fig. 17-21); bridging with feet on unstable surface (Fig. 17-22); and bilateral unsupported alter-

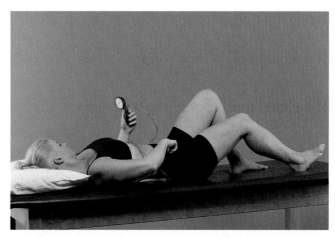

FIGURE 17-18 Drawing-in maneuver with single leg slide with contralateral leg support.

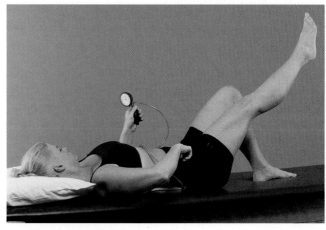

FIGURE 17-19 Drawing-in maneuver with unsupported leg slide with single knee extension with contralateral leg support.

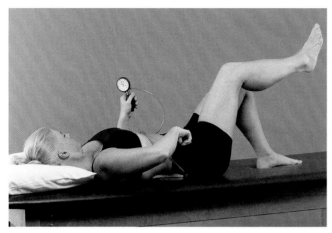

FIGURE 17–20 Drawing-in maneuver with single hip flexion with contralateral leg support.

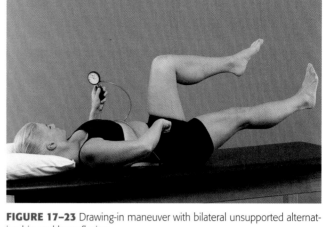

FIGURE 17–23 Drawing-in maneuver with bilateral unsupported alternating hip and knee flexion.

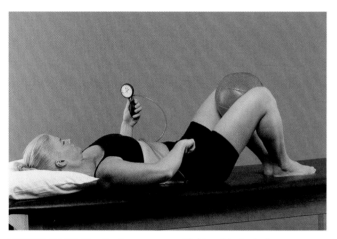

FIGURE 17–21 Drawing-in maneuver with hip adductor ball squeeze.

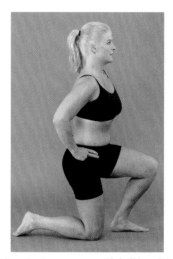

FIGURE 17–24 Drawing-in maneuver with half-kneeling.

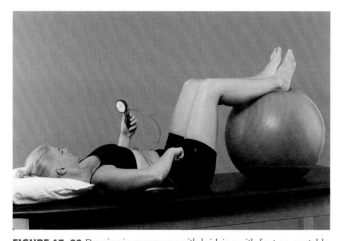

FIGURE 17–22 Drawing-in maneuver with bridging with feet on unstable surface.

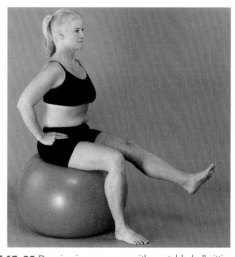

FIGURE 17–25 Drawing-in maneuver with unstable ball sitting with knee extension.

nating hip and knee flexion (Fig. 17-23). Once muscle recruitment in supported positions is accomplished, the patient is progressed to more challenging, unsupported positions such as half-kneeling (Fig. 17-24) and unstable ball sitting with knee extension (Fig. 17-25) and hip flexion (Fig. 17-26).[65]

In the cervical spine, endurance of the deep neck extensors may be developed through prone on elbow craniocervical flexion exercises (CCFE) with the cervical spine unsupported and through unsupported CCFE on stable and unstable surfaces (Figs. 17-27 and 17-28).

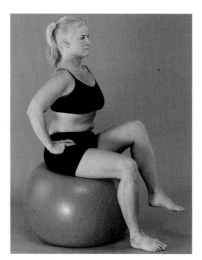

FIGURE 17–26 Drawing-in maneuver with unstable ball sitting with hip flexion.

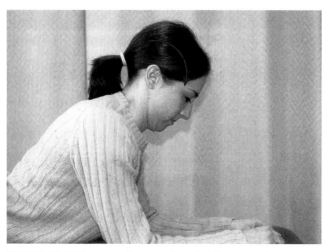

FIGURE 17–27 Prone on elbows craniocervical flexion exercise.

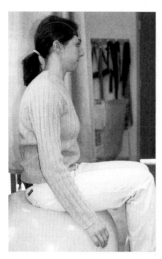

FIGURE 17–28 Craniocervical flexion exercise on unstable surface.

Intervention for Dyskinesia

Despite the absence of a gold standard and a clinically valid method for testing dyskinesia, the body of literature provides some common themes that may help to guide intervention.

NOTABLE QUOTABLE

"As movement specialists, physical therapists are uniquely trained to understand normal and abnormal movement and the difference between the two. As important as the amount of motion that is available at any given joint, the quality of motion is equally important. In intervention, the therapist often functions like a trainer seeking to reeducate the patient in the performance of more precise movement patterns."

C. Wise

Sahrmann et al[98,99] state that maintaining and restoring precise movement is the key to preventing or correcting musculoskeletal pain. Intervention must focus on neuromuscular retraining activities that seek to create precise movement patterns through specific exercise and, more importantly, through correction of aberrant functional activities.

THE MOVEMENT SYSTEMS BALANCE MODEL

The **movement systems balance (MSB) model** as espoused by *Shirley Sahrmann* and colleagues[98] is based on concepts first proposed by *Florence Kendall* et al.[100] The foundation of this approach includes the concept that movement imbalance results from the development of an altered **path of the instantaneous center of rotation (PICR)**.[98] Precise movement is the key to preventing impairment and pain results when the PICR becomes altered. In a multisegmental system, movement will take the path of least resistance, a concept referred to as **relative flexibility**.[98] For any segment, the path in which motion is least restricted is known as the **direction susceptible to movement (DSM)**.[98] The DSM leads to musculoskeletal

---

CLINICAL PILLAR

- Observing the patient's *path of the instantaneous center of rotation (PICR)* during movement is important in understanding alterations in movement precision.

- Alterations in the PICR may be due to aberrations in muscle length, muscle strength, and faulty alignment.

- The movement pattern that results from an altered PICR is the *direction susceptible to movement (DSM)* which produces cumulative trauma and impairment of the involved structures.

- The DSM is used to classify the patient's movement disorder.

impairment through cumulative trauma of associated structures, much like an unbalanced car tire will produce wear in a characteristic pattern through repeated movement around an altered center of rotation. Within this model, identification of the DSM is critical in allowing the therapist to classify and name the patient's movement disorder.

Several studies have shown that individuals with LBP demonstrate altered lumbo-pelvic rhythm when moving into and out of flexion.[101,102] To achieve optimal outcomes, addressing muscle length, strength, pattern of muscle recruitment, and observation of structural alignment is critical. It is most important for the manual therapist to consider the flexibility of each segment within a multisegmental movement system, not in isolation, but rather in relation to adjacent segments. Precise movement patterns are accomplished when all elements and components within a movement system achieve a balance that allows a variety of movements and postures. The following section is designed to provide an overview of the MSB model as it applies to disorders of the lumbar spine. Other sources are recommended for a more detailed exposition of this approach.[98]

Principles of Examination

Examination of Posture and Alignment

The first phase of examination includes examination of spinal alignment in standing and sitting. Three distinct measures are typically used to determine lumbo-pelvic alignment: the lumbar curve, deviation from the horizontal between the PSIS and the ASIS, and the hip joint angle. The strength and length of associated musculature is believed to exert a profound effect on static alignment and is presumed to be responsible for many issues related to faulty trunk alignment.[98]

Examination of Mobility

A detailed motion examination that attempts to determine the PICR is then performed. The location of the PICR will determine the moment exerted by trunk muscles on the spine. Altered spinal alignment will change the PICR and impact the subsequent moments which may cause cumulative trauma between segments during movement.[98]

During testing, identification of the final degree of lumbar curvature is of greater value than the total range of motion. Throughout testing, the examiner must observe the contribution of each segment to the overall motion. Hypomobile segments will often lead to compensatory hypermobility at adjacent regions. Furthermore, diminished contributions from other segments within this lumbo-pelvic-hip complex (i.e., hip, sacroiliac joint, etc.) may result in compensatory hypermobility. Identification of angulations, or areas around which motion appears to "hinge," is suggestive of segmental hypermobility.

Examination of Muscle Function

Examination of muscle function includes an appreciation of endurance and recruitment patterns. Testing involves observation of movement patterns in weight-bearing and non-weight-bearing movement. The role of muscles in facilitating normal kinesthesia and stabilization, as previously discussed, are concepts that are subsumed within this approach.

Like Kendall,[100] the MSB approach distinguishes between upper and lower abdominal muscle function. According to Sahrmann, isolated upper abdominal muscle recruitment is achieved through a contraction of the internal oblique and rectus abdominis, while the lower abdominals are tested by the ability to hold the pelvis flat against the supporting surface during bilateral leg lowering, which was first described by Kendall.[100] As the center of gravity moves from S2 to L4-L5 as the knees are flexed, forces transmitted to the spine will occur more proximally, highlighting the importance of individualized exercise recommendations.[103] Observation of an outward flare of the ribs during the trunk-curl sit-up occurs due to the action of the internal oblique muscle, whereas lower abdominal activity is more consistent with the action of the external oblique muscle.[97] With legs stabilized, the trunk-curl becomes a hip flexor rather than abdominal exercise. In lower abdominal testing, the examiner assists the patient in raising the patient's legs to a vertical position. The force exerted by the hip flexors upon lowering of the legs tends to tilt the pelvis anteriorly and acts as a strong resistance against the lower abdominal muscles.[100]

Classification of Lumbar Movement Impairment Syndromes

Classification of movement impairment syndromes involves a clustering of examination findings. The direction of motion in which symptoms are reproduced, or the DSM, is used to define the category of classification.[98] Therapists must consider the intensity of symptoms, reduction of symptoms with correction, and the consistency of the culpable movement direction when classifying patients. There is emerging evidence supporting the clinical utility of this classification system for individuals with LBP in the literature (Box 17-4). See Table 17-5 for a summary of the lumbar movement impairment syndromes, including symptoms, DSMs, and key features used for examination and paired intervention as outlined by Sahrmann and colleagues.[98]

CLINICAL PILLAR

Based on the examination findings provided, classify each of the following using the *MSB diagnostic classification categories* for the lumbar spine:

1. With return from forward bending, the back extensor musculature dominates over hip extensor muscle activity.

2. Symptoms are elicited with side bending that reduce when manual stabilization is provided above the iliac crest.

3. The lumbar spine contributes to forward bending more than the hips due to tight hamstrings.

4. Rocking forward in quadruped reveals a prominence that leads to a reduction in symptoms when force is applied to it.

Table 17–5	Summary of Lumbar Movement Impairment Syndromes

The clinical features of each syndrome are highlighted along with subsequent intervention. During intervention, the therapist pays strict attention that the primary movement is taking place without any compensatory movements or report of increased symptoms.

MSB SYNDROME	CHIEF COMPLAINT/DSM	EXAMINATION	INTERVENTION
Rotation-extension syndrome	Unilateral symptoms that increase with BB and ROT	*Standing*: Asymmetry, pain with return from FB, pain with SB with asymmetry and rotation *Sitting*: Increase with BB *Supine*: Pelvic rotation with hip/knee flexion, spine more flexible into ROT than hip is into abduction/ER, pain with hip/knee extension, pain with hip flexion/abducted ER *Side lying*: Pain but better with towel roll, hip ER causes pelvic ROT, hip adduction causes pelvic tilt *Prone*: Knee flexion increased pain, asymmetric pelvic ROT, hip extension with knee extension causes asymmetric spine ROT, hip rotation causes early spine ROT *Quadruped*: Pain with forward rocking, decreased with backward rocking	• Sit back in chair, hips/knees at same height with no lean, which produces ROT • Avoid sports where feet are fixed, which produce greater ROT in spine (i.e., golf) • Improve hip rotation mobility • Stand with slight posterior pelvic ROT, abdominals contracted, or against wall initially • Roll as a unit without pushing down with feet during movement • Avoid hip rotation and spine BB with sit to stand • Contract abdominals during stair climbing, lean forward while ascending if hip extensions motion is limited • Walk slowly with smaller steps to avoid anterior pelvic ROT
Extension syndrome	Symptoms associated with BB and decreased with movements away from BB	*Standing*: Hypertrophied extensors, increased lordosis, return from FB leads with BB and pain, better when hip motion elicited, against wall, less pain with posterior pelvic ROT *Prone*: Pain that increases with hip extension/knee extension *Sitting*: Increase with BB *Supine*: Pain with anterior pelvic ROT, spine BB, less pain with abdominal contraction, pain with hip/knee extension *Quadruped (Spine BB)*: Less pain with rock forward, more pain with rock back	• Correct increased lordosis and increase abdominal activity • Stretch hip flexors without producing anterior pelvic ROT and spine BB • Supine heel slides, hip/knee extension from hook-lying position and progress to oblique exercises to train abdominals and stretch hip flexors • Bilateral knee to chest • Hip abduction and ER from flexion improves abdominal control of pelvis • Shoulder flexion with spin stabilization • Hip abduction in side-lying position for posterior gluteus medius and lateral abdominals • Prone knee flexion with abdominals, hip ER with abdominals • Rocking backward in quadruped • Sitting back in chair, use a footstool • Stand against wall, spine flat, hips/knees flexed, contract abdominals and hips/knees are extended or shoulder flexion with abdominals

Table 17–5	Summary of Lumbar Movement Impairment Syndromes—cont'd		
MSB SYNDROME	**CHIEF COMPLAINT/DSM**	**EXAMINATION**	**INTERVENTION**
Rotation syndrome	Unilateral symptoms that increase with ROT	*Standing*: Asymmetry, pain with SB *Supine*: Pelvic ROT with hip or knee flexion, hip abduction/ER from flexion causes early spine ROT *Side lying*: Painful, better with towel roll, pelvic ROT with hip ER, pelvic tilt with hip adduction *Prone*: Asymmetrical pelvic ROT with knee flexion, asymmetric ER during hip extension with hip and knee extension, lumbo-pelvic ROT early with hip rotation *Quadruped*: Asymmetry, spine ROT with arm lift *Sitting*: lumbo-pelvic ROT with knee extension, spine ROT increases with rocking backward	• Prevent spine and pelvic ROT during work or in sports • Increase hip rotation mobility • Correct ROT malalignment with rocking backward exercise • Lower abdominal progression in supine, hip abduction/ER from flexion and hip adduction/IR with abdominals • Shoulder abduction at 135° diagonal with weight with return to 90° with abdominals • Hip ER in side lying with abdominals, hip abduction, or adduction without pelvic tilt • Prone knee flexion and hip ER with abdominals • Rock back without ROT, quadruped unilateral shoulder flexion with abdominals • Sitting knee extension without spine ROT • Standing side bending with support at trunk
Rotation-flexion syndrome	Unilateral symptoms that increase with sit to stand	*Standing*: Pain with FB and increased asymmetry, less pain into FB with greater degree of hip flexion *Supine*: With hip abduction/ER from flexion, spine rotates early and increased pain, lie with hips and knees extended without change in pain, better with towel support under spine, pelvic ROT with hip flexion *Side lying*: Pain, better with towel, pelvic ROT with hip ER, pelvic tilt with hip adduction *Prone*: Pain with hip rotation, with lumbo-pelvic ROT early *Quadruped*: Prefer FB, rock back produces spine ROT and pelvic tilt/ROT, arm lift produces ROT of spine *Sitting*: Pain with FB, knee extension if associated with lumbo-pelvic ROT	• Use abdominals to control ROT without FB • Improve back extensor function to prevent spine FB, improve motion of hip flexion, maintain spine flat in sitting • Supine hip/knee flexion without pelvic ROT • Contract abdominals while doing knee to chest to stretch hip extensors without spine FB • Hip abduction/ER from flexion with abdominals to prevent ROT • Hip ER without pelvic ROT and hip abduction and adduction without pelvic tilting in side lying • Prone knee flexion/hip rotation with abdominals while preventing spine ROT • Hip extension through limited range to improve glut function and decrease hamstring dominance • Shoulder flexion 90°–180° to improve back extensor function • Quadruped rock back while preventing FB and increase hip flexion without ROT • Standing FB with axis at hips allowing knees to flex, side bending with support at trunk

Continued

Table 17-5	Summary of Lumbar Movement Impairment Syndromes—cont'd			
MSB SYNDROME	**CHIEF COMPLAINT/DSM**	**EXAMINATION**		**INTERVENTION**
Flexion syndrome	Symptoms associated with movement into FB and decrease with movement away from FB	*Standing*: Greater contribution from spine with FB vs. hip, pain with FB that decreases with greater hip recruitment *Quadruped*: Rock back reveals more motion from spine vs. hip *Sitting*: Pain, spine FB with knee extension *Supine*: Pain during final phase of hip flexion with knees flexed, spine FB before 120° of hip flexion, lies with hip/knee extended without increased pain, towel under spine decreases pain.		• Teach proper sitting and move hips, not lumbar spine • Supine knee to chest without spine FB • Shoulder flexion with chest lift to improve length of abdominals • Prone arms overhead, shoulder flexion one at a time to improve back extensor function • Prone pillow under spine, unilateral hip extension • Quadruped rock back recruiting hip flexion, not spine FB • Sitting knee extension with isometric back extension • Hamstring stretching in sitting with leaning forward at hips • Standing FB from hips with knee flexion • Squatting without spine FB

FB, forward bending (flexion); BB, backward bending (extension); SB, side bending; ROT, rotation.

Box 17-4 MSB DIAGNOSTIC CLASSIFICATION CATEGORIES FOR THE LUMBAR SPINE

(Categories are listed from most to least prevalent.)

- Rotation-extension syndrome
- Extension syndrome
- Rotation syndrome
- Rotation-flexion syndrome
- Flexion syndrome

The muscle balance approach advocated by *Vladimir Janda*[103,104,106] is similar conceptually to the MSB model in the sense that deficits in the synchrony of movement patterns are thought to lead to imbalances. Janda,[103,104] a neurologist, founded the rehabilitation department at *Charles University Hospital* in Prague, Czechoslovakia. Janda's observations regarding muscle imbalances, faulty posture and gait, and their association with chronic pain syndromes, etiologically, diagnostically, and therapeutically, have profoundly influenced rehabilitation. Janda's approach involves the examination of postural versus phasic muscle actions and type I versus type II muscle fiber types.[103,104] Janda's approach to intervention, however, differs significantly from the MSB model. The Janda approach focuses on interventions that require vigorous manual stretching procedures,[103,104] whereas the MSB approach emphasizes correct alignment and proper muscle recruitment patterns. The MSB approach requires the performance of

gentle exercises designed to optimize recruitment of selected musculature while controlling for unwanted movement leading to more precise movement patterns. MSB intervention de-emphasizes the use of manual techniques and requires adherence to correct movement patterns during daily activities and regular performance of an independent exercise regimen.[97]

Janda observed that gluteal activation and pelvic stability are often decreased in individuals who are experiencing chronic LBP.[103,104] Bullock-Saxton et al[103] investigated the importance of motor control and programming in intervention. The authors investigated whether the gluteal muscles could be activated more effectively by stimulating the proprioceptive mechanism during walking. Electromyographic recordings of gluteus maximus and medius in 15 healthy subjects were made during barefoot and balance shoe walking before and after 1 week of facilitation. Significant increases ($P < 0.0002$) in gluteal activity and significant decreases ($P < 0.01$) in time to 75% maximum contraction demonstrated the value of sensorimotor elicitation of subconscious and automatic responses in muscles often weakened in back pain sufferers.[103]

Another tenant of Janda's approach is the influence that injury to a distal joint may have on the function of proximal muscles.[103] Bullock-Saxton et al[104] conducted a controlled study in which the function of muscles at the hip was compared between subjects who had suffered severe unilateral ankle sprains and healthy matched control subjects. The pattern of activation of the gluteus maximus, hamstring muscles, and erector spinae muscles was monitored through the use of surface electromyography during hip extension from prone lying. Analyses revealed that the pattern of muscle activation in subjects with previous injury differed markedly from normal control subjects and that changes appeared to occur on both the uninjured and the injured sides of the body. The most notable difference between the two groups was the delay in onset of activation of the gluteus maximus muscle in previously injured subjects.[104]

CLINICAL PILLAR

- *Postural, type I* muscles typically respond to injury by developing stiffness and resistance to movement and elongation.
- *Phasic, type II* muscles typically respond to injury by developing weakness and issues with muscle recruitment and force production.
- Understanding which muscle type is involved allows the manual therapist to better know how to direct intervention.
- Intervention for *postural, type I* muscles consists of *endurance* training.
- Intervention for *phasic, type II* muscles consists of *strength* training

---

Principles of Intervention

Within the MSB model, segmental hypomobility contributes to compensatory motion at adjacent segments but is not considered to be the region from which symptoms are originating.[98] This approach attributes most spine-related symptoms to the regions that have excessive relative flexibility (i.e., the DSM) as opposed to segments in which motion is reduced. Therefore, the focus of intervention is directed toward achieving and maintaining proper spinal alignment and the prevention of unwanted movement. To achieve these goals, trunk musculature must demonstrate proper neuromuscular performance. Intervention is focused on modifying daily activities to reduce repetitive stresses followed by an exercise regimen based on the test movements that were found to be positive. An emphasis is placed on the correct performance of each test movement to ensure that no symptoms are elicited and that precise movement patterns are adopted.[98]

Within the MSB approach, exercises are incorporated into the patient's daily routine, with an emphasis on self-intervention so movement patterns become habitual.[98] Close interaction between the therapist and the patient is critical initially to ensure proper performance of each exercise.

If individuals have difficulty performing an entire movement pattern, the activity may be broken down into smaller, more manageable components. Throughout intervention, an emphasis is placed on the precision of movement that is to be

Table 17–6	Similarities and Unique Features of Common Exercise Approaches in the Management of Spinal Disorders	
	EXERCISE PRESCRIPTION	**SIMILARITIES**
Mechanical diagnosis and therapy (McKenzie)	Exercise based on direction of preference	Focus on maintenance of posture may have stabilization effect; patient independence is encouraged for self-management
Medicine training therapy (Holten)	Exercise based on mobility testing and locking out of joint segments to isolate involved levels	Stabilization exercises focus on midrange exercise and proximal stability prior to distal mobility
Dynamic spinal stabilization (Richardson et al)	Exercise based on ability to contract deep spinal muscles; lower abdominal progression with isolation of transverse abdominus	Lower abdominal progression involves maintenance of pelvic position (proximal stability) during lower extremity movement.
Movement systems balance (Sahrmann)	Exercise based on ability to maintain pelvic position during single limb movement; lower abdominal progression focuses on contraction of external obliques	Lower abdominal progression involves maintenance of pelvic position (proximal stability) during lower extremity movement; patient independence is encouraged for self-management
Muscle balance (Janda)	Evaluation according to tonic vs. phasic muscle action, vigorous stretching techniques employed to lengthen shortened muscles	Proximal stability required for distal mobility

performed asymptomatically. Intervention involves instructing patients to move about proper joint axes and contract muscles and supporting structures that are excessively lengthened and weak. Rather than passively stretching shortened muscles, the antagonists of these muscles are contracted to create a lengthening effect.

SUMMARY AND CONCLUSIONS

This chapter focused on the review of several common TE approaches used in the care of individuals with spinal disorders. Principles of examination leading to classification and subsequent intervention were covered in light of the current best evidence.

Based on a review of the literature, McGill[105] offers several suggestions that can be applied to spinal exercise regimens, with an emphasis on the lumbar spine. McGill notes that, as of 1998, only 28 randomized controlled trials attempting to investigate the role of exercise regimens for LBP were identified.[105] Despite a greater emphasis on the investigation of these concepts in recent years, the disparities observed by McGill still exist today. Based on his review, he concluded that specific exercise regimens have a limited impact on acute LBP, that it is difficult to determine which patients are likely to respond to which exercise regimen, that the McKenzie regimen may produce short-term symptomatic relief, and that exercise is most effective within the first 6 weeks after injury.[105] He advocates incorporating lower extremity mobility and flexibility exercises and muscle endurance training while maintaining neutral postures. General aerobic training has been found to be helpful in controlling spine-related symptoms. This routine should include side support activities, known as plank exercises, and back extensor training, while avoiding prone extension and sit-up exercises to reduce increased spinal loads in an attempt to re-establish muscular balance. Most importantly, McGill concludes that exercise regimens should be patterned to each individual's distinct clinical presentation (Box 17-5).[105]

Regardless of the approach, incorporating an active exercise regimen guided by impairment-based classification that seeks to engender patient independence is critical in the comprehensive care of those suffering from spinal disorders. Such interventions serve as an ideal complement to OMPT interventions and, in some cases, become the primary feature in the management of these conditions. It is of paramount importance that the manual physical therapist understands the benefits as well as the limitations of OMPT. OMPT is not a panacea, but rather it is a valuable tool that may be used in combination with other valuable tools that collaboratively constitute an entire approach to addressing the individual needs of those whom we serve.

Box 17-5 GENERAL RECOMMENDATIONS FOR SPINAL EXERCISE REGIMENS

Specific exercise regimens have limited impact on acute LBP.

- It is difficult to determine which patients are likely to respond to which exercise regimen.
- The McKenzie regimen may produce short-term symptomatic relief.
- Exercise may be more effective in patients with chronic LBP; however, exercise that is initiated within the first 6 weeks after injury may serve to prevent the occurrence of a more chronic condition.
- Include exercises that begin with cycles of flexion and extension under minimal loads to reduce stiffness.
- Incorporate lower extremity mobility and flexibility exercises as a priority over specific flexibility exercises for the spine.
- Advance to training of specific muscles, beginning with abdominal muscles, followed by lateral trunk muscles, then extensor muscles in neutral postures.
- Exercise is most beneficial when performed daily and within pain tolerance.
- Aerobic training has been found to be helpful in controlling spine-related symptoms.
- Avoid full-range movements, particularly in the morning.
- Use neutral spine positioning versus pelvic tilting.
- Resistance training focuses on endurance versus strength.
- Include variations of the curl-up and side support activities for enhancing abdominal and quadratus lumborum muscle performance and back extensor strengthening through single leg extension exercises while avoiding prone extension and sit-ups.
- Reestablish balanced muscle performance between abdominal and paravertebral musculature.
- Most importantly, exercises should be patterned to the distinct clinical presentation of the patient.

CLINICAL CASE

CASE 1

History of Present Illness (HPI)

C.J. is a 27-year-old male who presents to your facility today with complaint of severe right lumbo-sacral pain at an 6/10+ level of intensity that occurred 2 days ago while performing repetitive lifting activities at work, involving lifting 50 lb boxes from the floor to overhead. Upon further questioning, he describes radiating pain and numbness into the posterior aspect of his right leg into his foot. His symptoms are constant in nature, and he has been unable to find significant relief with movement or position. Increased symptoms are noted with all motions, particularly when he attempts to stand erect. You notice his inability to sit in the waiting room, and while he is standing you observe a moderate left lateral shift and forward bent posture. He is currently out of work and on Worker's Compensation until further notice.

Review of systems: Denies hypertension (HTN), diabetes mellitus (DM), cardiac history. Reports no history of surgery.

Diagnostic imaging: Radiographs are negative. MRI has been ordered but not yet performed.

Self-assessed disability: Oswestry Disability Questionnaire score is 60%.

Active range of motion (AROM): Forward bending (FB) and repeated FB (10×) = 25% of full range of motion with an increase in his right lower extremity symptoms from 6/10+ to 8/10+ level. Backward bending (BB) and repeated BB (10×) = 50%, with a reduction in right lower extremity pain and paresthesia.

Neurological: Deep tendon reflexes (DTRs): Right Achilles = 3+, all else is within normal limits (WNL); light touch diminished at plantar aspect of the right foot only; myotomes reveal weakness into ankle plantarflexion.

1. Based on your examination findings, what is your current clinical hypothesis regarding the origin of C.J.'s condition? Classify C.J. using the system proposed by McKenzie as described in this Chapter.
2. What aspects of C.J.'s presentation were most useful in allowing you to confirm your differential diagnostic classification of this patient? Perform each procedure on your partner.
3. Briefly describe the three broad syndromes that constitute the mechanical diagnosis and therapy classification system.

Compare and contrast the mechanical diagnosis and therapy classification system with the other classification systems discussed in this chapter.
4. Based on the examination findings of this patient, implement an exercise regimen that ascribes to the direction of preference model. Include a progression of three to five specific exercises and instruct your partner in the performance of each.

CASE 2

HPI

A 65-year-old man reports to your office today with report of onset of LBP occurring gradually over the past 2 weeks that appears to be related to his present work duties, which involve prolonged awkward positions while painting ceilings. His symptoms consist of central lumbosacral pain that is at a 4/10+ level of intensity on the average and of the constant, dull ache variety with intermittent complaint of bilateral lower extremity (LE) pain that is most notable upon exertion. He also notes tingling into the posterior aspects of bilateral lower extremities and increased episodes of losing balance, which is affecting his job performance. He notes having significant difficulty with sleeping. He notes that his best position is sitting. This patient has experienced similar complaints in the past; however, this episode is much worse. He wishes to return to gainful employment, but, realistically, he is not sure how he will ever be able to get into the positions required of his job again.

Structure: Static posture in standing reveals a band of hypertrophy in the region of L5-S1 that reduces in prone-lying position with abdominal support. Increased lumbar lordosis with bilateral anterior pelvic rotation is noted. Patient demonstrates poor tolerance for static postures during history taking.

AROM: FB = 75%, decreased pain, poor lumbo-pelvic rhythm noted with increased lumbar contribution during FB and lumbar extension early in range with return to neutral. During FB AROM, patient demonstrates poor movement quality and control. Dominance of back extensor musculature noted with sustained recruitment throughout entire range of motion. BB = 25% with increase in LBP from 4/10+ to 8/10+. Side bending (SB) and rotation right = 50%; left = 75% bilaterally with an increase from 4/10+ to 5/10+ upon right SB. Symptoms resolve with manual stabilization of the iliac crest on the right with right SB.

Gait: Antalgic gait with excessive back extensor activity throughout. A reduction in LBP is noted with reducing step length and when eliciting an abdominal muscle contraction.

Special tests: Thomas test: B = +, bent knee fall out: B = +, quadruped rocking back = reduced pain, drawing-in maneuver in prone with Stabilizer reveals a decrease by 2 mm Hg maintained for 2 seconds only, segmental multifidus test in prone reveals poor selective recruitment of the multifidus.

1. Classify this patient according to the treatment-based classification (TBC) approach as espoused by Delitto et al[7,16] based on the examination findings presented. Discuss the stages that are used in this approach and the manner in which this classification system may be used to direct intervention. Compare and contrast this approach with the other classification systems discussed in this chapter. Based on this classification system what is the initial course of intervention for this patient?

2. Based on the movement systems balance model (MSB),[22,98] what syndrome is this patient most likely suffering from? What are the components of this examination that most clearly suggest the presence of this syndrome?

3. Based on the syndrome identified in question 2 above, develop an exercise regimen consisting of three to five specific exercises that would be most appropriate for this patient. Instruct your partner in the performance of these exercises.

4. Compare and contrast intervention based on the MSB model with intervention based on the direction of preference model for this patient. What are the primary objectives of each approach? How will you determine that a successful outcome has been achieved?

5. Based on the results of this examination, what signs of clinical instability are present? Discuss the difference between hypermobility and instability. Develop an exercise regimen that may be used to address suspected spinal segmental instability in this patient. Describe three specific exercises that you would implement and attempt to perform them while your partner monitors your performance and provides feedback.

CASE 3

HPI

A 25-year-old man presents to your office today noting onset of symptoms 2 weeks ago secondary to a rear-end collision that occurred while on his way home from work one evening. He was seen in the emergency room immediately following the motor vehicle accident and was seen for follow-up with his physician yesterday who referred him to PT with diagnosis of cervical whiplash to include modalities and gentle ROM. He presents with constant central pain that is noted at the lower cervical spine, which improves with use of a soft collar. He is unable to sleep and reports paresthesia into the posterior aspect of his right arm, which is intermittent in nature, and responds to motion and position of cervical spine. In addition, numbness is noted into the thenar eminence of the right hand which is constant in nature. Past medical history is noncontributory.

Self-assessed disability: *Numeric Pain Scale*: Best = 6/10+, Worst = 10+/10+, Neck Disability Index (NDI) = 75%, Visual Analog Scale (VAS) = 8 cm.

Structural examination/observation: The patient is in apparent distress while sitting in the waiting room, with restlessness observed, forward head, rounded shoulder posture, head postured in slight left SB and rotation. Atrophy of right thenar eminence noted.

Peripheral joint screen: Right temporomandibular joint (TMJ) examination reveals pain with opening, accompanied by reciprocal click and deviation to the right. Weakness in right thumb with overpressure noted.

Neurological examination: Dermatomes: Decreased light touch sensation along the posterior aspect of the right upper arm, and right thenar eminence, digits 1 to 3. Myotomes: Cervical spine is reduced secondary to pain, weakness in thumb flexion/adduction. DTR: Triceps = 1+, all else 2+.

AROM: FB = 50% with report of paravertebral muscle pull/pain and deviation to right, BB = 25% with pain on right and increased paresthesia into posterior upper arm, SB L = 25% with right upper trap/levator scapular muscle pull/pain, SB R = 10% with pain on right and increased paresthesia into posterior upper arm and ipsilateral rotation, ROT L = 75% with pull on right, ROT R = 10% with pain on right and increased paresthesia into posterior upper arm. Pain increased from 6/10+ to 9/10+ level following single repetition AROM. Slow, unsteady movement noted. Physiologic motions reveal improved motion and less pain. Repeated motion and overpressure not performed due to patient's level of pain.

Passive physiologic intervertebral mobility testing (PPIVM): Downglide/closing examination reveals segmental hypomobility at C6-C7 with local pain.

Manual muscle testing: Opponens pollicis, flexor pollicis brevis, longus=2/5; cervical N/T due to pain response with myotome testing.

Functional examination: Limitations with backing up in car, using bifocals on computer, putting in lightbulbs at home, difficulty in sleeping in favorite position of prone.

Special tests: Craniocervical flexion test (CCFT) reveals poor motor recruitment of deep neck flexors and extensors.

Palpation: General nonspecific pain throughout paravertebral musculature, exquisite tendernss to the touch, right greater than left at the anterior, middle scalene, articular pillar C6-T2, and right TMJ. Profound increase in tissue tone of the scaleni, suboccipital musculature, and of the upper trapezii and levator scapulae, right greater than left.

1. Classify this patient according to the McClure[20] system of classification. What is this patient's irritability classification, and what is his movement profile classification? What aspect of the examination was most useful in classifying this patient?
2. Based on this classification, into what direction of cervical motion would intervention be directed?
3. Classify this patient according to the Childs et al[45] system of classification. What is the primary focus of intervention according to this approach? Do you expect this patient to change categories during the course of intervention?
4. Do the results of AROM and PPIVM testing relate to one another, and do these findings correlate with the patient's subjective report?
5. To what degree do the results of the CCFT relate to the patient's symptoms? Describe a specific exercise regimen that would be effective in addressing the issues identified by the results of the CCFT.

HANDS-ON

With a partner, perform the following activities:

1 Instruct your partner in the following exercises based on the concepts discussed in this chapter. Identify the objective and challenges in performing each exercise.

EXERCISE	OBJECTIVE	CHALLENGES TO PERFORMANCE
Extension and flexion in lying		
Transverse abdominus progression		
Deep neck flexor progression		
Hip flexor and hamstring muscle stretching without stressing the lumbar spine		
A stabilization exercise based on medicine training therapy principles		
A mobilization exercise based on medicine training therapy principles		

2 Develop a TE progression based on the three models of TE discussed in this chapter by completing the following table.

Choose a progression of three exercises for each syndrome. Take turns instructing your partner in each progression.

MODEL	SYNDROME	EXERCISE PROGRESSION
Direction of preference model	McKenzie postural syndrome	1. 2. 3.
	McKenzie dysfunction syndrome	1. 2. 3.
	McKenzie derangement syndrome	1. 2. 3.
	Compression stress (low irritability)	1. 2. 3.
	Compression stress (high irritability)	1. 2. 3.
	Tension stress (low irritability)	1. 2. 3.
	Tension stress (high irritability)	1. 2. 3.
	Mixed stress (low vs. high irritability)	1. 2. 3.
Mobility impairment model	Hypomobility impairment	1. 2. 3.
	Hypermobility/instability impairment	1. 2. 3.
	Dyskinesia impairment	1. 2. 3.
Movement systems balance model	Lumbar rotation-extension syndrome:	1. 2. 3.
	Lumbar extension syndrome:	1. 2. 3.
	Lumbar rotation syndrome:	1. 2. 3.
	Lumbar rotation-flexion syndrome:	1. 2. 3.
	Lumbar flexion syndrome:	1. 2. 3.

3 Observe your partner perform lumbar AROM in all planes and identify the quantity and quality of each movement pattern as well as any reproduction of symptoms that may occur and identify the presence of clinical signs of instability. In addition, identify the path of the instantaneous center of rotation (PICR) and the direction susceptible to movement (DSM). Based on the nature of the reproduced symptoms, determine your partner's direction of preference.

MOTION	QUANTITY	QUALITY	SYMPTOMS	INSTABILITY	PICR/DSM	DIRECTION OF PREFERENCE
Forward bending						
Backward bending						
Side bending right						
Side bending left						
Rotation right						
Rotation left						
Combined motion						

4 With your partner, progress through an exercise and OMPT intervention progression that uses the Piva et al,[43] Wang et al,[44] and Childs et al[45] cervical spine algorithms. Discuss with your partner how you would integrate OMPT and TE into a comprehensive intervention scheme that may be used to address neck pain.

REFERENCES

1. Philadelphia panel evidence-based clinical practice guidelines on selected rehabilitation interventions for low back pain. *Phys Ther.* 2001;81:1641-1674.
2. Quebec Task Force on Spinal Disorders. Scientific approach to the assessment and management of activity-related spinal disorders. A monograph for clinicians. *Spine.* 1987;12:51-59.
3. Van Tulder M, Malmivaara A, Esmail R, Koes B. Exercise therapy for low back pain: a systematic review within the framework of the Cochrane Collaboration Back and Review Group. *Spine.* 2000;25:2784-2796.
4. Riddle D. Classification and low back pain: a review of the literature and critical analysis of selected systems. *Phys Ther.* 1998;78:708-735.
5. American Physical Therapy Association. Guide to physical therapist practice, 2nd ed. *Phys Ther.* 2001;81:42-47.
6. Borkan JM, Koes B, Shmuel R, Cherkin D. A report from the second international forum for primary care research on LBP: reexamining priorities. *Spine.* 1998;23:1992-1996.
7. Fritz JM, Delitto A, Erhard RE. Comparison of classification-based physical therapy with therapy based on clinical practice guidelines for patients with acute low back pain: a randomized clinical trial. *Spine.* 2003;28:1363-1371.
8. Leboeuf-Yde C, Lauritzen JM, Lauritzen T. Why has the search for causes of LBP largely been nonconclusive. *Spine.* 1997;22:877-881.
9. Zimny NJ. Diagnostic classification and orthopaedic physical therapy practice: what we can learn from medicine. *J Orthop Sports Phys Ther.* 2004;34:105-115.
10. Delitto A, Cibulka MT, Erhard RE, et al. Evidence for an extension/mobilization category in acute LBP: a prescriptive validity pilot study. *Phys Ther.* 1993;73:216-228.
11. Erhard RE, Delitto A, Cibulka MT. Relative effectiveness of an extension program and a combined program of manipulation and flexion and extension exercise in patients with acute low back syndrome. *Phys Ther.* 1994;74:1093-1100.
12. Sinaki M, Lutness MP, Ilstrup DM, et al. Lumbar spondylolisthesis: retrospective comparison and three-year follow-up of two conservative treatment programs. *Arch Phys Med and Rehabil.* 1989;70:594-598.
13. Stankovic R, Johnell O. Conservative treatment of acute LBP: a 5-year follow-up study of two methods of treatment. *Spine.* 1995;20:469-472.
14. Maluf KS, Sahrmann SA, Van Dillen LR. Use of a classification system to guide nonsurgical management of a patient with chronic low back pain. *Phys Ther.* 2000;80:1097-1111.
15. McKenzie RA. *The Lumbar Spine. Mechanical Diagnosis and Therapy.* Wellington, New Zealand: Spinal Publications Limited; 1981.
16. Delitto A, Cibulka MT, Erhard RE, et al. Evidence for an extension/mobilization category in acute LBP: a prescriptive validity pilot study. *Phys Ther.* 1993;73:216-228.
17. Spitzer WO. Scientific approach to the assessment and measurement of activity-related spinal disorders: a monograph for clinicians-report of the Quebec Task Force on Spinal Disorders. *Spine.* 1987;12(suppl):S1-S59.
18. Buchbinder R, Goel V, Bombardier C, Hogg-Johnson S. Classification systems of soft tissue disorders of the neck and upper limb: do they satisfy methodological guidelines? *J Clin Epidem.* 1996;49:141-149.
19. Newton W, Curtis P, Witt P, Hobler K. Prevalence of subtypes of LBP in a defined population. *J Family Pract.* 1997;45:331-335.
20. McClure P. The degenerative cervical spine: pathogenesis and rehabilitation concepts. *J Hand Ther.* 2000;4-6:163-174.
21. Binkley J, Finch E, Hall J, Black T, Gowland C. Diagnostic classification of patients with low back pain: report on a survey of physical therapy experts. *Phys Ther.* 1993;73:138-155.
22. Van Dillen LR, Sahrmann SA, Norton BJ, et al. Reliability of physical examination items used for classification of patients with low back pain. *Phys Ther.* 1998;78:979-988.
23. Petersen T, Thorsen H, Manniche C, Ekdahl C. Classification of non-specific low back pain: a review of the literature on classifications systems relevant to physiotherapy. *Phys Ther Rev.* 1999;4:265-281.
24. McCarthy CJ, Arnall FA, Strimpakos N, Freemont A, Oldham JA. The biopsychosocial classification of non-specific low back pain: a systematic review. *Phys Ther Rev.* 2004;9:17-30.
25. Laslett M, Oberg B, Aprill CN, McDonald B. Centralization as a predictor of provocation discography results in chronic low back pain, and the influence of disability and distress on diagnostic power. *J Spine.* 2005;5:370-380.
26. Donelson R, Aprill C, Medcalf R, Grant W. A prospective study of centralization of lumbar and referred pain: a predictor of symptomatic discs and annular competence. *Spine.* 1997;22:1115-1122.
27. Fritz JM, Delitto A, Vignovic M, Busse RG. Interrater reliability of judgments of the centralization phenomenon and status change during

movement testing in patients with low back pain. *Arch of Phys Med Rehabil.* 2000;81:57-61.
28. Clare HA, Adams R, Maher CG. Reliability of McKenzie classification of patients with cervical or lumbar pain. *J Man Physiol Ther.* 2005;28:122-127.
29. Razmjou H, Kramer JF, Yamada R. Intertester reliability of the McKenzie evaluation in assessing patients with mechanical low back pain. *J Orthop Sports Phys Ther.* 2000;30:368-369.
30. Kilpikoski S, Airaksinen O, Kankaanpaa M, et al. Interexaminer reliability of low back pain assessment using the McKenzie method. *Spine.* 2002;27:207-214.
31. Long AL. The centralization phenomenon: its usefulness as a predictor of outcome in conservative treatment of chronic low back pain (a pilot study). *Spine.* 1995;20:2513-2521.
32. Riddle DL, Rothstein JM. Intertester reliability of McKenzie's classifications of the syndrome types present in patients with low back pain. *Spine.* 1993;18:1333-1344.
33. Alexander AH, Jones AM, Rosenbaum Jr. DH. Nonoperative management of herniated nucleus pulposus: patient selection by the extension sign long-term follow-up. *Orthop Rev.* 1992;21:181-188.
34. Werneke MW, Hart DL. Categorizing patients with occupational low back pain by use of the Quebec Task Force classification system versus pain pattern classification procedures: discriminant and predictive validity. *Phys Ther.* 2004;84:243-254.
35. Karas R, McIntosh G, Hasll Hamilton, Wilson L, Melles T. The relationship between nonorganic signs and centralization of symptoms in the prediction of return to work for patients with low back pain. *Phys Ther.* 1997;77:354-360.
36. George SZ, Delitto A. Clinical examination variables discriminate among treatment-based classification groups: a study of construct validity in patients with acute low back pain. *Phys Ther.* 2005;85:306-314.
37. Werneke M, Hart DL. Discriminant validity and relative precision for classifying patients with nonspecific neck and back pain by anatomic pain patterns. *Spine.* 2003;28:161-166.
38. Werneke M, Hart DL. Centralization phenomenon as a prognostic factor for chronic low back pain and disability. *Spine.* 2001;26:758-765.
39. Atlas SJ, Deyo RA, Patrick DL, et al. The Quebec Task Force classification for spinal disorders and the severity, treatment, and outcomes of sciatica and lumbar spinal stenosis. *Spine.* 1996;21:2885-2892.
40. DeRosa CP, Porterfield JA. A physical therapy model for the treatment of low back pain. *Phys Ther.* 1992;72:261-272.
41. Fritz JM, George S. The use of a classification approach to identify subgroups of patients with acute low back pain: interrater reliability and short-term treatment outcomes. *Spine.* 2000;25:106-114.
42. Delitto A, Cibulka MT, Erhard RE, Bowling RW, Tenhula JA. Evidence for use of an extension-mobilization category in acute low back syndrome: a prescriptive validation pilot study. *Phys Ther.* 1993;73:216-228.
43. Piva SR, Erhard RE, Al-Hugail M. Cervical radiculopathy: a case problem using a decision-making algorithm. *J Orthop Sports Phys Ther.* 2000;30:745-754.
44. Wang WTJ, Olson SL, Campbell AH, Hanten WP, Gleeson PB. Effectiveness of physical therapy for patients with neck pain: an individualized approach using a clinical decision-making algorithm. *Am J Phys Med Rehabil.* 2003;82:203-218.
45. Childs JD, Fritz JM, Piva SR, Whitman JM. Proposal of a classification system for patients with neck pain. *J Orthop Sports Phys Ther.* 2004;34:686-700.
46. McKenzie, RA. *The Cervical and Thoracic Spine: Mechanical Diagnosis and Treatment.* Waikanae, New Zealand: Spinal Publications; 1990.
47. Ponte DJ, Jensen GL, Kent BE. A preliminary report on the use of the McKenzie protocol versus Williams protocol in the treatment of low back pain. *J Orthop Sports Phys Ther.* 1984;6:130-139.
48. Nwuga G, Nwuga V. Relative therapeutic efficacy of the Williams and McKenzie protocols in back pain management. *Physiother Prac.* 1985;1:99-105.
49. Schenk R, Jozefczyk C, Kopf A. A randomized trial comparing interventions in patients with lumbar posterior derangement. *J Man Manip Ther.* 2003;11:95-102.
50. Cook C, Hegedus E, Ramey K. Physical therapy exercise intervention based on classification using the patient response method: a systematic review of the literature. *J Man Manip Ther.* 2005;13:152-162.
51. Paris SV, Loubert PV. *Foundations of Clinical Orthopaedics.* St. Augustine, FL: Institute Press; 1990:24.
52. Paris SV, Nyberg R, Irwin M. *S2 Course Notes.* St. Augustine, FL: Institute of Physical Therapy; 1993.
53. Cook C, Brismee J-M, Fleming R, Sizer PS. Identifiers suggestive of clinical cervical spine instability: Delphi study of physical therapists. *Phys Ther.* 2005;85:895-906.

54. Panjabi MM. The stabilizing system of the spine. Part 1. Function, dysfunction, adaptation, and enhancement. *J Spinal Disorders*. 1992;5:383-389.

55. Fritz JM, Erhard RE, Hagen BF. Segmental instability of the lumbar spine. *Phy Ther*. 1998;78:889-896.

56. Gill KP, Callaghan MJ. The measurement of lumbar proprioception in individuals with and without low back pain. *Spine*. 1998;23:371-377.

57. Parkhurst TM, Burnett CN. Injury and proprioception in the lower back. *J Orthop Sports Phys Ther*. 1994;19:282-295.

58. Brooks VB. Motor control: how posture and movements are governed. *Phys Ther*. 1983;63:664-673.

59. Latash ML. *Neurophysiological Basis of Movement*. Champaign, IL: Human Kinetics; 1998.

60. Vleeming A, Pool-Goudzwaard AL, Stoeckart R, Van Wingerden J, Snijders CJ. The posterior layer of the thoracolumbar fascia: its function in load transfer from spine to legs. *Spine*. 1995;20:753-758.

61. Nies-Byl N, Sinnott PL. Variations in balance and body sway in middle-aged adults: subjects with healthy backs compared with subjects with low-back dysfunction. *Spine*. 1991;16:325-330.

62. Cholewicki J, Panjabi M, Khachatryan A. Stabilizing function of trunk flexor-extensor muscles around a neutral spine posture. *Spine*. 1997;22:2207-2212.

63. Granata KP, Marras WS. The influence of trunk muscle coactivity on dynamic spinal loads. *Spine*. 1995;20:913-919.

64. Paris SV. Physical signs of instability. *Spine*. 1985;3:277-279.

65. Richardson C, Jull G, Hodges P, Hides J. *Therapeutic Exercise for Spinal Segmental Stabilization in Low Back Pain. A Scientific Basis and Clinical Approach*. London, England: Churchill Livingston; 1999.

66. Bergmark A. Stability of the lumbar spine. A study in mechanical engineering. *Acta Orthopaedica Scandinavica*. 1989;230(suppl):20-24.

67. Parkhurst TM, Burnett CN. Injury and proprioception in the lower back. *J Orthop Sports Phys Ther*. 1994;19:282-295.

68. Hides JA, Richardson CA, Jull GA. Multifidus muscle recovery is not automatic after resolution of acute, first-episode low back pain. *Spine*. 1996;21:2763-2769.

69. Haggins M, Adler K, Cash M, Daugherty J, Mitriani G. Effects of practice on the ability to perform lumbar stabilization exercises. *J Orthop Sports Phys Ther*. 1999;29:546-555.

70. Childs JD, Whitman JM, Piva SR, Young B, Fritz JM. Lower cervical spine. *APTA Home Study Course 13.3.2, Physical Therapy for the Cervical Spine and Temporomandibular Joint*. LaCrosse, WI: APTA; 2003.

71. Jull G. Management of Neck Pain with Exercise. *J Man Manip Ther*. 2005;13: 177-188.

72. Taylor JL, McCloskey DI. Proprioceptive sensation in rotation of the trunk. *Exp Brain Res*. 1990;81:413-416.

73. Laskowski ER, Newcomer KL, Smith J. Refining rehabilitation with proprioceptive training: expediting return to play. *Phys Sportsmed*. 1997;25:89-102.

74. Kandel ER, Schwartz JH. *Principles of Neural Science*, 2nd ed. New York, NY: Elsevier; 1985.

75. McLain RF, Pickar JG. Mechanoreceptor endings in human thoracic and lumbar facet joints. *Spine*. 1998;23:168-173.

76. Yamashita T, Minaki Y, Oota I, Yokogushi K, Ishii S. Mechanosensitive afferent units in the lumbar intervertebral disc and adjacent muscle. *Spine*. 1993;18:2252-2256.

77. Cavanaugh JM, Kallakuri S, Ozaktay AC. Innervation of the rabbit lumbar intervertebral disc and posterior longitudinal ligament. *Spine*. 1995;20:2080-2085.

78. Roberts S, Eisenstein SM, Menage J, Evans EH, Ashton IK. Mechanoreceptors in intervertebral discs: morphology, distribution, and neuropeptides. *Spine*. 1995;20:2645-2651.

79. Newcomer KL, Laskowski ER, Yu B. Differences in repositioning error among patients with low back pain compared with control subjects. *Spine*. 2000;25:2488-2493.

80. Luoto S, Aalto H, Taimela S, et al. One-footed and externally disturbed two-footed postural control in patients with chronic low back pain and healthy control subjects: a controlled study with follow-up. *Spine*. 1998;23:2081-2089.

81. Radebold A, Cholewicki J, Polzhofer GK, Greene HS. Impaired postural control of the lumbar spine is associated with delayed muscle response

82. times in patients with chronic idiopathic low back pain. *Spine*. 2001;26: 724-730.

82. Nouwen A, Van Akkerveeken PF, Versloot JM. Patterns of muscular activity during movement in patients with chronic low-back pain. *Spine*. 1987;12:777-782.

83. Hodges PW, Richardson CA. Inefficient muscular stabilization of the lumbar spine associated with low back pain: a motor control evaluation of transversus abdominis. *Spine*. 1996;21:2640-2650.

84. Paquet N, Malouin F, Richards CL. Hip-Spine movement interaction and muscle activation patterns during sagittal trunk movements in low back pain patients. *Spine*. 1994;19:596-603.

85. Radebold A, Cholewicki J, Panjabi M, Patel T. Muscle response pattern to sudden trunk loading in healthy individuals and in patients with chronic low back pain. *Spine*. 2000;25:947-954.

86. Parnianpour M, Nordin M, Kahanovitz N, Frankel V. The triaxial coupling of torque generation of trunk muscles during isometric exertions and the effect of fatiguing isoinertial movements on the motor output and movement patterns. *Spine*. 1988;13:982-991.

87. Taimela S, Kankaanpaa M, Luoto S. The effect of lumbar fatigue on the ability to sense a change in lumbar position: a controlled study. *Spine*. 1999;24:1322-1335.

88. Brumagne S, Cordo P, Lysens R. The role of paraspinal muscle spindles in lumbosacral position sense in individuals with and without low back pain. *Spine*. 2000;25:989-994.

89. Solomonow M, Zhou B, Harris M, Lu Y, Baratta RV. The ligamento-muscular stabilizing system of the spine. *Spine*. 1998;23:2552-2562.

90. Indahl A, Kaigle A, Reikeras O, Holm S. Electromyographic response of the porcine multifidus musculature after nerve stimulation. *Spine*. 1995;20:2652-2658.

91. Gustavsen R. *Training Therapy Prophylaxis and Rehabilitation*. New York, NY: Thieme Inc.; 1985.

92. Jull G, Trott P, Potter H, et al. A randomized controlled trial of exercise and manipulative therapy for cervicogenic headache. *Spine*. 2002;27: 1835-1843.

93. O'Sullivan PB, Twomey LT, Allison GT. Evaluation of specific stabilizing exercise in the treatment of chronic low back pain with radiologic diagnosis of sponylosis or spondylolisthesis. *Spine*. 1997;22:2959-2967.

94. Miller ER, Schenk RJ, Karnes JL, Rousselle JG. A comparison of the McKenzie approach to a specific spine stabilization program for chronic low back pain. *J Man Manip Ther*. 2005;13:103-112.

95. O'Leary S, Falla D, Jull G. Recent advances in therapeutic exercise for the neck: implications for patients with head and neck pain. *Aust Endod J*. 2003;29:1338-1142.

96. Richardson CA, Jull GA. Muscle control-pain control. What exercises would you prescribe? *Manual Ther*. 1995;1:2-10.

97. McGill, SM. Low back stability: from formal description to issues for performance and rehabilitation. *Exer Sport Sci Rev*. 2001;29:26-31.

98. Sahrmann SA. *Diagnosis and Treatment of Movement Impairment Syndromes*. St. Louis, MO: Mosby; 2002.

99. Van Dillen LR, Sahrmann SA, Norton BJ, et al. Effect of active limb movements on symptoms in patients with low back pain. *J Orthop Sports Phys Ther*. 2001;31:402-418.

100. Kendall FP, McCreary EK, Provance PG. *Muscles Testing and Function*, 4th ed. Baltimore, MD: Williams & Wilkins, 1993.

101. Esola MA, McClure PW, Fitzgerald GK, Siegler S. Analysis of lumbar spine and hip motion during forward bending in subjects with and without a history of low back pain. *Spine*. 1996;21:71-78.

102. McClure PW, Esola M, Schreier R, Siegler S. Kinematic analysis of lumbar and hip motion while rising from a forward, flexed position in patients with and without a history of low back pain. *Spine*. 1997;22:552-558.

103. Bullock-Saxton JE, Janda V, Bullock MI. Reflex activation of gluteal muscles in walking. An approach to restoration of muscle function for patients with low-back pain. *Spine* 1993;18:704-708.

104. Bullock-Saxton JE, Janda V, Bullock MI. The influence of ankle sprain injury on muscle activation during hip extension. *Int J Sports Med*. 1994;15:330-334.

105. McGill SM. Low back exercises: evidence for improving exercise regimens. *Phys Ther*. 1998;78:754-765.

The Role of High-Velocity Thrust Manipulation in Orthopaedic Manual Physical Therapy

Ben Hando, PT, DSc, OCS, FAAOMPT

Timothy Flynn, PT, PhD, OCS, FAAOMPT

Chapter Objectives

At the conclusion of this chapter, the reader will be able to:

- Understand the history and evolution of thrust manipulation among disparate professions.
- Understand the role thrust manipulation plays in physical therapists' management of musculoskeletal disorders
- Identify patients with low back pain who are likely to respond to thrust manipulation.
- Explain the risks associated with cervical spine manipulation.
- Articulate best-evidence strategies for screening for vertebrobasilar insufficiency.
- Understand the appropriate medical screening procedures to perform prior to administering manipulation to the cervical spine.
- Articulate best-evidence strategies for screening for upper cervical spine instability.
- Understand the appropriate physical examination screening procedures to perform prior to administering manipulation to the cervical spine.
- Summarize the body of evidence that supports cervical thrust and nonthrust manipulation for individuals with neck pain.
- Identify individuals with neck pain who are likely to respond to cervical spine thrust manipulation.

- Identify individuals with neck pain who are likely to respond to thoracic spine thrust manipulation.
- Summarize the supportive evidence for thrust manipulation for osteoarthritis of the hip.
- Summarize the supportive evidence for glenohumeral translational manipulation under anesthesia for adhesive capsulitis.
- Describe the appropriate procedures to conduct prior to glenohumeral manipulation under anesthesia.
- Describe the postmanipulative care required following glenohumeral translational manipulation under anesthesia.
- Summarize the supportive evidence for manipulation of the wrist for lateral epicondylalgia.
- Describe the performance of the following techniques:
  - Supine lumbosacral regional thrust manipulation.
  - Side-lying lumbar thrust manipulation.
  - Seated cervicothoracic thrust manipulation.
  - Supine thoracic flexion/opening thrust manipulation.
  - Cervical flexion/opening thrust manipulation.
  - Hip joint distraction thrust manipulation.
  - Inferior glenohumeral manipulation.
  - Posterior glenohumeral manipulation.
  - Wrist/scaphoid extension thrust manipulation.

INTRODUCTION

Operational Definitions

There is considerable variability within physical therapy literature and practice regarding the terminology used to describe manipulative techniques. For the purposes of this chapter and text, **mobilization** refers to Grade I to IV nonthrust techniques, while **manipulation** refers to "high velocity, low amplitude thrust movements within or at the end range of motion."[1] In the literature and in practice, these terms may be used interchangeably (Box 18-1).

This chapter is not intended to be comprehensive but rather to provide the reader an evidence-based perspective of the role of thrust manipulation in the management of several musculoskeletal diagnoses commonly encountered by physical therapists. Detailed descriptions of the manipulative techniques used in the reviewed studies are provided. Every effort is made to describe the techniques in the manner in which they were performed in their respective studies. Based on the ever-evolving nature of evidence in this area of study, the reader is encouraged to consult the literature for the current best evidence. This chapter intends to highlight several of the important studies performed in this area; however, new evidence has emerged since the writing of this chapter.

Historical Overview

The use of thrust manipulation as a therapeutic intervention pre-dates the earliest medical writings (see Chapter 1). *Hippocrates* (460–357 BC), considered by many to be the father of modern medicine, wrote extensively on the methodology and benefits of manual medicine.[2] Since that time, countless groups have practiced manipulation, including American Indian tribes, Arabian physicians, European surgeons, and the bone setters of England and North America.[2–5]

Osteopathy

Manipulation gained popularity in the late nineteenth century in North America with the advent of osteopathic medicine in 1874 (see Chapter 4). The founder of osteopathy, *Andrew Still*, claimed that diseases were partly the result of "dislocated bones" that impeded vascular and neural "flow."[2–4] As the profession evolved, joint manipulation became a less critical skill set for the practicing doctor of osteopathy (DO). Although many DOs still practice manipulative therapy, the majority of joint manipulation that occurs within orthodox healthcare today is performed by physical therapists.[4]

Chiropractic

The profession most commonly associated with the practice of thrust is chiropractic, which was founded in 1895 by *Daniel*

Box 18-1 Quick Notes! MANIPULATION

Manipulation is:

a high-velocity, low amplitude thrust movement within or at the end range of motion.

Palmer.[2,4] Palmer believed that a major cause of pain and disease was malpositioned vertebral segments he termed "subluxations" that impinged neural, vascular, and lymphatic structures passing through the intervertebral foramen.[2,3] Spinal "adjustments" alleviated the impingement, thus facilitating organic healing of the diseased structures.[2,3] Additionally, Palmer stressed the importance of specific techniques in which he claimed to use the spinous and transverse processes as levers.[2,4] Unlike osteopathy, chiropractic has maintained its identity as a naturopathic discipline and has remained a distinct alternative to orthodox medicine.

Physical Therapy

Thrust manipulation has never been regarded as the centerpiece of physical therapy practice. Physical therapists have generally failed to subscribe to theories on the far-reaching benefits of manipulation for multiple body systems. The *American Physical Therapy Association Orthopedic Section's* position statement on mobilization/manipulation states that mobilization/manipulation techniques are "one component of the conservative management of the patient with a musculoskeletal disorder and are used in combination with a variety of physical therapy procedures to assist in the elimination of pain and improvement in function in activities of daily living and recreational and work settings."[6]

Physical therapists have used thrust manipulation in the treatment of neuromuscular and musculoskeletal impairments since the inception of the profession circa 1900.[1,3,5] Early physical therapists learned manipulation from medical doctors.[2,3] Throughout the early to mid-1900s prominent physicians such as James and John Mennell and Edgar and James Cyriax lectured and wrote extensively on manipulation, primarily to an audience of physical therapists.[3] Interestingly, physical therapists now frequently teach manipulation to physicians.[2,3]

By 1960, as physical therapy's subordinate relationship to orthodox medicine evolved to a more collaborative one, physical therapists began developing unique approaches to thrust manipulation as well as conducting research on the efficacy of manipulation in treating various musculoskeletal pathologies. As use of manipulation among physical therapists increased, so did competition with chiropractors.[3] Chiropractic responded to this competition with legislative and political efforts aimed at restricting physical therapists' ability to perform these procedures.[3,5] These efforts have continued to the present day, and despite countermeasures from physical therapists, chiropractors have succeeded in limiting the manipulation privileges of physical therapists in a small number of states.[3,5]

Today, manipulation remains an important element of physical therapy practice. Numerous high-quality research studies investigating the effectiveness of manipulation have validated the critical role that manipulation plays in the conservative management of many musculoskeletal diagnoses. Physical therapists have emerged as leading contributors in this area of research and are ideally positioned to solidify this role into the future.

- Which discipline was the first to adopt the principles and practice of manipulation?
- Should these techniques be considered as "belonging" to any one specific discipline?
- How does the training and practice of PTs make them uniquely qualified to provide this form of intervention?
- How is the practice of manipulation within physical therapy philosophically different from its practice within other disciplines?

THE ROLE OF THRUST MANIPULATION IN THE MANAGEMENT OF ACUTE LOW BACK PAIN

Low back pain (LBP) is the most common musculoskeletal complaint seen by physical therapists.[7] Although there is a growing body of evidence, very few interventions have demonstrated even a minimal degree of effectiveness when subjected to the rigors of scientific inquiry.[7-10] Some have suggested that the dearth of evidence may be the result of failing to identify homogeneous subgroups of patients who are likely to respond to specific interventions.[11-14]

CLINICAL PILLAR

Classification of patients with low back pain according to history and physical examination may do the following:

- Enable researchers to study more homogenous groups of patients
- Improve clinical decision making and ultimately patient outcomes by matching patients with interventions that are likely to be of benefit

Lumbosacral Regional Manipulation

Evidence Summary

Flynn and colleagues[13] developed a **clinical prediction rule (CPR)** to classify patients based on their likelihood of responding to a spinal manipulation technique. In this prospective cohort study, subjects referred to physical therapy with a diagnosis related to the lumbosacral spine received a standardized historical and physical examination followed by a maximum of two treatment sessions within a 1-week period. Treatment sessions consisted of a lumbosacral regional manipulation followed by a pelvic tilt range of motion exercise. A successful outcome was defined as a 50% or greater reduction in disability as measured by the *Modified Oswestry Disability Index*. A logistic regression analysis was conducted to identify findings from the historical and physical examination that could serve as predictors for a successful outcome.

CLINICAL PILLAR

CLINICAL PREDICTION RULE
For patients with LBP who are likely to benefit from manipulation[13]:

1. Duration of symptoms less than 16 days
2. At least one hip greater than 35 degrees of internal rotation (IR)
3. Hypomobility with lumbar spring testing in one or more segments
4. A score of less than 19 on a subscale of the FABQ
5. No symptoms distal to the knee

If the patient is positive on four of five variables, the probability of a successful outcome increased from 45% (pretest probability) to 95% (posttest probability)

The five criteria for the CPR were as follows: (1) duration of symptoms less than 16 days, (2) hypomobility with lumbar spring testing in one or more segments, (3) a score of less than 19 on a subscale of the Fear-Avoidance Beliefs Questionnaire (FABQ), (4) no symptoms distal to the knee, and (5) at least one hip with greater than 35 degrees of internal rotation. The CPR demonstrated a positive likelihood ratio of 24.4, indicating that individuals who were positive for at least four of the five variables increased their likelihood of a successful outcome with manipulation from 45% (pretest probability) to 95% (posttest probability).

Childs and colleagues[12] conducted a validation study to test this CPR in a variety of clinical settings and among clinicians with varying levels of experience. Successive patients referred to physical therapy with a primary complaint of low back pain were randomized to receive either spinal manipulation that was used in the prior study[13] or a lumbar stabilization program. Patients who met the criteria for the CPR (positive for four or more variables) and were treated with spinal manipulation demonstrated significantly better outcomes than did those who received spinal manipulation but did not meet the CPR or those who met the CPR and were treated with lumbar stabilization.[12,15] These results were maintained at the 6 month follow-up evaluation. The CPR demonstrated a positive likelihood ratio of 13.2, indicating that for those individuals meeting at least four of the CPR's five criteria, the likelihood of achieving a successful outcome from spinal manipulation increased from 44% (pretest probability) to 92% (posttest probability).[12] These studies represent the initial evidence supporting the use of CPRs in the use of manipulation for low back pain. Since the writing of this text, a myriad of CPRs have been developed to help guide the practitioner in identifying individuals who are most likely to benefit from manipulation. It is recommended that the reader consult the ever-evolving literature in this area.

Technique Description: Lumbosacral Regional Manipulation

The following example describes a right lumbosacral regional manipulation as used in the aforementioned studies. The patient is positioned supine with his or her arms at the side. The clinician stands to the left of the patient opposite the side that is being manipulated. Right side bending of the lumbar spine is initiated by translating the patient's pelvis to the left. The lower extremities are then positioned to the right to further laterally flex the spine (Fig. 18-1). The patient is instructed to interlock his or her fingers behind the neck or to fold the arms across the chest, and the lumbar spine is positioned in maximum right side bending and slight left rotation. This is achieved by introducing left lumbar rotation by propping the patient on his or her left shoulder (Fig. 18-2). The clinician next places the right hand on the right scapula of the patient and the left hand on the right anterior superior iliac spine (ASIS). The manipulation is carried out by rotating the torso of the patient to the left with the right hand while maintaining the position of the left hand on the right ASIS (Fig. 18-3). When the right side of the pelvis begins to elevate, a quick thrust is delivered through the right ASIS in a posteroinferior direction (Fig. 18-4).

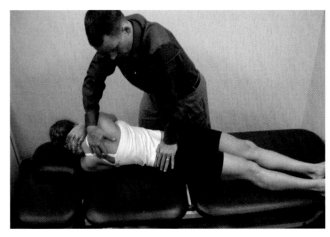

FIGURE 18–3 Right-sided sacroiliac regional manipulation (cont.). The patient's torso is rotated to the left while the clinician maintains contact with the right ASIS.

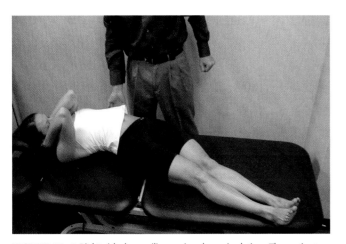

FIGURE 18–1 Right-sided sacroiliac regional manipulation. The patient interlaces his or her fingers behind the neck and approximates the elbows. The clinician stands on the left side of the patient and laterally flexes the lumbar spine to the right.

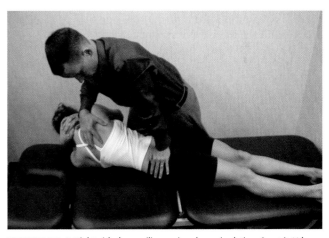

FIGURE 18–4 Right-sided sacroiliac regional manipulation (cont.). When the right side of the pelvis begins to elevate off the table, a quick thrust is delivered through the right ASIS in a posteroinferior direction.

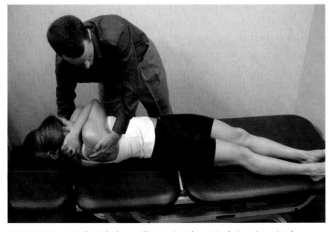

FIGURE 18–2 Right-sided sacroiliac regional manipulation (cont.). The clinician positions the patient in maximum right lumbar side bending and slight left lumbar rotation by propping the patient on his or her left shoulder.

Alternative Manipulative Techniques for Individuals Who Satisfy the CPR

Evidence Summary

Cleland and colleagues[16] explored the generalizability of the lumbosacral manipulation CPR to other manipulative techniques. In this randomized controlled trial, patients with lower back pain who met the CPR were randomized to receive either a supine lumbosacral thrust manipulation, a side-lying lumbar thrust manipulation, or a prone nonthrust lumbar manipulation. All subjects attended two sessions of manipulation and exercise followed by three sessions of a standardized exercise intervention. Follow-up evaluations were conducted at 1, 4, and 26 weeks following baseline examination. These results suggest that this CPR is generalizable to at least one additional thrust manipulation technique (lumbar side-lying thrust manipulation), but not to a nonthrust technique (prone lumbar nonthrust manipulation). For patients who meet the CPR, the clinician should expect similar clinical outcomes with using either the side-lying or supine thrust manipulation technique.[16]

Technique Description: Side-Lying Lumbar Rotational Manipulation

The patient is positioned in left side-lying position with his or her head resting on a pillow. The clinician stands in front of the patient and palpates the interspinous space of the targeted segment using the right hand. Using the left hand, the clinician flexes the patient's right hip until motion is perceived in the interspinous space, at which time the patient's right foot is placed in the popliteal fossa of the left knee (Fig. 18-5). The clinician then places the left hand in the interspinous space and grasps the patient's left shoulder and arm using the right hand. Right lumbar rotation and left lumbar side bending are then introduced by sliding the patient's left shoulder anteriorly until motion is again perceived in the interspinous space (Fig. 18-6). Next, the clinician loops his or her hand through the patient's arms and log rolls the patient toward the edge of the table. Both hands should now be monitoring the interspinous space as shown and providing a skin-lock over the segment to be mobilized. The clinician's right proximal forearm and elbow should be resting on the patient's right anterior shoulder, and the left forearm resting over the patient's right posterolateral hip. The manipulation is carried out using the clinician's arms

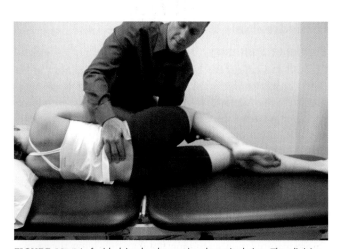

FIGURE 18–5 Left side-lying lumbar regional manipulation. The clinician flexes the patient's right hip while monitoring lumbar intervertebral motion with the right hand.

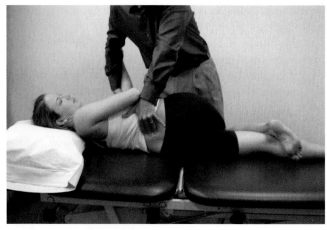

FIGURE 18–6 Left side-lying lumbar regional manipulation (cont.). The clinician introduces left lumbar side bending and right lumbar rotation while monitoring intervertebral motion with the left hand.

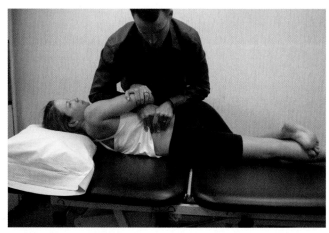

FIGURE 18–7 Left side-lying lumbar region manipulation (cont.). Using his or her arms and body, the clinician stabilizes the torso while translating the right side of the pelvis anteriorly.

and body to rotate the right side of the pelvis anteriorly while stabilizing the torso with the right forearm (Fig. 18-7). Once the restrictive barrier is engaged, a small-amplitude high-velocity thrust manipulation is delivered bringing the right side of the pelvis anteriorly.

THE ROLE OF THRUST MANIPULATION IN THE MANAGEMENT OF NECK PAIN

Neck pain is a common and costly malady with point prevalence of 10% to 22% in the general population and ranking second only to low back pain in annual U.S. Workers' Compensation costs.[17,18] Individuals with neck pain account for 15% to 25% of all patients receiving outpatient physical therapy services.[19] Physical therapy interventions for neck pain are highly variable, and evidence is generally lacking.[18,20,21] There is mounting evidence that manual therapy and exercise are most effective when used in combination.[22–26]

- Why is manipulation for the cervical spine used less frequently in the clinic?
- What is the actual versus perceived risk of cervical spine thrust manipulation?
- What are the most common side effects of cervical spine manipulation?
- What methods may be used by PTs to reduce the risk of adverse effects from manipulation?

Evidence Summary: Cervical Spine Manipulation and Risk of Adverse Side Effects

Much of the controversy surrounding cervical thrust involves vertebral artery accidents. The best available estimate of the incidence states that for every 100,000 persons 45 years of age who receive thrust, approximately 1.3 cases of vertebral artery dissection would be observed within 1 week of manipulative therapy.[27] Similar rates of stroke have been noted in patients seeking care from their physician, suggesting that in some cases patients with headache and neck pain are experiencing a vertebral artery dissection in progress.[28]

Rivett et al[29] performed a prospective study that investigated the complications of cervical spine manipulation. Twenty experienced therapists were asked to report any adverse response to cervical thrust. The incident rate reported in this study was 0.21% per manipulation and 0.42% per patient. No serious or significant complications were reported following nearly 500 cervical spine manipulations performed over a 3 month period.

In a commentary discussing the uncertainties that exist regarding the ability to identify the patients at risk for vertebrobasilar injury, Hurwitz et al[30] reported that the risk of serious complications resulting from cervical spine manipulation is approximately 6 per 10 million and the risk of death estimated at 3 in 10 million manipulations.

Although these estimates reflect a relatively low risk, clearly a consideration of precautionary measures is warranted for clinicians administering cervical thrust. Unfortunately, useful evidence to suggest that individuals at risk for *vertebral basilar insufficiency (VBI)* can be identified through historical or objective screening procedures does not exist.[31–33] Consequently, several authors have suggested simply avoiding the use of interventions that have been implicated as potential contributors to VBI and using in their place presumably safer techniques.[31,33,34]

The majority of documented cases of VBI reportedly induced by thrust have involved techniques incorporating either end-range cervical spine rotation or a combination of end range rotation and extension of the upper cervical spine.[31–33] Therefore, performing techniques in which the cervical spine is positioned closer to a neutral position could potentially reduce the risk of VBI associated with these procedures.[31,33] Another suggested alternative is to simply direct intervention toward other areas of the spine.[31,34–36] There is some evidence that patients with neck pain may benefit from thoracic spine manipulation.[34–36] Several authors have suggested substituting thoracic spine manipulation as a method of lowering the risk of VBI when treating neck pain.[34]

Screening Procedures for Cervical Spine Thrust Manipulation

Manual physical therapists should be aware of prudent screening procedures for both the cervical artery system (vertebral artery and carotid arteries) as well as the stabilizing structures of the neck. A baseline neurological examination should be considered as a minimum standard of care prior to cervical treatment. Contraindications to manual interventions of the cervical spine include multilevel nerve root pathology; worsening neurological function; unremitting, severe, nonmechanical pain; upper motor neuron lesions; and spinal cord damage.[37] Furthermore, a number of risk factors for cervical vascular disease have been proposed. Of particular note is the use of blood pressure screening for hypertension in patients with neck complaints. Readers are referred to Kerry and Taylor[38] for greater detail on this issue.

In addition to vascular pathology, the following risk factors suggest the potential for bony or ligamentous compromise of the upper cervical spine: history of trauma (e.g., whiplash, rugby neck injury); congenital collagenous compromise (syndromes such as Down's, Ehlers-Danlos's, Grisel's, Morquio's); inflammatory arthritis (rheumatoid arthritis, ankylosing spondylitis); and recent neck/head/dental surgery.[39] There are numerous clinical tests for cervical spine instability currently in use in clinical practice, and most are intended to assess the integrity of the alar and transverse ligaments. Unfortunately, most of these tests have not been validated in patients with neck pain and headaches, and the level of reliability of the tests varies. Following a thorough history and neurological examination, a reasoned approach to testing cervical stability involves systematically analyzing and progressing from active patient generated movements to passive therapist generated movements, to gentle passive overpressure of the movement, followed by accessory movement testing. Throughout the entire process, particular attention is paid to the patient's response to increases in motion or empty end-feel, reproduction of symptoms of instability, or production of lateral nystagmus and nausea. Ultimately, management of the cervical spine with physical therapy procedures requires prudent clinical reasoning and particular attention to the neurovascular system throughout examination and intervention.

METHODS FOR REDUCING THE RISK OF ADVERSE EVENTS FROM CERVICAL SPINE MANIPULATION[38]

1. Premanipulative screening of the vertebrobasilar arterial system
2. Premanipulative screening of the subcranial capsuloligamentous system

3. A detailed history to identify trauma or a systemic condition that may impact segmental stability

4. Blood pressure screening

5. Neurological screening

6. Diagnostic imaging in cases of trauma or previous history, most notably including an open mouth radiologic view of the subcranial spine

7. Response to active, passive, and accessory motions, including overpressure

8. Response to premanipulative positioning

Evidence Summary: Orthopaedic Manual Physical Therapy for Mechanical Neck Pain

Walker et al[22] compared the effectiveness of manual therapy and exercise versus minimal intervention in patients with mechanical neck disorders. Patients in the manual and exercise group received individualized *impairment based manual therapy* as well as a standardized exercise program. Manual therapy interventions were left to the discretion of the treating therapist and included high-velocity thrust techniques in addition to a variety of other soft tissue and joint techniques directed toward the cervical spine, thoracic spine, and costal cage. All patients receiving manual therapy also received a standardized home exercise program of cervical range of motion and deep neck cervical flexor strengthening exercises. Patients in the minimal intervention group received advice and encouragement to maintain cervical range of motion, carry on with normal activities of daily living, cervical active range of motion (AROM) exercises, and subtherapeutic pulsed ultrasound.

At 6-week and 1-year follow-up, patients in the manual and exercise group experienced significantly greater pain reduction and functional improvement than did individuals in the other group. It is important to note that nearly half of the patients in the manual group received thrust manipulation.

Hoving et al[40] recently demonstrated that therapists with advanced training in specific manipulation produced a 68% success rate in patients treated with nonthrust techniques and exercise compared to a 51% success rate for the patients treated by the physical therapists with more general training and 36% success rate for patients treated by a general medical practitioner. Korthals-de Bos et al[41] reported that manual physical therapy required fewer treatment sessions for a more favorable outcome, with the cost of these sessions being approximately one-third of the cost of the other two treatment groups that were used in the Hoving et al[40] study. The authors concluded that manual physical therapy was more cost effective for treating neck pain than general physical therapy or care provided by a general practitioner.[41] It is important to highlight that these favorable outcomes were obtained through the use of nonthrust manipulation techniques.

A clinical prediction rule has been developed to identify patients who are likely to report an immediate positive response to cervical thrust manipulation.[42] The six criteria are: (1) initial scores on the neck disability index (NDI) of less than 11.50, (2) the presence of a bilateral pattern of involvement, (3) not involved in the performance of sedentary work for more than 5 hours each day, (4) report of feeling better while moving the neck, (5) no report of feeling worse while extending the neck, and (6) the diagnosis of spondylosis without radiculopathy. If four or more of the six criteria are present, there is an 89% chance of an immediate positive response to the manipulation. Outcomes were measured as either a 50% reduction in their pain scale score, a 4-point change in their global perceived effect, or a report of being highly satisfied with the treatment.[42] This CPR has not yet been validated; however, it provides preliminary data to guide the clinician with appreciating those most likely to benefit from these procedures.[42]

More recently, Puentedura and colleagues[43] performed a study on 82 consecutive patients who presented to physical therapy with primary complaint of neck pain. After a clinical examination, all patients received a standardized treatment regimen, consisting of cervical manipulation for one or two sessions over 1 week. Thirty-nine percent of the patients had a successful outcome, as determined by a score of +5 or higher on the GROC scale. Variables retained in the regression model were used to develop a multivariate CPR, which included four criteria: (1) symptom duration less than 38 days, (2) positive expectation that manipulation will help, (3) side-to-side difference in cervical rotation range of motion of 10 degrees or greater, and (4) pain with posteroanterior spring testing of the midcervical spine. If three or more of the four attributes were present (+LR = 13.5), the probability of experiencing a successful outcome improved from 39% to 90%. Future studies are necessary to validate the results including long-term follow-up and a comparison group test.[43] The reader is referred to the current literature that has emerged regarding this topic since the writing of this chapter.

CLINICAL PILLAR

CLINICAL PREDICTION RULE

For patients with neck pain who are likely to benefit from cervical manipulation: [43]

1. Symptom duration less than 38 days

2. Positive expectation that manipulation will help

3. Side-to-side difference in cervical rotation range of motion of 10 degrees or greater

4. Pain with posteroanterior spring testing of the midcervical spine

If the patient is positive on three or more of the four variables, the probability of experiencing a successful outcome increases from 39% to 90% (+LR = 13.5).

Technique Description: High-Velocity, Mid-Range, Right Side-Bending Force to the Mid-Cervical Spine

The technique described below was frequently used by the treating clinicians in the Walker et al study.[22] The following example is intended to "open" the left C4/C5 segment. The patient lies supine, with the clinician standing at the head of the patient. Both hands are placed around the patient's head and neck, with the thumbs resting over the mandible and the right second metacarpophalangeal (MCP) joint positioned firmly over the right facet of the targeted segment (Fig. 18-8).[29] The right hand will deliver the mobilizing or manipulative force, while the left hand serves primarily to control motion of the neck. The head and neck are flexed by the clinician ulnarly, deviating both wrists. The neck is then translated from right to left, or left rotation is introduced, to engage the targeted segment, and final minor adjustments are made (Fig 18-9). When the motion segment has reached its restrictive barrier, a high-velocity, low-amplitude thrust is delivered from right to left. When performing this technique, attention should be given to ensure the right second MCP contact point remains posterior to the facet joint and not over the transverse process. Special attention should also be given to ensure the clinician's right forearm stays in line with the direction of the manipulative thrust.[29]

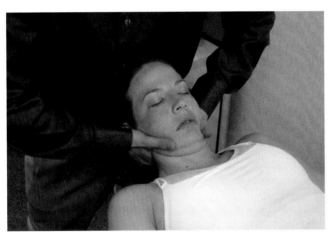

FIGURE 18–8 Left cervical opening/flexion manipulation. The clinician supports the patient's head and neck with the thumbs resting over the mandible and the right second MCP joint positioned firmly over the right facet of the targeted segment.

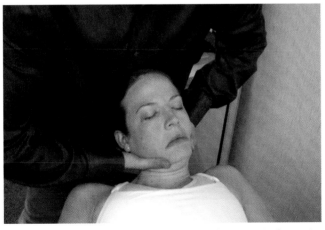

FIGURE 18–9 Left cervical opening/flexion manipulation (cont.). The restrictive barrier is engaged by translating the patient's neck from right to left.

Evidence Summary: Thoracic Spine Manipulation for Mechanical Neck Pain

Cleland and colleagues[34] investigated the immediate effects of thoracic spine manipulation on perceived pain levels in individuals suffering from neck pain. Participants between the ages of 18 and 60 years with a primary complaint of neck pain were randomized to either a manipulation group or a placebo manipulation group. A visual analog scale (VAS) was used to quantify patients' resting level of neck pain prior to and immediately following the intervention. A segmental mobility examination was performed and used to guide intervention. Each subject received an average of three manipulations.

Patients in the manipulation group demonstrated significantly greater immediate improvements in VAS scores than did individuals in the placebo manipulation group, leading the authors to conclude that thoracic spine manipulation may be an effective alternative in the management of patients with mechanical neck pain.

Cleland and colleagues[36] also conducted a prospective cohort study to develop a CPR to identify patients with neck pain who are likely to benefit from thoracic spine thrust manipulation. This study design was similar to that used by Flynn et al[13] in developing the CPR for patients with acute low back pain. Seventy-eight consecutive patients between the ages of 18 and 60, referred to physical therapy with a primary complaint of neck pain, with or without upper extremity symptoms, were recruited to participate in the study. Patients were excluded from the study if they were previously diagnosed with cervical spinal stenosis, were found to exhibit any medical red flags, had suffered a whiplash-associated disorder within the previous 6 weeks, showed evidence of central nervous system involvement, or demonstrated signs of nerve root compression during physical examination. Subjects received a standardized historical and physical examination followed by, at most, two intervention sessions within a 1-week period consisting of three distinct thoracic spine manipulation techniques and instruction in the performance of a cervical active range of motion exercise. A successful outcome was defined by a score of 5 or greater on the global rating of change scale (GROC). A logistic regression analysis was conducted to identify examination findings that could serve as predictors for a successful outcome following thoracic spine manipulation. Six variables were identified as predictors and together formed the CPR. The variables are as follows: (1) duration of symptoms less than 30 days, (2) no symptoms distal to the shoulder, (3) subject reporting that looking up does not aggravate symptoms, (4) a FABQ (physical assessment) score of less than 12, (5) diminished upper thoracic spine kyphosis (T3-T5), and (6) cervical extension range of motion less than 30 degrees. The CPR demonstrated a positive likelihood ratio of 12.0, indicating that individuals who were positive for at least four of the six variables increased their likelihood of a successful outcome with thoracic manipulation from 54% (pretest probability) to 93% (posttest probability). Although this CPR has failed to achieve validation, it may still be useful in identifying individuals with neck pain that may benefit from thoracic manipulation.

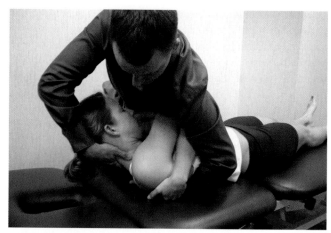

FIGURE 18–11 Supine right thoracic opening/flexion manipulation. The clinician supports the patient's head and neck while localizing motion to the desired segment through flexion, left side bending, and left rotation of the spine.

Technique Description: Supine Thoracic Spine Opening/Flexion Manipulation (Pistol Technique)

This technique was used by the treating clinicians in the two Cleland et al[34,36] studies previously described. The following example is intended to flex or "open" the right T4-T5 segment. The patient lies supine with his or her arms crossed over the chest, right over left. The clinician briefly rolls the patient onto the left shoulder and places the left hand over the vertebral level immediately caudal to the restricted segment using a "pistol grip" as shown (Fig. 18-10). In this example, the clinician's hand will make contact with the transverse processes of the T5 vertebra. The patient is then rolled supine, and the clinician supports the patient's head and neck with the right hand and localizes motion to the desired segment through flexion, left side bending, and left rotation of the spine from above downward (Fig. 18-11).[44] When motion is localized to the desired segment, the patient is instructed to take a deep breath in, and upon exhaling, the clinician delivers a high-velocity, low-amplitude thrust with his or her body in an anterior to posterior direction. This thrust is intended to introduce a flexion movement to open or flex the right zygapophyseal joint.[44]

Technique Description: Upper Thoracic Spine Traction Manipulation

The upper thoracic spine traction manipulation has been described in several case reports.[45-47] This technique is purportedly indicated for individuals with mechanical neck dysfunction, with or without radicular symptoms, that has decreased segmental mobility and localized pain in the upper thoracic segments.[45-47] Piva et al[45] report that this technique is particularly effective for individuals with the aforementioned findings that also exhibit limited cervical flexion active range of motion.

The patient is seated on a treatment table with his or her hands clasped behind the neck. The clinician stands behind the patient and raises the table until the top of the patient's shoulders are at a level even with the nipple line of the clinician. The clinician flexes his or her knees and loops the hands through the patient's arms, placing the hands on top of or just below the patient's hands, as shown (Fig. 18-12). The clinician's chest

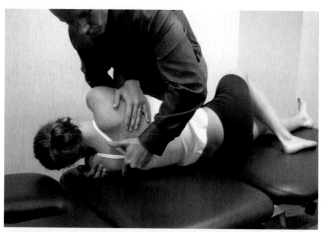

FIGURE 18–10 Supine right thoracic opening/flexion manipulation. The clinician makes contact with the transverse process of the thoracic vertebra immediately caudal to the restricted segment using a "pistol grip."

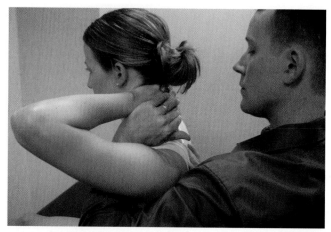

FIGURE 18–12 Seated upper thoracic traction manipulation. The clinician loops both hands through the patient's arms, placing the hands on top of or just below those of the patient.

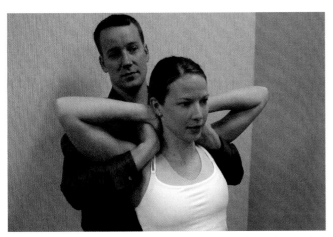

FIGURE 18–13 Seated upper thoracic traction manipulation (cont.). The clinician introduces bilateral shoulder retraction and spinal extension using his or her hands and chest. The mobilizing force is generated by the clinician pushing upward with the legs while simultaneously slightly extending the spine.

should contact the mid- to upper-thoracic segments. The patient is instructed to sit erect, and the clinician introduces bilateral shoulder retraction and spinal extension using his or her hands and chest.[45] The mobilizing force is initiated by the clinician gradually extending the knees to produce an axial traction force on the targeted segments. Once the restrictive barrier is engaged, the clinician performs a high-velocity thrust by quickly pushing upward with his or her legs while simultaneously extending the spine (Fig. 18-13). Special attention should be given to ensure the mobilizing force is generated from the legs and torso and not the arms and hands, which could produce unintended forced cervical flexion.

THE ROLE OF THRUST MANIPULATION IN THE MANAGEMENT OF HIP OSTEOARTHRITIS

Individuals suffering from hip *osteoarthritis (OA)* are frequently treated by physical therapists.[48] Several interventions for hip OA typically administered by physical therapists have been investigated in the medical literature. Included are land-based therapeutic exercise, aquatic therapy, and manual therapy.[49-54] Manual therapy of the hip typically consists of one or more of the following: graded mobilization, high-velocity thrust manipulation, and manual stretching of hip musculature.[55,56] Land-based exercise therapy and group-based aquatic therapy have been shown to reduce pain and disability in patients suffering from hip OA.[49,51,53] Unfortunately, recidivism occurs if compliance is not maintained.[50,56] Initial studies have shown manual physical therapy to be effective in reducing pain and increasing function in individuals with hip OA both in the short and long term.[54,56]

Evidence Summary: Manual Therapy for Hip Osteoarthritis

Hoeksma et al[54] compared the effectiveness of manual therapy and exercise in patients with hip OA. The exercise program consisted of a program found to be beneficial for patients with hip OA.[49] Manual therapy consisted of hip muscle stretching followed by a traction thrust manipulation technique. The treatment period for both groups consisted of nine sessions over a duration of 5 weeks. Subjects receiving manual therapy demonstrated greater improvements in hip function (measured with the Harris hip score), walking speed, hip range of motion, and pain at the conclusion of the 5-week treatment period. The majority of these improvements were maintained at 3- and 6-month follow-up, leading the authors to conclude that manual therapy is an effective option in the management of hip OA.

Technique Description: Hip Traction Manipulation

In the Hoeksma et al[54] study, the patient is positioned supine with the contralateral limb resting either flat on the table or flexed at the hip and knee to minimize slide during the procedure. The clinician's hands are positioned around the ankle, just proximal to the malleoli, and the hip is positioned in 15 to 30 degrees of abduction and flexion, deemed as the open-packed position (Fig. 18-14). The therapist stands in a straddled stance with elbows extended to encourage mobilizing force from the hips, which is initiated by applying distraction oscillations through the long axis of the limb to stretch the hip capsule. When capsular resistance is perceived, a distraction thrust manipulation is performed into the restriction. The manipulation may be repeated up to five times per session. For each subsequent manipulation, the joint is positioned in an increasingly limited position (which will vary for different patients), so that the final manipulation is performed with the hip in its most limited position. Active assisted hip range of motion exercises are performed between manipulations to aid in relaxation. The immediate effects of the manipulation are observed by assessing end-feel of hip distraction and passive hip flexion. When the end-feel of the involved hip approximates that of the contralateral hip, an optimal result has been achieved.[54,56]

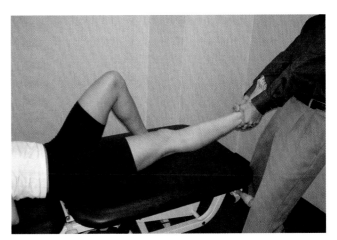

FIGURE 18–14 Hip distraction manipulation. The clinician's hands are positioned around the ankle, just proximal to the malleoli, and the hip is positioned in 15 to 30 degrees of abduction and flexion.

THE ROLE OF THRUST MANIPULATION IN THE MANAGEMENT OF GLENOHUMERAL ADHESIVE CAPSULITIS

Adhesive capsulitis (AC), also known as "frozen shoulder," is a relatively common, painful shoulder disorder that has an incidence of 2% to 5% in the general population and 10% to 20% in the diabetic population.[57] AC has been the subject of considerable disagreement and controversy in the medical literature.[58-61] Numerous interventions have been studied and subsequently recommended, including benign neglect, steroid injections, brisement or capsular distension, end-range joint mobilizations, self-stretching exercises, arthroscopic release, manipulation under general anesthesia, and translational manipulation under regional interscalene block.[57,61-74]

Despite the large number of interventional studies, there is little consensus among authors on the ideal course of intervention for patients suffering from frozen shoulder. In a review of interventions for shoulder pain conducted by the Cochrane collaboration, Green et al reported that "no conclusions can be drawn regarding the efficacy of the interventions studied for adhesive capsulitis."[75] More recently, a clinical practice guideline (CPG) related to management of AC was published by Kelley et al.[76] In this CPG, the intervention with the strongest evidence to support its use was corticosteroid injection. Patient education and stretching had moderate evidence and joint mobilization and translational manipulation under anesthesia (MUA) were both considered to possess weak evidence upon systematically reviewing the published literature.[76] Although most authors characterize frozen shoulder as a self-limiting disorder that has complete resolution within 1 to 3 years, several long-term studies have found a significant percentage of patients with symptoms and functional limitations up to 10 years after initial diagnosis.[58-60,77,78]

Patients with AC who are unresponsive to conservative measures often receive MUA.[58,61,79] In this procedure, while the patient is under general anesthesia, the humerus is grasped proximal to the elbow and forcefully mobilized through physiologic shoulder motions.[70-72,79] MUA has undergone criticism because of the documented bony and soft tissue injuries that have occurred during its performance.[61,73,79]

Evidence Summary: Glenohumeral Translational Manipulation under Regional Interscalene Block Anesthesia

To reduce the risk of injury associated with traditional glenohumeral manipulation, Roubal et al[73] developed a novel technique of translational manipulation following interscalene brachial plexus block. Forty-three patients treated with translational MUA have been reported in the medical literature.[57,73,74] The initial study by Roubal et al[73] followed eight patients for 1 month post-MUA and observed significant improvements in range of motion (ROM), function, and pain levels for all patients receiving the intervention.[73] Placzek et al[74] found the effectiveness of translational MUA on 31 individuals was maintained at 14 months. Boyles et al[57] conducted a case series of four patients treated with translational MUA and evaluated glenohumeral arthrokinematic motion

pre- and postmanipulation using video fluoroscopy. Improvements in range of motion, function, and pain levels were similar to previous findings.[73,74] Additionally, increased caudal translation of the humeral head during active shoulder abduction was noted when comparing pre- and post-video fluoroscopic images.[57] Furthermore, no adverse events were observed, leading both authors to conclude that glenohumeral translational manipulation under regional interscalene block appears to be a safe and effective intervention for the treatment of AC.[57,74]

The advantages of translational manipulation over traditional, or long lever, manipulation result from hand placement and the direction of applied forces.[80] Grasping the humeral head adjacent to the joint line minimizes the lever arm, eliminates the rotary forces, and produces linear translation across the joint.[80] This hand placement also permits the operator to isolate the manipulative force to the glenohumeral joint, therefore minimizing the risk of injury to adjacent structures.[74,75,80]

Technique Description: Glenohumeral Translational Manipulation under Regional Interscalene Block Anesthesia

Premanipulation Procedures

Once the patient has consented to undergo translational MUA, several steps must be taken in preparation for the procedure[57,73] The patient should first be evaluated by the referring physician to ensure agreement between providers concerning the diagnosis of AC, and the patient will also meet with the anesthesiologist to ensure there are no contraindications to undergoing the regional interscalene block. Placzek et al[74] recommend a short course of oral corticosteroids; specifically a Medrol 6-day dose pack (Upjohn Corp, Kalamazoo, MI), to begin the day prior to the manipulation.[74] In patients with certain comorbidities (i.e., diabetes), this medication may be contraindicated and, therefore, other pain medication should be considered. The only imaging requirement prior to the intervention is plain radiographs to rule out competing diagnoses (i.e., severe OA).[57] A pre-manipulation pathway proposed by Boyles et al[57] is displayed in Figure 18-15.

After the anesthesiologist has performed the regional interscalene block, the involved upper extremity is placed in a sling and the patient is transported to the physical therapy clinic. Prior to the manipulation, passive range of motion values are recorded under anesthesia to confirm the diagnosis of AC.[57]

Technique Description: Glenohumeral Translational MUA

Each glenohumeral translational MUA procedure consists of the application of three forces: a *stabilizing force*, a *traction force*, and a *mobilizing force*. The stabilizing force is provided by an assistant, the manipulator, or gravity. The traction force and the mobilizing force are provided to the humeral head by the manipulator. Each technique begins with slow, progressive, linear forces applied at the end range of glenohumeral movement. If shoulder range of motion has not improved after three such attempts, a high-velocity, low-amplitude thrust is performed at the end range of available motion. Up to three thrusts may be performed at the joint's newly established end range of movement.[80] The following is a description of a translational

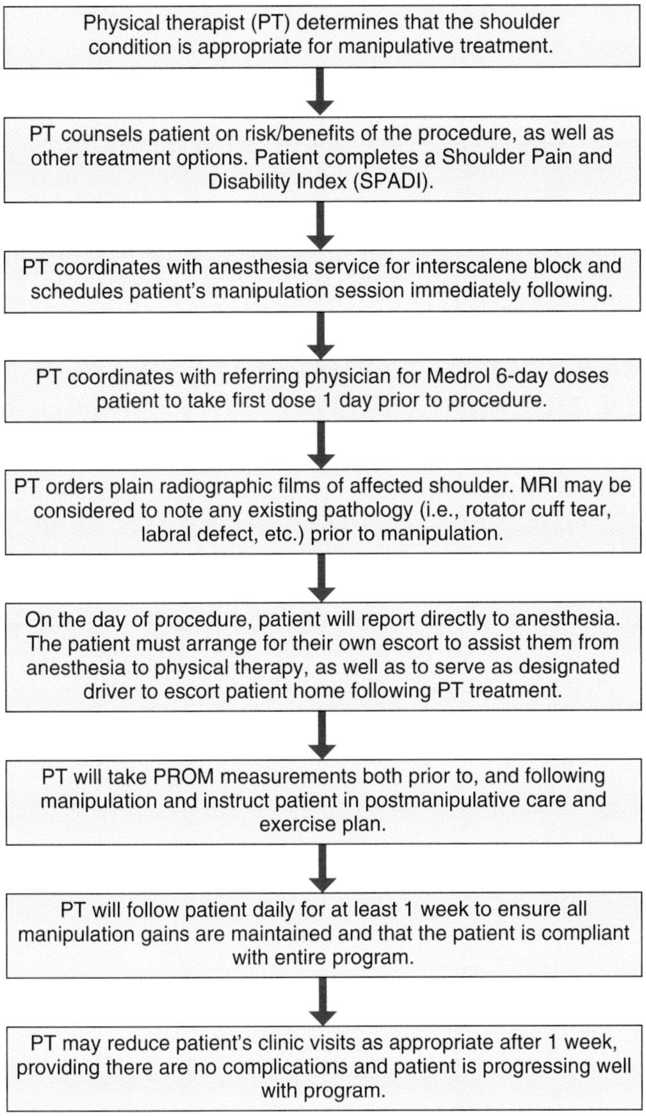

Physical therapist (PT) determines that the shoulder condition is appropriate for manipulative treatment.

↓

PT counsels patient on risk/benefits of the procedure, as well as other treatment options. Patient completes a Shoulder Pain and Disability Index (SPADI).

↓

PT coordinates with anesthesia service for interscalene block and schedules patient's manipulation session immediately following.

↓

PT coordinates with referring physician for Medrol 6-day doses patient to take first dose 1 day prior to procedure.

↓

PT orders plain radiographic films of affected shoulder. MRI may be considered to note any existing pathology (i.e., rotator cuff tear, labral defect, etc.) prior to manipulation.

↓

On the day of procedure, patient will report directly to anesthesia. The patient must arrange for their own escort to assist them from anesthesia to physical therapy, as well as to serve as designated driver to escort patient home following PT treatment.

↓

PT will take PROM measurements both prior to, and following manipulation and instruct patient in postmanipulative care and exercise plan.

↓

PT will follow patient daily for at least 1 week to ensure all manipulation gains are maintained and that the patient is compliant with entire program.

↓

PT may reduce patient's clinic visits as appropriate after 1 week, providing there are no complications and patient is progressing well with program.

FIGURE 18–15 A premanipulation pathway used for frozen shoulder patients by Boyles and colleagues.[57]

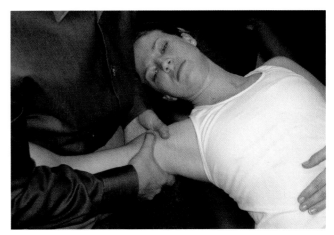

FIGURE 18–16 Left inferior glenohumeral manipulation. The clinician positions his or her hands immediately adjacent to the AC joint and externally rotates the humerus. Tension in the brachial plexus is reduced by placing the neck in ipsilateral side bending and the elbow midway between 90 degrees of flexion and full extension.

approximately midway between 90 degrees of elbow flexion and full extension (Fig. 18-16). The humerus is then abducted to its end range while maintaining external rotation in order to avoid subacromial impingement. A slight traction force is next applied perpendicular to the glenoid with the manipulator's right hand, while the translational or mobilizing force is applied to the humeral head with the left hand in an inferior direction, parallel to the glenoid (Fig. 18-17). Once the restrictive barrier is engaged, the manipulation is applied with a slow, progressively increasing force. As audible and/or palpable yielding of adhesions is perceived, the humerus is repositioned into its new end range of abduction and the technique is repeated. If three such attempts fail to improve glenohumeral range of motion, a high-velocity thrust is delivered into the restrictive barrier. If the restriction remains after the first thrust, up to three attempts may be performed at the new end range of motion. Care must be taken to mobilize the humeral head parallel to the treatment plane of the glenoid fossa, ensuring the proximal and distal humerus travel an equal distance inferiorly. Performing the technique in this manner will eliminate potentially injurious rotary forces at the joint.

MUA of the right shoulder, adapted from the works of Placzek et al[80] and Boyles et al.[57]

Inferior Manipulation

Inferior manipulation increases the humeral head's caudal translation during shoulder elevation and therefore effectively preserves the subacromial space. Thus, the inferior manipulation should be performed first to protect against traumatic subacromial impingement during subsequent techniques.

The patient is positioned supine with the cervical spine laterally flexed toward the involved extremity to limit stress placed on the brachial plexus. An assistant stabilizes the scapula by positioning the patient's thenar eminence just inferior to the glenoid rim and providing a medially and superiorly directed force to the lateral border of the scapula. This stabilizing action serves to limit inferior migration of the glenoid during the manipulation. The humerus is grasped with both hands by the manipulator adjacent to the joint line, then externally rotated. To further reduce tension in the brachial plexus, the elbow should be maintained

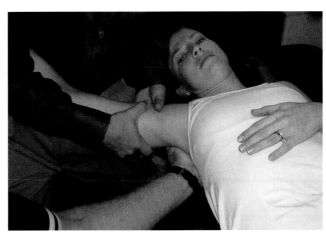

FIGURE 18–17 Left inferior glenohumeral manipulation (cont.). Using the right hand, the clinician applies a traction force to the humerus, while the mobilizing force is applied to the humeral head with the left hand in an inferior direction, parallel to the glenoid.

Posterior Manipulation

With the patient supine, the clinician stands at the head of the patient facing the patient's feet, with their right hand on the lateral border of the scapula applying a medial and slightly anteriorly directed stabilizing force. The patient's right arm is flexed to approximately 80 degrees, and the clinician's left hand grasps the anterior humerus. While maintaining the stabilizing force to the scapula, the humerus is brought into maximal horizontal adduction. The left hand provides a posterior translation force while simultaneously applying lateral traction (Fig. 18-18). As with the inferior manipulation, the mobilizing force is first applied in a slow, progressive fashion. If three such attempts fail to improve ROM, up to three applications of high-velocity thrusts are performed into the restriction.

Additional Manipulations

After performing the inferior and posterior manipulations as above, Boyles et al[57] recommend assessing the glenohumeral joint for additional restrictions, and if identified, additional manipulation(s) may be administered.[57] Glenohumeral joint mobility is assessed by grasping the humerus close to the joint line and performing anterior, posterior, inferior, and combined directional glides to detect joint hypomobility (see Chapter 22). This assessment is performed at various degrees of flexion, abduction, internal, and external rotation. Once a restriction is found, the therapist administers two or three 30-second, low-velocity oscillatory mobilizations (Maitland grade IV to IV+). If this fails to improve range of motion, up to three high-velocity thrusts are performed into the restriction.[57]

Postmanipulative Care

Following manipulation, passive range-of-motion (PROM) values are again recorded, and the patient's shoulder is wrapped in ice and the patient is positioned with his or her hand behind the head. The patient is discharged home the same day with the involved shoulder in a sling and instructions to perform 5 minutes of shoulder flexion active assisted range of motion (AAROM) exercises every 2 hours, followed by ice. Sling use

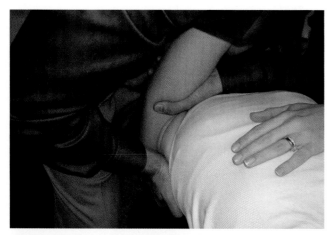

FIGURE 18–18 Left posterior glenohumeral manipulation. The clinician stabilizes the scapula with the right hand and introduces horizontal adduction, lateral traction, and posterior translation to the humerus with his or her rib cage and left hand.

may be discontinued once sensory and motor function return to the extremity. Boyles et al[57] recommend daily physical therapy for the first 5 days following the manipulation, consisting of exercise and ice.[57] The frequency of sessions can decrease to three times per week for the second and third week postmanipulation. Shoulder mobilizations should continue, and rotator cuff strengthening should gradually be incorporated into the patient's routine during week 2.[74] Discharge to a home exercise program should be considered at 3 to 4 weeks depending on the patient's recovery.[57]

THE ROLE OF THRUST MANIPULATION IN THE MANAGEMENT OF LATERAL EPICONDYLALGIA

Lateral epicondylalgia (LE) or "tennis elbow" as it is commonly referred to, is the most common overuse injury of the elbow.[81] It has a prevalence of 1% to 3% in the general population and afflicts up to 15% of workers in highly repetitive hand task industries.[82,83] Conservative management for LE is highly variable, and although numerous intervention strategies for LE have been reported in the literature, high level of evidence supporting the use of one intervention over another is nonexistent.[81-84] Conservative treatment options for LE include rest, ice, bracing, iontophoresis, ultrasound, electrotherapy, exercise therapy, corticosteroid injection(s), nonsteroidal anti-inflammatory drugs, extracorporeal shock-wave therapy, and manual therapy.[81,84-86] Common manual therapy interventions for LE include deep transverse friction massage, joint mobilizations, and high-velocity thrust techniques directed at the elbow, wrist, cervical spine, and thoracic spine.[81-84,87]

Evidence Summary: Manipulation of the Wrist for Lateral Epicondylalgia

Struijs et al[87] conducted a randomized controlled trial comparing the effectiveness of manipulation of the wrist to a combined treatment program of ultrasound, friction massage, and muscle stretching and strengthening in patients with tennis elbow. Twenty-eight patients were randomized to receive one of the two treatment protocols. Patients receiving the combined treatment approach underwent a total of nine sessions over a 6-week period, consisting of ultrasound and deep transverse friction massage followed by strengthening and stretching for wrist and elbow musculature. Patients in the combined treatment group were instructed to restrict use of their affected extremity according to their pain threshold. Subjects in the wrist manipulation group attended a maximum of nine sessions over a 6-week period. Treatment sessions consisted of repeated applications of a wrist/scaphoid manipulation. No restrictions regarding upper extremity use were placed on subjects in the manipulation group.

Subjects receiving manipulation demonstrated greater improvement in the primary outcome measure, which was "global measure of improvement," at initial 3-week follow-up. However, at 6 weeks no differences between groups were found in any of the outcome measures. Struijs et al[87] provides some evidence for the initial positive effects of wrist manipulation in the management of LE.

Technique Description: Wrist/Scaphoid Extension Manipulation

In the Struijs et al[87] study, the patient is seated with the forearm resting on the table with the palm facing down. The clinician sits facing the ulnar aspect of the subjects affected side and grips the patient's wrist with their thumb over the dorsal aspect of the scaphoid and the index finger over the volar aspect of the scaphoid (Fig. 18-19). This hand position is then reinforced with the thumb and index finger of the opposite hand. The wrist is brought into extension, and a high-velocity thrust is delivered to the scaphoid in a ventral direction (Fig. 18-20). The manipulation is repeated approximately 15 to 20 times per session, with forced passive wrist extension or active wrist extension against resistance briefly performed between manipulations.

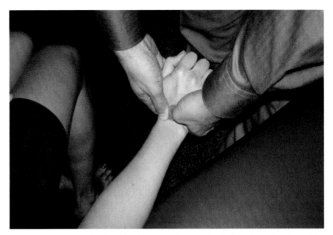

FIGURE 18–20 Wrist/scaphoid extension manipulation (cont.). The clinician extends the patient's wrist and delivers a high-velocity thrust to the scaphoid in a ventral direction.

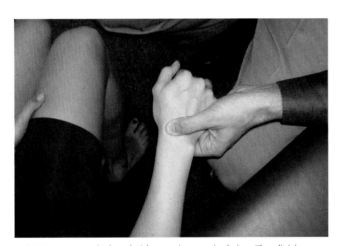

FIGURE 18–19 Wrist/scaphoid extension manipulation. The clinician grasps the patient's wrist, placing the thumb and index finger over the dorsal and volar aspects of the scaphoid.

SUMMARY AND CONCLUSIONS

Despite the long-term use of thrust manipulation for the management of musculoskeletal conditions over the centuries, the use of such techniques has not been traditionally considered to be part of standard physical therapy practice. More recent evidence has generated a renewed interest in the utilization of these procedures for individuals seeking physical therapy care. This chapter has attempted to provide a summary of the evidence along with descriptions of a variety of thrust manipulation techniques as outlined in the quoted studies. Given the information provided, the reader is encouraged to consider the implementation of these techniques into routine clinical practice and to become involved in the pursuit of additional evidence related to this area of clinical orthopaedic manual physical therapy practice.

CLINICAL CASE

History of Present Illness (HPI)

Mr. Jones presents today noting an incident which occurred 8 days ago at work. He reports that he was twisting to the left and reaching behind him while loading the truck, at which time the truck pulled forward quickly. He reports having immediate left lumbosacral pain at a 7/10 level of intensity and denies referral of symptoms into his lower extremities. He reports an increase in pain in the morning, which is mainly described as "stiffness" and an increase in pain after a long day at work. He reports pain with standing for more than 15 minutes. He notes that since his injury, he has been inactive and sitting or lying for long periods of time, which is his most comfortable position.

Self-assessed disability: FABQ (work) = 15.

Observation: He is in apparent distress with antalgic gait

Neurological: All within normal range (WNL)

Strength: He has 4/5 strength in proximal hip musculature with pain upon testing, which patient reports is due to a "pull on his low back."

Palpation: He is tender to touch over central and left midlumbar region, with palpable muscle hypertonicity within the left lumbar paravertebral musculature.

Passive accessory intervertebral mobility (PAIVM) testing: There is reproduction of symptoms and hypomobility with central posteroanterior (PA) glides at L2-L3 and L4-L5 regions.

AROM (% of full range): Forward bending = 75% with pain and deviation to left; backward bending = 50% with reproduction of pain; side bending right = 25% with contralateral muscle pull, left = 10% with reproduction of pain; rotation right = 10% with reproduction of pain, left = 25% with myofascial limitations. Repeated flexion in standing (RFIS) and lying (RFIL) reveals improved mobility and less pain, whereas repeated extension in standing REIS and lying (REIL) reveal an increase in pain after five repetitions.

Hip PROM: Extension = –5 degrees bilaterally, external rotation (ER) = 40 degrees bilaterally, internal rotation (IR) = 35 degrees bilaterally.

1. Based on the results of this examination, do you believe that Mr. Jones is a candidate for spinal high-velocity thrust manipulation? Is there any additional information that you need to know in order to make this decision? What aspects of his presentation allow you to feel confident that this patient will likely benefit from these techniques?

2. Are there any premanipulative screening procedures that you would like to test prior to performing these techniques? If so, practice the performance of these tests on a partner now.

3. What specific manipulation procedure would you use in this case, and what is your rationale for choosing this technique? Perform this technique on a partner now.

4. What instructions would you give the patient immediately following this technique, later that evening, and the following day?

5. How will you verify that you have been effective in the use of this technique? What outcome measures will you use to provide evidence of effectiveness? How will you determine poor tolerance and/or ineffectiveness?

6. What other manual or nonmanual interventions will you use to either prepare this patient for thrust manipulation or to support the patient following the procedure? Outline a comprehensive plan of care that describes the specific manual and nonmanual interventions that you might use that includes the sequence of implementation.

HANDS-ON

With a partner, perform the following activities:
Sequential partial-task practice (SPTP) lab activity:

1 Students are divided into two groups: a patient group and a therapist group. The patient group lies on the plinth, and the therapist group stands beside the patient and is prepared to rotate to the next patient after performance of each partial task. After completing the entire technique, the two groups switch places.

2 The instructor demonstrates a lumbopelvic technique as a whole task in real time using a student volunteer.

3 The instructor then breaks down each technique into three main parts: (1) patient set-up SPTP, (2) hand placement SPTP, and (3) force application SPTP

4 The instructor performs the **"patient set-up SPTP"** on a student volunteer with a clear verbal description of the task as each participant simultaneously performs the task on a "patient." The participant then moves to the next patient and performs the SPTP again, and so on until three to five repetitions of the same task have been performed on three to five different patients.

5 The instructor performs the **"hand placement SPTP"** on a student volunteer with a clear verbal description of the task as

each participant simultaneously performs the task on a "patient." The participant then moves to the next patient and performs the SPTP again, and so on until three to five repetitions of the same task have been performed on three to five different patients.

6 The instructor performs the **"force application SPTP"** on a student volunteer with a clear verbal description of the task as each participant simultaneously performs the task on a "patient." The participant then moves to the next patient and performs the SPTP again, and so on until three to five repetitions of the same task have been performed on three to five different patients.

7 The instructor, in conjunction with each participant, simultaneously performs the whole task of the technique in real time on a "patient," after which the participant moves to the next patient" and so on until three to five repetitions of the same task have been performed on three to five different patients.

8 Lab instructors are available to provide feedback during performance.

9 Partners then switch and the process is repeated.

REFERENCES

1. APTA. Manipulation Education Committee. *Manipulation Education Manual.* APTA Manipulation Task Force; 2004.
2. Harris JD, McPartland JM. Historical perspectives of manual medicine. *Phys Med Rehabil Clin N Am.* 1996;7:679-692.
3. Paris SV. A history of manipulative therapy through the ages and up to the current controversy in the United States. *J Man Manip Ther.* 2000;8:66-77.
4. Waddell G, Allan D. Back pain through history. In: Waddell G, ed. *The Back Pain Revolution.* Edinburgh, Scotland: Churchill Livingston; 1998:45-67.
5. Lomax E. Manipulative therapy: a historical perspective from ancient times to the modern era. In: Goldstein M, ed. *The Research Status of Spinal Manipulative Therapy.* (DREW Publication [NIA: 76-998. Bethesda, MD: US Department of Health, Education and Welfare; 1975.
6. APTA. *Manipulation Take Action Packet.* Alexandria, VA: APTA; 2006.
7. Mikhail C, Korner-Bitensky N, Rossignol M, et al. Physical therapists' use of interventions with high evidence of effectiveness in the management of hypothetical typical patient with acute low back pain. *Phys Ther.* 2005;85: 1151-1167.
8. Moffett JK, Mannion AF. What is the value of physical therapies for back pain? *Best Pract Clin Rheumatol.* 2005;19:623-638.
9. Assendelft JJ, Morton SC, Yu EI, et al. Spinal manipulative therapy for low-back pain: a meta-analysis of effectiveness relative to other therapies. *Ann Intern Med.* 2003;138:871-881.
10. Assendelft WJ, Morton SC, Yu EI, et al. Spinal manipulative therapy for low-back pain. *Cochrane Database of Sys Rev.* 2004;3.
11. Hicks GE, Fritz JM, Delitto A, et al. Preliminary development of a clinical prediction rule for determining which patients with low back pain will respond to a stabilization exercise program. *Arch Phys Med Rehabil.* 2005;86:1753-1762.
12. Childs JD, Fritz JM, Flynn TW, et al. A clinical prediction rule to identify patients with low back pain most likely to benefit from spinal manipulation: a validation study. *Ann Intern Med.* 2004;141:920-928.
13. Flynn T, Fritz J, Whitman J, et al. A clinical prediction rule for classifying patients with low back pain who demonstrate short-term improvement with spinal manipulation. *Spine.* 2002;27:2835-2843.
14. Fritz JM, Delitto A, Erhard RE. Comparison of a classification-based approach to physical therapy and therapy based on clinical practice guidelines for patients with acute low back pain: a randomized clinical trial. *Spine.* 2003;28:1363-1372.
15. Cleland J. *Orthopaedic Clinical Examination: An Evidence-Based Approach for Physical Therapists.* Carlstadt, NJ: Icon Learning Systems; 2005.
16. Cleland JA, Fritz JM, Kulig K, et al. Comparison of the effectiveness of three manual physical therapy techniques in a subgroup of patients with low back pain who satisfy a clinical prediction rule. *Spine.* 2009;34:2720-2729.
17. Hoving JL, Henrica CW, Koes BW, et al. Manual therapy, physical therapy or continued care by the general practitioner for patients with neck pain: long-term results from a pragmatic randomized clinical trial. *Clin J Pain.* 2006;22:370-377.
18. Childs JD, Fritz JM, Piva SR, et al. Proposal of a classification system for patients with neck pain. *J Ortho Sports Phys Ther.* 2004;34:686-696.
19. Jette AM, Smith K, Haley SM, et al. Physical therapy episodes of care for patients with low back pain. *Phys Ther.* 1994;74:101-110.
20. Kay TM, Gross A, Goldsmith C, et al. Exercises for mechanical neck disorders. *Cochrane Database of Syst Rev.* 2006;1.
21. Kroeling P, Gross A, Goldsmith CH. Electrotherapy for neck disorders. Cochrane Back Group. *Cochrane Database of Syst Rev.* 2006;1.
22. Walker MJ, Boyles RE, Young BA, Strunce JB, Garber MB, Whitman JM, Deyle G, Wainner RS. *The effectiveness of manual physical therapy and exercise for mechanical neck pain: a randomized clinical trial. Spine.* 2008;33(22):2371-2378.
23. Hoving JL, Koes BW, de Vet HC, et al. Manual therapy, physical therapy or continued care by a general practitioner for patients with neck pain. A randomized, controlled trial. *Ann Intern Med.* 2002;136:713-722.
24. Jull G, Trott P, Potter H, et al. A randomized controlled trial of exercise and manipulative therapy for cervicogenic headache. *Spine.* 2002;27:1835-1843.
25. Evans R, Bronfort G, Nelson B, et al. Two-year follow-up of a randomized clinical trial of spinal manipulation and two types of exercise for patients with chronic neck pain. *Spine.* 2002;27:2383-2389.
26. Gross AR, Hoving JL, Haines TA, et al. A Cochrane Review of manipulation and mobilization for mechanical neck disorders. *Spine.* 2004;29:1541-1548.
27. Rothwell DM, Bondy SJ, Williams I. Chiropractic manipulation and stroke: a population-based case-control study. *Stroke.* 2001;32:1054-1060.
28. Cassidy, JD, Boyle E, Cote P, et al. Risk of vertebrobasilar stroke and chiropractic care results of a population-based case-control and case-crossover study. *Spine.* 2008;33:S176-S183.
29. Rivett DA, Milburn P. A prospective study of the complications of cervical spine manipulation. *J Man Manip Ther* 1996;4:166-170.
30. Hurwitz EL, Aker PD, Adams AH, Meeker WC, Shekelle PG. Manipulation and mobilization of the cervical spine. A systematic review of the literature. *Spine.* 1996;21:1746-1760.
31. Childs JD, Flynn TW, Fritz JM, et al. Screening for vertebrobasilar insufficiency in patients with neck pain: manual therapy decision-making in the presence of uncertainty. *J Ortho Sports Phys Ther.* 2005;35:300-306.
32. Maitland GD, Hengeveld E, Banks K, et al. *Maitland's Vertebral Manipulation.* Oxford: Butterworth-Heinemann; 2000.
33. Di Fabio RP. Manipulation of the cervical spine: risks and benefits. *Phys Ther.* 1999;79:50-65.
34. Cleland JA, Childs JD, McRae M, et al. Immediate effects of thoracic manipulation in patients with neck pain: a randomized clinical trial. *Man Ther.* 2005;10:127-135.
35. Cleland JA, Whitman JM, Fritz JM, et al. Manual physical therapy, cervical traction and strengthening exercises in patients with cervical radiculopathy: a case series. *J Ortho Sports Phys Ther.* 2005;35:802-811.
36. Cleland JA, Childs JD, Fritz JM, et al. Development of a clinical prediction rule for classifying patients with neck pain who demonstrate short-term improvement with thoracic spine thrust manipulation. *Phys Ther.* 2007; 87:9-23.
37. Moore A, Jackson A, Jordan J, Hammersley S, et al. *Clinical Guidelines for the Physiotherapy Management of Whiplash Associated Disorder.* London, UK: Chartered Society of Physiotherapy; 2005.
38. Kerry R, Taylor A. Cervical arterial dysfunction: knowledge and reasoning for manual physical therapists. *J Ortho Sports Phys Ther.* 2009;39:378-387.
39. Cook C, Brismee JM, Fleming R, Sizer PS. Identifiers suggestive of clinical cervical spine instability: a Delphi study of physical therapists. *Phys Ther.* 2005;85:895-906.
40. Hoving JL, Koes B, DeVet HCW, et al. Manual therapy, physical therapy, or continued care by a general practitioner for patients with neck pain: a randomized, controlled trial. *Ann Int Med.* 2002;10:713-722.
41. Korthals-de Bos IBC, Hoving JL, van Tulder MW, et al. Cost effectiveness of physiotherapy, manual therapy, and general practitioner care for neck pain: economic evaluation alongside a randomized controlled trial. *BMJ.* 2003;326:911-914.
42. Tseng YL, Wang WTF, Chen WY, et al. Predictors for the immediate responders to cervical manipulation in patients with neck pain. *Man Ther.* 2006;11:306-315.
43. Puentedura EJ, Cleland JA, Landers MR, et al. Development of a clinical prediction rule to identify patients with neck pain likely to benefit from thrust joint manipulation to the cervical spine. *J Ortho Sports Phys Ther.* 2012;42:577-592.
44. Flynn TW, Whitman JM, Magel J. *Orthopaedic Manual Physical Therapy Management of the Cervical-Thoracic Spine and Ribcage.* Fort Collins, CO: Manipulations, Inc.; 2000.
45. Piva SR, Erhard RE, Al-Hugail M. Cervical radiculopathy: a case problem using a decision-making algorithm. *J Ortho Sports Phys Ther.* 2000;30:745-754.
46. Waldrop MA. Diagnosis and treatment of cervical radiculopathy using a clinical prediction rule and a multimodal intervention approach: a case series. *J Ortho Sports Phys Ther.* 2006;36:152-159.
47. Browder DA, Erhard RE, Piva SR. Intermittent cervical traction and thoracic manipulation for management of mild cervical compressive myelopathy attributed to cervical herniated disc: a case series. *J Ortho Sports Phys Ther.* 2004;34:701-712.
48. Cibulka M, Threlkeld J. The early clinical diagnosis of osteoarthritis of the hip. *J Ortho Sports Phys Ther.* 2004;34:462-467.
49. Van Baar ME, Dekker J, Oostendorp RA, et al. The effectiveness of exercise therapy in patients with osteoarthritis of hip or knee: a randomized clinical trial. *J Rheumatol.* 1998;25:2432-2439.
50. Van Baar ME, Dekker J, Oostendorp RA, et al. The effectiveness of exercise therapy in patients with osteoarthritis of hip or knee: nine months' follow-up. *Ann Rheum Dis.* 2001;60:1123-1130.
51. Tak E, Staats P, Van Hespen A, et al. The effects of an exercise program for older adults with osteoarthritis of the hip. *J Rheumatol.* 2005;32:1106-1113.
52. Hopman-Rock M, Westhoff MH. The effects of a health educational and exercise program for older adults with osteoarthritis of the hip or knee. *J Rheumatol.* 2000;27:1947-1954.
53. Cochrane T, Davey RC, Edwards SM. Randomised control trial of the cost-effectiveness of water-based therapy for lower limb osteoarthritis. *Health Technology Assessment.* 2005;9.
54. Hoeksma HL, Dekker J, Ronday HK, et al. Comparison of manual therapy and exercise therapy in osteoarthritis of the hip: a randomized clinical trial. *Arthritis Rheum.* 2004;51:722-729.

55. Hoeksma HL, Dekker J, Ronday HK, et al. Manual therapy in osteoarthritis of the hip: outcome in subgroups of patients. *Rheumatol.* 2005;44:461-464.

56. MacDonald C, Whitman JM, Cleland JA, et al. Clinical outcomes following manual physical therapy and exercise for hip osteoarthritis: a case series. *J Ortho Sports Phys Ther.* 2006;36:588-599.

57. Boyles R, Flynn T, Whitman J. Manipulation following regional interscalene anesthetic block for shoulder adhesive capsulitis: a case series. *Man Ther.* 2005;10:80-87.

58. Sandor R. Adhesive capsulitis: optimal treatment of "frozen shoulder." *Phys Sportsmed.* 2000;28:23-29.

59. Miller M, Wirth M, Rockwood C. Thawing the frozen shoulder: the "patient" patient. *Orthopedics.* 1996;19:849-853.

60. Ozaki J, Yoshiyuki N, Goro S, et al. Recalcitrant chronic adhesive capsulitis of the shoulder. *J Bone Joint Surg Am.* 1989;71:1511-1515.

61. Hannafin J, Strickland S. Frozen shoulder. *Curr Opin Ortho.* 2000;11:271-275.

62. Codman EA. *The Shoulder: Rupture of the Supraspinatus Tendon and Other Lesions in or about the Subacromial Bursa.* Boston: Thomas Todd Company; 1934.

63. van der Windt D, Koes B, Deville W, et al. Effectiveness of corticosteroid injections versus physiotherapy for treatment of painful stiff shoulder in primary care: randomized trial. *BMJ.* 1998;317:1292-1296.

64. Piotte F, Gravel D, Moffet H, et al. Effects of repeated distension arthrographies combined with a home exercise program among adults with idiopathic adhesive capsulitis of the shoulder. *Am J Phys Med Rehabil.* 2004;83:537-546.

65. Halverson L, Maas R. Shoulder joint capsule distension (hydroplasty): a case series of patients with "frozen shoulders" treated in a primary care office. *J Fam Pract.* 2002;51:61-63.

66. Vad VB, Sakalkale D, Warren RF. The role of capsular distension in adhesive capsulitis. *Arch Phys Med Rehabil.* 2003;84:1290-1292.

67. Vermeulen H, Obermann W, Burger H, et al. End-range mobilization techniques in adhesive capsulitis of the shoulder joint: a multiple-subject case report. *Phys Ther.* 2000;80:1204-1213.

68. Green A, Mariatis J. Influence of comorbidity on self-assessment instrument scores of patients with idiopathic adhesive capsulitis. *J Bone Joint Surg Am.* 2002;84:1167-1173.

69. Castellarin G, Ricci M, Vedovi E, et al. Manipulation and arthroscopy under general anesthesia and early rehabilitative treatment for frozen shoulders. *Arch Phys Med Rehabil.* 2004;85:1236-1240.

70. Kivimaki J, Pohjolainen T. Manipulation under anesthesia for frozen shoulder with and without steroid injection. *Arch Phys Med Rehabil.* 2001;82:1188-1190.

71. Hill JJ, Bogoumill HL. Manipulation in the treatment of frozen shoulder. *Orthopedics.* 1988;9:1255-1260.

72. Farell C, Sperling J, Cofield R. Manipulation for frozen shoulder: long-term results. *J Shoulder Elbow Surg.* 2005;14:480-484.

73. Roubal P, Dobritt D, Placzek J. Glenohumeral gliding manipulation following interscalene brachial plexus block in patients with adhesive capsulitis. *J Ortho Sports Phys Ther.* 1996;24:66-77.

74. Placzek J, Roubal P, Freeman D, et al. Long term effectiveness of translational manipulations for adhesive capsulitis. *CORR.* 1998;356:181-191.

75. Green S, Buchbinder R, Glazier R, et al. Interventions for shoulder pain. *Cochrane Database Syst Rev.* 2001;3:1-53.

76. Kelley MJ, Shaffer MA, Kuhn JE, Michener LA, Seitz AL, Uhl TL, Godges JJ, McClure PW. Shoulder pain and mobility deficits: adhesive capsulitis. *J Orthop Sports Phys Ther.* 2013:43(5);A1-A31.

77. Reeves B. The natural history of the frozen shoulder syndrome. *Scand J Rheumatol.* 1975;14:193-196.

78. Shaffer B, Tibone J, Kerlan R. Frozen shoulder: a long-term follow-up. *J Bone Joint Surg Am.* 1992;74-A:738-746.

79. Loew M, Heichel T, Lehner B. Intraarticular lesions in primary frozen shoulder after manipulation under general anesthesia. *J Shoulder Elbow Surg.* 2005;14:16-21.

80. Placzek J, Roubal P, Kulig K, et al. Theory and technique of translational manipulation for adhesive capsulitis. *Am J Ortho.* 2004;33:173-179.

81. Murphy K, Giuliani J, Freedman B. The diagnosis and management of lateral epicondylitis. *Curr Opin Ortho.* 2006;17:134-138.

82. Cleland JA, Whitman JM, Fritz JM. Effectiveness of manual physical therapy to the cervical spine in the management of lateral epicondylalgia: a retrospective analysis. *J Ortho Sports Phys Ther.* 2004;34:713-724.

83. Bisset L, Paungmali A, Vicenzino B, et al. A systematic review and meta-analysis of clinical trials on physical interventions for lateral epicondylalgia. *Brit J Sports Med.* 2005;39:411-422.

84. Stasinopoulos D, Johnson M. Cyriax physiotherapy for tennis elbow/lateral epicondylitis. *Scand J Rheumatol.* 2004;38:675-677.

85. Vicenzino B, Paungmali A, Buratowski S, et al. Specific manipulative therapy treatment for chronic lateral epicondylalgia produces uniquely characteristic hypoalgesia. *Man Ther.* 2001;6:205-212.

86. Pettrone F, McCall B. Extracorporeal shock wave therapy without local anesthesia for chronic lateral epicondylitis. *J Bone Joint Surg Am.* 2005;87-A:1297-1304.

87. Struijs P, Damen P, Bakker E, et al. Manipulation of the wrist for management of lateral epicondylitis: a randomized pilot study. *Phys Ther.* 2003;83:608-616.

The Theory and Practice of Neural Dynamics and Mobilization

Stephen John Carp, PT, PhD, GCS

Chapter Objectives

At the conclusion of this chapter, the reader will be able to:

- Understand the varying etiological factors associated with peripheral nerve injury.
- Understand the structural and cellular anatomy of the peripheral nervous system.
- Appreciate the varying signs and symptoms associated with injury to the peripheral nervous system.

- Understand the classification of peripheral nerve injuries.
- Develop a systematic algorithm for the clinical assessment of peripheral nerve injuries.
- Develop and modify physical therapy intervention strategies for peripheral nerve injuries.

STRUCTURAL AND FUNCTIONAL ANATOMY OF THE PERIPHERAL NERVOUS SYSTEM

Overview of Peripheral Nerve Anatomy

The *peripheral nerve* is a component of an intricate conduction system that serves as a mediator for bidirectional transport between the *central nervous system (CNS)* and other tissues. This conduction system is involved in regulation, homeostasis, repair, function, learning, posture, reproduction, mobility, and protection. For descriptive purposes, peripheral nerves are classified according to their function and site of CNS origin. *Cranial nerves* emerge from the base of the brain, *spinal nerves* originate in the spinal cord, and the autonomic system is intimately associated with the cranial and spinal nerves but differs in function, structure, and distribution (Figs. 19-1, 19-2).

The bidirectional movement of action potentials along the peripheral nerve enables afferent pathways, efferent pathways, and autonomic pathways. **Afferent pathways** are primarily sensory. The variability of sensory modalities are impressive, ranging from vision, hearing, smell, and taste to touch, pressure, and warmth, among others.[1] Neurologic symptoms related to impairment are typically described as sensations additive to normal perception such as burning,

tingling, hyperalgesia, or pain. Neurologic signs may consist of numbness, ataxia, orthostasis, loss of visual acuity, and dyskinesia. Fortunately, in humans there is a redundancy of sensory modalities that maintains function in the presence of sensory loss. Adequate balance, for example, requires the composite function of the visual, vestibular, and proprioceptive systems.

Efferent pathways are primarily motoric in function. This complex system requires a variety of both afferent and efferent neural tissues as well as contractile and noncontractile connective tissues. These structures work in harmony to provide coordinated movement patterns and locomotion (Table 19-1).

The *lower motor neuron* consists of a cell body located in the anterior gray column of the spinal cord or brain stem and an axon passing via the peripheral nerves to the motor end plate within the muscle. It is often referred to as the final common pathway because it is acted upon by the rubrospinal, olivospinal, vestibulospinal, corticospinal, and tectospinal tracts and their associated intersegmental and intrasegmental reflex neurons. It is the ultimate pathway through which neural impulses reach the muscle. Motor disturbances may be the result of lesions within the muscle, at the myoneural junction, within the peripheral nerve, or within the CNS. The specific nature of the patient's

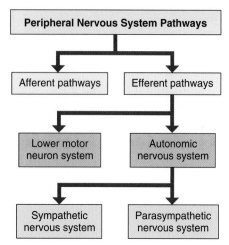

FIGURE 19–1 Divisions of the peripheral nervous system.

presenting signs and symptoms may lead the astute clinician to the specific etiology and serve to guide intervention (Table 19-2). Depending upon the site of injury, the predominate clinical signs of a lower motor neuron injury is weakness, reduced or absent deep tendon reflexes, and reduced or loss of sensation. The presence of myalgia or dyskinesia may also be present.

The **autonomic nervous system (ANS)** is a division of the peripheral nervous system that is distributed to glands and smooth muscle, whose primary functions are carried out below the level of conscious input. The cell body of the pre-ganglionic or presynaptic neuron, located within the CNS, sends its axon to one of the outlying ganglia from where the postganglionic axon extends to its terminal distribution. Cell bodies of presynaptic sympathetic nerve fibers lie in the ventral horn from cord segments T1-L3. Postganglionic fibers arise from the sympathetic trunk. The ANS is divided into the *sympathetic* and *parasympathetic* systems. With injury to a peripheral nerve, signs and symptoms related to an autonomic dysfunction may appear, which include aberrations in vascular flow, skin moisture, hair growth, trophic changes, nail loss, and delayed wound healing.

Although most peripheral nerves are considered to be mixed nerves, that consist of motor, sensory, and autonomic fibers, some mixed nerves have larger percentages of one type versus another. For instance, the *median* and *sciatic* nerves both have a greater concentration of autonomic fibers

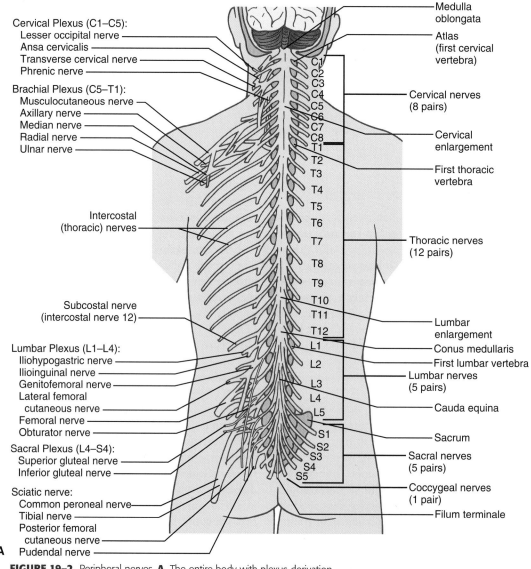

FIGURE 19–2. Peripheral nerves. **A.** The entire body with plexus derivation.

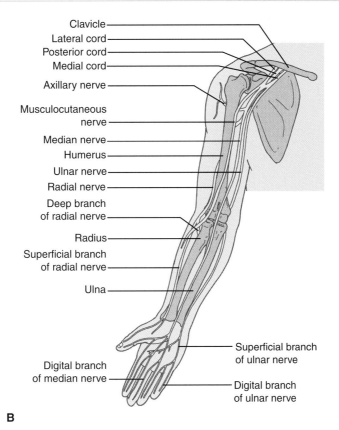

Clavicle
Lateral cord
Posterior cord
Medial cord
Axillary nerve
Musculocutaneous nerve
Median nerve
Humerus
Ulnar nerve
Radial nerve
Deep branch of radial nerve
Radius
Superficial branch of radial nerve
Ulna
Digital branch of median nerve
Superficial branch of ulnar nerve
Digital branch of ulnar nerve

B

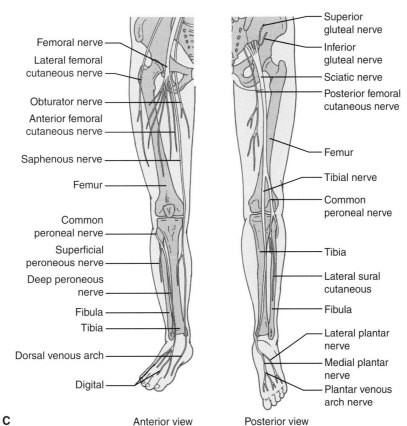

Femoral nerve
Lateral femoral cutaneous nerve
Obturator nerve
Anterior femoral cutaneous nerve
Saphenous nerve
Femur
Common peroneal nerve
Superficial peroneous nerve
Deep peroneous nerve
Fibula
Tibia
Dorsal venous arch
Digital

Superior gluteal nerve
Inferior gluteal nerve
Sciatic nerve
Posterior femoral cutaneous nerve
Femur
Tibial nerve
Common peroneal nerve
Tibia
Lateral sural cutaneous
Fibula
Lateral plantar nerve
Medial plantar nerve
Plantar venous arch nerve

C   Anterior view   Posterior view

FIGURE 19–2. B. Upper extremity. **C.** Lower extremity.

Table 19–1	Peripheral Nervous System Pathways				
PN PATHWAY	**CELL BODY LOCATION**	**DIRECTION**	**CLASS**	**PRIMARY FUNCTIONS**	**DYSFUNCTION**
Afferent	Dorsal root ganglion (DRG)	Toward CNS synapsing in the dorsal horn	Sensory	Vision, hearing, smell, taste, rotational acceleration, linear acceleration, verticality, touch, pressure, warmth, cold, pain, proprioception, kinesthesia, muscle length, muscle tension, arterial blood pressure, central venous pressure, inflation of lung, temperature of blood in the head, osmotic pressure of plasma and arteriovenous blood glucose difference	Related to the sensory modality that is being compromised. Positive signs are sensations additive to normal perception such as burning, tingling, hyperalgesia, pain, or temperature change. Negative signs are a reduction such as numbness, ataxia, orthostasis, loss of visual acuity, tracking degradation, dyskinesia
Lower Motor Neuron	Ventral horn of the spinal cord	Away from the CNS synapsing in the ventral horn	Motoric	Skeletal muscular contractions and subsequent joint movement	Weakness, dyskinesia, paralysis, and decrease or absent deep tendon reflexes and the addition of myalgias or muscle-specific pain as a result of lesions within the muscle, at the myoneural junction, within the peripheral nerve, or within the CNS
Autonomic Nervous System (ANS)	Presynaptic pathways located within the CNS to outlying ganglia where the postsynaptic axon extends to terminal distribution. Cell bodies of presynaptic sympathetic pathways lie in ventral horn from T1-L3. Postsynaptic pathways arise from the sympathetic trunk	Bidirectional	Subconscious	ANS is divided into the *sympathetic* and *parasympathetic* systems and functions are carried out below the level of conscious input.	Aberrations in vascular flow, aberrations in skin moisture, aberrations in hair growth, trophic changes, nail loss, and delayed wound healing

than do other extremity peripheral nerves. Although the *lateral femoral cutaneous* nerve is purely sensory, there are no pure motor nerves.

Structure of the Peripheral Nerve

Each nerve fiber represents the greatly elongated process of a nerve cell whose body lies within the CNS or one of the outlying ganglia. The nerve cell, or *neuron*, consists of a cell body and all of its processes. The cell body, which contains the nucleus, is the vital center controlling the metabolic activity of

the cell. Injury to the nerve fiber results in degeneration of the distal segment.

A typical spinal motor neuron has many processes called *dendrites* that extend out from the cell body and arborize greatly. It also has a long **axon** that originates from an area of the cell body, the *axon hillock*. Near its origin, the typical motor neuron develops a sheath of **myelin**, which is composed of a lipoprotein complex arranged in many layers. The myelin sheath envelops the axon except at its ending and at periodic constrictions that are approximately 1 mm apart. This arrangement of the myelin sheaths is known as the

Table 19-2	Criterion Related Differences Between Upper Motor Neuron, Lower Motor Neuron, and Myogenic Impairment		
CRITERION	**UPPER MOTOR NEURON**	**LOWER MOTOR NEURON**	**MYOGENIC**
Deep Tendon Reflex	Decreased or increased	Decreased	Decreased or unchanged
Muscle Wasting	Yes or no	Yes	Yes or no
Clonus	Yes	No	No
Babinski	Yes	No	No
Sensory Changes	Yes or no	Yes or no	No
Fasciculations	Rarely	Yes	No
Autonomic Changes	Yes	Yes	No
Pain	With activity and with rest	With activity and with rest	With activity, but decreases with rest

nodes of Ranvier. This discontinuity in the myelin sheath allows rapid impulse conduction as the action potential leaps from one node to the next. In nonmyelinated fibers, one *Schwann cell* is associated with a number of axons, whereas in the myelinated fibers, the ratio is one Schwann cell per axon. Unmyelinated axons are enveloped by Schwann cell cytoplasm and plasma membrane but do not have the multiple wrappings of Schwann cell plasma membranes as seen in myelinated axons.

The **dendritic zone** is the term used to refer to the receptor membrane of a neuron. The axon is a single elongated protoplasmic neuronal process with the specialized function of moving impulses away from the dendritic zone and ends in a number of *axon telodendria*. Typically, the cell body is located at the dendritic zone, but it may occasionally be located within the axon or attached to the side of the axon (Fig. 19-3).

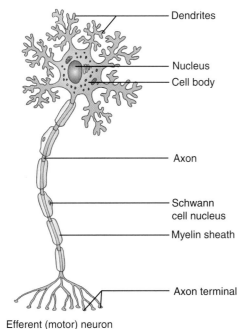

FIGURE 19-3 Diagram of a typical neuron.

The nerve fiber, which is the functional component of the peripheral nerve, is surrounded by connective tissue. Together, these connective tissues provide protection to the nerve fibers. Axons and the bundled nerve fibers, called *fascicles*, run an undulated course through the peripheral nerve that serves to resist tensile forces. In the peripheral nerve, the number of fascicles is greater proximally than distally.

The **mesoneurium** is a loose areolar tissue that surrounds peripheral nerve trunks and provides friction relief between the nerve and adjacent structures. The **epineurium** is the outermost connective tissue of the fascicles. Collagen bundles are arranged longitudinally.[2] External epineurium provides a definitive sheath among the fascicles.[3] Internal epineurium helps keep the fascicles apart and assists gliding between fascicles, a necessary adjunct to movement, especially when the nerve must move about a joint.[4] A lymphatic capillary network exists in the epineurium, drained by channels accompanying the arteries of the nerve trunk. The epineurial layer also includes bundles of type I and type III collagen fibrils, elastic fibers, as well as fibroblasts, mast cells, and fat cells.[5]

Bundles of nerve fibers are surrounded by a thin sheath known as the **perineurium**. Lundborg[6] describes the role of the perineurium as protecting the contents of the endoneural tubes, acting as mechanical barriers to external forces, and serving as a diffusion barrier. With a high ratio of elastin to collagen, the perineurium is thought to prevent neural damage from tensile forces.[4] Thomas[7] describes the perineurium as having elastin fibers running parallel to the nerve and to a lesser extent, oblique fibers running at an angle to the longitudinal fibers. It is hypothesized that the oblique fibers may assist in the prevention of kinking of the nerve as it flexes at the interior surfaces of joints.

The **endoneurium,** with its longitudinally arranged collagen fibers, is the membrane associated with the neural tube and maintains positive pressure around the neuron. Due to increased demands for protection, cutaneous sensory nerves have a greater percentage of endoneurium than motor nerves.[8]

The blood supply of the peripheral nervous system is called the **vasa nervorum**. Extrinsic vessels supply feeder arteries to the nerve. Once inside the nerve, there is a rich anastomotic intrinsic blood supply. The redundant blood supply to the nerve, necessary because of the high metabolic demands of neural tissue[9] and the mobility of the peripheral nervous system,[10] provides excellent perfusion. The intrinsic system is quite extensive, linking the mesoneurium, endoneurium, and perineurium. Intraneural blood vessels have autonomic innervation[11] that adjusts blood supply to meet the functional demands of the nerve.

Specialized cells for detecting changes in the environment are called receptors. **Exteroceptors** include those receptors affected by changes in the external environment. **Teleceptors** are receptors sensitive to distant stimuli. **Proprioceptors** receive impulses directly from muscle spindles, Golgi tendon organs, tendons, and periarticular tissues. **Interoceptors** are sensitive to changes within visceral tissues and blood vessels.

PERIPHERAL NERVE INJURY AND PATHOANATOMY
Peripheral Nerve Response to Injury

When the inflammation that is produced by repetitive activity, trauma, or infection is sufficient to alter the capabilities of the humoral components of the immune system, a nonspecific reaction termed, the **acute phase response (APR)**, is initiated.[12] This complex network of molecular and cellular responses amplifies or depresses the concentration of humoral defensive components, collectively referred to as **acute response proteins (ARPs).** In concert with other systemic features, the synthesis of these liver-derived ARPs by hepatocytes marks the characteristic and dramatic increase in serum levels of ARPs seen in the later stages (12 to 24 hours) of acute inflammation. **Cytokines** (Table 19-3) have a prominent role in regulation and contribute to the remediation of the signs and symptoms that are characteristic of inflammation. The APR process is designed to aid tissue repair and facilitate a return to physiologic homeostasis.

Cytokines are effector neuropeptide molecules produced by many cells, including monocytes/macrophages and lymphocytes, in response to injury. *Interleukin-1 (IL-1)* and *tumor necrosis factor-α (TNF-α)* are two cytokines that appear to control the amount and variety of cells that accumulate in inflamed tissue.[13] IL-1 and TNF-α are also able to induce major changes in adhesion molecule expression on endothelial cells. This allows the neutrophils to pass through capillary walls and into tissues.[14] As part of the APR, phagocyte and soluble antimicrobial substances are directed to the site of trauma. These same cytokines increase expression of adhesion molecules on monocytes, aiding in their infiltration into injured tissues. IL-1 and TNF-α, therefore, stimulate most mechanisms of inflammation.[15]

Al-Shatti et al[16] examined cytokines in rat median nerves following performance of a high repetition reaching and grasping task. They found increased immunoexpression of *IL-6* by week 3 and increases in all five cytokines by week 5. This response was transient as all cytokines returned to control levels by 8 weeks of performance of a high-repetition negligible force task. These findings suggest that cytokines are involved in the pathophysiology of repetitive motion injuries in peripheral nerves.

Table 19-3	**Cytokines Involved in the First and Second Wave of the Acute Phase Response**

First wave
  IL-1 family
    IL-α, IL-β
  TNF family
    TNF-α
  Important cells of origin
    Macrophage/monocyte
Second Wave
  Chemotaxis
    IL-8, MCP, MIP, RANTES
  Growth and differentiation/repair
    IL-6, colony-stimulating factors, FGF, EGF, TGF-β, PDGF
  Important cells of origin
    Macrophage/monocyte, activated stromal cells
  Immune response
    IL-2, IL-3, IL-4, IL-5, IL-7, IL-12
  Regulatory
    IL-4, IL-10, IL-13
  Important cells of origin
    Activated T cells, monocytes/macrophages

MCP, macrophage/monocyte chemotactic protein; MIP, macrophage inflammatory protein; RANTES, regulated upon activation normal T cell expressed and selected; FGF, fibroblast growth factor; EGF, epidermal growth factor; TGF, transforming growth factor; PDGF, platelet-derived growth factor; IL, interleukin; TNF, tumor necrosis factor
Adapted from Aggarwal BB, Puri RK. *Human Cytokines: Their Role in Disease and Therapy.* Ann Arbor, MI: Braun Brumfield; 1995.

Using the rat model, Clark et al[17] found median nerves at the level of the wrist demonstrating increases in macrophages, collagen, and connective tissue growth factor–positive cells. In addition, there was impaired sensation, motor weakness, and decreased median nerve conduction velocity. These effects were seen in both the reach and nonreach limbs. IL-1 and TNF-α have also been shown to produce a variety of systemic effects.[18] IL-6 has been found to possess many proinflammatory effects that overlap those of IL-1 and TNF-α.

QUESTION *for* REFLECTION
- Briefly describe the series of events that occurs during the *acute phase response* (APR), including each component and their specific roles in this process.
- What is the specific role of *cytokines* in the APR, and which are most involved?

Chromatolysis is the process of degeneration of the cell body, axon, and synapse after axonal injury. Histologically, the neuronal swelling after injury is accompanied by displacement of the *Nissl substance* to the periphery of the cell.[19] Enlargement of a neuron after its axon has been injured is representative of a regenerative rather than degenerative process.[20] In chromatolysis, the cytoplasm increases in volume, primarily because of an increase in *ribonucleic acid (RNA)* and associated enzymes. From 4 days after injury until a peak is reached at about 20 days, the amount of RNA increases, as does the cell's metabolic rate.[21]

From a clinical view, there are three basic ways in which nerve fibers may respond to injury. These categories of nerve injury were initially described by Seddon[22] and expanded upon by Sunderland.[23] Nerves are not homogeneous structures but rather considered to be *anisotropic*. Most nerve injuries result in a combination of the three primary categories of nerve injury.

Neurapraxia is defined as a segmental block of axonal conduction. The nerve can conduct an action potential above and below the blockage but not across the blockage. The conduction block is due to a physiologic process without histological change. There is no *Wallerian degeneration* present in neurapraxia. Etiology can include mild blunt blows, prolonged mild compression, or stretch. Stimulation proximal to the injury typically fails to produce a muscle contraction; however, stimulation distal to the injury provokes a muscle contraction. Typical neurapraxia affects the larger, myelinated fibers. Fine fibers innervating pain and autonomic function are often spared. Recovery is usually uncomplicated and occurs from minutes to months postinjury.

Axonotmesis is defined as a loss of continuity of the nerve axons with maintenance of the continuity of the connective tissue sheaths (Box 19-1). Axonotmesis leads to Wallerian degeneration of the distal portion of the nerve. An electromyogram (EMG) performed 2 to 3 weeks after injury shows fibrillations and denervation potentials distal to the injury.[24] Recovery occurs only through regeneration of the axon. The etiology of axonotmesis is similar to that of neurapraxia, with the difference being the severity of the injury. There is usually an element of additional retrograde nerve injury that must be overcome for complete recovery to occur.[25] The rate of axonal regeneration varies according to the presence of any comorbidities, activity at the site of the injury, and the distance between the injury site and the CNS.[26] Uncomplicated recovery rates vary from 1.5 mm/day to 3 mm/day.

Neurotmesis, like axonotmesis, involves destruction of the axons. In addition, the connective tissues are also injured. Neurotmesis is caused by a severe contusion, stretch, avulsion, or laceration. There are three basic types of neurotmesis. *Type one* involves a loss of the continuity of the axons and endoneurium, with an intact perineurium. *Type two* involves a loss of the continuity of the axons, endoneurium, and perineurium, with an intact epineurium. *Type three* involves a complete transection of the nerve. EMG examination of neurotmesis typically reveals the same findings as those seen with axonotmetic injury.[27] Spontaneous repair and recovery of function is much less likely to occur because regeneration axons produce a disorganized, impenetrable repair site. Regenerating axons may not function even after reaching distal end organs unless they arrive close to their original sites.[28] Regeneration of ulnar, median, and facial motor fibers have seldom been found to return to normal function.[29]

Histological changes typically occur in the denervated muscles by the third week. The muscle fibers kink and their cross-striations decrease.[30] With continued denervation and lack of movement or extrinsic muscle stimulation, the entire muscle may be replaced by fat or fibrous tissue within 2 to 4 years.

The Physiologic Basis for Biomechanical and Chemotaxic Nerve Injury

The three primary etiologies of neuropathy include mechanical, ischemic, and metabolic factors. Although consensus exists as to the biomechanical factors, there remains confusion as to the histological markers of such factors.

Box 19-1 THREE WAYS IN WHICH NERVES RESPOND TO INJURY

1. **Neuropraxia:** Segmental block of axonal conduction due to a physiologic process without histological change. Etiology can include mild blunt blows, prolonged mild compression, or stretch. Recovery is usually uncomplicated and occurs from minutes to months postinjury.

2. **Axonotmesis:** Loss of continuity of the nerve with continuity of the connective sheaths. Recovery occurs through regeneration of the axon. There is usually an element of retrograde nerve injury that must be overcome in order for complete recovery to occur. Uncomplicated recovery rates vary from 1.5 mm/day to 3 mm/day.

3. **Neurotmesis:** Involves destruction of the axons including the connective supporting tissues of the axon. Caused by a severe contusion, stretch, avulsion, or laceration. There are three basic types of neurotmesis. Stimulation above and below the injury site will not produce a muscle contraction. Spontaneous repair and recovery of function is much less likely to occur because the regeneration axons become entangled in a swirl of collagen and fibroblasts that produce a disorganized, impenetrable repair site.

QUESTION *for* REFLECTION

- What are the three primary etiologies of neuropathy?
- Which of the three etiological factors are best/least understood?
- How would knowledge of these factors influence the manner in which the manual therapist treats the patient and the recommendations for reducing the risk of reinjury?
- Briefly explain the process whereby a peripheral nerve becomes damaged in response to the application of biomechanical forces.

Nerves are relatively strong structures with substantial ability to resist tensile forces. However, tensile demands often produce symptoms prior to histological changes within the nerve. The median nerve at the level of the wrist can withstand 70 to 220 N of traction before complete transection occurs.[31] Ochs et al[32] reported an in vivo complete action potential block after 30 minutes of mild stretch with no apparent histological changes and postulated that the nerve block was due to vascular ischemia. Sunderland[4] believed that the majority of tensile resistance of the nerve is due to the perineurium. Therefore, as long as the perineurium remains intact, the tensile resisting function of the nerve remains sufficient.

With the application of a small tensile force, the intact nerve reacts with characteristics of an elastic material. As the linear limit is reached, the nerve fibers begin to rupture within the endoneurial tube. With ever-increasing load, the epineurium and perineurium begin to rupture; there is disintegration of the elastic properties of the nerve, and the nerve begins to react more like plastic material.[4,33,34] Sunderland[4] estimated that the elastic limit of a nerve is resting length plus 20% of resting length and that maximum elongation prior to rupture is resting length plus 30% resting length.

Dyck et al[35] assessed structural changes of nerves during compression of peroneal nerves in rats. The nerves were compressed at various pressures for various times. Clinically, the fact that nerve fiber rupture occurs prior to epineural and perineural rupture indicates that after a moderate stretch injury, the axons may have intact pathways to follow to their respective end organ. This bodes well for recovery of function. Epineural and perineural scarring, seen with chronic nerve compression and tension, may result in loss of nerve elasticity, resulting in early rupture. One must also question the effect of epineural and perineural scarring on blood flow. Such scarring may limit oxygen and nutrient uptake by the neural components, thus leading to a worsening of the injury and slower healing.

Cornefjord et al[36] used a porcine model to investigate the effects of chronic nerve compression. They identified inflammatory cells, nerve fiber damage, endoneurial hyperemia, and bleeding at the site of compression. Similar findings in a rat model of work-related musculoskeletal disorder were found by Barr et al.[37] Typically, the relationship between force of compression and time of compression is significant in defining the extent of the nerve injury. Pressures as low as 30 mm Hg have been shown to cause functional loss and intraneural edema with epineural scarring.[38] It was found that 80 mm Hg of pressure immediately caused local ischemia.[39] Indirect compression at very high pressures causes less of a functional loss than direct compression at much lower pressures.[40]

Compared with other tissues, peripheral nerves are relatively resistant to ischemic injury because of its abundant circulation. Impulse propagation is directly related to local oxygen supply.[10] A rich anastomosis provides a wide safety margin in the presence of a nerve transection. Lundborg and Dahlin[10] dissected the regional nutrient vessels from a 15 cm section of rabbit sciatic nerve and found no reduction in intrafascicular blood flow.

Rosen and Lundborg[41] showed that elongation of just 8% of resting length results in impaired venular flow. At elongations greater than 8% of resting nerve length, there was impaired arteriole flow until, at 15% greater than resting nerve length, all arteriole flow stopped completely. Studies of the rat sciatic nerve have demonstrated that blood flow is reduced by 50% with a strain of 11% and 100% with a sustained strain of 15.7%.[42] Mizisin and Weerasuriya[43] showed that epineural repair with a preoperative gap resulted in less favorable functional return than an epineural repair without a preoperative gap. From a clinical standpoint, care must be taken during passive stretching maneuvers that result in neurological symptoms so as not to interfere with normal healing.

QUESTION *for* REFLECTION

- Describe the blood supply to peripheral nerves.
- How does this vascular network provide resistance to ischemic injury?
- What are the typical neuropathic signs and symptoms of ischemia?

Barr and Barbe[44] have summated their recent work detailing the relationship between repetitive movements associated with *work-related musculoskeletal disease (WMSD)* and inflammation (Table 19-4). Barbe et al[45] have demonstrated a coincidental increase in the production of proinflammatory cytokines and the degradation of reach movements in rats that performed a high-repetition negligible-force task. Proinflammatory cytokines may induce the movement of macrophages into injured tissue. These macrophages secrete proinflammatory cytokines that further stimulate the secretion of cytokines. Barr et al,[46] using a rat model, compared the effects of high and low repetition exposures over an 8-week period on serum levels of proinflammatory cytokines and reach performance. The results showed a dose-related response between reach rate and both behavioral and physiological responses to a repetitive reaching and grasping task in rats. Dubner and Ruda[47] have shown that a sustained and chronic overstimulation of nociceptive afferents results in the release of excitatory neurotransmitters and neuropeptides such as *glutamate* and *substance P*. These neuropeptides act on the postsynaptic cell, resulting in a persistent hyperalgesia and *allodynia*. Studies such as these suggest a systemic component to local inflammation. Sakai et al[48] examined the expression of proinflammatory cytokines and basic fibroblast growth factor in the subacromial bursa of individuals with documented rotator cuff tears. A frequent etiology of rotator cuff tears is cumulative trauma. Finding inflammatory markers in the bursa may have a significant impact on future intervention strategies especially if the expression of these proinflammatory cytokines can be modulated.

Space occupying lesions may also result in significant biomechanical changes that may result in peripheral nerve injury. Bony exostoses caused by trauma have been associated with neuropathy. Tumors may also impinge on peripheral nerves

Table 19–4	**Summary of the Work of Barbe, Barr, and Clark Related to the Cytokine Network Involving WMSD in Rat Model**

AUTHORS	SUMMARY OF RESULTS
Barr et al., 2000[37]	A HR, negligible force task in rats increased ED1 immunoreactive macrophages in muscle, tendon, and radiocarpal ligaments. Tissue inflammation was evident by week three via levels of IL-1β, COX 2 and hsp72 (indicator of cellular injury). The degradation in reach movement patterns coincided with the tissue changes.
Barr et al., 2002[44]	In a comparison of HR and LR reaching and grasping task in rats, serum IL-1α and IL-1β were collected at 6 and 8 weeks. HR animals experienced an increase in serum IL-1α and a decrease in IL-1β. IL-1α and IL-1β both decreased in the LR group.
Barbe et al., 2003[45]	Inflammatory reactions resulting from a voluntary, HR, negligible force reaching and grasping task in rats over an 8-week period were studied. Elevated tissue macrophages (via ED1) were seen in all tissues examined bilaterally, especially at 6 and 8 weeks. Serum IL-1α increased significantly from week 0 to week 8.
Barr et al., 2003[46]	Investigated bone histological changes associated with a voluntary, HR, negligible force reaching and grasping task. ED1+ cells increased in the distal radius and ulna of the reach and nonreach limbs compared with the controls. Increases were the greatest at the muscle attachment and metaphyseal regions.
Clark et al., 2003	Motor degradation and anatomical and physiologic changes indicating inflammation were investigated in rats trained to perform an HR, negligible force reaching and grasping task. Elevated tissue macrophages were present in the median nerve at the level of the wrist by 6 weeks. NCV decreased in the reach limb by 9–12 weeks.
Clark et al., 2004[17]	Grip strength, nerve conduction velocity, macrophages, collagen, and connective-tissue growth factor-positive cells were assessed in rats trained to perform an HR, high-force repetitive task. Both reach rate and performance declined over the 12 weeks. Median nerves at the level of the wrist showed histological changes associated with inflammation with concomitant decreased NCV bilaterally. Forepaw sensation decreased bilaterally.

HR, high repetition; ED-1, macrophage specific antibody; IL, interleukin; COX 2, cyclooxygenase-2; hsp-72, heat shock protein 72; LR, low repetition; NCV, nerve conduction velocity.

leading to injury.[49] Degenerative arthropathies caused by connective tissue disorders may result in elongation or compression neuropathies.

In addition to biomechanical factors, there are a host of infectious and chemotaxic etiologies that may cause peripheral nerve injury. Diabetes mellitus is the most common cause of peripheral neuropathy. Fifty-nine percent of type II and 66% of type I individuals with diabetes have objective evidence of a sensory or motor neuropathy.[50] Although intervention is available for diabetic neuropathy, prevention of complications from diabetes through tight glycemic control from the onset of diagnosis (Table 19-5) remains at the forefront of effective therapies.

Diabetic nerves are more susceptible to tensile and compressive forces than are nondiabetic nerves. Commonly, injured nerves include the third and sixth cranial nerves, the median nerve at the wrist, the ulnar nerve at the elbow, the lateral femoral cutaneous nerve, truncal sensory neuropathy, and the common peroneal nerve at the head of the fibula.

Diabetic polyneuropathy is a systemic complication usually beginning at the feet and moving proximally that often involve the hands. *Neurological impotence* may also occur, which consists of an atonic bladder, hyper- or hypohidrosis of the skin, diarrhea, and gastric paresis. Richardson[50] discusses three

important clinical signs for diagnosing diabetic peripheral neuropathy. These include an absent Achilles reflex, even with a **Jendrassik maneuver,** diminished vibratory sense, and diminished proprioception.

Guillain-Barre syndrome (GBS) typically consists of a variety of acute peripheral nervous system disorders that are monophasic, with the peak neurological deficit reached within 2 weeks in most cases and frequently preceded by an

Table 19–5	**Criteria-Based Diagnosis of Diabetes Mellitus**

1. Symptoms of diabetes plus causal plasma glucose concentration of greater than 200 mg/dL with casual being defined as any time of day without regard to time since last meal.

or

2. Fasting plasma glucose equals 126 mg/dL or greater. Fasting is defined as no caloric intake for greater than 8 hours.

or

3. Two-hour plasma glucose equals 200 mg/dL or greater during an oral glucose tolerance test.

Adapted from World Health Organization: Diabetes Mellitus: Report of WHO Study Group. Tech Rep Ser No. 727. Geneva, Switzerland: World Health Organization, 1985.

antecedent event. Electrodiagnostic guidelines for the identification of peripheral nerve demyelination in patients with GBS have been established.[51]

Peripheral neuropathies may also be associated with *connective tissue diseases*. Examples include systemic lupus erythematosus, scleroderma, rheumatoid arthritis, and Sjogren's syndrome. An interesting hallmark is the related presentation of trigeminal sensory neuropathy. This entity appears to be associated with a lesion of the sensory ganglion of the fifth cranial nerve. Almost all of the connective tissue disorders are associated with a length-dependent sensorimotor neuropathy (Table 19-6).

QUESTION *for* **REFLECTION**

- What disease processes are known to lead to peripheral neuropathy?
- Explain the mechanism involved in each and the neuropathic effects.

Exposures to various environmental substances may also lead to neuropathy. Chronic exposure to *arsenic* leads to sensory neuropathy followed by distal motor neuropathy.[52] The other major environmental cause of neuropathy is *lead* intoxication. Lead can cause motor neuropathy in the upper limbs, but the presence of lead is not as common as it was in past decades. Those most at risk include children ingesting paint chips and manufacturers who routinely work with lead. Contaminated food may also be a source of lead intoxication.[53] The so-called alcoholic neuropathy may or may not exist. There are documented studies of alcoholics experiencing neuropathy, but it is unclear if the alcohol is the etiological agent or whether there is a nutritional component, such as thiamine deficiency, which has led to the neuropathic process.[54]

Nitrous oxide, an anesthetic commonly used in dental procedures, and gaining popularity as a recreational abuse drug, may cause a dose-dependent neuropathy.[55] *Phenytoin (Dilantin)* is one of the most commonly used antiseizure medications. It has been associated with a mild, predominantly sensory neuropathy. Approximately 18% of patients taking phenytoin for 5 years develop a neuropathy.[56] Table 19-7 provides a list of these neurotoxic agents that may cause peripheral neuropathy.

PRINCIPLES OF EXAMINATION
Chief Complaint and History of Present Illness

Perhaps more than any other major diagnostic category, the chief complaint and history of the present illness with regard to peripheral nerve injury are of tantamount importance in leading to a correct diagnosis. In many cases, the etiology of the injury is insidious, but with time and sensitive questioning, the patient and clinician together can come to understand causation.

CLINICAL PILLAR

When considering the origin of neuromusculoskeletal dysfunction, the manual therapist must adopt an impairment-based model of examination that includes a systems approach to rehabilitation with the knowledge that impairment is rarely an isolated event. The manual therapist must consider all interrelated systems.

CLINICAL PILLAR

The chief complaints of an individual with neuropathy typically consist of sensory disturbance, functional loss, or motor weakness.

Table 19-6	Neuropathies Associated With Major Connective Tissue Diseases				
	NEUROPATHIC SIGNS				
	Sensorimotor changes	**Dorsal root ganglionitis**	**Multiple mononeuropathy**	**CIDP**	**Trigeminal sensory neuralgia**
Systemic Lupus erythematosus	+	–	+	+	+
Scleroderma	+	–	–	–	+
Mixed connective tissue disease	+	–	–	–	+
Rheumatoid arthritis	+	–	+	–	+
Sjogren's syndrome	+	+	+	+	+

CIDP: chronic inflammatory demyelinating polyneuropathy.
Adapted from Lisak RP and Mendell JR. Peripheral neuropathies associated with connective tissue disease. In: Mendell JR, Kissel JT, Cornblath DR, eds. *Diagnosis and Management of Peripheral Nerve Disorders*. New York, NY: Oxford University Press, 2001.

Table 19–7 Drugs Causing Peripheral Neuropathy		
Almitrine	Amiodarone	Chloroquine
Cisplatin	Colchicine	Dapsone
Didanosine	Disulfiram	Doxorubicin
Ethambutol	FK 506	Gold salts
Isoniazid	Metronidazole	Mesonidazole
Nitrous Oxide	Nitrofurantoin	Taxol
Perhexiline	Phenytoin	Procainamide
Pyridoxine	Stavudine	Suramin
Thalidomide	Vinca alkaloids	Zalcitabine

Adapted from Mendell JR, Kissel JT, Cornblath DR, eds. *Diagnosis and Management of Peripheral Nerve Disorders*. New York, NY: Oxford University Press, 2001.

Detailed information is especially important in the presence of headache-related symptoms. In addition to routine questions regarding loss of consciousness and change in mental status, questions about cognitive processing acuity, and mood must also be included. During this portion of the examination, the therapist should also document the patient's current level of pain and the nature and type of sensory disturbances, including the adjectives used to describe his or her pain.

Past Medical History (PMH)

The past medical history interview should focus on four key areas. The patient should describe, in detail, all prior medical diagnoses and surgical interventions. Any history of obvious peripheral neuropathy-inducing diagnoses, along with any other possible etiologic factors from more esoteric causes such as renal or hepatic disease should be determined. A surgical history will include details regarding any specific procedures such as carpal tunnel release, ulnar nerve transposition, or lumbar laminectomy. The therapist should also be aware of any reported surgical stabilization procedures, such as triple arthrodesis that may reflect ankle instability due to nerve injury.

The second key area that must be reviewed during the PMH is medication. Ideally, the patient will bring a list of current medications and dosages. The therapist must also ask for a list of over-the-counter and herbal medications that the patient has used or is currently using.

The third key feature of the PMH is to inquire about any familial neuropathic illnesses. Examples include amyotrophic lateral sclerosis (ALS), Huntington's disease, and familial tremor.

CLINICAL PILLAR

The four key areas to be included in the past medical history are the following:

1. Prior medical diagnoses and surgical interventions, history of peripheral neuropathy–inducing diagnoses such as diabetes or connective tissue disorders, along

---

with any other possible etiological factors. A surgical history will include details regarding any specific procedures such as carpal tunnel release, ulnar nerve transposition, or lumbar laminectomy, as well as any surgical stabilization procedures that may reflect instability caused by nerve injury.

2. Current medications and dosages. The therapist should correlate these medications with current medical diagnoses. The therapist must also ask for a list of over-the-counter and herbal medications.

3. Familial neuropathic illnesses such as amyotrophic lateral sclerosis (ALS), Huntington's disease, and familial tremor.

4. A list of physicians, other than the primary care physician, whom they may have seen over the past 5 years.

The fourth key feature is to ask the patient for a list of physicians other than the primary care physician whom they have seen over the past 5 years. The therapist's knowledge of the patient's medical and surgical histories, medications, and recent caregivers will greatly assist in providing *triangulation* in regard to the patient's current medical status and will serve to improve the validity of the garnered information.

Social History

The primary purpose of taking a detailed social history is to learn of possible occupational or social habits that may cause or exacerbate the patient's presenting peripheral neuropathy. Dentists, dental hygienists, and dental office workers are routinely exposed to nitrous oxide.[57] Cabinetmakers, refinishers, carpenters, restorers, painters, and body and fender workers are commonly exposed to hexacarbons, which may contribute to the pathogenesis of peripheral neuropathy.[58] In addition, painters and restorers routinely encounter lead in older paints (Table 19-8).

The Physical Examination

The extraordinarily large number of etiologies and differential diagnoses associated with peripheral neuropathies makes a thorough review of systems a requirement. The patient should be asked to wear an examination gown and remove all clothing, including shoes and socks. This allows the therapist to easily inspect for loss of muscle bulk, gross structural abnormalities, scars, loss of skin integrity, orthoses, and abnormal shoe wear.

Mentation/Cognition Examination

Mental changes are sometimes encountered during the neurological examination. The therapist should note the patient's speech, appearance, level of cooperation, general attitude, mannerisms, and voluntary and involuntary motor behavior, degree of eye contact, lability, and relationship with family and friends.

The **Mini-Mental State Examination** is an excellent tool to assess intellectual capability, cognition, and orientation that may be used to ascertain the patient's level of intelligence.[59] This examination typically takes no longer than 15 minutes to complete.

Table 19–8	Occupational and Social Habits Predisposing to Peripheral Neuropathy

OCCUPATION	ASSOCIATED NEUROPATHIC TYPE/ETIOLOGY
Dentists, dental hygienists	Nitrous oxide–induced cobalamin deficiency
Cabinetmakers, painters	Hexacarbons
Farmers, nursery workers	Organophosphates
Dry cleaners, rubber workers	Trichloroethylene
Manufacturers of batteries, plastics, and paints; welders, roofers, printers, demolition crew, firearms instructors	Lead
Copper smelters, tree sprayers, taxidermists, farmers, jewelers, painters	Arsenic
Plastic industry workers	Acrylamide
Rayon industry workers	Carbon disulfide
HABIT	**BEHAVIOR**
Smoking	Paraneoplastic syndrome
Excessive alcohol	Nutritional/vitamin deficiency
Unprotected sex	HIV neuropathy
Intravenous drug use	HIV neuropathy
Vegetarian diet	Cobalamin deficiency
Nitrous oxide abuse	Cobalamin deficiency

Adapted from Mendell JR, Kissel JT, Cornblath DR, eds. *Diagnosis and Management of Peripheral Nerve Disorders*. New York, NY: Oxford University Press, 2001.

Postural Examination

Posture should be continuously assessed during the interview process. The therapist should note the presence of any protective posturing, lack of symmetry in gait and while sitting, any gait abnormalities, lack of coordination, dyskinesia, structural deformity, or alterations in skin integrity.

Vital Signs

Orthostatic hypotension is defined as a drop in systolic blood pressure of 30 mm Hg or more and a decrease in diastolic blood pressure of 15 mm Hg or more with positional change. Autonomic neuropathies affecting blood pressure are common in diabetes, Guillain-Barre syndrome, and the Shy-Drager complication of Parkinson's disease.[60] Oxygen saturation is often reduced with restrictive and obstructive lung disease. Elevated blood sugar may indicate glucose intolerance or diabetes mellitus.

Musculoskeletal Examination

Examination of Motor Function

Manual muscle testing (MMT) should be performed on at least one muscle for each myotomal segment of each extremity. The details related to the performance of these tests are described elsewhere by Cyriax[61] and Kendall and McCreary.[62] If weakness is found, the therapist should focus on the identified region to determine if the weakness is specific to a single muscle, involves one or more peripheral nerve distributions, follows a segmental myotome, or whether the entire extremity is involved. Symmetrical weakness is often characteristic of a *systemic polyneuropathy*. Focal weakness is often characteristic of a *mononeuropathy* or *multiple mononeuropathies*.

Range of Motion

The patient should be asked to perform functional movements such as "raise your hands above your head" and "squat down to the ground" so that the practitioner can identify any gross range of motion deficits. If a gross deficit is noted, a more specific range of motion examination should be performed. Neuropathic arthropathies and deformities such as *pes cavus*, which is associated with Charcot-Marie-Tooth disease, or the *intrinsic minus hand* deformity, which is observed with median and ulnar neuropathies, can best be identified during the range-of-motion examination.

Integumentary and Vascular Examination

Arterial vascular assessment should be performed in the anatomical position. Typically, the *radial pulses* are palpated in the upper extremity and the *dorsalis pedis pulse* in the lower extremity. In addition, the *positional vascular response* should be assessed as the therapist moves the upper extremity into flexion, abduction, and extension (Table 19-9). A reduction in the radial pulse may indicate an impingement of the subclavian artery within the thoracic outlet. The **thoracic outlet** is defined as the area between the intervertebral foramen and the insertion of the pectoralis minor muscle at the humerus. Gently pinching the fingertip and nail, then releasing pressure and assessing the speed at which the blanching disappears is a reasonable means of assessing capillary refill.

Impeded venous and lymphatic flow leads to edema. If edema is present, objective measures consisting of volumetric techniques are advised. An example of a neuropathy that is associated with decreased venous return is in the case of a mixed brachial plexopathy with concurrent *Paget-Schroetter syndrome*.

Painless, round, or oval, well demarcated calloused foot ulcers are typically either diabetic ulcers or autonomic sensory

neuropathies such as *Hanson's disease*. *Alopecia* is often a sign of hypothyroidism, systemic lupus erythematosus, or thallium intoxication. *Mees's lines*, the transverse white lines on nails, are seen with arsenic toxicity. *Fingertip clubbing* may be seen with neuropathy associated with Crohn's disease, liver disease, or pulmonary disease. *Trophic skin changes*, typically due to long axon neuropathies, include changes in hair growth in the extremities, hypohidrosis, mycotic-appearing nails, and the thinning of skin.

The presence of *Kaposi sarcoma* and *Kaposi lymphoma* are diagnostic of AIDS. The typical presentation is on the trunk or extremities, but early presentation may be on the oral mucosa.[63] Dry eyes are a common manifestation of Sjogren's syndrome. In advanced cases, corneal ulcers may appear.[64] Patients with **uveitis**, signs of inflammatory bowel disease, chronic inflammatory demyelinating polyneuropathy, or rheumatoid arthritis, often complain of decreased visual acuity, pain with pressure applied to the eye, and pain with eye movements.[65]

Sensory Examination

Valid assessment of the complex sensory system is an art that requires therapist knowledge of the peripheral and segmental dermatomal map, the sensory tract location in the spinal cord, and a general mapping of the sensory cerebral cortex. In addition, sensory assessment requires the complete cooperation of the patient (Fig. 19-4). At a minimum, testing should include light touch, pinprick, vibration, temperature, proprioception,

Table 19–9	Scoring of Pulse Assessment	
SCORE	**EXPLANATION**
0 with Doppler	No pulse audible with Doppler
+ with Doppler	Pulse audible with Doppler but not with palpation
+1	Faint pulse palpable
+2	Strong pulse palpable

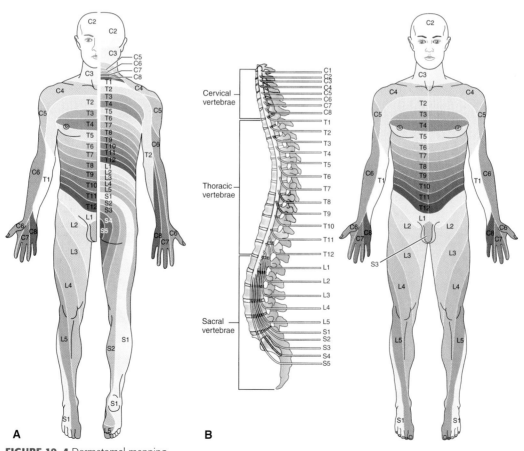

FIGURE 19–4 Dermatomal mapping.

and pain. Additional testing of *stereognosis, two-point discrimination, topognosis,* and *double stimulation* may be performed if indicated.

The patient is asked to offer an area of his or her body with no subjective sensory deficits. The therapist then touches this area with a sensory stimulant (pin, cold, etc.), asking the patient to describe the sensation perceived. If the response is what the therapist expects, the therapist then asks the patient to use the sensation perceived as "normal" and compare it to other areas. The therapist completes testing with one modality before beginning another. Documentation of the sensory examination findings should be both narrative and noted on a corporal sensory diagram. Vibratory testing should be performed over bony prominences only.

Neurodynamic Testing

Peripheral nerves exhibiting signs of inflammation or injury present with an increased subjective response to mechanical loading.[66] *Electroneuromyographic (ENMG)* testing can reveal abnormalities in significantly inflamed and injured nerves. Therapists routinely test for the mechanosensitivity of peripheral nerves during the clinical examination through the use of tapping, palpation, stretching, and compression (Table 19-10).

Lower limb and upper limb **neurodynamic testing** and peripheral nerve tension testing, (also known as ULNT/LLNT or ULTT/LLTT for upper and lower limb tension testing).[67] have been developed and popularized in recent years. Researchers such as Elvey and Elvey and colleagues,[68–70] Kenneally,[71] Totten and Hunter,[72] and Pechan[73] have added greatly to our present understanding of these clinical diagnostic maneuvers, and recent studies have added to the validity and reliability of testing.[67,68,70,73–77] Some, including the *sign of Brudzinski,*[78] the *straight leg raising test,* and the *prone knee bend (or flexion) test* are quite familiar, but others, especially those involving the upper limb, are often confusing.

Historically, the poor reliability associated with these tests is due to the complexity of the patient and therapist positional requirements and the inability of the patient to reliably differentiate whether the provoked symptoms are *neural* in nature versus the more generalized *soft tissue* complaints. Generally speaking, neurodynamic tests are deemed to be positive only when the exact

symptoms that brought the individual to seek care are reproduced. Ancillary symptoms that are dissimilar or in addition to the patient's presenting symptoms are duly noted and may be addressed at a later stage of intervention but are insufficient for the determination of a positive test. Asymptomatic individuals often experience symptoms from performance of these procedures. These tests are often considered to be very sensitive, yet not very specific, in detecting the presence of deficits in neural mobility. A positive test suggests a reduction in neural mobility, but the test itself is unable to specifically determine the exact location of injury or entrapment. Nerve tension tests are, therefore, considered to be good screening tools for the practicing clinician in identifying the extent to which neuropathic mechanisms are contributing to the patient's presenting complaints. However, more specific testing is required to determine the exact location and nature of the suspected neuropathy.

CLINICAL PILLAR

Neurodynamic tests are deemed positive *only* when the exact symptoms that brought the individual to seek care are reproduced. Ancillary symptoms that are dissimilar, or in addition, to the patient's presenting symptoms are duly noted and may be addressed at a later stage of intervention, but they are insufficient for determination of a positive test. These tests are often considered to be very sensitive, yet not very specific, in detecting the presence of deficits in neural mobility. A positive test suggests a reduction in neural mobility, but the test itself is unable to specifically determine the exact location of injury or entrapment.

The Sign of Brudzinski

The sign of Brudzinski (Fig. 19-5) was first described by Brudzinski in 1909.[79] It is commonly used as one of the clinical signs of *meningitis*. The patient is placed supine with the head flat and arms at the sides. The therapist asks the patient to raise his or her head off the bed. Once the head is off the bed, the

Table 19-10	Signs and Symptoms Differentiating Neural Versus Non-Neural Sites During Tension Testing	
SIGN/SYMPTOM	**NEURAL TISSUE**	**NON-NEURAL TISSUE**
Tissue example	Median nerve	Biceps tendon
Description of pain	"Unusual, never felt anything like this, deep, uncomfortable, toothache like, numbness, pins and needles"	"A pulled muscle, like I worked out too much, a sharp pain"
Constancy of pain	Prolonged perception after stretch; does not immediately decrease	Once tension removed, symptoms decrease rapidly.
Palpation symptoms	Causes radicular symptoms in specific innervation pattern	Local pain and tenderness occasionally with myotomal or dermatomal reference
Visualization	Therapist may see muscle fasciculations	Occasional muscle spasms.

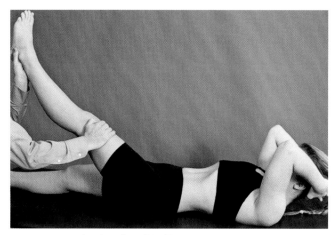

FIGURE 19–5 The sign of Brudzinski.

therapist passively flexes the neck chin toward chest or overpressure is provided by the patient. A description by the patient of radicular symptoms down the back and into the legs is considered a positive test. Care must be taken by the practitioner not to infer definitive meningitis from this test. Breig and Troup[80] found positive signs of Brudzinski in 35% of industrial workers with low back injuries referred to hospital emergency rooms.

The Straight Leg Raise Test

The *straight leg raise (SLR)* test has a long, yet unclear, history. Most textbooks refer to the originator of this test as Leseague in 1864,[80] hence the occasional reference in the literature to the *Leseague Test*. The patient is supine, arms at the side without a pillow. The therapist places one hand under the Achilles and the other over the patella. While preventing knee flexion, the examiner lifts the patient's leg off the bed. Magee[81] describes the first 35 degrees of motion as taking up the slack in the sciatic nerve. From 35 to 70 degrees, tension is placed through the sciatic nerve root. Symptoms above 70 degrees are attributed to sacroiliac joint pain. Comparison is then made with the contralateral leg. The SLR is deemed positive only when the exact symptoms that brought the individual to seek care are reproduced.

It is often challenging to differentiate between a positive SLR and an inflexible hamstring since both are often present concurrently. Comparing findings with the contralateral limb and basing the determination of a positive test on the reproduction of neurologic-type symptoms will help in differentiating between a hamstring strain and a restriction in neural mobility.

Over the years, many variations in performance and interpretation of the SLR have been adopted. The practitioner may add further tension along the sciatic nerve by passively dorsiflexing the ankle or flexing the cervical spine during performance of the SLR.[80] These variations are often referred to as the *Leseague* and the *Kernig* maneuvers, respectively.

Some have advocated the ability to differentiate between which division of the sciatic nerve appears most involved. This process begins with the baseline test followed by adjustment of various components of the test position to place additional stresses through the selected nerve. The baseline *sciatic nerve bias test* (Fig. 19-6a) is designed to place maximal tension through the sciatic nerve and consists of passive hip flexion, adduction, internal rotation, knee extension, and ankle dorsiflexion. The *tibial nerve bias test* (Fig. 19-6b) involves the baseline test with the ankle in dorsiflexion and the foot in eversion. The *common peroneal nerve bias test* (Fig. 19-6c) includes the baseline test with the ankle in plantarflexion and the foot in inversion. Lastly, the *sural nerve bias test* (Fig. 19-6d) consists of the baseline test with ankle dorsiflexion and foot inversion.

Palpation transversely across the sciatic nerve or any of its divisions may also be performed and is sometimes referred to as the *bowstring maneuver*. Palpation may occur at the apex of the SLR,[82] or palpation may be performed after a positive SLR has been elicited and tension along the nerve has been reduced. The sciatic nerve may be palpated prior to its division within the popliteal fossa, the tibial nerve is best palpated within the tarsal tunnel, and the common peroneal nerve may be palpated along its superficial location over the fibular head. The therapist takes note of any additional symptoms or return of symptoms that may occur upon direct palpation of these nerves.

The *well, or crossed, leg raise* is the term used to describe the process of symptom reproduction that occurs on the involved side when the contralateral, asymptomatic limb is raised during the SLR. These symptoms are attributed to a space-occupying lesion such as tumor or large central disc herniation.[81] Symptoms produced with a unilateral SLR that do not occur during performance of a *bilateral SLR* are attributed to sacroiliac joint pain that occurs in response to torsional forces placed through the joint during unilateral straight leg raising.

The Prone Knee Bend

The *prone knee bend (PKB)* test is the anterior corollary of the SLR and assesses the mobility of the upper lumbar nerve segments. First described by Wasserman in 1919,[83] this test is not as commonly performed as the SLR, most likely due to the infrequency of upper lumbar radiculopathies as compared with lower lumbar radiculopathies. To perform this test, the patient lies prone with the head turned toward the involved leg. The therapist stands on the involved side of the patient. The therapist grasps the patient's ankle and slowly flexes the knee, garnering a subjective response from the patient. As with all testing, the contralateral extremity is tested for comparison. As with the SLR, a positive test is indicated by reproduction of the patient's presenting symptoms.

Like the SLR, many clinicians advocate the use of small alterations in test position as a method of differentiating which nerve is most involved. The baseline test, or *femoral nerve bias test* (Fig. 19-7a), consisting of prone lying with the hip in neutral, or extended, and passive flexion of the knee, is first performed. The *lateral femoral cutaneous nerve bias test* (Fig. 19-7b) includes prone lying with passive hip extension, adduction, and knee flexion. The *saphenous nerve bias test* (Fig. 19-7c) includes prone-lying hip extension, abduction, and external rotation with knee extension, ankle dorsiflexion, and foot eversion.

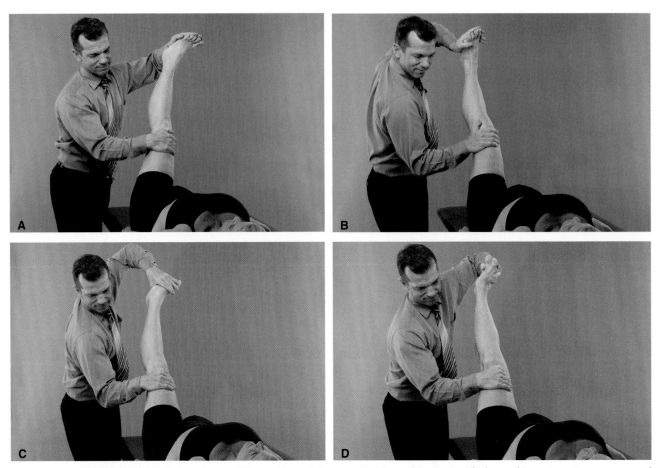

FIGURE 19–6 Straight leg raise neurodynamic test with nerve bias variations. **A.** Sciatic nerve bias test. **B.** Tibial nerve bias test. **C.** Common peroneal nerve bias test. **D.** Sural nerve bias test.

The Slump Test (Fig. 19-8)

Many have contributed to the development of the slump test; however, the refinement of this maneuver and it's utility in the process of differential diagnosis is attributed primarily to the work of Maitland.[84] See Chapter 8 for a summary of the evidence and details regarding the performance of this test. Unlike the other lower-limb neurodynamic tests, the slump test is performed in a weight-bearing, seated position. From an erect sitting posture, the patient is first guided by the therapist into trunk flexion without pelvic rotation. The patient's chin is brought to his or her chest, followed by passive knee extension and ankle dorsiflexion. Once this position is achieved, the cervical flexion component may be altered by moving the patient in and out of flexion while ascertaining the effect of these altered positions on the patient's reported symptoms. The cervical component of the test is called the *sensitizing maneuver* because it assists in differentiating between restrictions in neural versus non-neural tissue. As aforementioned, a positive test is achieved when symptom reproduction occurs. Each component of the test is elicited only after the patient denies onset of symptoms. To avoid injury, the therapist must position himself or herself in such a way (i.e., sitting or kneeling to the side of the patient) as to elicit each component of the maneuver passively without compromising his or her own well-being.

As mentioned, confusion regarding the correct performance and interpretation of neurodynamic testing impacts the reliability and validity of upper extremity testing as well. Unlike the straight leg raise and the prone knee bend tests, upper limb tension testing requires complex movement patterns affecting all upper extremity joints. In addition, the varying nomenclature is confusing. "Hunter,"[72] "Elvey,"[69,70,74] "High Hunter,"[72] "Low Hunter,"[72] "ULTT 1,"[83] "upper limb tension test,"[71] "military press,"[85] "Roos,"[85,86] and "stress abduction"[86] are all examples of common terms used in the literature and in the clinic to identify these maneuvers. Based on our review of the literature, which included cadaveric studies, we propose the following tests and nomenclature. Each test, with its preferred name, will be described with alternate names that are commonly used in the literature in parentheses.

The Median Nerve Traction Test (Median Nerve Bias, ULTT 1, ULTT 2a, ULNT 1) (Fig. 19-9)

Patient: With the patient in supine, the involved extremity is placed at the very edge of the plinth. The neck is relaxed with the head in a neutral position in all planes. The plinth stabilizes the scapula.

Therapist: The therapist stands on the involved side of the patient facing cephalad. One hand grasps the patient's hand,

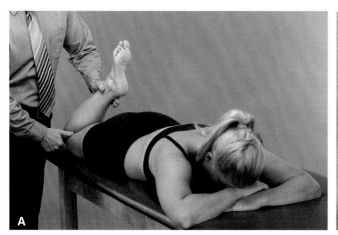
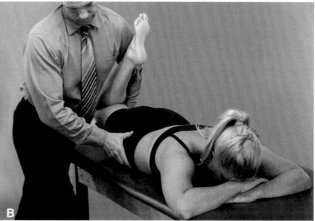
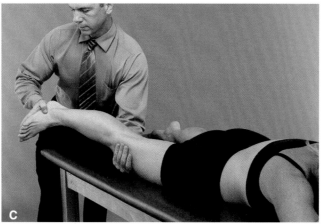

FIGURE 19–7 Prone knee bend neurodynamic test with nerve bias variations. **A.** Femoral nerve bias test. **B.** Lateral femoral cutaneous nerve bias test. **C.** Saphenous nerve bias test.

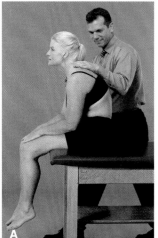
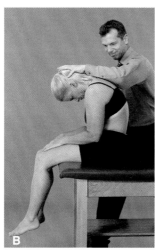
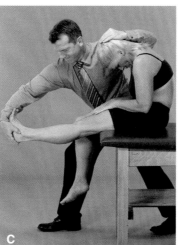
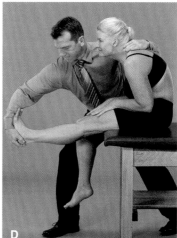

FIGURE 19–8 (A–D) The slump test for examination of sciatic nerve neurodynamics. Progressive tension is placed through the nerve during passive movement of each joint from proximal to distal. Cervical flexion and extension is the last component and is used as the sensitizing maneuver that serves to differentiate between deficits in mobility of neurological versus non-neurological tissue.

being sure to maintain the ability to control hand, finger, and thumb position. The therapist applies a slight downward force to the scapula that is maintained by placing the closed fist on the table at the superior border of the scapula.

Procedure: The patient is asked to report when the exact symptoms are reproduced. The therapist externally rotates the humerus until a soft end-feel is achieved (approximately 60 degrees). The therapist lifts the patient's arm a few inches off the plinth to allow passive extension of the elbow, wrist, thumb, fingers, and supination of the forearm. Finally, in approximately 30 degrees of abduction, the therapist gently, passively, and slowly extends the shoulder while monitoring end-feel.

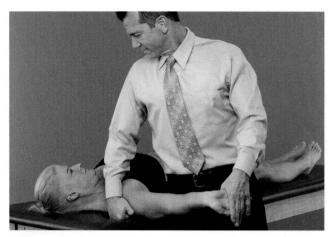

FIGURE 19–9 The median nerve traction test (median nerve bias, ULTT 1, ULTT 2a, ULNT 1).

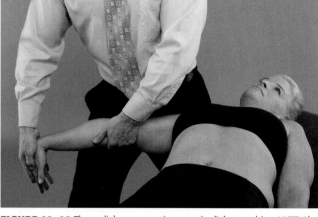

FIGURE 19–10 The radial nerve traction test (radial nerve bias, ULTT 2b, ULNT 2).

The therapist stops the test at the reproduction of neurological symptoms. The shoulder and/or elbow position at which point symptoms were reproduced are measured and recorded.

An alternate method of performing this test includes the sequential process of placing tension through this system from a proximal to distal fashion, beginning with scapular depression, followed by shoulder abduction to 90 to 110 degrees, elbow extension, forearm supination, and wrist, finger, and thumb extension. Typically, the process involves scapular depression and shoulder abduction, followed by taking up maximal motion in each of the distal joints (i.e., forearm, wrist, fingers, thumb), with elbow extension occurring last. The therapist may choose any one of the joints used in this test as the gauge for measuring the degree of tension in the system that precipitates symptoms. In the latter example, elbow extension is recruited last and is easily used to measure the degree of tension within the nerve. Regardless of the process used, it is vital that reliable measurements of joint angles are obtained using a goniometer so that progress subsequent to intervention can be accurately documented.

The therapist can add reliability to the test by "releasing" the median nerve by flexing the elbow or wrist and again monitoring symptoms. The therapist may also choose to engage in sensitizing maneuvers that involve the passive positioning of the patient's cervical spine into contralateral side bending or rotation. The patient may be prepositioned in contralateral side bending followed by recruitment of the distal segments as previously mentioned. Once a positive test is identified, the patient is then passively brought into ipsilateral side bending to assess an expected reduction in symptoms through lessening the tension on the nerve. A lessening or exacerbation of neurological symptoms during testing adds important information that serves to differentiate between neurologically induced symptoms and symptoms produced from soft tissue stretch.

The Radial Nerve Traction Test (Radial Nerve Bias, ULTT 2b, ULNT 2) (Fig. 19-10)

Patient: Supine on the plinth, the involved extremity is placed at, or slightly beyond, the edge of the plinth as described above for the median nerve test.

Therapist: The therapist stands on the involved side of the patient facing cephalad and grasps the patient's arm as described above. An alternate therapist position involves facing caudally. With the patient positioned obliquely on the table, the therapist's thigh provides slight scapular depression as it contacts the patient's shoulder, which is positioned slightly over the edge of the plinth. This position allows the therapist to use both hands to control motions throughout the remainder of the test.

Procedure: The patient is asked to note when their exact symptoms are reproduced. The therapist internally rotates and abducts the humerus until a soft end-feel is achieved. The therapist lifts the patient's arm a few inches off the plinth to allow passive extension of the elbow, flexion of wrist, thumb, and fingers, as well as forearm pronation and wrist ulnar deviation. Finally, in approximately 30 degrees of abduction, the therapist gently, passively, and slowly extends the shoulder, monitoring end-feel and all the while querying the patient for symptomology. The therapist stops the test when reproduction of the patient's neurological symptoms occur. The shoulder and/or elbow position at which point symptoms were reproduced are measured and recorded. As with the median nerve test, an alternate method of performing this test includes the sequential process of placing tension through this system in a proximal to distal fashion. The therapist may choose any one of the joints used in this test as the gauge for measuring the degree of tension in the system that precipitates symptoms. Typically, the therapist recruits maximal positioning in all distal joints, after which the shoulder is brought into abduction and the degree of abduction at the point of symptom provocation is then goniometrically measured and used as the baseline measurement for subsequent testing. Regardless of the process used, it is vital that reliable measurements of joint angles are obtained using a goniometer so that progress subsequent to intervention can be sufficiently documented.

As described for the median nerve test, sensitizing maneuvers can be used, including cervical side bending/rotation positioning during performance of these procedures. The therapist can add reliability to the test by "releasing" the nerve by extending the wrist and again monitoring symptoms.

The Ulnar Nerve Traction Test (Ulnar Nerve Bias, ULTT 3, ULNT 3) (Fig. 19-11)

Patient: Supine on the plinth, the involved extremity is placed at the edge of the plinth as described above for the median and radial nerve tests.

Therapist: The therapist stands on the involved side of the patient facing cephalad and grasps the patient's arm as described above. An alternate hand position may include the therapist applying a slight downward force to the scapula, which is maintained by the therapist placing his or her closed fist on the table just superior to the superior border of the scapula as for the median nerve test.

Procedure: The patient is asked to note when the exact neurological symptoms are reproduced. The therapist externally rotates the humerus until a soft end-feel is achieved. The therapist gently flexes the elbow fully while simultaneously pronating the forearm and extending the wrist, fingers, and thumb. The therapist gently abducts the humerus to 90 degrees while maintaining the shoulder in a neutral horizontal abduction/adduction position. The therapist monitors end-feel all the while querying the patient for symptomology. The shoulder and/or elbow position at which point symptoms were reproduced are measured and recorded. An alternate method of performing this test includes the sequential process of placing tension through this system from a proximal to distal fashion, beginning with scapular depression, followed by shoulder abduction and external rotation, elbow flexion, forearm pronation, and wrist, finger, and thumb extension. Typically, the process involves scapular depression and shoulder abduction, followed by taking up maximal motion in each of the distal joints (i.e., forearm, wrist, fingers, thumb), with elbow flexion occurring last. The therapist may choose any one of the joints used in this test as the gauge for measuring the degree of tension in the system that precipitates symptoms. In the latter example, elbow flexion is recruited last and is easily used to measure the degree of tension within the nerve. Regardless of the process used, it is vital that reliable measurements of joint angles are obtained using a goniometer so that progress subsequent to intervention can be sufficiently documented. As described

above, sensitizing maneuvers can be used including cervical side bending/rotation positioning during performance of these procedures.

Special Neurological Tests

Deep tendon reflexes (DTR) include the biceps reflex, the brachioradialis reflex, the triceps reflex, the patellar reflex, the hamstring reflex, and the ankle (more commonly known as Achilles tendon) reflex. When testing the *biceps DTR* (musculoskeletal; C5-C6), the patient is positioned with the elbow flexed to 90 degrees and in a supinated position (Table 19-11). The therapist strikes the thumb that has been positioned over the biceps tendon distally at the elbow. The *triceps DTR* (radial; C6, C7, C8) is tested in a similar fashion. The shoulder is internally rotated to allow the forearm to hang downward with the elbow flexed at 90 degrees. The therapist taps the thumb that has been positioned over the triceps tendon distally at the elbow. The *brachioradialis DTR* (radial; C5, C6, C7) is tested with the elbow flexed to 90 degrees and neutral with regard to pronation and supination. The wrist is allowed to hang into ulnar deviation. The forearm is supported by the examiner who strikes the wrist just proximal to the radial styloid. To test the *patellar DTR* (femoral; L3, L4) the patient is seated on a high examination table that allows the knees to swing freely. The therapist taps the thumb, which has been placed over the patellar tendon at the knee. The *hamstring DTR* (sciatica; L5, S1, S2) is tested with the patient prone, with the examiner supporting the leg with the knee in 20 degrees of flexion. The examiner taps the medial and lateral hamstring tendons just proximal to their insertions. The *ankle DTR* (tibial; S1-S2) is best tested with the patient kneeling on a chair with both ankles hanging over the chair or in sitting with the legs hanging freely. The therapist taps the thumb, which has been placed over the Achilles tendon at the ankle.

Three superficial reflexes should also be routinely tested. The **abdominal reflex** (T6-T12), is tested with patient lying supine with relaxed abdominal musculature. The skin of each quadrant of the abdomen is briskly stroked with a pin toward the umbilicus. Normally, the local abdominal muscles contract,

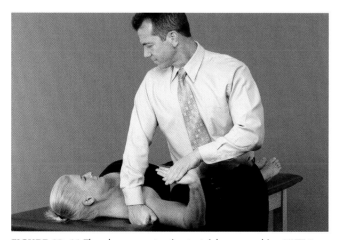

FIGURE 19–11 The ulnar nerve traction test (ulnar nerve bias, ULTT 3, ULNT 3).

Table 19–11	Scoring of Deep Tendon Reflex Assessment
0 with Jendrassik maneuver	No response to tendon tap with Jendrassik maneuver
+ with Jendrassik maneuver	Response to tendon tap with Jendrassik maneuver only
+1	Palpable response to tendon tap but no joint movement
+2	Small amount of joint movement in response to tendon tap
+3	Large amount of joint movement in response to tendon tap
+4	Synergistic muscle response to tendon tap

moving the umbilicus toward the quadrant tested. A negative response is determined if there is no visible or palpatory muscle contraction when the abdomen is stroked. A negative bilateral response may indicate a spinal pathological level, and a negative unilateral response may indicate a unilateral pathology such as a multilevel spinal stenosis caused by scoliosis. Negative responses are, however, often seen in anxious or overweight patients and in 12% of healthy patients.[87]

The plantar response, often called the **Babinski reflex**, is tested with the patient supine with the knees and hips extended and the ankle relaxed. With a wooden applicator, the skin of the sole of the foot is stroked in a parenthetical motion from the heel toward the base of the fifth toe and to the base of the first toe. Normal response is a slight flexion of all toes. In abnormal responses, there may be extension of the great toe with fanning and flexion of the lesser toes. This response is suggestive of an upper motor neuron lesion.

Clonus, defined as a repeated unidirectional joint movement caused by an involuntary muscle contraction of the agonist, is assessed by a quick agonist stretch. To test for clonus of the wrist flexors, for example, the wrist is quickly passively moved into extension. To test for clonus of the gastrocnemius-soleus complex, the ankle is quickly passively moved into dorsiflexion.

During the First World War, Wilkins and Brody[88] detailed a tingling response predicated by the tapping of an entrapped nerve. The tingling was felt to represent axonal regeneration and nerve healing indicating that further treatment was not needed. In current clinical practice, the **Tinel sign** is believed to be elicited over an area of focal demyelination that accompanies nerve entrapment. A positive Tinel sign is noted when manual tapping over a suspected area of nerve entrapment produces paresthesia or reproduction of symptoms along the distal distribution of the culpable nerve. Katz et al[89] demonstrated a limited sensitivity and specificity of 60% and 67% of the Tinel sign, making the clinical relevance of this test questionable.

Functional Examination

From an observational standpoint, the therapist observes the patient donning and doffing articles of clothing, transferring from stand to sit and supine to sit, and through gross movements. Formal gait analysis should be performed with the patient ambulating on level surfaces, curbs, and stairs. Common gait deviations caused by neuropathy are noted, such as drop foot, a compensated or uncompensated gluteus medius lurch (Trendelenburg), and recurvatum. Shoes should be examined for abnormal or excessive wear. A fall history should also be obtained, as well as balance assessment tests such as the *Tinetti*,[90] *timed up-and-go*,[91] and the *Berg balance test*.[92] Although technically not considered to be a formal balance test, the *Rhomberg* and *sharpened Rhomberg tests*,[93–95] are typically performed during the functional testing portion of the clinical examination. With the Rhomberg, the patient is asked to stand quietly for 30 seconds, with heels and toes together, arms crossed over the chest, and eyes closed. Sway commonly occurs in patients with proprioceptive loss in the trunk or lower extremities, cerebellar dysfunction, posterior white column

diseases, and diseases of the vestibular system. The sharpened Romberg is essentially the same test except that the feet are placed one in front of the other.

Adjunctive Diagnostic Tests

Electrodiagnostic Examination

Electrodiagnostic studies provide relevant information that should not replace the results of the clinical examination, but rather provide important adjunctive information that may aid in fully developing the history of present illness and prognosis.

According to Cornblath and Chaudhry,[96] the electrodiagnostic examination in conjunction with the clinical neurological examination assists in arriving at a differential diagnosis, determines the need for further testing, defines the site of the lesion, identifies the nature of the predominant pathological process, and assists in determining a prognosis. Typical electrodiagnostic procedures include sensory and motor *nerve conduction studies (NCS)*, *electromyography (EMG)*, and quantitative sensory testing, which is often referred to as *evoked potentials (EP)*.

Sensory and motor nerve conduction studies (NCS) are one of the most important, and more commonly used, components of the electrodiagnostic examination. The time required to traverse the segment nearest the muscle is known as the *distal latency*. The time for an impulse to travel a measured length of nerve determines the *conduction velocity*. Similar measurements are made for both motor and sensory nerves.

Electromyography (EMG) is concerned with the study of the electrical activity arising from muscles and associated muscle activity. It is most useful to the clinician in the diagnosis of lower motor neuron conditions. Needle electrodes are inserted into skeletal muscle to detect variations of potential. Less invasive surface electrodes over the target muscle may also be used. The electrical activity may be displayed on a cathode ray oscilloscope and played on a loudspeaker for simultaneous visual and auditory analysis. Clinically, normal muscle at rest should demonstrate absence of any action potentials. Denervated muscle fibers are recognized by their increased insertional and abnormal spontaneous activity. Particular aberrant potentials are diagnostic of specific neurological or muscular diseases. Although information related to the timing and recruitment patterns of muscle can be obtained, EMG data does not provide accurate information regarding the force-producing capability of the target muscle.

Radiographic Examination

Plain film radiographs may be useful in detecting bony or articular changes that may result in nerve impingement (Box 19-2). *Computerized tomography (CT)* and *magnetic resonance imaging (MRI)* are used to examine hard and soft tissue structures in the extremities, back, neck, and head. *Bone scintigraphy* or *scans* may assist in determining sites of inflammation subsequent to fracture, infection, or tumor, which may be associated with nerve damage or injury. *Positron emission tomography (PET) scans*, which examine the uptake of tracer amounts of radioisotopes to measure blood flow, glucose, and oxygen metabolism in the brain and other tissues, may also be used.

Box 19-2 RADIOGRAPHIC EXAMINATION USED IN THE DIAGNOSIS OF NERVE INJURY

1. **Plain Film Radiography**: Useful in detecting bony or articular changes that may result in nerve impingement.

2. **Computerized Tomography (CT)** and **Magnetic Resonance Imaging (MRI)**: Used to examine hard and soft tissue structures in the extremities, back, neck, and head.

3. **Bone Scintigraphy/Scans**: Assist in determining sites of inflammation subsequent to fracture, infection, or tumor that may be associated with nerve damage or injury.

4. **Positron Emission Tomography (PET)**: Examines the uptake of tracer amounts of radioisotopes to measure blood flow, glucose, and oxygen metabolism in the brain and other tissues.

Laboratory Studies

Laboratory studies are an important adjunct to the neurological clinical examination. Specific algorithms are used to determine what tests to order. Commonly ordered tests are detailed in Table 19-12.

PRINCIPLES OF INTERVENTION
Clinical Indications for Neural Mobilization

All articular movement produces some degree of nerve gliding to accommodate nerve length changes induced by angular rotation.[95–97] Several factors may limit the ability of a nerve to glide. A peripheral nerve may demonstrate limitations in normal mobility that results from restrictions in either the *extraneural tissues* (i.e., connective tissue structures around the nerve or between the nerve and surrounding tissues) or restrictions in the *intraneural tissues* (i.e., nerve tissue that composes the nerve itself). Neural mobilization, or neurodynamic, techniques are used in both acute or chronic conditions to develop or remodel extraneural and intraneural scarring into an alignment that facilitates normal physiologic nerve gliding (Table 19-13).

Neural mobilization techniques[67,70,71,94] typically include the practice of fixing the proximal portion of the nerve while the distal elements are stretched in a controlled fashion (Box 19-3). By fixing the proximal end and stretching the distal end, most of the excursion will occur at the distal end. The rationale for this approach agrees with the in vivo findings of Shaw et al,[98] who found that the greatest excursion of

Table 19-12   Commonly Ordered Laboratory Tests to Assist With Diagnosing Peripheral Neuropathy

TEST	RATIONALE
Albumin	Decreases in malnutrition, nephrosis, metastatic carcinoma, hepatic failure
Alkaline phosphatase	Increases in bone metastases, Paget's disease, rickets, healing fracture, heart failure, pregnancy
Creatinine	Increases in renal failure, urinary obstruction, dehydration, hyperthyroidism
Eosinophilic sedimentation rate	Increases with inflammation, such as infection, rheumatological diseases, cancer
Ethanol	Increases after alcohol ingestion
Glucose	Increases in diabetes mellitus, use of corticosteroids, Cushing's syndrome
Hemoglobin	Decreases in anemia, chronic illness, bleeding
Hemoglobin A1C	Increases in long-term hyperglycemia
PbB	Increases after lead ingestion
Rapid plasma reagin	Diagnostic for syphilis
Total protein	Decreases in burns, cirrhosis, malnutrition, malabsorption, nephrosis
White blood cell count	Increases in acute infection, decreases with chronic infection and with immunocompromise

Table 19-13   Acute Conditions Benefiting From Neural Mobilization

Carpal tunnel syndrome	Posterior interosseous nerve syndrome	Tarsal tunnel syndrome
Cervical strain	Lumbar radiculopathy	Lateral femoral cutaneous nerve syndrome
Herniated disk	Peroneal nerve entrapment	Proximal tibial neuropathy
Lumbar strain	Anterior interosseous nerve syndrome	Guillain-Barre syndrome
Parsonage-Turner syndrome	Ulner nerve entrapment at elbow	Whiplash
Pronator teres syndrome	Radial tunnel syndrome	Femoral neuropathy
Traumatic brachial plexopathy	Guyon's canal syndrome	Cervical radiculopathy

the upper extremity long nerves during functional movement patterns occurs distally at the level of the wrist.

Empirically, along with neural gliding, there is also neural sliding that occurs during neurodynamic intervention. This technique, not yet fully developed, encompasses the movement of the proximal end of the nerve toward the distal end while simultaneously elongating the distal end. This is immediately followed by moving the distal end of the nerve toward the proximal end while the proximal end is elongated. This technique would incur a *sliding* movement of the entire nerve, not unlike the motion used when flossing your teeth. Neural sliding, or sometimes called *flossing*, has a potentially high probability of performance error.

Manual Physical Therapy Interventions for Peripheral Nerve Disorders

General Guidelines and Specific Recommendations for Neural Mobilization

Neural mobilization is not a panacea and should be combined with other therapies to maximize its effectiveness. These therapies include those traditionally used by physical therapists. General principles of intervention have been established to guide the manual physical therapist when working with this unique cohort of patients (Box 19-4).[91,92]

Regardless of the indicated therapeutic interventions, the therapist must remain acutely aware of the need to avoid any additive inflammation through undue stresses. Based on its anatomical configuration, the nervous system is inherently mobilized with any degree of joint movement or movement related to intervention. Due to the reactive nature of neural tissue to imposed stresses, the utmost care should be taken to ensure that only the specifically prescribed mobilization is being performed and that all extraneous joint movement is controlled.

When considering technique aggressiveness, the excursion should be limited to the onset of symptoms, held for a short period of time (1-5 seconds initially), and then released. Proper daily reexamination occurs pre- and postintervention and is required in order to keep the therapist informed regarding the stage of healing. This is especially important during the early stages of therapy. Incorporation of a home self-management regimen is often delayed until the therapist has incorporated similar techniques during formal therapy sessions and is quite sure of the patient's ability to handle such stresses.

In general, specific neural mobilization techniques adopt the positions used for testing of the specific nerve in question. Therefore, the examination becomes the intervention. Specific recommendations for the use of neural mobilization techniques for peripheral neuropathies include the following.

1. When developing a home program that includes neural glides, give only one to two exercises to the patient at one time and be sure that the patient can fully demonstrate tolerance and competency.

2. Use a digital camera or video camera to photograph the patient performing the exercises properly.

3. The area of the neural glide should be heated before performing the exercise. This may be done externally with a shower, bath, or hot packs, or internally, via aerobic exercise such as walking, bicycling, or using an ergometer that does not compromise the injured area. A good rule of thumb is if the arms are injured, aerobically exercise the legs; if the legs are injured, aerobically exercise the arms.

4. The patient must understand that he or she needs to accept good pain and avoid bad pain with regard to neural glides. Good pain is muscle, ligament, or skin stretch. Bad pain is neural pain or reproduction of the presenting symptoms.

5. The patient should attempt to expose as much of the injured area as possible. Tight or bulky clothes may inhibit active motion and also limit the appreciation of the sensation produced by the movement.

6. The patient should be taught to exercise only with good back and neck alignment. The back and neck should be straight and without rotation. The nerve to be glided will determine the body's position.

7. Proper breathing is important. Inhale while at rest and exhale as the nerve glides away from the body. Inhale upon return to the initial starting position.

8. The movement should be quite slow. Typical guidelines initially consist of pausing for 1 to 2 seconds at the onset of symptoms for three to five repetitions maximum, with gradual progression to holding the provocative position for 10 seconds or longer.

9. Ten repetitions four times per day are prescribed as a starting point. The patient should perform the exercises in the clinic for the first time prior to performance at home. Pain lasting more than 1 hour indicates significant acuity, and the number of repetitions and frequency should be reduced.

Upper and Lower Quadrant Neural Mobilization Techniques

The General Median Nerve Glide

If the patient has sufficient scapular intrinsic and extrinsic strength to stabilize the scapulohumeral complex, then the exercises are best done standing in front of a mirror. The mirror provides excellent visual feedback. Using a skateboard on a tabletop can accommodate weak proximal musculature (Fig. 19-12). Very weak or paralyzed proximal musculature requires supine positioning and assistance of another individual to provide the range of motion. The patient begins the glide in position one with the palm facing the face and the shoulder abducted at 45 degrees. The patient is told to hold the position in which neurological symptoms develop. In position two, the shoulder is gently extended to 0 degrees flexion. In position three, the elbow is fully extended. In position four, the wrist is extended. In position five, the fingers and thumb are extended. If symptoms have not yet developed, the patient can further extend the shoulder (position six). Lastly, in the absence of symptoms, the patient can move to position seven by side bending the neck to the contralateral side. The position that marks the beginning of neurological symptoms is considered to be the provocative position, and if tolerated should be held for 10 seconds. After holding, it is important for the patient to return to the starting position before performing the next repetition.

The Median Nerve Glide at the Wrist

The median glide nerve at the wrist is indicated for conservatively treated and surgically treated carpal tunnel syndrome.

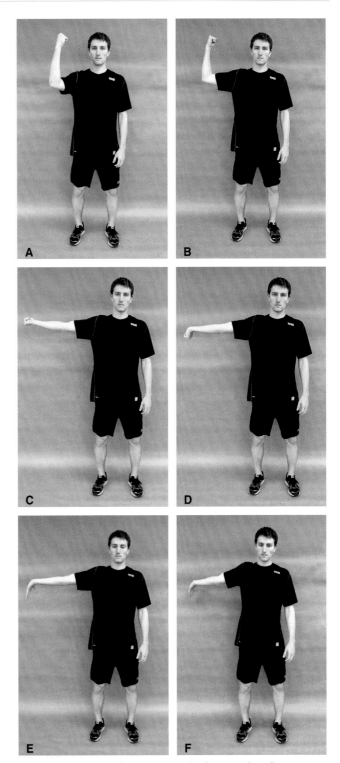

FIGURE 19–12 (A–F) The six positions for the general median nerve glide performed in standing.

The starting point, position one, for the median nerve glide at the wrist is sitting or standing with the elbow flexed to 90 degrees, the shoulder adducted, and the forearm neutral. The hand is clenched into a fist with the thumb outside the hand. Position two is the opening of the hand with the fingers and thumb adducted. In position three, the wrist is extended. Position four is the thumb extended. In position five, the wrist is supinated. In position six, the thumb is passively extended to the full available range of motion. The position, which marks the beginning of neurological symptoms, should be held for 10 seconds. The hand is then slowly brought back to the starting position.

The Radial Nerve Glide

The starting position for this glide is with the open palm in front of the face. In position two, the shoulder is extended to a 0 degree flexion position (Fig. 19-13). In position three, the shoulder is internally rotated. In position four, the wrist is flexed (the waiter's tip position). If symptoms do not appear, the shoulder can be extended further (position five). Lastly, in the absence of symptoms, the patient can laterally flex the neck to the contralateral side (position six). The position that marks the beginning of neurological symptoms should be held for 10 seconds. The hand is then slowly brought back to the starting position.

The Ulnar Nerve Glide

The starting position is with the open palm in front of the face. The shoulder is flexed to 90 degrees and fully horizontally abducted (Fig. 19-14). The shoulder is externally rotated. The elbow is fully flexed (position two). The wrist and fingers are extended (position three). Lastly, in the absence of symptoms, the patient can laterally flex the neck to the contralateral side (position three). The position that marks the beginning of neurological symptoms should be held for 10 seconds. The hand is then slowly brought back to the starting position.

The General Brachial Plexus Gliding Program

In position one, the patient faces the wall and places the palm, fingers abducted and thumb extended, against the wall. The shoulder is externally rotated 90 degrees (position two) (Fig. 19-15). By keeping the hand firmly against the wall and the elbow extended, the patient rotates the contralateral side away from the wall, causing the involved shoulder to horizontally abduct. The position that marks the beginning of neurological symptoms should be held for 10 seconds. The hand is then slowly brought back to the starting position.

The Lumbar Plexus Glide

The three anterior divisions of L2, L3, and L4 form the obturator nerve. The three posterior divisions unite to form the femoral nerve and the upper two give off twigs that form the lateral femoral cutaneous nerve (Fig. 19-16). Nerve glides influencing the roots, divisions, or peripheral nerves of L2-L4 are performed prone (position one), with the hips in a neutral rotation position and the knees extended. Using the hamstrings, the knee is actively flexed (position two). In position three, the patient's hand grasps the ankle to assist the knee into full flexion. In position four, the trunk is raised onto the contralateral elbow to provide increased hip extension. The position that marks the beginning of neurological symptoms should be held for 10 seconds. The ankle is then slowly brought back to the starting position.

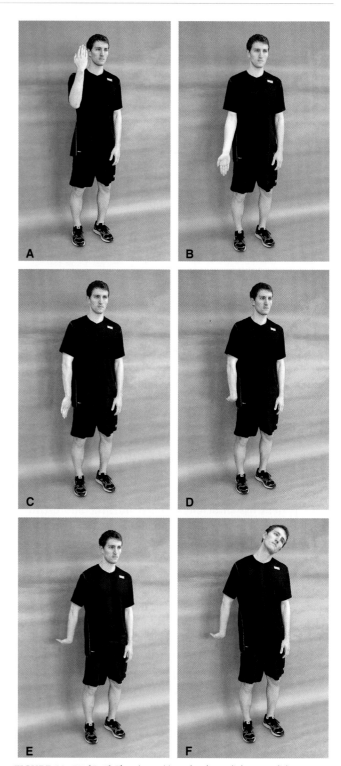

FIGURE 19–13 (A–F) The six positions for the radial nerve glide performed in standing.

The Sacral Plexus Glide

Typically, the sacral portion of the lumbosacral plexus arises by the five plexus roots formed by the anterior primary divisions of the fifth and part of the fourth lumbar nerves (lumbosacral trunk) and the first and parts of the second and third sacral nerves (Fig. 19-17). The main terminal branch is

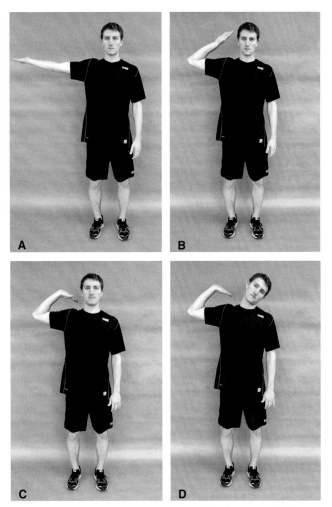

FIGURE 19–14 (A–D) The four positions of the ulnar nerve glide performed in standing.

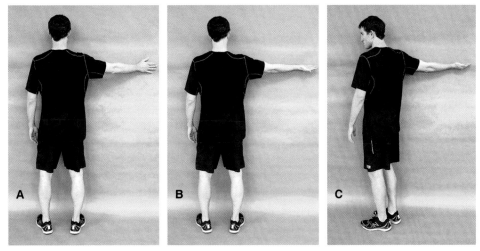

FIGURE 19–15 (A–C) The three positions of the general brachial plexus nerve glide.

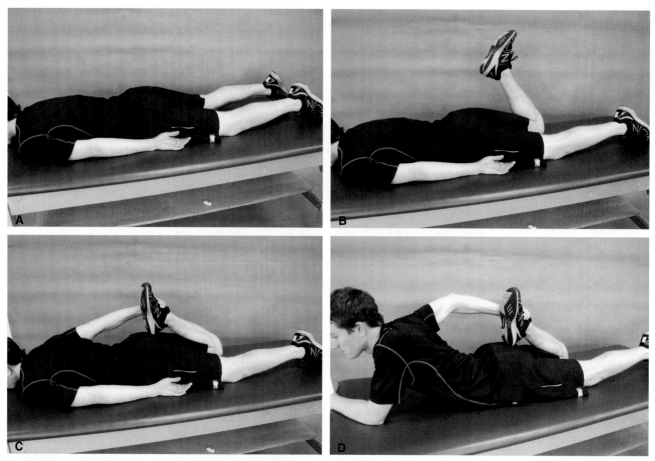

FIGURE 19–16 (A–D) The four positions of the lumbar plexus glide.

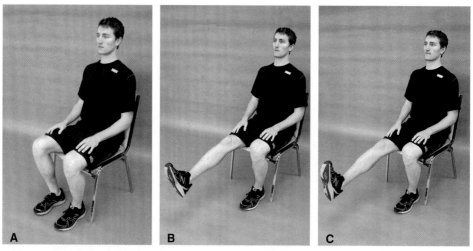

FIGURE 19–17 (A–C) The three positions of the sacral plexus glide.

the sciatic nerve. The upper four posterior divisions (L4-S2) join to form the common peroneal nerve. The anterior divisions form the tibial nerve. In the thigh, the peroneal and tibial nerves are fused as the sciatic nerve. To glide the sciatic, tibial, and common peroneal nerves, the starting position is sitting in a firm chair with the hands on the thighs, feet on the ground, and a lumbar roll supporting the low back. The involved knee is extended (position 2). In position three, the knee is maintained in extension while the ankle is actively dorsiflexed. The position that marks the beginning of neurological symptoms should be held for 10 seconds. The leg is then slowly brought back to the starting position.

SUMMARY AND CONCLUSIONS

In summary, neurodynamic testing and neural gliding are two important components of the neurological evaluation and clinical intervention approach, respectively. Neural tissue, like ligament, tendon, and muscle, is subject to postinjury, acute-phase cellular inflammatory response. This response eventually leads to scarring and real or apparent connective tissue passive insufficiency. Neurodynamic testing, when coupled with the neurological assessment and correlation with radiograph and electrodiagnostic testing, allows the therapist to develop a hypothesis, specifically, as

to which nerves are involved in the pathology. Neurodynamic testing also directs the therapist in clinical treatment program development and offers feedback as to progress. Neural gliding is a therapeutic modality that enables the therapist and patient to gradually mobilize and lengthen shortened neural and peri-neural structures. As such, these procedures, when indicated, should be included within the armamentarium of the manual physical therapist. Additional research is needed in vivo and in vitro at the histological, histochemical, and clinical levels to better objectify neurodynamic testing and to determine outcome standards for neural gliding techniques.

CLINICAL CASE

D.C. is a 52-year-old heating, ventilation, and air-conditioning mechanic. Eighteen months ago, he was involved in an explosion at work. The explosion caused his right (dominant) arm to violently horizontally abduct and externally rotate. Radiographs in the emergency department were consistent with an anterior dislocation of the right glenohumeral joint, a mid-shaft fracture of the right clavicle, and a concussion. Physical examination at the time revealed the aforementioned dislocation and fractures along with significant sensory and motor loss in the right C5-T1 myotomes and dermatomes. He was treated with closed reduction of the glenohumeral dislocation and a figure eight clavicular strapping. He was given a sling to wear for 3 weeks and scheduled for electrodiagnostic testing.

The electroneuromyograph was consistent with a motor and sensory neuropraxia of the C5-T1 nerve roots. Based upon the neuropraxic findings, the patient was told his prognosis was good for a complete recovery. He received outpatient physical therapy for gentle active assisted range of motion (AAROM) and motor facilitation techniques.

After 6 months, there was little improvement in strength or sensation. MMT revealed 2/5 proximal strength to 1/5 distal strength. Functionally, the patient had limited use of his right arm and was using only the left arm for daily activities. He was developing shoulder pain from capsular laxity owing to the dependent arm weight. He was not able to return to work. He had his car modified to allow left-hand driving. The electroneuromyograph now revealed denervation potentials in the C5-T1 myotomes. The decision was made to perform a supraclavicular dissection of the brachial plexus to identify any impediments to reinnervation.

The surgery reveled gross extraneural scarring of the entire brachial plexus with attachment of the plexus to the first rib, scalene muscles, and subclavian artery. The brachial plexus was carefully dissected free. Physical therapy was ordered postoperatively for brachial plexus gliding exercises.

Clinical Examination Questions

1. Postoperatively, on which nerves should the clinician perform upper limb neurodynamic testing?
2. Since there was involvement of the subclavian artery, how should the clinician assess arterial function?

3. Would the clinician expect hypo- or hyperactive deep tendon reflexes in the involved limb? In the contralateral limb?
4. What are the implications of 2/5 scapular muscle strength on glenohumeral stability and function?

Clinical Intervention Questions

1. For which nerves should the clinician teach nerve gliding exercises?
2. In which position should the patient perform these exercises?

3. Practice explaining to a partner the frequency, duration, and precautions for performing these exercises.

Advanced Clinical Decision-Making

1. If the patient has more than 3/5 strength in the involved upper extremity, how should the therapist counsel the patient to do the exercises at home?

2. The patient reports postoperative loss of bladder function. Is this a concern, and if so, why?

HANDS-ON

With a partner, perform the following activities:

1 Practice performing the major nerve glides as described in this chapter.

2 Practice teaching your partner how to perform the nerve glides described in this chapter.

3 List the expected symptoms that may be produced when performing nerve glides. List expected symptoms produced by non-neural contractile tissue stretch. How would you make the determination clinically between a positive test of neural tension versus a negative test?

4 List five possible etiologies of neuropathy.

REFERENCES

1. Ganong WF. *Review of Medical Physiology*. Los Altos, NM: Lange Medical; 1977.
2. Thomas PK, Olson Y. Microscopic anatomy and the function of the connective tissue components of the peripheral nerve. In: Dyck PJ, Thomas PK, Lambert EH, Bunge R, eds. *Peripheral Neuropathy*. 2nd ed. Philadelphia, PA: Saunders; 2001:128-143.
3. Millesi H. The nerve gap: theory and clinical practices. *Hand Clin*. 1986;4:651-663.
4. Sunderland S. *Nerve and Nerve Injuries*. Baltimore, MD: Williams & Wilkins; 1986.
5. Stolinski C. Structure and composition of the outer connective tissue sheaths of the peripheral nerve. *J Anat*. 1995;186:123-130.
6. Lundborg G. Nerve Injury and Repair. Edinburgh, Scotland: Churchill Livingstone; 1988.
7. Thomas PK. The connective tissue of a peripheral nerve; an electron microscope study. *J Anat*. 1963;97:35-44.
8. Gamble HJ, Eames RA. An electron microscope study of the connective tissues of human peripheral nerve. *J Anat*. 1964;98:655-663.
9. Dommisse GF. The blood supply of the spinal cord. In: Grieve GP, ed. *Modern Manual Therapy of the Vertebral Column*. Edinburgh, Scotland: Churchill Livingstone; 1986:44-92.
10. Lundborg G, Dahlin LB. Anatomy, function and pathophysiology of peripheral nerve and nerve compression. *Hand Clin*. 1996;12:185-193.
11. Appenzeller O, Dithal KK, Dowan T, Burnstock G. The nerves to blood vessels supplying blood nerves; the innervation of the vaso nervorum. *Brain Res*. 1984;304:383-386.
12. Yudkin JS, Kumari M, Humphries SE, Mohamed-Ali V. Inflammation, obesity, stress and coronary artery heart diseases, is interleukin-6 the link? *Atherosclerosis*. 2001;48:209-214.
13. Schall TJ. Biology of the RANTES/SIS cytokine family. *Cytokine*. 1991;3:1-18.
14. Xing Z, Jordana M, Kirpalani H, et al. Cytokine expression by neutrophils and macrophages in vivo; endotoxin induces TNF alpha, macrophage inflammatory protein-2, interleukin-1 beta, and interleukin-6, but not RANTES or transforming growth factor β1 mRNAs expression in lung inflammation. *Am J Respir Cell Mol Biol*. 1994;10:148-153.
15. Ruminy P, Gangneux C, Claeyssens S, et al. Gene transcription in hepatocytes during the acute phase of a systemic inflammation: from transcription factors to target organ. *Inflamm Res*. 2001;50:383-390.
16. Al-Shatti T, Barr AE, Safadi FF, Amin M, Barbe MF. Increase in inflammatory cytokines I median nerves in a rat model of repetitive motion injury. *J Neuroimmunol*. 2005;167:13-22.
17. Clark BD, Al-Shatti TA, Barr AE, Amin M, Barbe MF. Performance of a high-repetition, high-force task induces carpal tunnel syndrome in rats. *J Orthop Sports Phys Ther*. 2004;34:244-253.
18. Scuderi S, Gift TE. Thiothixene induced edema. *Psychiatr Med*. 1986;4:249-252.
19. Barr ML, Hamilton JD. A quantitative study of certain morphological changes in spinal motor neurons during axon reaction. *J Comp Neurol*. 1999;89:93-121.
20. Brattgard SO, Edstrom JE, Hyden H. The productive capacity of the neuron in retrograde reaction. *Exp Cell Res*. (suppl):1958;1:85.
21. Ducker TB, Kaufman FC. Metabolic factors in the surgery of peripheral nerves. *Clin Neurosurg*. 1977;24:406-424.
22. Seddon HJ. Three types of nerve injury. *Brain*. 1943;66:237.
23. Sunderland S. The relative susceptibility to injury of the medial and lateral popliteal divisions of the sciatic nerve. *Br J Surg*. 1953;41:51-64.
24. Blau JN, Critchley M, Gilliat RW, et al. Ergotamine tartrate overdosage. *Br Med J*. 1979;6158:265-266.
25. Aitken JT, Thomas PK. Retrograde changes in fiber size following nerve section. *J Anat*. 1962;96:121-129.
26. Sunderland S. Rate of regeneration in human peripheral nerves. *Arch Neurol Psychiatry*. 1947;58:251-295.
27. Horsch KW. Central responses of cutaneous neurons to peripheral nerve crush in the cat. *Brain Res*. 1978;151:581-586.
28. Zalewski A. Effects of neuromuscular reinnervation on denervated skeletal muscle by axons of motor, sensory and sympathetic neurons. *Am J Physiol*. 1970;219:1675-1679.
29. Hubbard IJ. *The Peripheral Nervous System*. New York: Plenum, 1974.
30. Rydevik B, Lundborg G, Bagg U. Effects of graded compression on intraneural blood flow. *J Hand Surg*. 1981;6:3-12.
31. Denny-Brown D. Clinical problems in neuromuscular physiology. *Am J Med*. 1953;15:368.
32. Ochs S, Pourmand R, Si K, Friedman RN. Stretch of mammalian nerve in vitro: effect on compound action potential. *J Peripheral Nerve*. 2000;5:227-235.
33. Lundborg G, Rydevik B. Effects of stretching the tibial nerve of the rabbit. A preliminary study of the intraneural circulation and barrier function of the perineurium. *J Bone Joint Surg*. 1973;55B:3390-3401.
34. Haftek J. Stretch injury to peripheral nerves. Acute effects of stretching rabbit nerve. *J Bone Joint Surg*. 1970;52B:354.
35. Dyck PJ, Giannini C. Pathological alterations in diabetic neuropathies of humans: a review. *J Neruoathol Exp Neruol*. 1996;55:1181-1193.
36. Cornefjord M, Sato K, Olmarker K, Rydevik B, Nordborg CA. Model for chronic nerve root compression studies. Presentation of a porcine model for controlled, slow-onset compression with analyses of anatomic aspects, compression onset rate, and morphological and neurophysiologic effects. *Spine*. 1997;22:946-957.
37. Barr AE, Safadi FF, Garvin RP, Popoff SN, Barbe MF. Evidence of progressive tissue pathophysiology and motor behavior degradation in rat model of work related musculoskeletal disease. In: *Proceedings of the IEA/HFES Congress*; San Diego, CA. 2000.
38. Rydevik B, Lundborg G, Myrhage R. The vascularization of human flexor tendons within the digital synovial sheath region-structural and functional aspects. *J Hand Surg Am*. 1977;6:417-427.

39. Lundborg G, Nordborg C, Rydevik B, Olsson Y. The effect of ischemia and the permeability of the perineurium to protein tracers in rabbit and tibial nerve. 1973;49:287-294.

40. Widerberg A, Lundborg G, Dahlin LB. Nerve regeneration enhancement by tourniquet. *J Hand Surg Br*. 2001;26:347-351.

41. Rosen B, Lundborg G. The long term recovery curve in adults after median or ulnar nerve repair: a reference interval. *J Hand Surg Br*. 2001;26: 196-200.

42. Ogata K, Naito M. Blood flow of the peripheral nerve effects of dissection, stretching and compression. *J Hand Surg Br*. 1986;18:149-155.

43. Mizisin AP, Weerasuriya A. Homestatic regulation of the endoneural microenvironment during development, aging, and in response to trauma, disease and toxic insult. *Acta Neuropathol*. 2010;14:291-312.

44. Barr AE, Barbe MF. Pathophysiology tissue changes associated with repetitive movement: a review of the evidence. *Phys Ther*. 2002;82:173-187.

45. Barbe MF, Barr AE, Gorzelany I, et al. Chronic repetitive reaching and grasping results in decreased motor performance and widespread tissue responses in a rat model of MSD. *J Ortho Res*. 2003;21:167-176.

46. Barr AE, Safadi FF, Gorzelany I, et al. Repetitive, negligible force reaching in rats induces pathological overloading of upper extremity bones. *J Bone Miner Res*. 2003;18:2023-2032.

47. Dubner R, Ruda MA. Activity dependent neuronal plasticity following tissue injury and inflammation. *Trends Neurosci*. 1992;15:154-161.

48. Sakai H, Fujita K, Sakai Y, Mizumo K. Immunolocalization of cytokines and growth factors in subacromial bursa of rotator cuff tear patients. *Kobe J Med Sci*. 2001;47:25-34.

49. Levin KH, Wilbourn AJ, Jones HR. Childhood peroneal neuropathy from bone tumors. *Pediatr Neurol*. 1991;4:308-309.

50. Richardson JK. The clinical identification of peripheral neuropathy among older persons. *Arch Phys Med*. 2002;83:1553-1558.

51. Hadden RDM, Cornblath DR, Hughes RAC, et al. Electrophysiological classification of Guillain Barre syndrome: clinical associations and outcomes. *Ann Neurol*. 1998;44:780-788.

52. Kyle RA, Pease GI. Hematologic aspects of arsenic intoxication presenting as Guillain-Barre Syndrome. *N Engl J Med*. 1965;273:218.

53. Selander S, Cramer K. Interrelationships between lead in blood, lead in urine and AKA in urine during lead work. *Br J Ind Med*. 1970;27:28-39.

54. Victor M. Polyneuropathy due to nutritional deficiency and alcoholism. In: Dyck PJ, Thomas PK, Lambert EG, eds. *Peripheral Neuropathy*. Philadelphia, PA: WB Saunders; 1975:1030-1066.

55. Layzer RB, Fishman RA, Schafer JA. Neuropathy following abuse of nitrous oxide. *Neurology*. 1978;28:504-506.

56. Lovelace RE, Horwitz SJ. Peripheral neuropathy in long-term diphenyl-hydantoin therapy. *Arch Neurol*. 1968;18:69-77.

57. Seidberg BH, Sullivan TH. Dentists' use, misuse, abuse or dependence of mood-altering substances. *NY State Dent J*. 2004;70:30-33.

58. Seppalainen AM, Husman K, Martenson C. Neurophysiological effects of long-term exposure to a mixture of organic solvents. *Scand J Work Environ Health*. 1978;4:304-314.

59. Molloy DW, Standish TI. Guide to the standardized Mini-Mental State Examination. *Int Psychogeriatr*. 1997;9(Suppl)1:87-94.

60. Mathias CJ. Autonomic disorders and their recognition. *N Engl J Med*. 1997;36:721-724.

61. Cyriax J. *Textbook of Orthopaedic Medicine*. Vol. 1. *Diagnosis of Soft Tissue Lesions*. London, UK: Balliere Tindall; 1978.

62. Kendall FP, McCreary EK. *Muscles Testing and Function*. Philadelphia, PA: Williams & Wilkins; 1983.

63. Hales M, Bottles K, Miller T, Donegan E, Lhung BM. Diagnosis of Kaposi's sarcoma by fine needle aspiration biopsy. *Am J Clin Pathol*. 1987;88:20-25.

64. Theander E, Andersson SI, Manthorpe R, Jacobsson LT. Proposed core set of outcome measures in patients with primary Sjogren's syndrome: 5 year follow-up. *J Rheumatol*. 2005;32:1495-1502.

65. Bonofioli AA, Orefice F. Sarcoidosis. *Semin Opthalmol*. 2005;20:177-182.

66. Calvin WH, Devor M, Howe JF. Can neuralgias arise from minor demyelination? Spontaneous firing, mechanosensitivy and afterdischarge from conducting axons. *Exp Neurol*. 1982;75:755-763.

67. Copieters MW, Stapaerts KH, Everaert DG, Staes FF. Addition of test components during neurodynamic testing: effect of ROM and sensory responses. *J Orthop Sports Phys Ther*. 2001;31:226-237.

68. Elvey RL. Painful restriction of shoulder movement: a clinical observational study. In: *Proceedings, Disorders of the Knee, Ankle and Shoulder*. Perth, Australia: Western Australian Institute of Technology; 1979.

69. Elvey RL, Quintner JL, Thoma AN. A clinical study of RSI. *Aust Fam Physician*. 1986;15:1314-1322.

70. Elvey RL. Treatment of arm pain associated with abnormal brachial plexus tension. *Aust J Physiother*. 1986;32:224-229.

71. Keneally M. The upper limb tension test. In: *Proceedings, Manipulative Therapists Association of Australia, 4th Biennial Conference*. Brisbane, Australia; 1985.

72. Totten PA, Hunter JM. Therapeutic techniques to enhance nerve gliding in thoracic outlet and carpal tunnel syndromes. *Hand Clin*. 1991;7:505-510.

73. Pechan JL. Ulnar nerve maneuver as a diagnostic aid in pressure lesions in the cubital region. *Czechoslovakia Neuroligie*. 1973;36:13-19.

74. Elvey R. Brachial plexus tension tests and the patho-anatomical origin of arm pain. In: Idczak R, ed. *Aspects of Manipulative Therapy, Proceedings of a Multidisciplinary International Conference on Manipulative Therapy*. Melbourne, Australia: Churchill Livingstone; 1979:105-110.

75. George SZ. Characteristic of patients with lower extremity symptoms treated with slump stretching: a case series. *J Orthop Sports Phys Ther*. 1998;32:39-42.

76. Turl SE, George KP. Adverse neural tension: a factor in repetitive hamstring strain? *J Orthop Sports Phys Ther*. 1998;27:16-20.

77. Coppieters M, Stappaerts K, Janssens K. Reliability and detecting 'onset of pain' and 'submaximal pain' during neural provocation testing of the upper quadrant. *Phys Res Int*. 2002;7:34-42.

78. Wartenberg R. The signs of Brudzinski and of Kernig. *J Pediatr*. 1950;37:679-684.

79. Troup JDG. Straight leg raising (SLR) and the qualifying tests for increased root tension. *Spine*. 1986:5;526-527.

80. Breig A, Troup JG. Biomechanical considerations in the straight leg-raising test. *Spine*. 1979;4:242-250.

81. Magee DT. *Orthopedic Physical Assessment*. St. Louis, MO: Elvesier Saunders; 2006.

82. McNabb I. *Backache*. Baltimore, MD: Williams & Wilkins; 1977.

83. Estridge MN, Rouhe SA, Johnson NG. The femoral stretching test. A valuable sign in diagnosing upper lumber disc herniations. *J Neurosurg*. 1982;57:813-817.

84. Koury MJ, Scarpelli E. A manual approach to evaluation and treatment of a patient with a chronic lumbar nerve root irritation. *Phys Ther*. 1994;74:548-560.

85. Roos DB. Historical perspectives and anatomical considerations. Thoracic outlet syndrome. *Semin Thorac Cardiovasc Surg*. 1996;8:183-189.

86. Toomingas A, Hagberg M, Jorulf L, et al. Outcome of the abduction external rotation test among manual and office workers. *Am J Ind Med*. 1991;19:214-227.

87. Dick JP. The deep tendon and abdominal reflexes. *J Neurol Neurosurg Psychiatry*. 2003;74:150-153.

88. Wilkins RH, Brody IA. Tinel's sign. *Arch Neurol*. 1971;24:573-575.

89. Katz JN, Larson MG, Subra A. The carpal tunnel syndrome: diagnostic utility of the history and physical findings. *Ann Intern Med*. 1990;112:321-327.

90. Tinetti ME, Liu WL, Claus EB. Predictors and prognosis of inability to get up after falls among elderly persons. *JAMA*. 1993;269:65-70.

91. Mathias S, Nayak US, Isaacs B. Balance in elderly patients: the "get up and go" test. *Arch Phys Med Rehabil*. 1986;67:387-389.

92. Harada N, Chiu V, Damron-Rodriguez J, et al. Screening for balance and mobility impairment in elderly individuals living in residential care facilities. *Phys Ther*. 1995;6:462-469.

93. Iverson BD, Grossman MR, Shaddeau SA, Turner ME. Balance performance force production and activity levels in noninstitutionalized men 60–90 years of age. *Phys Ther*. 1990;70:348-355.

94. Heitman DK, Gosman MR, Shaddeau SA, Jackson JR. Balance performance and step width in noninsitutionalized elderly, female fallers and nonfallers. *Phys Ther*. 1989;11:923-931.

95. Briggs RC, Gossman MR, Birch R, Drews JE, Shaddeau SA. Balance performance among noninsitutionalized elderly women. *Phys Ther*. 1989;69:748-756.

96. Cornblath DR, Chaudhry V. Electrodiagnostics and the peripheral neuropathy patient. In: Mendel JR, Kissel JT, Cornblath DR, eds. *Diagnosis and Management of Peripheral Nerve Disorders*. New York, NY: Oxford University Press; 2001.

97. McClellan DL, Swash M. Longitudinal sliding of the median nerve during movements of the upper limb. *J Neurol Neurosurg Psychiatr*. 1976;39: 566-569.

98. Shaw WE, Wilgis EF, Murphy R. The significance of longitudinal excursion in peripheral nerves. *Hand Clin*. 1986;2:761-766.

The Feldenkrais Method of Somatic Education

Jim Stephens, PhD, PT, CFP

Chapter Objectives

At the conclusion of this chapter, the reader will be able to:

- Identify the key factors that led to the development of the Feldenkrais method.
- Describe the key philosophical tenants of the Feldenkrais method.
- Define what constitutes normal motion and appreciate methods, within this paradigm, that might be used to restore normal motion.

- Understand the application of this paradigm to clinical physical therapy through appreciating key aspects of examination and intervention.
- Apply principles of the Feldenkrais method to clinical physical therapy.

HISTORICAL PERSPECTIVES
Moshe Feldenkrais's Life and Work

Moshe Feldenkrais was an eclectic thinker who incorporated a variety of disciplines into a method of thinking and acting in relation to the development and restoration of human function. These approaches included gestalt psychology,[1] progressive relaxation,[2] bioenergetics,[3] sensory awareness,[4] the hypnosis of Milton Erickson,[5] an ecological perspective on the mind[6] and human perception,[7] and the physiologic studies of Sherrington, Magnus, Pavlov, Fulton, and Schilder.[8]

Feldenkrais was born in Russia in 1904. At the age of 14, he traveled to Palestine, where he later developed a form of hand-to-hand combat that was used by the settlers for self-defense. He described these techniques in his book *Ju-Jitsu and Self Defense*, which was published in 1929.[9]

Feldenkrais studied mechanical and electrical engineering and physics in Paris in the late 1920s. During this time, he also studied the works of Freud and Coue. In 1930, he published a translation with commentary of Coue's work *Autosuggestion*. He met *Jigaro Kano,* originator of judo, in Paris and became the first European trained to the level of black belt in judo.[9] As an athlete, he played soccer with a French club and tore the meniscus of his left knee. His observations of how he learned

to walk and move without pain led to the development of his theories related to the role of awareness in restoring function.[8]

Feldenkrais spent World War II in England working to develop antisubmarine technology and continuing to study judo. He taught judo classes to his fellow engineers. This formed the beginning of his thinking about what later became known as awareness through movement.[10] During this time, he wrote several volumes on judo.[11,12] After World War II, he continued his study of psychology and neuroscience and learned about

Box 20-1 THE FELDENKRAIS METHOD

The Feldenkrais Method incorporates:
- Gestalt psychology
- Progressive relaxation
- Bioenergetics
- Sensory awareness
- Erickson hypnosis
- Ecological perspective on the mind
- Human perception
- Physiological concepts of Sherrington, Magnus, Pavlov, Fulton, and Schilder

the work of Alexander, Gindler, and Gurdieff, all of whom emphasized the importance of cultivating self-awareness for the purposes of personal and professional development. This wide-ranging study led to his publication of ***Body and Mature Behavior.*** [10,13] This book was his first attempt at the expression of the philosophy, science, and experience that provided the foundation for his evolving paradigm.

Feldenkrais returned to Israel and began teaching a small group of students about his work.[14] This training lasted for 3 years and became the foundation for his first American teaching in San Francisco in 1975. Another training began in the United States in 1981, but Feldenkrais died before it was finished. Students from Israel and San Francisco finished that training and have continued his work, forming the ***Feldenkrais Guild of North America*** and a number of other professional organizations around the world.

NOTABLE QUOTABLE

Philosophical and Theoretical Basis

"The human brain is such as to make . . . acquisition of new responses a normal and suitable activity. . . . The active pattern of doing is, therefore, essentially personal. This great ability to form individual nervous paths and muscular patterns makes it possible for faulty patterns to be learned. . . . The faulty behavior will appear in the executive motor mechanisms, which will seem later . . . to be inherent in the person and unalterable. It will remain largely so unless the nervous paths producing the undesirable pattern of motility are undone and reshuffled into a better configuration."

Moshe Feldenkrais, 1949

PHILOSOPHICAL FRAMEWORK
Central Theme

The central idea of Feldenkrais's work is that, as humans, the capacity to learn is inherent in our nervous systems. This capacity is physical as well as intellectual. It is through this process of physical learning that we are able to make adjustments and adaptations that allow us to move more effectively and to overcome obstacles such as fear, pain, injury, and disability, both physically and psychologically. Awareness of how actions are and can be performed in different ways is the key to this process. It is the process of finding new ways of doing familiar actions that is the transformational element of this approach.

To Feldenkrais, maturity meant that a person would live in his or her physical and psychological reality of the moment and bring to bear on present circumstances only those past experiences that would be useful.[13] Part of this understanding was borrowed from two concepts central to judo: (1) *posture from which a person could initiate movement in any direction with equal ease and without preliminary adjustments* and (2) *performance of movements with the minimal amount of effort and maximum efficiency.* These conditions would create a relaxed state of

Box 20-2 THE FELDENKRAIS METHOD'S CENTRAL THEME

- The capacity to learn is inherent in our nervous systems.
- This capacity is physical as well as intellectual.
- It is through a process of physical learning that we are able to make adjustments and adaptations in our lives.
- These adaptations allow us to move more effectively and to overcome obstacles such as fear, pain, injury, and disability both physically and psychologically.
- Awareness of how actions can be performed in different ways is the key to this process. The primary objective is to find new ways of doing familiar actions.

readiness, which would allow good recovery from any kind of challenge or trauma. This process relies on a well-developed kinesthetic sense, which is also necessary for learning, and a clear intention for action.

CLINICAL PILLAR

- What starting posture may be considered ideal for allowing the initiation of movement without requiring adjustment for the following activities: (1) sit to stand, (2) kneeling to stand, (3) stepping up a curb, (4) throwing a ball, (5) looking behind while sitting, (6) initiation of gait.
- Perform the activities just described in a manner that requires the minimal amount of effort with maximum efficiency. Perform each activity several times, making minor adjustments in your performance until the minimal amount of effort is used.

Definitions of Learning

Learning is defined as an organic process in which the mental and physical aspects are fully integrated. It proceeds at its own pace; is completely individualized, and is guided by the perception of an action occurring with greater ease. It occurs most readily in short, focused intervals of attention and when the learner is in a good mood. The outcome of this process is the development of self-knowledge and the awareness of how we do an action. "Learning is the acquisition of the skill to inhibit parasitic action (components of the action which are unrelated to the intention of the action resulting from some secondary intention) and the ability to direct clear motivations as a result of self-knowledge."[15] Initially, when learning a new skill, many components of movement interfere with the overall intention of the new skill. One by one the parasitic movements are eliminated, leaving only the essential, differentiated action. This learning is different from training, practice, or exercise. It involves the search to discover new ways to do activities that one already knows how to do.[16]

This description of learning has many similarities to the early, coordination stage of motor learning described by Newell and the stages of learning described by Bernstein.[17] Bernstein suggested that learning a new pattern of coordinated movement first involved freezing degrees of freedom, then step-by-step releasing degrees of freedom to allow appropriate and effective movements, and finally incorporating inertial forces from other moving segments of the body and reactive forces in the environment into the control process. Available patterns of movement that are well learned have been defined as **attractors**. With learning (i.e., skill development), the attractor dynamics change, usually in the direction of becoming more simplified or unified.[18]

Over the course of development, there is a broadening of the repertoire of behavior to give multiple options for doing any particular activity. Children develop this capacity naturally. Each person learns to satisfy basic needs in his or her own individual way.[15] Adult intervention in life experience may interfere with the child's process of organic learning, limiting the development of skill in acquiring multiple options for performing any activity. Feldenkrais believed that anxiety would be produced when our options were removed without alternative ways of acting.[13]

QUESTIONS *for* REFLECTION

- How is learning defined within the Feldenkrais paradigm?
- What is the expected outcome of learning?
- How does learning differ from training, practice, or exercise?
- What are the ways in which one can demonstrate that motor learning has occurred?
- What are the primary obstacles to the process of individualized motor learning?

Feldenkrais clearly conceived of the process of learning as producing new pathways, associations, and connections in the central nervous system. The various patterns of innervation involved in the control of voluntary movement develop as the control of action is being learned. Thus, the control of movement is integrated into what Feldenkrais called the, "vast background of vegetative and reflexive activity of the nervous system."[13] The imposition of anxiety, compulsion, or cross-motivation on this process of learning created what Feldenkrais called "faulty learning." The child learned to produce the behavior that was expected, the posture that was approved of, the expression that was acceptable, or learned to fear the outcome of an action and did not learn to test behavior against present reality. This kind of behavior is commonly observed in many people who act in protective ways, as if they were in danger, without testing the reality of their perception. In the adult, habitual patterns that were formed over years have molded the body to produce, for example, flat feet, stiff shoulders, a neck that won't turn, or a painful low back. Feldenkrais suggested that the problem may not be in the region of symptoms but rather the result of parasitic neuromuscular patterns that have been formed in conjunction with the loss of ability to adapt to new situations by learning.[13]

Interaction With History of Injury and Pathology

Later in his career, Feldenkrais recognized that physical injury and malfunction of the nervous system interacted significantly with the process of neuromuscular habit formation. If the nervous system does not work properly in its motor, sensory, or integrative/cognitive components, it becomes difficult or impossible to produce the normal functional control patterns used in everyday life. A musculoskeletal injury creates pain and interferes with normal function. A person who possesses rigid and maladaptive neuromuscular patterns is more likely to be injured and less likely to recover from injury.[8]

PRINCIPLES OF EXAMINATION AND INTERVENTION
The Subjective Examination

The examination begins with a conversation regarding the client's primary complaints. The practitioner asks the client to describe the nature of the concern, when he or she first experienced it, and information about the history of this issue. The practitioner inquires about what the client does during a normal day, what movements and functions are limited, and how these limitations affect performance of work, family, and leisure activities. The practitioner inquires about beliefs and attitudes concerning any limitations related to the condition. The practitioner asks the client what he or she would like to improve or perform more effectively and discusses the client's goals for the intervention. It is also important for the therapist to ascertain a description of pain and its intensity as well as any limitations in joint or whole body mobility.

The Objective Examination

The physical examination covers three primary areas: postural configuration and control, control and differentiation of movement intersegmentally and in relation to the environment, and the effort required to maintain posture and control movement. To ascertain this information, the therapist observes both static postures and normal active movements. Frequently, less common movements, such as lateral or diagonal tilting of the pelvis in a sitting position or a full turn of the body to look behind while the feet remain fixed, are used to assess the integration of the trunk and pelvis into movements of the whole body.

The physical examination includes the following:

- Assessment of postural configuration and control
- Control and differentiation of movement intersegmentally and in relation to the environment
- Identification of the amount of effort that goes into maintaining posture and controlling movement

Postural assessment focuses on understanding the ability of an individual to use the skeleton in relation to gravity and support surfaces in the context of the task being performed. The skeleton is thought to possess two main functions: resisting gravity and providing surface attachments and articulations for the muscles to execute movement. The therapist must consider whether or not skeletal structures are in proper alignment such that gravitational forces are translated optimally through the bones and joints for the purpose of minimizing the amount of muscular work required. In addition, a consideration of whether or not the support surface is being fully and effectively appreciated and used must be done. It is important to determine if the mass of the body is being projected through the skeleton into the support surface as compared to being held away from the support surface by increased muscular effort. Is the mass of the body being maintained within the base of support in an efficient manner? Feldenkrais recognized that posture is a dynamic neuromuscular state that allows a person to be prepared for action. He coined the term **acture** to describe this state.[15] The concept of acture raises the question of whether the current posture provides the person with the most efficient base from which to initiate any action.

Acture: A term that recognizes that posture is a dynamic neuromuscular state that allows a person to be prepared for action. This concept raises the question of whether the current posture provides the person with the most efficient base from which to initiate any action.

Questions used when assessing posture include the following:

- Are the bones maintained in an alignment, in any position, such that gravitational forces are translated optimally through the bones to minimize amount of muscular work is required?
- Is the support surface being fully and effectively appreciated and utilized?

- Is the mass of the body being projected through the skeleton into the support surface as compared to being held away from the support surface by increased muscular effort?
- Is the mass of the body being maintained within the base of support is an efficient manner?

Assessment of *movement control* has several dimensions, including differentiation and integration, coordination, and completeness of body image. The therapist must assess whether movements are fully *differentiated*. A person may be able to elevate the shoulder independently but when raising the arm, he or she may habitually elevate the scapula, demonstrating a lack of motion differentiation. Conversely, a person may be able to extend the neck and extend the back independently, but when the person looks overhead, he or she may extend only the back or the neck, and the other area may remain rigid. This movement pattern demonstrates a lack of *integration*. This approach recognizes that patterns of movement that distribute force over a greater number of segments are considered to be more biomechanically efficient than others and, therefore, are more desirable for effective function.

Assessment of *coordination* is designed to determine smoothness of control. The therapist seeks to determine if changes in position and velocity are smoothly controlled. Deficits in motion quality can be observed and felt and suggest a control process that is inefficient in relation to the intended movement. The therapist also determines whether the movement is reversible at any point along its trajectory. Such movement is possible as long as the velocity is not too great and the mass has not moved outside of the base of support.

Finally, the therapist considers the individual's ability to perceive a complete and accurate body image. Individuals who have major perceptual deficits from a stroke or other pathology may have deficits in perception of their body image. Feldenkrais proposed that faulty learning may also create gaps in internal body image. The proprioceptive image that Gallagher[19] demonstrated is the basis for automatic, spontaneous movement. These gaps create blank spots in our awareness of our body and simultaneously a reduction in the quality of motor control. Feldenkrais advocated enhancement in the awareness of the movement control processes of the body and in the position and motion of the body in its surrounding environment.

- Define the terms *differentiation, integration, and coordination.*
- In what ways might deficits in these three aspects of movement lead to impairment?
- How would deficits in these three features be identified and subsequently corrected?
- Discuss the value of assessing effort as it relates to movement and why less effort is deemed to be optimal?

The *effort* used to produce posture and movement is also assessed. This is done in several ways. Areas of muscle that are excessively contracted or habitually hyperactive are identified. These muscles can be palpated and occasionally observed. These may be muscles that are contracting unnecessarily in relation to the intended action. Feldenkrais identified such actions as *parasitic activity*.[13] The therapist should ask if the postural configurations, or underlying acture,[13] are effectively supporting the intended movement and whether inertial forces and momentum have become effectively integrated into the process of control. If they have not been integrated, there will be excessive muscular contraction required to direct force and produce stability. These forces may be unbalanced across joints and lead to the development of pain syndromes. The pain syndrome may be addressed by simply changing the motor control process/biomechanics. Another, more subtle area of effort is in relation to breathing. Feldenkrais proposed that normal motor control should be accompanied by continuous regular breathing, the rate and volume of which should be appropriately related to the level of muscular work that is occurring. It is not unusual for people to stop breathing or breath in very irregular ways when making excessive efforts or when engaged in cognitively challenging, attention-demanding activities. Irregular breathing is considered to be another indication that the motor control process is not being fully integrated.

Analytical Assessment and Documentation of Findings

Postural findings are documented in traditional ways in terms of alignment but also in terms of the appropriateness of a particular posture to support the intended movement that emerges from it. The position of the center of mass in relation to the base of support is noted. Joint position in relation to the flow of force through the skeleton and the muscular effort involved in an activity are also noted. The smoothness and ease of movement is described, and the presence of limitations of differentiation or integration of active movements, as described above, are also documented. Judgments related to completeness of body image may be documented, along with a description of excessive muscle contraction or parasitic activity. These findings are often communicated in relation to specific postural configurations (sitting, lying, supine) or activities (walking, running). Abnormal control of breathing may also be documented in relation to these activities.

PRINCIPLES OF INTERVENTION
Principles and Definitions

Conceptually, both the examination and intervention engage the client and the practitioner into a unitary process of exploration. The goals of the intervention process, which have emerged in examination and discussion between the client and the practitioner, are broadly bringing specific limitations into awareness and exploring alternative strategies for organizing movement that might be the basis for improving function. Beyond the specific findings of the examination process, there

are two questions that guide the development of the intervention process: (1) What kind of exploratory process will be most useful? (2) In what areas can movement be used to develop awareness that will allow expanded function? In the Feldenkrais method, there are two approaches for developing the exploratory movement process. **Awareness through movement (ATM)** is a process in which the practitioner provides verbal guidance for the client to actively explore many facets of a movement, thereby discovering ways of doing things that may have never occurred to the client or a movement that he or she has not done for many years. Throughout ATM, the movement done by the client is entirely voluntary. The other style of developing the exploratory movement process is **functional integration (FI),** in which the practitioner uses his or her hands to produce gentle force vectors through the client's skeleton in a seemingly passive process. The client is asked to attend to sensory dimensions of this process and track the evolving movements using available kinesthetic and proprioceptive information. They may also be covertly following the movements produced by a very low-level active movement process or may be asked during the process to reproduce a movement or segment of movement just experienced.

Selection of Techniques

The decision of whether to use ATM or FI is made on the basis of which would provide the most useful experience for the client as a way toward expanding his or her awareness and function. The process may frequently begin with FI. Safety and comfort are the primary considerations. It must be determined if the client possesses adequate strength, endurance, and range of motion to assume or maintain a particular posture and if the client's awareness of his or her body is poor. If pain is an issue, it is often best to begin in a more neutral position like supine or side lying with the person supported for maximum comfort and relaxation. Functional Integration is a more general approach to exploration of muscle tone and control. Using this approach, it is possible to quickly explore a wide range of issues related to muscle activity and skeletal alignment. ATM

Box 20-3 TWO APPROACHES TO INTERVENTION

1. **Awareness Through Movement (ATM)** is a process in which the practitioner provides verbal guidance for the client to actively explore many facets of a movement. The client discovers ways of moving that may never have occurred to him or her or that the client may not have performed for many years. In ATM, the client's movement is entirely voluntary.

2. **Functional Integration (FI)** is a process in which the practitioner uses his or her hands to produce gentle force vectors through the client's skeleton in an apparently passive process. The client is asked to attend to sensory dimensions of this process and track the evolving movements.

requires the client to listen and translate verbal suggestions into active movement and postural control. The verbal guidance of the ATM process, while needing to be precise enough to provide proper guidance, is also intended to be somewhat vague to allow people to solve the movement impairment in a variety of ways and to identify the optimal solution more independently. Occasionally, this limited feedback leads to frustration and difficulty in executing the desired movement. Many people want to have precise instructions and to know that they are "doing it right." However, even with precise instructions, the client may be unable to perform the desired movements. Feldenkrais attributed this inability to a lack of refinement or understanding of one's body image.[13] For this reason, FI may be a more optimal place to begin.

Through FI, some progress may be made in changing the habitual patterns of muscle contraction and postural control, and a range of possibilities for movement may be opened up that did not previously exist. When this point is reached, a decision to begin using ATM may be made. An ATM lesson usually involves the exploration of a specific set of movements surrounding a specific movement problem. In a sitting pelvic clock lesson, for example, a person is asked to explore a range of movements of the pelvis and lumbar spine over the hip joints while maintaining upright posture of the trunk and fairly constant position of the head in space. While the process of learning specific movements is enhanced within the context of voluntary control, the principle of specificity suggests that generalization of motor learning and carry over to other types of movement is minimal.[17] Clinical observation suggests that changes in body image seem to "enable" a wide range of movements, which may not have been learned in the intervention but may have been part of an earlier movement repertoire. Thus, a series of ATM lessons may follow Functional Integration to optimize the learning in specific functional activities.

Application of Techniques
Functional Integration

FI is intended to simultaneously address the complexity of the nervous system linked to control of the muscles through the skeleton within an environment that has been developed by the client over a lifetime. Through this process, the client learns to inhibit muscular effort that may be unintended and interferes with intended movement, until an orderly, effective and more differentiated/integrated version of the movement emerges.[8]

Functional Integration is generally a one-on-one process with minimal verbal interaction between the client and practitioner so that the client's full attention may be available to the kinesthetic and proprioceptive information of the session. Initially, a reference movement or function is assessed related to the expressed goals for improvement of the client. This reference movement may be returned to several times over the course of the session. The client is then made to feel as comfortable as possible by supporting the body to reduce muscular effort in the position of choice, lying, sitting, or standing in some manner. The session begins with the gentle, noninvasive

exploration of the limits of joint motion and continues with slow small movements produced by the practitioner within each joint's neutral range. The intention for the practitioner is to discover limitations and obstacles that are skeletal or muscular in nature and to bring these into the awareness of the client experientially. The practitioner works by directing gentle forces through the skeleton either by pulling or pushing with the hands or by substituting support from outside for the excessive muscular effort made by the client. The intention is to discover the habitual organization of the client's neuromuscular control process. The practitioner will first go with movements that are habitual and then, as muscle tone reduces, begin to explore, in a nonjudgmental way, other potential movement patterns. Multiple repetitions of movements are made incorporating minor variations, not for the purpose of practice, but rather to allow the client's nervous system to sense different possibilities. Artificial constraints may be used, such as placing the client's palm on his or her forehead and rotating the head, thus invoking a less differentiated movement of turning the head by involving the shoulder and upper extremity. Muscles of the shoulder can then be more easily differentiated in the process of turning the head. The types of intervention that the practitioner employs are in turn exploratory, conforming, and finally leading, with the intention of providing a comfortable, nonthreatening environment and eventually to create new options for movement that can be both perceived and produced by the client. The practitioner may choose to provide the client with an ATM lesson to further consolidate these new movement patterns or allow the client to explore these new movement patterns within the context of daily functional activities.[8,20–22]

Awareness Through Movement

ATM is a verbally directed movement process that can be done with one person or in large groups, as space allows. ATM lessons may be found at www.OpenATM.com. Different people respond in very individualized ways to any particular lesson using the material of that lesson at a level that they can manage.[23] One of the skills of the practitioner is to select an appropriate level of any lesson as a starting point and then to progress to higher levels of function.

An ATM lesson is a structured movement exploration that makes use of common movement forms to explore how the individual organizes his control of movement. A lesson may be done in supine, prone, sitting, or standing and involves small turns, bends, or weight shifts. The client is instructed to move with minimal effort and remain in control of the intended movement. The attention of the client is directed to areas of the body where tension and effort may be elicited. The role of the practitioner is to recognize limitations and patterns of control and begin to explore the boundaries of the movement in a dynamic way within the capability of the client. This movement process is used to generate changes in posture and patterns of control that the client can sense and reproduce and eventually to discover more efficient and comfortable patterns of movement and posture to replace habitual patterns.

Slow, small, simple movements are performed first to reduce effort and optimize awareness. The **Weber-Fechner principle** in sensory physiology supports the idea that excessive effort interferes with our ability to detect small changes.[24] A lesson might begin with a very small movement involving external rotation of the hip with flexion of the knee in the supine position. This movement would be repeated in slightly different ways 10 to 20 times. During this process, awareness is directed to involvement of other areas of the body in this movement, such as rotation of the spine, noticing whether the opposite hip may be lifting from the floor, a change in the pattern of breathing, a stiffening of the opposite leg or foot, or pressing into the floor with the opposite leg. When this simple movement is performed most clearly and with the least effort, then the opposite leg will be fully relaxed and the spine able to turn as weight is transferred laterally. Other parts of the body would be free to move in other directions: turning or nodding of the head for example should be easy. If the client discovers that he or she is holding the leg or foot stiffly, holding his or her breath, or not experiencing rotation and weight shift through the pelvis and spine, then the client has discovered that he or she is performing parasitic activity that is extraneous to the desired movement.

The practitioner looks for how a client organizes weight through the skeleton in relation to the base of support and whether or not the use of the skeleton is optimal. Additional questions may include: How much effort does the client make to hold a position or to transition from it? Is the intention of the movement clear? Are all the body segments organized to participate appropriately in the intended movement, or is one leg possibly anchoring a different intention, thus making the movement less efficient and potentially dangerous? Is the timing of control of one body segment contributing optimally to the movement of others? The better that the client is able to reduce effort and discriminate small changes, the more precise he or she may be in controlling each action. This type of observation forms the basis of continual assessment that is performed during the process of ATM.

ATM lessons commonly make use of novelty. Lessons can be structured in such a way that the outcome of the movement (rolling over, standing up) may not be obvious during the process. This use of novelty allows the client to maintain better awareness of the details of the movement in progress without reverting back to habitual movement patterns. In this way, new patterns of motor control can be developed. To assist in this process, artificial constraints may be used. This can be done either by placing an obstacle in the path of the movement or by requiring that the movement be done in a specific way, such as locking the pelvis in a posterior tilt. The constraints help create awareness of how movements are made and where alternative patterns may develop when the constraints are removed.

DIFFERENTIATING CHARACTERISTICS

In summary, the *Feldenkrais method (FM)* of somatic education is an approach to learning focused on developing body image, awareness of action, and new patterns of motor control. The component approaches of FI and ATM may or may not be considered manual approaches. FI is more commonly thought of as a manual approach, and ATM a process of verbal guidance, but both are subservient to the larger goals of creating an experiential process of physical learning. However, its emphasis on the establishment of more optimal movement patterns is consistent with the goals of manual physical therapy and, as such, may be considered to be an alternative form of manual therapy, or it may be used as an adjunct to the use of manual therapy. Depending on the practitioner and the issues of the client, the manual aspect of FI may be either a starting point or a transitional process at critical points in the development of differentiation and integration of new patterns of motor control. Often the process will weave back and forth between guided active movement and manual facilitation. In either case, the goal is to develop self-awareness, improve problem solving, and in other ways empower the client to become more effectively responsible for his or her own mobility and well-being. The process of the ongoing examination is embedded in the activity of the intervention, with the responses of the client determining the progression by the practitioner. In this way, every session with a client is fully individualized and focused on the identification of movement problems, functional problems, and individual goals.

At this point in the development of the FM, no diagnostic classification processes or categories have been established. The reference is always to normal movement and the most effective biomechanics, economy of movement, and comfort that the client's musculoskeletal and neurological systems are able to produce at the time. Learning is understood as a set of successive approximations, each with increasingly optimal patterns of movement supported by changes in body image and motor control.

As an individualized process, neither the examination nor intervention aspects are proscribed, so the process requires that the practitioner be very creative in continuing to develop a learning environment for the client. Another unique aspect is that the process is exploratory. Both ATM and FI progress by presentation of a variety of different movement suggestions to provide the opportunity to experience the differences in closely related repeated movements and thus appreciate that there are subtle, controllable differences and choices possible regarding how to move and act. Through this process both the client and the practitioner are searching for a control process and action that is as easy and comfortable as possible.

The modalities of ATM and FI are unique and very different from each other. On the one hand, ATM can be thought of in terms of specific sequences of suggestion for movement exploration and, as such, may be presented intact to large groups of people or through audio or video media. Even in this context, however, the experience of ATM is still very individual, and the process of presentation stresses the individual nature of the exploration. FI, on the other hand, is a completely spontaneous process that unfolds uniquely between the practitioner and the client on a moment-to-moment basis, merging the client's responses to the practitioner's probing and the practitioner's experience in interpreting those responses as they might lead to new functional relationships in movement control.

EVIDENCE SUMMARY

Search Strategy and Method of Evaluation

To complete this summary of evidence, the following databases were explored: Medline, CINAHL, PsychINFO, SPORTDiscus. Reviews were searched using the search terms *Feldenkrais, awareness through movement, ATM, and functional integration.* Due to the ever-evolving nature of clinical research, this summary is not intended to represent a comprehensive exposition of all of the evidence published on this topic. It is recommended that the reader explore the more recent literature related to this topic.

The Feldenkrais Guild of North America maintains a bibliography of all research done on the FM worldwide. This bibliography contains links to international sites and all research that has been done using a recognized research design, from case report to control group, that is double blinded, and that is published as a master's thesis, doctoral dissertation, or journal article. This list is updated annually and available at www.feldenkrais.com/research/res_bibliography.htm.[25]

Summary of Results and Clinical Implications

Much of the published work on this topic is in the form of single or multiple case studies. These reports contain detailed information about interventions that have been highly successful in producing functional gains. Examples of this type of literature include a report of improved functional mobility in a group of people with spinal cord injury,[26] the reduction of stuttering in three people using FI,[27] dramatic functional improvements in two women who had traumatic brain injury,[28] resolution of back pain,[29,30] reduction of pain and improved mobility in four women with rheumatoid arthritis,[31] improved mobility and well-being in four women with multiple sclerosis,[23] and improved function in patients with Parkinson's disease.[32] In two separate papers,[33,34] Stephens has reported outcomes from clinical practice that demonstrate a greater than 80% rate of clients achieving 100% of initial goals and a greater than 90% rate of clients achieving at least 75% of initial goals over a total of nearly 200 clients and 90 different ICD-9 diagnostic codes. The number of visits per episode of care fell well within the guidelines suggested by the **Guide to Physical Therapist Practice.**[35]

Ives and Shelly[36] reviewed the research published through 1996 and noted that in many cases well-controlled research designs were not used or there were other flaws in the experimental procedures. However, they concluded that further research was warranted because of the "sheer number of positive reports that fit within a sound theoretical framework." More recently, a number of studies incorporating more effective methods, larger groups, and random assignment control studies have been performed. The review that is to follow will discuss the effectiveness of this approach as it relates to four general areas of clinical outcomes: pain management, motor control, mobility, and psychological/quality of life effects.

The Effectiveness of the Feldenkrais Method in Pain Management

DeRosa and Porterfield[37] included FM among a number of intervention methods that would most successfully address the motor control elements underlying much of the presenting back pain seen in physical therapy clinics. More than 50% of clients seeking Feldenkrais Intervention came with an initial complaint of pain interfering with function.[34] Fibromyalgia is an increasingly common diagnosis. In a study with five women with fibromyalgia using ATM twice weekly for 2 months, Dean et al[38] showed a significant decrease in pain and improved posture, gait, sleep, and body awareness. In an attempt to replicate this work, Stephens et al,[39] using a repeated measures design with 16 people with fibromyalgia, observed changes in pain and mobility variables, but these were overshadowed by the high variability of repeated baseline measures. Bearman and Shafarman[40] found large decreases in pain perception, improvements in functional status, reduction in use of pain medication, and a 40% reduction in the cost of medical care during a 1-year follow-up period for a group of seven chronic pain patients following an 8-week intensive FM intervention paradigm. Working with 34 chronic pain patients in a retrospective study, Phipps et al[41] showed that FM helped to reduce the pain and improve function and that ATM methods that were learned were still used independently by patients 2 years postdischarge. In another study working with 12 people aged 35 to 67 with back pain who performed ATM lessons over a 5-week period, Alexander[42] found significant reductions in pain using the visual analog pain scale and Oswestry Disability Index measures. In a study of 97 auto workers in Sweden, Lundblad, Elert, and Gerdle[43] found significant decreases in complaints of neck and shoulder pain and in disability during leisure activity in the Feldenkrais intervention group compared to randomly assigned physical therapy and no intervention control groups. The Lundblad study is the best experimental design done to date in the area of pain management. When considered collectively, the literature suggests that the FM can be effectively used to reduce pain and improve performance in people who have pain of biomechanical origin.

The Effectiveness of the Feldenkrais Method in Motor Control and Postural Control

In the area of motor control, three kinds of problems have been explored: changes in activity of a muscle group during a standard task, changes in postural control related to breathing, and postural control related to standing balance and mobility. In a study involving 21 subjects, an ATM lesson exploring flexion led to a decrease in abdominal electromyographic activity and a perception of the standardized supine flexion task being performed with greater ease. A second group was used to control for the possible effects of imagery and suggestion used during the ATM process, indicating that the changes noted were a result of the exploratory movements alone.[44] Another study using 30 subjects reported an increase in supine neck flexion range of motion and a decrease in perceived effort in this movement compared to a control group.[45] Several groups have been interested in studying the effects of FM on hamstring length. In studies looking at hamstring function, James et al[46] and Hopper, Kolt, and McConville[47] reported no change in hamstring length following a single ATM lesson designed to lengthen hamstrings compared to relaxation and normal activity control groups. However, these studies looked at effects of ATM following a single lesson. Stephens et al[48] studied effects of a set of hamstring-lengthening ATM lessons used over a period of 3 weeks. There was a large and significant increase in hamstring length compared to a normal activity control group. This result suggests that a period of time longer than a single lesson may be required for adequate learning in most people.

Saraswati[49] showed changes in the pattern of breathing involving increased movement of the abdomen, postural changes involving increased use of erector spinae muscles, and increased peak flow rates compared to a matched group of young healthy controls following a series of ATM lessons. The use of ATM to improve breathing, mobility, and postural control has also been reported in people with Parkinson's disease.[50]

In an initial study of four women with multiple sclerosis, Stephens et al[23] documented improvements in transfers and a subjective report of generally improved control of balance and movement. In a follow-up study, Stephens et al,[51] using a randomized control group design, found significant improvements in balance performance and balance confidence compared to a group meeting for educational purposes only. In a similar study with 59 elderly women randomly divided into three groups, Hall et al[52] found improvements in activities of daily living score, timed up-and-go test, Berg balance assessment, and three of eight scales on the SF-36 following a 10-week series of ATM lessons. The results of this study were confirmed in a larger follow-up study by Vrantsidis et al.[53] Seegert and Shapiro[54] have also reported changes in static standing control in healthy young subjects. These studies suggest that ATM and FI can be used effectively to improve discrete aspects of motor control as well as broader aspects of motor control such as posture and balance. These improvements in control can then be translated into improved functional mobility.

The Effectiveness of the Feldenkrais Method in Functional Mobility

Several studies have shown improvements in functional mobility using timed up-and-go and other measures. These studies have been done with well elderly people[52,55,56] and people with multiple sclerosis.[23]

The Effectiveness of the Feldenkrais Method in Quality of Life and Body Image

As noted earlier, Feldenkrais's thinking was driven by theory from psychology as well as physiology. An overriding interest was to find a method of improving the level of maturity with which people function in their lives. This suggests that changes in psychological variables such as life satisfaction should be studied. In a qualitative study of 10 people who had prolonged experience

with FI, Steisel[57] found improvements in body awareness, motivation, self-esteem, and levels of anxiety. In a randomly assigned, cross-over design, Johnson et al[58] found a significant decrease in perceived stress and anxiety following Feldenkrais sessions in a group of 20 people with multiple sclerosis.

Dunn and Rogers[59] used an ATM lesson involving sequences of sensory imagery of brushing soft bristles over half the body to produce a reposted sense of lightness and lengthening in that side of the body. In an interesting study using analysis of clay figures, Deig[60] described expansion in the detail and form of body image after a series of ATM lessons. This work was extended by Elgelid[61] who found improvements in body image resulting from a series of ATM lessons using the Jourard-Secord Cathexis Scale. Hutchinson[62] also used this scale and reported improvements in body image in a group of overweight women. The best-designed study in this area involved a matched control group study with 30 patients with eating disorders. Laumer et al[63] used standardized psychological testing to measure outcomes. They concluded that a 9-hour course of ATM improved the level of acceptance of the body and self, decreased feelings of helplessness and dependence, increased self-confidence, and facilitated a general process of maturation of the whole personality in the experimental group. In a pilot study with people 2 years or more after cerebrovascular accident (CVA), Batson and Deutsch[64] reported large improvements in dynamic gait, Berg Balance Scale, and stroke impact scale following ATM lessons two times per week for 6 weeks. In the follow-up study, a larger group of subjects post-CVA also reported significant improvements in the Berg Balance Scale and elements of the Timed Movement Battery. This study also found that subjects improved their ability to image movement, using the Movement Imagery Questionnaire, and that there was a strong correlation between ability to image movement and improvement of balance.[65]

Gutman et al[66] did the first research involving the Feldenkrais method in a well elderly population divided into three matched groups: 6 weeks ATM, 6 weeks standard exercise, and a no exercise control. Although they were unable to show additional benefits of Feldenkrais sessions in functional or physiological measures compared to exercise and no exercise control groups because of measurement and design problems, they did find a trend toward improvement in overall perception of health status in the Feldenkrais group. Similar findings have been reported in people with multiple sclerosis. Well-being was reported to be improved in a controlled study of 50 participants with multiple sclerosis[67] and in a group of 4 women with multiple sclerosis using the index of well-being.[23]

Suggestions for Future Research

Based on the evidence presented in this chapter, the following questions are offered as suggestions to guide further critical inquiry in this area of specialization. These suggestions have been previously summarized elsewhere in the literature.[68]

- Does decreasing trunk and upper body muscle tone lower the center of gravity and improve control of balance?
- Does FI or ATM actually increase a person's awareness of his or her body?

- What is the relationship between improving body image and improving motor control?
- Do these methods produce long-term changes in biopsychosocial variables like fear of reinjury, confidence in performing activities, and quality of life?
- Is it possible to capture the changes in kinds of motor control processes occurring during practice of Feldenkrais method by assessment of brain plasticity using functional magnetic resonance imaging (fMRI) or some other similar technology?

patterns that are problematic and to provide multiple choices and a process for framing solutions to these problems on their own. The underlying philosophy of the approach is to empower the client by developing and incorporating an improved awareness of actions and their consequences and a process of generating choices for changing behavior in concrete physical ways.

SUMMARY AND CONCLUSION

The client typically enters the learning session with an interest in managing pain or resolving difficulties that are then framed within the context of specific daily activities. The processes of FI and ATM can be used within the postures (actures) and actions of those specific activities and the learning of body segment organization, coordination, and motor control established in that functional context. Embedded in this process is an expectation of learning by the client of ways to recognize

Box 20-4 DIFFERENTIATING CHARACTERISTICS
- The Feldenkrais Method seeks to empower a client by developing and incorporating an improved awareness of actions and their consequences through a process of generating choices for changing behavior in concrete physical ways.
- Imbedded in this process are the client's expectations of learning to recognize problematic patterns and, through multiple choices, finding a process for framing their own solutions to these problems.

CLINICAL CASE

Initial Examination

History of Present Illness: J.C. is a 55-year-old woman who presented with a primary complaint of low back pain (LBP) focused on the left side. There was a dull pain radiating into the buttock on the left and also pain radiating up to her shoulder and neck. She presented with a diagnosis of sacroiliac (SI) joint instability, which had been chronic since an injury 12 years before. She described this injury as occurring during a fall down some stairs in which she landed on her ischial area and back and "jammed the left side" of her pelvis. She reinjured this area again 2 years later while working out on some exercise equipment and again a year later due to a fall in the supermarket, at which time she again landed on her buttocks. She describes the left SI region as a "weak spot" that is very sensitive to disruption. A week before presenting for therapy, her SI joint "slipped out" when she bent forward to close a drawer. This had become a common problem and efforts to realign and stabilize her left SI joint through chiropractic care over the course of several years had not been successful. J.C. also reported a number of other falls and indicated that she thought that her balance was generally "not good." J.C. is a psychotherapist and spends a majority of her working time sitting at a computer keyboard.

Observation:
- Observation of sitting and standing posture, revealed an excessive amount of lumbar lordosis. When lumbar muscle tone was examined by palpation, the left low back extensors were hard and shortened even in prone and in supine so that her back arched away from the table.
- Bilateral tibias were externally rotated (torsioned) at the knee, with the right more rotated than the left. In standing and in gait, this created the impression of the hips being externally rotated although they were not.
- Observation of gait revealed a decrease in trunk rotation, increased step frequency, decreased step length, a relatively wide base of support, and a decrease in adduction on the stance leg bilaterally. Gait revealed a slow cadence, with difficulty increasing her speed significantly.
- J.C. was unable to sit on a 16-inch diameter therapy ball in a reversible, controlled manner and rise again from the ball. Assistance was needed, which required placing her upper extremities on her body or assistance from an external object to transfer from sitting to standing on the ball. She was also unable to do a full squat to the floor.

Range of Motion:

- Hip flexion was limited bilaterally, with the left (100°) greater than the right (110°). Flexion and rotation in the lumbar spine were also limited so that J.C. was unable to assume a quadruped on elbows and knees position. When asked if she was limited in quadruped due to pain, she said that she had no pain but felt tension in her left low back region and was afraid that if she flexed further she would hurt herself.
- Hamstring length measured with hip flexed to 90°: left = 45°, right = 60°.
- Quadriceps were shortened bilaterally, measuring 105° knee flexion from a prone position.
- Dorsiflexion was actively and passively limited to 5° bilaterally.
- Neck flexion was limited to 45°; rotation left less than right, approximately 50% or normal range.
- Shoulder flexion = 140°, abduction = 135°, external rotation = 70°, internal rotation = 60° bilaterally with mild forward head noted.

Strength:

- Upper extremity strength was normal.
- Trunk and lower extremity (LE) strength were impaired. Trunk strength was 4−/5 in both flexors and extensors. LE strength was 3+ in hip extensors, 4− in abductors, and 4− in quads.

Neurological: Sensory and reflex screening was normal.

Special Tests: Three tests for sacroiliac joint dysfunction were positive and consistent for identifying the presence of SI joint dysfunction on the painful side.[69]

- Compression test
- Sitting forward bend test
- Supine to long-sitting test
- SF-36 at initial exam and 5 weeks[70]
- OPTIMAL Baseline and Follow-up Instrument[71]

Radiographs: Radiographs were unavailable.

Clinical Decision-Making Process

1. This patient appears to have compensated for chronic (and bouts of acute) SI joint pain and dysfunction by co-contracting and stiffening through the low back, across the hips, and up the back into the shoulders and neck.
2. The most relevant data from the examination are positive diagnosis of SI joint dysfunction; increased muscle tone in the left lumbar spine; limitation of a set of functional movement activities including floor transfer, quadruped, forward flexion, and walking; initiation of SI dysfunction by simple movements like bending or reaching forward and fear of doing many movements involving trunk/hip flexion.
3. Acute correction of the SI alignment problem was not the goal. This was done easily in the first session using a muscle energy technique approach.
4. Maintaining the stability of the SI joint over time and expanding functional levels were deemed to be important long-term goals.

5. Limitation of movement by fear of reinjury is a common problem,[72] so some comprehensive approach to treatment involving biopsychosocial dimensions is important, thus suggesting an indication to utilize the Feldenkrais Method. After realignment of the SI joint, the plan was to address the low back muscle tension using Functional Integration.
6. Each treatment session would begin with a process of Functional Integration that was then followed by some active movements using the ATM process. (See below for specific descriptions.)
7. Exploratory ATM will be used to discover and learn ways of improving functional movements that were initially limited or impossible and at the same time address issues of strength, range of motion, balance, and coordination.
8. New patterns of movement and muscle function will support the SI joints, thus reducing the risk of exacerbation.

Intervention

1. Initial correction of the left SI joint malalignment was done using muscle energy technique (see Chapters 4 and 28), resisting hip extension at positions progressively flexed from 90° in the supine position. This was done during the first session, repeated in the second, and again at the beginning of the third session, after which further correction was not required.

2. Representative Functional Integration lessons:
   - ***Prone lumbar extension***: This lesson was done at the beginning of sessions 2, 3, and 4. J.C. was positioned in prone on the mat table with a soft roller under her hips and another under her ankles. She was free to position her arms and head, however was most comfortable for her. The roller at the hips created a passive extension of

the lumbar spine, which shortened the muscles crossing the low back to the ilium, allowing them to relax. These muscles were further shortened by manually gently accommodating the ends of the tightened muscles, slightly increasing the extension or lateral flexion of the lumbar spine. This process led to a relaxation and softening of the muscles through the lower back and was accompanied by spontaneous deep breathing and sighing by J.C. suggesting that a significant amount of tension was being released.

- *Compression through the head, shoulders, and ribs:* This lesson was done at the beginning of the third session. J.C. was positioned in supine with a roller under her knees for comfort. Gentle sustained pressure was applied manually through the first rib on each side independently and through the skull down into the spine in different directions, creating compressive forces to relax the muscles along the spine. During this lesson, J.C. inhaled deeply and exhaled deeply releasing muscle tension several times. After this lesson, J.C. talked about feeling taller, straighter, and breathing more fully.

- *Side lying trunk and shoulder:* During these lessons, J.C. was positioned in side-lying position with hips and knees flexed, a soft roller between her legs, and a foam support under her **head**. The organization of her rib cage with breathing, the movements of her trunk into extension and rotation, the rotation of her head and neck, and all movements of the scapula were explored using gentle pushing and pulling movements. This lesson was done first in right side lying and then at the next session in left side lying. After this lesson, J.C. talked about having a feeling of length first on the left side (right-side-lying lesson) and then on the right side (left-side-lying lesson) and feeling more freedom in turning movements.

- *Cervical movements:* For this lesson, J.C. was positioned in supine with a roller under her knees for comfort. After preparing her by providing gentle compression and rotation through the lower extremities, J.C. was approached at the head and neck. Initially, residual tension in trunk muscles caused stiffness in the neck, resulting in decreased turning range and a feeling of heaviness when attempting to lift the head. Movements of extension through the neck and upper back were explored, as were movements of rotation and then flexion. Combined movements were then explored. At the end of this lesson, the head and neck turned easily through its full range and felt much lighter when it was lifted. After this lesson, an ATM lesson using these movements was done. (See below.)

3. ATM sessions: Four basic ATM lessons were done with J.C. Each was developed over time as she was able to more easily perform the movements suggested.
- *Pelvic clock:* This lesson was done sitting on the edge of the mat table with feet flat on the floor and arms relaxed and resting on the legs. The basic idea is to develop differentiated, active control and awareness of movements

of the pelvis using the image of a clock on the sitting surface. Movements of the pelvis through cardinal planes of the clock (e.g., 6–12) and diagonal planes (e.g., 10–4), movements in short arcs, and finally whole circular movements around the outside of the clock were explored. Initially, it was useful to manually suggest some of these directions of movement. This type of lesson has been described in great detail elsewhere.[73]

- *Sitting on a therapy ball:* The pelvic clock lesson was a precursor for this lesson. Initially, J.C. had to be assisted to sit on a 17-inch diameter ball. This lesson was developed in several ways over a period of five sessions: (1) starting with pelvic clock movements on the ball, which resulted in rolling the ball in a circle under her; (2) forward bending, eventually to touch the floor; (3) moving from sit to stand and back again done in small and reversible movements to the point that she could lift her weight up slowly without losing contact with the ball and then sit back down; (4) abducting and adducting the legs while standing to reorganize the habit of internally rotating and adducting the legs to stabilize during standing; and (5) a progressive decrease in the size of the ball from 17-inch to 15-inch to 13-inch diameter to make the whole process more challenging by requiring more strength and better control. J.C. was given a 15-inch therapy ball to use at home to continue developing skill in these movements.

- *Supine extension and bridging:* (Fig. 20-1 and Fig. 20-2) J.C. was prepared for this lesson by the cervical movements FI above. J.C. initially lay on the floor in supine. Initial movements included exploration to find a way to place the hands palms down on the floor beside her shoulders to help support her head. Movements of pushing through a hand to lift that shoulder and pushing through a foot to lift that hip were explored. Tilting the neck into extension was explored to find a way to comfortably and safely press the head into the floor to lift the shoulders and trunk. This movement needs to be done very carefully, with the hands assisting in weight bearing as necessary. Initially,

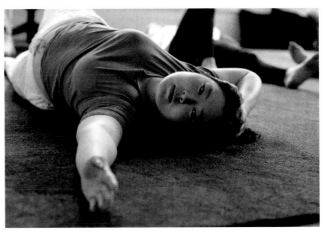

FIGURE 20–1 Supine extension.

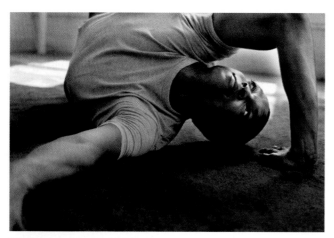

FIGURE 20–2 Supine bridging.

J.C. was manually guarded and assisted in this movement until she was safe on her own. Finally, all the extension movements—neck, arms and legs—were organized together until J.C. was able to lift her whole body up into a bridge between her hands, head, and feet. This lesson was done over a period of about 30 minutes. The idea was not to develop a high level of skill but rather to develop a concept of the control and strength of the back of her body. After this lesson she spoke about feeling taller and lighter and her chest being more expansive across the front.

• *New walking-old walking:* As her balance and control became greater, her gait changed from one that was slow, wide based, externally rotated, stiff, with reduced arm swing, and decreased stance adduction to a gait that was much faster, with narrower base, hips and arms swinging, and head upright. The ATM lesson here was to give each of these a name and to voluntarily, consciously, on command go back and forth from walking the old way to walking the new way. This brought all the elements of gait into her awareness so that she learned the restrictions of the "old walking," how they were produced, how to recognize them when they were happening, and how to change them to the "new walking" configuration. This lesson was done briefly at the end of several later sessions until she reported that she was doing 100% "new walking" in her daily life.

Outcomes
• After the second session, low back and buttock pain were gone, but some upper body pain remained.
• After the third session, the SI joint remained stable. On follow-up report, this lasted for at least 3 months.
• She felt taller and lighter so that friends remarked to her that she was standing straighter.
• She reported feeling more stable on her feet, "stuck into the ground," so that she did not have the frequent episodes of loss of balance that were previously characteristic for her.
• She spontaneously felt safe to do reaching, lifting, and carrying of things that she had not felt safe to do for many years. She also described much easier turning of her head and neck, which was most clearly noticeable in driving where she no longer needed to use mirrors exclusively when backing up.
• Her gait changed so dramatically that she began to call it her "new walking," which was summarized by her saying that she felt "athletic." This was a radical shift in her self-perception to a much earlier time in her life. Gait speed was not measured; however, gait was clearly faster and more fluid. Other changes in gait are described above. As a game and a challenge, J.C. was asked to switch back and forth between doing "new walking" and "old walking" on command to demonstrate that she was fully aware of both forms of organization. She was able to do this. She now had a choice that she didn't have before and could recognize when she was not walking the way she wanted.
• Changes in OPTIMAL scores:
  • Initial: Difficulty, 2.81/5 of 5 is high; confidence, 3.14 or 2.86/5 if 5 is high.
  • Follow-up: Difficulty, 1.95/5 if 5 is high; confidence, 2.36 or 3.80, if 5 is high.
  • A 21.5% decrease in difficulty level; 23.5% increase in confidence level.

HANDS-ON

Perform the following activities in lab with a partner:

1 FI: – Prone lumbar extension, described above

2 ATM 1: Pelvic clock, described above

3 ATM 2: Sitting on a therapy ball, described above

4 ATM 3: Supine extension, described above

5 Switch partners and perform these techniques on one other person. Teach your chosen techniques to one other person and provide that person with feedback regarding his or her performance.

6 If possible, videotape your performance of these techniques. Self-assess your performance of the chosen techniques by writing down three areas of deficiency and three areas of

proficiency when using these techniques. Focus on such factors as therapist position, patient position, hand placement, force direction, instruction to the patient, etc. Critique the performance of others in a similar fashion.

ACKNOWLEDGMENTS

The pictures illustrating the ATM lessons were obtained from the Feldenkrais Guild of North America public relations department and are used by permission.

REFERENCES

1. Kohler W. *Gestalt Psychology*. Paperbound ed. New York, NY: Liveright; 1970.
2. Jacobson E. *Progressive Relaxation*. Chicago, IL: University of Chicago Press; 1938.
3. Lowen A. *Bioenergetics*. New York, NY: Coward, McCann and Geoghegan; 1975.
4. Brooks CVW. *Sensory Awareness: The Rediscovery of Experiencing*. Great Neck, NY: Felix Morrow; 1974.
5. Erickson M. *Hypnotic Realities*. New York, NY: Irvington; 1976.
6. Bateson G. *Mind and Nature*. New York, NY: EP Dutton; 1979.
7. Gibson JJ. *The Senses Considered as a Perceptual System*. Boston, MA: Houghton Mifflin; 1966.
8. Feldenkrais M. *The Elusive Obvious*. Cupertino, CA: Meta Publications; 1981.
9. Hanna T. Moshe Feldenkrais: the silent heritage. *Somatics*. 1985;5:8-15.
10. Newell G. Moshe Feldenkrais: a biographical sketch of his early years. *Somatics*. 1992;7:33-38.
11. Feldenkrais M. *Higher Judo*. London, UK: Frederick Warne; 1942.
12. Feldenkrais M. *Judo*. London, UK: Frederick Warne; 1942.
13. Feldenkrais M. *Body and Mature Behavior: A Study of Anxiety, Sex, Gravitation, and Learning*. New York, NY: International Universities Press; 1949.
14. Talmi A. First encounters with Feldenkrais. *Somatics*. 1980;3:18-25.
15. Feldenkrais M. *The Potent Self. A Guide to Spontaneity*. San Francisco, CA: Harper and Row; 1985.
16. Shafarman S. *Awareness Heals: The Feldenkrais Method for Dynamic Health*. Reading, MA: Addison Wesley; 1997.
17. Schmidt RA, Lee TD. *Motor Control and Learning*. 4th ed. Champaign, IL: Human Kinetics; 2005.
18. Newell K, Vaillancourt DE. Dimensional change in motor learning. *Hum Mov Sci*. 2001;20:695-715.
19. Gallagher S. *How the Body Shapes the Mind*. Oxford, UK: Clarendon Press; 2005.
20. Rywerant Y. *The Feldenkrais Method: Teaching by Handling*. San Francisco, CA: Harper and Row; 1983.
21. Ginsburg C. Body-image, movement and consciousness: examples from a somatic practice in the Feldenkrais Method. *Consciousness Studies*. 1999;6:79-91.
22. Stephens J, Miller TM. Feldenkrais Method: learning to move through your life with grace and ease. (Or optimizing your potential for living). In: Davis C., ed. *Complimentary Therapies in Rehabilitation: Evidence for Efficacy, Prevention and Wellness*. 2nd ed. Thorofare, NJ: Slack Publishers; 2009.
23. Stephens JL, Call S, Evans K, et al. Responses to ten Feldenkrais Awareness Through Movement lessons by four women with multiple sclerosis: improved quality of life. *Phys Ther Case Rep*. 1999;2:58-69.
24. Kandel ER, Schwartz JH, Jessell TM. *The Principles of Neural Science*. 4th ed. Norwalk, CT: Appleton and Lange; 2000.
25. Feldenkrais Guild of North America. *The FGNA Research Bibliography* page. www.feldenkrais.com/resources/bibliography/
26. Ginsburg C. The Shake-a-Leg body awareness training program: dealing with spinal injury and recovery in a new setting. *Somatics*. 1986;Spring/Summer:31-42.
27. Gilman M, Yaruss JS. Stuttering and relaxation: applications for somatic education in stuttering treatment. *J Fluency Disord*. 2000;25:59-76.
28. Ofir R. A heuristic investigation of the process of motor learning using Feldenkrais Method in physical rehabilitation of two young women with traumatic brain injury [unpublished doctoral dissertation], New York, NY: Union Institute; 1993.
29. Lake B. Acute back pain: treatment by the application of Feldenkrais principles. *Aust Fam Physician*. 1985;14:53-77.
30. Panarello-Black D. PT's own back pain leads her to start Feldenkrais training. *PT Bull*. 1982;4:9-10.
31. Narula M, Jackson O, Kulig K. The effects of six-week Feldenkrais Method on selected functional parameters in a subject with rheumatoid arthritis [abstract]. *Phys Ther*. 1992;72(suppl):S86.
32. Johnson M, Wendell LL. Some effects of the Feldenkrais Method on Parkinson's symptoms and function. Paper presented at the annual conference of the Feldenkrais Guild of North America, San Francisco, CA: October, 2001.
33. Wildman F, Stephens J, Aum L. Feldenkrais Method. In: Novey DW, ed. *Clinician's Complete Reference to Complementary and Alternative Medicine*. St. Louis, MO: Mosby; 2000.
34. Stephens J. Feldenkrais Method: background, research and orthopedic case studies. *Orthop Phys Ther Clin N Am*. 2000;9:375-394.
35. APTA. *Guide to Physical Therapist Practice*. Rev., 2nd ed. Alexandria, VA: American Physical Therapy Association; 2003.
36. Ives JC, Shelley GA. The Feldenkrais Method in rehabilitation: a review. *Work*. 1998;11:75-90.
37. DeRosa C, Porterfield J. A physical therapy model for the treatment of low back pain. *Phys Ther*. 1992;72:261-272.
38. Dean JR, Yuen SA, Barrows SA. Effects of a Feldenkrais ATM sequence on fibromyalgia patients. Poster session presented at the annual conference of the Feldenkrais Guild of North America; Tamiment, PA: August, 1997.
39. Stephens J, Herrera S, Lawless R, Masaitis C, Woodling P. Evaluating the results of using Awareness Through Movement with people with fibromyalgia: comments on research design and measurement. Paper presented at the annual conference of the Feldenkrais Guild of North America: Evanston, IL: September, 1999.
40. Bearman D, Shafarman S. Feldenkrais Method in the treatment of chronic pain: a study of efficacy and cost effectiveness. *Am J Pain Manag*. 1999;9:22-27.
41. Phipps A, Lopez R, Powell R, Lundy-Ekman L, Maebori D. A functional outcome study on the use of movement re-education in chronic pain management [master's thesis]. Forest Grove, Oregon: Pacific University, School of Physical Therapy; 1997.
42. Alexander A. Perceived pain and disability decreases after Feldenkrais Awareness Through Movement [master's thesis]. Northridge, CA: California State University at Northridge; 2006.
43. Lundblad I, Elert J, Gerdle B. Randomized controlled trial of physiotherapy and Feldenkrais interventions in female workers with neck-shoulder complaints. *J Occupa Rehab*. 1999;9:179-194.
44. Brown E, Kegerris S. Electromyographic activity of trunk musculature during a Feldenkrais Awareness Through Movement lesson. *Isokinet Exerc Sci*. 1991;1:216-221.
45. Ruth S, Kegerreis S. Facilitating cervical flexion using a Feldenkrais method: Awareness Through Movement. *J Orthop Sports Phys Ther*. 1992;16:25-29.
46. James ML, Kolt GS, Hopper C, McConville JC, Bate P. The effects of a Feldenkrais program and relaxation procedures on hamstring length. *Aust J Physiother*. 1999;44:49-54.

47. Hopper C, Kolt GS, McConville JC. The effects of Feldenkrais Awareness Through Movement on hamstring length, flexibility and perceived exertion. *J Body Mov Ther.* 1999;3:238-247.

48. Stephens J, Davidson J, Derosa J, Kriz M, Saltzman N. Lengthening the hamstring muscles without stretching using Awareness Through Movement. *Phys Ther.* 2006;86:1641-1650.

49. Saraswati S. Investigation of human postural muscles and respiratory movements [master's thesis]. Sidney, Australia: University of New South Wales; 1989.

50. Shenkman M, Donovan J, Tsubota J, et al. Management of individuals with Parkinsons disease: rationale and case studies. *Phys Ther.* 1989;69: 944-955.

51. Stephens J, DuShuttle D, Hatcher C, Shmunes J, Slaninka C. Use of awareness through movement improves balance and balance confidence in people with multiple sclerosis: a randomized controlled study. *Neurology Report.* 2001;25:39-49.

52. Hall SE, Criddle A, Ring A, et al. Study of the effects of various forms of exercise on balance in older women [unpublished manuscript]. Nedlands, Western Australia: Dept. of Rehabilitation, Sir Charles Gairdner Hospital; 1999. Healthway Starter Grant, File no.7672.

53. Vrantsidis F, Hill KD, Moore K, et al. Getting grounded gracefully: effectiveness and acceptability of Feldenkrais in improving balance and related outcomes for older people: a randomized trial. *J Aging Phys Act.* 2009; 17:57-76.

54. Seegert EM, Shapiro R. Effects of alternative exercise on posture. *Clinical Kinesiology.* 1999;53:41-47.

55. Bennett JL, Brown BJ, Finney SA, Sarantakis CP. Effects of a Feldenkrais-based mobility program on function of a healthy elderly sample. Poster session Boston, MA: Combined Sections Meeting of the American Physical Therapy Association; February, 1998.

56. Learning to improve mobility and quality of life in a well elderly population: the benefits of awareness through movement. IFF Academy. *Feldenkrais Research Journal* 2005;2. http://www.iffresearchjournal.org/.

57. Steisel SG. The client's experience of the psychological elements in functional integration. *Dissertation Abstracts International.* Ann Arbor, MI: Massachusetts School of Professional Psychology; 1993.

58. Johnson SK, Frederick J, Kaufman M, Mountjoy B. A controlled investigation of bodywork in multiple sclerosis. *J Altern Complementary Med.* 1999;5:237-243.

59. Dunn PA, Rogers DK. Feldenkrais sensory imagery and forward reach. *Percept Mot Skills.* 2000;91:755-757.

60. Deig D. Self image in relationship to Feldenkrais Awareness Through Movement classes [master's thesis]. Indianapolis, IN: University of Indianapolis, Krannert Graduate School of Physical Therapy; 1994.

61. Elgelid HS. Feldenkrais and Body Image [master's thesis]. Conway, AK: University of Central Arkansas; 1999.

62. Hutchinson MG. *Transforming Body Image. Learning to Love the Body You Have.* Freedom, CA: The Crossing Press; 1985.

63. Laumer U, Bauer M, Fichter M, Milz H. Therapeutic effects of Feldenkrais Method Awareness Through Movement in patients with eating disorders. *Psychother Psychosom Med Psychol.* 1997;47:170-180.

64. Batson G, Deutsch JE. Effects of Feldenkrais Awareness Through Movement on balance in adults with chronic neurological deficits following stroke: a preliminary study. *Complementary Health Prac Rev.* 2005;10: 203-210.

65. Batson G, Duetsch J, Stephens J. Feasibility and outcomes of group-delivered Feldenkrais Awareness Through Movement on balance in adults post-stroke: preliminary findings [submitted]. *Arch Phys Med.* 2010.

66. Gutman G, Herbert C, Brown S. Feldenkrais vs conventional exercise for the elderly. *J Gerontol.* 1977;32:562-572.

67. Bost H, Burges S, Russell R, Ruttinger H, Schlafke U. Feldstudie zur wilksamkeit der Feldenkrais-Methode bei MS–betroffenen [unpublished manuscript]. Saarbrucken, Germany: Deutsche Multiple Sklerose Gesellschaft; 1994.

68. Thoughts on future research on Feldenkrais Method: 12 views from around the world. IFF Academy. *Feldenkrais Research Journal.* 2007;3. www.iffresearchjournal.org/index2007.htm

69. Cibulka MM, Koldehoff R. Clinical usefulness of a cluster of sacroiliac joint tests in patients with and without low back pain. *J Ortho Sports Phys Ther.* 1999;29:83-92.

70. Resnik L, Dobrykowski E. Outcomes measurement for patients with low back pain. *Orthop Nurs.* 2005;24:14-24.

71. Guccione AA, Mielenz TJ, DeVellis RF, et al. Development and testing of a self-report instrument to measure actions: Outpatient Physical Therapy Improvement in Movement Assessment Log (OPTIMAL). *Phys Ther.* 2005;85:515-530.

72. Vlaeyen JWS, Kole-Snijders AMJ, Heuts HTG, van Eek H. Behavioral analysis, fear of movement/(re)injury and behavioral rehabilitation in chronic low back pain. In: Vleeming A, et al, eds. *Movement, Stability and Low Back Pain.* New York, NY: Churchill Livingstone, 2005: 435-444.

73. Feldenkrais M. *Awareness Through Movement.* Paperback edition. New York, NY: HarperCollins; 1990:115-122.

The Theory and Practice of Therapeutic Yoga

Mary Lou Galantino, PT, PhD, MSCE

Heather Walkowich, DPT

Chapter Objectives

At the conclusion of this chapter, the reader will be able to:

- Define complementary and alternative medicine (CAM) therapy, therapeutic yoga, Patanjali's eightfold path to enlightenment, hatha yoga, pranayama, dhyana, pratyahara, dharana.
- Recognize the expanding role of CAM therapy in traditional Eastern medicine.
- Identify the major components of yoga.
- Identify the importance of psychological and spiritual well-being on the healing process.
- Recognize the potential impact of therapeutic yoga on the physiological, psychological, and spiritual aspects of well-being.

- Identify situations in which therapeutic yoga may enhanc recovery when used as an adjunctive treatment to traditional physical therapy treatment.
- Identify and describe some of the different postures and their influence on the body.
- Identify and use various clinical assessment tools to evaluate and integrate yoga into clinical practice.
- Apply the basic principles of yoga to various clinical orthopaedic cases.

HISTORICAL PERSPECTIVES

Complementary and alternative medicine (CAM), as defined by the *National Center for Complementary and Alternative Medicine (NCCAM)*, is a group of diverse medical and health care systems, practices, and products that are not presently considered to be part of conventional medicine. Techniques include, but are not limited to, meditation, prayer, guided imagery, acupuncture, mental healing, and therapies that use creative outlets such as art, music, or dance.[1] *Therapeutic yoga* is one form of movement therapy that has gained increasing popularity over the past decade.[2] A recent survey revealed that of those who used yoga specifically for therapeutic purposes, 21% did so because it was recommended by a conventional medical professional, 31% did so because conventional therapies were ineffective, and 59% thought it would be an interesting therapy to explore.[3]

Yoga is a form of CAM therapy that combines theory with practice and is designed to promote both physical, as well as emotional, health and well-being.[1,4] Conceptually, yoga is complex, even to define. The word *yoga* has several translations

and comes from the root *yug* (to join), or *yoke* (to bind together). Essentially, yoga describes a method of discipline or a means of uniting the body and mind.

For centuries, the virtues of yoga as a therapeutic modality have been extolled in traditional Indian medicine.[5] More recently, yoga has gained popularity in Western culture and is now the most common mind-body therapy in Western complementary medicine.[6] Its unique ability to facilitate both physical and psychological benefits, makes yoga appealing as a cost-effective alternative to conventional interventions.[7,8] Therapeutic yoga is an emerging field that demands a closer look; however, before it can be fully adopted and integrated into standard practice; additional evidence is required.[9]

Despite its long history, only recently have investigators begun to subject yogic concepts to empirical scrutiny. The effects of yoga have been explored in a number of patient populations, including individuals with asthma,[10,11] cardiac conditions,[12,13] arthritis,[14,15] kyphosis,[16] multiple sclerosis,[17] epilepsy,[18] headaches,[19] depression,[20] diabetes mellitus,[21] pain disorders,[22] and gastrointestinal disorders,[23] as well as in healthy individuals.[24] This chapter will focus on the use of yoga in the management of musculoskeletal disorders as a potential adjunct to orthopaedic manual physical therapy (OMPT).

PHILOSOPHICAL FRAMEWORK
Guiding Concepts and Origins

The concept of yoga originated around 1500 BC with the introduction of **Brahmanism**, the precursor to modern-day **Hinduism**.[25] Over the next several hundred years, the practice of yoga underwent numerous transformations as new concepts and beliefs were adopted and others were abandoned. As additional branches developed, each retained its own unique characteristics and functions, and stressed its own particular approach to life. Although each approach is different, the basic tenet of all branches of yoga focuses on uniting the mind and body, as well as promoting physical, psychological, and spiritual health.[2]

CLINICAL PILLAR

The basic tenet of all branches of yoga focuses on uniting the body and mind, as well as developing physical, psychological, and spiritual health.

The basic philosophy of yoga can be traced back nearly 2000 years to **Yoga Sutras**, a text written by the philosopher **Patanjali**, whom many consider to be the father of modern yoga.[25] In his treatise, Patanjali emphasized an eightfold path to enlightenment designed to help individuals transform themselves and gain control over their mind and emotions (Fig. 21-1).[25] Each limb of Patanjali's model acts as a guideline for living a meaningful and purposeful life and emphasizes moral and ethical conduct as well as self-discipline.[26] Patanjali's eight paths on the road to enlightenment include moral precepts (*yama*), personal behavior concepts (*niyama*), physical postures (*asana*), conscious regulation of breathing (*pranayama*), focusing the senses inward (*pratyahara*), concentration (*dharana*), meditation (*dhyana*), and ecstasy (*samadhi*).[2] With the attainment of each path, the individual is led to the next path until total enlightenment is eventually achieved.

Yoga, in the traditional sense, is a spiritual way of life that extends well beyond complex poses and controlled breathing. Traditionally, yoga has been considered a spiritual discipline encompassing a vast array of physical and mental exercises with the ultimate aim of transforming oneself through coalescence of the mind, body, and spirit. The practice of yoga combines rigorous spiritual discipline with a vast array of physical and mental exercise in addition to philosophical, moral, and nutritional adherences. As such, yoga truly embodies a holistic approach to life and health, often taking even the most dedicated a lifetime to master. Since its introduction into Western culture in the late 1880s, there has been a gradual shift from spiritually based forms of practice to more physically based forms.[2] It may be suggested that this shift toward more physically based forms of yoga is the result of an ever-increasing health-conscious society. Table 21-1 compares the features that characterize the Eastern and Western views of yoga.[27]

It is not possible to explore the totality of yoga within this chapter. The reader is referred to additional resources that may be procured to further explore yoga's history, philosophy, and practice. Texts written by George Feuerstein[9] are highly

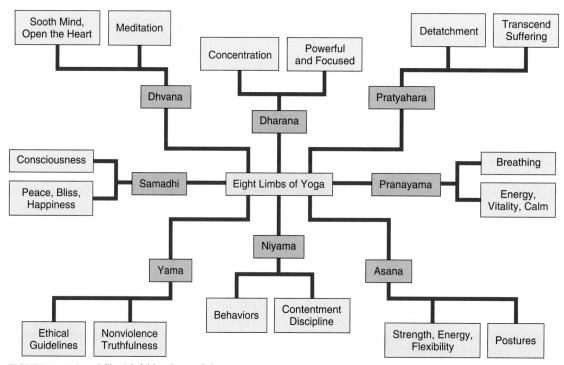

FIGURE 21–1 Patanjali's eightfold path to enlightenment.

Table 21–1	Generalizations That Characterize the Eastern and Western Views of Yoga Practice	
	EASTERN	**WESTERN**
Mental Focus	Internal	External
Heart Rate	Little change	80% predicted maximum heart rate
Speed	Slow	Fast
Cardiac Expenditure	Low	High
Muscle Tone	Soft, relaxed	Hypertrophy, firm
Breath	Synchronized with movement	Unrelated

Adapted from Magee D. *Orthopaedic Physical Therapy Clinics of North America.* Philadelphia, PA: W.B. Saunders; 2000.

recommended and widely praised to be the most complete works on the history and philosophy of yoga.

The Practice of Yoga

At present, there are six main classifications of yoga: *raja yoga, karma yoga, bhakti yoga, janana yoga, tantra yoga,* and *hatha yoga,* each containing numerous subcategories and extensions. What is commonly referred to as yoga in the West is actually *hatha yoga,* also known as *yoga of activity,* which focuses on physical postures, deep breathing, and meditation. These practices are in contrast to other forms of yoga that focus more on ethics, meditation, or diet. Hatha's popularity is attributed to its experiential nature that allows individuals to appreciate the physical components of yoga without requiring adoption of the spiritual aspects. All styles of yoga, however, are believed to lead to the same path to spiritual enlightenment through self-transformation.[9]

The word *hatha* is a combination of the Sanskrit words for sun *(ha)* and moon *(tha)* and refers to the positive and negative forces acting on the body.[28] When performing this type of yoga, all exercises are performed slowly, without straining, and within one's own limits. A desirable feature of Hatha is that each pose can be modified depending on the participant's abilities and flexibility. These characteristics make it an ideal form of exercise for all age groups, contributing further to its popularity. Overall, hatha yoga stresses the importance of physical postures *(asanas),* deep breathing *(pranayama),* and meditation *(dhyana)* with the goal of developing optimal flexibility, health, and vitality.[28]

QUESTIONS *for* REFLECTION

- What makes *hatha yoga* the predominant form of yoga in the United States?
- What are the distinguishing aspects of this form of yoga?
- Why is this form of yoga ideal for individuals with impairments?

Asanas (ā·sa·nas), or physical postures, may be used as a form of exercise promoting cardiovascular fitness, strength, and flexibility.[14] Each posture contributes to increased body awareness and proper positioning of the body in space both at rest and during movement. There are more than 200 asanas, each with its own unique purpose. Standing poses are emphasized early on for the purpose of building strength and ease of movement, to increase general vitality, and to improve circulation, coordination, and balance. Postures for deep relaxation are introduced from the beginning as well in order to facilitate the mind-body connection. Sitting and reclining postures, forward bends, inversions, backbends, twists, arm balance, and flowing sequences are gradually introduced over time.[29] Each pose is designed to elicit the activity of certain muscle groups while, at the same time, stretching others for the purpose of promoting relaxation and improving flexibility. In order to maximize the benefit from each exercise, yoga positions are typically held for a period of time. Maintenance of selected postures allows for the elongation of muscles, ligaments, and tendons safely and naturally.[2] Table 21-2 provides a brief description of five yoga postures that are in common use.

CLINICAL PILLAR

Yoga postures proceed in the following manner:

- Standing
- Sitting
- Reclining
- Forward bends
- Inversions
- Backward bends
- Twists
- Arm balance
- Flowing sequences

Procedures are followed for entering into, holding, and emerging from each pose, along with a recommended sequence of poses. Movements are typically slow and coordinated with controlled breathing so that full inhalation is achieved upon entering the pose. The pose and breath are briefly held, and then both released, simultaneously, so that the starting point is reached at full exhalation. Every pose has a counterpose to balance its effects.

During the course of a particular session, a variety of poses are often used. Most poses involve the muscles of the back and abdomen. Standing poses are designed for centering and alignment. Seated poses are designed to be more calming than the standing poses. Forward bends, with flexion in the hips, rather than the spine, can be done in seated, standing, supine, twisting, balancing, or inverted positions. *Balancing* postures are designed to develop the body's coordination and strength. *Twisting* poses help activate the spine, internal organs, and

Table 21–2	Goals of Yoga Asanas	
YOGA POSTURES	**DESCRIPTION**
Standing asanas	Help to build a strong foundation and develop strength, stamina, and determination. Help to develop awareness of the body.
Seated asanas	Improve flexibility of the hips, knees, and ankles. Reduce tension in the diaphragm and throat, making breathing smoother.
Twists	Extend and rotate the spine (ideal for relieving backache and stiffness in the neck and shoulders). Turning of the trunk stimulates the internal organs, aiding in digestion. As the spine becomes more supple, blood flow to the nerves in the spine improves, raising energy levels.
Inverted asanas	Revitalize the entire body system. The brain is nourished by the blood that flows toward it. With no weight on the lower body, inversions also bring relief to tired legs (i.e., headstands).
Supine or prone asanas	Stretch the abdomen and increase flexibility in the spine and hips. Some are restful, while others strengthen the back, arms, and legs.

Adapted from Smith, J. et al. *Pilates and yoga: A high-energy partnership of physical and spiritual exercise techniques to revitalize the mind and body.* London: Hermes House, 2005.

muscles. *Backbends* are meant to strengthen the extensor muscles, stretch the flexor muscles, and stimulate the entire nervous system. *Inversion* postures are designed to strengthen the cardiovascular system by reversing the effects of gravity.

Some methods of hatha use fast, flowing asana movements, called **ashtanga**. Others, like **iyengar**, use poses held for longer durations, with attention to specific performance. Iyengar is one of the most popular styles of hatha in the West and uses props to accommodate the special needs of the practitioner. **Viniyoga** is another popular form that allows poses to be customized to the individual, thus proving useful for those with physical limitations.

Along with asanas, **pranayama** (prā·Nā·yā·ma), or regulated breathing, is another key aspect of yogic practice. There are over one hundred different combinations of yoga breathing patterns that may be enacted[27]; each designed to gain conscious control of this most basic bodily function.[2] Breathing techniques in yoga are used as energy management tools to help curb the effects of increased stress.[27] These patterns of deep, rhythmic inhalation and exhalation through the nose bridge the connection between breathing, the mind, and emotions.[9]

Dhyana (dhy·ān·a), or meditation, is described as a conscious mental process that induces a set of integrated physiological changes.[1] The practice of meditation results in uninterrupted concentration aimed at quieting the mind and body. The mental focus required for yogic practice serves to increase awareness of movement and to enhance the perception of any aberrant movement patterns that may exist.[14,30] This increased awareness may serve to promote muscle relaxation and encourage the adoption of more beneficial postures and patterns of movement, resulting in the prevention of misalignment, cumulative stress, and pain.[14] Furthermore, the relaxation component of yogic practice is believed to counteract the negative effects induced by prolonged stress and chronic pain.[31]

Two other aspects of yogic practice, **pratyahara** (prut-yah-hah-ruh) (withdrawing of the senses) and **dharana** (dhah-ruh-nah) (concentration) are important skills that increase attention and awareness. Practicing these two paths helps to enhance awareness during attainment of the postures. These practices may also allow one to sense one's own physical limitations.[9] By drawing attention inward, these practices allow the individual to recognize habitual thought patterns and natural body rhythms. These concepts differ from the practice of dhyana, which results in uninterrupted concentration aimed at quieting the mind and body and is commonly used in practice apart from the other yogic practices.[9]

QUESTIONS *for* **REFLECTION**

- How might regulated breathing, meditation, withdrawing of the senses, and concentration serve to enhance the effects of standard interventions in physical therapy practice?
- Would these strategies work best when implemented before or after other interventions?

PRINCIPLES OF EXAMINATION AND INTERVENTION IN SELECTED POPULATIONS

Yogic practice has been shown to have a positive effect on the cardiovascular, musculoskeletal, and pulmonary systems.[32] Patel et al[33,34] found that yogic practice that incorporated relaxation and biofeedback techniques had the potential to reduce average mean blood pressure. Subsequently, the participants were able to reduce their use of antihypertensive drugs. After a 12 month follow-up period, the researchers found that the reductions in blood pressure had been maintained, ruling out a placebo effect and lending further support to the use of yoga as an alternative therapeutic modality.[33]

The *Guide to Physical Therapist Practice* advocates the role of the therapist in prevention and enhancement in performance of both impaired and nonimpaired individuals.

Some studies have looked at the efficacy of yoga on pulmonary conditions such as *asthma*. Unfortunately, many of these studies outlined only short-term effects and produced dubious findings.[32] However, some authors have attempted to determine the long-term effects of yoga on the number of attacks of airway obstruction, the severity of the attacks, drug dosages required to counteract the attacks, and peak expiratory flow.[32] Patients were followed for 4.5 years and showed significant improvements in each of the aforementioned variables.[32]

In the past, yoga and relaxation techniques have been used to address numerous musculoskeletal conditions.[15,22,30–32,35–39] Many orthopaedic conditions are the result of misaligned osseous structures, muscle imbalances, and overuse leading to significant morbidity in those afflicted.[15,30–32,35–39] Since yoga is designed to promote proper alignment and awareness of the body in space, the use of yoga in the management of musculoskeletal impairment has become the subject of great interest. The current best evidence promotes the use of exercise to treat orthopaedic conditions, placing an emphasis on the aerobic, strength, and mobility components of exercise as key factors that facilitate improvement. As yoga incorporates all of these aspects, it may be argued that yogic practice may be beneficial in restoring improved function for those individuals suffering from musculoskeletal impairment.

QUESTIONS *for* **REFLECTION**

- Why have the therapeutic effects of yoga been most studied in orthopaedic-related conditions?
- Why has the use of therapeutic yoga become popular in the management of musculoskeletal conditions?
- What aspects of therapeutic yoga make it effective in the care of such conditions?

The emphasis on precision of movement, which is an important aspect of yoga, is facilitated through careful concentration and control of specific movement patterns. The relationship between the distal and proximal segments of the extremities and the relationship between the extremities and the spine are vital aspects of yogic practice. With each motion, certain structures are lengthened while others are used for maintaining the posture. Thus, yoga has the potential to facilitate improvements in strength, coordination, and flexibility. These characteristics can be of great importance to those suffering from painful musculoskeletal conditions.

Therapeutic Yoga for Chronic Low Back Pain and Hyperkyphosis

General Principles

Low back pain (LBP) is one of the leading causes of disability in society today and is defined as any pain in the back that originates at the ribs and terminates just superior to the legs.[30,33,37,40] Although a wide variety of intervention options for the care of LBP exist, there are few interventions that have been shown to demonstrate efficacy as this condition becomes more chronic in nature. Recent evidence agrees on the notion that a more active approach that incorporates progressive activity and exercise is favored over an approach that emphasizes inactivity and rest.[41,42] LBP is among the most commonly reported indications for the use of CAM therapy. In 2002 alone, more than 1 million individuals used yoga as an intervention for LBP.[28]

Rationale and Efficacy

While there have been many studies on the effectiveness of interventions for the treatment of LBP, a recent **American College of Physicians (ACP)** journal review revealed that most of the literature related to the management of LBP was of poor methodological quality.[42] Two interventions that have shown promise in the literature include the use of NSAIDs and muscle relaxants in the care of these individuals.[43,44] The literature on the use of OMPT, back school, and exercise for LBP have also been shown to be efficacious.[43,45,46] No one intervention has been shown to be universally effective for all LBP patients.[41,46] Activity-related studies evaluating the success of specific interventions, including back exercises and alterations in activities of daily living (ADLs), have not all demonstrated good long-term effects.[47,48] Among the studies that explore various types of exercise for LBP, there are even fewer that examine nontraditional interventions, such as tai chi and yoga.

A multidimensional approach to managing pain that incorporates biopsychosocial factors has gained recent acceptance in Western medicine. This type of approach emphasizes the importance of psychological factors in the realm of pain research and practice.[49,50] It is generally accepted that chronic pain is comprised of at least three dimensions (biological, psychological, and social), which are equally important determinants of an individual's experience of pain.[49] CAM therapies, which routinely incorporate the concept of treating the mind as well as the body, focus on interventions that address more than one aspect of LBP and should be considered an important area worthy of further investigation.

One pilot study looked at the effects of a 6-week modified hatha yoga program on 22 patients with LBP.[51] Although potentially important trends in functional measurement scores showed improved balance and flexibility, as well as decreased disability and depression, the small sample size limited detection of significant changes. Preliminary data from a study by Williams et al[37] found that the majority of individuals with mild, chronic LBP who completed an iyengar therapeutic yoga regimen reported improvement in medical and functional pain-related outcomes.[30] This was confirmed in the published study, which also illustrated the benefit of a significant decrease in depression and a trend of reduced pain medication usage in the participants when compared to standard medical care 6-months postintervention.[52] Subjects presenting with nonspecific, chronic LBP received 16 weeks of iyengar yoga therapy and were compared to a control group who received education only. The results of medical and functional outcome measures revealed significant reductions in pain intensity (64%), functional disability (77%), and pain medication usage (88%) in the yoga group at discharge and upon 3-month follow-up.

CLINICAL PILLAR

Iyengar yoga is most frequently used in the management of LBP because it uses precise movements and alignment and employs a vast range of postures and supportive props.

A randomized controlled trial by Sherman et al[30] sought to determine whether yoga was more effective than conventional therapeutic exercise or a self-care booklet over 12 weeks for patients with chronic LBP. Back-related function in the yoga group was superior to the book and exercise groups at 12 weeks and improvements persisted at 26 weeks, revealing that yoga was more effective than traditional standard of care interventions.[36] Saper et al[53] conducted a 10-week pilot randomized controlled trial of hatha yoga in a mostly minority population of 30 participants with chronic LBP.[53] There were several statistically significant results in this study, including a decrease in mean pain scores (on a scale of 0 to 10); a decrease in the amount of overall pain medicines taken, especially NSAID and opiate usage; and overall improvement.[53] A reduction in mean *Roland-Morris Disability Questionnaire* scores was also noted.[53]

Current best evidence supports the use of exercise as a primary intervention that has been proven to be effective in reducing the symptoms associated with this entity (see Chapter 17).[30] Yoga couples positional exercise with breathing and mental focus, thus suggesting the potential benefit of incorporating yoga into the care of those suffering from LBP. Some studies have compared the effects of yoga with conventional exercise programs and found that, while yoga was beneficial, there were no statistically significant differences in outcomes when comparing yoga to conventional exercise regimens.[30] The use of flexion or extension exercises that concentrate on strengthening and/or lengthening of spinal musculature is routinely used in the care of individuals with LBP.[54] Therapeutic yoga often combines flexion and extension postures within each session and aspires to tailor movement and postures to each individual's specific presentation.

Improving one's level of general fitness is often associated with a decreased incidence of LBP and decreased level of disability.[55] Poor muscle function has long been associated with the incidence and perpetuation of LBP.[56–58] A return of complete muscle function, joint movement, and endurance is necessary for recovery of full function.[54] Strengthening and lengthening of the paraspinals, psoas, and hamstring musculature to achieve optimal physiologic balance of the lumbosacral spine is believed to lead to improved outcomes (see Chapter 17).[59]

In general, there are three types of exercises used in the management of LBP: mobility and strengthening exercise, flexion-biased exercise regimens, and extension-biased exercise regimens. Data demonstrating the efficacy of one type over another are conflicting.[60,61] Flexion exercises may be used to open the intervertebral foramina and facet joints, elongate the back extensor muscles, and strengthen the abdominal musculature.[62,63] Extension exercises are used to improve the muscle performance of the back extensors while elongating the trunk flexors. They are also routinely used in the early stages of rehabilitation for discogenic pathology (see Chapter 9).[54] Individuals with strong paraspinal extensor musculature have less postural fatigue and pain, greater capacity to lift weights, and greater ability to withstand axial compressive loads. Evidence has demonstrated the effectiveness of using extension exercises to strengthen the extensor muscles of the lumbar spine.[64,65]

The physical postures used in the asana practice of yoga combine flexion and extension for the purpose of improving flexibility and muscle function of the spine and associated structures.[66] Therefore, despite a lack of overwhelming evidence on its behalf, it seems plausible that various yogic postures may serve to be quite beneficial in the overall management of chronic LBP. To date, only two clinical trials on the benefits of yoga in LBP have used optimal clinical research methodology. Nevertheless, therapeutic yoga has been found to be effective in managing pain, strengthening paraspinal musculature, and improving motor performance.[67,68]

There is little research on the mechanisms by which yoga may relieve back pain.[30] Of the information available, there is no consistency regarding the type of yoga performed, the positions used, and the frequency with which a given protocol was used. Agreement does exist, however, on the exclusion of back-bending sustained poses to reduce the risk of reinjury in this population.[30,37] Such poses may place increased loads through the musculoskeletal system and, when performed incorrectly, may cause harm.[37]

Many of the published studies examining the correlation between yoga and LBP use postures that lengthen the muscles attaching to the spine and pelvis in positions where the spine is fully supported.[37] By maintaining support of the spine, stresses are decreased and the potential for injury is reduced. Standing poses require coordination between the extremities and the spine. These postures are often incorporated to educate individuals in the use of their extremities to lengthen pelvic and spinal tissues.[37]

The spine, legs, and hips are pivotal components that help to provide stability and support to the body during static and dynamic motion. Therefore, any imbalance or impairment in any of these areas can greatly affect the rest of the body.[29] These issues become especially important in the elderly population. Within this age group, there is a tendency to see increases in vestibular and visual impairments and a generalized decrease in coordination. Consequently, this may lead to increases in loss of balance and subsequent falls.[29]

Under normal conditions, most individuals undergo a process of *postural sway*. Even during static standing, most people experience a slow, continual shifting of body weight.[69] This shifting is believed to be due, in part, to cardiac dynamics and a lack of absolute proprioception.[69] Typically, this weight shift occurs 5 mm in a lateral direction and 8 mm in an anterior direction. Yoga may be effective at decreasing excessive postural sway and may help to improve balance, especially in the elderly population.[27] By using such poses as balancing on one foot or even concentrated standing on two feet, it may be possible to increase the strength of the knee, hip, and abdominal musculature, which may contribute to increased postural control and balance.[29]

If individuals are suffering from LBP secondary to misaligned vertebrae (either from osseous deformity or muscle imbalance) rotational movements or twists may be beneficial in alleviating symptoms. *Twists* are believed to produce contraction and relaxation of the deep back musculature, helping to realign the vertebra and decrease the potential for impingement of nerve roots. However, twists should be performed with caution, particularly in the case of intervertebral disc pathology. Finally, *inversions* may be included to reverse the compressive effects of gravity acting on the intervertebral disc space.[37] Performance of these asanas has contributed to reductions in pain medication usage, self-reported pain, and disability in some populations.[30,37] Additionally, yogic practice has also been found to be beneficial in increasing awareness of the body and in the reduction of stresses acting on the body during movement.[30,37]

At least one study has investigated the use of yoga therapy as an intervention for hyperkyphosis in women.[16] *Hyperkyphosis* is believed to result from vertebral fractures, poor posture, and/or muscular weakness.[16] In this study, a series of four different poses were used. Each series was modified to accommodate for the physical limitations of the kyphotic women. A more difficult series of new poses was introduced every 3 weeks.[16] As the poses progressed, the muscles and joints of the shoulders, erector spinae, abdominals, and cervical spine were closely monitored.[16] The results revealed an increase in baseline height and postural awareness. Additionally, 63% of the participants reported enhanced well-being, while 58% perceived an improvement in physical function.[14] A randomized controlled trial by Greendale et al. explored the use of yoga to decrease kyphosis in older men and women with adult-onset hyperkyphosis and had promising results.[70] Participants in the yoga group attended 1-hour classes 3 days per week for 24 weeks and experienced some statistically significant results, including a 4.4% improvement in flexicurve kyphosis angle ($P = 0.006$) and a 5% improvement in kyphosis index ($P = 0.004$).[(70)] Figure 21-2 displays a series of yoga asanas that are believed to be beneficial in the management of LBP.

Much of the research on yoga in the management of LBP has focused on the use of iyengar yoga protocols.[30,37] As previously described, this form of yoga allows for individual variation[14] and is practiced by a large portion of the U.S. population, making it an ideal topic for investigation.[37] This

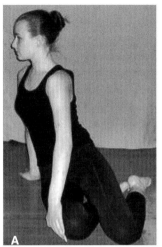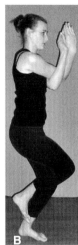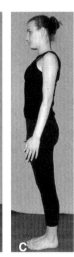

FIGURE 21–2 Asanas believed to be effective in the management of low back pain. **A.** *Bharadvajasana I* (Bharadvaja's twist). **B.** *Bharadvajasana I* (Bharadvaja's twist). **C.** *Tadasana* (mountain pose).

method of yoga emphasizes precision of movement and alignment and employs a vast range of postures and supportive props.[37] These props serve to enhance alignment, flexibility, mobility, and stability of all muscles and joints that affect spinal alignment and posture.[37] In regard to LBP, props may be used to provide external support, facilitate relaxation, provide traction, and bring awareness to specific regions of the body.[37] All of these aspects are critical components in the management and prevention of LBP.

Clearly, more evidence is needed to determine the effects of yoga on acute and chronic LBP that includes larger randomized sample sizes, group and individualized formats, and longer follow-up periods. Although much of the research on the efficacy of yoga as a therapeutic intervention for the reduction of LBP is encouraging, additional research is required to establish the efficacy and to identify specific intervention parameters required to achieve optimal outcomes. Despite the disparity of evidence, it is important to note that no evidence of harm from the use of yoga in patients with LBP has been reported in the few studies found.

QUESTIONS *for* REFLECTION

- How does an individual's ability to manage stress play a role in the incidence and perpetuation of chronic low back pain?
- What tools are available to allow manual therapists to reliably measure pain and disability?
- What role does yoga play in allowing individuals to better handle stress?

Indicators of Efficacy

Evidence supporting the efficacy of yoga in the management of LBP is sparse. Nearly all research has focused on the effectiveness of yoga on symptoms associated with regional LBP, failing to consider individuals with concomitant neurological signs and symptoms. At present, there is no one protocol that has been proven to be the most effective in controlling the symptoms associated with LBP.

Based on the current best evidence, individuals suffering from mechanical LBP for any duration of time, ranging from as little as 3 months to as long as 10 or more years, may benefit from some form of therapeutic yoga.[30,33,37,40] Additionally, individuals whose functional ability has been compromised, on any level, may find yoga extremely beneficial.[30,33,37,40] Even individuals with less severe symptoms presenting with visual analog scores (VAS) as low as 2 or 3 have reported reductions or abolishment of pain with the use of yoga.[37]

Although there are many measurement scales and other tools to evaluate levels of pain, discomfort, and functional ability, it is ultimately the patient's goals for therapy that dictate the use of CAM therapies. For individuals with high stress levels and/or poor stress management skills, the patient may consider trying therapeutic yoga as a means to manage overall stress and pain and as an aid in the resolution of symptoms.[5] Although yoga has been shown to reduce stress during intervention sessions, carry over to daily life is questionable.[5] Addressing stress and improving coping strategies is an important part of rehabilitative care (Table 21-3).[5] The relaxation and breathing aspects of yogic practice may help to relieve the stress associated with chronic pain conditions. For individuals for whom flexibility and strengthening of the thoracolumbar and abdominal musculature is indicated, yogic practice may be worth exploring.[5]

Therapeutic Yoga for Osteoarthritis
General Principles

Osteoarthritis (OA) is the most common form of arthritis and among the leading causes of disability in the United

Table 21-3	Coping Strategies That Can Help Alleviate Pain, Confusion, or Depression
COPING STRATEGY	**DESCRIPTION AND EXAMPLES**
Distraction	Trying to think of pleasant experiences. Doing something enjoyable.
Catastrophizing	Believing that something is awful and that it is never going to get better. Feeling that life isn't worth living.
Ignoring pain	Pretending that pain is not present. Acting as if nothing has happened.
Cognitive coping	Telling oneself that one can overcome anything. Reinforcing in oneself the idea that one can carry on, that things will be okay.
Distancing	Imagining that pain is outside the body.
Praying	Praying for the pain to go away. Relying on faith to get through the tough times.

Williams KA, et al. Effect of Iyengar yoga therapy for chronic low back pain. *Pain.* 2005;115(1-2):107-17.

States.[14,35,36,71] The standard of care for OA is aimed at decreasing pain and improving function by focusing intervention on periarticular tissues through exercise or external support.[14] Management of this condition typically involves correcting or supporting abnormal stresses, mobilizing hypomobility, and managing other joint symptoms.[40] While medications may be helpful in allowing individuals to cope with the symptoms of OA, it should be noted that pharmacological agents also carry potential side effects.[14] Consequently, researchers are looking for alternative methods to allow patients to better manage their symptoms.[14] The most promising intervention programs for OA include a combination of aerobic conditioning, strengthening, and techniques designed to increase range of motion (ROM).

Rationale and Efficacy

While yoga has the capacity to address OA-associated impairments, evidence regarding the effectiveness of yoga in the management of osteoarthritis is sparse. Much of the available information is limited to OA of the hands and knees.[14,35,72] These studies suggest that yoga may be beneficial in reducing pain and disability in individuals with OA.[14,35,72]

When individuals with OA present to the clinical setting, they typically complain of losses in ROM and function. In the advanced stages, chronic pain with all movements becomes the chief complaint. It is believed that the pain associated with mild to moderate OA is generally caused by contracture formation, while pain in the advanced stages is typically due to joint approximation and bony contact.[40] Clinically, the cause of pain may be distinguished easily by assessing whether pain increases with joint approximation or joint movement.[40]

In a pilot study on OA of the knees performed by Kolasinski et al,[14] the researchers used standing, sitting, and supine positions that focused on stretching and strengthening of the extremities. Participants were instructed to stretch as fully as possible without exceeding their own limits, and to use props when necessary. Props were used to provide support and balance during positions and transitional periods. For individuals with OA of the knees who are experiencing pain and/or discomfort, a prop may help to reduce weight-bearing forces through the knees. Additionally, individuals who are unsteady secondary to pain and/or discomfort may experience psychological comfort through knowing that the prop is there. Upon completion of the study, it was found that there were statistically significant improvements in levels of pain and disability.[14] Although failing to meet criteria for statistical significance, levels of stiffness were also reduced.[14]

A case-series study by Bukowski et al[73] compared the protocol used in the Kolasinski et al[14] study and compared the protocol to traditional exercise or no structured intervention. A group of 15 women and men had measurements of back and hamstring flexibility and quadriceps strength and function before and after the program. The *Western Ontario and McMaster Universities Osteoarthritis Index (WOMAC)* was used to assess subjective change after the 6-week intervention period.[73] A global assessment questionnaire was also completed by each participant and each instructor at the exit sessions to measure perceived changes in improvements since the initiation of the intervention.[73] This study found functional changes and improvement in quality of life in traditional exercise and a yoga-based approach that should encourage further comprehensive and carefully designed studies of yoga in osteoarthritis.[73] Figure 21-3 displays a commonly performed yoga asana that may be helpful in alleviating symptoms associated with OA of the lower extremity.

The mechanisms by which yoga is beneficial in the management of OA of the knees are not presently known.[14] However, several suggestions regarding such mechanisms have been made, including improvements in cardiovascular physical fitness, enhanced diaphragmatic breathing, strengthening, flexibility, and improvements in body awareness and positioning.[14]

In addition to these areas, research has also focused on psychological factors that may contribute to increased perception of symptoms such as pain and stiffness.[35,71] Stress and fatigue may cause psychological changes that may influence the manner in which an individual perceives the world around him or her. An individual who is depressed or extremely stressed may feel pain at a greater intensity than do those who are not experiencing such things. The meditation component of yoga practice may help in reducing some of these psychological influences, thus serving to regulate pain perception in this population.[29,33,35]

Indicators of Efficacy

Studies of OA of the knees by Kolasinski et al[14] and Bukowski et al[73] concluded that iyengar yoga may be "a feasible treatment option" for obese individuals greater than 50 years of age.[14,73] The researchers stated that this form of therapy has the potential to reduce pain and disability attributed to OA.[14,73] Based on the results of the Kolasinski et al[14] study, females greater than 50 years of age with a body mass index (BMI) of greater than 30 are ideal candidates for yoga therapy.[14] The Bukowski et al[73] study found functional changes and improvement in quality of life in traditional exercise and a yoga-based

approach, thus providing various therapeutic options for this population.[73]

Additionally, these researchers used several self-assessment disability scales to assess changes in symptoms over time. Although they did not provide the starting and ending data for each participant, statistically significant improvements were seen in the areas of pain, physical function, and affect.[14] Self-assessment instruments may be useful in monitoring the progress of individuals participating in therapeutic yoga and should be the focus of further investigation.

Therapeutic Yoga for Carpal Tunnel Syndrome

General Principles

Carpal tunnel syndrome (CTS) is one of the most clinically prevalent and most researched peripheral nerve entrapment neuropathies.[40] CTS is commonly associated with complications from repetitive activities, such as working on a keyboard, and may cause significant morbidity in those affected.[38]

Traditionally, CTS has been treated with wrist splints, anti-inflammatory agents, restructuring of occupational duties, injection therapy, and surgery.[38] The functional impact of CTS is profound, and current intervention strategies are often ineffective. The inability of current interventions to produce favorable outcomes has precipitated the search for alternative strategies to deal with the functional limitations and disability associated with CTS.

It is important to note that other serious conditions may present in a manner that is similar to CTS, making differential diagnosis challenging. Radiculopathy, central nervous system (CNS) lesions, vascular disorders, complex regional pain syndrome (CRPS), and other generalized peripheral neuropathies may all mimic CTS. Table 21-4 outlines the important clinical features necessary for the differential diagnosis of CTS.

Rationale and Efficacy

Yoga has been proposed as a potential intervention for CTS for a variety of reasons. It is believed that practicing better positioning and joint posture may help to decrease intermittent compression of the median nerve, while the stretching involved during performance of asanas may help to relieve compression in the carpal tunnel.[38] Finally, this relief of compression may help to improve blood flow, thus decreasing any ischemic effects on the median nerve.[38]

Of the studies that have been performed on the use of yoga for CTS, the majority of them naturally use a yoga program that focuses primarily on the upper body and extremities.[35,38] The poses adopted during therapeutic yoga regimens may help to improve flexibility and correct the alignment of the hands, wrists, arms, and shoulders and may increase awareness of optimal joint position during the performance of tasks.[38] Any poses that maintain the wrist in a flexed state for a period of time should be avoided because it places stress on the structures running through the carpal tunnel. A study by Sequeira[74] found that a posture as simple as *namaste* (prayer) serves to gently extend and stretch wrist and finger musculature, as well as

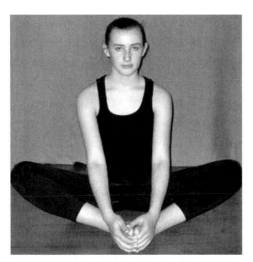

FIGURE 21–3 Asana believed to be effective in the management of osteoarthritis. *Baddha konasana* (bound angle pose/cobbler's pose).

Table 21-4	Differential Diagnosis of CTS

It is important to differentially diagnose CTS from other conditions that present with similar symptoms. The conditions, or CTS mimickers, below should be ruled out prior to initiating intervention.

CTS MIMICKERS	DIFFERENTIAL DIAGNOSTIC SYMPTOMS	
	(-) CTS	**(+) CTS**
Radiculopathy of sixth cervical nerve root	• Neck and shoulder pain • Pain with coughing, sneezing, Valsalva maneuver • Quiet night and daytime pain with use of arm • Weakness of muscles proximal to wrist	• Neck and shoulder pain are unusual with CTS. • Pain from CTS is typically relieved by massaging, shaking or immersing hand in water. • Nighttime symptoms
CNS lesions	• Typically Painless • (+) Hawkman and Babinski tests	• Pain with paresthesia • (-) CNS testing
Vascular disorders	• Symptoms in all digits	• Symptoms in median nerve distribution only
CRPS	• Generalized aching, burning with paresthesias of the entire hand	• Symptoms in median nerve distribution only
Generalized peripheral neuropathies	• Malnutrition • Toxic exposure to drugs/chemicals • Uremia • Diabetes • Leprosy	• Specific symptoms in specific neurologic distribution without widespread involvement

provide isometric resistance for the extensors and flexors.[74] Figure 21-4 displays yoga asanas that may be beneficial in reducing symptoms associated with CTS.

Indicators of Efficacy

The nonsurgical management of CTS is the first course of intervention for those with mild to moderate symptoms.[35,74,75] Most of the evidence related to the nonsurgical management of CTS is questionable due to the small number of well-controlled studies, variability in duration of symptoms and disability, and the broad range of reported outcome measures that were used. The current best evidence seems to demonstrate significant short-term benefit from oral steroids, splinting, ultrasound, carpal bone mobilization, and yoga.[2]

The literature examining the effects of yoga on CTS is particularly sparse. The only randomized controlled trial to date is a study performed by Garfinkel et al.[38] This study compared the effectiveness of iyengar yoga with the use of splinting for patients with CTS. The researchers used 11 yoga postures that were designed for strengthening, stretching, and balancing each joint in the upper body. Each posture was held for 30 seconds and followed by relaxation poses. In order for participants to be considered for this study, they had to present with at least two of five possible inclusion criteria. These criteria included a positive Tinel's sign, positive Phalen's test, pain in the median nerve distribution, sleep disturbances resulting from hand symptoms, and numbness or paresthesia in the median nerve distribution. Additionally, all participants were required to have

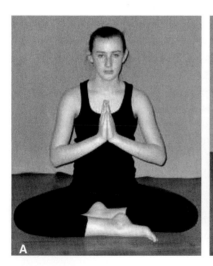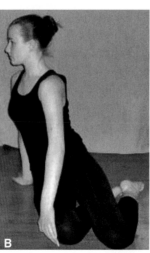

FIGURE 21-4. Asanas believed to be effective in the management of carpal tunnel syndrome. **A.** *Anjali mudra* (salutation seal). **B.** *Bharadvajasana I* (Bharadvaja's twist).

abnormal median nerve conduction latencies upon neuroelectrical testing. After 8 weeks, the results revealed that the yoga-based group had greater improvement in hand-grip strength as well as symptoms (pain) and signs (Phalen's test) associated with CTS compared to either the wrist splinting or no intervention control groups.[38] There was improvement in motor and sensory nerve conduction tests for all groups, and the difference between them was not statistically significant.[38]

It is interesting to note that a systematic review of the literature in 2002 showed yoga to be ineffective in providing short-term symptom relief for CTS.[2] A more recent review of this evidence, however, determined that there is significant short-term benefit from the use of yoga.[2] Another systematic review in 2004 found that yoga was, *"possibly effective"* and recommended yoga as the primary intervention choice in selected cases.[2] In order to further this case, more intervention trials are needed that seek to compare yoga to other management options.[2]

QUESTIONS *for* **REFLECTION**

- For each of the following selected musculoskeletal conditions, list the specific objectives for incorporation of yoga into the plan of care, additional examination procedures that may be used, and specific yoga techniques that may be used:
- Therapeutic yoga for *LBP*
- Therapeutic yoga for *OA*
- Therapeutic yoga for *CTS*

Yoga Across the Lifespan

Along with the management of neuromusculoskeletal impairment, the manual therapist must also be concerned with prevention of injury and enhancement of performance. The ***Guide to Physical Therapist Practice***[76] has clearly delineated the important role of physical therapists in the area of injury prevention. Possessing the keen ability to appreciate the finer nuances of movement, the manual physical therapist is uniquely positioned to facilitate the adoption of more normal movement patterns in the healthy, uninjured population.

Improvements in muscle power, dexterity, and visual perception in female athletes trained in yoga have shown greater results than traditional training.[77] Yoga has also demonstrated significant improvement in the running performance of high school students. Although the effect size was small in these studies, yoga demonstrated the ability to enhance athletic performance.[77]

The ancient system of **kundalini yoga (KY)** includes a vast array of meditation techniques. Elements of the KY protocol may have applications for psycho-oncology patients.[78] Case studies have been conducted in the use of KY as an adjunctive therapy. **Mindfulness-based stress reduction** is a clinically valuable, self-administered intervention for cancer patients with orthopaedic-related conditions.[78] Modifications to the traditional mindfulness-based stress reduction program makes comparisons

between studies difficult and a lack of well-controlled studies precludes the development of any firm conclusions regarding efficacy. Further research into the efficacy, feasibility, and safety of this approach for cancer patients is still needed.

Studies have also examined the use of yoga in the elderly population. Yoga was found to produce improvement in physical measures including the timed unilateral standing test and forward flexibility. In addition, improvement was found in a number of quality-of-life measures that were specifically related to a sense of well-being, energy, and fatigue compared to controls.[24] There were no relative improvements in cognitive function among healthy seniors in the yoga or exercise group compared to the wait-list control group. In another study, yoga was shown to improve sleep quality, depression, and daytime dysfunction in elders in assisted living facilities.[79]

A comprehensive, but not systematic, review of the literature on complementary and alternative interventions, specifically mind-body therapy, on musculoskeletal disease was conducted at Stanford University.[80] The goals of the review were to establish a comprehensive literature review and provide a rationale for future research on the theme of *successful aging*. Mind-body techniques were found to be efficacious, primarily as complementary interventions, for musculoskeletal disease and related disorders.[80] Studies provided evidence for treatment efficacy; however, the need for additional well-controlled research was established.[80]

Therapeutic Yoga as an Adjunct to Orthopaedic Manual Physical Therapy

Throughout this chapter we have attempted to introduce the philosophy and practice of therapeutic yoga as it applies to specific populations suffering from neuromusculoskeletal dysfunction. As for most interventions designed to address musculoskeletal impairment, therapeutic yoga is presumed to be most effective when combined with other intervention strategies. The effective use of OMPT interventions is based on a clear understanding of normal joint kinematics and the manual physical therapist's ability to identify aberrant movement patterns. By definition, OMPT emphasizes a "hands-on" approach to the management of musculoskeletal dysfunction; however, OMPT is not a panacea. Management of musculoskeletal conditions through OMPT relies on other interventions to enhance its effectiveness.

QUESTIONS *for* **REFLECTION**

- How might yoga be used as an adjunct to orthopaedic manual physical therapy?
- Consider how yoga may be used prior to the application of OMPT techniques or following techniques to prepare or support the patient, respectively.
- How does the use of yoga compare with other physical therapy interventions typically used as adjuncts to OMPT?

The beneficial effects of therapeutic yoga in promoting relaxation and reducing stress has been well-documented.[33,34] Individuals suffering from musculoskeletal impairment often present with pain, or fear of pain, that prohibits the manual physical therapist from implementing techniques designed to promote movement. The use of yogic postures and movements prior to, or immediately following, the application of OMPT techniques may serve to reduce voluntary muscle guarding and enhance the patient's willingness to move and/or be moved. More specifically, engaging in a yogic therapy regimen that incorporates concentration (dharana), meditation (dhyana), focusing inward (pratyahara), and the use of regulated breathing (pranayama) prior to OMPT may serve to control the fear often associated with movement of painful structures, thus allowing manual interventions to have a more optimal effect.

As previously described, the attainment of yogic postures and movements requires individuals to focus on the task at hand in a manner that allows them to "experience" each posture physically, mentally, and spiritually. Intense concentration (dharana) during the performance of slowly performed movements and static postures may allow individuals to engage in a process of motor learning that leads to more efficient, pain-free, and functional movement patterns. Teaching individuals to learn how to move efficiently within a newly acquired movement pattern is important for enhancing the effects of OMPT while preventing recidivism.

As the manual physical therapist endeavors to restore normal movement patterns, the principles of hatha yoga may prove to be effective. As described, this form of yoga allows the individual to experience the physical aspects of yoga through exploration of various multiplanar postures and movements. These procedures are effective at stretching tight muscles while improving the recruitment patterns of other muscles through the incorporation of functional movement. These movements may serve to reduce myofascial contributions to restricted movement prior to OMPT, thus allowing manual interventions to be more effective in reducing intra-articular restrictions. Other principles of hatha yoga that may enhance the effects of OMPT include sessions that involve a variety of poses, use of counterposes for each pose that is introduced, and a progression from basic to more advanced postures. The practice of ashtanga involves the use of flowing asana movements. These movements allow individuals to experience, use, and maintain functional movements that have been newly achieved through OMPT interventions.

Additionally, iyengar poses that use prolonged positioning may be a useful adjunct to OMPT. These poses are held for prolonged periods of time with strict attention to performance and the use of props to accommodate for individual impairments. Viniyoga poses are customized for the unique physical limitations of individuals. These poses may serve to facilitate more normal muscle recruitment patterns and enhance stability through cocontraction facilitated by sustained isometric contractions. The development of endurance in core-stabilizing musculature through a concentrated focus on static postures is an important feature of yoga that is also considered to be a necessary adjunct to OMPT as well.

EVIDENCE SUMMARY

A search of the **Cochrane Collection** evidence-based medicine databases for critical reviews published on existing and definitive controlled trials using the keyword *yoga*, and a search in the **Database of Abstracts of Reviews of Effects** resulted in only four critical reviews on this topic.

A search in the **Cochrane Database of Systematic Reviews** yielded 14 systematic reviews. One such review was on the nonsurgical management (other than steroid injection) for CTS.[81] This systematic review concluded that the current evidence demonstrates significant short-term benefit of yoga on symptoms of pain related to CTS and notes that more trials are needed to compare interventions and to ascertain the duration of benefit. In addition to limited evidence for the use of yoga for CTS, the efficacy of yoga for other musculoskeletal conditions, such as LBP, is also lacking. The high prevalence of chronic low back pain coupled with the lack of relevant literature indicates that more rigorous investigation into the use of therapeutic yoga for individuals with LBP is necessary.

Relevant studies were identified using several databases: **PubMed** (January 1960 to 2008), **CAM on PubMed** (January 1960 to July 15, 2004), **MEDLINE** (January 1966 to July 15, 2004), **CINAHL** (January 1983 to July 2004), and **PsychINFO** (January 1960 to July 15, 2004). English-only studies were included, which may likely have created some bias in the results. Some would argue, however, that this bias was minimized, as a recent assessment reported that non-English papers were likely of low quality and may, themselves, introduce bias.[82]

Currently, some 45 Indian medical journals are indexed in MEDLINE; we also searched the **Indian MEDLARS Center's IndMED** database (January 1985 to July 2004), which contains additional Indian journals. Results that were published in Indian journals are not discussed here largely because of their questionable quality and full-text inaccessibility.

Using various keywords, each database was searched, and when possible, searches were limited to *clinical trial, randomized controlled trial, review,* and *meta-analysis*. The PsychINFO and IndMED databases do not have the option of searching with limitations, and CINAHL does not limit studies to randomized controlled trials or meta-analyses. In order to determine the depth of research regarding two of the specific conditions and interventions discussed in this chapter, the keywords *carpal tunnel syndrome* and *low back pain* were searched, separately. Adding *therapy* to these two searches further refined the field, showing many review articles on these two subjects. A search using *yoga* yielded quite a few studies, but a cursory review revealed that most of these studies investigated the use of yoga for asthma, epilepsy, diabetes, multiple sclerosis, stress management, and psychotherapy, among others. Combining *yoga* with the additional keywords *pain, low back pain, carpal tunnel syndrome,* or *musculoskeletal* resulted in very few studies. That there are few studies on yoga and CTS and yoga and LBP is surprising. It is obvious that much work still needs to be done to scientifically demonstrate the potential preventative and therapeutic role of yoga on the neuromusculoskeletal system.

Lastly, since psychoemotional stress has been shown to be one of the factors leading to musculoskeletal disorders such as

LBP and CTS,[83] the literature concerning yoga's role in managing stress was also investigated. We used the keyword *yoga* paired with *stress, anxiety, or coping*. As expected, a large body of evidence was found that investigated yoga's role in managing stress and anxiety. Addressing stress and improving coping strategies is an important aspect of care that must routinely accompany OMPT interventions.

A more recent systematic review concluded that yoga was potentially effective and recommends its use as the first choice of management in selected cases.[84] Additional high-quality trials are necessary in order to fully delineate the role and efficacy of mind-body therapies, particularly yoga, in the management of musculoskeletal conditions. Future research should focus on identifying specific patient characteristics for which therapeutic yoga may be efficacious. Additional evidence is also required to outline which specific poses are most effective and what factors may be used to predict favorable outcomes in the management of these conditions. Future research initiatives should also focus on developing a greater understanding regarding the mechanisms of action, methods of evaluating outcomes, and on establishing the use of therapeutic yoga as an adjunct to OMPT and other, more traditional, interventions (Table 21-5).

SUMMARY AND CONCLUSIONS

The factor that makes yoga so promising as a therapeutic intervention worthy of consideration is its adaptability and applicability to a variety of different populations. Yogic postures and movements are routinely adapted to facilitate ease of performance and better tolerance for individuals across the life span who present with a variety of impairments ranging from cardiovascular to musculoskeletal to neurological in nature. Since yoga can be conducted in a group setting, it is a relatively inexpensive form of physical conditioning that may prove to be a cost-effective alternative in the management of musculoskeletal disorders. The reported benefits in nonspecific musculoskeletal syndromes have been sufficiently large and the incidence of serious side effects negligible.[85] These factors combine to promote therapeutic yoga as a potentially viable option for the innovative manual physical therapist and certainly an approach that warrants further investigation.

Studies are beginning to demonstrate that therapeutic yoga can help to decrease stress levels, thus decreasing an individual's perception of pain or discomfort.[19,20,23,29,78] In order for yoga to be optimally effective, it is important that all three domains (psychological, physical, and emotional) are being adequately addressed. Unlike other CAM therapies, such as acupuncture, yoga encompasses not only the physical domain, but the spiritual and psychological domains as well. All three realms are believed to play an important role in the healing process and in restoring individuals to optimal health.[24,77,78,86]

While in the past, the focus of yoga was primarily spiritual, in today's society yoga has found its niche in new and different areas of everyday life.[27] By expanding upon the basic application of yoga, some studies are finding that stress-related ailments are responding positively to this newly recognized intervention approach.[19,20,23,29,78] While there is not a great deal of evidence for yoga as a sole intervention, therapeutic yoga as a complement to more traditional approaches, may be effective in the alleviation of symptoms and in the promotion of optimal health and well-being.

Table 21–5   Results of Literature Search

DATABASE	PUBLICATION TYPE	YOGA AND BACK PAIN	YOGA AND OSTEOARTHRITIS	YOGA AND CTS
PubMed	Clinical Trials	3	2	0
	RCT	6	1	1
	Reviews	4	4	8
	Surveys	3	0	0
	Pilot Studies	1	0	0
	Case Reports	0	1	0
	Meta-Analysis	0	0	1
Health Source / Nursing Edition	Review	5	0	2
	RCT	3	0	1
	Survey	1	0	0
	Case Reports	1	0	0
	Pilot Studies	0	1	0
	Meta-Analysis	0	1	0
Elsevier Science Direct	RCT	2	0	0
	Reviews	1	0	1
	Surveys	1	0	0
PEDro	Clinical Trials	3	1	1
	Reviews	0	1	2
Database of Abstracts of Reviews of Effectiveness	Reviews	1	2	1

CLINICAL CASE

Examination

History of Present Illness: A 25-year-old graduate student with past medical history of chronic low back pain for 2 years presents to your facility with a more recent onset of bilateral wrist pain. He is currently undergoing work-up for CTS. He describes pain in his wrists that is most notable upon awakening, usually lasting for up to 1 hour. Intermittent pain is noted throughout the day after prolonged computer work. Pain is currently at a 7/10 level bilaterally. Furthermore, this patient also reports radiating pain, numbness, and paresthesia proximally and distally from the wrists. He has undergone a previous attempt at physical therapy for his low back pain approximately 2 years ago with only fair results. He was referred to your facility by his physician to begin a course of intervention designed to manage his newly acquired upper extremity pain and his chronic LBP complaints.

Patient Goals: "To decrease pain so that I can better tolerate a regular exercise program and daily activities."

Employment: Patient is a graduate student with no outside employment.

Recreational Activities: Prior to his recent LBP and wrist pain, he engaged in strength training, skiing, hiking, camping.

General Health: Good

Medications: None

Diagnostic Tests: Recent radiographs of the lumbosacral spine reveal a grade 2 anterior spondylolisthesis at L5-S1. Magnetic resonance imaging (MRI) reveals the presence of an anterior herniated nucleus pulposus (HNP) at L4-5. He is currently scheduled for nerve conduction velocity (NCV) and electromyogram (EMG) studies next week.

Musculoskeletal: Assisted range of motion (AROM): Trunk limited in full extension and flex, bilateral upper and lower extremities within normal limits except for bilateral wrists: −5 degrees of extension. Posture: Patient presents with forward head and shoulders. Cervical ROM: restricted in side bending and rotation at end range, bilaterally.

Neuromuscular: Force generation: Trunk: 4/5; bilateral extremities 5/5 throughout. Sensation: Decrease at C6-7 dermatomes, right greater than left. Tests for CTS: + Tinel's sign and Phalen's tests, bilaterally. Neural Tension Tests: + C5-7 nerve root involvement.

Function: Pain: LBP 4/10 in the seated position; 6/10 after moderate physical activity, including ambulation for more than 0.5 hour, repetitive forward flexion and extension. CTS pain: 7/10 on the right and 6/10 on the left.

Self-Assessed Disability: Short Form 36 Health Survey (SF 36) = 30 (below the standard norm); Oswestry Disability Index (ODI) = 38% (indicating moderate disability); Life Stress Inventory = 225 (implying a 50% chance of a major health challenge within the next 2 years).

Intervention

This patient attended eight physical therapy sessions over the course of a month that incorporated OMPT, including soft tissue mobilization and intervertebral joint mobilization of the lumbosacral spine, as well as therapeutic exercise designed to improve spinal mobility with a focus on core stabilization. He has continued with the prescribed exercise program with moderate compliance. He also incorporated the use of proper ergonomics in his workspace and was given wrist splints for his CTS pain, which he wears nightly.

After eight sessions, improvement in trunk ROM and flexibility was improved and an overall reduction in his wrist symptoms was noted; however, the relief that he experienced was brief in duration, and his symptoms still prohibited him from certain daily activities. A reexamination demonstrated an improvement in trunk ROM and flexibility by 30% overall. He reported improvement in LBP, which was at a 3/10 level, and CTS symptoms at a 4/10 level. Due to his persistent symptoms, transcutaneous electrical stimulation (TENS) was attempted but found to be too cumbersome to use on a regular basis and was, therefore, discontinued. Results of NCV and EMG studies revealed mild CTS. ODI score = 30%, revealing moderate disability.

Based on the presented information answer or discuss the following:

1. What are some of the potential reasons why the typical standard of care interventions for LBP and CTS were not completely successful in this case?

2. What aspects of this patient's presentation suggest that this individual may benefit from incorporating therapeutic yoga into the plan of care?

3. What aspects of yoga do you believe would be most beneficial for this patient? Outline how this patient may benefit from a course of therapeutic yoga that incorporates the following: self-awareness, relaxation and stress relief, controlled respiration, enhanced self-understanding and self-acceptance, increased body awareness and control, performance of precise movement patterns, sustained postures, and group and social support.

4. What asanas do you believe would be safest and most efficacious in the care of this patient? Choose a progression of asanas from Figures 21-2, 21-3, and 21-4 and provide rationale for your choices.

5. What props may be used during this individual's therapeutic yoga to increase patient tolerance leading to more favorable outcomes?

HANDS-ON

With a partner, perform the following activities:

1 Perform each asana listed in Figures 21-2, 21-3, 21-4. While performing each posture, identify which muscles are undergoing elongation, which muscles are contracting, and which muscles are most involved in maintaining the posture. While maintaining each posture, take note of any areas that are uncomfortable and the relative ease with which each position is achieved. Now, instruct your partner in the performance of each posture.

2 While maintaining each asana as recommended above, engage in deep breathing (pranayama) and concentrate (dharana) on the proper performance of each movement and attainment of each posture.

3 Identify one area of muscular inflexibility on your partner and choose an asana designed to address the area of tightness. Be sure to use specific instructions to maintain proper postures, and encourage concentration and regulated breathing. Reexamine the area of inflexibility immediately following your intervention to identify any changes.

REFERENCES

1. National Center for Complementary and Alternative Medicine (NCCAM). Home page. http://nccam.nih.gov/health/
2. Galantino ML, Musser J. Evidence-based yoga for chronic low back pain. In: Deutsch J, ed. *Complementary Therapies for Physical Therapists: A Clinical Decision-Making Approach*. St. Louis, MO: Saunders Elsevier; 2008.
3. Barnes PM, Powell-Griner E, McFann K, Nahin RL. Complementary and alternative medicine use among adults: United States, 2002. In: *Advance Data from Vital and Health Statistics*. Hyattsville, MD: National Center for Health Statistics; 2004.
4. Reid MC, Papaleontiou M, Ong A, et al. Self-management strategies to reduce pain and improve function among older adults in community settings: a review of the evidence. *Pain Med*. 2008;9:409-424.
5. Farrell SJ, Ross AD, Sehgal KV. Eastern movement therapies. *Phys Med Rehabil Clin N Am*. 1999;10:617-629.
6. Wolsko PM, Eisenberg DM, Davis RB, Phillips RS. Use of mind–body medical therapies: results of a national survey. *J Gen Intern Med*. 2004;19:43-50.
7. Sobel DS. Mind matters, money matters: the cost-effectiveness of mind-body medicine. *JAMA*. 2000;284:1705.
8. Sobel D. The cost-effectiveness of mind-body medicine interventions. *Prog Brain Res*. 2000;122:393-412.
9. Feuerstein G. *The Deeper Dimension of Yoga: Theory and Practice*. Boston, MA: Shambhala Publications; 2003.
10. Sabina AB, Williams AL, Wall HK, et al. Yoga intervention for adults with mild-to-moderate asthma: a pilot study. *Ann Allergy Asthma Immunol*. 2005;94:543-548.
11. Vempati R, Bijlani RL, Deepak KK. The efficacy of a comprehensive lifestyle modification programme based on yoga in the management of bronchial asthma: a randomized controlled trial. *BMC Pulm Med*. 2009;9:37.
12. Shannahoff-Khalsa DS, Sramek BB, Kennel MB, et al. Hemodynamic observations on yogic breathing technique claimed to help eliminate and prevent heart attacks: a pilot study. *J Altern Complementary Med*. 2004;10:757-766.
13. Jayasinghe SR. Yoga in cardiac health (a review). *Eur J Cardiovasc Prev Rehabil*. 2004;11:369-375.
14. Kolasinski SL, Garfinkel M, Tsai AG, et al. Iyengar yoga for treating symptoms of OA of the knees: a pilot study. *J Altern Complementary Med*. 2005;11:689-693.
15. Zaman T, Agarwal S, Handa R. Complementary and alternative medicine use in rheumatoid arthritis: an audit of patients visiting a tertiary care centre. *Natl Med J India*. 2007;20:236-239.
16. Greendale GA, McDivit A, Carpenter A, Seeger L, Huang M. Yoga for women with hyperkyphosis: results of a pilot study. *Am J Public Health*. 2002;92:1611-1614.
17. Oken BS, Kishiyama S, Zajdel D, et al. Randomized controlled trial of yoga and exercise in multiple sclerosis. *Neurology*. 2004;62:2058-2064.
18. Yardi N. Yoga for control of epilepsy. *Seizure*. 2001;10:7-12.
19. Benson H, Malvea BP, Graham JR. Physiologic correlates of meditation and their clinical effects in headache: an ongoing investigation. *Headache*. 1973;13:23-24.
20. Pilkington K, Kirkwood G, Rampes H, Richardson J. Yoga for depression: the research evidence. *J Affect Disord*. 2005;89:12-24.

21. Malhotra V, Singh S, Tandon OP, et al. Effect of yoga asanas on nerve conduction in type 2 diabetes. *Indian J Physiol Pharmacol.* 2002;46:298-306.
22. Hanada EY. Efficacy of rehabilitative therapy in regional musculoskeletal conditions. Best practice and research. *Clin Rheumatol.* 2003;17:151-166.
23. Shannahoff-Khalsa D. Complementary healthcare practices. Stress management for gastrointestinal disorders: the use of Kundalini yoga meditation techniques. *Gastoenterol Nurs.* 2002;25:126-129.
24. Oken BS, Zajdel D, Kishiyama S, et al. Randomized, controlled, six-month trial of yoga in healthy seniors: effects on cognition and quality of life. *Altern Ther Health Med.* 2006;12:40-47.
25. Sparrowe L. *Yoga: A Yoga Journal Book.* Fairfield, CT: Hugh Lauter Levin Associates; 2004.
26. Carrico M. Patanjali's eight-fold path offers guidelines for a meaningful and purposeful life. *Yoga J.* www.yogajournal.com/newtoyoga/158_1.cfm
27. Magee D. *Orthopaedic Physical Therapy Clinics of North America.* Philadelphia, PA: WB Saunders; 2000:341-359.
28. Marx I. *Yoga and Common Sense.* New York, NY: Bobbs-Merrill; 1970.
29. Smith J, Kelly E, Monks J. *Pilates and Yoga: A High-energy Partnership of Physical and Spiritual Exercise Techniques to Revitalize the Mind and Body.* London: Hermes House; 2005.
30. Sherman KJ, Cherkin DC, Erro J, Miglioretti DL, Deyo RA. Comparing yoga, exercise, and a self-care book for chronic low back pain: a randomized, controlled trial. *Ann Intern Med.* 2005;143:849-856.
31. Garfinkel MS, Singhal A, Katz WA, Allan, DA et al. Yoga-based intervention for carpal tunnel syndrome: a randomized trial. *JAMA.* 1998;280:1601-1603.
32. Eisenberg D, Post D, Davis RB, et al. Addition of choice of complementary therapies to usual care for acute low back pain: a randomized controlled trial. *Spine.* 2007;32:151-158.
33. Patel CH, North WR. Randomized control trial of yoga and bio-feedback in the management of hypertension. *Lancet.* 1973;2:1053-1055.
34. Patel C. 12-month follow-up of yoga and bio-feedback in the management of hypertension. *Lancet.* 1975;2:93-95.
35. Garfinkel MS. *The Effect of Yoga and Relaxation Techniques on Outcome Variables Associated with Osteoarthritis of the Hands and Finger Joints* [doctoral thesis]. Philadelphia: Temple University; 1992.
36. Van Baar ME, Dekker J, Lemmens JA. Pain and disability in patients with osteoarthritis of hip or knee: the relationship with articular, kinesiological, and psychological characteristics. *J Rheumatol.* 1998;25:125-133.
37. Williams KA, Petronis J, Smith D, et al. Effect of Iyengar yoga therapy for chronic low back pain. *Pain.* 2005;115:107-117.
38. Garfinkel MS, Singhal A, Katz WA, et al. Yoga-based intervention for carpal tunnel syndrome: a randomized trial. *JAMA.* 1998;280:1601-1603.
39. Bosch PR, Traustadottir T, Howard P, Matt KS. Functional and physiological effects of yoga in women with rheumatoid arthritis: a pilot study. *Altern Ther Health Med.* 2009;4:24-31.
40. Tomberlin JP, Saunders HD. *Evaluation, Treatment, and Prevention of Musculoskeletal Disorders.* 3rd ed.Minneapolis, MN: The Saunders Group; 1994.
41. Deyo RA, Walsh NE, Martin DC, Schoenfield LS. A controlled-trial of transcutaneous electrical nerve stimulation (TENS) and exercise for chronic low back pain. *N Engl J Med.* 1990;322:1627-1634.
42. Evans C, Gilbert JR, Taylor W, Hildebrand A. A randomized controlled trial of flexion exercises, education, and bed rest for patients with acute low back pain. *Physiother Can.* 1987;39:96-101.
43. Malanga GA, Nadler SF. Non-operative treatment of low back pain. *Mayo Clin Proc.* 1999;74:1135-1148.
44. Koes BW, Scholten RJ, Mens JM, Bouter LM. Efficacy of non-steroidal anti-inflammatory drugs for low back pain: a systematic review of randomised clinical trials. *Ann Rheum Dis.* 1997;56:214-223.
45. Shekelle PG, Adams AH, Chassin MR, Hurwitz EL, Brook RH. Spinal manipulation for low-back pain. *Ann Intern Med.* 1992;117:590-598.
46. Hurwitz EL, Morgenstern H, Harber P, et al. A randomized trial of medical care with and without physical therapy and chiropractic care with and without physical modalities for patients with low back pain: 6-month follow-up outcomes from the UCLA low back pain study. *Spine.* 2002;27:2193-2204.
47. Mannion AF, Muntener EA. A randomized clinical trial of three active therapies for chronic low back pain. *Spine.* 1999;24:2435-2448.
48. Frost H, Klaber Moffett JA, Moser JS, Fairbank JCT. Randomized controlled trial for evaluation of fitness programme for patients with chronic low back pain. *Brit Med J.* 1995;310:151-159.
49. Spelman MR. Back pain: How health education affects patient compliance with treatment. *Occup Health Nurs.* 1984;32:649-651.
50. Jacobson L, Marino AJ. General considerations of chronic pain. In: Loeser JD, ed. *Bonica's Management of Pain.* 3rd ed. Philadelphia, PA: Lippincott Williams & Wilkins; 2001.
51. Linton SJ. A review of psychological risk factors in back and neck pain. *Spine.* 2000;25:148-156.
52. Williams K, Abildso C, Steinberg L, et al. Evaluation of the effectiveness and efficacy of Iyengar yoga therapy on chronic low back pain. *Spine.* 2009;34:2066-2076.
53. Saper RB, Sherman KJ, Cullum-Dugan D, et al. Yoga for chronic low back pain in a predominantly minority population: a pilot randomized controlled trial. *Altern Ther Health Med.* 2009;6:18-27.
54. Galantino ML, Bzdewka TM, Eissler-Russo JL, et al. The impact of modified hatha yoga on chronic low back pain: a pilot study. *Altern Ther Health Med.* 2004;10:56-59.
55. Borenstein DG, Wiesel SW, Boden SD. Medical therapy. In: Borenstein DG, Wiesel SW, Boden SD, eds. *Low Back and Neck Pain: Comprehensive Diagnosis and Management.* 3rd ed. Philadelphia, PA: Elsevier; 2004:785-793.
56. Cady LD, Bischoff DP, O'Connell ER, Thomas PC, Allan JH. Strength and fitness and subsequent back injuries in firefighters. *J Occup Med.* 1979;21:269-272.
57. De Vries H. EMG fatigue nerve in postural muscles: a possible etiology for idiopathic low back pain. *Am J Phys Med.* 1968;47:175.
58. Magora A. Investigation of the relation between low back pain and occupation: IV. *Scand J Rehabil Med.* 1974;6:81-88.
59. Poulsen E. Back muscle strength and weight limits in lifting. *Spine.* 1981;6:73-75.
60. Nachemson A. The possible importance of the psoas muscle for stabilization of the lumbar spine. *Acta Othop Scand.* 1968;39:47-57.
61. Raghuraj P, Telles S. Muscle power, dexterity skill and visual perception in community home girls trained in yoga or sports and in regular school girls. *Indian J Physiol Pharmacol.* 1997;41:409-415.
62. Donohue B, Miller A, Beisecker M, et al. Effects of brief yoga exercises and motivational preparatory interventions in distance runners: results of a controlled trial. *Br J Sports Med.* 2006;40:60-63.
63. Williams P. Lesions of the lumbosacral spine. I. *J Bone Joint Surg.* 1937;19:343.
64. Williams P: Lesions of the lumbosacral spine. II. *J Bone Joint Surg.* 1937;19:690.
65. Pollock ML, Leggett SH, Graves JE, et al. Effect of resistance training on lumbar extension strength. *Am J Sports Med.* 1989;17:624-629.
66. Pauley J. EMG analysis of certain movements and exercise: some deep muscles of the back. *Anat Rec.* 1966;155:223.
67. Tran MD, Holly RG, Lashbrook J, Amsterdam EA. Effects of hatha yoga practice on the health-related aspects of physical fitness. *Prev Cardiol.* 2001;4:165-170.
68. Taylor MJ, Majundmar M. Incorporating yoga therapeutics into orthopaedic physical therapy. In: Galantino ML, ed. *Orthopaedic Physical Therapy Clinics of North America.* Philadelphia, PA: W.B. Saunders; 2000: 341-352.
69. Nespor K. Pain management and yoga. *Int J Psychosom.* 1991;38:76-81.
70. Greendale GA, Huang M-H, Karlamangla AS, Seeger L, Crawford S. Yoga decreases kyphosis in senior women and men with adult-onset hyperkyphosis: results of a randomized controlled trial. *J Am Geriatr Soc.* 2009;57:1569-1579.
71. Perry J. *Gait Analysis: Normal and Pathological Function.* Thorofare, NJ: SLACK, Inc.; 1992.
72. Towheed TE. Systematic review of therapies for osteoarthritis of the hand. *Osteoarthritis Cartilage.* 2005;13:455-462.
73. Bukowski E, Conway A, Glentz LA, Kurland K, Galantino ML. The effect of yoga and strengthening exercises for people living with osteoarthritis of the knee: a case series. *Int Q Community Health Educ.* 2007;26:287-305.
74. Sequeira W. Yoga in treatment of carpal tunnel syndrome. *Lancet.* 1999;353:689-690.
75. Wolfe F. Determinants of WOMAC function, pain and stiffness scores: evidence for the role of low back pain, symptom counts, fatigue and depression in OA, RA and fibromyalgia. *Rheumatology.* 1999;38:355-361.
76. APTA. *Guide to Physical Therapist Practice.* Rev., 2nd ed. Alexandria, VA: American Physical Therapy Association; 2003.
77. Raghuraj P, Telles S. Muscle power, dexterity skill and visual perception in community home girls trained in yoga or sports and in regular school girls. *Indian J Physiol Pharmacol.* 1997;41:409-415.
78. Shannahoff-Khalsa DS. Patient perspectives: Kundalini yoga meditation techniques for psycho-oncology and as potential therapies for cancer. *Integrative Cancer Therapy.* 2005;4:87-100.

79. Chen KM, Chen MH, Lin MH, et al. Effects of yoga on sleep quality and depression in elders in assisted living facilities. *J Nurs Res.* 2010;18:53-61.
80. Smith JE, Richardson J, Hoffman C, Pilkington K. Mindfulness-based stress reduction as supportive therapy in cancer care: systematic review. *J Adv Nurs.* 2005;52:315-327.
81. O'Connor D, Marshall S, Massy-Westropp N. Non-surgical treatment (other than steroid injection) for carpal tunnel syndrome. *Cochrane Database Syst Rev.* 2004;CD003219.
82. Egger M, Juni P, Bartlett C, Holenstein F, Sterne I. How important are comprehensive literature searches and the assessment of trial quality in systematic reviews? Empirical study. *Health Technol Assess.* 2003;7:68.
83. Gura ST. Yoga for stress reduction and injury prevention at work. *Work.* 2002;19:3-7.
84. Goodyear-Smith F, Arroll B. What can family physicians offer patients with carpal tunnel syndrome other than surgery? A systematic review of nonsurgical management. *Ann Fam Med.* 2004;2:267-273.
85. Luskin FM, Newell KA, Griffith M, et al. A review of mind/body therapies in the treatment of musculoskeletal disorders with implications for the elderly. *Altern Ther Health Med.* 2000;6:46-56.
86. Donohue B, Miller A, Beisecker M. Effects of brief yoga exercises and motivational preparatory interventions in distance runners: results of a controlled trial. 2006;40:60-63.

Practice of Orthopaedic Manual Physical Therapy

CHAPTER
22

Orthopaedic Manual Physical Therapy of the Shoulder Joint Complex

Christopher H. Wise, PT, DPT, OCS, FAAOMPT, MTC, ATC

Chapter Objectives

At the conclusion of this chapter, the reader will be able to:

- Identify the key anatomical and biomechanical features of the shoulder and their impact on examination and intervention.
- List and perform key procedures used in the orthopaedic manual physical therapy (OMPT) examination of the shoulder.
- Demonstrate sound clinical decision-making in evaluating the results of the OMPT examination.

- Use pertinent examination findings to reach a differential diagnosis and prognosis.
- Discuss issues related to the safe performance of OMPT interventions for the shoulder.
- Demonstrate basic competence in the performance of a skill set of joint mobilization techniques for the shoulder.

FUNCTIONAL ANATOMY AND KINEMATICS

Introduction

Normal function of the shoulder joint complex requires the precise synchronization of four distinct articulations. The *sternoclavicular, acromioclavicular, scapulothoracic,* and *glenohumeral joints* compose a system of interdependent joints that serve a preeminent role in the function of the upper extremity. Cyriax[1] describes the primary function of the shoulder as positioning the hand in space so as to allow an individual to interact with his or her environment and to perform fine motor functional tasks. See Table 22-1 for shoulder motions that are typically required to perform common functional activities.

The Sternoclavicular Joint

The *sternoclavicular (SC) joint* is generally considered to be a **saddle joint**[2,3] that operates about three axes of motion (Fig. 22-1). The head of the clavicle is larger than the

articulating surface of the sternum, thus predisposing the joint to instability, particularly in response to medially directed forces. The sternal articular surface is concave in the frontal plane and convex in the sagittal plane, which corresponds to the medial articular surface of the clavicle. An *intra-articular disc* divides the joint into two individual synovial cavities and resists medial migration of the clavicle and provides shock absorption. The medial clavicle also articulates inferiorly with the costal cartilage of the first rib, which contributes to the stability of the SC joint.

Stability of the SC Joint

The synovial capsule of the SC joint is considered to be least extensive at its inferior aspect.[4] The *sternoclavicular ligaments (SCL)* reinforce the weak capsule and provide restraint for anterior and posterior glide. Providing the primary restraint to superior and lateral displacement is the *interclavicular ligament (ICL)*, which spans the sternal notch extending from one SC joint to its contralateral counterpart. The extracapsular *costoclavicular ligament (CSCL)* lies lateral to the SC joint and provides a restraint to elevation of the clavicle.

Table 22–1	Shoulder Motions Required for Functional Activities
FUNCTIONAL ACTIVITY	**REQUIRED ROM**
Brushing hair	120 degrees of abduction 90 degrees of external rotation
Tuck in shirt	30 degrees extension 90 degrees internal rotation 60 degrees adduction
Eating	60 degrees abduction 45 degrees horizontal adduction
Apply deodorant	45 degrees flexion 60 degrees horizontal adduction
Clean ear	110 degrees abduction 80 degrees external rotation

Adapted from Magee DJ. *Orthopedic Physical Assessment*, 4th ed. Philadelphia, PA: WB Saunders; 2002.

Mobility of the SC Joint

There are three degrees of freedom available at the SC joint. *Elevation* and *depression* occur within the *frontal plane*. Elevation requires inferior accessory glide, which typically occurs between the medial clavicle and intra-articular disc (Fig. 22-2).[5] This motion is restrained by the CSCL.[4-6] Only 5 degrees of depression is expected; however, more movement may occur in cases of interclavicular ligament or suspensory muscle compromise.[7] *Protraction* and *retraction* generally occur in the *transverse plane*; however, the axis of motion is more commonly considered to be oblique in orientation.[2] Therefore, protraction is accompanied by depression and retraction by elevation.[2,4] Protraction and retraction are facilitated by anterior and posterior gliding between the sternal articular surface and the intra-articular disc, respectively (Fig. 22-3).[5] Protraction is limited by the posterior CSCL, ICL, and SC capsule[5,4] and retraction is limited by the anterior CCL and SC capsule.[4] *Upward* and *downward rotation* occur in the *sagittal plane* about the long axis of the clavicle.[8] The reference point for rotation is the anterior aspect of the clavicle.

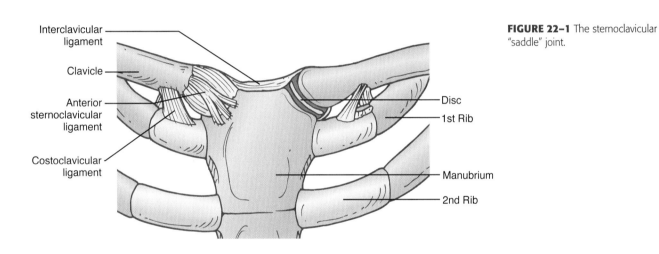

Interclavicular ligament
Clavicle
Anterior sternoclavicular ligament
Costoclavicular ligament
Disc
1st Rib
Manubrium
2nd Rib

FIGURE 22–1 The sternoclavicular "saddle" joint.

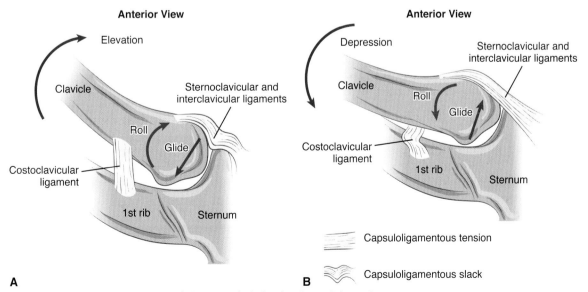

Anterior View

Elevation
Clavicle
Sternoclavicular and interclavicular ligaments
Roll
Glide
Costoclavicular ligament
1st rib
Sternum

Anterior View

Depression
Sternoclavicular and interclavicular ligaments
Clavicle
Roll
Glide
Costoclavicular ligament
1st rib
Sternum

Capsuloligamentous tension

Capsuloligamentous slack

A   **B**

FIGURE 22–2 A, B Accessory motion during sternoclavicular elevation and depression.

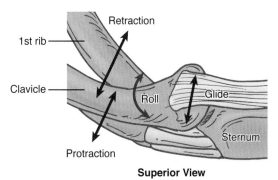

Superior View

FIGURE 22-3 Accessory motion during sternoclavicular protraction and retraction.

Upward rotation begins at approximately 90 degrees of arm elevation and is produced from an increase in tension of the *coracoclavicular ligament (CRCL)*.[8] A compensatory increase in scapular movement during elevation may cause the SC joint to engage in early and excessive upward rotation during shoulder elevation. The manual physical therapist may detect SC joint laxity through astute palpation of the clavicle during elevation.

The axis of motion for SC joint movement is generally believed to be just lateral to the clavicular head. The frame of reference used to describe SC physiologic movement is the lateral one-third of the clavicle. The total excursion of movement for the SC joint is generally considered to be *50 to 60 degrees* for elevation/depression,[2,7] *30 to 60 degrees* for protraction/retraction,[2,9] *25 to 55 degrees* for upward rotation[4,8,9] and less than *10 degrees* for downward rotation (Fig 22-4).[8]

The Acromioclavicular Joint

The *acromioclavicular (AC) joint's* primary functions are to allow the scapula additional ranges of rotation on the thorax, to allow for scapular adjustments in positions that are outside of the typical planes of motion during arm movement, and to transmit forces from the upper extremity to the clavicle and axial skeleton. The AC joint is considered to be a **planar joint** with flat, or slightly reciprocal, joint surfaces.[2] Both surfaces are enrobed in fibrocartilage and interposed with a fibrocartilaginous disc (Fig. 22-5).

Stability of the AC Joint

The weak AC joint capsule is reinforced by both the intraarticular *acromioclavicular ligament (ACL)* as well as accessory ligaments. The CRCL is particularly valuable for providing stability to the AC joint. The *conoid* portion of this ligament runs vertically, limiting the superior migration of the distal end of the clavicle, and the *trapezoid* portion runs vertically and laterally, serving to resist inferior and medial forces that may

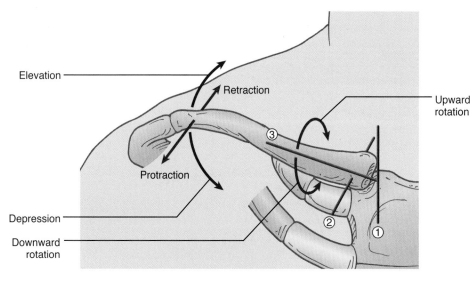

FIGURE 22-4 Physiologic motions of the sternoclavicular joint.

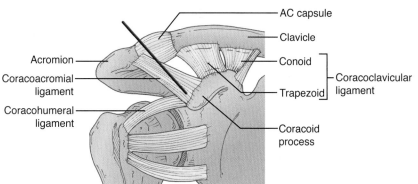

FIGURE 22-5 The acromioclavicular "planar" joint.

occur from a direct blow to the shoulder. The *coracoacromial ligament (CAL)* crosses no joint and serves as a restraint for superior migration of the humerus in cases of instability.

Mobility of the AC Joint

Although three degrees of freedom are available, including both translational and angular motion, rarely do they occur in isolation at the AC joint.[7] The largest contribution of the AC joint to shoulder complex motion occurs at the end range of elevation (Figure 22-6).[10]

There is approximately *30 degrees* of combined *internal* and *external rotation* that takes place about a vertical axis as the scapula moves over the convex costal cage during protraction and retraction, thus bringing the glenoid fossa anteromedially during internal rotation and posterolaterally during external rotation.[5] *Anterior* and *posterior tilting* occurs about a frontal plane axis and is approximately *30 to 40 degrees* during the full range of active movement from flexion to extension.[11] Anterior tilting leads to a tipping forward of the acromion, while the inferior angle of the scapula tips backward and the reverse occurs during posterior tilting. Anterior tilting occurs during glenohumeral extension and scapulothoracic elevation and posterior tilting accompanies glenohumeral flexion and scapulothoracic depression.

Lastly, the AC joint moves through an oblique anteroposterior axis that is perpendicular to the plane of the scapula. In vivo, *30 degrees* of *upward rotation* and *17 degrees* of *downward rotation* are available, which are limited by the CRCL.[12] Upward rotation at the SC joint releases tension on the CRCL, which inserts into the posterior aspect of the clavicle and releases the AC joint thus enabling it to move.

The Scapulothoracic Joint

As a "functional pseudoarticulation," the scapulothoracic (ST) joint relies on the integrity and movement capacity of the SC and AC joints. The SC and AC joint motions are best appreciated indirectly and, therefore, often documented through astute observation of ST joint movement.

In the anatomical position, the medial border of the scapula is located approximately 2 inches from the spine, with the *superior angle* at the level of T2 and the *inferior angle* at approximately T7. In the normal anatomic position, the scapula is internally rotated approximately 30 to 45 degrees anterior to the frontal plane, tilted anteriorly 10 to 20 degrees from vertical, and upwardly rotated 10 to 20 degrees from the horizontal.[13] The normal resting position of the scapula impacts movement of the glenohumeral joint. When glenohumeral movement occurs in alignment with the scapula, this motion is referred to as movement in the **plane of the scapula (POS)**. The POS, which is determined by the resting position of the scapula on the thorax, may vary slightly between individuals but is generally thought to be 30 to 45 degrees anterior to the frontal plane.

Mobility of the ST Joint

Elevation of the upper extremity requires synchronous recruitment of both the scapulothoracic and scapulohumeral muscles. The function of the scapulothoracic muscles in determining the position of the scapula determines the length and subsequent tension-producing capability of the scapulohumeral muscles. In addition, these muscles serve to secure the scapula so as to provide a stable base from which the scapulohumeral muscles may function.

Scapulothoracic *elevation* and *depression* involves frontal plane movement of the scapula relative to the thorax with the axis of motion located within the SC joint (Fig. 22-7). The excursion into elevation and depression is normally *4 to 6 cm*[10] and *1 to 2 cm*,[14] respectively. Elevation of the scapula requires concomitant elevation of the clavicular head and minor translation of the AC joint.[15] Depression of the ST joint typically occurs with associated anterior tilting when the *pectoralis minor* muscle predominates and posterior tilting when the *lower trapezius* muscle predominates.

Abduction and *adduction* are often referred to as *protraction* and *retraction*, respectively; however, the latter terms more specifically refer to movement of the SC joint in the transverse plane, as previously described (Fig. 22-8). The excursion for

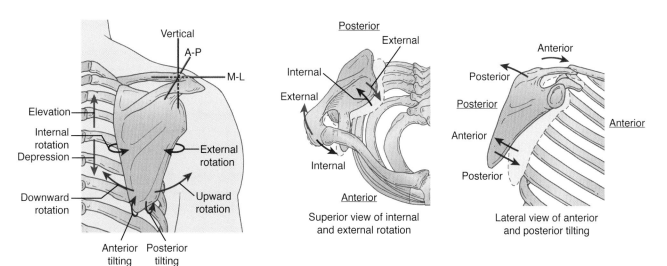

FIGURE 22–6 Physiologic motions of the acromioclavicular joint.

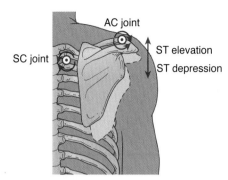

FIGURE 22–7 Scapulothoracic elevation and depression with component sternoclavicular and acromioclavicular joint motion.

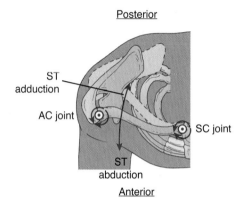

FIGURE 22–8 Scapulothoracic abduction and adduction with component sternoclavicular and acromioclavicular joint motion.

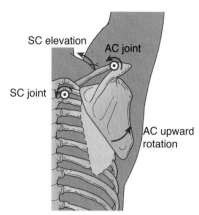

FIGURE 22–9 ST Scapulothoracic upward rotation with component sternoclavicular and acromioclavicular joint motion.

normal abduction is *7.5 to 10 cm and 4 to 5 cm* for adduction.[10] These motions are accompanied by anterior and posterior tilting due to the convexity of the thoracic wall.

Upward and *downward rotation* describe movement of the inferior angle of the scapula away from or toward the spine, respectively (Fig. 22-9). The normal amount of motion for upward and downward rotation is considered to be *60 degrees* and *20 degrees*, respectively. The axis of scapular rotation is believed to be near the root of the *spine of the scapula*, which shifts toward the glenoid during elevation.[15,16]

The Glenohumeral Joint

The glenohumeral (GH) joint lacks osteoarticular stabilizing support, with only 25% of the humeral head engulfed by the glenoid fossa. The disparity that exists at the interface between the glenoid and the humerus suggests that pure rotation predominates over translation at this joint.[17–19]

Glenoid *retroversion* of approximately 7.4 degrees serves to discourage anterior humeral translation. Therefore, individuals with glenoid anteversion or humeral retroversion may experience anterior instability.[20] The superior tilt of the glenoid inhibits inferior humeral migration. The ability of the scapula to reposition the glenoid during movement compensates for the deficiencies in the osseous framework of this joint.

The depth of the shallow glenoid fossa is enhanced by a 2-mm rim of fibrocartilage, known as the *glenoid labrum*. Invested into this wedge-shaped structure are the GH

ligaments, biceps tendon, and *capsuloligamentous complex (CLC)*. The labrum is most important as an anterior stabilizing structure and may dissociate from the glenoid in cases of traumatic anterior dislocation, in a condition known as the *Bankart lesion*.

The capsule of the GH joint is reinforced by the *coracohumeral ligament (CHL)* and the *glenohumeral ligament (GHL)*. The CHL is composed of two bands that reinforce the supraspinatus muscle, both superiorly and inferiorly. This ligament connects the supraspinatus with the subscapularis, forming the *rotator cuff interval (RCI)*, which is the primary restraint to posterior and inferior translation of the shoulder when in adduction. The CHL becomes taut during external rotation and extension with the arm adducted. As part of the RCI, the CHL is most valuable as a stabilizer in neutral and in combination with the superior GHL (Table 22-2).

The GHL is divided into three individual bands that span the anterior aspect of the GH joint. Along with the CHL, the *superior glenohumeral ligament (SGHL)* resists inferior humeral translation and external rotation in neutral and extension (Fig. 22-10).[21–23] The *middle glenohumeral ligament (MGHL)* stabilizes the GH joint from 0 to 45 degrees of abduction and becomes increasingly taut when external rotation is added leading to a restriction of anterior translation. However, full external rotation, as well as 90 degrees of abduction, both reduce tension within the MGHL.[20–22]

The *inferior glenohumeral ligament (IGHL)* with its broad axillary pouch is the most substantial. This ligament restrains both anterior and posterior humeral translation and limits both external and internal rotation at 90 degrees of abduction. The IGHL becomes most taut at 90 degrees of abduction with full external rotation.[21–24] The IGHL is, therefore, the primary restraint to anterior displacement in greater ranges of abduction, whereas the MGHL, subscapularis, and superior band of the IGHL are all involved in restraining anterior translation in neutral. The manual physical therapist may gain an appreciation for the integrity and function of these individual structures through examination of motion in various positions (Fig. 22-11).

The GH joint relies heavily on the periarticular musculature for *dynamic stability* and support, within the midranges of movement. The subscapularis is particularly important in restraining anterior shear when the shoulder is externally rotated

Table 22–2	Restraints to External and Internal Rotation of the Shoulder	
LIMITED MOTION	**JOINT POSITION**	**RESTRAINT**
External Rotation	0 degrees abduction	Subscapularis, superior glenohumeral, and coracohumeral ligament
	45 degrees abduction	Subscapularis, middle glenohumeral ligament
	90 degrees abduction	Inferior glenohumeral ligament
Internal Rotation	0 degrees abduction	Inferior glenohumeral ligament, teres minor, posterior capsule
	45 degrees abduction	Inferior glenohumeral ligament
	90 degrees abduction	Inferior glenohumeral ligament, posterior capsule

Adapted from Dutton M. *Orthopaedic Examination, Evaluation, and Intervention.* New York: McGraw-Hill; 2004.

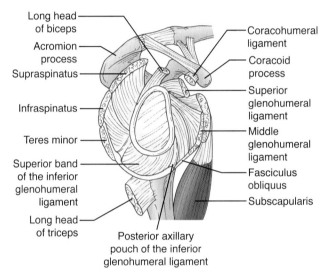

FIGURE 22–10 The capsular ligaments, muscular insertions, bursa, and osteological structure of the glenohumeral joint.

from the neutral position.[23] Through posterior translation of the humeral head during contraction, the infraspinatus and teres minor muscles serve to provide a restraint to anterior instability. These muscles, along with the posterior deltoid, also serve as restraints for posterior humeral translation. The collective line of pull of the rotator cuff muscles inferiorly serves to maintain the humeral head in an ideal positional relationship with the fossa during elevation.

Mobility of the GH Joint

Any discussion regarding mobility of the GH joint must begin with an appreciation of **scapulohumeral rhythm (SHR).** In its ideal form, SHR has been defined as the "synchronous culmination of shoulder girdle joint harmony."[25] The *setting phase*, which occurs during the first 30 degrees of active abduction and the first 60 degrees of active flexion, possesses a great deal of variability.[8] After the setting phase, normal SHR is believed to occur at a ratio of 2:1, resulting in 120 degrees of overall humeral excursion and 60 degrees of scapular excursion (Fig. 22-12). The initial resting position of the scapula may profoundly influence the SHR and GH joint restrictions and poor recruitment patterns of the scapulothoracic musculature may also lead to aberrations.

During GH joint motion, exceptions to the **convex-concave theory** are common (Fig. 22-13). During active elevation, the humeral head center of rotation remains relatively constant. The point of contact on the humerus and glenoid varies depending on the type of motion taking place (Fig. 22-14).[16,24,26] In order for the humeral head to remain centered during elevation, the rotator cuff musculature produces an inferiorly directed force (Fig. 22-15). Despite disparate opinions, evidence suggests that external rotation produces an increase in tension of the anterior CLC, which results in posterior translation, not anterior translation as the convex-concave theory would suggest (Fig. 22-16).[27,28] Conversely, internal rotation results in anterior accessory glide.

External and *internal rotation* are considered pure movements by virtue of the fact that they occur solely within the GH joint. Normal range is generally considered to be *90 degrees* for ER and *70 to 90 degrees* for IR, however, the quantity of motion will vary depending on the position of the shoulder. In cases of GH hypomobility, the scapula may compensate by tilting posteriorly or anteriorly during external and internal rotation, respectively.

Flexion in the sagittal plane is accompanied by internal rotation, and frontal plane *abduction* requires external rotation in order to prevent the greater tuberosity from contacting the coracoacromial arch.[18,29–32] During these complex motions, the CLC and associated tendons experience tension as they spiral around the rotating humerus. Elevation may, therefore, be restricted and symptomatic if GH rotation is limited. In addition to component rotation, elevation also requires contributions from the other joints within the shoulder complex. Normal range of flexion and abduction, albeit atypical, is considered to be *165 to 180 degrees*. By virtue of the associated component motions, accessory anterior glide and posterior glide accompany flexion and abduction, respectively.

A variation of abduction that must also be considered is abduction within the POS, often referred to as **scaption**. Although variability exists, the POS is described as existing between 30 and 45 degrees anterior to the frontal plane. Unlike elevation in other planes, scaption does not require component GH rotation.[33] Therefore, scaption is considered to be the least provocative manner in which to achieve elevation, and as such, it is often the preferred plane when introducing elevation. Migration toward the POS often occurs inadvertently

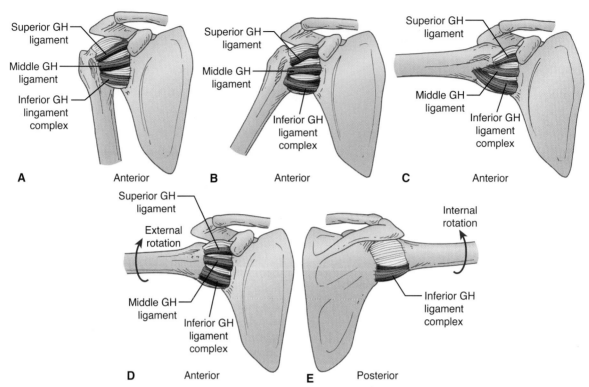

FIGURE 22–11 Influence of position on the ligaments of the glenohumeral joint at **A.** neutral, **B.** 45 degrees of abduction without rotation, **C.** 90 degrees of abduction without rotation, **D.** 90-degree abduction with ER, **E.** 90-degree abduction with IR.

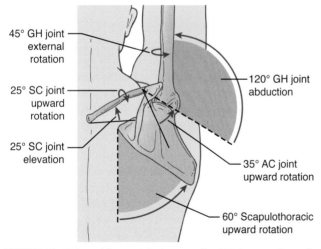

FIGURE 22–12 Scapulohumeral rhythm revealing 120 degrees of overall glenohumeral abduction, 45 degrees of ER, and 60 degrees of scapulothoracic upward rotation with component motions from the SC and AC joints.

during elevation as the joint seeks to take the path of least resistance. The POS is considered to be the **open-packed position** of the shoulder joint complex . Forward elevation (FE) is believed to be the position in which most individuals function overhead. This position is described as anterior to the POS but posterior to sagittal plane flexion. Normal range of FE is considered to be *150-160 degrees.*

Extension primarily occurs within the GH joint with ST downward rotation and ST elevation and anterior tilting occurring at end range.[10] Approximately *60 degrees* of extension is considered to be normal.[34]

EXAMINATION

The Subjective Examination

Self-Reported Disability Measures

The **Simple Shoulder Test (SST)** is a standardized self-report instrument that consists of 12 yes/no questions and has been found to have high test and retest reliability and sensitivity to a variety of shoulder pathologies.[35] Due to its simplicity, the SST is easy and quick to perform and has been found to be useful for documenting the effectiveness of intervention.[36]

The **Shoulder Pain and Disability Index (SPADI)** is a 13-question, pain-related tool designed to be completed within 3 minutes. This tool consists of five visual analog scales (VASs) to measure pain and 8 VASs to measure function of the shoulder. The total score is calculated by first summing the pain VAS, dividing by 55, then multiplying by 100, followed by taking the sum of the functional VAS, dividing by 8, then multiplying by 100, and adding the two scores.[37,38] The current best evidence suggests that the SPADI has demonstrated validity.[39,40]

The **Disability of The Arm, Shoulder, and Hand (DASH)** and Quick DASH are instruments used to measure self-reported upper extremity disability. These instruments consist of a 30-item disability scale with optional modules for sports/music and heavy work. There is also an additional questionnaire that may be used to assess the patient's level of perceived disability relative to office-related work. Each item is scored from 0 to 100, with higher scores representing greater levels of disability.[41,42] The two domains addressed within the DASH include symptoms and functional status. The categories included within the symptom

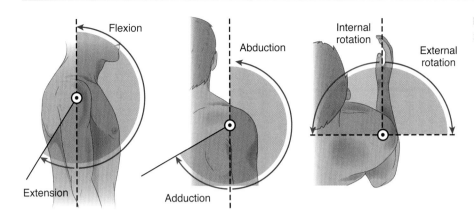

FIGURE 22–13 Physiologic motions of the glenohumeral joint.

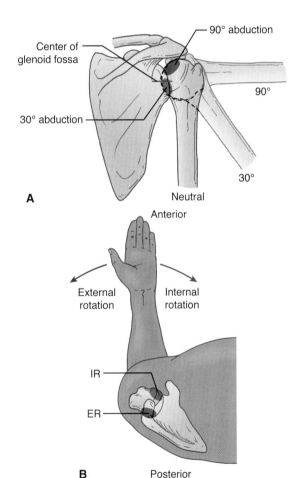

A

B   Posterior

FIGURE 22–14 A, B Contact points of the head of the humerus within the glenoid fossa during various positions of elevation in the plane of the scapula, during external rotation, and during internal rotation. IR, internal rotation; ER, external rotation.

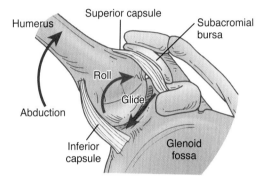

Anterior View of the Right Glenohumeral Joint
FIGURE 22–15 Accessory motion during glenohumeral abduction.

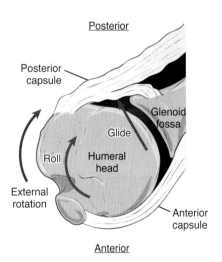

Superior View of the Right Glenohumeral Joint
FIGURE 22–16 Accessory motion during glenohumeral external rotation.

domain include weakness, pain, tingling/numbness, and stiffness. The functional domain includes physical, social, and psychological status.[43] This tool is not specific to the shoulder and has been validated on individuals with a wide range of upper extremity impairments.[44]

The **Constant Shoulder Score**[45] is divided into a subjective component that uses numeric ratings to determine the patient's pain during function, daily level of work, and the ability to work at specific heights. The objective component assigns numeric values that correlate with specific ranges of shoulder

motion and strength. The **Academy of Sport and Exercise Science** has also developed a standardized assessment form for the shoulder.[46] This form contains a VAS for pain coupled with a numeric pain score that correlates with activities of daily living.

Review of Systems

The most common nonmusculoskeletal condition that results in a referral of symptoms to the left shoulder is *myocardial infarction (MI)*.[47] Along with shoulder pain, an MI also leads to chest pain, nausea, sweating, and dyspnea, among other symptoms. Regardless of the nature, intensity, mechanism, and time since onset, unremitting pain in the shoulder is uncommon except in the case of tumors.

Shoulder pain is often the primary and most significant symptom resulting from what is known as *Pancoast's tumor*. This malignant tumor, which is located in the upper apices of the lung, places pressure upon the C8 and T1 nerve roots as well as the subclavian artery and vein, thus producing symptoms that mimic thoracic outlet syndrome, cervical disc disorder, or shoulder pathology. The symptoms related to this tumor progress over time and eventually produce muscle atrophy of the hand intrinsics and venous distention.[47] Due to the fact that this condition often goes misdiagnosed, a male patient over the age of 50 years who has a history of smoking should be referred back to the physician for further investigation if no improvement is noted after several bouts of physical therapy intervention.

Neural irritation may produce unyielding pain and can be easily differentiated through the neurological examination. Many individuals with shoulder pathology have difficulty tolerating overhead positions. However, individuals with nerve root compromise at the C6-7 segment may experience relief from placing the arm in this position (known as the *Bakody sign*). A checklist of the common red flags that must be ruled out in individuals presenting with shoulder pain is presented in Table 22-3.

Table 22-3	Medical Red Flags for the Shoulder	
MEDICAL CONDITION	**RED FLAGS**
Spinal Accessory Nerve Palsy	Weak shoulder abduction Unable to perform shoulder shrug Poor stabilization of scapula
Suprascapular Nerve Palsy	Weakness and atrophy of supraspinatus Weak abduction and external rotation
Long Thoracic Nerve Palsy	Weak serratus anterior Scapular winging
Axillary Nerve Palsy	Weak abduction and flexion
Pancoast's Tumor	Men older than 50 Tobacco use Pain at vertebral border of scapula Pain into ulnar nerve distribution
Myocardial infarction	Angina Dyspnea, pallor History of coronary artery disease, hypertension, diabetes, tobacco, increased cholesterol Men over age 40, women over age 50

Adapted from Boissonnault WG. *Primary Care for the Physical Therapist: Examination and Triage*. St. Louis, MO: Elsevier Saunders; 2005.

History of Present Illness

As the therapist progresses through the examination, every attempt should be made to correlate examination findings with the patient's presenting condition. Primary and secondary factors must be differentiated from common incidental findings that are unrelated to the patient's presenting impairment(s).

The two most common conditions of the shoulder are lesions of the *rotator cuff*[48,49] and *GH instability*.[50–52] Factors such as a decrease in tendon tensile strength and reduced vascularity render the tendons of the rotator cuff susceptible to dysfunction in the population over 40 years of age. Conversely, GH instability is more commonly seen in the population under the age of 30.[52–54] *Degenerative changes* of the rotator cuff typically occur in patients between the ages of 40 and 60. Conversely, partial or full-thickness rotator cuff tears caused from a single traumatic event are more prevalent in the younger population. Primary *adhesive capsulitis* is often observed in the population between the ages of 45 and 60.[55]

Acromioclavicular joint degeneration with subsequent osteophyte formation is often observed upon radiographic imaging in the older population, while acute *acromioclavicular joint separation* is typically found in the younger population subsequent to falling onto the superior shoulder. Shoulder impairment is common in individuals who engage in repeated or sustained overhead use, particularly if these activities are performed with heavy loads.[56]

As mentioned, falling on the superior aspect of the shoulder suggests acromioclavicular pathology whereas a *fall on an outstretched hand (FOOSH)* may lead to fracture of the humerus along with GH dislocation. The position of the shoulder at the time of injury may provide useful information regarding the structures that may be implicated.

Cumulative trauma involves a myriad of structures that include both primary and secondary compensatory impairments. Over time, a reduction in inferior humeral glide during elevation may result in *subacromial bursitis* and *supraspinatus tendonopathy*.

Acute or cumulative trauma that leads to pathology of the rotator cuff immediately puts the shoulder at risk for instability. Acute injury often results in what is known as a **TUBS** type of instability (**t**raumatic onset, **u**nidirectional anterior with a **B**ankart lesion responding to **s**urgery). With a TUBS instability, as its name implies, immediate surgical repair is often optimal.[14] Instability that results from atraumatic causes are more difficult to diagnose and often have less favorable outcomes. This type of instability is known as an **AMBRI** (**a**traumatic cause, **m**ultidirectional with **b**ilateral shoulder findings with **r**ehabilitation as appropriate treatment, and rarely **i**nferior capsular shift surgery). In order of prevalence, *anterior instability* is followed closely by *inferior* and *posterior instability*. Outcomes are presumably less favorable in cases of *multidirectional instability*.

Individuals with impingement have poor tolerance for overhead activities and may report a painful arc between 60 and 120 degrees of elevation. Individuals with injury or degeneration of the AC joint have local pain between 170 and 180 degrees and pain with horizontal adduction.

The levator scapula and upper trapezius often respond to cervical or shoulder impairment by developing associated *trigger points* (see Chapter 16).[57] The influence of cervical spine movement on shoulder symptoms and a *neurological upper quarter screen* may be helpful in ruling out cervical spine contributions.

Due to patterns of embryological development, pathology that involves structures of the shoulder may lead to *referred pain patterns*. Lateral deltoid pain may be caused by GH joint dysfunction, and such a condition may lead to referred pain into the C5 and C6 dermatomes distally. Supraspinatus tendonopathy may lead to pain over the lateral deltoid and into the C5 dermatome. Pain over the AC or SC joints often produce local pain over the involved joint or more diffuse pain within the C4 dermatome.

A feeling of heaviness, weakness, fatigue, or the presence of edema, pallor, or temperature changes are all indications of *vascular compromise*. **Thoracic outlet syndrome**, which involves entrapment of the brachial plexus and subclavian artery and vein, may lead to both neurological and/or vascular compromise.

The Objective Physical Examination
Examination of Structure

It is best to perform observation of structure without the patient's knowledge in order to ascertain the patient's true *preferred posture*. Although the chief indicator of normalcy during the structural examination is symmetry, deviations are common in the normal population.

It is typical for the shoulder of the dominant hand to posture slightly inferior to the nondominant shoulder. Palpation of the acromion process is often useful in determining relative height, as is the angle of the clavicles to the horizontal. Asymmetry of shoulder height will also produce a change in the **thoracobrachial angle**, which is the angle between the arm and the thorax. In addition to bony landmarks, observation of muscle bulk is important for identifying nerve involvement.

Often in concert with a forward head posture is the typical *rounded shoulder posture*. There are several variations of this posture that may be observed. Laterally, thoracic kyphosis is assessed, with normal determined to be approximately 40 degrees.[58] Rounded shoulders may also be the result of protracted, elevated, and downwardly rotated scapulae. Alterations in scapular positioning often serve as contributors to the onset of shoulder impingement.

Palpation of the inferior scapular angle (level of T7) and space between the spine and medial border (5 to 9 cm) is useful for bilateral comparison of scapular position.[57,59] The scapula may be in a position of medial winging, from serratus anterior deficiency, or elevation and downward rotation with anterior displacement, from pectoralis minor tightness and poor function of the middle and lower trapezii.[25]

Screening of Adjacent Structures

To fully appreciate the movement capability of the shoulder girdle, a detailed examination of both the cervical spine and the thoracic spine, including the costal cage, must be performed routinely. Aberrations in normal movement patterns of the shoulder girdle may be the result of subtle deficits in cervicothoracic or costal cage mobility, and the influence of these regions on shoulder function must not be underestimated.

Examination of Mobility
Active Physiologic Movement Examination

Active physiologic movement, or active range of motion (AROM), testing serves as the initial pass, or screen, during which aberrations in the quantity and quality of motion and any reproduction of symptoms are assessed. The motions that are tested include the traditional cardinal plane motions, as previously described. Combined extension, adduction, and internal rotation may be assessed via the *scratch test*, where the patient reaches behind his or her back to achieve the highest spinal level possible. This is sometimes referred to as functional IR. Abduction and external rotation is measured by the ability of the patient to reach the back of his or her head, referred to as functional ER (Fig. 22-17).[60]

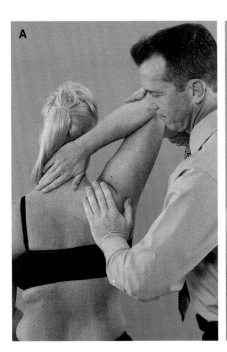
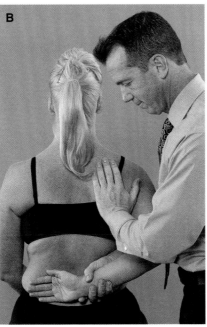

FIGURE 22–17 Movement testing of **A.** functional ER and **B.** functional IR.

Examination of *functional movement* may include diagonal patterns of functional reach or may involve specific tasks that the patient may be required to perform at home or work. This examination often incorporates the use of patterns. Active performance of **proprioceptive neuromuscular facilitation (PNF)** *diagonal patterns* provide an efficient method for examining combined movements (see Chapter 12).

Observation of movement quality into elevation is best obtained from the posterior view, which is performed bilaterally for single and repeated (5 to 10 repetitions) motions. In the presence of pain, weakness, or limitations, the patient may take the path of least resistance by migrating into the plane of the scapula (Fig. 22-18).

When observing the SHR, it is important to appreciate not only the active elevation phase, which requires concentric muscle activity, but also observation of the eccentric lowering phase. Full active physiologic motion requires at least *fair* grade *(3/5)* strength in order to move the weight of the extremity through its full range of movement against gravity. Comparing the results of active movement testing to passive movement testing serves to provide information regarding muscle function. Deficits in the supraspinatus and/or deltoid will impact elevation and may result in compensatory upper trapezius and levator scapula activity leading to scapular elevation. Serratus anterior deficits may lead to medial scapular winging, which is often more apparent with elevation in the sagittal (ie. flexion), versus elevation in the frontal (ie. abduction), plane. The clinical relevance of observed movement deficits is accomplished through correlating the patient's movement patterns with the patient's chief complaint. The patient's level of reactivity will dictate his or her tolerance for intervention.

During performance of active physiologic movement, it is critical to identify the specific movement, or combination of movements, that most reproduces the patient's chief complaint. If single and repeated cardinal plane movements do not reproduce symptoms, the manual physical therapist must explore the use of multiplanar movements and combined movements involving both physiologic and accessory motion.

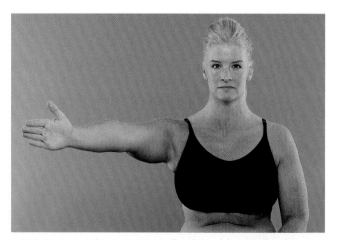

FIGURE 22–18 Active movement in the plane of the scapula (also known as scaption), which may occur in the presence of glenohumeral capsular restrictions.

Passive Physiologic Movement Examination

During passive physiologic movement testing, or PROM, goniometric measurement of each of the cardinal plane motions is performed.[61] During testing, it is critical to move the joint to its maximum available range while disallowing compensatory movement, which is common.

Lesions within the CLC presumably produce a characteristic loss of motion, known as a **capsular pattern**, that should be differentiated from other potential causes. Cyriax[1] described the capsular pattern of the shoulder to be a preferential loss of external rotation, followed by abduction, with the least amount of restriction into internal rotation *(external rotation>abduction> internal rotation)* (see Chapter 5). Noncapsular patterns are attributed to extra-articular restrictions, internal GH derangements, and isolated restrictions within the CLC.[25] The variability identified among capsular patterns may best be explained by the fact that isolated and combined lesions of the capsule and other extra-articular structures may exist.[62,63] Therefore, the capsular pattern concept must be considered in light of its limitations. Table 22-4 displays the physiologic motions of the shoulder, including normal ranges of motion, open and closed-packed positions, and normal and abnormal end-feels.

External/Internal Rotation

Inflation of external rotation/internal rotation (ER/IR) measurements occur when the scapula is inadequately stabilized. The degree to which restrictions within the GH joint may contribute to a loss of elevation can be determined by measuring ER and IR. If no loss is noted in these motions, the GH joint is not considered to be the primary restricted region.

To comprehensively evaluate the integrity of the CLC, it is best for the manual physical therapist to examine ER and IR in varying degrees of abduction, as previously noted. The greatest and least amount of ER is typically noted at 90 degrees abduction and 0 to 30 degrees abduction, respectively. ER places increased tension across the anterior aspect of the joint, leading to the necessary posterior translation of the humeral head. Therefore, restrictions in the anterior capsule may result in an increase in the amount of posterior glide. Conversely, laxity of the anterior capsule, which is a common finding, may lead to a reduction in posterior glide or a humeral head that has migrated anterior to its corresponding glenoid fossa.

The posterior capsule is the chief limiting structure for internal rotation. With increasing degrees of abduction, the inferior capsule is most restricted. Pathologic tightness of the posterior capsule, which is common, may lead to excessive anterior translation of the humeral head relative to the glenoid fossa. The natural tendency toward anterior CLC laxity and posterior CLC tightness may result in an overall inclination toward abnormal anterior migration of the humeral head.

When measured at 90 degrees of abduction, internal rotation is generally less than that expected for external rotation. It is common for therapists to overestimate the range of internal rotation; therefore, avoidance of compensation from the scapulothoracic joint is critical.

The final component of passive movement testing is assessment of combined accessory and physiologic motion. Based on a foundational knowledge of shoulder kinematics, the therapist

Table 22–4	Physiologic (Osteokinematic) Motions of the Shoulder					
JOINT	**NORMAL ROM**	**OPP**	**CPP**	**NORMAL END-FEEL**	**ABNORMAL END-FEEL**
Sternoclavicular	50°-60° elevation, depression (4-6cm elevation, 1-2cm depression) 30°-60° protraction, retraction (7-10cm protraction, 4-5cm retraction) 25°-55° upward rotation <10° downward rotation	30°-45° anterior to the frontal plane	Maximal abduction & ER	Flexion= elastic, firm Abduction= elastic Scaption= elastic IR / ER= elastic, firm Horizontal adduction = soft tissue Extension= firm Horizontal abduction = firm, elastic	Empty = subacromial bursitis, tendonopathy, RC lesion Capsular = Adhesive capsulitis Capsular Pattern= ER > abduction > IR
Acromioclavicular	30° internal, external rotation 30°-40° anterior, posterior tilting 30° upward rotation 17° downward rotation	Same for all	Same for all	Same for all	Same for all
Scapulothoracic	4-6cm elevation 1-2cm depression 7.5-10cm abduction 4-5cm adduction 60° upward rotation 20° downward rotation	Same for all	Same for all	Same for all	Same for all
Glenohumeral	90° ER 70°-90° IR 165°-180° Flexion 165°-180° Abduction 60° Extension	Same for all	Same for all	Same for all	Same for all

ROM, range of motion; OPP, open-packed position; CPP, close-packed position; IR, internal rotation; ER, external rotation; RC, rotator cuff. Adapted from: Wise CH, and Gulick DT. *Mobilization Notes: A Rehabilitation Specialist's Pocket Guide*. Philadelphia, PA: FA Davis; 2009.

provides accessory glides that correlate with the physiologic movement being tested. ER and IR may be measured during the application of a gentle anteroposterior and posteroanterior glide, respectively. During this process, the manual physical therapist identifies any change in range or symptoms. The information gleaned from this process may prove to be invaluable, acting as a form of trial intervention, the results of which will be used to determine subsequent care.

Flexion

Throughout passive testing of *flexion*, the manual physical therapist must use caution to avoid trunk extension, excessive scapular posterior tilt, or migration toward the POS. Under normal conditions, flexion requires movement of all of the joints within the shoulder girdle complex. The previously described scapulohumeral rhythm applies to active motion only. Passively, scapular motion may not be detected until 80 degrees of elevation as tension in the CLC is engaged. Premature scapular motion suggests the presence of CLC restrictions. The middle GH ligament is primarily responsible for limiting flexion. The contribution of both the SC and AC joints may be assessed by palpating the anterior border of the clavicle as

it upwardly rotates, along with elevation of the lateral clavicle and depression of the clavicular head during elevation. Passive inferior or posteroanterior accessory glides during physiologic movement testing may also be performed.

Abduction

During passive testing of abduction, substitution is observed as contralateral trunk lean and excessive scapular upward rotation. Restrictions in the CLC may produce premature recruitment of scapulothoracic motion. The specific range at which symptoms are reported and the nature of such symptoms must also be fully documented.

Passive physiologic abduction in both the frontal plane and in the POS may be measured with superimposed accessory glides. For frontal plane abduction, either an inferior or anteroposterior glide may be used. Combined glides, glides in multiple directions, distraction, and/or compression accessory movements may also be attempted.

Passive Accessory Movement Examination

Upon identifying physiologic movement loss, therapists often infer accessory motion loss. Although more challenging to perform, accessory movement loss is best appreciated through direct assessment as opposed to indirectly assuming accessory motion loss from identified deficits in physiologic motion. During performance of each glide, the therapist evaluates the quantity, end-feel, and onset of symptom reproduction. When such procedures impact motion or symptoms, the examination becomes the intervention.

Initial testing often occurs in the open-packed position; however, testing in multiple positions, including end range, may provide useful information. The mobilization techniques that follow later in this chapter will provide details regarding the performance of accessory glides and may be used for both examination and intervention of passive accessory movement. Table 22-5 displays the accessory motions of the shoulder.

Examination of Muscle Function

Examination of muscle function must be performed in a manner that is *specific* and *functional* for the muscle in question. When examining muscle function, the examiner must consider each muscle's dominant *type of contraction* (isometric, concentric, eccentric), dominant *length* (early range, midrange, late range) in which

it functions, dominant *plane* of function (frontal, transverse, sagittal), and its dominant role as either a *postural* muscle (slow twitch muscle used primarily for endurance and maintenance of posture) or *phasic* muscle (fast twitch muscle used primarily to create movement and produce force) muscle.[64,65]

Standard manual muscle testing (MMT) uses *break testing* as the preferred method for determination of normalcy (5/5).[66] However, this form of testing fails to consider the force-producing capability of the muscle throughout the entire range of motion.

The ST muscles tether the scapula to the spine and largely consist of type I, slow twitch, or postural-type muscles. The ST muscles maintain static position of the scapula and control the scapula during active movement, which serves to reduce impingement and optimize the length of the prime movers throughout motion. The *scapulohumeral (SH)* muscles attach the humerus to the scapula and primarily consist of type II, fast twitch, or phasic-type muscles.

A detailed description of the formal procedure for MMT of each muscle within the shoulder girdle has been well described in the literature.[66] An appreciation of the specific positions and

Table 22–5 Accessory (Arthrokinematic) Motions of the Shoulder

	ARTHROLOGY		ARTHROKINEMATICS
Sternoclavicular Joint	Convex surface: Clavicular head Concave surface: Disc & manubrium	*To facilitate elevation:* Lateral clavicle rolls upward & medial clavicle glides inferior on disc & manubrium	*To facilitate depression:* Lateral clavicle rolls downward & medial clavicle glides superior on disc & manubrium
	Concave surface: Medial clavicle & disc Convex surface: Manubrium	*To facilitate retraction:* Medial clavicle & disc rolls & glides posterior on manubrium	*To facilitate protraction:* Medial clavicle & disc rolls & glides anterior on manubrium
Acromioclavicular Joint	Planar surface: Clavicle Planar surface: Acromion	*To facilitate upward/downward rotation:* Scapula (acromion) glides superior & lateral OR inferior & medial on clavicle *To facilitate internal/external rotation:* Scapula (acromion) glides anterior & medial OR posterior & lateral on clavicle	*To facilitate anterior/posterior tilting:* Scapula (acromion) glides superior & anterior OR inferior & posterior on clavicle
Scapulothoracic Joint	Convex surface: Thorax Concave surface: Scapula	*To facilitate elevation:* Scapula glides superior on thorax *To facilitate abduction:* Scapula glides lateral around thorax *To facilitate upward rotation:* Inferior angle of scapula glides superior & lateral around thorax	*To facilitate depression:* Scapula glides inferior on thorax *To facilitate adduction:* Scapula glides medial around thorax *To facilitate downward rotation:* Inferior angle of scapula glides inferior & medial around thorax
Glenohumeral Joint	Concave surface: Glenoid fossa Convex surface: Humeral head	*To facilitate flexion:* Humeral head rolls superior & glides inferior and anterior on glenoid *To facilitate IR:* Humeral head rolls/spins posterior & glides anterior on glenoid *To facilitate horizontal adduction:* Humeral head rolls medial & glides lateral on glenoid *To facilitate elevation in POS:* Humeral head rolls superior & glides inferior on glenoid	*To facilitate abduction:* Humeral head rolls superior & glides inferior and posterior on glenoid *To facilitate ER:* Humeral head rolls/spins anterior & glides posterior on glenoid *To facilitate horizontal abduction:* Humeral head rolls lateral & glides medial on glenoid *To facilitate extension:* Humeral head rolls/spins anterior & glides anterior on glenoid

ER, external rotation: IR, internal rotation. From: Wise CH, and Gulick DT. *Mobilization Notes: A Rehabilitation Specialist's Pocket Guide.* Philadelphia, PA: FA Davis; 2009.

contacts used during MMT is important when attempting to isolate muscles when prescribing progressive resistance exercise regimens.

Closed Chain Functional Examination

Although the ST and SH muscles of the shoulder girdle function primarily in an open chain fashion, there are occasions when these muscles must function in closed chain. Athletes and individuals who perform certain occupations, such as bricklayers and housekeepers, may require the prolonged use of these muscles in a closed chain fashion. Although not part of the routine examination, the ability of these muscles to perform in this manner may need to be determined.

Closed chain function of the entire shoulder joint complex can be tested through performance of the *bilateral static push-up test*. With this test, the manual physical therapist monitors through observation and palpation both ST as well as SH muscle function. The test is discontinued when either the patient is no longer able to hold the position or when form fatigue has occurred. For example, if the patient is no longer able to exhibit scapular control, the medial border of the scapula may wing, at which time the test is brought to a conclusion and the amount of time in which the push-up was held is documented. An alternative to this test is the *active push-up test*. During this procedure, the patient is asked to perform as many push-ups as possible as the therapist records the quantity and monitors quality. For both procedures, it is important to standardize the parameters of the test, including hand and foot position.

The *one arm hop test* has been described in the literature as a method of testing the functional status of athletes prior to return to competition.[67] The patient maintains the one arm push-up position and then hops from the floor to a 4-inch step and back for five repetitions. The patient is asked to perform this activity as quickly as possible, and the time required to do so is compared with the uninvolved extremity. A time of less than 10 seconds is considered to be normal.[67]

Palpation

In addition to identification of tenderness, palpation may also be used to detect changes in temperature, tissue texture and tone, atrophy, and edema. Edema of the shoulder joint often leads to temperature changes that may be best appreciated by using the back of the hand. Swelling and/or atrophy may be palpated over the greater tuberosity as well as gaps in the continuity of the tendons in cases of large rotator cuff insertion tears or bicep tendon tears.

The manual physical therapist must appreciate that some structures about the shoulder are tender under normal conditions. Joint *audibles* or *crepitus* may also be identified upon palpation during movement testing. Such audibles may be considered typical variations but may suggest the presence of pathology. Clinical relevance is attributed to findings of tenderness and joint audibles when these findings correlate with the patient's chief complaint.

Osseous Palpation

To gain purchase of the *medial border* of the scapula, the patient is placed in side-lying position and the shoulder is moved posteriorly, which allows complete palpation from the *inferior* to the *superior angle*. Access may be enhanced by having the patient place the arm behind his or her back while they are seated or lying.[68]

As the manual physical therapist follows the spine of the scapula laterally, the spine eventually terminates as the prominent *acromion process*. The borders of the acromion can be easily palpated, along with its articulation with the lateral clavicle. The *s-shaped* clavicle is palpated with an appreciation of its acromial end, which rises superiorly, and its sternal end, which curves inferiorly. Both the *AC* and *SC joints* are then fully palpated for relative position and potential tenderness (Fig. 22-19).

The final bony landmark on the scapula that must be palpated is the *coracoid process*. This landmark is found between the fibers of the deltoid and pectoralis major and is often tender to the touch. To palpate, find the lateral clavicle and move inferiorly 1.5 inches, until the tip of the coracoid is identified. The coracoid is an important insertion site for the short head of the biceps brachii, coracobrachialis, as well as the pectoralis minor muscles, and may be tender in cases of impairment within any of these structures.

Palpation of the humerus begins at the *greater tuberosity (GT)*, the *lesser tuberosity (LT)*, and the corresponding *intertubercular*, or *bicipital*, *groove*. By virtue of the fact that three of the four rotator cuff muscles attach to the GT and the other rotator cuff muscle attaches to the LT, these bony landmarks are of extreme importance during palpation. Palpation of these structures begins by identifying the GT, which is found by locating the acromion and then moving laterally and inferiorly approximately 1 inch. Confirmation is achieved by internally and externally rotating the shoulder (Fig. 22-20).[68] On external rotation, the therapist will come upon the intertubercular groove and the more medially located LT.

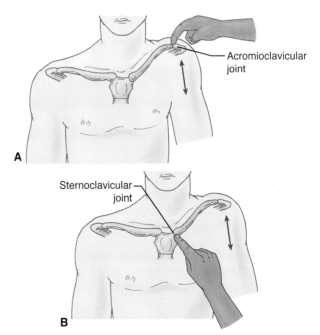

FIGURE 22–19 Palpation of the **A.** acromioclavicular and **B.** sternoclavicular joints.

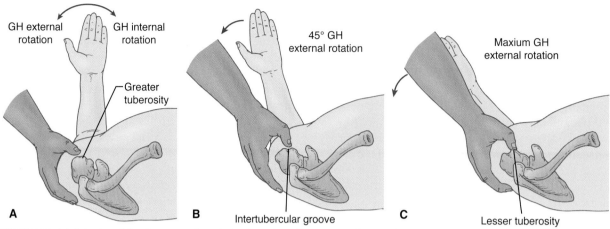

FIGURE 22-20 Palpation of the **A.** greater tuberosity, **B.** intertubercular groove, **C.** lesser tuberosity.

Moving distally, the therapist should attempt to come upon the *deltoid tuberosity*, which is located on the lateral aspect of the shaft of the humerus approximately halfway between the shoulder and the elbow. Confirmation is obtained by resisting abduction and palpating the fibers of the deltoid inserting into this region.[68]

Soft Tissue Palpation

Inserting into the sternum and clavicle are the two heads of the *sternocleidomastoid (SCM)* muscle. This muscle is palpated along its full length as it inserts into the mastoid process and is recruited unilaterally through resistance of *ipsilateral side bending* or bilaterally through resistance of *forward bending* with the head in midline. The SCM is differentiated from the adjacent *anterior* and *middle scalene* muscles, which dive beneath the clavicle to insert into the first and second ribs, by resisting *contralateral rotation*, which selectively recruits the SCM. Once locating the clavicular head of the SCM, the broad anterior scalene is located just lateral to it and superior to the clavicle. Moving laterally, the smaller middle scalene, separated from its anterior counterpart by a septum, is smaller and more challenging to identify.[68]

The *upper trapezius (UT)* and *levator scapula (LS)* are responsible for elevation of the scapula and may be overused as a compensation for deficits in scapulohumeral muscle function during elevation. The UT is palpated along its length from the spinous processes of cervical vertebrae 2–7 to the lateral one-third of the clavicle and acromion process, while the LS is palpated from the transverse processes of cervical vertebrae 2–7 to the superior angle of the scapula. The LS is best palpated just anterior to the upper border of the UT within the posterior triangle of the neck. These muscles may be differentiated from one another during palpation by resisting *contralateral cervical rotation*, which recruits the UT, and compared with resistance of *ipsilateral rotation*, which recruits the LS.[68]

The *middle trapezius* is best palpated by locating the spine of the scapula and moving medially off the medial border. The *lower trapezius* is located by drawing a line between the spine of the scapula and T12. To confirm palpation of the middle and lower fibers of the trapezius, the patient performs scapular adduction against isometric resistance (Fig. 22-21). The lower trapezius is isolated by resisting scapular depression. Running in an oblique direction beneath the trapezius muscle are the *rhomboids*. By palpating through the trapezius, the manual physical therapist is able to feel this muscle between the spine of the scapula and the inferior angle just off its medial border. Palpation is confirmed through gentle resistance of bringing the elbow up and thus producing scapular adduction, elevation, and downward rotation through the *"chicken wing"* position.

One of the more prominent and easily palpated muscles of the shoulder is the *deltoid* muscle. The deltoid is located between the acromion process and the deltoid tuberosity.[68] During palpation, attempts to isolate the *anterior*, *middle*, and *posterior* fibers of this muscle may be made through slight alterations in shoulder rotation.

The *supraspinatus (SS)* muscle must be palpated through the UT. For optimal palpation of the belly of the SS, the patient is placed in side-lying position on the uninvolved side or prone in order to place the extremity in a gravity-lessened position. The involved extremity is placed in 60 degrees of abduction, with the back of the patient's hand placed on his or her buttocks as the therapist palpates the muscle belly of the SS through the silent UT (Fig. 22-22A). The optimal position for palpating the tendon of the SS is with the patient's arm behind his or her back with the shoulder in extension and internal

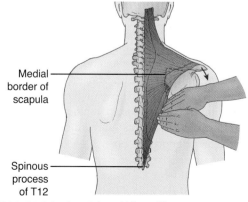

FIGURE 22-21 Palpation of the middle and lower trapezius.

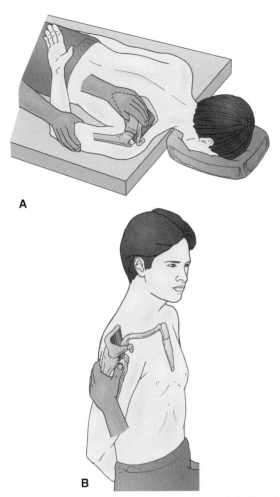

FIGURE 22–22 Palpation of the **A.** supraspinatus muscle belly and **B.** suprspsinatus tendon.

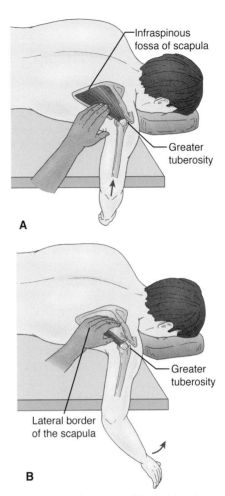

FIGURE 22–23 Differential palpation of the **A.** infraspinatus and **B.** teres minor.

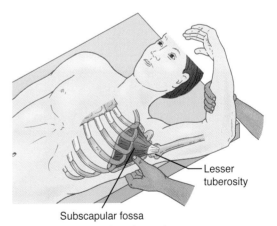

FIGURE 22–24 Palpation of the subscapularis.

rotation. The therapist begins by first palpating the anterolateral aspect of the acromion. Approximately 2 cm inferior to this landmark the tendon and tenoperiosteal junction of the SS can be easily palpated (Fig. 22-22B). This position is also optimal for palpation of the subacromial bursa.[25]

For palpation of the *infraspinatus (IS)*, the patient is sitting with the shoulder in 90 degrees of flexion, horizontal adduction, and external rotation. The tendon is found distal to the muscle belly approximately 1 cm inferior to the posterolateral acromion.[25] With the patient in prone with the shoulder abducted, the IS belly can be identified in the fossa as the patient lifts the elbow upward slightly (Fig. 22-23A). The IS can be differentiated from the *teres minor* by moving laterally off the lateral border of the scapula.[68] The muscle belly is grasped by reaching into the axilla and confirmed by asking the patient to gently externally rotate (Fig. 22-23B). The *teres major* is located just inferior to the minor.

Palpation of the *subscapularis (SB)* muscle is challenging given its location at the anterior aspect of the scapula and confirmed by eliciting gentle resistance to internal rotation. In supine, the shoulder is brought into 90 degrees of abduction to move the scapula away from the costal cage. The SB belly is then palpated through the latissimus dorsi within the patient's axilla (Fig. 22-24). For palpation of the SB tendon, the therapist identifies the insertion into the lesser tuberosity by internally and externally rotating the shoulder. In 50 degrees of external rotation, the tendon can be fully palpated approximately 2 cm below the anterolateral acromion. The *latissimus dorsi* is best palpated with the patient supine and the arm positioned in flexion. The manual physical therapist resists shoulder extension and palpates the muscle along the lateral border of the scapula.[68]

Through ER and IR with the arm at the side, the bicipital groove is palpated. It is difficult to palpate the *long head of the biceps (LHB) tendon* within the groove since the deltoid lies over it. This tendon is commonly uncomfortable to the touch, even in asymptomatic individuals.[25] The muscle belly of the biceps can be easily palpated, and attempts should be made to assess its function compared to the other elbow flexors, as will be discussed in Chapter 23.

Special Testing

Special tests for the shoulder have been clearly described in many other texts and in the literature; therefore, only a brief description of selected special tests will be provided here. Table 22-6 provides the sensitivity, specificity, and likelihood ratios for the more commonly performed special tests used in the examination of the shoulder joint complex. The reader is encouraged to consult other sources for additional information regarding the performance of these useful confirmatory tests.

Table 22-6	Special Tests for the Shoulder				
TEST	**SENSITIVITY**	**SPECIFICITY**	**+LR**	**-LR**	**REFERENCE**
Hawkins-Kennedy Test	71.5-92%	25-66.3%	NA	NA	Michener LA et al.[69] Hawkins RJ, et al.[70] MacDonald PB et al.[71] Calis M et al.[72] Park HB et al.[73] Tomberlin J.[74]
Neer Test	68-95%	25-68%	1.29-1.44	0.35-0.52	Michener LA et al.[69] Neer CS et al.[75] Valadic AL et al.[76] Buchberger DJ et al.[77] MacDonald PB et al.[71] Calis M et al.[72] Park HB et al.[73] Post M et al.[78] Tomberlin J.[74]
Yergason Test	9-37%	86-96%	NA	NA	Park HB et al.[73]
Apprehension Sign and Relocation Test	30-63%,	61-99%	0.53-3.08	0.47-1.11	Matsen FA et al.[79] Gerber C et al.[80] Kvitne RS et al.[81] Luime JJ et al.[82] Hawkins RJ et al.[83] Lo IK et al.[84] Speer KP et al.[85] Mok DWH, et al.[78] Guanche CA et al.[87]
Jerk Test	NA	NA			Kim SH et al.[88]
Sulcus Sign	17%	93%	2.43	0.89	Matsen FA et al.[79] Gerber C et al.[80] Bigliani LU et al.[89] McClusky GM.[90] Nakagawa S et al.[91]
External Rotation Lag (Dropping) Sign	20-100%	69-100%	NA	0.0-0.64	Ludewig P.[92] Tomberlin J.[74] Michener LA.[69] Neer CS et al.[75] Hertel R et al.[93] Walch G et al.[94]
Hornblower Sign	92-100%	30-93%	14.3	0.0	Ludewig P.[92] Tomberlin J.[74] McClusky CM.[90] Walch G et al.[94]
Drop Arm Test	15%	100%	NA	NA	Calis et al.[72]

Table 22–6	Special Tests for the Shoulder—cont'd				
TEST	**SENSITIVITY**	**SPECIFICITY**	**+LR**	**-LR**	**REFERENCE**
Lift Off Test	62-89%	98-100%			Chao S et al.[95] Rigsby R et al.[96] Ludewig P.[92] Tomberlin J.[74] Ticker JB et al.[97] Greis PE et al.[98] Gerber C et al.[99] Lyons RP et al.[100] Ostor AJ et al.[101]
Full Can/Empty Can Test	FC: 66-86% EC: 63-89%	FC: 57-74% EC: 55-68%	FC: 1.83-2.96 EC: 1.40-2.41	FC: 0.25-0.53 EC: 0.22-0.67	Itoi E et al.[102] Ostor AJ et al.[103] Ludewig P.[92] Tomberlin J.[74] Michener LA et al.[69] Park HB et al.[73]
Speed Test	Biceps: 9-100% SLAP: 9-44%	Biceps: 55.5-87% SLAP: 74-75%			Guanche CA et al.[103] Calis M et al.[72] Holtby R et al.[104] Park HB et al.[73] Tomberlin J.[74]
Biceps Load Test	78-91%	97%	26.38-30	0.11	Kim SH et al.[105] Lewis CL et al.[106] Kim SH et al.[107] Wilk KE et al.[108] Myers TH et al.[109]
O-Brien Test	47-100%	11-98%	0.78-2.33	0.51-1.48	Burkhart SS et al.[110] O'Brien SJ et al.[111] Myers TH et al.[109] Wilk KE et al.[108] Stetson WB et al.[112]
Crank Test	9-91%	56-100%	1.04-13	0.10-2	Liu SH et al.[113] Lewis CL et al.[106] Walsworth, MK et al.[114] Guanche CA et al.[87] Stetson WB et al.[112] Mimori K et al.[115] Parentis MA et al.[116] Myers TH et al.[109]
Kim Test	80-82%	86-94%	NA	NA	Kim SH et al.[105] Lewis CL et al.[106]
SLAP Prehension Test	50% for Type I lesions & 87.5% for Type II, III, IV lesions	NA	NA	NA	Berg EE et al.[117]
Anterior Slide Test	8-78%	84-92%	0.56-9.75	0.24-1.1	Kibler WB.[118] Kibler WB.[119] Andrews JR et al.[120] Parentis MA et al.[116] McFarland EG et al.[121]
Adson Test	32-87%,	74-100%	NA	NA	Adson AW et al.[122] Marx RG et al.[123] Lee AD et al.[124] Plews MC et al.[125] Rayan GM et al.[126]

Continued

Table 22-6	Special Tests for the Shoulder—cont'd				
TEST	**SENSITIVITY**	**SPECIFICITY**	**+LR**	**-LR**	**REFERENCE**
Allen Test	NA	18-43%	NA	NA	Gillard J et al.[127] Marx RG et al.[123]
Roos Test	82-84%	30-100%	NA	NA	Roos DB.[128] Gillard J et al.[127] Howard M et al.[129]
Wright Test	Pulse: 70% Pain: 90% With Roos: 83%	Pulse: 53% Pain: 29% With Roos: 47%	NA	NA	Wright IS.[130]
Military Press Test	NA	53-100%	NA	NA	Gillard J et al.[127] Plews MC et al.[125] Rayan GM et al.[126]
Acromioclavicular Shear Test	100%	97%	NA	NA	Davies GJ et al.[131]
Cross Body Adduction Test					Powell JW et al.[132] Axe MJ.[133] Clark HD et al.[134] Shaffer BS.[135] Chronopoulus E et al.[136] Calis M et al.[72] Park HB et al.[73] Ostor AJ et al.[101]

SPECIAL TESTS FOR THE SHOULDER

Special Tests for Impingement

Hawkins-Kennedy Test (Fig. 22-25)

Purpose:	To test for the presence of subacromial impingement
Patient:	Sitting
Clinician:	Standing in front of the patient
Procedure:	Passively place shoulder in 90 degrees of flexion and maximal internal rotation.
Interpretation:	The test is positive if there is a reproduction of shoulder pain indicating impingement of the supraspinatus.

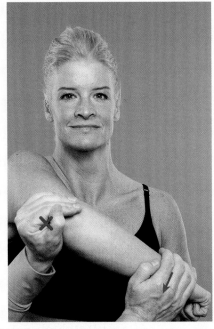

FIGURE 22–25 Hawkins-Kennedy test.

Neer Test (Fig. 22-26)

Purpose:	To test for the presence of subacromial impingement
Patient:	Sitting or supine, with the table providing additional scapular stabilization
Clinician:	Standing behind the patient
Procedure:	Passively move the shoulder into flexion with internal rotation as the therapist holds down the scapula from behind, using the forearm over the scapula or holding down the anterior lateral border of the scapula if the patient is supine.
Interpretation:	The test is positive if there is a reproduction of shoulder pain indicating impingement of supraspinatus or the long head of the biceps tendon. Further confirmation may be obtained if relief is noted upon application of an inferior glide.

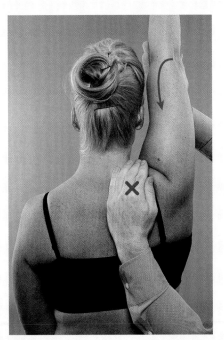

FIGURE 22–26 Neer test.

Yergason Test (Fig. 22-27)

Purpose: To test for the presence of bicipital tendonopathy or transverse humeral ligament rupture

Patient: Sitting with the elbow flexed to 90 degrees and pronated with arm at the side

Clinician: Standing to the side of the patient

Procedure: Clinician resists forearm supination.

Interpretation: The test is positive if there is pain and weakness experienced upon resistance at the anterior shoulder region.

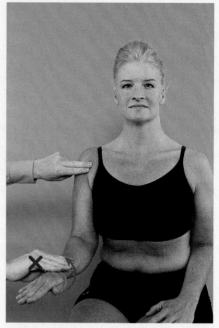

FIGURE 22–27 Yergason test.

Special Tests for Instability
Apprehension Sign and Relocation Test
(Fig. 22-28)

Purpose: To test for the presence of anterior glenohumeral instability

Patient: Supine with the arm at 90 degrees of abduction and full external rotation

Clinician: Sitting on involved side with one hand placed as a fulcrum just posterior to the humeral head

Procedure: Passively move the shoulder into maximal external rotation against the fulcrum of the other hand.

Interpretation: The test is positive if there is a reproduction of shoulder pain or apprehension to further movement. Further confirmation may be obtained if relief is noted upon application of a posteriorly directed force over the anterior humeral head.

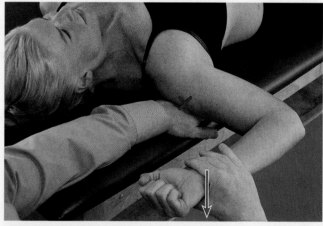

FIGURE 22–28 Apprehension sign and relocation test.

Jerk Test (Fig. 22-29)

Purpose:	To test for the presence of posterior gleno-humeral instability
Patient:	Sitting with the shoulder at 90 degrees of flexion and internal rotation with elbow flexed
Clinician:	Standing in front of the patient, one hand on flexed elbow and the other stabilizing at scapula
Procedure:	Axial compression through the humerus is applied while passively moving the shoulder into horizontal adduction.
Interpretation:	The test is positive if there is a reproduction of shoulder pain with a joint audible.

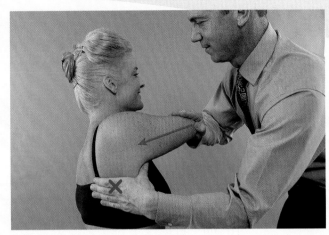

FIGURE 22–29 Jerk test.

Sulcus Sign (Fig. 22-30)

Purpose	To test for the presence of inferior gleno-humeral instability
Patient:	Sitting with the arm at the side
Clinician:	Sitting or standing at the side of the patient
Procedure:	Palpation of the superior aspect of the glenohumeral joint as inferior distraction is provided.
Interpretation:	The test is positive if greater than a one finger-width gap is palpated.

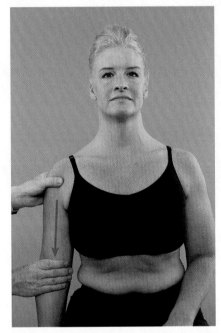

FIGURE 22–30 Sulcus sign.

Special Tests for Rotator Cuff Dysfunction

External Rotation Lag (Dropping) Sign (Fig. 22-31)

Purpose: To test for the presence of a rotator cuff tear, namely the infraspinatus

Patient: Sitting with the arm at the side and elbow flexed to 90 degrees

Clinician: Standing to the side of the patient

Procedure: Passively place the shoulder in the maximal amount of external rotation and ask the patient to hold that position.

Interpretation: The inability to hold the externally rotated position suggests the presence of a large rotator cuff tear.

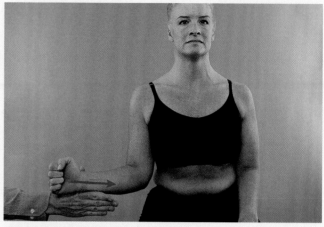

FIGURE 22–31 External rotation lag sign.

Hornblower Sign (Fig. 22-32)

Purpose: To test for the presence of a rotator cuff tear, namely the teres minor

Patient: Sitting

Clinician: Standing to the side of the patient

Procedure: Passively move the shoulder into elevation in the plane of the scapula or in flexion with maximal external rotation and ask the patient to hold that position.

Interpretation: The inability to hold the externally rotated position suggests the presence of a rotator cuff tear.

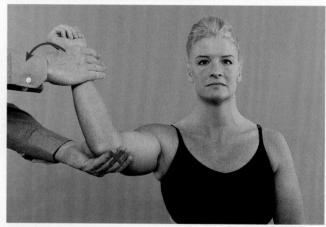

FIGURE 22–32 Hornblower sign.

Drop Arm Test (Fig. 22-33)

Purpose: To test for the presence of a rotator cuff tear, namely the supraspinatus

Patient: Sitting

Clinician: Standing to the side of the patient

Procedure: Passively move the shoulder into 90 degrees of abduction and ask the patient to hold and slowly lower the arm.

Interpretation: The inability to hold and lower the arm in a controlled fashion suggests the presence of a rotator cuff tear of the supraspinatus.

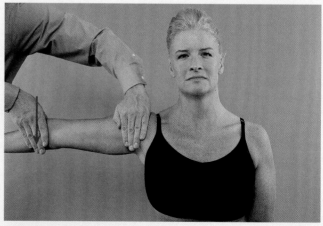

FIGURE 22–33 Drop arm test.

Lift-Off Test (Fig. 22-34)

Purpose:	To test for the presence of a rotator cuff tear, namely the subscapularis
Patient:	Sitting with the arm behind the back in an extended and internally rotated position
Clinician:	Standing behind the patient
Procedure:	Passively move the hand away from the patient's back.
Interpretation:	The inability to hold the lift-off position suggests a rotator cuff tear of the subscapularis.

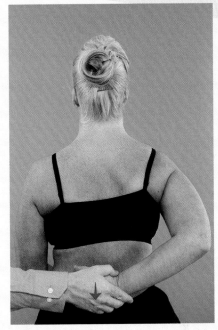

FIGURE 22–34 Lift-off test.

Full Can/Empty Can Test (Fig. 22-35 A, B)

Purpose:	To test for the presence of a rotator cuff tear, namely the supraspinatus
Patient:	Sitting
Clinician:	Standing in front of patient
Procedure:	Patient elevates the shoulder in the plane of the scapula or flexion in the sagittal plane with ER (thumb up) then IR (thumb down). The clinician resists elevation in both positions for full can test, then places arm with thumb down for the empty can test and resists elevation.
Interpretation:	The inability to hold against resistance suggests the presence of a rotator cuff tear of the supraspinatus.

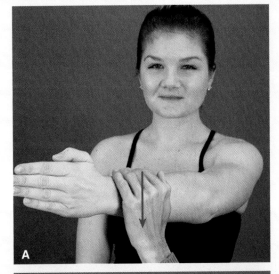

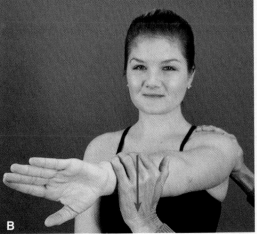

FIGURE 22–35 A. Full can test. **B.** Empty can test. (Courtesy of Bob Wellmon Photography, BobWellmon.com)

Special Tests for Glenoid Labrum Dysfunction

Speed Test (Fig. 22-36)

Purpose: To test for the presence of bicipital tendonopathy or glenoid labral pathology

Patient: Sitting with the arm flexed to 90 degrees, elbow extended, forearm supinated

Clinician: Standing in front of the patient

Procedure: Apply a downward force.

Interpretation: The test is positive if pain and weakness is experienced upon resistance at the anterior shoulder region.

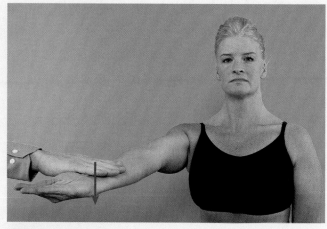

FIGURE 22–36 Speed test.

Biceps Load Test (Fig. 22-37)

Purpose: To test for the presence of a labral tear

Patient: Supine with the shoulder at 90 degrees of abduction, full external rotation, elbow flexed to 90 degrees, and forearm supinated

Clinician: Standing to the side of the patient

Procedure: Resist elbow flexion and supination.

Interpretation: The test is positive if there is reproduction of pain upon resistance. Provocation may also be noted if clinician passively moves forearm into pronation and elbow extension.

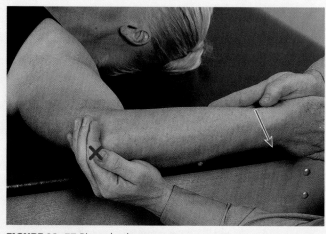

FIGURE 22–37 Biceps load test.

O'Brien Test (Fig. 22-38 A, B)

Purpose: To test for the presence of a labral tear or pathology of the acromioclavicular joint

Patient: Sitting with shoulder at 90 degrees, slight horizontal adduction and internal rotation

Clinician: Standing to the side of the patient

Procedure: Resist elevation with arm in internal rotation followed by resistance with arm in external rotation.

Interpretation: The test is positive if there is pain and weakness experienced on resistance with the arm in internal rotation that exceeds the pain and weakness noted in external rotation, suggesting a labral tear or acromioclavicular joint pathology.

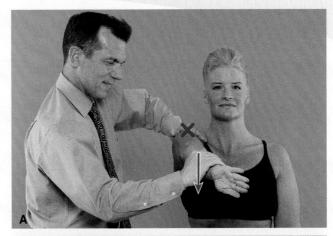

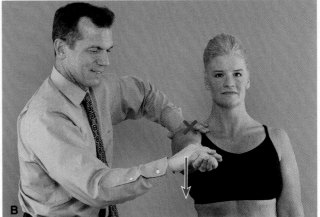

FIGURE 22–38 O'Brien test. **A.** Resist with shoulder in IR. **B.** Resist with shoulder in ER.

Crank Test (Fig. 22-39)

Purpose: To test for the presence of a labral tear

Patient: Sitting with the shoulder at 160 degrees and elbow flexed with the hand on the head

Clinician: Standing to the side of the patient

Procedure: Provide axial compression while the shoulder is externally and internally rotated.

Interpretation: The test is positive if there is reproduction of pain with clicking or clunking.

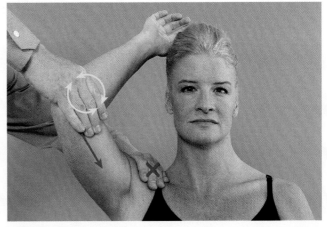

FIGURE 22–39 Crank test.

Kim Test (Fig. 22-40)

Purpose: To test for the presence of a labral tear

Patient: Sitting with the shoulder elevated to approximately 130 degrees in the plane of the scapula and the elbow flexed to 90 degrees

Clinician: Standing to the side of the patient

Procedure: Apply a compressive force through the humerus.

Interpretation: The test is positive if there is pain or clicking.

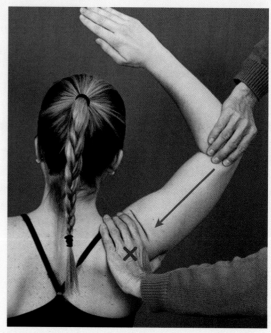

FIGURE 22–40 Kim test (Courtesy of Bob Wellmon Photography, BobWellmon.com.)

SLAP Prehension Test (Fig. 22-41 A, B)

Purpose: To test for the presence of a labral tear

Patient: Sitting

Clinician: Standing in the front of the patient

Procedure: Horizontally adduct the patient's arm across the chest with elbow extended, forearm pronated, and shoulder internally rotated (thumb down). Repeat horizontal adduction with the patient's arm supinated and shoulder externally rotated (thumb up).

Interpretation: The test is positive if there is pain in the area of the bicipital groove with or without an audible or palpable click when in pronation greater than supination.

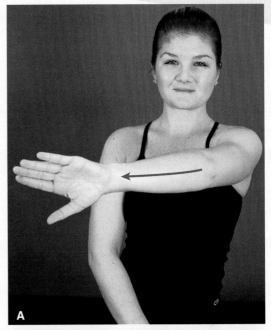

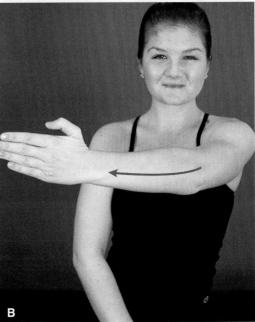

FIGURE 22–41 SLAP prehension. **A.** Position in shoulder internal rotation and **B.** external rotation. (Courtesy of Bob Wellmon Photography, BobWellmon.com.)

Anterior Slide Test (Fig. 22-42)

Purpose: To test for the presence of a labral tear

Patient: Sitting with hands on hips and thumbs pointing posteriorly

Clinician: Standing to the side of the patient

Procedure: Clinician places one hand on top of affected shoulder and the other hand on the olecranon. Clinician applies a forward and superior force through the elbow.

Interpretation: The test is positive if there is pain over the anterior shoulder or a joint audible.

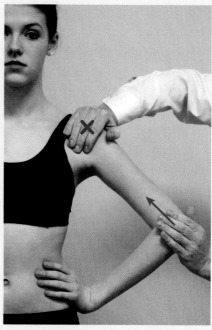

FIGURE 22–42 Anterior slide test.

Special Tests for Thoracic Outlet Syndrome
Adson Test (Fig. 22-43)

Purpose: To assess for the presence of thoracic outlet syndrome at the scalene triangle

Patient: Sitting

Clinician: Standing behind the patient

Procedure: Palpate the radial pulse; move the shoulder into abduction, extension, and ER; rotate the head toward involved side; then take a deep breath and hold.

Interpretation: The test is positive if symptoms are reproduced or if there is an absent or diminished pulse.

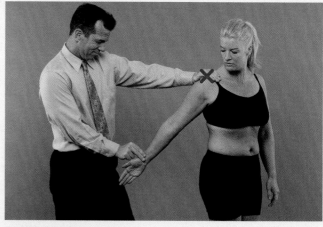

FIGURE 22–43 Adson test.

Allen Test (Fig. 22-44)

Purpose:	To assess for the presence of thoracic outlet syndrome at the pectoralis minor muscle
Patient:	Sitting
Clinician:	Standing behind the patient
Procedure:	Palpate the radial pulse, move the shoulder into 90 degrees of abduction and 90 degrees of elbow flexion; turn the head away, and take a deep breath and hold.
Interpretation:	The test is positive if symptoms are reproduced or if there is an absent or diminished pulse.

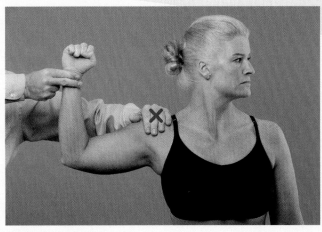

FIGURE 22–44 Allen test.

Roos Test (Fig. 22-45)

Purpose:	To assess for the presence of thoracic outlet syndrome
Patient:	Sitting with both arms at 90 degrees of shoulder abduction, ER, and elbow flexion
Clinician:	Standing/sitting in front of the patient
Procedure:	Open and close hands for 3 minutes; record time of onset of symptoms.
Interpretation:	The test is positive if symptoms are reproduced, or if there is an absent or diminished pulse.

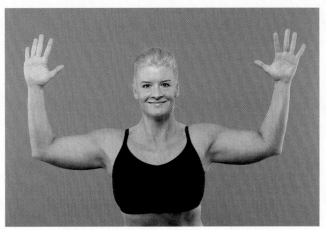

FIGURE 22–45 Roos test.

Wright Test (Fig. 22-46)

Purpose:	To assess for the presence of thoracic outlet syndrome at the coracoid/rib and pectoralis minor muscle
Patient:	Sitting
Clinician:	Standing behind the patient
Procedure:	Palpate the radial pulse, passively abduct the shoulder to 180 degrees, and ER; take a deep breath and hold.
Interpretation:	The test is positive if the symptoms are reproduced or if there is an absent or diminished pulse.

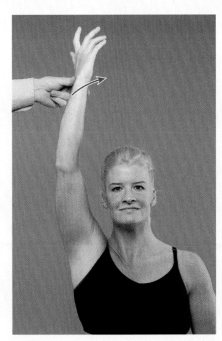

FIGURE 22–46 Wright test.

Military Press Test (Fig. 22-47)

Purpose: To assess for the presence of thoracic outlet syndrome at the first rib and clavicle

Patient: Sitting

Clinician: Standing behind the patient

Procedure: Palpate the radial pulse, retract the shoulders into extension and abduction with the neck in extension (exaggerated military posture).

Interpretation: The test is positive if symptoms are reproduced or if there is an absent or diminished pulse.

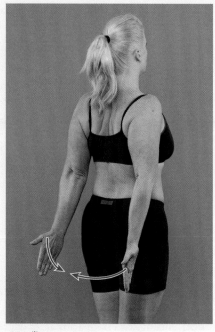

FIGURE 22–47 Military press test.

Special Tests for Acromioclavicular Joint Dysfunction

Acromioclavicular Shear Test (Fig. 22-48)

Purpose: To test for the presence of acromioclavicular joint dysfunction

Patient: Sitting with the arm at the side

Clinician: Standing to side of the patient with hands over the acromioclavicular joint

Procedure: Provide compression to the joint.

Interpretation: The test is positive if there is reproduction of pain at the AC joint.

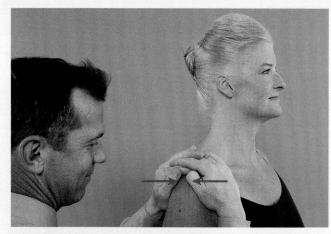

FIGURE 22–48 Acromioclavicular Shear test.

Cross-Body Adduction Test (Fig. 22-49)

Purpose: To test for the presence of acromioclavicular joint dysfunction

Patient: Standing or sitting

Clinician: Sitting or supine

Procedure: Flex the shoulder to 90 degrees and horizontally adduct the arm across the body.

Interpretation: The test is positive if there is reproduction of pain at the AC joint.

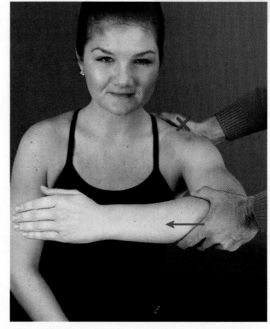

FIGURE 22–49 Cross-body adduction. (Courtesy of Bob Wellmon Photography, BobWellmon.com.)

JOINT MOBILIZATION OF THE SHOULDER JOINT COMPLEX

Note: The indications for the joint mobilization techniques described in this section are based on expected joint kinematics. Current evidence suggests that the indications for their use are multifactorial and may be based on direct assessment of mobility and an individual's symptomatic response.

Scapulothoracic Joint Mobilizations

Scapulothoracic Glides and Distractions

Indications:
- *Scapulothoracic Glides and Distractions* are indicated for any condition in which mobility of the scapula relative to the thoracic wall is reduced and/or painful. Perform *lateral glide* for protraction and elevation, *medial glide* for retraction, *upward rotation glide* for elevation, *downward rotation glide* for return to neutral, *superior glide* for elevation, and *inferior glide* for depression.

Accessory Motion Technique (Figs. 22-50, 22-51, 22-52)
- **Patient/Clinician Position:** The patient is side lying with the arm at the side and the scapula being mobilized in neutral. The shoulder may be pre-positioned at the point of restriction. Stabilization is provided through the patient's body weight. Stand facing the patient.
- **Hand Placement:** Place your caudal hand beneath the patient's arm capturing the inferior angle of the scapula and your cephalad hand at the superior angle of the scapula. Place your chest or abdomen in contact with the patient's anterior shoulder to provide another point of contact for the mobilization.

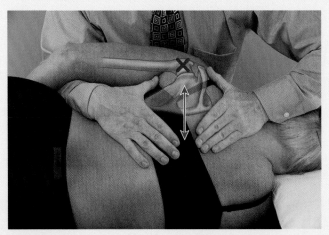

FIGURE 22–50 Scapulothoracic medial and lateral glide.

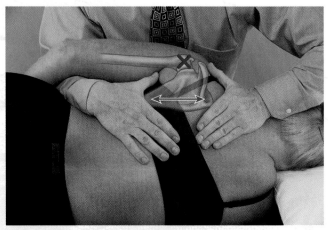

FIGURE 22–51 Scapulothoracic superior and inferior glide.

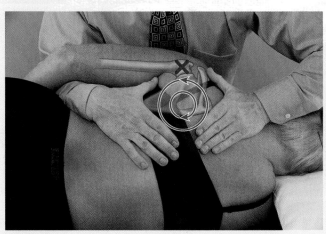

FIGURE 22–52 Scapulothoracic upward and downward rotation.

- **Force Application:** Through your hand contacts at the superior and inferior angles of the scapula, produce a distraction force as if lifting the scapula away from the thoracic wall. Both mobilization hands work in unison to mobilize the scapula in a superior, inferior, lateral, medial, or up/downward rotation direction while maintaining distraction.

Accessory With Physiologic Motion Technique (Fig. 22-53)
- **Patient/Clinician Position:** The patient is sitting. Stand on the contralateral side of the shoulder being mobilized.
- **Hand Placement:** Place the mobilization hand over the posterior aspect of the scapula, at either the inferior angle or medial border, and the stabilization hand over the mid-clavicle.
- **Force Application:** Apply force as the patient actively moves into the direction of greatest restriction, either

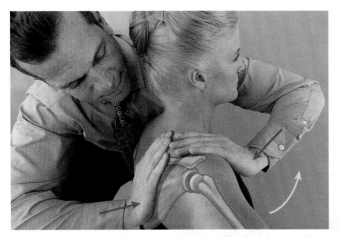

FIGURE 22–53 Scapulothoracic compression with physiologic motion.

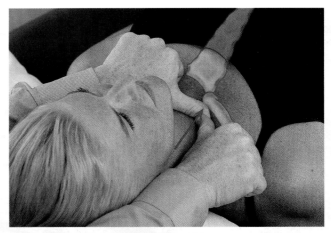

FIGURE 22–55 Sternoclavicular inferior glide.

abduction or flexion. Maintain force throughout the entire range of motion and sustain force at end range.

Sternoclavicular Joint Mobilizations

Sternoclavicular Glides

Indications:

- *Sternoclavicular glides* are indicated for any condition in which the mobility of the scapula relative to the thoracic wall is reduced and/or painful. Perform a *posterior glide* for horizontal abduction, *inferior glide* for elevation, and *superior glide* for return to neutral.

Accessory Motion Technique: (Figs. 22-54, 22-55, 22-56)

- **Patient/Clinician Position:** The patient is supine with the arm in neutral and supported by pillows with hand placed over the abdomen. The shoulder may be pre-positioned at the point of restriction with the arm in elevation for

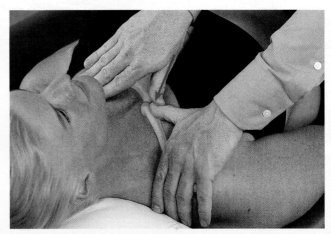

FIGURE 22–56 Sternoclavicular superior glide.

inferior glides or horizontal abduction for posterior glides. Stabilization is provided by the patient's body weight. Stand on the ipsilateral side of the shoulder being mobilized.

- **Hand Placement:** Place thumb over thumb or hypothenar eminence over thumb of your mobilization hand in contact with the anterior aspect of the clavicular head for posterior glides, the superior aspect for inferior glides, and the inferior aspect for superior glides.
- **Force Application:** Take up the slack in the joint and apply force through your mobilization hand contacts in a posterior, inferior, or superior direction.

Accessory With Physiologic Motion Technique (Fig. 22-57)

- **Patient/Clinician Position:** The patient is sitting. Stand on the contralateral side of the shoulder being mobilized.
- **Hand Placement:** Place your mobilization hand contacts in the same position as for the accessory motion technique. Thumb over thumb or hypothenar over thumb contacts may be used at the clavicular head or force may be applied through the thenar or hypothenar eminence of the mobilization hand while the stabilization hand is placed at the scapula.

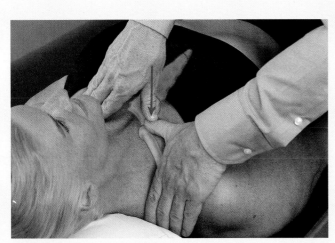

FIGURE 22–54 Sternoclavicular posterior glide.

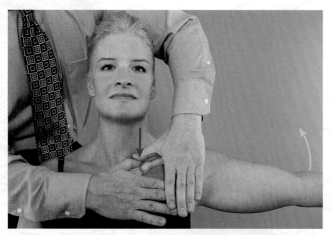

FIGURE 22–57 Sternoclavicular inferior glide with physiologic motion.

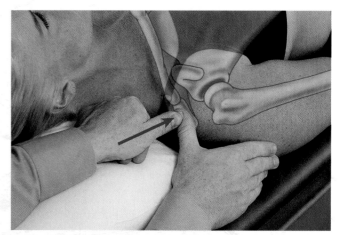

FIGURE 22–58 Acromioclavicular inferior glide.

- **Force Application:** Apply force through your mobilization hand contacts as the patient actively moves into the direction of greatest restriction. Maintain force throughout the entire range of motion and sustain force at end range.

Acromioclavicular Joint Mobilizations

Acromioclavicular Glides

Indications:
- *Acromioclavicular glides* are indicated for any condition in which mobility of the scapula is reduced and/or painful. Perform an *anterior* or *posterior glide* for internal and external rotation, respectively. Perform a *medial* or *lateral glide* for upward and downward rotation, respectively. Perform an *inferior glide* for elevation.

Accessory Motion Technique (Fig. 22-58)
- **Patient/Clinician Position:** The patient is supine, with the arm in neutral and supported by pillows with hand placed over the abdomen. The shoulder may be pre-positioned with arm in elevation to point of restriction during inferior glides. Stabilization is provided by the patient's body weight. Stand at the head of the patient.
- **Hand Placement:** Place thumb over thumb or hypothenar eminence over thumb contact at the superior, posterior, or anterior aspect of the acromion process.
- **Force Application:** Take up slack in the joint and apply force through the mobilization hand contacts.

Accessory With Physiologic Motion Technique (Not pictured)
- **Patient/Clinician Position:** The patient is sitting. Stand behind the patient.
- **Hand Placement:** Place your mobilization hand contacts in the same position as for the accessory motion technique.

- **Force Application:** Apply force through your mobilization hand contacts as the patient actively moves into the direction of greatest restriction. Maintain force throughout the entire range of motion and sustain force at end range.

Glenohumeral Joint Mobilizations

Glenohumeral Distraction

Indications:
- *Glenohumeral distractions* are indicated when there is a loss of mobility in all directions.

Accessory Motion Technique: (Fig. 22-59)
- **Patient/Clinician Position:** The patient is in the supine or sitting position with the shoulder in neutral. The shoulder may be pre-positioned at the point of restriction. Sit or stand on the ipsilateral side of the shoulder being mobilized facing cephalad.
- **Hand Placement:** Your stabilization hand grasps the distal aspect of the patient's humerus. Your mobilization hand is draped by a towel and placed within the patient's axilla. A mobilization strap may be applied to the patient's proximal humerus and around your gluteal folds.
- **Force Application:** After taking up the slack in the joint, apply a laterally directed force through your mobilization hand or strap at the patient's proximal humerus as your stabilization hand provides counterforce at the distal humerus, thus producing a short-arm lever.

Accessory With Physiologic Motion Technique (Fig. 22-60)
- **Patient/Clinician Position:** The patient is supine. Stand on the ipsilateral side of the shoulder being mobilized.
- **Hand Placement:** Grasp the patient's distal humerus or just proximal to the wrist with both hands.

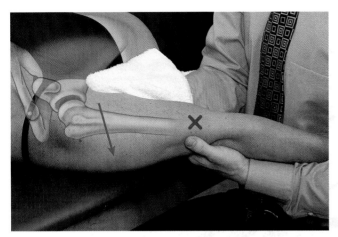

FIGURE 22–59 Glenohumeral distraction.

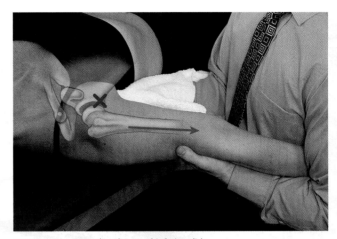

FIGURE 22–61 Glenohumeral inferior glide.

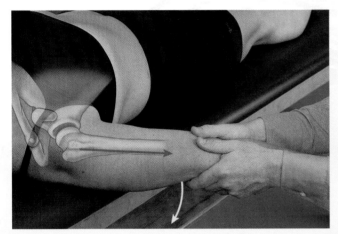

FIGURE 22–60 Glenohumeral distraction with physiologic motion.

hand, grasp the distal humerus with the patient's forearm firmly held between your forearm and body. Be sure that your forearm is in line with the direction of force
- **Force Application:** While maintaining all contacts, rotate your trunk away from the patient, take up the slack in the joint, and apply an inferior glide against pressure from the stabilizing contact. When mobilizing out of neutral, apply inferiorly directed force over the superior aspect of the proximal humerus while providing stabilization at the elbow with the patient in the supine or sitting position.

Accessory With Physiologic Motion Technique (Figs. 22-62, 22-63)

- **Force Application:** Apply a long axis distraction force as the patient actively moves into the direction of greatest restriction. Maintain force throughout the entire range of motion and sustain force at end range. Be prepared to follow the extremity through its excursion of motion.

Glenohumeral Inferior Glide

Indications:
- *Glenohumeral inferior glides* are indicated for restricitons in elevation of the GH joint. The functional IR mobilization is indicated when there are restrictions and/or pain with this combined movement pattern.

Accessory Motion Technique: (Fig. 22-61)
- **Patient/Clinician Position**: The patient is in the supine or sitting position with the shoulder in neutral. The shoulder may be pre-positioned at the point of restriction. Sit or stand on the ipsilateral side of the shoulder being mobilized facing cephalad.
- **Hand Placement:** Place the towel-draped stabilization hand within the patient's axilla. Using your mobilization

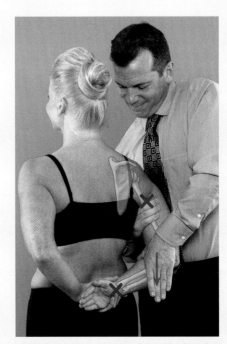

FIGURE 22–62 Glenohumeral inferior glide with physiologic motion into extension, internal rotation, and adduction.

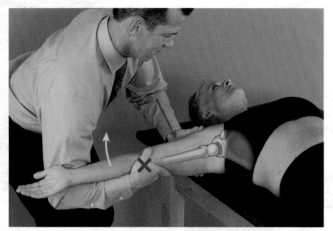

FIGURE 22–63 Glenohumeral inferior glide with physiologic motion into abduction.

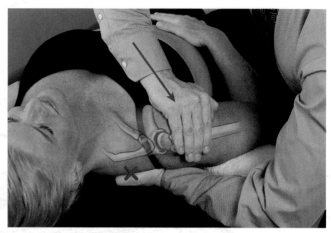

FIGURE 22–64 Glenohumeral posterior glide.

Technique 1:
- **Patient/Clinician Position:** The patient is sitting or standing with the shoulder in extension, adduction, and internal rotation with the elbow flexed and firmly held behind the back by the uninvolved hand. Stand on the ipsilateral side of the shoulder being mobilized.
- **Hand Placement:** Place the stabilization hand within the patient's axilla to block scapular motion and localize the inferior glide to the glenohumeral joint. Place the mobilization hand or belt on the patient's forearm, just distal to the flexed elbow. Be sure to maintain this contact throughout the entire range of motion with the forearm in line with the direction of force.
- **Force Application:** Take up the slack in the joint and apply an inferior glide while the patient moves into greater degrees of motion with your assistance and the assistance of the uninvolved hand. Maintain force throughout the entire range of motion and sustain force at end range.

Technique 2:
- **Patient/Clinician Position:** The patient is in the supine or sitting position with her shoulder in neutral. The shoulder may be pre-positioned at the point of restriction. Stand near the patient's head facing caudally.
- **Hand Placement:** Place your mobilization hand on the superior aspect of the proximal humerus.
- **Force Application:** Impart an inferior glide as the stabilization hand brings the shoulder into greater ranges of elevation with assistance from the patient. Maintain force throughout the entire range of motion and sustain force at end range.

Glenohumeral Posterior Glide

Indication:
- *Glenohumeral posterior glides* are indicated for restrictions in ER and abduction of the GH joint. NOTE: Traditionally, posterior glides have been used for restrictions in IR.

More recent evidence and clinical practice suggests its use for restrictions in ER. Posterior glides have the potential to enhance mobility in both directions.

Accessory Motion Technique (Fig. 22-64)
- **Patient/Clinician Position:** The patient is in the supine position with the shoulder in the open-packed position with a bolster supporting the elbow in a flexed position and the patient's hand on the abdomen. The shoulder may be pre-positioned with the arm at the point of restriction. Stand on the ipsilateral side of the shoulder being mobilized facing cephalad.
- **Hand Placement:** Place your open hand, or folded towel, beneath the patient's scapula with the thenar and hypothenar eminences positioned just proximal to the glenohumeral joint to provide scapular stabilization. Place the palm of the mobilization hand on the anterior aspect of the humeral head with your forearm in line with the direction of force.

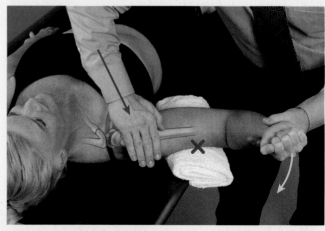

FIGURE 22–65 Glenohumeral posterior glide with physiologic motion into external rotation.

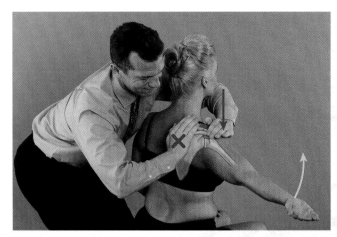

FIGURE 22–66 Glenohumeral posterior glide with physiologic motion into abduction.

- **Force Application:** With hand contacts in place, take up the slack in the joint and apply a postero-lateral glide as the scapula is stabilized.

Accessory With Physiologic Motion Technique (Figs. 22-65, 22-66)
Technique 1:
- **Patient/Clinician Position:** The patient is in the supine position with the shoulder in the open-packed position with a bolster supporting the elbow in a flexed position. The shoulder may be pre-positioned with the arm at the point of restriction. Stand on the ipsilateral side of the shoulder being mobilized facing cephalad.
- **Hand Placement:** Place the palm of the mobilization hand on the anterior aspect of the humeral head with your forearm in line with the direction of force while the stabilization hand guides the shoulder into external rotation. No hand contact is made at the scapula, however, a small towel roll may be used for stabilization.
- **Force Application:** With the mobilization hand in place at the anterior aspect of the humeral head, apply a postero-lateral glide as the shoulder is moved into external rotation. Maintain the force throughout the entire range of motion with a sustained hold at end range.

Technique 2:
- **Patient/Clinician Position:** The patient is sitting or standing. Stand on the contralateral side of the shoulder being mobilized.
- **Hand Placement:** Place the palm of the mobilization hand, or mobilization strap, over the anterior aspect of the humeral head with the forearm in line with the direction of force. Place the palm of the stabilization hand over the posterior aspect of the scapula.
- **Force Application:** The patient actively moves into elevation in the direction of greatest restriction. During active movement, take up the slack in the joint and apply a postero-laterally

directed force over the anterior aspect of the humerus while simultaneously stabilizing the scapula posteriorly throughout the entire range of motion. Maintain the force throughout the entire range of motion with a sustained hold at end range.

Glenohumeral Anterior Glide

Indications:
- *Glenohumeral anterior glides* are indicated for restrictions in IR, flexion, and extension. NOTE: Traditionally, anterior glides have been used for restrictions in ER. More recent evidence and clinical practice suggests its use for restrictions in IR. Anterior glides have the potential to enhance mobility in both directions.

Accessory Motion Technique: (Fig. 22-67)
- **Patient/Clinician Position:** The patient is prone with a wedge stabilizing the scapula anteriorly. The shoulder may be pre-positioned at the point of restriction. Stand on the ipsilateral side of the shoulder being mobilized and face cephalad.
- **Hand Placement:** Place the forearm of the stabilization arm over the scapula and reach anteriorly moving the scapula into a neutral position. Contact the posterior aspect of the humeral head with the hyopthenar eminence of your mobilization hand. Be sure your forearm is in line with the direction of force
- **Force Application:** With contacts in place, take up the slack in the joint and apply an antero-medial glide with the arm in neutral, or at the point of greatest restriction.

Accessory With Physiologic Motion Technique (Fig. 22-68)
- **Patient/Clinician Position:** The patient is sitting or standing. Stand on the contralateral side of the shoulder being mobilized.
- **Hand Placement:** Place your mobilization hand at the posterior humerus while your stabilization hand contacts the distal clavicle.

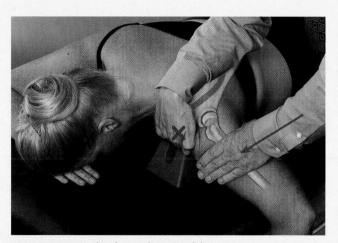

FIGURE 22–67 Glenohumeral anterior glide.

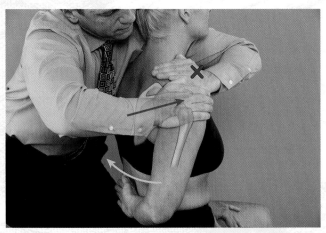

FIGURE 22–68 Glenohumeral anterior glide with physiologic motion into internal rotation, extension, adduction.

- **Force Application:** The patient actively moves in the direction of greatest restriction, primarily functional IR (IR, extension, adduction), or extension. During active movement, take up the slack in the joint and apply an antero-medially directed force over the posterior aspect of the humerus while simultaneously stabilizing over the clavicle. Maintain the force throughout the entire range of motion with a sustained hold at end range.

CLINICAL CASE

CASE 1

Subjective Examination

History of Present Illness

A 29-year-old right-hand-dominant female presents to your office today with chronic complaint of right lateral shoulder pain with onset 3 years ago. The most recent exacerbation is 3 weeks ago and is of insidious onset. She reports that she was a competitive swimmer in high school and since that time regularly swims laps (100 laps, two to three times per week) at the local health club. She spends long hours sitting at the computer at work and notes no difficulty in performing these activities. Her symptoms increase from an average 2/10 level to 6/10 level when she reaches overhead, with occasional increased pain in the morning when she has slept on the right side or when she awakens with her arms in an overhead position. She reports intermittent minimal pain in her left shoulder as well.

Objective Physical Examination

Examination of Structure

In sitting, this patient presents with broad shoulders, including symmetrical hypertrophic deltoid musculature. Severe rounded shoulder and forward head posture is apparent.

Examination of Mobility

Physiologic mobility testing: All motions are within functional limits for AROM and PROM. On the right a painful arc is noted from 80 to 120 degrees. Capsular end-feel is noted at the end range of all motions on the right, with report of pain at end range and for elevation only on the left.

Accessory mobility testing: Reduced inferior glide and posterior glide is noted on the right when examined in the open-packed position, which increases in severity when tested in elevation. In both cases, resistance is experienced prior to pain. An increase from 90 to 130 degrees with less pain is noted when an accessory posterior glide is applied to active abduction in sitting.

Examination of muscle function: Examination yields 5/5 bilaterally using break testing in midrange with the exception of right ER = 4/5 and flexion = 4/5 with pain.

Palpation: There is tenderness to the touch over the long head of the biceps tendon within the intertubercular groove and at the most superior aspect of the greater tuberosity.

Special Testing: Hawkins = +, Neer = +, Speed = +, Empty Can/Full Can = +, Drop Arm = −, Hornblower = −, ER Lag = −, Lift Off = −, Apprehension/Relocation = − .

1. Based on this presentation, what is your differential diagnosis? Is this patient in need of a referral for additional medical testing? Which portion(s) of the clinical examination was most helpful in allowing you to reach these conclusions?
2. What structural factors may be contributing to the onset and perpetuation of this condition? What behavioral factors may be playing a role?
3. Explain the clinical significance of the painful arc? For this patient, what are the three R's (see Chapter 2)? What is the patient's reproducible sign, region of origin, and level of reactivity?
4. How will your intervention be guided by your findings from accessory mobility testing? What is the clinical significance of engaging initial resistance (R1) and final resistance (R2) prior to the first onset of pain (P1) and final onset of pain (P2)?
5. Develop a prioritized problem list that goes from the most significant to the least significant impairment. Match each impairment with a specific manual and nonmanual intervention.
6. Describe the three most important interventions that you would implement with this patient at the time of her next visit. Practice these manual interventions on a partner.
7. What is your prognosis and expected outcome for this patient? What aspects of the examination have been most helpful in determining these outcomes.

CASE 2

Subjective Examination

History of Present Illness

A 62-year-old right-hand-dominant female presents today having sustained a fracture of her left proximal humerus at the region of the surgical neck 4 months ago for which she was immobilized for 8 weeks with good radiological union as noted upon recent radiographs. She enters your clinic today with complaint of pain at a 2/10 level of intensity and describes her pain as dull and achy in nature. She reports significant deficits in performing most functional activities such as brushing her hair and clasping her brassiere, which cause an increase in pain to a 6/10 level. She notes that her symptoms awaken her at night.

Self-reported disability measures: Disability of arm, shoulder, and hand (DASH) score = 62.

Past Medical History: History of osteoporosis, non-insulin-dependent diabetes mellitus, and osteoarthritis.

Diagnostic Imaging: Arthrography reveals reduced left glenohumeral joint volume with an absent axillary fold.

Objective Physical Examination

Examination of Structure: In sitting, the patient is observed to posture her left upper extremity at her side in adduction, internal rotation, and elbow flexion. Her left shoulder and scapula are elevated compared to the left side.

Examination of Mobility

Physiologic mobility testing: Right shoulder is within normal limits (WNL). The left shoulder is as follows:

MOTION	AROM	PROM	END-FEEL	SYMPTOM REPRODUCTION	QUALITY
Flexion	110 degrees	125 degrees	Empty	P1, P2 before R1, R2. Anterior, axilla	Deviation into plane of scapula at 80 degrees. Poor eccentric control of ST muscles from 30 to 0 degrees
Abduction	85 degrees	95 degrees	Empty	P1, P2 before R1, R2. Anterior, axilla anterior, axilla	Deviation into plane of scapula at 45 degrees with associated pain and excessive scapular elevation with increased activation of upper trapezius
External Rotation	20 degrees	35 degrees	Capsular	P1 before R1, but R2 before P2	Compensatory arching of back at end range
Internal Rotation	65 degrees	65 degrees	Capsular	R1, R2 before P1, P2	Scapular protraction as evidenced by shoulder lifting off table

Accessory mobility testing: Reduced accessory glides in all directions which are most notable in the inferior and lateral directions.

Examination of muscle function: Grossly 4+/5 strength throughout upon manual muscle testing of the scapulohumeral muscles in midrange, with pain noted and 4−/5 strength when tested at the end of available range. Scapulothoracic muscle testing is 4−/5 and pain free throughout.

Palpation: No significant tenderness to the touch noted throughout. Increased tissue tension and tone within the muscle bellies of the upper trapezius and levator scapula on the left.

Neurological scan: All WNL throughout.

Special testing: All special tests for labrum, instability, rotator cuff integrity are negative.

1. How will the patient's score on the DASH influence your plan of care?
2. What do the results of your movement examination tell you about this patient's condition? How will this information guide your choice of manual and nonmanual interventions?
3. Do the results of diagnostic imaging confirm your diagnosis?
4. Provide rationale for the deficits noted in the quality of this patient's movement patterns. What physiologic processes might contribute to such findings?
5. Are the results of muscle function testing consistent with the rest of the examination? What do the results of this patient's muscle function examination tell you about the contribution of these deficits to this patient's condition and how might these findings serve to guide intervention?
6. Based on the results of this examination, what are this patient's reproducible sign, region of origin, and reactivity level? How will this determination guide your intervention?
7. Describe, in detail, the type and manner in which you would initiate intervention at the time of this patient's next visit to physical therapy. Consider the integration of both manual and nonmanual interventions as well as the sequencing of specific interventions.

HANDS-ON

With a partner, perform the following activities:

1 Consider the key indicators that may be revealed during the history and interrogation of your partner that may suggest the presence of the following conditions. These indicators may include such things as the mechanism of injury and pain pattern. Based on these indicators, what examination procedures might you use to rule in or rule out the presence of each particular condition? Complete the grid.

DYSFUNCTION	HISTORICAL INDICATORS	CONFIRMATORY SIGNS
AC Joint Degeneration		
Adhesive Capsulitis		
Multidirectional Instability		
Impingement Syndrome		
Rotator Cuff Tear		
AC Joint Separation		
Nerve Palsy (Suprascapular, Dorsal Scapular, Long Thoracic, Radial, Axillary, Spinal Accessory)		
Peripheral Nerve Entrapment		
Nonmechanical Pathologic Condition		

2 Observe your partner as he or she performs active physiologic movements over single and repeated repetitions and single and multiplane directions, and identify the quantity, quality, and any reproduction of symptoms that may be produced. Compare these active movements with performance of these same movements passively.

3 In an attempt to relate each impairment to a structural cause, provide several possible pathoanatomical etiologies for each of the movement impairments identified during active and passive physiologic movement testing above. Complete the grid.

ACTIVE PHYSIOLOGIC MOVEMENT IMPAIRMENT	PASSIVE PHYSIOLOGIC MOVEMENT IMPAIRMENT	POSSIBLE PATHOANATOMIC ORIGIN

4 Perform passive physiologic movement testing in all directions followed by passive accessory movement testing in all planes, and determine the relationship between the onset of pain (P1 and P2, if present) and stiffness or resistance (R1 and R2). Determine the end-feel in each direction. Compare your findings bilaterally and on another partner.

5 Perform passive accessory movement testing in all planes with the shoulder in the neutral, or open-packed, position. Then perform the same tests with the shoulder in other non-neutral and close-packed positions. Identify any changes in the quantity and quality of available motion and report any reproduction of symptoms. Consider which anatomical structures are most responsible for limiting motion in each position. Complete the grid.

PASSIVE ACCESSORY MOVEMENT	QUANTITY, QUALITY, REPRODUCTION IN NEUTRAL	QUANTITY, QUALITY, REPRODUCTION IN NON-NEUTRAL	LIMITING STRUCTURES
SC Joint Superior Glide			
SC Joint Inferior Glide			
SC Joint Posterior Glide			
ST Joint Upward Glide			
ST Joint Downward Glide			
ST Joint Medial Glide			
ST Joint Lateral Glide			
ST Joint Upward Rotation			
ST Joint Downward Rotation			
GH Inferior Glide			
GH Posterior Glide			
GH Anterior Glide			

6 Perform muscle testing for the key muscles about the shoulder using isometric break testing, static testing, and active testing based on the functional preference of each muscle during normal activity. That is, the manner in which the muscle most typically functions (isometrically, concentrically, eccentrically, or all). Complete the grid.

MUSCLE TESTED	FUNCTIONAL PREFERENCE/ MANNER OF TESTING	RESULTS

7 Through palpation, attempt to identify the primary soft tissue and bony structures of the shoulder and compare tissue texture, tension, tone, and location bilaterally.

8 Based on your movement examination as identified above, choose two mobilizations. Perform these mobilizations on your partner and identify any immediate changes in mobility or symptoms in response to these procedures.

9 Perform each mobilization described in the intervention section of this chapter bilaterally on at least two individuals. Using each technique, practice Grades I to IV. Then switch and allow your partner to mobilize your shoulder. Provide input to your partner regarding set-up, technique, comfort, and so on. When practicing these mobilization techniques, utilize the Sequential Partial Task Practice Method, in which students repeatedly practice one aspect of each technique (i.e., position, hand placement, force application) on multiple partners each time adding the next component until the technique is performed in real time from beginning to end. (Wise CH, Schenk RJ, Lattanzi JB. A model for teaching and learning spinal thrust manipulation and its effect on participant confidence in technique performance. *J. Man. Manip. Ther.*, August 2014.)

REFERENCES

1. Cyriax J. *Textbook of Orthopaedic Medicine*. Vol. 1. 8th ed. London, UK: Bailliere Tindall; 1982.
2. Steindler A. *Kinesiology of the Human Body under Normal and Pathological Conditions*. Springfield, IL: Charles C. Thomas; 1955.
3. Williams P, Bannister L, Berry M, et al. *Gray's Anatomy, The Anatomical Basis of Medicine and Surgery*. London, UK: Churchill Livingstone; 1995.
4. Bearn JG. Direct observations on the function of the capsule of the sternoclavicular joint in clavicular support. *J Anat*. 1967;101:159-170.
5. Dempster WT. Mechanisms of shoulder movement. *Arch Phys Med Rehabil*. 1965;46:49.
6. Cave AJ. The nature and morphology of the costoclavicular ligament. *J Anat*. 1961;95:170.
7. Mosely HF. The clavicle: its anatomy and function. *Clin Orthop*. 1968;58:17.
8. Inman VT, Saunder JR, Abbott LC. Observations on the function of the shoulder joint. *J Bone Joint Surg*. 1944;26:1.
9. Pronk GM, van der Helm FCT, Rozendaal LA. Interaction between the joints in the shoulder mechanism: the function of the costoclavicular, conoid and trapezoid ligaments. *Proceedings Institute of Mechanical Engineering*. 1993;207:219-229.
10. Bateman JE. *The Shoulder and Neck*. Philadelphia, PA: WB Saunders; 1971.
11. McClure P. Direct 3-dimensional measurement of scapular kinematics during dynamic movements in vivo. *J Shoulder Elbow Surg*. 2001:10; 269-277.
12. Conway A. Movements at the sternoclavicular and acromioclavicular joints. *Phys Ther Rev*. 1961;41;421-432.
13. Ludewig P, Cook T. Alterations in shoulder kinematics and associated muscle activity in people with symptoms of shoulder impingement. *Phys Ther*. 2000:80;276-291.

14. Dvir Z, Berme N. The shoulder complex in elevation of the arm: a mechanism approach. *J Biomech*. 1978;11:219.
15. Rowe CR, Sakellarides HT. Factors related to recurrences of anterior dislocation of the shoulder. *Clin Orthop*. 1961;20:41.
16. Poppen NK, Walker PS. Normal and abnormal motion of the shoulder. *J Bone Joint Surg*. 1976;58A:195.
17. Kaltenborn FM. Mobilization of the extremity joints: examination and basic treatment techniques. Oslo, Norway: Olaf Bokhandel; 1980.
18. MacConail MA, Basmajian JV. Muscles and movements: a basis for human kinesiology. Baltimore, MD: Williams & Wilkins; 1969.
19. Soslowsky LJ, Flatow EL, Bigliani LU, Mow VC. Articular geometry of the glenohumeral joint. *Clin Orthop*. 1992;295:181.
20. Saha AK. Mechanism of shoulder movements and a plea for the recognition of the "zero position" of glenohumeral joint. *Ind J Surg*. 1950;12:153.
21. O'Connell PW, Nuber GW, Mileski RA, Lautenschlager E. The contribution of the glenohumeral ligaments to anterior stability of the shoulder joint. *Am J Sports Med*. 1990;18:579.
22. Terry GC, Hammon D, France P, Norwood LA. The stabilizing function of the passive shoulder restraints. *Am J Sports Med*. 1991;19:26.
23. Turkel SJ, Panio MW, Marshal JL. Stabilizing mechanisms preventing anterior dislocation of the glenohumeral joint. *J Bone Joint Surg*. 1981;63A:1208.
24. Kelkar R, Flatow EL, Bigliani LU, et al. A stereophotogrammetric method to determine the kinematics of the glenohumeral joint. *Advanced Bioengineering*. 1992;19:143.
25. Kelley MJ, Clark WA. *Orthopedic Therapy of the Shoulder*. Philadelphia PA: Lippincott Williams & Wilkins; 1995.
26. Nobuhara K. *The Shoulder: Its Function and Clinical Aspects*. Tokyo, Japan: Igaku-Shoin; 1977.
27. Howell SM, Galinat BJ, Renzi AJ, Marone PJ. Normal and abnormal mechanics of the glenohumeral joint in the horizontal plane. *J Bone Joint Surg*. 1988;70A:227.
28. Harryman DT, Sidles JA, Harris SZ, Matzen FA III. The role of the rotator internal capsule in passive motion and stability of the shoulder. *J Bone Joint Surg*. 1992;74A:53.
29. Blakely RL, Palmer ML. Analysis of rotation accompanying shoulder flexion. *Phys Ther*. 1984;64:1214.
30. Duchenne GB. *Physiology of Motion*. EB Kaplan, trans. Philadelphia, PA: JB Lippincott; 1949.
31. Codman EA. *The Shoulder*. Boston, MA: Thomas Todd; 1934.
32. DePalma AF. *Surgery of the Shoulder*. Philadelphia,PA: JB Lippincott, 1973.
33. Johnston TB. The movements of the shoulder joint: a plea for the use of the "plane of the scapula" as the plane of reference in movements occurring at the humero-scapular joint. *Br J Surg*. 1937;25:252.
34. American Academy of Orthopaedic Surgeons. *Joint Motion: Method of Measuring and Recording*. Chicago, IL: American Academy of Orthopaedic Surgeons; 1965.
35. Lippitt SB, Harryman DT, Matsen FA. A practical tool for evaluating function. The simple shoulder test. In: Matsen FA, Fu FH, Hawkins RJ, eds. *The Shoulder: A Balance of Mobility and Stability*. Rosemeont, IL: American Academy of Orthopaedic Surgeons; 1993:501.
36. Matsen FA, et al. Shoulder motion. In: Matsen FA, et al, eds. *Practical Evaluation and Management of the Shoulder*. Philadelphia, PA: WB Saunders; 1994:19.
37. Michener LA, Leggin BG. A review of self-report scales for the assessment of functional limitation and disability of the shoulder. *J Hand Ther*. 2001;14:68.
38. Williams JW, Holleman DR, Simel DL. Measuring shoulder function with the shoulder pain and disability index. *J Rheumatol*. 1995;22:727.
39. Cook KF, Gartsoman GM, Roddey TS, Olson SL. The measurement level and trait-specific reliability of 4 scales of shoulder functioning: an empiric investigation. *Arch Phys Med Rehabil*. 2001;82:1558.
40. Beaton D, Richards R. Measuring function of the shoulder. A cross-sectional comparison of five questionnaires. *J Bone Joint Surg Am*. 1996;78:882.
41. Hudak PL, Amadio PC, Bombardier C. Development of an upper extremity outcome measure: the DASH. The Upper Extremity Collaborative Group. *Am J Ind Med*. 1996;29:602.
42. MacDermid JC, Tottenham V. Responsiveness of the disability of the arm, shoulder, and hand (DASH) and patient-rated wrist/hand evaluation in evaluating change after hand therapy. *J Hand Ther*. 2004;17:18.
43. Dutton M. *Orthopaedic Examination, Evaluation, and Intervention*. New York, NY: McGraw-Hill, 2004.
44. Gummesson C, Atroshi I, Ekdahl C. The disabilities of the arm, shoulder, and hand (DASH) outcome questionnaire: longitudinal construct validity and measuring self-rated health change after surgery. *BMC Musculoskelet Disord*. 2003;4:11.
45. Constant CR, Murley AHG. A clinical method of functional assessment of the shoulder. *Clin Orthop Rel Res*. 1987:214;160.
46. Richards RR, Bigliani LU, et al. A standardized method for the assessment of shoulder function. *J Shoulder Elbow Surg*. 1994:3;347.
47. Boissonnault WG. *Primary Care for the Physical Therapist: Examination and Triage*. St. Louis, MO: Elsevier Saunders; 2005.
48. Brewer BJ. Aging of the rotator cuff. *Am J Sports Med*. 1979:7;102.
49. Booth RE, Marvel JP. Differential diagnosis of shoulder pain. *Orthop Clin North Am*. 1975:6;353.
50. Hovelius L. Recurrences after initial dislocation of the shoulder. *J Bone Joint Surg*. 1983;65:343.
51. Hovelius L. Anterior dislocation of the shoulder in teenagers and young adults: five-year prognosis. *J Bone Joint Surg*. 1987;69:393.
52. Kazar B, Relovsky E. Prognosis of primary dislocation of the shoulder. *Acta Orthop Scand*. 1969;40:216.
53. McLaughlin HL, Cavallaro WU. Primary anterior dislocation of the shoulder. *Am J Surg*. 1950;80:615.
54. Rowe CR. Prognosis in dislocations of the shoulder. *J Bone Joint Surg*. 1956;8:957.
55. Magee DJ. *Orthopedic Physical Assessment*. 4th ed. Philadelphia, PA: WB Saunders; 2002.
56. Herberts D, Kadefors R, Andersen G, Petersen I. Shoulder pain in industry: an epidemiological study in welders. *Acta Orthop Scand*. 1981;52:299.
57. Laumann U. Kinesiology of the shoulder joint. In: Kolbel R, Helbig B, Blauth W, eds. *Shoulder Replacement*. Berlin, Germany: Springer-Verlag; 1987.
58. Levangie PK, Norkin CC. *Joint Structure and Function: A Comprehensive Analysis*. 4th ed. Philadelphia, PA: FA Davis, 2005.
59. Kapandji I. *The Physiology of the Joints*. Vol. 1. Baltimore, MD: Williams & Wilkins; 1970.
60. Woodward T, Best T. The painful shoulder: part II. Acute and chronic disorders. *Am Fam Phys*. 2000:61;3291-3300.
61. Norkin CC, White DJ. *Measurement of Joint Motion: A Guide to Goniometry*. 3rd ed. Philadelphia, PA: FA Davis; 2003.
62. Mitsch J, Casey J, McKinnis R, Kegerreis S, Stikeleather J. Investigation of a consistent pattern of motion restriction in patients with adhesive capsulitis. *J Man Manipulative Ther*. 2004;12:153.
63. Rundquist P, Ludewig PM. Patterns of motion loss in subjects with idiopathic loss of shoulder range of motion. *Clin Biomech*. 2004;19:810.
64. Janda V. Muscle spasm–a proposed procedure for differential diagnosis. *J Manual Med*. 1991;6:136-130.
65. Janda V. Muscles and back pain: assessment and intervention, movement patterns, motor recruitment. Course notes, 2nd ed. Edinburgh, UK: Churchill Livingstone; 1994.
66. Kendall FP, McCreary EK. *Muscle Testing and Function*. 3rd ed. Baltimore, MD: Williams & Wilkins; 1982.
67. Falsone SA. One-arm hop test: reliability and effects of arm dominance. *J Orthop Sports Phys Ther*. 2002:32;98-103.
68. Biel A. *Trail Guide to the Body*. Boulder, CO: Andrew Biel, LMP, 1997.
69. Michener LA, Walsworth MK, Doukas WC, Murphy KP. Reliability & diagnostic accuracy of 5 physical examination tests & combination of tests for subacromial impingement. *Arch Phys Med Rehabil*. 2009;90:1898-1903.
70. Hawkins RJ, Kennedy JC. Impingement syndrome in athletics. *Am J Sports Med* 1980;8:151-163.
71. MacDonald PB, Clark P, Sutherland K. An analysis of the diagnostic accuracy of the Hawkins & Neer subacromial impingement signs, *J Shoulder Elbow Surg*. 2000;9:299-301.
72. Calis M, Akgun K, Birtane M, et al. Diagnostic values of clinical diagnostic tests in subacromial impingement syndrome. *Ann Rheum Dis*. 2000;59:44-47.
73. Park HB, Yokota A, Gill HS, El Rassi G, McFarland EG. Diagnostic accuracy of clinical tests for the different degrees of subacromial impingement syndrome. *J Bone Joint Surg*. 2005;87-A:1446-1455.
74. Tomberlin J. Physical diagnostic tests of the shoulder: an evidence-based perspective. In: *Home Study Course 11.1.2 Solutions to Shoulder Disorders*. LaCrosse, WI: American Physical Therapy Association, Orthopaedic Section; 2001.
75. Neer CS, Welsh RP. The shoulder in sports. *Orthop Clin N Am*. 1977;8:583-591.
76. Valadic AL, Jobe CM, Pink MM, et al. Anatomy of provocative tests for impingement syndrome of the shoulder. *J Shoulder Elbow Surg*. 2000;9:36-46.
77. Buchberger DJ. Introduction of a new physical examination procedure for the differentiation of acromioclavicular joint lesions & subacromial impingement. *J Manip Physio Ther*. 1999;22:316-321.
78. Post M, Cohen J. Impingement syndrome: a review of late stage II & early stage III lesions. *Clin Orthop*. 1986;207:127-132.

79. Matsen FA, Thomas SC, Rockwood CA. Glenohumeral instability. In: Rockwood CA, Matsen FA, eds. *The Shoulder*. Philadelphia, PA: WB Saunders; 1990.

80. Gerber C, Ganz R. Clinical assessment of instability of the shoulder. *J Bone Joint Surg Br*. 1984;66:551-556.

81. Kvitne RS, Jobe FW. The diagnosis and treatment of anterior instability in the throwing athlete. *Clin Orthop*. 1993;291:107-123.

82. Luime JJ, Verhagen AP, Miedema HS, et al. Does this patient have instability of the shoulder or a labrum lesion? *JAMA*. 2004;292:1989-1999.

83. Hawkins RJ, Mohtadi NG. Clinical evaluation of shoulder instability. *Clin J Sports Med*. 1991;1:59-64.

84. Lo IK, Nonweiler B, Woolfrey M, Litchfield R, Kirkley A. An evaluation of the apprehension, relocation, & surprise tests for anterior shoulder instability. *Am J of Sports Med*. 2004;32:301-307.

85. Speer KP, Hannafin JA, Altchek DW, Warren RF. An evaluation of the shoulder relocation test. *Am J Sports Medicine*. 1994;22:177-183.

86. Mok DWH, et al. The diagnostic value of arthroscopy in glenohumeral instability. *J Bone Joint Surg*. 1990;72-B:698-700.

87. Guanche CA, Jones DC. Clinical testing for tears of the glenoid labrum. *Arthroscopy*. 2003;19:517-523.

88. Kim SH, Park JS, Jeong WK, et al. The Kim test: a novel test for posteroinferior labral lesion of the shoulder—a comparison to the jerk test. *Am J Sports Med*. 2005;33:1188-1191.

89. Bigliani LU, Codd TP, Conner PM, et al. Shoulder motion and laxity in the professional baseball player. *Am J Sports Med*. 1997;25:609-613.

90. McClusky GM. Classification and diagnosis of glenohumeral instability in athletes. *Sports Med Artho Rev*. 2000;8:158-169.

91. Nakagawa S, Yoneda M, Hayashida K, et al. Forced shoulder abduction & elbow flexion test: a new simple clinical test to detect superior labral injury in the throwing shoulder. *Arthroscopy*. 2005;21:1290-1295.

92. Ludewig P. Functional anatomy and biomechanics. In: *Home Study Course 11.1 Solutions to Shoulder Disorders*. LaCrosse, WI: American Physical Therapy Association, Orthopaedic Section; 2001.

93. Hertel R, Ballmer FT, Lambert SM, et al. Lag signs in the diagnosis of rotator cuff rupture. *J Shoulder Elbow Surg*. 1996;5:307-313.

94. Walch G, Boulahia A, Calderone S, et al. The "dropping" & "Hornblower's" signs in evaluating rotator cuff tears. *J Bone Joint Surg Br*. 1998;80:624-628.

95. Chao S, Thomas S, Yucha D, et al. An electromyographic assessment of the bear hug: an examination for the evaluation of the subscapularis muscle. *Arthroscopy*. 2008;24:1265-1270.

96. Rigsby R, Sitler M, Kelly JD. Subscapularis tendon integrity: an examination of shoulder index tests. *J Athl Train*. 2010;45:404-406.

97. Ticker JB, Warner JJ. Single-tendon tears of the rotator cuff: evaluation & treatment of subscapularis tears. *Orthop Clin North Am*. 1997;28:99-116.

98. Greis PE, Kuhn JE, Schultheis J, et al. Validation of the lift-off sign test & analysis of subscapularis activity during maximal internal rotation. *Am J Sports Med*. 1996;24:589-593.

99. Gerber C, Krushell RJ. Isolated ruptures of the tendon of the subscapularis muscle. *J Bone Joint Surg Br*. 1991;73:389-394.

100. Lyons RP, Green A. Subscapularis tendon tears. *J Am Acad Ortho Surg*. 2005;13:353-363.

101. Ostor AJ, Richards CA, Prevost AT, Hazleman BL, Speed CA. Interrater reproducibility of clinical tests for rotator cuff lesions. *Ann Rheum Dis*. 2004;63:1288-1292.

102. Itoi E, Kido T, Sano A, Urayama M, Sato K. Which is more useful, the "full can test" or the "empty can test" in detecting the torn supraspinatus tendon. *Am J Sports Med*. 1999;27:65-68.

103. Guanche CA, Jones DC. Clinical testing for tears of the glenoid labrum. *Arthroscopy*. 2003;19:517-523.

104. Holtby R, Razmjou H. Accuracy of the Speed's & Yergason's tests in detecting biceps pathology & SLAP lesions: comparison with arthroscopic findings. *Arthroscopy*. 2004;20:231-236.

105. Kim SH, Ha KI, Han KY. Biceps load test: a clinical test for superior labrum anterior & posterior lesions in shoulder with recurrent anterior dislocations. *Am J Sports Med*. 1999;27:300-303.

106. Lewis CL, Sahrmann SA. Acetabular labral tears. *Phys Ther*. 2006;86:110-121.

107. Kim SH, Ha KI, Ahn JH, Kim SH, Choi HJ. Biceps load test II: a clinical test for SLAP lesions of the shoulder. *Arthroscopy*. 2001;17:160-164.

108. Wilk KE, Reinold MM, Dugas JR, et al. Current concepts in the recognition & treatment of superior labral (SLAP) lesions. *J Orthop Sports Phys Ther*. 2005;35:273-291.

109. Myers TH, Zemanovic JR, Andrews JR. The resisted supination external rotation test. *Am J Sports Med*. 2005;33:1315-1320.

110. Burkhart SS, Morgan CD, Kibler WB. The disabled throwing shoulder: spectrum of pathology, part two: evaluation & treatment of SLAP lesions in throwers. *Arthroscopy*. 2003;19:531-539.

111. O'Brien SJ, Pagnoni MJ, Fealy S, et al. The active compression test: a new & effective test for diagnosing labral tears & acromioclavicular joint abnormality. *Am J Sports Med*. 1998;26:610-613.

112. Stetson WB, Templin K. The crank test, the O'Brien test, & routine magnetic resonance imaging scans in the diagnosis of labral tears. *Am J Sports Med*. 2002;30:806-809.

113. Liu SH, Henry MH, Nuccion SL. A prospective evaluation of a new physical examination in predicting glenoid labral tears. *Am J Sports Med*. 1996;24:721-725.

114. Walsworth MK, Doukas WC, Murphy KP, Mielcarek BJ, Michener LA. Reliability & diagnostic accuracy of history and physical examination for diagnosing glenoid labral tears. *Am J Sports Med*. 2008;36:162-168.

115. Mimori K, Muneta T, Nakagawa T, Shinomiya K. A new pain provocation test for superior labral tears of the shoulder. *Am J Sports Med*. 1999;27:137-142.

116. Parentis MA, Mohr KJ, El Attrache NS. Disorders of the superior labrum: review & treatment guidelines. *Clin Orthop Relat Res*. 2002:77-87.

117. Berg EE, Ciullo JV. A clinical test for superior glenoid labral or "SLAP" lesions. *Clin J Sports Med*. 1998;8:121-123.

118. Kibler WB. Clinical examination of the shoulder. In: Pettrone FA, ed. *Athletic Injuries of the Shoulder*. New York, NY: McGraw-Hill; 1995.

119. Kibler WB. Specificity & sensitivity of the anterior slide test in throwing athletes with superior glenoid labral tears. *Arthroscopy*. 1995;11:296-300.

120. Andrews JR, Gillogly S. Physical examination of the shoulder in throwing athletes. In: Zarins B, Andrews JR, Carson WG, eds. *Injuries to the Throwing Arm*. Philadelphia, PA: WB Saunders; 1985.

121. McFarland EG, Kim TK, Savino RM. Clinical assessment of three common tests for superior labral anterior-posterior lesions. *Am J Sports Med*. 2002;30:810-815.

122. Adson AW, Coffey JR. Cervical rib: a method of anterior approach for relief of symptoms by division of the scalenus anticus. *Ann Surg*. 127;85:839-857.

123. Marx RG, Bombardier C, Wright JC. What do we know about the reliability & validity of physical examination tests used to examine the upper extremity? *J Hand Surg*. 1999;24A:185-193.

124. Lee AD, Agarwal S, Sadhu D. Doppler Adson's test: predictor of outcome of surgery in non-specific thoracic outlet syndrome. *World J Surg*. 206;30:291-292.

125. Plews MC, Delinger M. The false-positive rate of thoracic outlet syndrome shoulder maneuvers in healthy patients. *Acad Emerg Med*. 1998;5:337-342.

126. Rayan GM, Jensen C. Thoracic outlet syndrome: provocative examination maneuvers in a typical population. *J Shoulder Elbow Surg*. 1995;4:113-117.

127. Gillard J, Pérez-Cousin M, Hachulla E, et al. Diagnosing thoracic outlet syndrome: contribution of provocative tests, ultrasonography, electrophysiology, & helical computed tomography in 48 patients. *Joint Bone Spine*. 2001;68:416-424.

128. Roos DB. Historical perspectives & anatomical considerations. Thoracic outlet syndrome. *Semin Thorac Cardiovasc Surg*. 1996;8:183-189.

129. Howard M, Lee C, Dellon AL. Documentation of brachial plexus compression utilizing provocative neurosensory & muscle testing. *J Reconstr Microsurg*. 2003;19:303-312.

130. Wright IS. The neurovascular syndrome produced by hyperabduction of the arms. *Am Heart J*. 1945;29:1-19.

131. Davies GJ, Gould JA, Larson RL. Functional examination of the shoulder girdle. *Phys Sports Med*. 1981;9:82-104.

132. Powell JW, Huijbregts PA. Concurrent criterion-related validity of acromioclavicular joint physical examination tests: a systematic review. *J Man Manip Ther*. 2006;14:E19-E29.

133. Axe MJ. Acromioclavicular joint injuries in the athlete. *Sports Med Artho Rev*. 2000;8:182-191.

134. Clark HD, McCann PD. Acromioclavicular joint injuries. *Orthop Clin North Am*. 2000;31:177-187.

135. Shaffer BS. Painful conditions of the acromioclavicular joint. *J Am Acad Orthop Surg*. 1999;7:176-188.

136. Chronopoulus E, Kim TK, Park HB, et al. Diagnostic value of physical tests for isolated chronic acromioclavicular lesions. *Am J Sports Med*. 2004;32:655-661.

Orthopaedic Manual Physical Therapy of the Elbow and Forearm

Christopher H. Wise, PT, DPT, OCS, FAAOMPT, MTC, ATC

Chapter Objectives

At the conclusion of this chapter, the reader will be able to:

- Identify the key anatomical and biomechanical features of the elbow and forearm and their impact on orthopaedic manual physical therapy (OMPT) examination and intervention.
- List and perform key procedures used in the OMPT examination of the elbow and forearm.
- Demonstrate sound clinical decision-making in evaluating the results of the OMPT examination.

- Use pertinent examination findings to reach a differential diagnosis and prognosis.
- Discuss issues related to the safe performance of OMPT interventions for the elbow and forearm.
- Demonstrate basic competence in the performance of a skill set of joint mobilization techniques for the elbow and forearm.

FUNCTIONAL ANATOMY AND KINEMATICS

Introduction

The elbow joint complex is comprised of the *humeroulnar*, *humeroradial*, and the proximal and distal *radioulnar joints*, all of which serve the primary function of positioning the hand in space. The elbow joint proper (humeroulnar and humeroradial joints) functions as a *loose hinge joint* with one degree of freedom that permits movement in the sagittal plane about a frontal plane axis (Fig. 23-1). A small degree of frontal and transverse plane movement that serves to enhance function is also available. The proximal and distal radioulnar joints function collaboratively to provide transverse plane rotation about a longitudinal axis.

The Humeroulnar (HU) Joint

Positioned between the medial and lateral epicondyles of the distal humerus is the spherical *capitulum*, which comprises lateral one-third of the humeral articulating surface. Occupying the middle two-thirds of the humeral articulating surface is the larger, spool-shaped *trochlea*, with its obliquely oriented

central *trochlear groove*. Both the capitulum and the trochlea are covered by articular *hyaline cartilage*. Observation of bone density reveals that the distal humerus sustains its greatest loads anteriorly and distally.[1] The trochlea protrudes anteriorly in relation to the humerus and the medial aspect of the trochlea extends more distally than its lateral counterpart. Orientation of the trochlea results in a valgus angulation of the forearm. The **carrying angle** is defined as the angle between the long axis of the humerus and the long axis of the ulna when the elbow is extended and fully supinated. The average carrying angle is considered to be 10 to 15 degrees in the frontal plane (Fig. 23-2).[2] The *coronoid fossa*, which is just proximal to the trochlea, accommodates the *coronoid process* of the ulna when the elbow is fully flexed. The larger *olecranon fossa* receives the *olecranon process* of the ulna, thus producing the hard end-feel at terminal range of elbow extension.

Forming the distal aspect of this articulation is the ulna, which consists of the hyaline cartilage-enrobed *trochlear notch* that corresponds to the trochlea of the humerus. The trochlea does not contact the notch in the central portion except when loaded.[3] The lateral aspect of the coronoid process is occupied by the *radial notch*, which serves as an elliptical facet for articulation with the radial head.

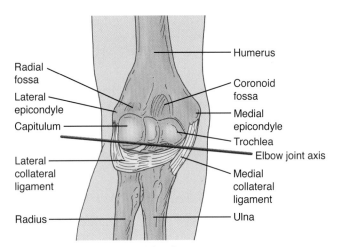

FIGURE 23–1 Anterior view of the elbow.

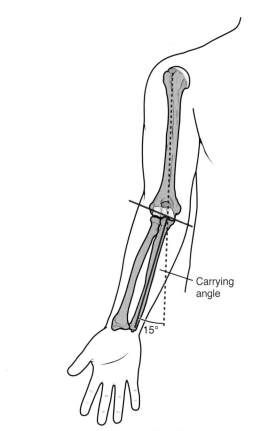

FIGURE 23–2 The carrying angle of the elbow.

The Humeroradial (HR) Joint

The proximal aspect of the radius includes the radial head, neck, and tuberosity. The most proximal aspect of the *radial head*, the *fovea*, is concave and articulates with the convex capitulum of the humerus forming a joint that allows transverse plane movement around a longitudinal axis. The *radial neck* lies just distal to the head. Its smaller diameter serves as an ideal location for the *annular ligament*. The *radial tuberosity* is an important insertion site for the biceps brachii muscle and can be palpated distal to the neck at the anteromedial aspect of the radius. The greatest degree of articular cartilage and subchondral

bone density is found at the central portion of the fovea, suggesting its important role in sustaining forces.[4] The convex capitulum is slightly smaller than the radial fovea, thus rendering this joint somewhat incongruous.[5] It is most congruent when the elbow is flexed. With the elbow in extension, only the posterior capitulum articulates with the radius.[1]

The Proximal and Distal Radioulnar (RU) Joints

The proximal and distal RU joints are mechanically linked and interdependent. Optimal congruency occurs when the forearm is in neutral between pronation and supination. Conversely, minimal articular contact is noted when the joints are in either maximal pronation or supination.

Although not considered as part of the elbow joint proper, the proximal radioulnar joint is enclosed within the capsule of the elbow joint, thus making it an important contributor to elbow function. The proximal RU joint is comprised of the ulnar radial notch, head of the radius, and the capitulum of the humerus. The radial notch, which is located at the lateral aspect of the proximal ulna, is concave and lined with articular cartilage. The annular ligament, which is also lined with articular cartilage, encircles the radial head and provides stability for the joint thus controlling transverse plane motion (Fig. 23-3A). Although located at some distance from the elbow, the distal RU joint must possess adequate mobility in order to facilitate normal forearm pronation and supination and sufficient joint glide is necessary for enabling the full range of elbow flexion and extension. The distal RU joint must, therefore, routinely be considered in the management of the elbow and forearm (Fig. 23-3B).

Stability of the Elbow Joint Complex

Although not perfectly congruent, the articular surfaces of the humerus, radius, and ulna create a limitation to medial-lateral joint play and serve to guide flexion and extension.[1] To allow mobility, the capsule possesses several folds that distend during movement. The capsule demonstrates its greatest degree of laxity posteriorly. Isolated resection of the capsule does not selectively alter stability of the joint.[6]

Medially and laterally, the elbow joint capsule is reinforced by the extensive *medial (ulnar) collateral ligament (MCL)* and *lateral (radial) collateral ligament (LCL)*, respectively. The MCL resists valgus forces while the LCL resists varus forces. Selective resection of the MCL reveals that the anterior portion resists valgus forces between extension and moderate flexion,[7-10] whereas the posterior portion is the primary restraint in flexion.[7-9]

The LCL may also be divided into individual portions, each of which are responsible for providing the primary restraint to varus forces.[11] Although taut throughout the entire range of motion, the anterior aspect is a primary restraint in extension, while the posterior aspect is taut when the elbow is flexed. The annular ligament prevents subluxation of the joint in the presence of traction forces. The *interosseous membrane* is a thin band of connective tissue that transfers forces between the radius and ulna.[12]

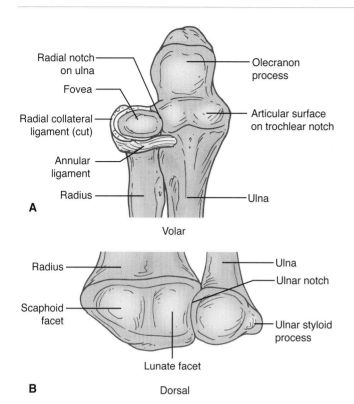

FIGURE 23-3 The **A.** proximal and **B.** distal radioulnar joints.

Mobility of the Elbow Joint Complex

The axis of motion for the HU and HR joints is not fixed and demonstrates significant variation among individuals with most variability occurring within the frontal plane.[13] As the forearm is moved away from the fully supinated position, a reduction in the quantity of flexion is observed. As the concave trochlear notch of the ulna moves into flexion on the convex trochlea of the humerus, accessory joint glide occurs anteriorly in the same direction as the roll (Fig. 23-4). On the lateral aspect of the elbow joint, the concave fovea of the radius moves upon the convex capitulum of the humerus about an axis through the capitulum, requiring anterior accessory glide during flexion (Fig. 23-5).

Pronation and supination are the result of the combined effect of both the proximal and distal radioulnar joints. During these motions, the radius moves on a relatively fixed ulna.

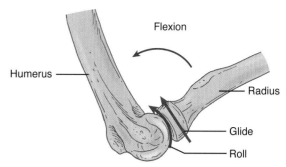

FIGURE 23-5 Physiologic and accessory motion of the humeroradial joint during flexion (ulna removed).

However, the distal ulna moves slightly and in the opposite direction to radial movement.[14] To maintain the hand in a static position, the ulna must also have the ability to radially deviate during these movements.[15,16] During supination and pronation, the majority of accessory glide occurs at the distal radioulnar joint. During supination, roll and glide of the radius on a relatively fixed ulna occurs posteriorly and in the same direction as osteokinematic motion at the distal RU joint. At the proximal RU joint, the radius rotates, or spins, around a longitudinal axis (Fig. 23-6A). Conversely, during pronation, the radius rolls and glides anteriorly in the same direction as osteokinematic motion on the ulna at the distal RU joint and the radius rotates, or spins, at the proximal RU joint (Fig. 23-6B).

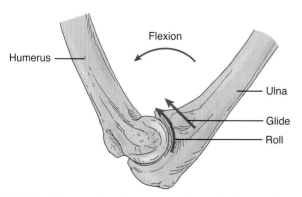

FIGURE 23-4 Physiologic and accessory motion of the humeroulnar joint during flexion (radius removed).

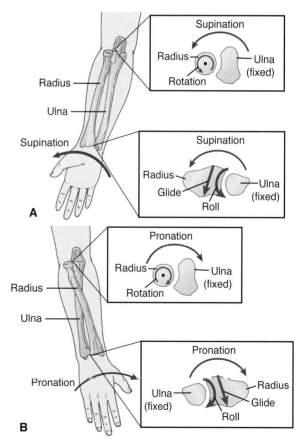

FIGURE 23-6 Physiologic and accessory motion of the proximal and distal radioulnar joints during **A.** supination and **B.** pronation.

It is important to note that the starting position for these motions is neutral, midway between supination and pronation. Evidence suggests that most functional activities require a range of flexion-to-extension motion from 30 to 130 degrees and 50 degrees of pronation to 50 degrees of supination.[1]

EXAMINATION
The Subjective Examination
Self-Reported Disability Measures

The instrument most commonly used to assess the self-perceived functional status of the elbow is the **Disabilities of the Arm, Shoulder, and Hand (DASH)** self-assessment questionnaire. The DASH provides an outcome measure regarding the functional status of the upper extremity.[17] The DASH has been described in detail in Chapter 22 of this text.

Another instrument that has been used to determine elbow function involves a combination of patient-generated subjective items and therapist-tested objective items. The **clinical evaluation elbow form** as proposed by Morrey et al[18] consists of four main sections that are designed to provide important information regarding the functional status of the elbow. The first section is designed to correlate symptoms with movement. The second section contains a strength-testing component. The third section is designed to rule out the presence of joint instability. The fourth section requires testing of specific activities in which the elbow is involved. The patient's response to each of these categories is graded and summed, leading to an overall functional assessment score (95–100 = excellent function, 80–95 = good function, 50–80 = fair function, <50 = poor function).

Review of Systems

Tendon and ligamentous ruptures may result from innocuous stresses in individuals who have a history of chronic steroid use.[19] Differentiation of a full versus partial thickness tear may be identified by a palpable defect. Postmenopausal females often experience *osteopenia*, and a variety of systemic disease processes may result in bone demineralization. A fall on an outstretched hand or direct trauma onto the elbow may cause fracture. Fracture of the radial head will result in limitations of pronation and supination and result in maintenance of the elbow in the open-packed position. Fracture of the prominent olecranon may result in pain with elbow extension.[19]

History of Present Illness

The age of the patient may provide pertinent data that suggests a greater likelihood of one etiology over another in cases of elbow pain. A young child with elbow pain, as evidenced by splinting the arm, may be the result of dislocation. This is particularly true if the patient also lacks supination and the mechanism of pulling or swinging by the arms is reported. Adolescents reporting pain following a fall on an outstretched hand may also complain of elbow pain as a result of fracture of the distal radius or ulna and/or elbow dislocation, which may be impacting motion and function. Middle-age individuals, particularly those involved in repetitive tasks at work or recreation, often develop elbow pain from tendinosis of the common flexor or extensor tendons of the elbow. *Panner's disease* may occur until age 10 and *osteochondrosis dissecans* is typically present between the ages of 15 and 20.[20]

Adolescent and elite baseball pitchers may present with single event or progressive onset of elbow pain. For these individuals, pain is often associated with the end range of the cocking phase due to substantial valgus forces and during the follow-through phase that exerts excessive eccentric shoulder and forearm muscular forces. In the throwing athlete, a "pop" with subsequent pain and inflammation suggests an ulnar collateral ligament sprain. Hyperextension injuries of the elbow may present with a variety of complaints, including neurological symptoms.[20]

Neurological compromise from elbow dysfunction may involve the median, ulnar, or radial nerves. Peripheral nerve entrapment syndromes are common in the elbow. These nerves may be individually or collectively involved at one or multiple locations throughout the upper extremity (Table 23-1). In the presence of neurological symptoms, the cervical spine must be ruled out.

Pain and limitation noted during pronation and supination may suggest dysfunction of the radioulnar joint. Locking of the joint suggests the presence of a loose body within the joint. Local pain and edema over the olecranon suggests *olecranon bursitis*. The inability to fully extend the elbow suggests the possibility of *synovitis*.[21]

Lateral or medial elbow pain suggests the presence of *lateral epicondyle tendonopathy* (tennis elbow) and *medial epicondyle*

Table 23–1	Nerve Injuries of the Elbow and Their Associated Functional Loss
NERVE	**FUNCTIONAL LOSS**
Median Nerve (C6-C8, T1)	Loss of pronation
	Loss of wrist flexion, radial deviation
	Loss of thumb flexion, abduction, opposition
	Loss of gripping
	Ape hand deformity (loss of pinch)
Ulnar Nerve (C7-C8, T1)	Loss of wrist flexion, ulnar deviation
	Loss of fifth digit PIP flexion
	Loss of finger abduction and adduction
	Benediction hand deformity (loss of extension of PIP and DIP of digits four and five)
Radial Nerve (C5-C8, T1)	Loss of supination
	Loss of wrist extension
	Loss of gripping
	Loss of wrist stabilization
	Loss of finger extension
	Loss of thumb abduction

PIP, proximal interphalangeal; DIP, distal interphalangeal. Adapted from Magee DJ. *Orthopedic Physical Assessment*. 4th ed. Philadelphia, PA: WB Saunders; 2002.

tendonopathy (golfer's elbow), respectively. Medial elbow pain may also be present in cases of ulnar collateral sprains and subsequent to compression of the ulnar nerve.[17] Severe pain within the anterior aspect of the elbow that occurs in response to forceful hyperextension of the elbow often denotes a brachialis or biceps brachii muscle rupture or capsular adhesions.[17] Posterior elbow pain is suggestive of triceps tendonopathy, which often results from repetitive and forceful elbow extension.

The Objective Physical Examination
Examination of Structure

The manner in which the patient postures the upper extremity when observed without his or her knowledge may yield important information regarding the patient's level of reactivity and dysfunction. In the case of pain, the extremity is often splinted across the abdomen with an unwillingness to move. Facial grimacing may be noted during active or passive motion.

Upon inspection of the extremity, the therapist must document any areas of deformity, edema, ecchymosis, or muscle atrophy. Neurological conditions involving the elbow may result in atrophy of forearm and hand musculature or hand deformity. Edema may be the result of elbow joint complex trauma or pathology that may be best observed in the region between the lateral epicondyle and olecranon. Intra-articular edema at the elbow may cause the joint to posture in its open-packed position, which is approximately 70 degrees of flexion with the forearm in neutral. A distinct region of local edema is often observed over the olecranon process in cases of olecranon bursitis, the result of direct trauma.[22]

For measurement of the carrying angle, the stationary arm of a large goniometer is placed at the midline of the humerus and the mobile arm is place at the midline of the ulna while the axis is floating. In addition, sagittal plane elbow position is obtained through using standard landmarks for flexion/extension measurements using a large goniometer. In cases of systemic hypermobility, both elbows may posture in excessive degrees of hyperextension. The clinical relevance of observed elbow hyperextension is accomplished through bilateral comparison, reproduction of pain upon attaining the end range position, and later checking end-feel and ligamentous joint play. A carrying angle that is greater than 15 degrees is referred to as **cubitus valgus.** An angle that is less than 5 to 10 degrees is a **cubitus varus.**

Posteriorly, with the patient's elbow at 90 degrees of flexion and full pronation, the examiner may observe a triangle formed by the medial epicondyle, olecranon process, and lateral epicondyle (see Fig. 23-8). These points fall in line as the elbow is extended. This observation, which may be identified clinically or upon radiography, provides a quick assessment of elbow structure. In cases of dislocation or fracture, alterations in this triangular configuration may be observed.

Upper-Quarter Screen

Due to the potential for referred symptoms from the cervical spine, this region must be fully screened. In addition, symptoms may be referred and compensatory movement patterns adopted in the presence of shoulder or wrist and hand dysfunction must be ruled out. Gross active movement testing provides information regarding the patient's muscle function and the patient's neurological status. Myotomal resistance testing is performed for C1-T1 using isometric break testing. Deep tendon reflexes for *biceps (C5-C6), brachioradialis (C6), and triceps (C7)* are performed. If deficits are noted during the upper-quarter screen, a more detailed inspection of the identified structures must be performed with an attempt to explore any association with the individual's presenting chief complaint.

Examination of Mobility
Active Physiologic Movement Examination

The quantity, quality, and reproduction of the patient's primary symptoms are noted during performance of active physiological motion, which, in the elbow, occurs predominantly within the sagittal plane. Transverse plane motion, which takes place at the radioulnar joints, as previously described, is also an important consideration when evaluating elbow function.

When performing bilateral AROM, visual estimation may be used and asymmetry of motion is appreciated through bilateral comparison. When quantifying elbow motion, the patient is asked to perform single movements, then repeated (5–10 times) movements, both unilaterally as well as bilaterally. Bilateral movement is useful for allowing immediate comparison between sides.

The motions that are tested include the traditional cardinal plane motions of flexion/extension in the sagittal plane and forearm supination/pronation in the transverse plane. A functional movement examination that uses patient-specific movements based on reported deficits must also be performed. Examination of mobility often involves the use of combined movement patterns across multiple joints. Pronation of the forearm is considered to be an adjunctive movement associated with elbow extension, and supination occurs in conjunction with elbow flexion.[23] **Overpressure** is provided at the end range of all motions, and the relationship between symptoms and tissue resistance is noted. **Counterpressure** may also be used to block one or more adjacent joints during active movement. The use of counterpressure, or blocking, may serve to isolate the most culpable joint within the elbow joint complex. *Proprioceptive neuromuscular facilitation (PNF)* patterns of movement are often adopted as an efficient method for examining combined movement across multiple joints during active performance of functionally relevant motions (see Chapter 12). Throughout motion testing, it is critical that the manual physical therapist obtain an understanding of the patient's level of **reactivity**, which is procured through understanding the relationship between the onset of symptoms and end range resistance. As previously discussed, determination of reactivity guides the aggressiveness with which intervention may be initiated.

Passive Physiologic Movement Examination

For quantification of passive physiologic elbow movement, *goniometry* is most commonly used. The manual physical therapist must attend to astute palpation of bony landmarks so as to ensure proper placement of the goniometer. Supine, with the humerus supported, is ideal for goniometric measurement of passive movement. The humerus supported at the patient's side, with the elbow flexed to 90 degrees, is the ideal position for eliminating shoulder substitution during measurement of pronation and supination.

Comparing the differences in elbow range of motion in response to alterations in forearm and shoulder positioning may be beneficial in determining the primary source of limitation, thus guiding intervention, for example, if the degree of elbow extension significantly reduces when the forearm is pronated and when the shoulder is extended. The manual physical therapist may presume tightness of the biceps to be the culpable structure. In such cases, intervention designed to stretch and reduce the tissue tension tone of the biceps may be preferred over joint mobilization techniques. At the end range of passive movement, end-feel may be appreciated. The elbow is brought to its end range of flexion followed by extension, at which time overpressure is provided. Table 23-2 displays the physiologic motions of the elbow, including normal ranges of motion, open and close-packed positions, and normal and abnormal end-feels.

Humeroulnar and Humeroradial Passive Physiologic Movement

The axis of the elbow is traditionally believed to be a fixed axis passing horizontally through the trochlea and capitulum and bisecting the longitudinal axis of the humerus. This fixed-axis hypothesis has more recently been challenged in favor of a more loosely arranged hinge joint, which allows some degree of both frontal plane and transverse plane movement.

Although the primary plane of motion for flexion and extension is sagittal, it is important to appreciate that concomitant frontal plane motion also occurs due largely to the configuration of the trochlear groove. The capsular pattern of both the humeroulnar and humeroradial joints is generally considered to be a greater limitation in flexion followed by extension (flexion > extension). For the humeroulnar joint, the open-packed position is considered to be 70 to 90 degrees of elbow flexion and 10 degrees of supination, and the close-packed position is extension with supination. For the humeroradial joint, the

open-packed position is 70 degrees of flexion and 35 degrees of supination, while the close-packed position is considered to be 90 degrees of flexion and 5 degrees of supination.

Flexion

Normal range of passive motion for elbow flexion is generally considered to be *150 to 160 degrees*. The path of the ulna as the elbow moves from full extension to full flexion is dependent largely on the shape of the trochlea. Although variations exist, the most common shape of the trochlear groove dictates that the ulna is guided progressively in a medial direction during movement from full extension to full flexion. As the elbow flexes, the carrying angle disappears and the ulna comes to lie in the same plane as the humerus.

The normal end-feel for elbow flexion is considered to be soft tissue approximation as the biceps brachii contacts the muscles of the forearm. In children and those with less muscle mass, the end-feel may be firmer as the coronoid process comes into contact with the fossa of the humerus.

Any deviations or limitations in this path of motion must be observed. Edema in the elbow joint as a result of trauma or pathology will typically produce a reduction in the range of elbow flexion. The magnitude of this limitation is thought to be approximately 2 degrees of decreased motion for every millimeter of intra-articular edema.[24]

Extension

Elbow extension range of motion is generally considered to be *5 to 10 degrees* of hyperextension. As noted, the fully extended position of the elbow is the most stable and least mobile position (i.e., close-packed position). Normal end-feel for elbow extension is hard, or bone-to-bone, end-feel as the olecranon process of the ulna approximates the olecranon fossa of the humerus.

Proximal and Distal Radioulnar Joint
Passive Physiologic Movement

The axis of motion for supination/pronation extends from the center of the radial head to the center of the ulnar head distally. In supination, the ulna and radius are parallel. In pronation, the radius rolls over the ulna anteriorly. The ulna moves on the radius

Table 23-2	Physiologic (Osteokinematic) Motions of the Elbow				
JOINT	**NORMAL ROM**	**OPP**	**CPP**	**NORMAL END-FEEL**	**CAPSULAR PATTERNS**
Humeroulnar	150°-160° flexion	70°-90° flexion, 10° supination	Full extension, Full supination	Flexion = soft tissue approximation or hard	Flexion > Extension
Humeroradial	5°-10° extension	70° flexion, 35° supination	90° flexion, 5° supination	Extension = hard	
Proximal radioulnar	80°–90° pronation 80°–90° supination	70° flexion, 35° supination	5° supination	Pronation = capsular, tissue stretch Supination = capsular, tissue stretch	Pronation = Supination (equally limited)

ROM, range of motion; OPP, open-packed position; CPP, close-packed position. Adapted from Wise CH, Gulick DT. *Mobilization Notes: A Rehabilitation Specialist's Pocket Guide.* Philadelphia, PA: F.A. Davis; 2009.

minimally during both supination and pronation. Conversely, the head of the radius spins around its long axis, which is sustained by osteoligamentous structures, including the annular ligament. Maximal congruency between the radius and ulna is present at the midrange of supination and pronation, with only minimal surface contact when the joint is fully supinated or fully pronated.

For the proximal radioulnar joint, the open-packed position is considered to be 35 degrees of supination and 70 degrees of elbow flexion and the close-packed position is 5 degrees of supination. The capsular pattern of the proximal radioulnar joint is believed to be an equal limitation of both supination and pronation (supination = pronation).

Supination

Forearm supination is a functionally important movement by virtue of its influence on hand position. Forearm supination results in tissue stretch, or capsular, end-feel under normal conditions. The normal expected range of motion for forearm supination is considered to be *80 to 90 degrees*. Supination may be pathologically limited by tightness of the *pronator quadratus* or *pronator teres*, with the latter being a less substantial imitation when the elbow is flexed compared to the former, which limits supination in both extension and flexion equally.

Pronation

Like supination, normal range of pronation is expected to be approximately *80 to 90 degrees*. The range of pronation may be pathologically limited by tightness of the biceps brachii when the elbow is extended, which may reduce upon flexing the elbow. Restrictions in the posterior fibers of the medial collateral ligament may also be involved in limiting pronation.

Passive Accessory Movement Examination

Humeroulnar Joint Passive Accessory Movement

During active and/or passive elbow flexion and extension with the distal end of the extremity free to move (open kinetic chain), the ulna has the propensity to glide posteriorly during extension and anteriorly during flexion. However, due to the osteological framework and congruency of this joint, glides are challenging and do not occur in their purest form. The olecranon process and trochlear notch of the ulna, which encompasses the trochlear groove of the humerus, makes performance of accessory glides at this joint challenging. Assessment of medial and lateral glides easily translates into mobilization that may be used during intervention.

Humeroradial Joint Passive Accessory Movement

Accessory movement testing and subsequent mobilization of the HR joint is initially performed with the patient supine and with the joint in the open-packed position of full extension and full supination. The treatment plane for the HR joint is determined by the concave fovea of the radius. Anterior and posterior glide that accompanies elbow flexion and extension, respectively, are assessed. Rotation about a longitudinal axis primarily occurs during supination and pronation at this joint. Nevertheless, posterior and anterior glides are assessed as accessory motions of supination and pronation, respectively.

Proximal Radioulnar Joint Passive Accessory Movement

Examination begins with the joint in the open packed position which is 35 degrees of supination and 70 degrees of elbow flexion. The manual physical therapist must exercise caution when performing these techniques since the radial head may be tender to pressure.

Examination of accessory motion becomes the intervention when restrictions are identified. The mobilization techniques that follow later in this chapter will provide details regarding the performance of accessory glides for all of the joints of the elbow joint complex and may be used for both examination and intervention of passive accessory movement. Table 23-3 displays accessory motions of the elbow.

Examination of Muscle Function

Examination of elbow muscle function must be performed in a manner that is specific and functional for the muscle in question. Muscles about the elbow should be tested in a way that resembles

Table 23-3	Accessory (Arthrokinematic) Motions of the Elbow		
	ARTHROLOGY	**ARTHROKINEMATICS**	
Humeroulnar	**Concave surface:** Trochlear notch of ulna **Convex surface:** Trochlea of humerus	*To facilitate flexion:* Radius and ulna roll and glide anterior on humerus	*To facilitate extension:* Radius and ulna roll and glide posterior on humerus
Humeroradial	**Concave surface:** Fovea of radial head Convex surface: Capitulum of humerus	Same as above.	Same as above.
Proximal radioulnar	**Concave surface:** Radial notch of ulna Convex surface: Radial head	*To facilitate pronation:* Radius spins medially on ulna. Radius glides anterior. Ulna glides posterior.	*To facilitate supination:* Radius spins laterally on ulna. Radius glides posterior, Ulna glides anterior.

Adapted From Wise CH, Gulick DT. *Mobilization Notes: A Rehabilitation Specialist's Pocket Guide.* Philadelphia, PA: F.A. Davis; 2009.

the manner in which the muscle predominantly functions. When testing muscles of the elbow isometrically, the extensors possess 60% of the strength of the flexors, and the pronators are generally 85% of the strength of the supinators.[25] Due to close functional relationships, muscle testing of the entire upper extremity should be performed when examining the elbow. Typically, isometric break testing is initially used to provide a general profile of muscle function, after which specific testing may be performed that is designed to more closely approximate actual function. Testing of combined movement patterns and functional movements are also encouraged, particularly if standard muscle testing reveals normal findings. Although the muscles of the upper extremity are primarily designed to function in an **open chain** fashion, under certain circumstances it may be important to test these muscles in **closed chain** positions as well. Athletes, such as weight lifters and bikers, who are involved in a significant amount of closed chain function, should be examined in closed chain. The reader is referred to other sources for a more detailed exposition of formal manual testing of the muscles of the elbow.[26]

The three primary flexors of the elbow are the biceps brachii, brachialis, and brachioradialis. Based on length-tension relationships and angle of pull, the greatest degree of force generated by these flexors, collectively, occurs between 90 and 110 degrees of elbow flexion with the forearm in supination.[27] In this position, the brachialis and the biceps brachii are both in optimal positions to exert force. The one-joint brachialis muscle can be easily differentiated from the multijoint biceps brachii muscle by testing elbow flexion with the forearm in pronation, thus inhibiting the contribution of the biceps brachii, which attaches to the radius, without changing the angle of pull of the brachialis (Fig. 23-7).

As a multijoint muscle, the biceps also plays a key role in the production of supination, making its greatest contribution to this movement at 90 degrees of elbow flexion,[28] as well as flexion of

the shoulder. To produce shoulder flexion, both the long and the short heads of the biceps are active, yet the long head is involved to a greater degree.[29] The ability of this muscle to produce force at the elbow is reduced (particularly within the long head) if elbow flexion is occurring when the shoulder is flexed. Conversely, the biceps demonstrates an increased ability to generate flexion force at the elbow if the shoulder is slightly extended.[30]

The third flexor of the elbow, the brachioradialis, may be preferentially recruited by placing the forearm midway between supination and pronation, providing an optimal angle of pull for this muscle to produce flexion. Although this muscle receives innervation from the radial nerve which also innervates the extensors of the wrist, it is primarily a flexor of the elbow and may have a slight contribution to supination and pronation in the neutral position under resistance.[29]

A less-considered flexor of the elbow is the *pronator teres* muscle, which, as its name implies, is generally accepted as a pronator of the forearm, a function that is unrelated to elbow position.[29] The contribution of this muscle to both forearm pronation and elbow flexion appears to be most significant when these motions are performed under resistance, as in using a screwdriver.[29] Tightness of this muscle is most apparent when the elbow is extended and the forearm is supinated. As a muscle that crosses several articulations, the pronator teres may be considered a likely contributor to a limitation of elbow extension if elbow extension range improves as the forearm is pronated, thus placing this muscle on slack.[1]

The extensors of the elbow are less numerous than those designed to produce flexion. The *triceps brachii* muscle, composed of a long, lateral, and medial head, is located along the entire posterior aspect of the arm and is considered to be the primary extensor of the elbow. In addition to its vital role as an elbow extensor, this muscle also functions to produce shoulder extension and adduction. The role of the triceps at the shoulder, however, has not been clearly delineated in the literature, and its true functional significance as a shoulder extensor and adductor has not been confirmed.[30] By virtue of its insertion into the ulna, this muscle produces extension independent of forearm position. Peak torque for the triceps has been found to occur between 70 and 90 degrees of elbow flexion.[25,31] Due to the small cross-sectional size of the long head, this portion of the muscle is believed to contribute up to 25% of the total extensor moment.[32] Unlike elbow flexion, where other muscles in addition to the biceps contribute significantly to movement, elbow extension moments are almost exclusively the responsibility of the triceps.

The *anconeus* muscle serves to assist the triceps brachii with elbow extension. This relatively small muscle, however, is believed to contribute no more than 10% to 15% of the total extensor torque.[32] It has been suggested that the primary role of the anconeus is to prevent impingement of the posterior capsule of the elbow during active extension.[1] These muscles may be collectively tested with the patient in prone and with the arm abducted to 90 degrees while resistance to elbow extension is provided. Differentiation between these muscles may be accomplished by altering the position of the shoulder. With the patient in prone, with arm at side in extension, isolated testing of the lateral and medial heads of the triceps can be performed.

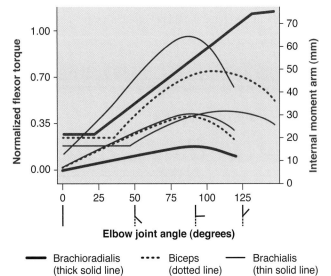

FIGURE 23–7 Elbow flexion force through the range of elbow motion. (Adapted from An, KN, Kauffman KR, Chao EY. Physiological considerations of muscle force through the elbow joint. *J Biomech.* 1989;22:1249; Amis AA, Dowson D, Wright V. Muscle strengths and musculoskeletal geometry of the upper limb. *Eng Med.* 1979;8:41.)

As mentioned, the biceps brachii is a major contributor to the motion of supination. As a single-joint muscle, the *supinator's* role in producing supination is unchanged by elbow position. However, this muscle appears to be most active when the elbow is fully extended, as in turning a door knob, presumably to compensate for a reduction in the contribution from the biceps. It is also the first muscle to engage with recruitment of the biceps occurring later as resistance is added to this motion.[29]

Palpation

Osseous Palpation

The most prominent osteological structure posteriorly is the *olecranon process* of the ulna. During flexion, the olecranon moves out of its corresponding *fossa*, and a portion of this fossa can be easily palpated through the triceps tendon as a small crescent-shaped orifice just proximal to the tip of the olecranon.[25] This is a common area of tenderness in cases of direct trauma resulting from hyperextension forces or in the presence of olecranon bursitis. In this region, the tendon of the triceps can also be palpated as it inserts onto the olecranon.

Often involved in cumulative trauma disorders of the elbow resulting in tenderness to palpation are the medial and lateral epicondyles of the humerus. Once the olecranon has been identified, the manual physical therapist migrates medially, contacting the large medial epicondyle. The lateral epicondyle, although smaller, remains the distinctive osseous landmark occupying the lateral compartment of the elbow. Both epicondyles remain stationary during flexion and extension. Serving as the common insertion site for the forearm flexors and extensors, respectively, the medial and lateral epicondyles are commonly tender in response to activities that involve excessive or repetitive wrist and hand motion or gripping. The relationship between the olecranon and the humeral epicondyles is triangular when observed posteriorly with the elbow flexed (Fig. 23-8).

From the olecranon, the ulna is palpated along its full length. At the most distal aspect of the ulna, the ulnar head, with its knob-like configuration, may be palpated before contacting the small spike-like ulnar styloid process (Fig. 23-9).

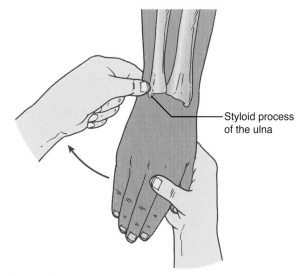

FIGURE 23–9 Palpation of the styloid process of the ulna.

This structure may be more easily palpated by ulnarly deviating the wrist. The radial styloid is larger than the ulnar styloid and extends more distally. From the styloid, the shaft of the radius is palpated, and lying just distal to the lateral epicondyle is the head of the radius (Fig. 23-10). This fairly prominent landmark lies just distal to the lateral epicondyle and can be palpated through the surrounding musculature and confirmed with the performance of passive supination and pronation.

Soft Tissue Palpation

The biceps brachii is best palpated at the elbow by resisting flexion, at which time the superficial biceps tendon becomes prominent as it courses distally and medially to its insertion into the radial tuberosity (Fig. 23-11A). This muscle may be

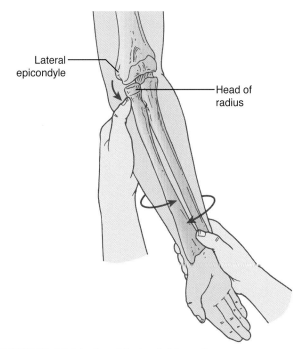

FIGURE 23–10 Palpation of the head of the radius.

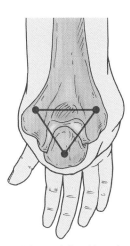

FIGURE 23–8 Palpation of the medial and lateral epicondyles which form a triangle with the olecranon process when the elbow is flexed to 90 degrees.

differentiated from the one-joint brachialis by resisting supination, which will differentially recruit the biceps, or by resisting elbow flexion with the forearm pronated, which inhibits bicep brachii activation (Fig. 23-11B). The brachialis can be easily palpated by first locating the tendon of the biceps. The brachialis may be identified on either the medial or lateral side of the biceps tendon, as its broad expanse occupies the plane beneath. The brachioradialis is palpated by resisting flexion with the forearm in neutral.

Palpation of the triceps brachii is best accomplished with the patient in prone with the shoulder abducted to 90 degrees and the arm positioned beyond the table. The tendon is palpated proximally as it transitions into the medial and lateral heads of the triceps, eventually diving deep to the posterior belly of the deltoid. The long head of the triceps courses proximally along the medial aspect of the arm. This tendon splits the teres minor and teres major muscles, which can be located by resisting shoulder external and internal rotation, respectively. The triceps can be differentiated from these muscles by resisting elbow extension (Fig. 23-12).

Special Testing

Special tests for the elbow have been clearly delineated in many other texts and in the literature. Therefore, only a brief description of selected special tests will be provided here. Table 23-4 provides an overview of the sensitivity, specificity, and likelihood ratios for the more commonly performed special tests used in the examination of the elbow joint complex.[33-39] The reader is encouraged to consult other sources for additional information regarding the performance of these useful confirmatory tests.

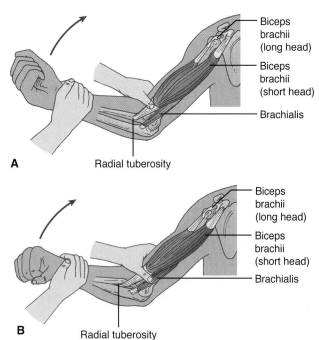

FIGURE 23-11 Palpation of the **A.** biceps brachii, which is isolated by resisting elbow flexion with the forearm supinated and palpation of the **B.** brachialis, which is isolated by resisting elbow flexion with the forearm pronated.

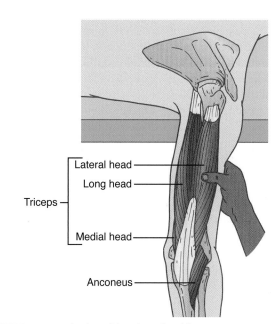

FIGURE 23-12 Palpation of the triceps brachii.

Table 23-4	Special Tests of the Elbow					
TEST	**SENSITIVITY**	**SPECIFICITY**	**+LR**	**−LR**	**REFERENCE**
Moving Valgus Stress Test	100%	75%	4.0	0.00	O'Driscoll et al.[33]
Varus Stress Test	NA	NA	NA	NA	Regan et al.[34]
Valgus Stress Test	NA	NA	NA	NA	O'Driscoll et al.[33] Regan et al.[34]
Tinel Sign	68%–70%	76%–98%	2.8–3.5	0.31–0.42	Novak et al.[35] Kingery et al.[36] Goldman et al.[37]
Compression Test	30 sec = 91%; 60 sec = 89%–98%	30 sec = 97%; 60 sec = 95%–98%	44.5	0.11	Novak et al.[35] Goldman et al.[37]
Cozen Sign	NA	NA	NA	NA	Magee[38]
Mill Test	NA	NA	NA	NA	Magee[39]

SPECIAL TESTS FOR THE ELBOW

Special Tests for Ligamentous Integrity
Moving Valgus Stress Test (Fig. 23-13)

Purpose: To test for the presence of ulnar collateral ligament dysfunction

Patient: Sitting with the shoulder abducted to 90 degrees and the elbow in maximal flexion

Clinician: Standing behind the patient

Procedure: Apply a constant valgus force while the shoulder is externally rotated and the elbow is quickly extended from a flexed position.

Interpretation: The test is positive if there is reproduction of medial elbow pain between 120 and 70 degrees of elbow flexion

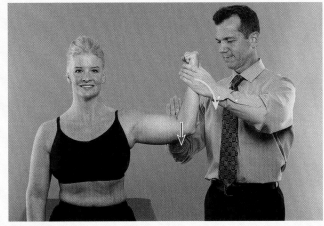

FIGURE 23–13 Moving valgus stress test.

Varus and Valgus Stress Test (Fig. 23-14 A, B)

Purpose: To test for the presence of radial and ulnar collateral ligament pathology

Patient: Sitting with the elbow in 20 degrees of flexion

Clinician: Standing in front of the patient

Procedure: Apply varus (Fig. 23-14A) then valgus (Fig. 23-14B) stress to the elbow while stabilizing the distal forearm

Interpretation: The test is positive if there is increased laxity compared to the uninvolved side and reproduction of symptoms.

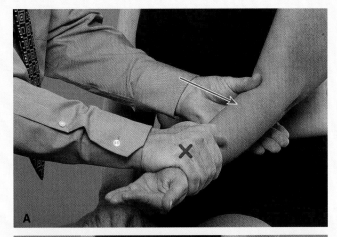

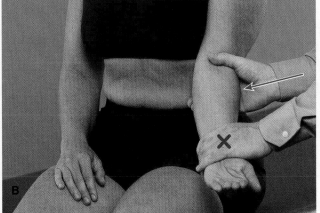

FIGURE 23–14 A. Varus stress test. **B.** Valgus stress test.

Special Tests for Neural Provocation
Tinel Sign and Compression Test (Fig. 23-15)

Purpose: To test for the presence of ulnar or median nerve involvement

Patient: Sitting with the elbow flexed between 70 and 90 degrees. For compression test, 20 degrees of flexion is optimal.

Clinician: Standing in front of the patient

Procedure: Apply four to six taps where the nerve is most superficial within the cubital tunnel for the ulnar nerve and just proximal to the pronator teres for the median nerve. For compression test, apply and maintain firm pressure just proximal to the cubital tunnel for 60 seconds.

Interpretation: The test is positive if there is reproduction of neurological symptoms along the nerve distribution.

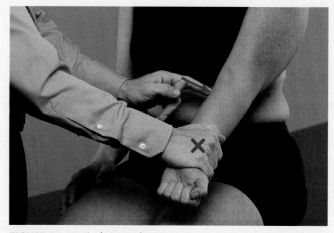

FIGURE 23–15 Tinel sign and compression test.

Special Tests for Epicondylalgia
Cozen Sign (Fig. 23-16)

Purpose: To test for the presence of lateral epicondylalgia

Patient: Sitting with the elbow flexed to 90 degrees and the wrist extended

Clinician: Standing to the side of the patient

Procedure: Resist wrist extension and supination with elbow flexed or resist third digit extension with elbow extended for testing of the extensor digitorum.

Interpretation: Test is positive if there is reproduction of pain over the lateral epicondyle.

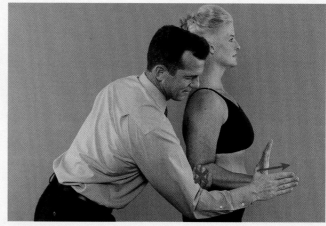

FIGURE 23–16 Cozen sign.

Mill Test (Fig. 23-17)

Purpose: To test for the presence of lateral epicondylalgia

Patient: Standing with the shoulder and elbow extended and the wrist flexed

Clinician: Standing behind the patient

Procedure: Passively move the wrist into flexion and the forearm and elbow into pronation and extension.

Interpretation: The test is positive if there is reproduction of pain over the lateral epicondyle.

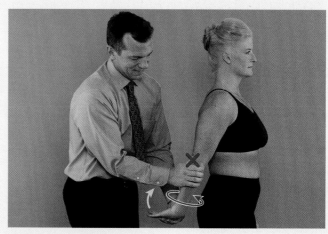

FIGURE 23–17 Mill test.

JOINT MOBILIZATION OF THE ELBOW JOINT COMPLEX

Note: The indications for the joint mobilization techniques described in this section are based on expected joint kinematics. Current evidence suggests that the indications for their use are multifactorial and may be based on direct assessment of mobility and an individual's symptomatic response.

Humeroulnar Joint Mobilizations

Humeroulnar Distraction

Indications:
- *Humeroulnar distraction* is indicated for restrictions in elbow flexion and extension.

Accessory Motion Technique (Fig. 23-18)
- **Patient/Clinician Position**: The patient is in the supine position with the upper arm resting on the table or folded towel and the dorsal forearm resting on the clinician's shoulder. The elbow is in the humeroulnar open-packed position. The elbow may be pre-positioned with the arm at the point of restriction. Sit on the ipsilateral side of the elbow being mobilized.
- **Hand Placement:** Your stabilization hand holds the upper arm in contact with the table. Your mobilization hand grasps the anterior aspect of the proximal ulna. Be sure that your forearm is in line with the direction of force.
- **Force Application:** While stabilizing the upper arm, force is exerted through the ulnar contact in a caudal direction. This technique may be progressed by moving the elbow in the direction of greatest restriction.

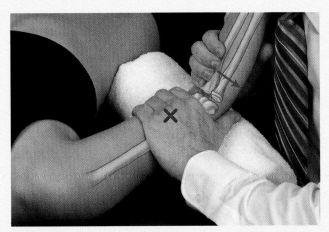

FIGURE 23–18 Humeroulnar distraction. (Photo from Wise CH, Gulick DT. *Mobilization Notes: A Rehabilitation Specialist's Pocket Guide.* Philadelphia, PA: F.A. Davis; 2009).

Accessory With Physiologic Motion Technique (Fig. 23-19)
- **Patient/Clinician Position:** The patient is in the supine position. Stand on the ipsilateral side of the elbow being mobilized.
- **Hand Placement:** Your mobilization hand is as described above. Your stabilization hand is on the posterior aspect of the distal forearm.
- **Force Application:** The patient actively moves into the direction of greatest restriction while you apply a distraction force that is perpendicular to the olecranon against the stabilizing force at the distal forearm. Be prepared to move during the mobilization to ensure correct force application. Force is maintained throughout the entire range of motion and sustained at end range.

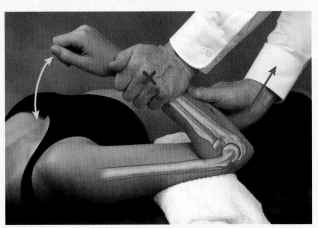

FIGURE 23–19 Humeroulnar distraction: accessory with physiologic motion technique (Photo from Wise CH, Gulick DT. *Mobilization Notes: A Rehabilitation Specialist's Pocket Guide.* Philadelphia, PA: F.A. Davis; 2009.)

Humeroulnar Medial and Lateral Glide

Indications:
- *Humeroulnar medial glides* are indicated for restrictions in elbow flexion, and *lateral glides* are indicated for restrictions in elbow extension. Medial and lateral glides are also indicated in cases where pain and/or symptoms are present with gripping.

Accessory Motion Technique (Fig. 23 20)
- **Patient/Clinician Position**: The patient is supine or sitting with the elbow flexed to approximately 90 degrees with the arm at the side or pre-positioned with the elbow at the point of restriction. Stand on the ispilateral side of the elbow being mobilized.

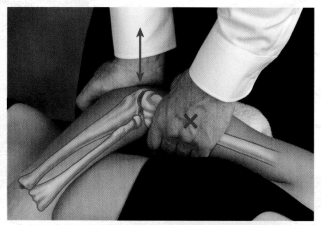

FIGURE 23–20 Humeroulnar medial and lateral glide. (Photo from Wise CH, Gulick DT. *Mobilization Notes: A Rehabilitation Specialist's Pocket Guide.* Philadelphia, PA: F.A. Davis; 2009)

- **Hand Position**: Your stabilization hand contacts the distal humerus. Using a lumbrical grip contact, the thenar eminence of your mobilization hand is placed posteriorly over the olecranon and proximal ulna. Be sure that your forearm is in line with the direction of force.
- **Force Application:** Using a lumbrical gripping motion, perform a medial or lateral glide to the olecranon and ulna.

Accessory With Physiologic Motion Technique (Fig. 23-21)

- **Patient/Clinician Position:** The patient is supine or sitting with the elbow flexed to 90 degrees. Stand of the ipsilateral side of the elbow being mobilized.
- **Hand Placement:** Place your stabilization hand as described above and your mobilization hand, or mobilization belt, at the proximal radius and ulna.
- **Force Application:** The patient actively moves into the direction of greatest restriction or performs repeated gripping. During active movement, apply force in a medial or lateral direction through hand contacts, or belt. Be prepared to move during the mobilization to ensure correct force

application. Force is maintained throughout the entire range of motion and sustained at end range.

Humeroradial Joint Mobilizations

Humeroradial Anterior and Posterior Glide

Indications:
- *Humeroulnar anterior glides* are indicated for restrictions in elbow flexion and pronation. *Humeroulnar posterior glides* are indicated for restrictions in elbow extension and supination.

Accessory Motion Technique (Fig. 23-22)
- **Patient/Clinician Position**: The patient is in a supine position with the arm on the table and the elbow in the open-packed position. You may pre-position the elbow at the point of restriction. Sit on the ipsilateral side of the elbow being mobilized.
- **Hand Placement:** Grasp the distal aspect of the humerus with your stabilization hand. Using a three-jaw pinch contact, grasp the proximal radius with your mobilization hand. Be sure that your forearm is in line with the direction of force.
- **Force Application:** Apply force in an anterior or posterior direction on the stabilized humerus.

Accessory With Physiologic Motion Technique (Not pictured)
- **Patient/Clinician Position:** The patient is in a supine position. Sit on the ipsilateral side of the elbow being mobilized.
- **Hand Placement:** Use the same hand placement as described above

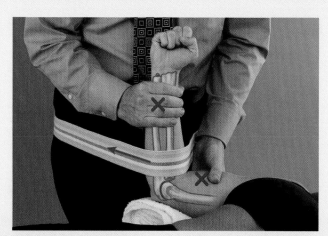

FIGURE 23–21 Humeroulnar medial or lateral glide: accessory with physiologic motion technique.

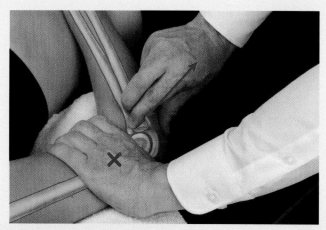

FIGURE 23–22 Humeroradial anterior and posterior glide. (Photo from Wise CH, Gulick DT. *Mobilization Notes: A Rehabilitation Specialist's Pocket Guide.* Philadelphia, PA: F.A. Davis; 2009.)

- **Force Application:** The patient actively moves into the direction of greatest restriction. During active movement, apply force in an anterior or posterior direction through the same hand contacts for flexion/pronation and extension/supination, respectively. Be prepared to move during the mobilization to ensure correct force application. The force is maintained throughout the entire range of motion and sustained at end range.

Proximal Radioulnar Joint Mobilizations

Proximal Radioulnar Anterior and Posterior Glide

Indications:

- *Anterior radioulnar glides* of the radius on a fixed ulna or the ulna on a fixed radius are indicated for restrictions in elbow flexion/pronation and elbow flexion/supination, respectively. *Posterior radioulnar glides* of the radius on a fixed ulna or the ulna on a fixed radius are indicated for restrictions in elbow extension/supination and elbow extension/pronation, respectively.

Accessory Motion Technique (Fig. 23-23)

- **Patient/Clinician Position:** The patient is in a supine position, with the upper arm resting on the table with the elbow in the open-packed position. You may pre-position with the arm at point of restriction. Sit on the ipsilateral side of the elbow being mobilized.
- **Hand Placement:** Using a lumbrical grip contact, grasp the proximal ulna or radius with your stabilization hand. Using a three-jaw pinch contact, grasp the proximal radius or ulna with your mobilization hand. Be sure that your forearm is in line with the direction of force.

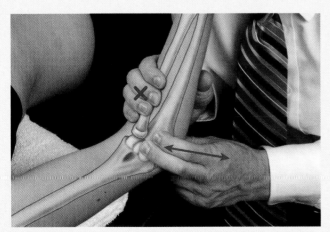

FIGURE 23–23 Proximal radioulnar anterior and posterior glide. (Photo from Wise CH, Gulick DT. *Mobilization Notes: A Rehabilitation Specialist's Pocket Guide.* Philadelphia, PA: F.A. Davis; 2009.)

- **Force Application:** For anterior glides, anterior force is applied to the proximal radius as the ulna is stabilized or anterior force is applied to the proximal ulna as the radius is stabilized. For posterior glides, posterior force is applied to the proximal radius as the ulna is stabilized or posterior force is applied to the proximal ulna as the radius is stabilized.

Accessory With Physiologic Motion Technique (Fig. 23-24)

- **Patient/Clinician Position:** The patient is in a supine position with the arm at the side and the elbow flexed to 90 degrees. Stand on the ipsilateral side of the elbow being mobilized.
- **Hand Placement:** Grasp the wrist with your stabilization hand. Your mobilization hand contact is the same as that described above.
- **Force Application:** Apply an anterior or posterior force to the radius as the patient actively moves into elbow flexion/pronation or elbow extension/supination, respectively. Be prepared to move during the mobilization to ensure correct force application. Force is maintained throughout the entire range of motion and sustained at end range.

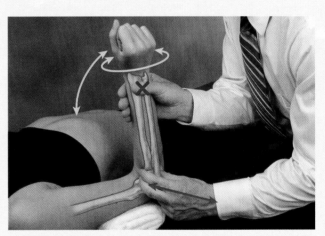

FIGURE 23–24 Proximal radioulnar anterior and posterior glide: accessory with physiologic motion technique. (Photo from Wise CH, Gulick DT. *Mobilization Notes: A Rehabilitation Specialist's Pocket Guide.* Philadelphia, PA: F.A. Davis; 2009.)

Proximal Radioulnar Inferior Glide

Indications:

- *Proximal radioulnar inferior glides* are indicated for restrictions in elbow extension and wrist flexion. This technique may also be used for *distraction of the humeroradial joint*, which is indicated for restrictions in any of the physiologic motions of the elbow.

Accessory Motion Technique (Fig. 23-25)

- **Patient/Clinician Position:** The patient is in a supine position with the upper arm resting on table and the elbow in the open-packed position. You may pre-position the elbow at the point of restriction. Stand on the ipsilateral side of the elbow being mobilized.

- **Hand Placement:** Your stabilization hand secures the distal humerus on the table. Using a "golfer's grip" contact, the mobilization hand grasps the distal aspect of the radius being sure to remain proximal to the wrist. Be sure that your forearm is in line with the direction of force.
- **Force Application:** While maintaining all hand contacts, rotate your body away from the patient, imparting an inferiorly directed force of the radius on the stabilized humerus.

Accessory With Physiologic Motion Technique (Fig. 23-25)

- **Patient/Clinician Position:** The patient is in a supine position as described above. Stand on the ipsilateral side of the elbow being mobilized as described above.
- **Hand Placement:** Utilize all hand contacts as described above.
- **Force Application:** The patient actively moves into progressively greater ranges of elbow extension. During active movement, apply an inferiorly-directed force. Be prepared to move during the mobilization to ensure correct force application. Force is maintained throughout the entire range of motion and sustained at end range.

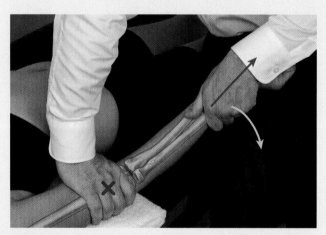

FIGURE 23–25 Proximal radioulnar inferior glide: accessory motion technique and accessory with physiologic motion technique. (Photo from Wise CH, Gulick DT. *Mobilization Notes: A Rehabilitation Specialist's Pocket Guide.* Philadelphia, PA: F.A. Davis; 2009.)

Proximal Radioulnar Superior Glide

Indications:

- *Proximal radioulnar superior glides* are indicated for restrictions in elbow flexion and wrist extension.

Accessory Motion Technique (Fig. 23-26)

- **Patient/Clinician Position:** The patient is in a supine position, with the upper arm resting on the table and the elbow in the open-packed position. You may pre-position the elbow at the point of restriction. Stand on the ipsilateral side of the elbow being mobilized facing cephalad.

- **Hand Placement:** Your stabilization hand secures the distal humerus on the table. Using a "saw grip" contact, the patient's wrist is positioned into extension for the purpose of providing support for compressive forces. Be sure that your forearm is in line with the direction of force.
- **Force Application:** While stabilizing the distal humerus, apply a superiorly directed force through the "saw grip" hand contact.

Accessory With Physiologic Motion Technique (Fig. 23-26)

- **Patient/Clinician Position:** The patient is in a supine position as described above. Stand on the ipsilateral side of the elbow being mobilized as described above.
- **Hand Placement:** Use all hand contacts as described above.
- **Force Application:** The patient actively moves into progressively greater ranges of elbow flexion with some pronation and supination. During active movement, apply a superiorly-directed force. Be prepared to move during the mobilization to ensure correct force application. Force is maintained throughout the entire range of motion and sustained at end range.

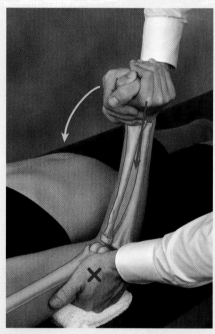

FIGURE 23–26 Proximal radioulnar superior glide: accessory motion technique and accessory with physiologic motion technique.. (Photo from Wise CH, Gulick DT. *Mobilization Notes: A Rehabilitation Specialist's Pocket Guide.* Philadelphia, PA: F.A. Davis; 2009.)

Proximal Radioulnar Anterior High-Velocity Thrust (Mill Manipulation) (Fig. 23-27)

Indications:

- *High-velocity thrust* is indicated for the purpose of altering positional relationships of the radioulnar joint, to increase mobility, or to reduce pain. The Mill manipulation may be effective for chronic cases of recalcitrant lateral epicondylalgia.

Patient/Clinician Position:

- The patient is in a standing position with the elbow in 20 degrees of flexion, the forearm fully pronated, and the wrist flexed and ulnarly deviated. Stand behind the patient and on the ipsilateral side of the elbow being mobilized.

Hand Placement:

- Place the thumb of your mobilization hand at the posterior aspect of the radial head as your other hand flexes and ulnarly deviates the patient's wrist and controls the position of the elbow.

Force Application:

- Apply an anteriorly directed force through the radial head contact as you bring the elbow toward end-range extension with your other hand. At end range, apply a short amplitude, high velocity thrust to the radial head while maintaining wrist flexion and ulnar deviation.

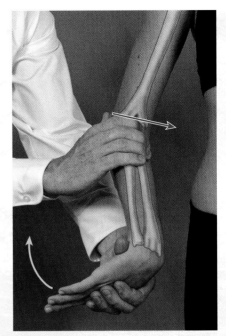

FIGURE 23–27 Proximal radioulnar anterior high-velocity thrust (Mill manipulation). (Photo from Wise CH, Gulick DT. *Mobilization Notes: A Rehabilitation Specialist's Pocket Guide*. Philadelphia, PA: F.A. Davis; 2009.)

CLINICAL CASE
Subjective Examination

Self-Reported Disability Measure

The clinical evaluation elbow form, as proposed by Morrey et al,[23] revealed a score of 65.

History of Present Illness

A 20-year-old male intercollegiate competitive tennis player presents today reporting gradual onset of left lateral elbow pain, with onset approximately 4 years ago when he was in college, with intermittent pain since that time. He reports an overall increase in symptoms during tennis season and upon performance of gripping activities. Numeric pain rating scale reveals pain at present at 5/10, best past 30 days at 2/10, and worst past 30 days at 8/10.

Objective Physical Examination

Examination of Structure: Observation reveals no signs of edema or deformity. Carrying angle is 12 degrees.

Upper Quarter Screen: Cervical spine and shoulder is within normal limits (WNL), and motion has no effect on symptoms.

Examination of Mobility

Physiologic Mobility Testing: Active range of motion and passive range of motion are all WNL, with the exception of pronation, which is 60 degrees actively and passively. All end-feels are also WNL. An increase in symptoms is reported from 5/10 to 7/10 during passive end-range pronation. (R2 = P2).

Accessory Mobility Testing: Reduced anterior glide of the humeroradial joint is noted with resistance (R1) identified prior to the initial onset of pain (P1).

Examination of Muscle Function: The following tests reproduce the patient's chief complaint of pain over the lateral epicondyle. Left wrist extension (in elbow extension) = 4/5, radial deviation = 4−/5, pronation = 3/5. Weakness and pain is noted with resisted third digit extension with the elbow extended. All else is 5/5.

Palpation: Exquisite tenderness to the touch noted over the lateral epicondyle and within the muscle belly of the extensor carpi radialis.

Special Testing: Cozen Test = +; Mill Test = +

Note: R1—the point in the range where the initial onset of tissue resistance is noted; R2—the point in the range where further motion is limited by tissue resistance; P1—the point in the range where the initial onset of pain is noted; P2—the point in the range where further motion is limited by pain.

Discuss the following:

1. Based on your examination findings, what is your differential diagnosis? Briefly explain how this condition occurs, the histological basis for its existence, and why it often presents as a chronic problem. Why do standard interventions used to reduce symptoms from inflammatory conditions often fail to yield positive outcomes in this condition?
2. What is the significance of the accessory motion restrictions that were identified during the examination? Have these restrictions contributed to the onset of this condition, or are these restrictions considered to be sequelae?
3. What is the sensitivity and specificity of the special tests that were used during the examination?
4. What type of manual interventions would you implement in the care of this patient? When would you begin strength training? Would you use bracing or splinting in this patient's plan of care? When would you consider soliciting a surgical consult?

HANDS-ON

With a partner, perform the following activities:

1 Consider the key indicators that may be revealed during the history and "interrogation" of your partner that may suggest the presence of the following conditions. These indicators may include such things as the mechanism of injury or pain pattern. Based on these indicators, what examination procedures might you use to rule in or rule out the presence of each particular condition that is listed? Complete the grid.

DYSFUNCTION	HISTORICAL INDICATORS	CONFIRMATORY SIGNS
Medial Epicondylalgia		
Lateral Epicondylalgia		
Olecranon Bursitis		
Ulna, Radius Fracture		
Elbow Dislocation		
Radial Collateral Ligament Sprain		
Ulnar Collateral Ligament Sprain		

2 Observe your partner as he or she performs active physiologic movements for single and repeated repetitions and single and multiplane directions, and identify the quantity, quality, and any reproduction of symptoms that may be identified. Compare these active movements with performance of the same movements passively.

3 In an attempt to relate each impairment to a structural cause, attempt to provide several possible pathoanatomical etiologies for each of the movement impairments identified during active and passive physiologic movement testing in the clinical case study that was previously presented. Complete the grid.

ACTIVE PHYSIOLOGIC MOVEMENT IMPAIRMENT	PASSIVE PHYSIOLOGIC MOVEMENT IMPAIRMENT	POSSIBLE PATHOANATOMIC ETIOLOGY

4 Perform passive physiologic movement testing in all directions followed by passive accessory movement testing in all planes, and determine the relationship between the onset of pain, if present (P1 and P2) and resistance, if present (R1 and R2). Determine the end-feel in each direction. Compare your findings bilaterally and on another partner.

5 Perform passive accessory movement testing in all planes with the elbow in the neutral, or open-packed, position. Then perform the same tests with the elbow in other non-neutral and close-packed positions. Identify any changes in the quantity and quality of available motion and report any reproduction of symptoms. Consider which anatomical structures are most responsible for limiting motion in each position. Complete the grid.

PASSIVE ACCESSORY MOVEMENT	QUANTITY, QUALITY, REPRODUCTION IN OPEN-PACKED	QUANTITY, QUALITY, REPRODUCTION IN CLOSE-PACKED	LIMITING STRUCTURES
HU Distraction			
HU Medial Glide			
HU Lateral Glide			
HR Distraction			
HR Compression			
HR Anterior Glide			
HR Posterior Glide			
RU Anterior Glide			
RU Posterior Glide			

6 Perform muscle testing for the key muscles about the elbow using isometric break testing, static testing, and active testing, based on the functional preference of each muscle during normal activity. Complete the grid.

MUSCLE TESTED	FUNCTIONAL PREFERENCE/ MANNER OF TESTING	RESULTS

7 Through palpation, attempt to identify the primary soft tissue and bony structures of the elbow and compare tissue texture, tension, tone, and location bilaterally.

8 Based on your movement examination within the clinical case study above, choose two mobilizations. Perform these mobilizations on your partner and identify any immediate changes in mobility or symptoms in response to these procedures.

9 Perform each mobilization described in the intervention section of this chapter bilaterally on at least two individuals. Using each technique, practice Grades I to IV. Then switch and allow your partner to mobilize your elbow. Provide input to your partner regarding patient/clinician position, hand placement, force application, comfort, and effectiveness, and so on. When practicing these mobilization techniques, utilize the Sequential Partial Task Practice Method, in which students repeatedly practice one aspect of each technique (i.e., position, hand placement, force application) on multiple partners each time adding the next component until the technique is performed in real time from beginning to end. (Wise CH, Schenk RJ, Lattanzi JB. A model for teaching and learning spinal thrust manipulation and its effect on participant confidence in technique performance. *J. Man. Manip. Ther.*, August 2014.)

REFERENCES

1. Oatis CA. *Kinesiology: The Mechanics and Pathomechanics of Human Movement.* Philadelphia, PA: Lippincott Williams & Wilkins; 2004.
2. Stroyan M, Wilk KE. The functional anatomy of the elbow complex. *J Orthop Sports Phys Ther.* 1993:17;279-288.
3. Eckstein F, Lohe F, Schulte E, et al. Physiological incongruity of the humeroulnar joint: a functional principle of optimized stress distribution acting upon articulating surfaces? *Anat Embryology.* 1993:188;449-455.
4. Eckstein F, Muller-Gerbl M, Steinlechner M. Subcondral bone density in the human elbow assessed by computed tomography osteoabsorptiometry: a reflection of the loading history of the joint surfaces. *J Orthop Res.* 1995:13;268-278.
5. Putz R, Milz S, Maier M, et al. Functional morphology of the elbow joint. *Orthopade.* 2003:32;684.
6. Nielsen KK, Olsen BS. No stabilizing effect of the elbow joint capsule. A kinematic study. *Acta Orthop Scand.* 2000:70;6-8.
7. Fuss FK. The ulnar collateral ligament of the human elbow joint. Anatomy, function, and biomechanics. *J Anat.* 1991:175;203-212.
8. Callaway GH, Field LD, Deng XH, et al. Biomechanical evaluation of the medial collateral ligament of the elbow. *J Bone Joint Surg.* 1997: 79;1223-1231.

9. Regan WD, Korinek SL, Morrey BF, An KN. Biomechanical study of ligaments around the elbow joint. *Clin Orthop.* 1991:271;170-179.
10. Eygendaal D, Olsen BS, Jensen SL, et al. Kinematics of partial and total ruptures of the medial collateral ligament of the elbow. *J Shoulder Elbow Surg.* 1999:8;612-616.
11. Olsen BS, Sojbjerg JO, Dalstra M, Sneppen O. Kinematics of the lateral ligamentous constraints of the elbow joint. *J Shoulder Elbow Surg.* 1996:5; 333-341.
12. Birckbeck DP. The interosseous membrane affects load distribution in the forearm. *J Hand Surg.* 1997:22;975-980.
13. Ericson A, Arndt A, Stark A, et al. Variation in the position and orientation of the elbow flexion axis. *J Bone Joint Surg Br.* 2003:85;538.
14. Linscheid RL. Biomechanics of the distal radioulnar joint. *Clin Orthop.* 1992:275;46.
15. Weinberg AM, Pietsch IT, Helm MB, et al. A new kinematic model or pro- and supination of the human forearm. *J Biomech.* 2000:33;487-491.
16. Kapandji IA. *The Physiology of the Joints. Volume I. The Upper Limb.* Edinburgh, UK: Churchill Livingstone; 1982.
17. Hudak PL, et al. Development of an upper extremity outcome measure: the DASH (disabilities of the arm, shoulder, and hand). *Am J Ind Med.* 1995:29;602-608.
18. Morrey BF, An KN, Chao EYS. Functional evaluation of the elbow. In: Morrey BF, ed. *The Elbow and Its Disorders.* Philadelphia, PA: WB Saunders; 1985:88-89.
19. Boissonnault WG. *Primary Care for the Physical Therapist: Examination and Triage.* St. Louis, MO: Elsevier Saunders; 2005.
20. Dutton M. *Orthopaedic Examination, Evaluation, & Intervention.* New York, NY: McGraw-Hill; 2004.
21. Watrous BG, Ho G. Elbow pain. *Prim Care.* 1988:15;725-735.
22. Magee DJ. *Orthopedic Physical Assessment.* 3rd ed. Philadelphia, PA: WB Saunders; 1997.
23. Morrey BF, Askew LJ, Chao EYS. A biomechanical study of normal functional elbow motion. *J Bone Joint Surg.* 1981:63;872-877.
24. McGuigan FX, Bookout CB. Intra-articular fluid volume and restricted motion in the elbow. *J Shoulder Elbow Surg.* 2003:12;462.
25. Askew LJ, An KN, Morrey BF, Chao EYS. Isometric elbow strength in normal individuals. *Clin Orthop.* 1987:261-266.
26. Kendall FP, McCreary EK, Provance PG. *Muscle Testing and Function.* Baltimore, MD: Williams & Wilkins; 1993.
27. Kapandji AI. *The Physiology of the Joints, Volume 1: Upper Limb.* New York, NY: Churchill Livingstone; 1970.
28. Ramsey ML. Distal biceps tendon injuries: diagnosis and management. *J Am Acad Orthop Surg.* 1999:7;199-207.
29. Basmajian JV, DeLuca CJ. *Muscles Alive. Their Function Revealed by Electromyography.* Baltimore, MD: Williams & Wilkins; 1985.
30. Hislop HJ, Montgomery J. *Daniel's and Worthingham's Muscle Testing: Techniques of Manual Examination.* Philadelphia, PA: WB Saunders; 1995.
31. Knapik JJ, Wright JE, Mawdsley RH, Braun J. Isometric, isotonic, and isokinetic torque variations in four muscle groups through a range of joint motion. *Phys Ther.* 1983:63;938-947.
32. Zhang LQ, Nuber GW. Moment distribution among human elbow extensor muscles during isometric and submaximal extension. *J Biomech.* 2000:33;145-154.
33. O'Driscoll SWM, et al. The "moving valgus stress test" for medial collateral ligament tears of the elbow. *Am J Sports Med.* 2005;33:231-239.
34. Regan WD, Morrey BF. The physical examination of the elbow. In: Morrey BF, ed. *The Elbow & Its Disorders.* Philadelphia, PA: WB Saunders; 1993.
35. Novak CB, Lee GW, Mackinnon SE, Lay L. Provocation testing for cubital tunnel syndrome. *J Hand Surg Am.* 1994;19:817-820.
36. Kingery WS, Park KS, Wu PB, Date ES. Electromyographic motor Tinel's sign in ulnar mononeuropathies at the elbow. *Am J Phys Med Rehabil.* 1995;74:419-426.
37. Goldman SB, Brininger TL, Schrader JW, Koceja DM. A review of clinical tests & signs for the assessment of ulnar neuropathy. *J Hand Ther.* 2009;22:209-220.
38. Magee DJ. *Orthopedic Physical Assessment.* 5th ed. Philadelphia, PA: WB Saunders; 2008.
39. Magee DJ. *Orthopedic Physical Assessment.* 4th ed. Philadelphia, PA: WB Saunders; 2002.

Orthopaedic Manual Physical Therapy of the Wrist and Hand

Christopher H. Wise, PT, DPT, OCS, FAAOMPT, MTC, ATC

Chapter Objectives

At the conclusion of this chapter, the reader will be able to:

- Identify the key anatomical and biomechanical features of the wrist and hand and their impact on examination and intervention.
- List and perform key procedures used in the orthopaedic manual physical therapy (OMPT) examination of the wrist and hand.
- Demonstrate sound clinical decision-making in evaluating the results of the OMPT examination.

- Use pertinent examination findings to reach a differential diagnosis and prognosis.
- Discuss issues related to the safe performance of OMPT interventions for the wrist and hand.
- Demonstrate basic competence in the performance of a skill set of joint mobilization techniques for the wrist and hand.

FUNCTIONAL ANATOMY AND KINEMATICS

Introduction

The wrist-and-hand complex provides an extraordinary example of both the complexity and the precision with which human motion can occur. The compound *radiocarpal* and *midcarpal* joints collectively form the wrist-joint complex;[1] however, the proximal and distal *radioulnar* joints also exert an important influence on wrist function. This complex accumulation of bones, muscles, and articulations provides function that ranges from fine motor tasks to the production of substantial force, all of which are accompanied by a great degree of individual variability.[1]

The Distal Radioulnar (RU) Joint

The distal RU joint forms a compound articulation with the proximal RU joint, which collectively provides the motions of pronation and supination. Although external to the wrist joint proper, the distal RU joint contributes greatly to hand function

and is commonly involved in dysfunction of the hand and wrist.[2,3] This joint is classified as a *pivot joint*; however, on closer inspection, one can see that a substantial amount of gliding occurs at this joint as well.[3] The degree of joint glide afforded at this joint is due largely to the mismatch in curvature between the *ulnar head* and the corresponding *radial sigmoid notch*.[2,4]

Stability of the Distal Radioulnar Joint

The distal RU joint relies heavily on its noncontractile soft tissue structures for support, with minimal support osteologically.[5] The joint capsule and the *triangular fibrocartilage complex (TFCC)* provide direct support, while the *annular ligament*, as well as the *interosseous membrane*, provide indirect support. The joint capsule is more substantial distally and may contribute to axial stability of this joint.[6] Although this capsule is weak anteriorly, it contains folds that distend to allow for full supination and to guard against excessive supination.[7]

The TFCC serves an important role in attenuating axially loaded forces by distributing these forces to the ulna, increasing the articular surface of the wrist, and stabilizing the entire wrist complex.[7,8] The TFCC is composed of fibrocartilage, the *dorsal* and *volar radioulnar ligaments*, the *ulnar collateral ligament*, and a *meniscus*.[7] The base of the TFCC inserts into the sigmoid notch of the radius, and its apex loosely connects to the styloid process of the ulna. Its central portion is thin, lending to its propensity toward rupture. Thus, communication between the distal RU and radiocarpal joints is created, which can be viewed through the migration of contrast dye during performance of an *arthrogram*. The meniscus of the TFCC, running from the radius to the volar aspect of the *triquetrum*, is composed of vascularized loose connective tissue.[3,9] As with most joint capsules, the radioulnar ligaments blend with the joint capsule of the RU joint and TFCC.[6] These ligaments primarily serve to stabilize by limiting the degree of rotation and gliding that occurs during pronation and supination.[9]

Mobility of the Distal Radioulnar Joint

When the hand is free to move in space, pronation and supination occurs through rotation of the radius about a relatively fixed ulna. However, when the hand is fixed (as in grasping a doorknob), as the radius rotates about the ulna during pronation the ulna migrates dorsally and radially.[10,11]

The Wrist Joint Complex

The Radiocarpal (RC) Joint

By definition, the RC joint is the articulation between the radius and the proximal row of carpal bones. Closer inspection, however, reveals that only the scaphoid and lunate directly articulate with the radius (Fig. 24-1 A, B). The joint surfaces, consisting of the concave distal radius and the corresponding convex row of carpal bones, appear congruent. The average inclination of the distal radius is 23 degrees as a result of the radius demonstrating greater length. The distal radius is also tilted volarly 11 degrees as a result of the dorsal aspect of the radius being slightly longer than its volar counterpart.[12] The length of the ulna relative to the radius is an important factor that impacts wrist function.[13] An ulna that is shorter or longer than normal relative to the distal radius is identified as a **negative** or **positive ulnar variance**, respectively.[14] Ulnar-sided wrist pain, especially during ulnar deviation and pronation, may result from the presence of an ulnar variance.[15] More specifically, TFCC derangement has been associated with a positive ulnar variance[16]. Conversely, RC joint damage,[13] and avascular necrosis of the lunate, a condition known as *Kienbock's disease*, may result from a negative ulnar variance.[15]

Within the RC joint, the surface contact area increases when the joint is loaded, and the congruency between the scaphoid and radius is greater than that which is between the lunate and radius.[17] The RC joint capsule encloses each of these bones, whose articular surfaces are covered by articular cartilage. The RC joint capsule also inserts into the TFCC, which serves as the "roof" of the RC joint.[7]

The Midcarpal (MC) Joint

The MC articulation formed between the proximal and distal rows of carpal bones is structurally and functionally divided

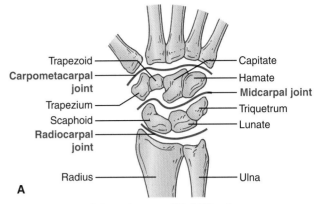

Dorsal Aspect of the Right Wrist and Hand

A

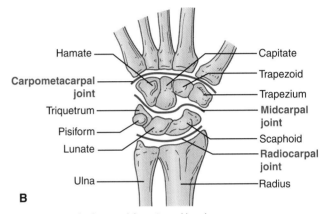

Palmer Aspect of Right Hand

B

FIGURE 24–1 The bones of the wrist and hand.

into a lateral and a medial compartment (Fig. 24-1). The lateral compartment has been classified as a *planar joint*[18] or *saddle joint*[19] due to the relatively level articular surfaces of the *scaphoid, trapezoid,* and *trapezium*. The medial compartment consists of the concave *scaphoid, lunate,* and *triquetrum* articulating with the convex *capitate* and *hamate*. Each of these articular surfaces is covered with articular hyaline cartilage, and the capsule of the MC joint is irregular, enclosing the joint spaces between the proximal and distal rows as well as between individual carpal bones. Reinforcing the joint capsule are numerous intrinsic and extrinsic ligaments.[7] The MC joint is inextricably linked to the RC joint both structurally and functionally.

Stability of the Wrist Joint Complex

The ligaments of the wrist may be classified as either *extrinsic* or *intrinsic*.[7] The intrinsic ligaments, found between each of the carpal bones, rely on synovial fluid for their nutrition and are stronger than the extrinsic ligaments, which span several of the carpal bones.[20] Both extrinsic and intrinsic ligaments are more substantial volarly, suggesting the requirement for greater stability at the end ranges of extension. Of all extrinsic ligaments, the *collaterals* are the least significant, and the *flexor retinaculum* is the most extensive.[19] The majority of wrist ligaments converge on either the capitate or the lunate.[7]

The *volar carpal ligaments*, which are divided into the *radiocarpal* and *ulnocarpal ligaments* exert their greatest influence at end range of wrist extension.[11] The volar RC ligament has three distinct bands.[21] The *radial collateral ligament* invests into the RC ligament and capsule.[22] The ulnocarpal ligament complex includes both the TFCC and the *ulnar collateral ligaments*.[22] The *scapholunate interosseous ligament* is an important stabilizing structure for the scaphoid and, consequently, for the wrist in general.[23] The *lunotriquetral interosseous ligament* is another intrinsic ligament that, when injured, may contribute to instability of the lunate.[24]

The *dorsal carpal ligaments*, which exert their greatest influence during wrist flexion,[11] consist primarily of the *dorsal radiocarpal ligament*. This ligament runs obliquely across the wrist, ultimately terminating on the triquetrum along with the *dorsal intercarpal ligament*.[21,25] These two ligaments create a V-type configuration at the medial aspect of the wrist, which promotes scaphoid stability during movement.[25] An important component of injury prevention is the fact that these ligaments have the ability to sustain a greater degree of deformation compared to most other ligaments throughout the body.[26]

Mobility of the Wrist Joint Complex

The capitate is traditionally considered to be the center of rotation for wrist complex motion in both the sagittal plane and the frontal plane (Fig. 24-2).[27] More recent evidence suggests that the axes of motion for the wrist are not constant and that a significant degree of variability exists between individuals.[28]

The proximal row of carpal bones serves as a "mechanical coupler" between the distal aspect of the radius and distal row of carpals and metacarpals, acting as the middle segment of a three-segment chain. In response to compressive loads, the proximal row of carpal bones collapses and migrates in the direction opposite that of the distal segment.[29] The ligamentous stabilizing structures provide the necessary support for the proximal row during movement. It is believed that the intercarpal ligaments mechanically link the bones of the proximal row, causing them to move together in a direction that is opposite that of the distal row. This counterrotation between the two rows of carpal bones produces an increase in tension through the ligamentous structures, resulting in increased stability.[30]

Wrist Flexion and Extension

Much controversy exists regarding the relative contribution of the RC and MC joints to overall wrist *flexion* and *extension* mobility.[17,31–35] There is some consensus that the distal row of carpal bones moves as a unit into flexion and extension on the proximal row, indicating a greater contribution from the midcarpal joint.[17,31,33,34] However, some suggest that the RC joint exhibits a greater contribution to these movements.[34,35] Regardless, movement of both segments is required to achieve normal wrist mobility.

Conwell[36] has proposed and Levangie and Norkin[1] have summarized the movements that occur at the RC and MC joints during wrist movement. The wrist extensors initiate movement of the distal carpal bones and metacarpals in the same direction as that of the hand until neutral, at which time the capitate and scaphoid are drawn into a close-packed position by the intercarpal ligaments. At approximately 45 degrees of extension, the remaining proximal carpals (lunate and triquetrum) engage, and both rows of carpals then move as one unit. The remainder of wrist extension occurs as the proximal row moves on the radius.

As the convex proximal row of carpal bones moves upon the concave radius, it is generally considered that the direction of joint glide is opposite to the direction of hand motion and that the distal row of carpals glides in the same direction as hand motion (Fig. 24-3). Research related to patterns of contact, however, have brought into question whether or not this assumption is universally true.[37] Some studies also suggest that movement of individual carpal bones may occur in a multiplanar fashion

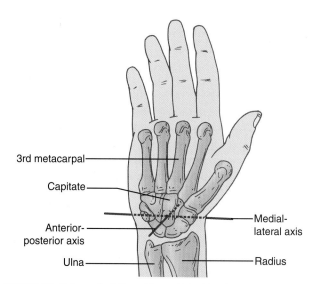

FIGURE 24–2 Axes of rotation of the wrist and hand.

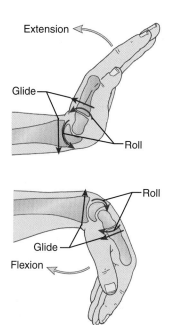

FIGURE 24–3 Movement of the proximal and distal row of carpal bones during wrist extension and flexion denoting the important contributions from both the radiocarpal and midcarpal joints during global wrist movement.

during cardinal plane wrist movements. The scaphoid and triquetrum have been shown to pronate and supinate during wrist flexion and extension, respectively.[17]

Wrist Radial Deviation and Ulnar Deviation

Radial deviation (RD) and *ulnar deviation (UD)* have been shown to involve multiplanar carpal bone movement to a greater extent than that identified for flexion and extension.[7] These motions, however, more closely follow the expected direction of joint glide during movement. During RD, the proximal carpals glide in an ulnar direction, with the opposite occurring during UD. Simultaneous flexion/extension of the proximal row with motion in the opposite direction occurs at the distal row of carpal bones.[38] The greatest degree of RD and UD are present with the wrist in neutral[39] and most agree that the largest contribution to RD and UD motion comes from the distal row[17,29,31] (Fig. 24-4).

Oatis[7] has summarized several aspects of wrist motion in which there is agreement. In general, the wrist functions as two individual rows, with the distal row functioning more as a unit and the bones of the proximal row demonstrating greater variability and independence. To achieve full range of motion at the wrist, both the RC and MC joints must contribute. There is no single axis about which motion occurs, and motion is often multiplanar in nature. Full *radial deviation and/or wrist extension* is considered to be the close-packed position of the wrist. The open-packed position is considered to be approximately 0 to 20 degrees of wrist flexion/extension. See Table 24-2 for the open- and close-packed positions for each joint within the wrist and hand complex.

The Hand Complex

This complex structure of 19 bones and an equal number of joints demonstrates a unique balance between power and dexterity. Each of the five digits are structured as columns of bone supported by inert ligamentous guy wires and powered by multijoint intrinsic and extrinsic musculature.

The Carpometacarpal (CMC) Joint

The position of the trapezium relative to the hand results in a slight rotation of the thumb toward the fifth digit.[40] The CMC joint of the thumb, which is formed by the saddle-shaped trapezium and first metacarpal, allows a motion unique to humans that is known as *opposition*.[41] The uniquely shaped trapezium is concave in the direction of CMC abduction and adduction and convex in the directions of flexion and extension.[19,42]

This joint is typically described as a synovial *saddle-type joint*[42] that provides abduction, adduction, flexion, and extension. Opposition is a composite motion that consists of flexion, abduction, and medial rotation, in which the thumb moves toward the palm of the hand.

The CMC joints of digits 2 to 5 are considered to be *gliding joints*,[42] with the second digit possessing the least mobility and the fifth possessing the most.[42] The relative immobility of the second and third CMC joints provides a stable axis around which each of the other digits move.[43]

Within the hand, there are three distinct arches designed to conform to objects that are being grasped.[1] The trapezoid, trapezium, capitate, and hamate form a palmer concavity, known as the *proximal transverse (carpal) arch*. The *distal transverse arch*, at the level of the metacarpal heads, maximizes the motion available through the first, fourth, and fifth CMC joints. The *longitudinal arch*, as its name implies, courses the entire length of the digits.

Stability of the Carpometacarpal Joint

The primary supporting structures of the CMC joint of the thumb include the *dorsal and volar oblique ligaments*, the *joint capsule*, and the *radial CMC ligament*.[44] The CMC joints of the fingers are supported by both longitudinal and transverse ligamentous structures.[45] Several of the intrinsic muscles of the hand insert into the transverse carpal ligament, which may enhance its stabilizing function by tensing this inert structure under certain conditions.[1]

Mobility of the Carpometacarpal Joint

As previously described, the CMC joint of the thumb dictates the position of the thumb, and movement of this joint is often synonymous with thumb motion. The CMC of the thumb performs *flexion* and *extension*, which occurs in the frontal plane toward and away from the hand, respectively. *Adduction* and *abduction* is movement in the sagittal plane with the thumb moving toward and away from the palm, respectively. *Medial and lateral rotation* involves transverse plane movement toward and away from the palm. *Opposition*, as aforementioned, involves the combined movements of flexion, abduction, and medial rotation (Fig. 24-5).[7]

The CMC joints of digits 2, 3, and 4 are able to perform *flexion* and *extension*; however, the second and third CMC joints are virtually immobile.[27] The fifth CMC joint is able to flex and extend as well as *abduct* and *adduct*. Mobility of this joint is important in facilitating opposition with the thumb.[18,43]

The Metacarpophalangeal (MCP) Joint

The MCP joint of the hand is best described as the *convex metacarpal head* articulating with the *concave base of the proximal phalanx*. The MCP joints of the thumb and digits 2 to 5 are classified as biaxial synovial joints; however, some discount the often minimal amount of abduction/adduction and refer to the

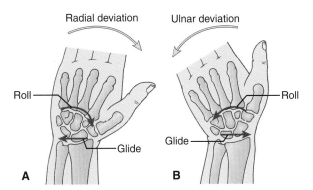

FIGURE 24–4 Movement of the carpal bones during **A.** radial deviation and **B.** ulnar deviation.

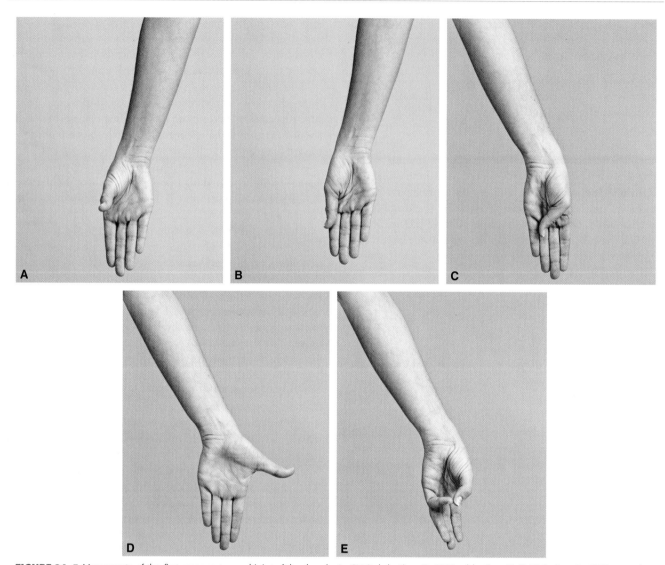

FIGURE 24–5 Movements of the first carpometacarpal joint of the thumb. **A.** CMC abduction, **B.** CMC adduction, **C.** CMC flexion, **D.** CMC extension, and **E.** CMC opposition.

joint as a simple hinge joint.[46] The MCP joint of the thumb differs only slightly from the MCP joints of digits 2 to 5.

The *volar plate* is a fibrocartilaginous structure that is loosely adhered to the base of the proximal phalanx.[24] Its loose association with the phalanx allows the plate to migrate distally and proximally with MCP extension and flexion, respectively.[1] When the MCP joint is in extension, the volar plate increases the degree of surface contact between the proximal phalanx and the large metacarpal head.[47] The volar plate increases joint congruency, enhances joint stability by limiting hyperextension, and serves as protection from compressive forces.[11,47]

Stability of the Metacarpophalangeal Joint

The metacarpal heads of digits 2 to 5 are interconnected by the *deep transverse metacarpal ligament*. *Sagittal bands* attach the volar plates to the extensor muscle expansion on the dorsal side of the hand, which maintains the position of the plates.[19] The MCP joints of all five digits include collateral and accessory ligaments and joint capsules.

As primary restraints, the collateral ligaments become taut with MCP flexion, thus disallowing abduction and adduction.[48,49] In addition, at 70 degrees of flexion, the shape of the volar surface of the metacarpal head provides an additional bony block to abduction/adduction.[50]

Mobility of the Metacarpophalangeal Joint

Mobility of the MCP joint of the thumb is less than that of the other MCP joints.[19,42] MCP joints are biaxial, allowing flexion, extension, abduction, and adduction. Some hold the opinion that the axis of MCP motion is stationary, lying within the metatarsal head,[7] while others contend that the axis moves volarly with flexion and dorsally with extension.[51] The complexity of MCP movement is fully recognized by appreciating the manner in which the fingers converge upon the scaphoid when moving from a fully opened hand position to a closed fist position.

Ranges of *flexion* of the MCP joint vary from *50 degrees* in the thumb to up to nearly *100 degrees* in the MCP of the fifth digit. The quantity of *extension* is cited as ranging from *30 degrees* to *60 degrees.* Generally, the amount of *abduction* is considered to be greater than the degree of *adduction;* however, these ranges have not been fully determined in the literature.[18] As noted, abduction and adduction is greatest when the joint is in extension and least when the joint is in flexion.

The Proximal Interphalangeal and Distal Interphalangeal Joints

Each *proximal interphalangeal (PIP)* and *distal interphalangeal (DIP)* joint comprises the head of one phalanx and the base of the next distal phalanx, which results in a hinge joint with one degree of freedom into flexion and extension. The base of each middle and distal phalanx has two concave facets divided by a ridge, which articulates with the convex head of the phalanx that is proximal to it, creating a concave-on-convex structural arrangement.

Stability of the Interphalangeal Joints

The supporting noncontractile structures of the interphalangeal (IP) joints consist of the volar plates, the joint capsule, and two collateral ligaments. The volar plates serve the primary function of limiting the degree of joint hyperextension through its insertion into the capsule of the joint.[52] The collateral ligaments comprise both cord-like bands and fan-shaped expansions that extend across each IP joint, much like the collateral ligaments of the MCP joints. These supporting structures are interconnected through fibrocartilaginous projections that extend from the extensor mechanism, collateral ligaments, and volar plates to the base of each phalanx.

Mobility of the Interphalangeal Joints

Much like the MCP joints, movement of the IP joints consists primarily of sagittal plane motion (flexion/extension); however, a slight degree of frontal plane and transverse plane motion also exists, which allows the digits to angle toward the thumb when moving from the open-hand to a closed-fist position. As with the MCP joints, there is a progressive increase in the degree of IP mobility from the radial to the ulnar side of the hand.[7] Fifth-digit PIP flexion may achieve up to *135 degrees* of flexion, and the fifth-digit DIP joint may achieve up to *90 degrees* of flexion. The increased amount of motion that is available in the ulnar-side digits produces an angulation of the digits toward the centrally located scaphoid bone. Generally, the DIP joints allow greater ranges of extension, while the PIP joints allow greater ranges of flexion.[7]

EXAMINATION

The Subjective Examination

Self-Reported Disability Measures

The Hand Disability Index[53] is a self-assessment questionnaire that requires patients to rate their ability to perform seven specific functionally relevant tasks, such as opening car doors, opening jars, and turning on a faucet, on a scale from 0 to 3, where 0 = inability to perform the task and 3 = ability to perform the task normally. The **Disability of the Arm, Shoulder,** *and Hand Instrument (DASH)* and **Quick DASH,** described in Chapter 22, are also commonly used to assess self-perceived disability in individuals who are experiencing functional limitations of the wrist and hand.

Review of Systems

Injuries to the wrist and hand are common subsequent to falls or repetitive trauma. Those suffering from conditions that lead to demineralization of bone, or *osteopenia,* may be more inclined to experience bone fracture in response to seemingly low levels of force.[54] Individuals with compromised immune systems owing to systemic pathology may experience localized *infections* within the hand.[54] The hand is often the locus of infection in immunosuppressed individuals because of the significant number of open spaces. The classic signs of hand infection include swelling, local tenderness, and erythema. Infection within the hand often leads to deformity as bones and joints become malaligned in the presence of space-occupying edema. Intervention for infection often includes drainage and aggressive organism-specific antibiotic therapy. Table 24-1 provides the red flags for a variety of conditions often experienced at the elbow, wrist, and hand.[54]

History of Present Illness

Arthrosis, often referred to as arthritis, should be suspected in the population over the age of 40 who have an insidious onset of symptoms that consist primarily of stiffness that improves with active movement. Certain occupations lead to a higher propensity toward various disorders; therefore, a complete review of the critical demands of the patient's occupation must be obtained. Individuals who engage in repetitive activities are more susceptible to *cumulative trauma disorders (CTD).* Perhaps the most frequently described CTD involving the hand is *carpal tunnel syndrome (CTS).* The repeated use of the muscles of the hand with the wrist in extension or while resting on firm surfaces, as experienced during keyboarding, are often precipitating factors. Bakers and cake decorators who perform an excessive amount of gripping activities are also susceptible to CTS.

Injuries to the hand and wrist that occur in response to single traumatic events must also be explored. A *fall on an outstretched hand (FOOSH),* for example, may lead to fractures of the distal radius and ulna with or without displacement or wrist dislocation. The force experienced by such an injury, however, may also result in more discrete injuries such as volar *subluxation* of the lunate or *fracture* of the scaphoid. The former condition may lead to encroachment of the carpal tunnel and the latter may result in delayed union and avascular necrosis by virtue of its precarious blood supply.

The Objective Physical Examination

Examination of Structure

Examination of structure begins immediately as the patient enters the facility. General posturing of the hand in a relaxed fashion with progressively greater degrees of finger flexion from the radial to the ulnar side of the hand is expected. The

Table 24-1	Medical Red Flags for the Elbow, Wrist, and Hand
MEDICAL CONDITION	**RED FLAGS**
Fracture	Recent fall or history of direct trauma
	Exquisite pain, tenderness, edema, ecchymosis
	Chronic use of steroids
	History of bone demineralization
Tendon rupture	Grade I, II: Pain with motion and passive stretch, edema, tenderness
	Grade III: Total loss of motion, palpable defect, edema, tenderness
Infection	History of recent open injury
	Presence of an abscess
	Signs of edema
	Chills, fever, malaise
Complex regional pain syndrome (CRPS)	History of traumatic event
	Hypersensitivity
	Pitting edema
	Trophic changes including brittle nails, course hair growth, erythema
	Poor response to analgesics
Raynaud's phenomenon	Blanching and redness in response to cold
	Pain and paresthesia to cold
	History of rheumatoid arthritis, vascular disease, use of beta-blockers, tobacco use

Adapted from Boissonnault WG. *Primary Care for the Physical Therapist: Examination and Triage.* St. Louis, MO: Elsevier Saunders; 2005.

presence of any protective patterns, such as splinting the hand close to the side, should be noted.

Close inspection of the hand must be performed in a sequential fashion, and it is recommended to proceed proximally from the tips of the fingers toward the elbow. Overall appearance is first considered. The contour of both volar and dorsal aspects of the wrist and hand must be evaluated including assessment of the arch structure of the hand. Loss of hand arches may signify neurological compromise. Alignment of the hand relative to the wrist and forearm will also provide information regarding dislocation, fracture, or instability of the radiocarpal or distal radioulnar joints. A patient with a **Colle's fracture** may present with a dorsal displacement of the distal radius, known as a "dinner fork deformity," secondary to falling on a hand with the wrist in extension. As a result of falling on a flexed wrist, a patient having sustained a **Smith's fracture** may present with volar displacement of the distal radius.

Due to the structural nature of the hand, observation of edema is often easily identifiable. Whether the edema is localized or generalized, hard or soft, pitting or nonpitting, it is critical to the examination and must be noted. Localized edema with tenderness and erythema is suggestive of a localized infection that demands immediate medical attention. Edema following trauma that persists for more than a week after onset is suggestive of bony or joint trauma, such as a fracture or dislocation. Localized edema of the MCP and IP joints is consistent with either *osteoarthritis (OA)* or *rheumatoid arthritis (RA)*.

Observation is often the first step toward diagnosing the presence of peripheral nerve entrapment syndromes. Along with a combination of motor and sensory impairments of the wrist and hand, *median nerve entrapment* at the wrist may result in atrophy of the thenar eminence, which is easily observable. *Ulnar nerve entrapment* at the wrist may result in atrophy of the hypothenar eminence and atrophy of the interossei spaces, since this nerve innervates both dorsal and palmer interossei. *Radial nerve entrapment* at the wrist will result in sensory changes in the hand without any motor involvement.

When considering the basic structure of each digit as a column of bone that is profoundly influenced by its contractile supporting structures, it is not difficult to appreciate the presence of deformity as a sequela of tendon rupture, nerve palsy, or a systemic condition that impacts the function of this complex musculotendinous system. A **mallet finger**, which is a rupture of the extensor tendon at its insertion into the distal phalanx, may occur at any digit and is easily identified by observing the DIP resting in a flexed position (Fig. 24-6A).[55] A rupture of the central tendon of the extensor hood mechanism may result in a flexion deformity of the PIP and extension deformity of the DIP in a condition known as **boutonniere deformity** (Fig. 24-6B).[55] Deformity involving PIP extension, DIP flexion, as well as MCP flexion, may result from tendon rupture or contracture of the intrinsic hand muscles in a condition known as **swan-neck deformity** (Fig. 24-6C).[55] Peripheral entrapment of the median and ulnar nerves will impact the function of the hand intrinsics and, if severe, may result in an

intrinsic minus hand. This condition results in a loss of the hand arches, atrophy of the hand intrinsics, and unchecked extrinsic muscle activity resulting in the **classic claw hand deformity** composed of MCP extension and PIP/DIP flexion (Fig. 24-6D).[55] Palsy of the median nerve alone may lead to **ape hand deformity**, where the thumb falls into the frontal plane with the other digits, along with atrophy of the thenar eminence and the inability to engage in thumb opposition (Fig. 24-6E).[55] In cases of radial nerve palsy, the patient may develop **drop-wrist deformity**, in which not only wrist and hand extension is limited, but wrist and hand flexion may be limited as well. Perhaps, the most debilitating of the nerve palsies is involvement of the ulnar nerve. Wasting of muscles on the ulnar side of the hand will result in the characteristic **bishop's hand deformity**, which includes flexion of digits 4 and 5 (Fig. 24-6F).[55] Atraumatic, non-neurologic conditions may also occur at the wrist and hand. A **Dupuytren's contracture** involves the atraumatic formation of nodules, primarily at digits 3 to 5, which impacts hand function.[55,56] In the presence of OA, observation may reveal deformity, which includes **Heberden's nodes** of the DIPs and **Bouchard's nodes** of the PIPs (Fig. 24-6G). Rheumatoid arthritis often manifests itself as deformity in the smaller joints of the wrist and hand, which includes PIP and DIP joint deformity and **ulnar drift** of the MCP and IP joints (Fig. 24-6H).

Peripheral nerve injury that influences the sympathetic nervous system may also result in *trophic changes*. These changes may include brittle fingernails; hand diaphoresis; red, shiny skin appearance; loss of hair on the hand; radiographic evidence of bone demineralization; and temperature changes. Such effects may also be present in response to neurovascular disease, *peripheral vascular disease*, *Raynaud's syndrome*, and *diabetes mellitus*. In such cases, a combination of *vasomotor*, *sudomotor*, and *pilomotor* effects may be observed in conjunction with trophic changes.

A detailed observation of nail appearance is critical in understanding the presence of any potential underlying pathology that may be present. **Beau's lines**, for example, are transverse ridges that reveal disruptions in nail growth secondary to nutritional deficiency or systemic disease. A decrease in nail rigidity may be experienced secondary to chronic arthritis, endocrine disease, or syphilis. Individuals presenting with nail appearance that is out of the ordinary should be referred to their medical physician for further testing.

Screening of Adjacent Structures

As the most distal segment of the upper extremity kinetic chain, the wrist and hand is often influenced by mobility impairments within the proximal segments. Identification and restoration of normal mobility within these proximal structures may be necessary for resolution of the presenting condition. Bilateral mobility and muscle function screening of the entire upper quarter is necessary to ensure that the manual physical therapist is not missing any key contributors to the problem.

Examination of Mobility

Mobility testing typically proceeds from proximal to distal and from lateral to medial, beginning with examination of the

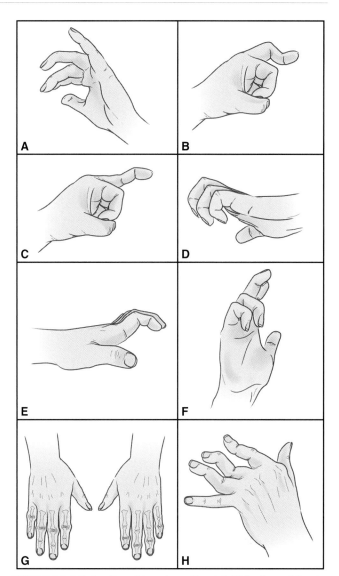

FIGURE 24–6 Deformities of the wrist and hand. **A.** Mallet finger deformity. **B.** Boutonniere deformity. **C.** Swan-neck deformity. **D.** Claw hand deformity. **E.** Ape hand deformity. **F.** Bishop's hand deformity. **G.** Bouchard's nodes of the PIPs and Heberden's nodes of the DIPs. **H.** Ulnar drift.

thumb. Prior to goniometric measurement, screening of finger motion can be performed by observing the hand as it moves from a maximally open to a maximally closed position. Due to both *active insufficiency* and *passive insufficiency*, it is important to be aware that wrist position impacts hand and finger mobility and, likewise, hand and finger position will impact wrist mobility. For example, a greater degree of passive wrist extension is expected with the MCP and IP joints in flexion than that which might be expected if the fingers were in an extended position.

Active Physiologic Movement Examination

Due to the large quantity of joints in the hand, active motion testing may serve to screen the joints that require more detailed assessment, thus improving the efficiency of the examination. Determination of movement *quantity*, *quality*, and any *reproduction* of symptoms is documented.

To reliably measure wrist and hand movement, a medium and small goniometer is used. The optimal position for measuring wrist motion is in sitting with the patient's forearm supported on the table. Examining both single and repeated movement (5 to 10 times) is recommended in order to provide a more reliable movement profile that truly demonstrates the patient's movement capacity.

During normal function, it is rare for the joints of the wrist and hand to move in isolation; therefore, examination of *combined movement* patterns is considered to be an important aspect of the examination. Tightness of the hand intrinsic muscles is suspected if the PIP joint moves better with the MCP in flexion, and joint capsular restrictions are suspected if the PIP joint is unable to flex in either position. This procedure is often referred to as the **Bunnell-Littler** test. Testing wrist flexion/extension in conjunction with radial/ulnar deviation may also be performed to assess mobility.

Perhaps the most functionally important combined movement pattern performed by the hand is movement of the hand into a fist. A *standard fist* requires maximal flexion of the MCP, PIP, and DIP joints. The *hook fist* tests extension of the MCP joints and flexion of the PIP and DIP joints. Lastly, the *straight fist*, also known as the *roof hand position*, requires flexion of the MCP and extension of the PIP and DIP joints.[57] Testing and comparing mobility of these three fist positions provides important information regarding mobility and muscle function. These fist positions may also be used when performing tendon gliding exercises.

The wrist and hand serves as the terminal extent of the upper extremity. Testing **proprioceptive neuromuscular facilitation (PNF)** patterns for the entire extremity may be useful in understanding the function of the wrist and hand complex relative to its proximal counterparts. Lastly, **overpressure** may be added at end range of all motions for the purpose of determining the quality of resistance at end range, which is known as **end-feel**.

During gross finger flexion, all of the digits should converge upon the same point, which is near the region where the radial pulse may be palpated. Movement that occurs in a cogwheel-type fashion may suggest the presence of *tenosynovitis*, as in the case of *trigger finger*. Movement of the wrist into extension with resultant finger flexion known as **tenodesis grip**, may be used to grasp objects by individuals without volitional finger flexor function.

The clinical significance of observed mobility restrictions is established if the movement in question reproduces the patient's chief presenting complaint. Establishing the patient's level of reactivity serves to dictate the aggressiveness with which intervention may be initiated.

Passive Physiologic Movement Examination

In order to improve efficiency, passive physiologic testing primarily focuses on the movements that were found to be deficient during active movement testing. During joint mobility testing, it is important to reduce the impact of muscular influences on movement. For example, when measuring MCP and IP flexion, the wrist should be placed in extension, and when measuring IP flexion, the MCP joints should be slightly extended. As noted, application of overpressure at the end of available range of motion to ascertain end-feel is critical in determining the nature of the observed restriction. Pronation and supination at the distal radioulnar joint reveals an *elastic end-feel*. Radiocarpal flexion and extension exhibits an *elastic end-feel*, RD has *a hard end-feel*, and UD a *firm end-feel*. Motions of the first CMC joint reveal an *elastic end-feel*. The metacarpophalangeal joints reveal a *firm end-feel* for flexion and extension at the thumb but an *elastic end-feel* for the same motions and a *firm end-feel* for abduction at MCP joints 2-5. Both PIP and DIP joints exhibit *firm end-feels* for both flexion and extension.

In addition, the manual physical therapist attempts to identify the presence of any capsular patterns. The capsular pattern of the distal radioulnar joint is full motion, with pain on performance of pronation and supination.[55] For the wrist, the capsular pattern is an equal limitation of flexion and extension *(flexion = extension)*.[55] The capsular pattern of the MCP and IP joints is that flexion is more limited than extension *(flexion > extension)*.[55] The capsular pattern of the CMC joint of the thumb is that abduction is more limited than extension *(abduction > extension)*. Table 24-2 displays the physiologic motions of the wrist and hand, including normal ranges of motion, normal end-feels, and capsular patterns.

Passive Physiologic Movement Examination of the Wrist
Movement of the distal RU joint follows movement of its proximal counterpart in providing pronation and supination. Some authors support the notion that the axis for wrist complex motion lies in close proximity to the capitate,[31,35] whereas others believe the axis is mobile.[33] Therefore, clinical measurement of wrist complex movement must be viewed as an oversimplified approximation of true motion, which involves a complex interplay between all of the joints of the carpus. Normal values for flexion range from *60 to 98 degrees*; for extension, *50 to 74 degrees*; for radial deviation, *20 to 35 degrees*; and for ulnar deviation, *26 to 37 degrees*.[7]

Passive Physiologic Motion Carpometacarpal and Metacarpophalangeal
Thumb CMC joint mobility dictates its position and the terms used to describe these movements are used synonymously with thumb movement. Movement of this joint, however, is probably most easily appreciated through examination of the combined movement of opposition. Normal opposition is determined by the ability of each finger to touch the thumb. Normal first (thumb) CMC motion is expected to reveal flexion equal to *15 degrees*, extension equal to *70 to 80 degrees*, and abduction equal to approximately *70 degrees*.[7] CMC mobility of digits 2 through 5 demonstrate a progressive increase in mobility from the radial to the ulnar-sided digits, which is important for opposition.

Mobility of the CMC joint is often measured as a component motion of MCP motion. During goniometric measurement, the hand and proximal joints are fully supported in a position that reduces the influence of the extrinsic musculature. The quantity of MCP flexion ranges from approximately *90 to 110 degrees* and MCP extension from approximately *30 to 50 degrees*, with a progressive increase in mobility from digits 2 through 5.[7]

Table 24–2	Physiologic (Osteokinematic) Motions of the Wrist and Hand				
JOINT	**NORMAL ROM**	**OPP**	**CPP**	**NORMAL END-FEEL(S)**	**CAPSULAR PATTERNS**
Distal radioulnar	90° pronation 90° supination			Pronation = elastic Supination = elastic	Full ROM, pain with pronation and supination
Radiocarpal	60°–98° flexion 50°–74° extension 20°–35° RD 26°-37° UD	0°-20° flexion or extension slight UD	Full RD and extension	Flexion = elastic Extension = elastic RD = hard UD = firm	Restrictions in all directions, Flexion = Extension
Intercarpal	60°–98° flexion with RC joint 50°–74° extension with RC joint 20°–35° RD with RC joint 26°-37° UD with RC joint				
CMC thumb	15° flexion 70°-80° extension 70° abduction Opposition= contact with 5th distal phalanx	Mid-range flexion/ extension and abduction/ adduction	Maximal opposition	Flexion, Extension, Abduction = elastic	Abduction > Extension
MCP thumb	75°–90° flexion 10°-15° extension	Slight flexion	Maximal extension	Flexion = firm Extension = firm	Flexion > Extension
MCP 2–5	90°-110° flexion 30°-50° extension	20° flexion	Maximal flexion	Flexion = elastic Extension = elastic Abduction = firm	Flexion > Extension
PIP 1–5	70°-110° flexion 5°-20° extension	Slight flexion	Maximal extension	Flexion = firm Extension = firm	Flexion > Extension
DIP 1-5	80°-90° flexion 15°-20° extension	Slight flexion	Maximal extension	Flexion = firm Extension = firm	Flexion > Extension

ROM, range of motion; OPP, open-packed position; CPP, close-packed position; RD/UD, radial deviation/ulnar deviation; RC, radiocarpal; CMC, carpometacarpal; MCP, metacarpophalangeal; PIP, proximal interphalangeal; DIP, distal interphalangeal. Adapted from Wise CH, Gulick DT. *Mobilization Notes: A Rehabilitation Specialist's Pocket Guide.* Philadelphia, PA: FA Davis Company; 2009.

Passive Physiologic Motion Interphalangeal

Passive Physiologic Movement

The PIP and DIP joints contain a small degree of frontal plane translation; however, motion at these articulations occurs almost exclusively within the sagittal plane. As with the MCP joints, the degree of IP motion increases from the radial to the ulnar side of the hand. As when measuring the degree of motion, all proximal joints are supported and stabilized in an attempt to isolate motion to the joint being measured. Normal PIP flexion ranges from *70 to 90 degrees* at the thumb to greater than *110 degrees* at the fifth digit, while PIP extension ranges from *5 degrees* at the thumb to over *20 degrees* at the fifth digit.[7] Normal DIP flexion averages around *80 to 90 degrees*, and extension averages around *15 to 20 degrees*.[7]

Passive Accessory Movement Examination

The large number of articulations present within the wrist and hand complex makes examination of accessory motion challenging. To reduce external influences, the therapist seeks to examine these movements with the joint in the open-packed position. Within the joints of the fingers, the direction in which gliding is presumed to occur is based primarily on a biomechanical model that appreciates the reciprocal concave-convex joint relationships. Some evidence suggests that true joint translation may be of little consequence within the joints of the fingers, bringing into question the value of examining and treating deficits in accessory mobility within these joints.[7] As deficits in accessory mobility are identified, the procedures used during examination may become the intervention. The mobilization techniques that follow later in this chapter will provide details regarding the performance of accessory glides and may be used for both examination and intervention of passive accessory movement. Table 24-3 provides a description of wrist and hand arthrology and the expected accessory (arthrokinematic) motions for each joint within the wrist and hand complex.

Examination of Muscle Function

Extrinsic muscles are those that originate outside of the hand yet exert an influence on hand function by virtue of their insertion

Table 24-3	Accessory (Arthrokinematic) Motions of the Wrist and Hand		
	ARTHOLOGY	**ARTHROKINEMATICS**	
Radiocarpal	Concave surface: Radius & radio-ulnar disc	*To facilitate wrist flexion:* Proximal carpus rolls volarly and Glides dorsally on radius	*To facilitate extension:* Proximal carpus rolls dorsally and glides volarly on radius
	Convex surface: Proximal carpus	*To facilitate radial deviation:* Proximal carpus rolls lateral and glides medial on radius	*To facilitate ulnar deviation:* Proximal carpus rolls medial and glides lateral on radius
Distal radioulnar	Concave surface: Ulnar notch of radius	*To facilitate pronation:* Radius rolls and glides volarly on a fixed ulna	*To facilitate supination:* Radius rolls and glides dorsally on a fixed ulna
	Convex surface: Head of ulna	Ulna rolls volarly and glides dorsally on a fixed radius	Ulna rolls dorsally and glides volarly on a fixed radius
CMC thumb	Concave surface: Base of the 1st metacarpal	*To facilitate thumb flexion:* Metacarpal rolls & glides medial on trapezium	*To facilitate thumb extension:* Metacarpal rolls & glides lateral on trapezium
	Convex surface: Trapezium	*To facilitate thumb abduction:* Metacarpal rolls proximal and glides distal on trapezium	*To facilitate thumb adduction:* Metacarpal rolls distal and glides proximal on trapezium
MCP 2-5	Concave surface: Base of proximal phalanx	*To facilitate flexion:* Proximal phalanx rolls and glides volarly on metacarpal	*To facilitate extension:* Proximal phalanx rolls and glides dorsally on metacarpal
		To facilitate abduction 2nd MCP: Proximal phalanx rolls and glides laterally on metacarpal	*To facilitate adduction 2nd MCP:* Proximal phalanx rolls and glides medially on metacarpal
	Convex surface: Head of metacarpal	*To facilitate abduction 4th and 5th MCP:* Proximal phalanx rolls and glides medially on metacarpal	*To facilitate adduction 4th and 5th MCP:* Proximal phalanx rolls and glides laterally on metacarpal
MCP thumb	Concave surface: Base of proximal phalanx	*To facilitate thumb flexion:* Phalanx rolls and glides volarly on metacarpal	*To facilitate thumb extension:* Phalanx rolls and glides dorsally on metacarpal
	Convex surface: Head of metacarpal		
IP 2-5	Concave surface: Base of more distal phalanx	*To facilitate flexion:* More distal phalanx rolls and glides volarly on the more proximal phalanx	*To facilitate extension:* More distal phalanx rolls and glides dorsally on the more proximal phalanx
	Convex surface: Head of more proximal phalanx		

Adapted from Boissonnault WG. *Primary Care for the Physical Therapist: Examination and Triage.* St. Louis, MO: Elsevier Saunders; 2005.

into the hand. *Intrinsic muscles* of the hand both originate and insert within the hand.

Extrinsic Muscles of the Wrist and Hand

The group of superficial muscles that are located along the anterior aspect of the forearm share the primary responsibility for flexing the wrist. This group consists of five muscles that have a common insertion, known as the *common flexor tendon*, on the medial epicondyle of the humerus. By virtue of this attachment, these muscles also serve to pronate the forearm and flex the elbow. However, their role in the production of the latter is believed to be minimal.

Based on its distal insertion into the metacarpals on the lateral aspect of the hand, the *flexor carpi radialis (FCR)* is able to produce radial deviation in addition to the motions just described. Functionally, this muscle is only minimally active across the elbow.[58] During examination, the best method for assessing recruitment of this muscle is by resisting the combined movements of flexion and radial deviation.[59]

The *palmaris longus (PL)* is an extremely small, yet superficial, muscle that is absent in 10 percent of the population.[58] Along with production of wrist flexion, this muscle is also able to produce a cupping motion of the hand and it is not routinely differentially examined. The largest of the wrist flexor muscles is the *flexor digitorum superficialis (FDS)*. This muscle has the ability to perform wrist flexion, radial and ulnar deviation, as well as flexion of the MCP and PIP joints, but it may be distinguished by its ability to flex the PIP joints without flexing the DIP joints.[60] More specifically, testing isolated flexion of the PIP of the third digit is the ideal method for differentially evaluating this muscle.[58] Due to the location of the FDS tendon, which traverses the capitate, this muscle may be active during both radial and ulnar deviation, depending on the position of the wrist during testing.

The most medial boundary of this muscle group and the muscle with the largest cross-sectional area is the *flexor carpi ulnaris (FCU)*. The FCU is an important muscle for stabilizing the wrist during most functional activities that place lateral forces through the wrist.[61] This muscle is analogous to the FCR and best tested through the combined movements of flexion and ulnar, rather than radial, deviation.

The superficial extensors of the wrist insert via the *common extensor tendon* upon the lateral epicondyle of the humerus. The *extensor carpi radialis longus (ECRL)* and *extensor carpi radialis brevis (ECRB)* are intimately related, yet perform distinctly different actions. When attempting to differentiate between function of the ECRL and ECRB, the manual physical therapist should be aware that the ECRB seems to contribute more to the production of wrist extension[62] while the ECRL contributes slightly more to radial deviation.[58]

Analogous to the FDS, the *extensor digitorum (ED)* is composed of tendon slips that extend to digits 2 to 5. The distal attachments of the ED have received considerable attention in the literature. The ED splits into a central tendon, which inserts at the base of the middle phalanx, and two lateral slips, which converge at the base of the distal phalanx in an arrangement referred to as the **extensor hood mechanism**.

The extensor hood receives insertions from the hand intrinsics, and the four tendons are interconnected by a fibrous expansion known as the *juncturae tendinae*, which restricts independent movement.[7] Differentiating ED function is accomplished through testing MCP extension with the IP joints flexed.[63]

The *extensor digiti minimi (EDM)* function specifically at the fifth digit and contributes to ulnar deviation. The *extensor carpi ulnaris (ECU)* is the ulnar-sided counterpart of the ECRB, producing wrist extension and ulnar deviation. As the wrist moves from flexion to extension, an accompanying degree of ulnar to radial deviation occurs, due in part to the muscles of the forearm.[7,62]

The remainder of the extrinsic muscles are located deep to the muscles just described. Anteriorly, the *flexor digitorum profundus (FDP)* is located immediately adjacent to the *flexor pollicis longus (FPL)*. To selectively test the FDP, flexion of the DIP is resisted. Due to its force-producing capabilities, the FDP is preferentially used for gripping activities; however, when more independent finger motion is desirable, the FDS is the muscle of choice.[58,63]

The FPL is the only muscle capable of flexing the IP joint of the thumb via its insertion into the base of the distal phalanx. This unique function of the FPL is best accomplished in conjunction with stabilizing moments performed by the hand intrinsic muscles at the CMC and MCP joints.[58]

The deep posterior extrinsic muscles of the forearm include the supinator, three muscles that dictate function of the thumb, and one muscle dedicated to providing movement of the index finger. The *supinator* is most active in its role of supinating the forearm when the elbow is extended. The *abductor pollicis longus (APL)*, which serves as the anterior border of the *anatomical snuffbox*, is considered to be a better extensor than abductor of the CMC joint of the thumb.[60,64] Movement of the thumb serves to alter the repertoire of possible moment arms that this muscle may adopt. The *extensor pollicis brevis (EPB)* shares the same tendon sheath and functions in a fashion that is similar to the APL. The distinguishing characteristic of the EPB is its ability to extend the MCP of the thumb.[42] The *extensor pollicis longus (EPL)* inserts into the base of the distal phalanx of the thumb after angulating around *Lister's tubercle* and acts with the EPB to extend the MCP joint; however, it is distinguished from the EPB in its action as extensor of the thumb's IP joint. At the CMC joint, the EPL has a better moment arm to adduct rather than extend the thumb.[65] The final extrinsic muscle of the posterior forearm is the *extensor indicis (EI)*, whose differentiating role is in providing index finger extension independently.

Intrinsic Muscles of the Wrist and Hand

During normal function, the wrist and hand adopt a pattern of movement that minimizes the effects of both active insufficiency and passive insufficiency. The prime intrinsics of the thumb are the *abductor pollicis brevis (APB)*, *flexor pollicis brevis (FPB)*, *opponens pollicis (OP)*, and *adductor pollicis (AP)*. Collectively, these muscles are responsible for directing the function of the thumb as their names suggest.

Analogous to the intrinsic muscles of the thenar eminence are those of the hypothenar eminence, consisting of the *abductor digiti minimi (ADM), flexor digiti minimi brevis (FDMB),* and the *opponens digiti minimi (ODM),* which direct function of the fifth digit in much the same fashion.

There are four *dorsal interossei (DI)* and either three or four *palmar interossei (PI).* The DI diminish in cross-sectional area from the first to the fourth, with the first being the second largest hand intrinsic muscle. The fifth digit does not possess a dorsal interossei since this role is fulfilled by the ADM, but the third digit possesses two dorsal interossei on both the medial and laterals aspects. As a group, the DI perform abduction and flexion of the MCP joints. The PI are generally smaller than the DI. These muscles collectively provide MCP adduction and flexion. Like the DI, the PI also serve to extend the PIP and DIP joints of the fingers to which they attach (digits 3 to 5).

The *lumbricals* are the smallest of the hand intrinsics and are unique in that they possess no bony attachment. These muscles run from the FDP tendons and insert upon the radial side of the extensor hood mechanism. Collectively, this muscle group is responsible for producing flexion of the MCP joints and extension of the PIP and DIP joints, a position often referred to as the *roof hand position* or *lumbrical grip position.*

Functional Hand Examination

Assessment of Grip

Examination of grip allows the manual physical therapist to gain insight into both the movement and force-producing capabilities of the hand. An important tool for measurement of grip is the **Jamar hand-grip dynamometer** (Asimow Engineering Co., Santa Monica, CA).[66] Hand grip and pinch dynamometry have been found to be a valid and reliable method for assessing grip strength.[67]

Assessment of Fine and Gross Motor Coordination

The ability of the hand to function in a coordinated fashion to perform fine motor tasks is often referred to as *dexterity.* Perhaps the most well-known test of dexterity is the **Purdue Pegboard Test.** During this test, the patient is timed during performance of small object manipulation. Bilateral comparison and comparison with documented normal values allow a quantitative determination of fine motor coordination.[68,69]

Similar to the Purdue Pegboard Test, the **Nine-Hole Peg Test** involves the manipulation of small pegs for the purpose of testing fine motor dexterity of the hand and fingers. The time it takes for each hand to perform placement and removal of the pegs is compared to the other hand and documented normal values.[68,70]

To test gross motor coordination, the **Minnesota Rate of Manipulation Test** may be used. In this test, the patient is timed in the manipulation of checker-like pieces that are placed and turned unilaterally and bilaterally.[68,70]

Palpation

Osseous Palpation

Beginning on the medial side of the forearm, the manual physical therapist carefully palpates the *shaft of the ulna* distally as it terminates as the *head of the ulna* and the *ulnar styloid process.*

On the lateral side of the wrist, the broad distal radius with its large *radial styloid process* can be palpated. On the dorsal aspect of the radius, the small projection known as Lister's tubercle may be palpated (Fig. 24-7). To confirm its location, the EPL is tested by resisting IP extension of the thumb. The distal radioulnar joint may also be palpated.

Moving distally, the manual physical therapist must attempt to palpate each of the carpal bones in a systematic and efficient manner. Once Lister's tubercle located at the dorsal aspect of the radius is palpated, the therapist then palpates the base of the third metacarpal. An imaginary line that connects the tubercle with the base of the metacarpal is drawn. Along this line, within the proximal and distal row of carpals lies the lunate and capitate, respectively. The lunate is identified as a hollow region just distal to the radius. Confirmation is obtained by flexing and extending the wrist, which produces movement of the lunate in a dorsal and volar direction, respectively. Just distal to the lunate, the capitate is the largest of the carpal bones and is quite prominent dorsally (Fig. 24-8).

Moving laterally, the therapist elicits active thumb extension and adduction, which increases the prominence of the snuffbox muscles. Located between the EPB and the EPL and forming the floor of the snuffbox is the scaphoid bone, which lies immediately adjacent to the lunate and trapezium within the proximal row of carpal bones (Fig. 24-9).

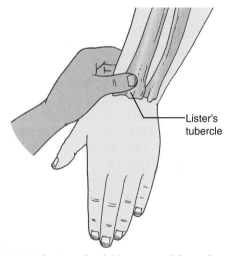

FIGURE 24–7 Palpation of styloid process of the radius and Lister's tubercle.

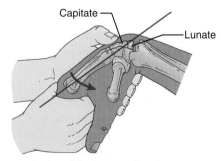

FIGURE 24–8 Palpation of the lunate and capitate.

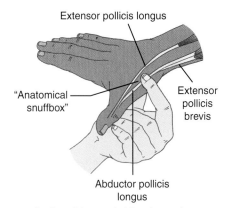

FIGURE 24–9 Palpation of the scaphoid and trapezium.

The lunate is relocated, and the examiner moves medially and identifies the *pisiform*, a superficial bony prominence to which the FCU is attached. When this muscle is placed on slack during wrist flexion and ulnar deviation, the pisiform can be moved in all directions. A line is drawn between the lunate and the pisiform on which the small triquetrum bone within the proximal row is located.

Just distal and lateral to the pisiform is a small tooth-like projection of the hamate bone, known as the hook of the hamate. This structure is best found by moving three-quarters of an inch toward the base of the index finger. From the hamate, the capitate can be palpated by moving laterally. The base of the second metacarpal is located and followed proximally. In line with the second metacarpal is the trapezoid, and immediately adjacent and lateral is the larger trapezium. The remainder of the hand is palpated by moving distally into the metacarpals and *phalanges*.

Soft Tissue Palpation

Using the palm of the therapist's hand on the medial epicondyle with the fingers directed distally, the thumb represents the location of the *pronator teres (PT)*, followed in sequential order from the second to the fifth digit by the FCR, PL, FDS, and FCU (Fig. 24-10). Confirmation of these muscles as a group is accomplished through resisting wrist flexion. The superficial FDS and its deeper counterpart, the FDP, may be palpated along the anterior and medial aspect of the forearm by resisting MCP and PIP flexion and DIP flexion, respectively.

In a similar fashion, the extensors of the wrist may also be palpated along the posterior aspect of the forearm. The *extensor carpi radialis longus and brevis (ECRL, ECRB), extensor digitorum (ED)*, and *extensor carpi ulnaris (ECU)* insert via the common extensor tendon upon the lateral epicondyle (Fig. 24-11). Moving lateral and posterior from the *brachioradialis*, the first muscle identified is the ECRL and ECRB. With the therapist placing the palm of the hand over the lateral epicondyle and the forearm pronated, the therapist's thumb and fingers represent sequentially, from medial to lateral, the ECRL, ECRB, ED, and ECU. This group may be palpated together by resisting wrist extension. The brachioradialis is differentiated from the ECRL and ECRB by resisting radial deviation, which does not recruit the brachioradialis and does not cross the wrist.

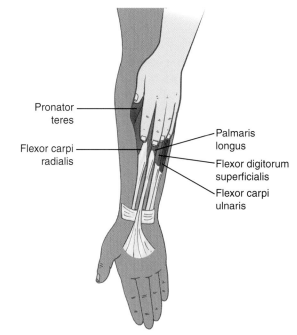

FIGURE 24–10 Palpation of the forearm flexor muscles.

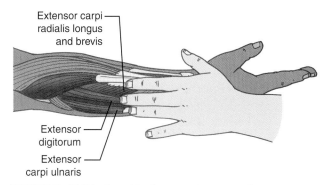

FIGURE 24–11 Palpation of the forearm extensor muscles.

To palpate the extrinsic muscles of the thumb, which include the APL, the EPB, and the EPL, the thumb is actively brought into extension. This position will allow visualization of the tendons that comprise the anatomical snuffbox (Fig. 24-12). The intrinsic muscles of the thumb, including the APB, FPB, and OP, occupy the thenar eminence of the hand. These muscles are collectively recruited through resistance to opposition. A

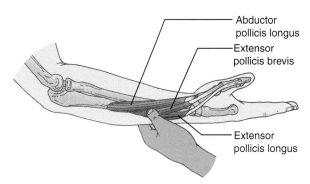

FIGURE 24–12 Palpation of the tendons of the anatomical snuffbox muscles.

fourth thumb intrinsic muscle, the AP, a broad muscle located within the web space between the thumb and index finger, is recruited through resistance of adduction of the thumb.

The muscles of the hypothenar eminence of the hand, which include the ADM, FDM, and ODM, are arranged in much the same manner as those of the thenar eminence. The most substantial of these muscles, which is located most laterally, is the ADM. From lateral to medial, the FDM and ODM are immediately adjacent to the ADM.

The remainder of the hand intrinsic muscles, namely the lumbricals and interossei, are difficult to selectively palpate. The interossei are located within the intermetacarpal region. Palpation of the first dorsal interosseus is easiest to palpate due to its size and more prominent location between the web space of the thumb and index finger. For the remaining interossei, the examiner may place the palpating finger between each metacarpal and elicit abduction (movement away from the long

finger) followed by adduction (movement toward the long finger) of each digit, during which a swelling of the dorsal and palmar interossei will occur, respectively.

Special Testing

The manual physical therapist's choice of special tests to use during the course of any given examination is dependent upon the results of the examination findings that have preceded testing. These tests serve to confirm suspicions regarding culpable structures. If positive, they suggest that the pathology in question exists. However, false positives may be common. Table 24-4 provides the sensitivity, specificity, and likelihood ratios for the more commonly performed special tests used in the examination of the wrist and hand.[71-104] The reader is encouraged to consult other sources for additional information regarding the performance of these useful confirmatory tests.

Table 24-4	Special Tests for the Wrist and Hand					
TEST	**SENSITIVITY**	**SPECIFICITY**	**+LR**	**−LR**	**RELIABILITY**	**REFERENCE**
Phalen Test	34%–88%	40%–100%	1.29–9.88	0.12–0.89	kappa = 0.53–0.88	LaStayo et al.[71] Wainner et al.[72] Marx et al.[73] Ahn[74] Heller et al.[75] Szabo et al.[76] Gonzalez del Pinto et al.[77] Hansen et al.[78] Gunnarsson et al.[79] Katz et al.[80] Tetro et al.[81]
Reverse Phalen Test	88%	93%	NA	NA	NA	LaStayo et al.[71] Wainner et al.[77]
Carpal Compression Test	0.42%–0.75%	0.84%–0.95%	5.6–10.7	0.13–0.26	kappa = 0.77 (95% CI)	LaStayo et al.[71] Wainner et al.[72]
Tinel Sign	68%–70%	76%–98%	2.8–35	0.31–0.42	NA	Marx et al.[73] Ahn[74] Heller et al.[75] Szabo et al.[76] Gonzalez del Pinto et al.[77] Hansen et al[78] Tetro et al.[81] Moldaver[82]
Froment Sign	NA	NA	NA	NA	NA	Blacker et al.[83] Goldman et al.[84]

Table 24-4	Special Tests for the Wrist and Hand—cont'd					
TEST	SENSITIVITY	SPECIFICITY	+LR	−LR	RELIABILITY	REFERENCE
Wartenberg Test	NA	NA	NA	NA	NA	Wartenberg[85] Bradshaw et al.[86] Feindel et al.[87] Miller[88] Posner[89] Regan et al.[90]
TFCC Load Test	100%	NA	NA	NA	NA	LaStayo et al.[71]
TFCC Press Test	100%	NA	NA	NA	NA	LaStayo et al.[71] Lester et al.[91]
Gripping Rotatory Impaction Test	NA	NA	NA	NA	NA	LaStayo et al.[92]
Watson Scaphoid Instability Test	69%	64%–68%	2.03	0.47	NA	LaStayo et al.[71] Marx et al.[73] Watson et al.[93] Watson et al.[94] Young et al.[95] Young et al.[96] Lan[97] Taleisnik[98]
Axial Loading Test	89%	98%	49	0.02	NA	Waeckerle[99]
Clamp Sign	52%–100%	34%–100%	1.52	0	NA	Powell et al.[100]
Murphy Sign	NA	NA	NA	NA	NA	Booher et al.[101]
Finkelstein Test	81%–100%	50%–100%	1.62	0.38	NA	Finkelstein[102] Batteson et al.[103] Alexander et al.[104]

NA, not available; CI, confidence interval. Adapted from Wise CH, Gulick DT. *Mobilization Notes: A Rehabilitation Specialist's Pocket Guide*. Philadelphia, PA: FA Davis Company; 2009.

SPECIAL TESTS FOR THE WRIST AND HAND

Special Tests for Carpal Tunnel Syndrome

Phalen Test (Fig. 24-13)

Purpose:	To test for the presence of carpal tunnel syndrome
Patient:	Sitting with the dorsum of both hands in contact with one another
Clinician:	Standing in front of the patient
Procedure:	The patient brings hands together, flexing both wrists and then holding for 60 seconds.
Interpretation:	The test is positive if there is a reproduction of symptoms within the median nerve distribution.

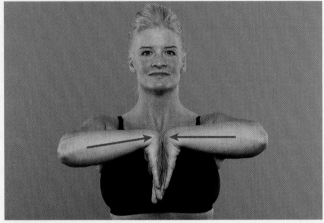

FIGURE 24–13 Phalen test.

Reverse Phalen Test (Fig. 24-14)

Purpose:	To test for the presence of carpal tunnel syndrome
Patient:	Sitting with the palms of both hands in contact with one another
Clinician:	Standing in front of the patient
Procedure:	The patient brings hands together, extending both wrists and then holding for 60 seconds.
Interpretation:	The test is positive if there is a reproduction of symptoms within the median nerve distribution.

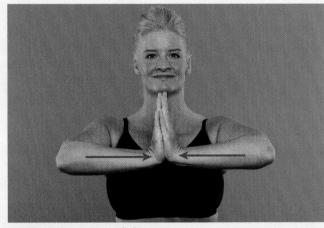

FIGURE 24–14 Reverse Phalen test.

Carpal Compression Test (Fig. 24-15)

Purpose:	To test for the presence of carpal tunnel syndrome
Patient:	Sitting with the hand supported on table with the palmer side up. Wrist flexion to 60 degrees may be added.
Clinician:	Sitting in front of the patient
Procedure:	Apply compression over the carpal tunnel for 30 seconds.
Interpretation:	The test is positive if there is a reproduction of symptoms within the median nerve distribution.

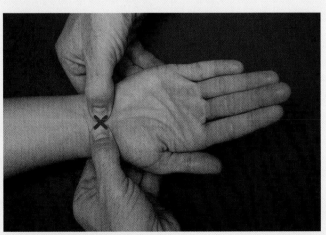

FIGURE 24–15 Carpal compression test.

Tinel Sign (Fig. 24-16)

Purpose: To test for the presence of carpal tunnel syndrome

Patient: Sitting with the hand supported on the table with the palmer side up and the hand in neutral

Clinician: Sitting in front of the patient

Procedure: Using the long finger, apply four to six gentle taps over the carpal tunnel.

Interpretation: The test is positive if there is a reproduction of symptoms within the median nerve distribution.

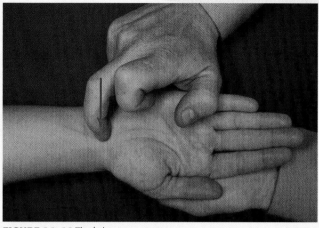

FIGURE 24–16 Tinel sign.

Special Tests for Neurological Compromise

Froment Sign (Fig. 24-17 A, B)

Purpose: To test for the presence of ulnar nerve compromise

Patient: Sitting with paper held between the index finger and thumb

Clinician: Sitting in front of the patient

Procedure: Gently pull the paper away while the patient holds the paper.

Interpretation: The test is positive if there is an inability to hold the paper or if DIP or MCP flexion occurs as the FPL compensates for weakness of the adductor pollicis from nerve compromise.

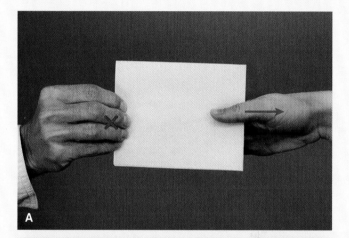

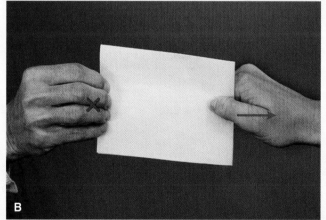

FIGURE 24–17 Froment sign. (Courtesy of Bob Wellmon Photography, BobWellmon.com.)

Wartenberg Sign (Fig. 24-18)

Purpose: To test for the presence of ulnar nerve compromise

Patient: Sitting with the hand on the table

Clinician: Sitting in front of the patient

Procedure: Resist fifth MCP adduction.

Interpretation: The test is positive if weakness of fifth MCP adduction is present.

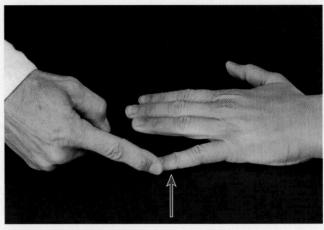

FIGURE 24–18 Wartenberg sign. (Courtesy of Bob Wellmon Photography, BobWellmon.com.)

Special Tests for Triangular Fibrocartilage Complex Dysfunction
Triangular Fibrocartilage Complex Load Test (Fig. 24-19)

Purpose: To test for the presence of TFCC pathology

Patient: Sitting with the wrist in ulnar deviation

Clinician: Sitting in front of the patient

Procedure: Apply overpressure into ulnar deviation with long axis compression.

Interpretation: The test is positive if there is a reproduction of pain in the region of the TFCC.

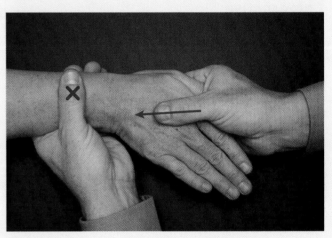

FIGURE 24–19 Triangular fibrocartilage complex load test.

Triangular Fibrocartilage Complex
Press Test (Fig. 24-20)

Purpose: To test for the presence of TFCC pathology

Patient: Sitting in a chair with both hands on the arm rests

Clinician: Sitting in front of the patient

Procedure: The patient lifts his or her body weight by pushing down through the arms.

Interpretation: The test is positive if there is a reproduction of pain in the region of the TFCC.

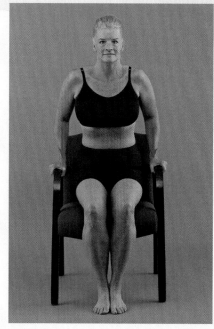

FIGURE 24–20 Triangular fibrocartilage complex press test.

Gripping Rotatory Impaction Test (Fig. 24-21 A, B)

Purpose: To test for the presence of TFCC pathology

Patient: Sitting with a hand dynamometer or blood pressure cuff

Clinician: Sitting in front of the patient

Procedure: Using a hand dynamometer or blood pressure cuff, compare grip strength in both pronation and supination.

Interpretation: The test is positive if grip strength in supination is greater than grip strtength in pronation.

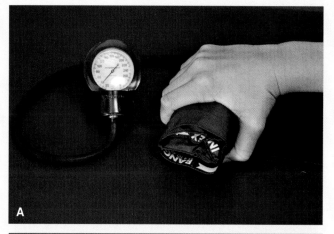

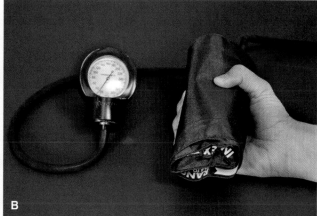

FIGURE 24–21 Gripping rotatory impaction test. Using a hand dynamometer or blood pressure cuff, compare grip strength in both **A.** pronation and **B.** supination. (Courtesy of Bob Wellmon Photography, BobWellmon.com.)

Special Tests for Instability, Fracture, and Tendonopathy
Watson Scaphoid Instability Test (Fig. 24-22 A, B)

Purpose:	To test for the presence of intercarpal instability
Patient:	Sitting with the hand on the table with the palm facing upward
Clinician:	Sitting in front of the patient, apply pressure over the scaphoid tubercle with your thumb while the other hand grasps the metacarpals
Procedure:	Beginning in ulnar deviation and extension, passively move the wrist into radial deviation and flexion.
Interpretation:	The test is positive if the scaphoid subluxes as pressure is applied.

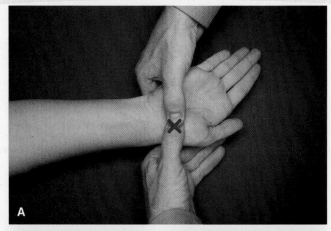
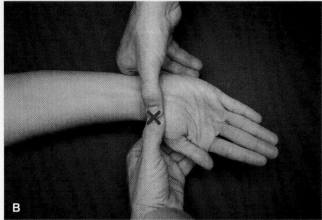

FIGURE 24–22 Watson scaphoid instability test.

Axial Loading Test (Fig. 24-23)

Purpose:	To test for the presence of a scaphoid fracture
Patient:	Sitting with the forearm on the table
Clinician:	Sitting in front of the patient
Procedure:	Passively abduct and extend the MCP joint of the thumb, after which axial compression is applied through the first CMC joint.
Interpretation:	The test is positive if there is a reproduction of pain at the base of the thumb.

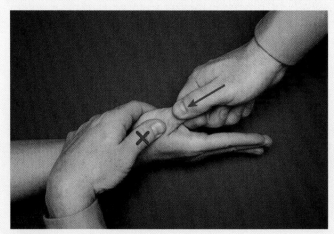

FIGURE 24–23 Axial loading test.

Clamp Sign (Fig. 24-24)

Purpose: To test for the presence of a scaphoid fracture

Patient: Sitting with the forearm on the table

Clinician: Sitting in front of the patient

Procedure: Passively pronate, extend, and ulnarly deviate the wrist, then apply a longitudinal load.

Interpretation: The test is positive if there is a reproduction of symptoms within the median nerve distribution.

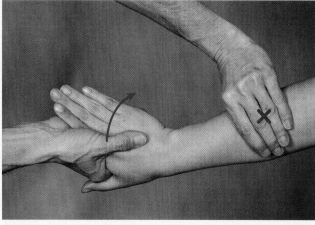

FIGURE 24–24 Clamp sign. (From: Gulick D. Ortho Notes. Philadelphia PA: F.A. Davis Company; 2010.)

Murphy Sign (Fig. 24-25)

Purpose: To test for the presence of a lunate dislocation

Patient: Sitting

Clinician: Standing or sitting in front of the patient

Procedure: Observe alignment of the MCP joints as the patient forms a fist.

Interpretation: The test is positive if the third MCP is level with the second and fourth, indicating proximal displacement

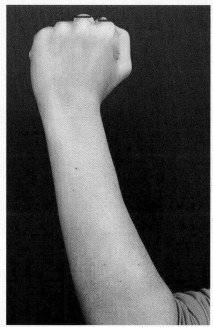

FIGURE 24–25 Murphy sign. (Courtesy of Bob Wellmon Photography, BobWellmon.com.)

Finkelstein Test (Fig. 24-26)

Purpose: To test for the presence of DeQuervain's syndrome, which is tenosynovitis of the abductor pollicis longus and extensor pollicis brevis tendons.

Patient: Sitting with the arm unsupported, making a fist with the thumb placed between the palm and fingers

Clinician: Sitting in front of the patient

Procedure: Stabilize the patient's forearm with one hand while passively ulnarly deviating the patient's wrist.

Interpretation: The test is positive if there is reproduction of pain over the radial styloid process.

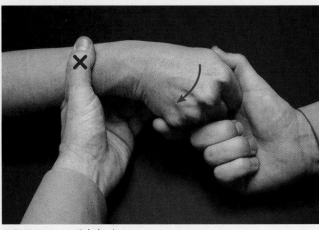

FIGURE 24–26 Finkelstein test.

JOINT MOBILIZATION OF THE WRIST AND HAND

Note: The indications for the joint mobilization techniques described in this section are based on expected joint kinematics. Current evidence suggests that the indications for their use are multifactorial and may be based on direct assessment of mobility and an individual's symptomatic response.

Distal Radioulnar Joint Mobilizations

Distal Radioulnar Dorsal and Volar Glides

Indications:

- *Distal radius on ulna dorsal and volar glides* are indicated for restrictions in forearm supination and pronation, respectively, as well as wrist flexion and extension. *Distal ulna on radius dorsal and volar glides* are indicated for restricitons in forearm pronation and supination, respectively, as well as wrist flexion and extension.

Accessory Motion Technique (Figs. 24-27, 24-28)

- **Patient/Clinician Position**: The patient is in the sitting position with the forearm supported on the table, or elbow flexed on table with the dorsum of the hand facing the clinician. The wrist may be pre-positioned at the point of restriction. Sit on the ipsilateral side of the wrist being mobilized.

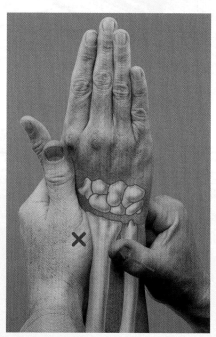

FIGURE 24–28 Distal radioulnar dorsal and volar glide, technique 2.

- **Hand Placement**: Using the fingers and thumb of the stabilization hand, grasp the distal ulna or radius or use a lumbrical grip over the radial side of the wrist and hand. Using the fingers and thumb or *lateral pinch grasp* of the mobilization hand grasp the distal ulna and ulnar head. Be sure to place your forearm in line with the direction of force.

- **Force Application**: For technique 1, while stabilizing the ulna, apply a dorsal or volar glide to the radius for supination and pronation, respectively. While stabilizing the radius, apply a dorsal or volar glide to the ulna for pronation and supination, respectively. For technique 2, the thumb places volar force at the ulnar head as the flexed second digit of the mobilization hand is positioned over the pisiform to stabilize the proximal row of carpal bones. The stabilization hand stabilizes the distal radius and radial aspect of the wrist. Alternately, stabilize the radial side of the wrist and hand using a lumbrical grip while the ulna is mobilized volarly against a stabilized triquetrum.

Accessory With Physiologic Motion Technique (Fig. 24-29)

- **Patient/Clinician Position:** The patient is in a sitting or supine position with the elbow flexed to 90 degrees and the forearm in full pronation for volar glides and supination for dorsal glides. Sit on the side ipsilateral to the elbow being mobilized.

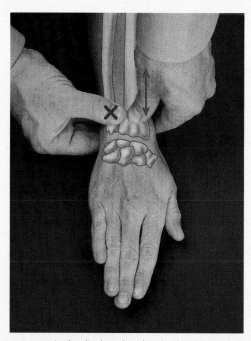

FIGURE 24–27 Distal radioulnar dorsal and volar glide, technique 1.

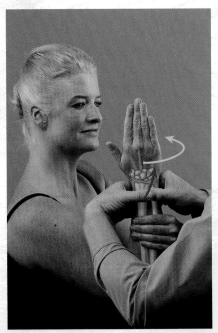

FIGURE 24–29 Distal radioulnar dorsal and volar glide accessory with physiologic motion.

- **Hand Placement:** Thumb over thumb contact at the distal aspect of the radius or ulna with the fingers of both hands grasping the wrist to guide the forearm into pronation or supination.
- **Force Application:** As the patient actively moves from full pronation to full supination or the reverse, maintain a volarly directed or dorsally directed force, respectively. As the patient provides overpressure into supination or pronation, maintain force throughout the entire range of motion and sustain the force at end range. Be prepared to move during the mobilization to ensure correct force application.

Radiocarpal Joint Mobilizations

Radiocarpal Distraction

Indications:
- *Radiocarpal distractions* are indicated when there is a loss of mobility in all directions.

Accessory Motion Technique: (Fig. 24-30)
- **Patient/Clinician:** The patient is in a sitting position with the forearm supported by the table, the wrist in neutral, and the hand over the edge of the table. The wrist may be pre-positioned at the point of restriction. Sit on the ipsilateral side of the wrist being mobilized.
- **Hand Placement:** With your stabilization hand grasp the distal radius and ulna. Place your mobilization hand immediately adjacent to the stabilization hand just distal to the

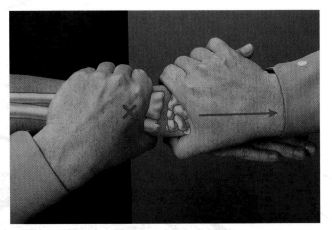

FIGURE 24–30 Radiocarpal distraction.

patient's wrist over the proximal row of carpal bones. Be sure that your forearm is in line with the direction of force.
- **Force Application:** After taking up the slack in the joint, apply force in the direction of the long axis of the forearm.

Accessory With Physiologic Motion Technique (Not pictured)
- **Patient/Clinician Position:** The patient is in a sitting position as described above. You are sitting in the same position as described above.
- **Hand Placement:** Your hand contacts are the same as that described above.
- **Force Application:** As the patient actively flexes and extends the wrist, apply a distraction force. Be prepared to move during the mobilization to ensure correct force application. Force is maintained throughout the entire range of motion and sustained at end range.

Radiocarpal Dorsal and Volar Glide

Indications:
- *Radiocarpal dorsal glides* are indicated for restricitons in wrist flexion. *Radiocarpal volar glides* are indicated for restrictions in wrist extension.

Accessory Motion Technique: (Figs. 24-31, 24-32)
- **Patient/Clinician Position:** The patient is sitting with the elbow flexed to 90 degrees and forearm pronated with the wrist in neutral and the hand over the edge of table. You may pre-position the patient with the wrist at the point of restriction. Sit on the ipsilateral side of the wrist being mobilized.
- **Hand Placement:** With your stabilization hand grasp the distal radius and ulna. Place your mobilization hand immediately adjacent to the stabilization hand just distal to the patient's wrist over the proximal row of carpal bones. Be sure that your forearm is in line with the direction of force.

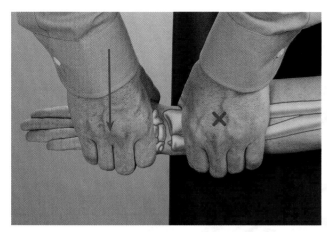

FIGURE 24–31 Radiocarpal dorsal glide.

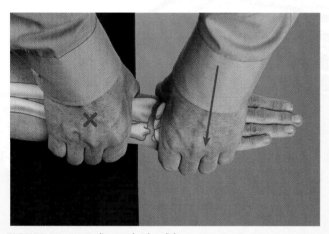

FIGURE 24–32 Radiocarpal volar glide.

- **Force Application:** Take up the slack in the joint, and apply force in an upward direction for dorsal glides and apply force in a downward direction for volar glides.

Accessory With Physiologic Motion Technique (Not pictured)

- **Patient/Clinician Position:** The patient is in a sitting position as described above. You are sitting in the same position as described above.
- **Hand Placement:** Your hand contacts are the same as that described above.
- **Force Application:** As the patient actively flexes the wrist, apply a dorsal glide. As the patient actively extends the wrist, apply a volar glide. Be prepared to move during the mobilization to ensure correct force application. Force is maintained throughout the entire range of motion and sustained at end range.

Radiocarpal Medial and Lateral Glide

Indications:

- *Radiocarpal medial and lateral glides* are indicated for restrictions in RD and UD, respectively.

Accessory Motion Technique: (Figs. 24-33, 24-34)

- **Patient/Clinician Position**: The patient is sitting with her elbow flexed to 90 degrees and her forearm between pronation and supination with her hand over the edge of the table. You may pre-position the patient with her wrist at the point of restriction. Sit on the ipsilateral side of the wrist being mobilized.
- **Hand Placement:** Grasp the distal radius and ulna with your stabilization hand. Place your mobilization hand immediately adjacent to your stabilization hand, just distal to the patient's wrist over the proximal row of carpal bones.
- **Force Application:** Force is applied in a downward direction for medial glides and an upward direction for lateral glide.

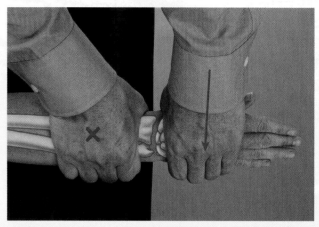

FIGURE 24–33 Radiocarpal medial glide.

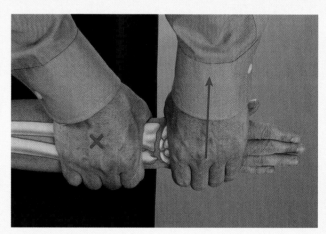

FIGURE 24–34 Radiocarpal lateral glide.

Accessory With Physiologic Motion Technique (Fig. 24-35)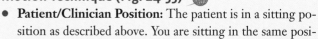

- **Patient/Clinician Position:** The patient is in a sitting position as described above. You are sitting in the same position as described above.
- **Hand Placement:** Your hand contacts are the same as that described above.
- **Force Application:** The patient actively moves into wrist flexion, extension, radial deviation or ulnar deviation as you apply a medial or lateral glide through the mobilization

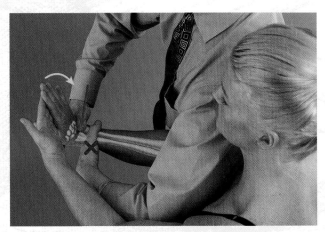

FIGURE 24–35 Radiocarpal medial or lateral glide accessory with physiologic motion.

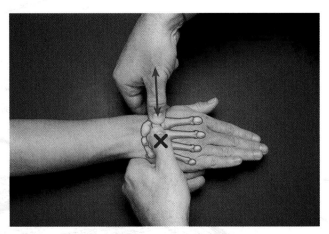

FIGURE 24–36 Midcarpal and intercarpal multiplanar glide.

hand. The patient applies overpressure at end range. Be prepared to move during the mobilization to ensure correct force application. Force is maintained throughout the entire range of motion and sustained at end range.

Midcarpal and Intercarpal Joint Mobilizations

Midcarpal and Intercarpal Multiplanar Glide

Indications:
- *Midcarpal and intercarpal dorsal and volar glides* of the proximal row of carpal bones are indicated for restrictions in wrist flexion and extension, respectively. *Midcarpal and intercarpal dorsal and volar glides* of the distal row of carpal bones are indicated for restrictions in wrist extension and flexion, respectively. *Multiplanar glides* are indicated for intercarpal mobility in all directions.

Accessory Motion Technique (Fig. 24-36)
- **Patient/Clinician Position:** The patient is in a sitting position with the forearm fully pronated and supported on table. You may pre-position the elbow at the point of restriction. Sit on the ipsilateral side of the elbow being mobilized.
- **Hand Placement:** *Tip-to-tip pinch grasp* contacts two adjacent carpal bones.
- **Force Application:** Force is applied in a dorsal, volar, or multiplanar fashion in the direction of greatest restriction.

Accessory With Physiologic Motion Technique (Not pictured)
  Patient/Clinician Position: The patient is in a sitting position as described above. You are sitting in the same position as described above.
  Hand Placement: Your hand contacts are the same as that described above.

Force Application: The patient actively performs wrist movement in any direction as stabilization and mobilization contacts are maintained throughout the range of motion and sustained at end range.

Carpometacarpal Joint Mobilizations

Carpometacarpal Distraction and Glide

Indications:
- *Carpometacarpal distractions* are indicated when there is a loss of mobility in all directions.
- At the first CMC joint, *glides* toward palm of hand are indicated for restrictions in abduction, and *glides* away from the palm are indicated for restrictions in adduction.
- *Lateral glides* of the first CMC joint are indicated for restrictions in extension, and *medial glides* are indicated for restrictions in flexion.
- For second to fifth CMC joint, *glides* toward the palm of hand are indicated for restrictions in flexion and *glides* away from the palm are indicated for restrictions in extension.

Accessory Motion Technique (Figs. 24-37, 24-38)
- **Patient/Clinician Position:** The patient is in a sitting position with the forearm fully pronated and the palm facing downward. You may pre-position the hand with the joint at the point of restriction. Sit on the ipsilateral side of the hand being mobilized.
- **Hand Placement:** Grasp the distal row carpal bone between the finger and thumb of the stabilization hand. With your mobilization hand, grasp the base of the metacarpal immediately adjacent to the stabilizing hand.
- **Force Application:** Take up the slack in the joint and apply force in the direction of the long axis of the metacarpal. For volar glides, apply downward force. For dorsal glides, apply upward force.

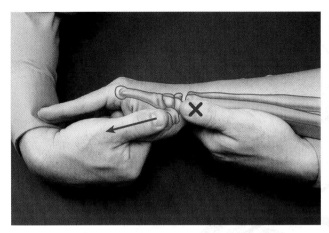

FIGURE 24–37 Carpometacarpal distraction.

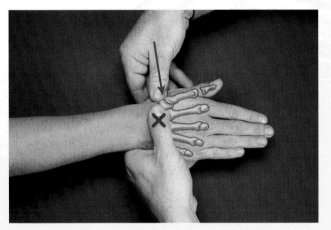

FIGURE 24–38 Carpometacarpal glide.

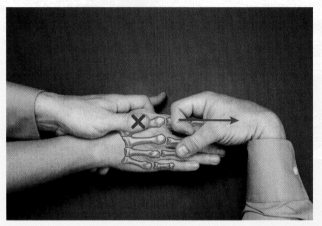

FIGURE 24–39 Metacarpophalangeal distraction.

Accessory Motion Technique (Fig. 24-39)

- **Patient/Clinician Position**: The patient is in a sitting position with the forearm fully pronated and the palm facing downward. The MCP joint is in 20 degrees of flexion. You may pre-position the hand with the joint at the point of restriction. Sit on the ipsilateral side of the hand being mobilized.
- **Hand Placement:** Grasp the metacarpal head between the thumb and index finger of the stabilization hand. Grasp the proximal phalanx immediately adjacent to the stabilization hand using a *hook grasp* or *pinch grasp* of your mobilization hand.
- **Force Application:** Take up the slack in the joint and apply force in the direction of the long axis of the phalanx.

Accessory With Physiologic Motion Technique (Not pictured)

- **Patient/Clinician Position:** The patient is in a sitting position as described above. You are sitting in the same position as described above.
- **Hand Placement:** Your hand contacts are the same as that described above.
- **Force Application:** As the patient actively performs MCP flexion and extension, apply distraction that is maintained throughout the entire range of motion and sustained at end range. Adjust the direction of force to remain in line with the long axis of the phalanx.

Metacarpophalangeal Dorsal and Volar Glide

Indications:

- *Metacarpophalangeal dorsal glides* are indicated for restrictions in MCP extension. *Metacarpophalangeal volar glides* are indicated for restrictions in MCP flexion.

Accessory Motion Technique (Fig. 24-40)

- **Patient/Clinician Position**: The patient is in a sitting position with the forearm fully pronated and the palm facing

Accessory With Physiologic Motion Technique (Not pictured)

- **Patient/Clinician Position:** The patient is in a sitting position as described above. You are sitting in the same position as described above.
- **Hand Placement:** Your hand contacts are the same as that described above.
- **Force Application:** As the patient actively performs CMC flexion, extension, abduction, and adduction, distraction or glide of the joint is maintained throughout the entire range of motion and sustained at end range. Adjust the direction of force to remain in line with the long axis of the phalanx.

Metacarpophalangeal Joint Mobilizations

Metacarpophalangeal Distraction

Indications:

- *Metacarpophalangeal distractions* are indicated when there is a loss of mobility in all directions.

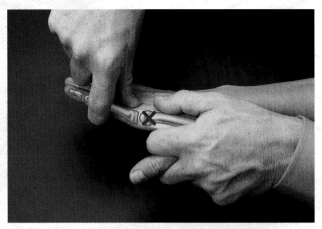

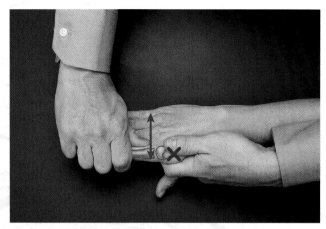

FIGURE 24–40 Metacarpophalangeal dorsal and volar glide.

FIGURE 24–41 Metacarpophalangeal medial and lateral glide.

downward. The MCP joint is in 20 degrees of flexion. You may pre-position the hand with the joint at the point of restriction. Sit on the ipsilateral side of the hand being mobilized.

- **Hand Position:** To stabilize, grasp the metacarpal head between the thumb and index finger. Grasp the base of the proximal phalanx immediately adjacent to the stabilization hand.
- **Force Application:** Take up the slack in the joint and apply force in a downward direction for volar glides and an upward direction for dorsal glides.

Accessory With Physiologic Motion Technique (Not pictured)

- **Patient/Clinician Position:** The patient is in a sitting position as described above. You are sitting in the same position as described above.
- **Hand Placement:** Your hand contacts are the same as that described above.
- **Force Application:** As the patient actively performs MCP flexion and extension, apply volar and dorsal glides that are maintained throughout the range of motion and sustained at end range. Adjust the direction of force to ensure proper force application.

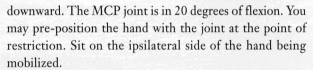

Metacarpophalangeal Medial and Lateral Glide

Indications:

- *Metacarpophalangeal medial glides* are indicated for restrictions in MCP abduction. *Metacarpophalangeal lateral glides* are indicated for restrictions in MCP adduction.

Accessory Motion Technique (Fig. 24-41)

- **Patient/Clinician Position**: The patient is in a sitting position with the forearm fully pronated and the palm facing downward. The MCP joint is in 20 degrees of flexion. You may pre-position the hand with the joint at the point

of restriction. Sit on the ipsilateral side of the hand being mobilized.

- **Hand Placement:** To stabilize, grasp the metacarpal head between the thumb and index finger. Grasp the base of the proximal phalanx immediately adjacent to the stabilization hand.
- **Force Application:** Apply force in a medial and lateral direction as indicated.

Accessory With Physiologic Motion Technique (Fig. 24-42)

- **Patient/Clinician Position:** The patient is in a sitting position as described above. You are sitting in the same position as described above.
- **Hand Placement:** Your hand contacts are the same as that described above.
- **Force Application:** As the patient actively performs MCP flexion and extension, lateral and medial glides are maintained throughout the range of motion and sustained at end range.

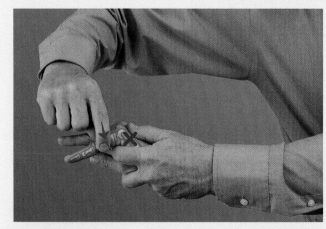

FIGURE 24–42 Metacarpophalangeal medial or lateral glide accessory with physiologic motion.

Proximal/Distal Interphalangeal Joint Mobilizations

Proximal/Distal Interphalangeal Distraction

Indications:
- *Proximal/distal interphalangeal distractions* are indicated when there is a loss of mobility in all directions.

Accessory Motion Technique (Fig. 24-43)
- **Patient/Clinician Position**: The patient is in a sitting position with the forearm fully pronated and the palm facing downward. The IP joint is in 20 degrees of flexion. You may pre-position the hand with the joint at the point of restriction. Sit on the ipsilateral side of the hand being mobilized.
- **Hand Placement:** To stabilize, grasp the proximal phalanx between the thumb and index finger. Contact the base of the distal phalanx immediately adjacent to the stabilization hand using a hook or pinch grasp.
- **Force Application:** Apply force in the direction of the long axis of the phalanx.

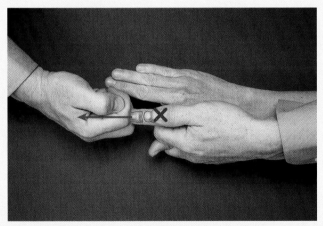

FIGURE 24–43 Proximal/distal interphalangeal distraction.

Accessory With Physiologic Motion Technique (Not pictured)
- **Patient/Clinician Position:** The patient is in a sitting position as described above. You are sitting in the same position as described above.
- **Hand Placement:** Your hand contacts are the same as that described above.
- **Force Application:** As the patient actively performs IP flexion and extension, distraction is maintained throughout the entire range of motion and sustained at end range. Adjust the direction of force to ensure proper force application.

Proximal/Distal Interphalangeal Dorsal and Volar Glide

Indications:
- *Proximal/distal interphalangeal dorsal and volar glides* are indicated for restrictions in IP extension and flexion, respectively.

Accessory Motion Technique (Fig. 24-44)
- **Patient/Clinician Position:** The patient is in a sitting position with the forearm fully pronated and the palm facing downward. The IP joint is in 20 degrees of flexion. You may pre-position the hand with the joint at the point of restriction. Sit on the ipsilateral side of the hand being mobilized.
- **Hand Placement:** To stabilize, grasp the proximal phalanx between the thumb and index finger. Grasp the distal phalanx immediately adjacent to the stabilization hand.
- **Force Application:** Apply force in an upward or downward direction for dorsal and volar glides, respectively.

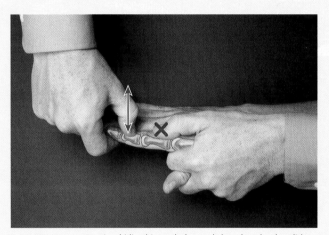

FIGURE 24–44 Proximal/distal interphalangeal dorsal and volar glide.

Accessory With Physiologic Motion Technique (Not pictured)
- **Patient/Clinician Position:** The patient is in a sitting position as described above. You are sitting in the same position as described above.
- **Hand Placement:** Your hand contacts are the same as that described above.
- **Force Application:** As patient actively performs IP flexion and extension, glide is maintained throughout the entire range of motion and sustained at end range.

Intercarpal Joint Mobilizations

Intercarpal Volar/Dorsal Glide High Velocity Thrust

Indications:

- *Intercarpal dorsal/volar glide high velocity thrusts* are indicated for the purpose of altering positional relationships, breaking through adhesions that may be restricting motion, or to facilitate general improvements in mobility at any of the intercarpal joints.

Accessory Motion Technique (Fig. 24-45 A, B)

- **Patient/Clinican Position:** The patient is in a sitting position with the wrist in approximately 20 degrees of flexion with fingers relaxed for volar glides and 20 degrees of extension for dorsal glides. You are standing facing the patient.
- **Hand Placement:** Both hands grasp the patient's hand. Thumb over thumb contact is placed on the dorsal aspect of the carpal bone to be mobilized for volar glides and on the volar aspect of the carpal bone for dorsal glides. Fingers wrap around hand and control wrist motion.
- **Force Application:** From the starting position, the wrist is brought toward extension or flexion, and at end range a short-amplitude, high-velocity thrust is applied in a volar or dorsal direction through the thumb contacts.

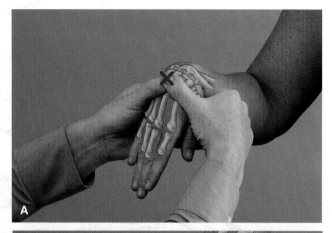

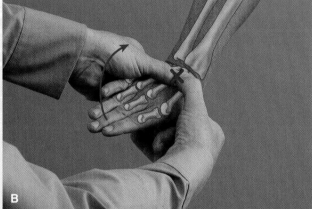

FIGURE 24–45 Intercarpal volar or dorsal glide high velocity thrust.

CLINICAL CASE

CASE 1

Subjective Examination

History of Present Illness

A 55-year-old, right-hand dominant, postmenopausal administrative assistant presents to your office today reporting paresthesia and occasional numbness into the first three digits of her right hand, which increases after a particularly busy day at work. Her symptoms appear to worsen at night and often prohibit her from obtaining a full night's sleep. She denies complaint of pain at this time and denies history of trauma or injury to her cervical spine or upper extremity, with the exception of a fall on outstretched hand with palm open approximately 3 months ago.

Past Medical History: Positive for noninsulin dependent diabetes mellitus.

Objective Physical Examination

Examination of Structure: Absence of edema, erythema. Slight atrophy of the thenar eminence is noted upon bilateral comparison.

Upper Quarter Screen: Cervical spine and shoulders are within normal limits (WNL), with no change in existing symptoms upon testing.

Examination of Mobility

Physiologic Mobility Testing: Active range of motion (AROM) and passive range of motion (PROM) of the right wrist and hand are grossly within normal limits at this time, with the exception of active thumb opposition, which reveals the inability to perform opposition between the thumb and fifth digit. Passive opposition is WNL.

Accessory Mobility Testing: Reduced intercarpal dorsal glide of the right lunate is noted. Volar glide of the lunate reveals hypermobility, with reproduction of thenar paresthesia.

Examination of Muscle Function: Right thumb opposition, abduction, and flexion are all 3+/5. Five-position Jamar dynamometer hand grip testing reveals the following:

1: Right = 25 lb, Left = 33 lb
2: Right = 46 lb, Left = 57 lb
3: Right = 67 lb, Left = 84 lb
4: Right = 43 lb, Left = 52 lb
5: Right = 27 lb, Left = 36 lb

Neurological Testing: DTRs at biceps, triceps, brachioradialis = 2+. Diminished light touch sensation and two-point discrimination at digits 1 to 3, volar and dorsal.

Palpation: Slight tenderness to the touch over the volar wrist and proximal row of carpal bones. The lunate on the right is volarly displaced compared to the left.

Special Testing: Right Phalen test is positive, right Tinel sign at wrist is positive, Allen and Adson tests are negative, cervical quadrant sign is negative.

Discuss the following:

1. Based on your examination findings, what is your initial working hypothesis regarding the cause of this patient's symptoms? What is your differential diagnosis? Briefly review the anatomical structures typically involved in this condition.

2. Do you believe that this condition is isolated to the wrist and hand? How have you or would you rule out contributions from proximal structures?

3. Identify the pertinent aspects of this patient's history that contribute to your initial hypothesis? Do you believe this patient's report of falling has contributed to her condition? If so, how?

4. How might your structural examination findings relate to this condition? How do your structural examination findings impact your assessment of time since onset and prognosis?

5. Provide rationale for your findings upon mobility testing. How do your AROM findings impact your assessment of time since onset and prognosis? How might the results of your mobility examination serve to guide intervention?

6. Should the results of hand grip testing be considered normal? How might hand grip testing be used to guide intervention and document progress and outcomes?

7. Based on the results of your examination, develop a prioritized problem list and briefly describe your plan of care, including all manual and nonmanual interventions.

CASE 2

Subjective Examination

History of Present Illness

A 32-year-old, left-hand dominant male presents to your office today with report of falling on an outstretched hand and landing on the dorsum of the left hand 9 weeks ago. After radiographic imaging that revealed a Smith's fracture, a closed reduction was performed, followed by application of a short arm cast that was removed 2 days ago. This patient is a carpenter with no light duty available and is currently out of work until further notice.

Past Medical History: Unremarkable.

Objective Physical Examination

Examination of Structure: Observation reveals significant atrophy of the entire forearm, with some erythema and flaky skin. Edema is observed within the left hand.

Upper Quarter Screen: Cervical spine and shoulder is WNL, with no effect on symptoms.

Examination of Mobility

Physiologic Mobility Testing: Left upper extremity reveals the following:

MOTION	AROM	PROM	END-FEEL
Pronation	46 degrees	65 degrees	Capsular
Supination	70 degrees	75 degrees	Capsular
Wrist Flexion	15 degrees	22 degrees	Empty
Wrist Extension	11 degrees	14 degrees	Empty
Radial Deviation	27 degrees	40 degrees	Empty
Ulnar Deviation	40 degrees	50 degrees	Capsular
MCP Flexion	65 degrees	75 degrees	Soft
MCP Extension	45 degrees	60 degrees	Soft

Accessory Mobility Testing: Reduced radiocarpal dorsal and volar glide and medial and lateral glide. Reduced distal radioulnar superior glide. Reduced MCP dorsal glide. All glides are nonpainful, revealing a stiffness-dominant condition.

Examination of Muscle Function: Grossly 4/5 throughout left wrist and hand, with the exception of wrist flexion and extension, which is 4–/5 and painful.

Neurological Testing: WNL throughout.

Palpation: Moderate tenderness to the touch over both the volar and dorsal aspects of the distal radius and ulna.

Discuss the following:

1. What is the difference between a Colles's fracture and a Smith's fracture? Describe the mechanism of injury for each. What is the typical sequelae of distal wrist fractures, and how might you curtail this process?

2. Given the nature of this injury, what physiologic and accessory movements would you expect to be limited, and why? Is this patient's movement profile consistent with your expectations?

3. Describe in detail and practice on your partner the specific mobilizations that you would use to restore normal range of motion and provide rationale for each. Use accessory mobilization only and accessory mobilization with physiologic movement procedures to treat this patient.

4. What other nonmanual intervention strategies might you employ when working with this patient? Briefly discuss the manner in which you would sequence these interventions to facilitate optimal outcomes and provide rationale.

HANDS-ON

With a partner, perform the following activities:

1 Consider the key indicators that may be revealed during the history and "interrogation" of your partner that may suggest the presence of the following conditions. These indicators may include such things as the mechanism of injury or pain pattern. Based on these indicators, what examination procedures might you use to rule in or rule out the presence of each particular condition? Complete the grid.

DYSFUNCTION	HISTORICAL INDICATORS	CONFIRMATORY SIGNS
Colles's Fracture vs. Smith's Fracture vs. Scaphoid/Lunate Fracture		
Carpal Tunnel Syndrome		
Rheumatoid Arthritis vs. Osteoarthritis		
DeQuervain's Syndrome		
Dupuytren's Contracture		
Boutonniere Deformity vs. Swan-Neck Deformity vs. Mallet Finger		
TFCC Lesions		
Peripheral Neuropathies		
Complex Regional Pain Syndrome (CRPS)		

2 Observe your partner as he or she performs active physiologic movements over single and repeated repetitions and single and multiplane directions, and identify the quantity, quality, and any reproduction of symptoms that may be produced. Compare these active movements with performance of these same movements passively.

3 In an attempt to relate each impairment to a structural cause, provide several possible pathoanatomical etiologies for each of the movement impairments identified during active and passive physiologic movement testing above. Complete the grid.

ACTIVE PHYSIOLOGIC MOVEMENT IMPAIRMENT	PASSIVE PHYSIOLOGIC MOVEMENT IMPAIRMENT	POSSIBLE PATHOANATOMIC ETIOLOGY

4 Perform passive physiologic movement testing in all directions followed by passive accessory movement testing in all planes, and determine the relationship between the onset of pain (Pain 1 or P1 and Pain 2 or P2, if present) and stiffness or resistance (Resistance 1 or R1 and Resistance 2 or R2). Determine the end-feel in each direction. Compare your findings bilaterally and on another partner.

5 Perform passive accessory movement testing in all planes with the wrist and hand in the neutral, or open-packed, position. Then perform the same tests with the wrist/hand in other non-neutral and close-packed positions. Identify any changes in the quantity and quality of available motion and report any reproduction of symptoms. Consider which anatomical structures are most responsible for limiting motion in each position. Complete the grid.

PASSIVE ACCESSORY MOVEMENT	QUANTITY, QUALITY, REPRODUCTION IN NEUTRAL	QUANTITY, QUALITY, REPRODUCTION IN NON-NEUTRAL	LIMITING STRUCTURES
Distal RU Dorsal/Volar Glide			
Distal RU Inferior Glide			
Distal RU Superior Glide			
RC Distraction			
RC Dorsal/Volar Glide			
RC Medial/Lateral Glide			
MC, IC Multiplanar Glides			
CMC Distraction/Glides			
MCP Distraction/Glides			
PIP, DIP Distraction/Glides			

6 Perform muscle testing for the key muscles about the wrist and hand using isometric break testing, static testing, and active testing based on the functional preference of each muscle during normal activity. Complete the grid.

MUSCLE TESTED	FUNCTIONAL PREFERENCE/ MANNER OF TESTING	RESULTS

7 Through palpation, attempt to identify the primary soft tissue and bony structures of the wrist and hand and compare tissue texture, tension, tone, and location, bilaterally.

8 Based on your movement examination as identified above, choose two mobilizations. Perform these mobilizations on your partner and identify any immediate changes in mobility or symptoms in response to these procedures.

9 Perform each mobilization described in the intervention section of this chapter bilaterally on at least two individuals. Using each technique, practice Grades I to IV. Then switch and allow your partner to mobilize your elbow. Provide input to your partner regarding setup, technique, comfort, and so on. When practicing these mobilization techniques, utilize the Sequential Partial Task Practice Method, in which students repeatedly practice one aspect of each technique (i.e., position, hand placement, force application) on multiple partners each time adding the next component until the technique is performed in real time from beginning to end. (Wise CH, Schenk RJ, Lattanzi JB. A model for teaching and learning spinal thrust manipulation and its effect on participant confidence in technique performance. *J. Man. Manip. Ther.*, August 2014.)

REFERENCES

1. Levangie PK, Norkin CC. *Joint Structure and Function: A Comprehensive Analysis*. 4th ed. Philadelphia, PA: FA Davis; 2005.
2. Ekenstam FA. Anatomy of the distal radioulnar joint. *Clin Orthop*. 1992;275:14-18.
3. Jaffe R, Chidgey LK, LeStayo PC. The distal radioulnar joint: anatomy and management of disorders. *J Hand Ther*. 1996;9:129-138.
4. Linscheid RL. Biomechanics of the distal radioulnar joint. *Clin Orthop*. 1992;275:46-55.
5. Schuind F, An KN, Berglund L, et al. The distal radioulnar ligaments: a biomechanical study. *J Hand Surg*. 1991;16A:1106-1114.
6. Kleinman WB, Graham TJ. The distal radioulnar joint capsule: clinical anatomy and role in posttraumatic limitation of forearm rotation. *J Hand Surg*. 1998;23A:588-599.
7. Oatis CA. *Kinesiology: The Mechanics and Pathomechanics of Human Movement*. Philadelphia, PA: Lippincott Williams & Wilkins; 2004.
8. Shaw JA, Bruno A, Paul EM. Ulnar styloid fixation in the treatment of posttraumatic instability of the radioulnar joint: a biomechanical study with clinical correlation. *J Hand Surg*. 1990;15A:712-720.
9. Garcia-Elias M. Soft tissue anatomy and relationships about the distal ulna. *Hand Clin*. 1998;14:165-176.
10. Defrate LE, Li G, Zayontz SJ, Herndon JH. A minimally invasive method for the determination of force in the interosseous ligament. *Clin Biomech*. 2001;16:895-900.

11. Tubiana R, Thomine JM, Mackin E. *Examination of the Hand and Wrist.* Philadelphia, PA: WB Saunders; 1996.
12. Szabo RM, Weber SC. Comminuted intraarticular fractures of the distal radius. *Clin Orthop.* 1988;230:39-48.
13. Drobner WS, Hausman MR. The distal radioulnar joint. *Hand Clin.* 1992;8:631-644.
14. Palmer AK, Glisson RR, Werner FW. Ulnar variance determination. *J Hand Surg.* 1982;7:376-379.
15. Green D, Hotchkiss RN, Pederson WC. *Operative Hand Surgery.* 4th ed. New York, NY: Churchill Livingstone; 1999.
16. Palmer A, Glisson RR, Werner FW. Relationship between ulnar variance and triangular fibrocartilage complex thickness. *J Hand Ther.* 1984;9:681-682.
17. Kobayashi M, Berger RA, Linscheid RL, An KN. Intercarpal kinematics during wrist motion. *Hand Clin.* 1997;13:143-149.
18. Kapandji IA. *Physiology of the Joints.* Vol 1. *The Upper Limb.* Edinburgh, Scotland: Churchill Livingstone; 1982.
19. Williams P, Bannister L, Berry M, et al. *Gray's Anatomy, The Anatomical Basis of Medicine and Surgery.* London, UK: Churchill Livingstone; 1995.
20. Nowalk M, Logan S. Distinguishing biomechanical properties of intrinsic and extrinsic human wrist ligaments. *J Biomech Eng.* 1991;113:85-93.
21. Taleisnik J. The ligaments of the wrist. *J Hand Surg.* 1976;1:110-118.
22. Mizuseki T, Ikuta Y. The dorsal carpal ligaments: their anatomy and function. *J Hand Surg.* 1989;14:91-98.
23. Belvens A, Light T, Jablonsky W, et al. Radiocarpal articular contact characteristics with scaphoid instability. *J Hand Surg.* 1989;14:781-790.
24. Shin AY, Battaglia MJ, Bishop AT. Lunotriquetral instability: Diagnosis and treatment. *J Am Acad Orthop Surg.* 2000;8:170-179.
25. Vegas S, Yamaguchi S, Boyd N, et al. The dorsal ligaments of the wrist: anatomy, mechanical properties, and function. *J Hand Surg.* 1999;24:456-468.
26. Nowalk MD, Logan SE. Distinguishing biomechanical properties of intrinsic and extrinsic human wrist ligaments. *J Biomech Eng.* 1991;113:85-93.
27. Youm Y, McMurthy RY, Flatt AE, et al. Kinematics of the wrist. An experimental study of radial-ulnar deviation and flexion-extension. *J Bone Joint Surg.* 1978;60:423.
28. Neu CP, Crisco JJ, Wolfe SW. In vivo kinematic behavior of the radio-capitate joint during wrist flexion-extension and radio-ulnar deviation. *J Biomech.* 2001;34:1429-1438.
29. Ruby LK, Cooney WP, An KN, et al. Relative motion of selected carpal bones: a kinematic analysis of the normal wrist. *J Hand Surg.* 1988;13:1-10.
30. Garcia-Ellis M. Kinetic analysis of carpal stability during grip. *Hand Clin.* 1997;13:151-158.
31. Berger RA. The anatomy and basic biomechanics of the wrist joint. *J Hand Ther.* 1996;9:84-93.
32. Berger RA, Crowninshield RD, Flatt AE. The three-dimensional rotational behaviors of the carpal bones. *Clin Orthop.* 1982;167:303-310.
33. Patterson R, Nicodemus CL, Viegas SF, et al. Normal wrist kinematics and the analysis of the effect of various dynamic external fixators for treatment of distal radius fractures. *Hand Clin.* 1997;13:129-141.
34. Sarrafian SK, Melamed JK, Goshgarian GM. Study of wrist motion in flexion and extension. *Clin Orthop.* 1977;126:153-159.
35. Patterson R, Nicodemus CL, Viegas SF, et al. High-speed, three-dimensional kinematic analysis of the normal wrist. *J Hand Surg.* 1998;23A:446-453.
36. Conwell H. *Injuries to the Wrist.* Summit, NJ: CIBA Pharmaceutical; 1970.
37. Patterson R, Viegas S. Biomechanics of the wrist. *J Hand Ther.* 1995;8:97-105.
38. Taleisnik J. Current concepts review: carpal instability. *J Bone Joint Surg.* 1988;70:1262-1268.
39. MacConaill M. The mechanical anatomy of the carpus and its bearing on some surgical problems. *J Anat.* 1941;75:166.
40. Cooney WP, Lucca MJ, Chao EYS, Inscheid RL. The kinesiology of the thumb trapeziometacarpaal joint. *J Bone Joint Surg.* 1981;63A:1371-1381.
41. Harty M. The hand of man. *Phys Ther.* 1971;51:777-781.
42. Romanes GJE. *Cunningham's Textbook of Anatomy.* Oxford, England: Oxford University Press; 1981.
43. Ritt M, Berger R, Kauer J. The gross and histologic anatomy of the ligaments of the capitohamate joint. *J Hand Surg.* 1996;21:1022-1028.
44. Imaeda T, An KN, Cooney WP. Functional anatomy and biomechanics of the thumb. *Hand Clin.* 1992;8:9-15.
45. Nakamura K, Patterson RM, Viegas SF. The ligament and skeletal anatomy of the second through fifth carpometacrapal joints and adjacent structures. *J Hand Surg.* 2001;26:1016-1029.
46. Barmakian JT. Anatomy of the joints of the thumb. *Hand Clin.* 1992; 8:683-691.
47. Benjamin M, Ralphs J, Shibu M, et al. Capsular tissue of the proximal interphalangeal joint: normal composition and effects of Dupuytren's disease and rheumatoid arthritis. *J Hand Surg.* 1993;18:370-376.
48. Minami A, An KN, Cooney WP, et al. Ligament stability of the metacarpophalangeal joint. A biomechanical study. *J Hand Surg.* 1985;10A:255-260.
49. Minami A, An KN, Cooney WP, et al. Ligamentous structures of the metacarpophalangeal joint: a quantitative anatomic study. *J Orthop Res.* 1984;1:361-368.
50. Shultz R, Storace A, Kirshnamurthy S. Metacarpophalangeal joint motion and the role of the collateral ligaments. *Int Orthop.* 11:1987;149-155.
51. Fioretti S, Jetto L, Leo T. Reliable in vivo estimation of the instantaneous helical axis in human segmental movements. *IEEE Trans Biomed Eng.* 1990;37:398-409.
52. Bowers WH, Wolf JW, Nehil JL, et al. The proximal interphalangeal joint volar plate. I. An anatomical and biomechanical study. *J Hand Surg.* 1980;5:79-88.
53. Eberhardt K, Malcus Johnson P, Rydgren L. The occurrence and significance of hand deformities in early rheumatoid arthritis. *Brit J Rheumatol.* 1991;30:211-213.
54. Boissonnault WG. *Primary Care for the Physical Therapist: Examination and Triage.* St. Louis, MO: Elsevier Saunders; 2005.
55. Magee DJ. *Orthopedic Physical Assessment.* 5th ed. Philadelphia, PA: WB Saunders; 2008.
56. Saar JD, Grothaus PC. Dupuytren's disease: an overview. *Plast Reconstr Surg.* 2000;106:125-136.
57. Dutton M. *Orthopaedic Examination, Evaluation, & Intervention.* New York, NY: McGraw-Hill; 2004.
58. Brand P, Hollister A. *Clinical Mechanics of the Hand.* 3rd ed. St. Louis, MO: Mosby-Year Book; 1999.
59. Buchanan TS, Moniz MJ, Dewald JPA, Rymer WZ. Estimation of muscle forces about the wrist joint during isometric tasks using an EMG coefficient method. *J Biomech.* 1993;26:547-560.
60. Basmajian JV, DeLuca CJ. *Muscles Alive. Their Function Revealed by Electromyography.* Baltimore, MO: Williams & Wilkins; 1985.
61. Ryu JR, Cooney WP, Askew LJ, et al. Functional ranges of motion of the wrist joint. *J Hand Surg.* 1991;16A:409-419.
62. Loren GJ, Shoemaker SD, Burkholder TJ, et al. Human wrist motors: biomechanical design and application to tendon transfers. *J Biomech.* 1996;29:331-342.
63. Close JR, Kidd CC. The functions of the muscles of the thumb, the index, and the long fingers. *J Bone Joint Surg.* 1969;51A:1601-1620.
64. Brandsma JW, Oudenaarde EV, Oostendorp R. The abductors pollicis muscles: clinical considerations based on electromyographical and anatomical studies. *J Hand Ther.* 1996;9:218-222.
65. Cooney WP, An KN, Daube JR, Askew LJ. Electromyographic analysis of the thumb: a study of isometric forces in pinch and grasp. *J Hand Surg.* 1985;10A:202-210.
66. Bechtol CO. Grip test: the use of a dynamometer with adjustable hand spacings. *J Bone Joint Surg.* 1954;36A:820-824.
67. Mathiowetz V. Reliability and validity of grip and pinch strength evaluations. *J Hand Surg.* 11984;9A:222-226.
68. Fess EE. The need for reliability and validity in hand assessment instruments. *J Hand Surg.* 1986;11A:621-623.
69. Service Research Associates. *Purdue Pegboard Test of Manipulative Dexterity.* Chicago, IL: Service Research Associates; 1968.
70. Blair SJ, et al. Evalution of impairment of the upper extremity. *Clin Orthop.* 1987;221:42-58.
71. LaStayo P, Howell J. Clinical provocative tests used in evaluating wrist pain: a descriptive study. *J Hand Ther.* 1995;8:10-17.
72. Wainner RS, Fritz JM, Irrgang JJ, et al. Development of a clinical prediction rule for the diagnosis of carpal tunnel syndrome. *Arch Phys Med Rehabil.* 2005;86:609-618.
73. Marx RG, Bombardier C, Wright JC. What do we know about the reliability & validity of physical examination tests used to examine the upper extremity? *J Hand Surg.* 1999;24A:185-193.
74. Ahn D. Hand elevation: a new test for carpal tunnel syndrome. *Ann Plast Surg.* 2001;46:120-124.
75. Heller L, Ring H, Costeff H, Solzi P. Evaluation of Tinel's & Phalen's signs in diagnosis of the carpal tunnel syndrome. *Eur Neurol.* 1986;25:40-42.
76. Szabo RM, Slater RR. Diagnostic testing in carpal tunnel syndrome. *J Hand Surg.* 2000;25:184.
77. Gonzalez del Pinto, et al. Value of the carpal compression test in the diagnosis of carpal tunnel syndrome. *J Hand Surg Br.* 1997;22:38-41.
78. Hansen P, Mickelsen P, Robinson L. Clinical utility of the flick maneuver in diagnosing carpal tunnel syndrome. *Am J Phys Med Rehabil.* 2004;83:363-367.
79. Gunnarsson LG, Amilon A, Hellstrand P, Leissner P, Philipson L. The diagnosis of carpal tunnel syndrome. Sensitivity & specificity of some clinical & electrophysiological tests. *J Hand Surg.* 1997;22:34-37.

80. Katz J, Larson M, Sabra A, et al. The carpal tunnel syndrome: diagnosis utility of the history and physical examination findings. *Ann Interna Med.* 1990;112:321-327.
81. Tetro AM, Evanoff BA, Hollstien SB, Gelberman RH. A new provocation test for carpal tunnel syndrome. Assessment of wrist flexion & nerve compression. *J Bone Joint Surg.* 1998;80:493-498.
82. Moldaver J: Tinel's sign: its characteristics & significance. *J Bone Joint Surg Am.* 1978;60:412-414.
83. Blacker GJ, Lister GD. The abducted little finger in low ulnar nerve palsy. *J. Hand Surg.* 1991;16:967-974.
84. Goldman SB, Brininger TL, Schrader JW, Koceja DM. A review of clinical tests & signs for the assessment of ulnar neuropathy. *J Hand Ther.* 2009;22:209-220.
85. Wartenberg R. A sign of ulnar palsy. *JAMA.* 1939;112:1688.
86. Bradshaw DY, Shefner JM. Ulnar neuropathy at the elbow. *Neurol Clin.* 1999;17:447-461.
87. Feindel W, J Stratford J. Cubital tunnel compression in tardy ulnar palsy. *Can Med Assoc J.* 1958;78:351-353.
88. Miller RG. The cubital tunnel syndrome: diagnosis & precise localization. *Ann Neurol.* 1979;6:56-59.
89. Posner J. Compressive ulnar neuropathies at the elbow: I. Etiology & diagnosis. *J Am Acad Orthop Surg.* 1998;6:282-288.
90. Regan WD, Morrey BF. The physical examination of the elbow. In: Morrey BF, ed. *The Elbow & Its Disorders.* Philadelphia, PA: WB Saunders; 1993.
91. Lester B, et al. "Press test" for office diagnosis of triangular fibrocartilage complex tears of the wrist. *Ann Plast Surg.* 1995;35:41-45.
92. LaStayo P, Weiss S. The GRIT: a quantitative measure of ulnar impaction syndrome. *J Hand Ther.* 2001;14:173-179.
93. Watson HK, Ballet FL. The SLAC wrist: scapulolunate advanced collapse pattern of degenerative arthritis. *J Hand Surg Am.* 1984;9:358-365.
94. Watson HK, Ashmead D, Makhlouf MV. Examination of the scaphoid. *J Hand Surg Am.* 1988;13:657-660.
95. Young D, Papp S, Giachino A. Physical examination of the wrist. *Hand Clin.* 2010;26:21-36.
96. Young D, Giachino A. Clinical examination of scaphoid fractures. *Physician Sports Med.* 2009;37:97-105.
97. Lan LB. The scaphoid shift test. *J Hand Surg.* 1993;18A:366-368.
98. Taleisnik J: Carpal instability. *J Bone Joint Surg Am.* 1988;70:1262-1268.
99. Waeckerle JF. A prospective study identifying the sensitivity of radiographic findings & the efficacy of clinical findings in carpal navicular fractures. *Ann Emerg Med.* 1987;16:733-737.
100. Powell JM, Lloyd GJ, Rintoul RF. New clinical test for fracture of the scaphoid. *Can J Surg.* 1988;31:237-238.
101. Booher JM, Thibodeau GA. *Athletic Injury Assessment.* St. Louis, MO: CV Mosby; 1989.
102. Finkelstein H. Stenosing tendovaginitis at the radial styloid process. *J Bone Joint Surg.* 1930;12:509.
103. Batteson R, Hammond A, Burke F, Sinha S. The de Quervain's screening tool: validity and reliability of a measure to support clinical diagnosis and management. *Musculoskeletal Care.* 2008;6:168-180.
104. Alexander RD, Catalano LW, Barron OA, Glickel SZ. The extensor pollicis brevis entrapment test in the treatment of de Quervain's disease. *J Hand Surg.* 2002;27:813-816.

Orthopaedic Manual Physical Therapy of the Hip

Christopher H. Wise, PT, DPT, OCS, FAAOMPT, MTC, ATC

Chapter Objectives

At the conclusion of this chapter, the reader will be able to:

- Identify the key anatomical and biomechanical features of the hip, their relationship to the lumbo-pelvic-hip complex (LPHC), and their impact on physical therapy examination and intervention.
- List and perform key procedures used in the orthopaedic manual physical therapy (OMPT) examination of the hip.
- Demonstrate sound clinical decision-making in evaluating the results of the OMPT examination.

- Use pertinent examination findings to reach a differential diagnosis and prognosis.
- Discuss issues related to the safe performance of OMPT interventions for the hip.
- Demonstrate a basic level of proficiency in the performance of an essential skill set of joint mobilization techniques for the hip.

FUNCTIONAL ANATOMY AND KINEMATICS

Introduction

The hip joint is best defined as a *diarthrodial joint* that forms the articulation between the acetabulum of the pelvis and the head of the femur. The hip joint possesses three degrees of freedom and provides an important link between the axial skeleton and the lower extremity. Unlike the shoulder, the hip possesses the additional responsibility of bearing superincumbent forces from the *head, arm, and trunk (HAT)* as well as accommodating for *ground reaction forces* from the lower extremities. In this chapter, we will focus on the important kinematic and functional connections between the hip and the adjacent structures of the lower kinetic chain. As an integral part of the *lumbo-pelvic-hip complex (LPHC)*, the hip joint plays an important role in dictating the function of the trunk and lower quarter.

The *acetabulum* is formed by the fusion of the ilium, ischium, and pubis, which do not become fully ossified until the age of 25.[1] On the periphery of the acetabulum, the horseshoe-shaped *lunate surface*, which is covered with hyaline cartilage, serves as the primary articulating surface for the head of the

femur.[2] The inferior gap of the lunate is bridged by the *transverse acetabular ligament*. The *acetabular labrum* serves to increase the depth and enhance congruency between the acetabulum and the femur, thus adding to its overall stability. The *acetabular fossa*, which serves as a deep, fibrous tunnel for the passage of blood vessels, is located medially and represents the non-weight-bearing surface of the acetabulum.

The *femur* is the largest long bone in the body. The head of the femur is more regularly shaped than its acetabular counterpart, comprising nearly two-thirds of a complete sphere. The entire head is covered with articular cartilage, with the exception of a region at the posteromedial aspect, identified as the *fovea capitis*, which serves as the attachment site for the *teres ligament*, also known as the *ligament to the head of the femur*.

Stability of the Hip Joint

Osseous Stability

Critical to understanding stability of the hip is an appreciation of the orientation of the acetabulum and femur. The acetabulum is positioned so that it faces laterally, anteriorly, and slightly inferiorly. The head of the femur is directed medially, superiorly, and projects anteriorly within the acetabulum. The alignment of the femoral head with the acetabulum allows exposure of the superior and anterior aspects of the femoral head when the joint is in neutral, which facilitates flexion and limits extension (Fig. 25-1).[3]

The orientation of the acetabulum in an anterior direction is referred to as **acetabular anteversion**. This structural feature is an important determinant of hip joint stability (Fig. 25-2). Acetabular anteversion that is larger than the normal values of 18.5 degrees and 21.5 degrees[4] for males and females, respectively, may render the hip susceptible to anterior dislocation. The amount of inferior tilt of the acetabulum determines the degree of femoral head coverage and is referred to as the **center edge (CE) angle,** or **angle of Wiberg** (Fig. 25-3).[5] This angle is determined upon radiography by connecting a line drawn between the lateral rim of the acetabulum and the center of the femoral head, which forms an angle with the vertical.[5] The normal range of values for the CE angle have been listed as between 22 and 42 degrees.[4]

In addition to the position of the acetabulum, the orientation of the femur relative to the acetabulum must also be carefully considered. The **angle of inclination (AI)** is described as the angle formed by a line drawn through the femoral head

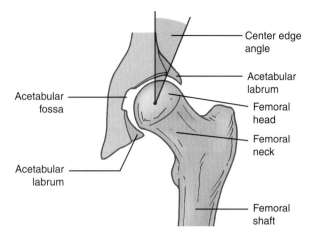

FIGURE 25–3 Center edge angle, which defines the extent to which the acetabulum contains the superior aspect of the femoral head.

and neck and the long axis of the femoral shaft in the frontal plane (Fig. 25-4). The average normal value for the AI is 125 degrees, ranging from 115 to 140 degrees in middle-aged adults.[1,5] Children typically possess a much greater angle, whereas the elderly typically have a smaller AI.[6] An angle of less than 125 degrees in an adult is referred to as **coxa vara**. A patient with a unilateral coxa vara deformity may present with a short leg on the involved side, prominent greater trochanters, genu valgus at the knees, and may be prone to compressive impairments resulting from an increased gluteus medius moment arm. Conversely, a **coxa valga** deformity, where the AI is greater than 125 degrees in the adult, will present with a long leg on the involved side, genu varus at the knees, and may be prone to hip subluxation by virtue of reduction in the moment arm of the gluteus medius. *Limb length discrepancies (LLD)* are of high prevalence in the normal population and may be associated with low back pain if they exceed greater than 5 mm.[7–10] Limb length discrepancies that are greater than 20 mm are considered to be clinically significant.[7]

Another femoral angle, which is referred to as the **angle of torsion (AT)**, exists within the transverse plane. This angle is best visualized by placing the femoral condyles in the frontal plane and measuring the angle between the frontal plane and a line drawn through the femoral head and neck. A normal range for the AT in adults is 15 to 25 degrees,[11] with the

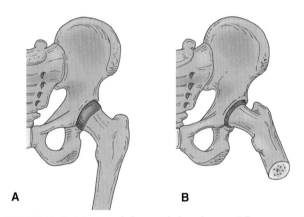

FIGURE 25–1 A. In neutral, the acetabulum does not fully accommodate the spherical femoral, therefore allowing exposure of the superior and anterior aspects of the femoral head. **B.** When the hip is flexed, abducted, and externally rotated, maximal joint congruency is achieved. (Adapted from Levangie PK, Norkin CC. *Joint Structure and Function: A Comprehensive Analysis.* 4th ed. Philadelphia: FA Davis; 2005.)

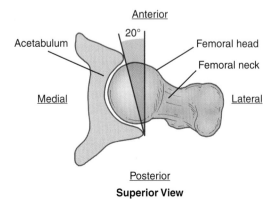

FIGURE 25–2 Acetabular anteversion angle, which defines the extent to which the acetabulum contains the anterior aspect of the femoral head.

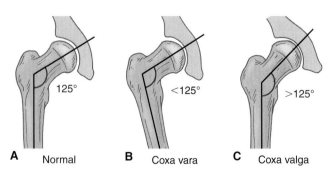

FIGURE 25–4 A. Angle of inclination of the femur with normal values between 115 and 140 degrees in a middle-aged adult. **B.** An angle of less than 125 degrees is defined as coxa vara. **C.** An angle of greater than 125 degrees is defined as coxa valga.

femoral head and neck torsioned anteriorly relative to the frontal plane; therefore, unimpaired adults possess a normal degree of anterior rotation in the transverse plane, which is known as **femoral anteversion**. However, a femur with an AT that is greater than 25 degrees is considered to possess pathological anteversion. A femur with an AT that is less than 15 degrees is considered to possess what is known as **femoral retroversion** (Fig. 25-5). When considering these structural impairments, it is necessary to be aware that these conditions are intrinsic to the femur yet often mimic impairments in hip mobility. An indicator of femoral anteversion or retroversion may be identified by observing foot position in weight bearing or by comparing hip rotational mobility from side to side (Fig. 25-6). Femoral anteversion and retroversion may mimic excessive hip internal rotation and external rotation, respectively. Using a three-dimensional computer model of the hip, Arnold et al[12] revealed that excessive femoral anteversion decreased the moment arm of the gluteus medius and concluded that internal rotation of the hip may occur as a compensation.

Capsuloligamentous Stability

The *capsuloligamentous complex (CLC)* of the hip spans from the rim of the acetabulum to the intertrochanteric line of the femur, thus encapsulating the entire femoral head and neck. The femoral neck is, therefore, considered to be intracapsular, whereas the trochanters are extracapsular. The CLC is best described as a dense fibrous structure that is most substantial anteroposteriorly, with multidirectional fibers that contribute greatly to hip joint stability.[13]

The *iliofemoral ligament*, known as the *Y ligament of Bigelow*, courses from the rim of the acetabulum and anterior inferior iliac spine (AIIS) in two sections toward its insertion into the

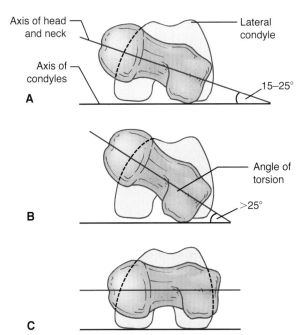

FIGURE 25–5 A. Angle of torsion of the femur with normal values between 15 and 25 degrees of anteversion. **B.** An angle of greater than 25 degrees is considered anteversion. **C.** An angle of less than 15 degrees is retroversion.

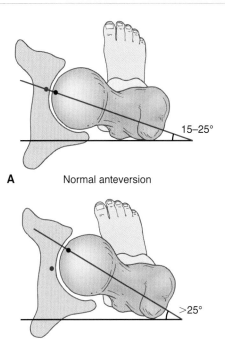

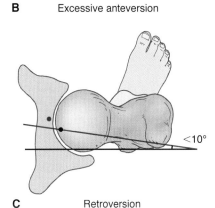

FIGURE 25–6 Femoral anteversion and retroversion of the femur may impact the position of the foot in weight-bearing. **A.** With a normal degree of anteversion, the foot is aligned with the leg. **B.** Excessive anteversion leads to misalignment between the acetabulum (red dot) and the femur (black dot), which may produce in-toeing. **C.** Retroversion leads to misalignment between the acetabulum (red dot) and the femur (black dot), which may produce out-toeing.

intertrochanteric line of the femur.[11] Forming a *z-shaped* configuration with the iliofemoral ligament at the anterior aspect of the hip joint is the *pubofemoral ligament*. This ligament is located between the anterior pubic ramus and the intertrochanteric line. Together, these ligaments effectively reinforce the anterior capsule of the hip joint, which collectively has the ability to support superincumbent body weight in standing. The iliofemoral ligament also limits external rotation and adduction, and the pubofemoral ligament limits abduction.

Reinforcing the capsule posteriorly is the *ischiofemoral ligament*. This obliquely oriented ligament spirals from the posterior acetabular rim to the femoral neck, where it blends with the capsule. This ligament is most involved in limiting extension, as well as internal rotation, and adduction when the hip is flexed.

The ligament to the head of the femur, or *ligamentum teres*, which runs from the acetabular notch to the fovea of the femur and is intra-articular but extrasynovial, serves as a conduit for the passage of blood vessels.

Mobility of the Hip Joint

Open Chain Mobility of the Hip

Values for normal ranges of open chain hip motion vary considerably in the literature.[14] The quantities given for normal ranges of motion of the hip are as follows: flexion is equal to *125 degrees*, extension is equal to *15 degrees*, abduction is equal to *45 degrees*, adduction is equal to *15 degrees*, and internal and external rotation are both equal to *45 degrees*.[15]

Open chain movement occurs with accessory glide that is in the opposite direction from the physiologic movement.[16,17] Due to the depth of the acetabulum, however, some propose that true glide is not possible, but rather a stretch, or deformation, of the capsule occurs in a direction opposite to the physiologic movement.[18,19] Frontal and transverse plane movements (i.e., abduction/adduction and internal/external rotation), however, are believed to possess a greater demand for gliding compared to motion in other planes (Fig. 25-7).[5]

A combination of extra- and intra-articular factors may contribute to limitations in hip movement. Even in the absence of impairment, the multiarticulate muscles of the hip such as the hamstrings and rectus femoris, may become *passively insufficient* and disallow the achievement of full range. The extensive anterior CLC or the architectural features of the joint's osteology may also contribute to motion restrictions. Astute assessment of hip mobility with the hip in neutral compared to assessment of hip mobility with the hip flexed or hip mobility with the knee flexed compared to extended may provide differentiation regarding the source of potential restrictions.

Several authors have attempted to study the relationship between hip mobility and low back pain (LBP).[20–22] Chesworth et al[20] found a significant difference in hip external and internal rotation active range of motion (AROM) in subjects with LBP compared to controls. In agreement with other authors[21,23] Ellison et al[24] revealed that patterns of hip rotation were altered in the presence of LBP, identifying that 48% of individuals with LBP had a general loss of hip internal rotation. Cibulka et al[21] observed that subjects with sacroiliac joint (SIJ)-related symptoms had reduced internal rotation on the side of the posteriorly-rotated pelvis.

Closed Chain Mobility of the Hip

During a typical gait cycle, the majority of time is spent in the unilateral stance phase as opposed to either the bilateral stance or swing phases.[25,26] Consequently, the ability of the hip to both sustain forces from the HAT and contralateral limb while attempting to generate movement requires a unique combination of stabilizing and mobilizing forces.

A variety of terms have been used to describe movement of the pelvis upon a relatively fixed femur. These terms are fully delineated in Chapter 28 of this text (Fig. 25-8). As the concave acetabulum is moving about the convex femoral head, glide or stretch will occur in the same direction as the physiologic movement.

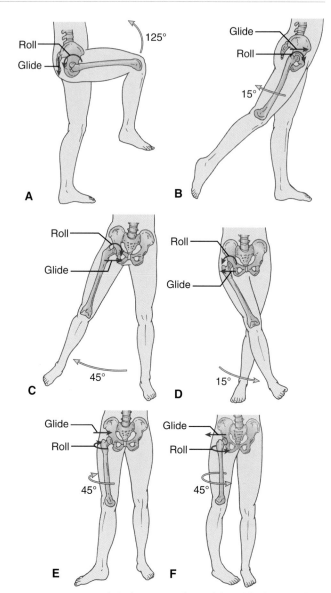

FIGURE 25-7 Open chain, femur on pelvis mobility of the hip in all three cardinal planes revealing **A.** open chain flexion, **B.** open chain extension, **C.** open chain abduction, **D.** open chain adduction, **E.** open chain external rotation, and **F.** open chain internal rotation. The black, red, and yellow arrows demonstrate motion of the femur. The yellow arrow reveals the normal amount of osteokinematic hip motion in open chain. During open chain motion of the femur on the relatively fixed pelvis, convex is moving on concave, thus joint glide (red arrow) is in the opposite direction and joint roll (green arrow) is in the same direction from osteokinematic motion (yellow arrow).

EXAMINATION

The Subjective Examination

Self-Reported Disability Measures

Perhaps, the most commonly used disability questionnaire when managing patients with hip pain is the ***Harris Hip Rating Scale***.[27] This tool is divided into a *pain section*; *function section*, which includes assessment of gait and functional activities; an *absence of deformity section*, which includes possible structural and functional impairments; and a *range of motion section*. This tool is useful for rating functional improvement in response to surgery. A successful result is described as a postoperative increase

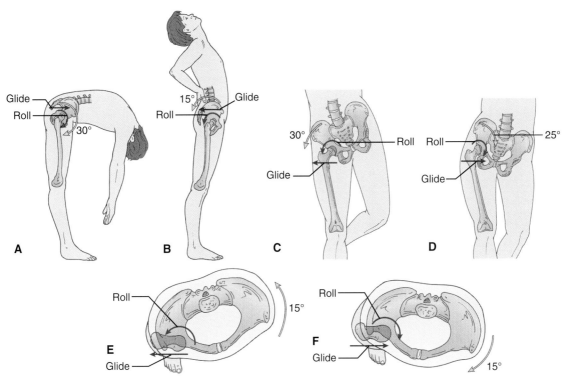

FIGURE 25–8 Closed chain, pelvis on femur mobility of the hip in all three cardinal planes revealing **A.** closed chain flexion, **B.** closed chain extension, **C.** closed chain abduction, **D.** closed chain adduction, **E.** closed chain external rotation, and **F.** closed chain internal rotation. The black, red, and yellow arrows demonstrate motion of the pelvis. The yellow arrow reveals the normal amount of osteokinematic hip motion in closed chain. During closed chain motion of the pelvis on the relatively fixed femur, concave is moving on convex, thus joint glide (red arrow) and joint roll (green arrow) are in the same direction as osteokinematic motion (yellow arrow). Please note, the convex femoral head glides in the opposite direction to the pelvis during these motions.

of greater than 20 points, along with a radiographically stable implant and no additional femoral reconstruction. Scoring is as follows: less than 70 is poor, 70 to 79 if fair, 80 to 89 is good, 90 to 100 is excellent.[28] The *Western Ontario and McMaster Universities Osteoarthritis Index (WOMAC)* is used to evaluate relevant changes in health status, primarily with arthroplasties of the hip and knee. This tool has three sections that are scored from 1 to 5, with a higher score suggesting greater disability.[29]

The *Oxford Hip Score* consists of 12 multiple choice questions that are scored as follows: 0 to 19 indicates severe hip arthritis, surgical intervention is likely; 20 to 29 indicates moderate to severe hip arthritis. See your family physician for an assessment and x-ray. Consider an orthopaedic consultation. A score of 30 to 39 indicates mild to moderate hip arthritis. You may benefit from nonsurgical treatment. A score of 40 to 48 indicates satisfactory joint function. You may not require any formal treatment.[30] Lastly, the *Lower Extremity Functional Scale (LEFS)* consists of a 20-item list of functional activities, which is scored from 0 to 4 regarding level of difficulty in the performance of each task. The sum of responses (80 possible points) composes the score. The minimum detectable change as well as the minimum clinically important difference for this tool is 9 points.[31]

Review of Systems

There are a variety of medical conditions that may impact the proximal femur, thus rendering it susceptible to *pathological facture* and injury. Individuals over the age of 50 years, particularly

postmenopausal females, are most at risk. *Osteoporosis* or *osteopenia* may lead to a reduction in the force-accepting capabilities of the femoral head and neck. Patients experiencing these issues often present with groin pain and/or lateral thigh pain, and the involved extremity is often postured in external rotation and may be slightly shorter than the other side.[32]

Other medical conditions that may impact the hip include *avascular necrosis*, which may occur subsequent to trauma or idiopathically at birth, in a condition known as *Legg-Calve-Perthes disease*. Individuals experiencing these conditions often experience pain in the groin, thigh, or knee, which worsens upon weight-bearing and ambulation, and a loss of internal rotation and abduction.[32]

One of the more common neoplasms that may refer pain to the pelvis and hip is *colon cancer*. As the third most common type of cancer in both males and females,[33] an individual with pelvis and hip pain that is unremitting and nonmechanical should be screened for the possibility of cancer. A list of medical red flags for the hip is displayed in Table 25-1.

History of Present Illness

Pain in the groin that leads to antalgic gait in the toddler may suggest the presence of Legg-Calve-Perthes disease or a *slipped capital femoral epiphysis (SCFE)*, particularly if the child is male. *Congenital hip dysplasia* involving failure of the acetabulum to fully develop renders the hip susceptible to dislocation, which may occur during the birthing process. The elderly population

Table 25-1	Medical Red Flags for the Hip
MEDICAL CONDITION	**RED FLAGS**
Slipped Capital Femoral Epiphysis (SCFE	Recent growth
	History of traumatic event
	Adolescent and overweight Posturing in hip external rotation
	Restricted ability to run
	Restricted hip mobility
	Groin pain that increases upon weight-bearing
Avascular Necrosis (AVN)	Traumatic event
	Fracture to the proximal femur
	Developmental dysplasia of the hip
	Young boys with groin pain
	Pain upon weight-bearing and hip movement
	Chronic steroid use
Fractures	History of traumatic event
	Constant pain that increases upon weight-bearing and movement
	Elderly females with groin or lateral hip pain
Cancer of the Colon	Unexplained weight loss
	Family history of colon cancer
	Unremitting pain
	Older than 50 years
	Rectal bleeding

(Adapted from Boissonnault WG. *Primary Care for the Physical Therapist: Examination and Triage.* St. Louis, MO: Elsevier Saunders; 2005.)

has a higher propensity of pathological fractures resulting from conditions such as osteoporosis, osteopenia, *osteomalacia*, or *Paget's disease*.

Lateral hip pain with tenderness to palpation suggests the presence of *greater trochanteric bursitis*. These patients often display a *gluteus medius lurch* or positive *Trendelenburg sign*. Groin and anteromedial thigh pain may result from several hip-related dysfunctions including osteoarthritis, avascular necrosis, and a slipped capital femoral epiphysis, among others. Osteoarthritis often causes morning stiffness that may improve with activity.

Buttock pain or pain in the region of the posterior superior iliac spine (PSIS) may be the result of *piriformis syndrome* or hypertonicity of the deep external rotators of the hip. These patients will exhibit pain and limitation of hip flexion, adduction, and internal rotation (FADIR). This syndrome is the most common peripheral nerve entrapment syndrome of the hip. Medial thigh/groin pain and lateral hip pain may suggest an L1-3 and L4 *radiculopathy*, respectively. In cases of hip pain, a quick screen for the lumbar spine should routinely be performed.

Joint audibles upon motion may be referred to as *snapping hip syndrome*. The most clinically significant cause of joint sounds are ruptures of the acetabular labrum, which most commonly occur in individuals between the ages of 20 and 40 years as a result of pivoting in closed chain and when moving the hip into adduction and external rotation.[34,35] It is fairly common for the tendon of the iliopsoas to snap over the lesser trochanter at 45 degrees as the hip moves from flexion to extension or when then hip is internally rotated during this movement.[34,36] Determining if the joint sound is intra- or extra-articular is of value in differentiating its origin.

The Objective Physical Examination

Examination of Structure

Observation of Gait

The therapist begins the process of observation upon the patient's entrance into the clinic, without his or her knowledge. A general sense of step length, cadence, weight acceptance, propulsiveness, and the presence of any symptoms may be noted. The trunk is often the first indicator of inadequate hip function during gait.

In the presence of gluteus medius weakness or hip pain, excessive lateral weight shifting is often adopted. Although counterintuitive, leaning over the impaired hip will move the *center of gravity (COG)* closer to the painful, or weak, hip and reduce the moment arm of gravity, thereby reducing the amount of gravitational torque acting over the involved hip (Fig. 25-9). The inability to maintain frontal plane stability of the pelvis in weight bearing is identified as a positive Trendelenburg sign, which is commonly referred to as a gluteus medius lurch during ambulation. Limitations in hip extension are common

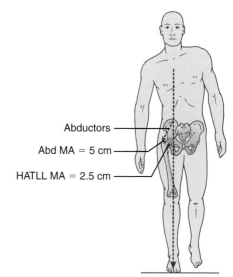

Abductors

Abd MA = 5 cm

HATLL MA = 2.5 cm

FIGURE 25–9 Biomechanical rationale for the gluteus medius lurch, which involves weight shifting of the trunk over the weight-bearing hip for the purpose of reducing the moment arm (MA) of gravitational forces of the head, arms, trunk, and left leg (HATLL) and thereby reducing the need for increased torque from the abductors. (Adapted from Levangie PK, Norkin CC. *Joint Structure and Function: A Comprehensive Analysis.* 4th ed. Philadelphia: FA Davis Company; 2005.)

among asymptomatic populations. Such limitations may lead to alterations in weight distribution, step length, and cadence. Limitations in hip internal and/or external rotation may result in transverse plane deviations and compensations.

The use of a cane on the unaffected side serves to reduce forces through the painful hip. Levangie and Norkin[5] propose that the downward force through the cane arrives at the pelvis through contraction of the latissimus dorsi, resulting in elevation of the pelvis and an abduction moment through the weight-bearing hip that counteracts the adduction moment resulting from gravity, which effectively reduces gluteus medius force.

Observation of Posture

In erect bipedal stance, the *line of gravity (LOG)* lies just posterior to the greater trochanter, which produces an extension moment at the hip. Likewise, the LOG should bisect the body when viewed in the frontal plane. Any deviation from midline will move the LOG in the direction of the deviation. Structural factors, such as a leg length discrepancy or scoliosis, may also produce a shift in the location of the LOG.

Postural deviations are common, even within the asymptomatic population. Therefore, the manual physical therapist should be careful not to make direct correlations between postural deviations and a patient's presenting symptoms (Table 25-2). Postural observation is best performed in a systematic fashion that takes into account anterior, posterior, and lateral views.

Examination of Mobility

When examining hip motion, it may be important to appreciate both open and closed chain function. The *close-packed position*

of the hip is considered to be full extension, internal rotation, and abduction. The more mobile *open-packed position* is considered to be approximately 30 degrees of flexion, 30 degrees of abduction, and slight external rotation (FABER position). In the neutral position of the hip, the anterosuperior portion of the femoral head is exposed.

Active Physiologic Movement Examination

The optimal position for measuring hip AROM will vary depending on the motion being tested. Hip flexion, abduction, and adduction are best measured in supine, extension in prone or side lying, and external and internal rotation in sitting. When measuring active or passive hip motion, it is critical to appreciate the effects of *passive and active insufficiency* as multijoint muscles cross this articulation. Comparing passive to active range serves to delineate the cause of the motion restriction.

Examination of both *single and repeated movements* (5 to 10 times) is recommended in order to provide a more reliable movement profile. In addition to single cardinal plane motions designed to isolate movement, *combined movements* that include multiplanar movement must also be assessed. Testing **proprioceptive neuromuscular facilitation (PNF)** patterns for the entire extremity may be useful in understanding the function of the hip relative to its distal counterparts. A *functional movement examination* that uses patient-specific movements based on reported deficits or functionally relevant movements must also be performed. These movement patterns include multiplanar motions that mimic the functional demands of the patient. Testing mobility in closed chain positions is extremely important for understanding functional mobility of the hip.

Table 25–2	Structural Impairments of the Hip and Common Compensatory Patterns
STRUCTURAL MALALIGNMENT	**COMPENSATORY PATTERNS**
Coxa vara	Ipsilateral foot plantarflexion and supination
	Contralateral foot dorsiflexion and pronation
	Contralateral genu recurvatum
	Contralateral hip and/or knee flexion
	Ipsilateral anterior pelvic rotation and/or contralateral posterior pelvic rotation in standing
Coxa valga	Ipsilateral foot dorsiflexion and pronation
	Contralateral foot plantarflexion and supination
	Ipsilateral genu recurvatum
	Ipsilateral hip and/or knee flexion
	Ipsilateral posterior pelvic rotation and/or contralateral anterior pelvic rotation in standing
Femoral anteversion (greater than 15–25 degrees)	Ipsilateral external tibial torsion
	Ipsilateral foot supination
	Ipsilateral knee extension
Femoral retroversion (less than 15–25 degrees of anteversion)	Ipsilateral internal tibial torsion
	Ipsilateral foot pronation
	Ipsilateral knee flexion

(Adapted from Reigger-Krugh C, Keysor JJ. Skeletal malalignments of the lower quarter: correlated and compensatory motions and postures. *J Orthop Sports Phys Ther*. 196;23:166-167.)

Comparison of *pure hip joint motion* with *hip complex motion* may provide evidence for identifying the most culpable structures. Examination of pure hip joint motion is best accomplished in open chain, as described above, for the purpose of precisely isolating motion within the hip. However, to fully appreciate the manner in which the hip joint normally functions, the manual physical therapist should examine the hip in closed chain. Assessment of what has been termed *lumbopelvic rhythm* is useful in understanding the contribution of the hip to closed chain function[37–41] (see Chapter 28).

Use of the *numeric pain rating scale (NPRS)* is important in establishing a baseline level of symptoms and documenting changes in symptoms in response to movement. Identifying the patient's reproducible symptom(s) can then be used during the course of intervention to gauge progress, establish the efficacy of chosen interventions, and verify outcomes. Establishing the patient's level of reactivity also serves to inform intervention.

In order to fully elucidate the locus of pathology during the mobility examination, the manual physical therapist may incorporate the use of *overpressure* and/or *counterpressure*. As mentioned, the first step is to establish the patient's baseline symptoms. Overpressure is then added at the end range of all motions for the purpose of determining end feel and the presence of any reproducible symptoms. Counterpressure may also be used when examining this complex for the purpose of isolating the specific region of symptomatic origin. A reduction in the reproducible symptom in response to a specifically localized counterpressure force may provide information regarding the specific locus of pathology that helps to guide subsequent intervention.

Passive Physiologic Movement Examination

Passive physiologic mobility testing is performed on the regions and movements that were found to be deficient during AROM testing. As with AROM, passive joint mobility testing endeavors to reduce the influence of the muscles that cross the hip.

The application of overpressure at the end of available range in order to ascertain the *end feel* provides additional information regarding the nature of the restriction. Normal end feels for the hip are generally considered to be *tissue stretch* or *elastic* for all motions, with the addition of *soft tissue approximation* for hip flexion and adduction.[36] The capsular pattern of the hip is generally believed to be a loss of *flexion, abduction,* and *internal rotation*; however, the relative magnitude of loss may vary substantially between individuals.[36]

During the passive physiologic movement examination, *goniometric* measurements of all cardinal plane motions are performed as described elsewhere.[42] During passive goniometric testing, the manual physical therapist carefully monitors the pelvis to disallow any extraneous movement, suggesting that the full extent of available hip motion has been exhausted. Hip flexion, abduction, and adduction are best tested in supine, hip extension in prone, and hip external and internal rotation in sitting or prone with the knee flexed. While moving the hip joint through its available range, the therapist is careful to appreciate the onset of tissue resistance (Resistance 1 or R1), the nature of this resistance, and its relationship to symptoms, particularly the patient's chief complaint.

There is much controversy and lack of normative data related to expected ranges of hip motion.[2] There appear to be minor difference in range of motion between genders and, contrary to popular belief, insignificant reductions in range of motion have been noted in the elderly.[14] Generally, the degree of hip flexion is often cited as ranging between *120 and 125 degrees*, normal hip extension ranges from *9 to 19 degrees*, hip abduction from *39 to 46 degrees*, hip adduction from *15 to 31 degrees*, hip external and internal rotation from *32 to 47 degrees*.[2] Table 25-3 displays the physiologic motions of the hip, including normal ranges of motion, open- and closed-packed positions, normal end feels, and capsular pattern.

Passive Accessory Movement Examination

Both direct and indirect testing of accessory movement may be performed, with the former being the most valid for truly revealing the extent of available accessory movement. Direct assessment is performed by the therapist passively moving the femur relative to the acetabulum while, as with passive range of motion (PROM), assessing the relationship between tissue resistance and the onset of symptoms. Extrapolating limitations observed during passive physiologic testing to deficits in accessory motion testing

Table 25-3	Physiologic (Osteokinematic) Motions of the Hip				
NORMAL ROM	**OPP**	**CPP**	**NORMAL END FEEL(S)**	**CAPSULAR PATTERN**
Flexion = 120–125°	30 degrees flexion	Maximum extension, IR, abduction	Extension, Abduction, ER, IR = tissue stretch or elastic	Flexion = Abduction = IR variable
Extension = 9-19°	30 degrees abduction and slight ER		Flexion and Adduction = soft tissue approximation and elastic	
Abduction = 39–46°				
Adduction = 15-31°				
ER, IR = 32–47°				

ROM, range of motion; OPP, open-packed position; CPP, close-packed position; IR, internal rotation; ER, external rotation.
(Adapted From Wise CH, Gulick DT. *Mobilization Notes: A Rehabilitation Specialist's Pocket Guide.* Philadelphia, PA: FA Davis Company; 2009)

without actually testing the accessory motion constitutes indirect testing. Although intervention may involve positioning of the joint at the boundaries of its available motion, initial testing should be performed in the open-packed position of flexion, abduction, and slight external rotation to reduce external influences. The mobilization techniques that follow later in this chapter will provide details regarding the performance of accessory glides and may be used for both examination and intervention of passive accessory movement. Table 25-4 displays the accessory motions of the hip.

Examination of Muscle Function

When examining muscle function of the hip, it is important to test each muscle in a manner that is both specific and functional in order to provide the therapist with information regarding hip muscle performance. Specificity of muscle testing is enhanced by testing each muscle in its dominant type of contraction (i.e., isometric, concentric, eccentric) and at the length (i.e., shortened, midrange, lengthened) and plane (i.e., frontal, sagittal, transverse) in which it typically functions. Muscles about the hip may function as prime movers that produce a substantial amount of force, which may be used to propel the body forward in space during activities such as ambulation and jumping. The muscles of the hip are often required to fulfill dichotomous functions within a short span of time. For example, during the single-limb stance phase of gait, the gluteus medius muscle on the weight-bearing side functions isometrically to maintain a level pelvis in the frontal plane. However, this same muscle may also work eccentrically in the late swing phase to allow the contralateral limb to approximate the floor.

An appreciation for the functional requirements of each of the muscles of the hip is necessary in order for the manual physical therapist to gain a complete understanding of muscle function. Some authors have attempted to develop functional testing procedures for the proximal muscles of the hip.[43,44] The *step-down test*, as described within the special testing portion of this chapter, is designed to assess the ability of the proximal hip muscles to control descent of the contralateral limb while stepping down from a step or stool. Normal performance is described as the ability to perform this activity while maintaining the knee in the sagittal plane.[43,44] Qualitative gait analysis may also yield important data regarding the closed chain function of these muscles.

During muscle function testing, it is critical to determine if true deficits exist or if the observed weakness is positional in origin; therefore, muscle function testing must be performed in a manner that reduces the effects of active insufficiency. Deficits in muscle force production that occur as a result of active insufficiency are an important consideration for the manual physical therapist who is attempting to reduce impairment and subsequent disability. Patient education and retraining of movement patterns may serve to enhance function by reducing the influence of active insufficiency on muscle force production.

Prior to embarking on formal muscle function testing, *selective tissue tension (STT)* testing, as described by Cyriax,[45] may be performed as a screening procedure to focus the examination. The joint is placed in neutral, and submaximal isometric testing is performed. Pain and/or weakness noted during testing serves to identify the suspected pathological muscle. For example, the sartorius is the only muscle that flexes the hip, externally rotates the hip, abducts the hip, and flexes the knee. If weakness or pain was noted when testing this unique combination of movements, the sartorius muscle would be suspected and more specific testing would be performed.

Delp[46] identified that the position of the hip influences the function of proximal hip musculature. When the hip is in the 0 degree neutral position, the majority of the gluteus maximus and medius function as external rotators, along with the deep rotators of the hip. However, when these same muscles are tested with the hip flexed to 90 degrees, all heads of the gluteus medius and nearly all heads of the gluteus maximus become internal rotators, as does the piriformis muscle (Fig. 25-10). Except for the piriformis, the deep rotators serve as external rotators regardless of hip position; therefore, when testing these muscles, it is important to consider that in neutral, the hip is able to generate more force into external rotation, than when the hip is flexed to 90 degrees.[46]

Generally, hip strength is greater in men and appears to diminish with age.[47] The hip flexors and extensors demonstrate nearly equal strength.[48] The hip adductor muscle group demonstrates greater force production than the hip abductor group when tested isometrically in both the neutral and abducted positions.[47,49] However, the disparity between the two muscle groups is less when tested with the hip in the neutral

Table 25-4	Accessory (Arthrokinematic) Motions of the Hip	
ARTHROLOGY	**ARTHROKINEMATICS**	
Concave surface: acetabulum	*To facilitate hip flexion:* Femur rolls anterior and glides inferior and posterior	*To facilitate hip extension:* Femur rolls posterior and glides anterior
Convex surface: femoral head	*To facilitate hip abduction:* Femur rolls lateral and glides medial	*To facilitate hip adduction:* Femur rolls medial and glides lateral
	To facilitate hip IR: Femur rolls medial and glides posterior and lateral	*To facilitate hip ER:* Femur rolls lateral and glides anterior and medial

IR, internal rotation; ER, external rotation.
(Adapted From Wise CH, Gulick DT. *Mobilization Notes: A Rehabilitation Specialist's Pocket Guide.* Philadelphia, PA: FA Davis Company; 2009)

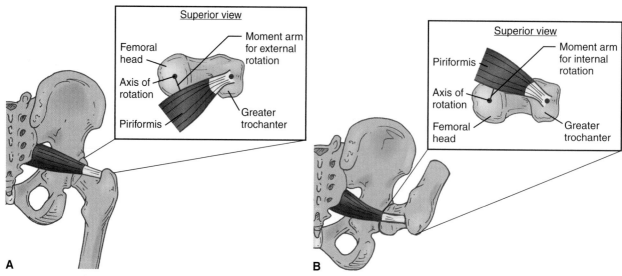

FIGURE 25–10 Change in piriformis function from an external rotator when the hip is **A.** extended to an internal rotator when the hip is **B.** flexed.

position.[47] There is inconclusive evidence regarding strength ratios between the hip external and internal rotators. Some consensus exists that suggests that the hip internal rotators are able to produce more force than the external rotators when tested in the standard hip and knee flexed position.[50,51]

Examination of Function

Functional testing may be viewed as a useful tool that can be used to screen for specific deficits that may be more fully considered during the physical examination (Table 25-5). These tests are often best performed early in the examination so that their results remain uninfluenced by the many procedures that are to follow. A quick screen for the hip, and entire lower extremity, is the *squat test*. Performance of this test may serve to direct the more specific mobility and muscle function testing. The patient is simply asked to squat to the floor from a standing position and then to return to standing. This quick test allows the therapist to assess the mobility of the hips, knees, and ankles, as well as the strength of the

muscles that work across each of these joints. The Functional Movement Screen (FMS) has been advocated as an efficient and systematic way to observe basic movement patterns that form the underlying properties of various sports. The FMS consists of seven specific activities that are scored based on the level of precision that the individual is able to demonstrate.[52]

Palpation

Osseous Palpation

After identifying the iliac crest, the therapist moves distally approximately 6 inches until the large prominence of the *greater trochanters* are identified and palpated in their entirety. Confirmation is achieved by having the patient externally and internally rotate his or her hip or shift body weight from side to side (Fig. 25-11).

Serving as the insertion for the hamstrings as well as the sacrotuberous ligament, the *ischial tuberosity* is an important landmark that warrants investigation. This prominent landmark

Table 25–5	Required Motion for Performance of Typical Functional Activities	
FUNCTIONAL TASK	**RANGE OF REQUIRED HIP MOTION**
Squatting	Flexion: 115 degrees
	Abduction: 20 degrees
	Internal rotation: 20 degrees
Sitting	Flexion: 115 degrees
Ascending stairs	Flexion: 70 degrees
Descending stairs	Flexion: 40 degrees
Donning pants	Flexion: 90 degrees
Crossing legs	Flexion: 120 degrees
	Abduction: 20 degrees
	External Rotation: 20 degrees

(Adapted from Magee DJ. *Orthopedic Physical Assessment.* 4th ed. Philadelphia, PA: W.B. Saunders Company; 2002.)

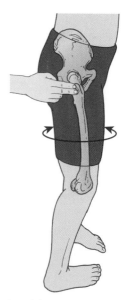

FIGURE 25–11 Palpation of the greater trochanter.

is best palpated in side lying with the hip flexed (Fig. 25-12). Confirmation is achieved by gently resisting knee flexion.

Soft Tissue Palpation

Beginning anteriorly, the examiner palpates the multijoint *rectus femoris* in supine with the hip slightly flexed over a bolster (Fig. 25-13). The examiner carefully palpates along a line that runs from the AIIS to the patella, gently strumming the fibers of this muscle, which is approximately three finger widths wide.[53]

In side lying, the adductor group of the bottom leg can be palpated by first identifying the *gracilis*. The *sartorius* angles toward its insertion on the ASIS while the gracilis runs toward the pubic bone. Immediately posterior to the gracilis is the *adductor magnus*, which possesses a much wider muscle belly and lies in a deeper plane than does the gracilis. The gracilis is once again identified, after which the examiner then migrates anteriorly to contact the *adductor longus*. This muscle can be differentiated from the gracilis by the manner in which it angles anteriorly as it runs distally (Fig. 25-14).

To appreciate the expanse of the gluteus medius muscle at the lateral hip, the heel of the examiner's hand is placed over the lateral aspect of the iliac crest with the fingers pointing distally toward the muscle's insertion into the greater trochanter (Fig. 25-15). The thumb of the hand represents the approximate location of the tensor fascia latae, the index finger, long, ring finger, and little finger represent the anterior, middle, and posterior bellies of the gluteus medius muscle, respectively.

In prone-lying position, the gluteus maximus and hamstrings are palpated. Gentle isometric resistance for hip extension with the knee flexed is performed. In prone, the hamstrings as a group can be easily palpated.

Special Testing

These tests have been described in detail within a variety of other sources; therefore, only brief descriptions of their performance will be included here.[36,54] Table 25-6 provides the sensitivity, specificity, and likelihood ratios for the more commonly performed special tests used in the examination of the hip. [55–82] The reader is encouraged to consult other sources for additional information regarding the performance of these useful confirmatory tests. [36,54]

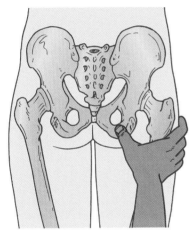

FIGURE 25–12 Palpation of the ischial tuberosity.

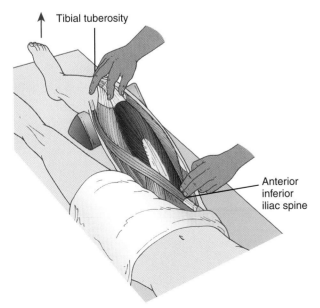

FIGURE 25–13 Palpation of the rectus femoris muscle.

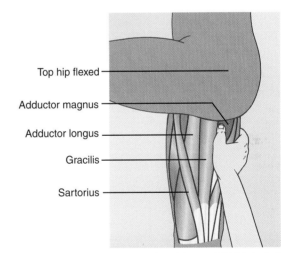

FIGURE 25–14 Palpation of the muscles of the medial thigh, including the gracilis, sartorius, adductor magnus, and adductor longus.

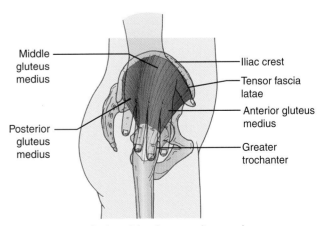

FIGURE 25–15 Palpation of the gluteus medius muscle.

Table 25-6	Special Tests for the Hip					
TEST	**SENSITIVITY**	**SPECIFICITY**	**+LR**	**−LR**	**RELIABILITY**	**REFERENCE**
Flexion abduction external rotation (FABER) test (Patrick's test)	41%–89%	16%–100%	0.82	0.23–1.94	ICC = 0.66– 0.96	Mitchell et al[55] Cliborne et al[56] Maslowski et al[57] Martin et al[58] Dreyfuss et al[59] Broadhurst et al[60] Flynn et al[61] Kokmeyer et al[62]
Flexion adduction internal rotation (FADIR) test	88%	83%	5.2	0.14	NA	Fishman et al[63]
Femoral grind (scour) test	75%–91%	43%	1.32	0.58	NA	Maitland[64] Narvani et al[65] Leuning et al[66]
Anterior labral test	75%	43%	1.32	0.58	NA	Narvani et al[65] Fitzgerald[67]
Posterior labral test	75%	43%	1.32	0.58	NA	Narvani et al[65] Fitzgerald[67]
Modified Thomas test	NA	NA	NA	NA	ICC = 0.50– 0.67	Peeler et al[68] Browder et al[69]
Trendelenburg sign	73%	77%	3.15	0.335	Kappa = 0.676	Trendelenburg[70] Bird et al[71]
Ely test	NA	NA	NA	NA	ICC = 0.69	Peeler et al[72] Offierski et al[73]
Step down test	NA	NA	NA	NA	NA	Powers et al[43,44]
Craig test	NA	NA	NA	NA	ICC = 0.85– 0.94	Reynolds et al[74] Crane[75] Ruwe[76] Staheli et al[77]
Sign of the buttock	NA	NA	NA	NA	NA	Greenwood et al[78] Burns et al[79]
Ortolani test						Ortolani[80] Tachdjian[81] Baronciani et al[82]
Barlow test						Tachdjian[81] Baronciani et al[82]

+LR, positive likelihood ratio; −LR, negative likelihood ratio; ICC, intraclass correlation coefficient; NA, not applicable.

SPECIAL TESTS FOR THE HIP

Special Tests for Symptom Reproduction

Flexion Abduction External Rotation (FABER) Test (Patrick Test) (Fig. 25-16)

Purpose: To test for the presence of hip pathology

Patient: Supine, with hip in FABER position

Clinician: Standing to the side of the patient

Procedure: Gentle force is applied to move the hip into external rotation by applying posterior force.

Interpretation: The test is positive if there is a reproduction of hip pain or limitation in range of motion.

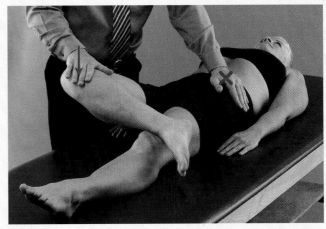

FIGURE 25–16 Flexion abduction external rotation (FABER) test (Patrick Test).

Flexion Adduction Internal Rotation (FADIR) Test (Fig. 25-17)

Purpose: To identify peripheral nerve entrapment of the sciatic nerve by the deep external rotators of the hip, known as piriformis syndrome

Patient: Supine, with hip in FADIR position

Clinician: Standing to the side of the patient

Procedure: Clinician passively moves the hip into the FADIR position.

Interpretation: The test is positive if there is a reproduction of pain within the mid-buttock region or referred symptoms into the leg.

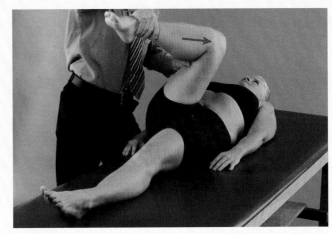

FIGURE 25–17 Flexion adduction internal rotation (FADIR) test.

Femoral Grind (Scour) Test (Fig. 25-18)

Purpose: To identify the presence of intra-articular derangement of the hip, including the acetabular labrum

Patient: Supine

Clinician: Standing to the side of the patient

Procedure: Passively flex the hip and provide a longitudinal compression force through the long axis of the femur while externally and internally rotating the hip

Interpretation: The test is positive if there is a reproduction of pain and clicking within the hip joint.

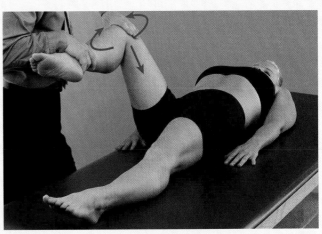

FIGURE 25–18 Femoral grind (scour) test.

Special Tests for Acetabular Labrum Dysfunction

Anterior Labral Test (Fig. 25-19)

Purpose: To identify the presence of an anterior acetabular labral tear

Patient: Supine

Clinician: Standing to the side of the patient

Procedure: Passively move the hip from abduction, ER, and flexion to adduction, IR, and extension while providing long axis compression.

Interpretation: The test is positive if this motion produces pain and/or a click.

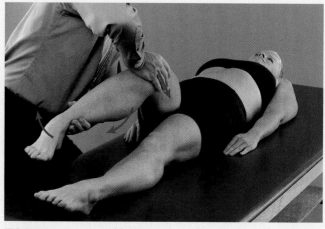

FIGURE 25–19 Anterior labral test

Posterior Labral Test (Fig. 25-20)

Purpose: To identify the presence of a posterior acetabular labral tear

Patient: Supine

Clinician: Standing to the side of the patient

Procedure: Passively move the hip from adduction, IR, and flexion to abduction, ER, and extension while providing long axis compression.

Interpretation: The test is positive if this motion produces pain and/or a click.

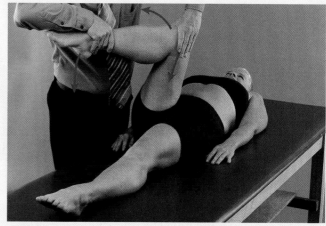

FIGURE 25–20 Posterior labral test

Special Tests for Muscle Function
Modified Thomas Test (Fig. 25-21)

Purpose: To identify the presence of a hip flexion contracture and tightness of the tensor fascia latae

Patient: Begin by leaning on table, then moving into supine while holding knees to chest

Clinician: Standing at the foot of the patient

Procedure: While holding one leg on chest, the other leg is lowered, and the angle between the hip and the table is measured.

Interpretation: The test is positive if there is an inability to achieve full range of hip extension. If the knee extends, and when flexed a reduction in hip extension is noted, then rectus femoris tightness is suspected. If the hip moves into abduction upon lowering, tensor fascia latae tightness is suspected.

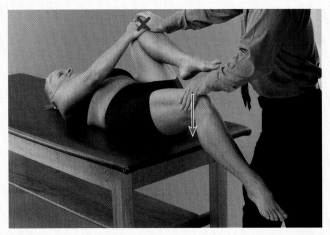

FIGURE 25–21 Modified Thomas test

Trendelenburg Sign (Fig. 25-22)

Purpose: To identify the presence of gluteus medius weakness

Patient: Standing

Clinician: Standing behind patient

Procedure: The patient is asked to stand on one leg while the clinician assesses the degree of pelvic drop.

Interpretation: The test is positive if there is an inability to keep the pelvis level during unilateral stance.

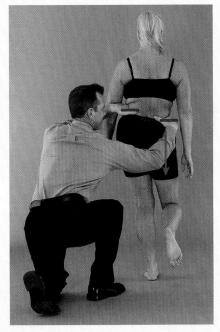

FIGURE 25–22 Trendelenburg sign.

Ely Test (Fig. 25-23)

Purpose: To assess for restrictions of the rectus femoris muscle

Patient: Prone without pillow support

Clinician: Standing to the side of the patient near the feet

Procedure: Passively flex the patient's knee with the hip in neutral and monitor movement of the hip

Interpretation: The test is positive if there is limited knee flexion or the hip flexes when the knee is flexed.

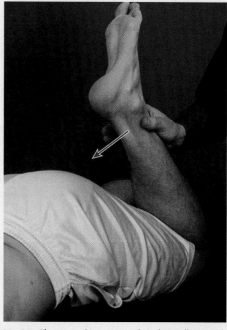

FIGURE 25–23 Ely test. (Courtesy of Bob Wellmon Photography, BobWellmon.com.)

Step Down Test (Fig. 25-24)

Purpose: To assess closed chain muscle function of proximal hip musculature

Patient: Standing on stool

Clinician: Standing in front of patient and providing support as needed

Procedure: Patient slowly lowers one foot toward the ground, followed by lowering the contralateral leg.

Interpretation: The test is positive if the weight-bearing leg migrates out of the sagittal plane during contralateral leg lowering.

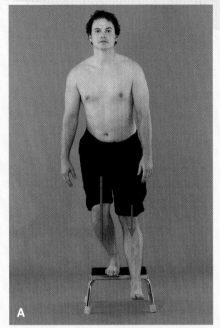

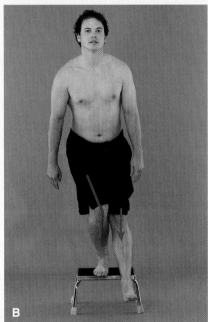

FIGURE 25–24 Step down test. **A.** Normal performance, and **B.** abnormal performance demonstrating impairment of the hip external rotators and abductors.

Special Tests for Structural Impairment
Craig Test (Fig. 25-25)

Purpose: To identify the presence of femoral anteversion or retroversion

Patient: Prone with knee flexed to 90 degrees

Clinician: Standing to the side of the patient

Procedure: While palpating the greater trochanter, internally and externally rotate the hip until the greater trochanter arrives at its most lateral position, after which the angle that the lower leg makes with the table is measured.

Interpretation: The test is positive if there is an angle of greater than 25 degrees between the tibia and the horizontal, suggesting femoral anteversion, or less than 15 degrees between the tibia and the horizontal, suggesting femoral retroversion.

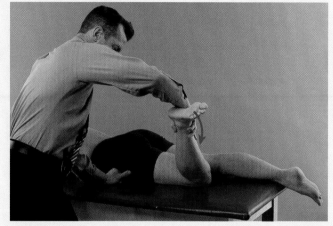

FIGURE 25–25 Craig test.

Sign of the Buttock (Fig. 25-26)

Purpose: To identify the presence of a lesion or pathology within the buttock, including the possibility of ischial bursitis, an abscess, or neoplasm within the buttock

Patient: Supine

Clinician: Standing at the foot of the patient

Procedure: Perform a straight leg raise test, and if a limitation is found, flex the knee then flex the hip again.

Interpretation: The test is positive if hip flexion does not increase when the knee is flexed.

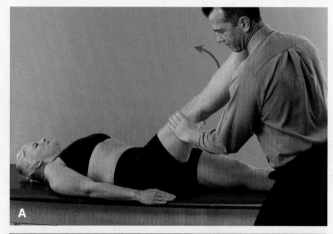

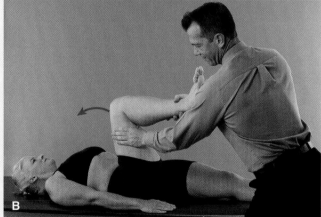

FIGURE 25–26 Sign of the buttock.

Ortolani Test (Fig. 25-27A)

Purpose: To assess for congenital hip dislocation

Patient: Supine

Clinician: Standing at the patient's feet

Procedure: The patient is supine, with hips and knees at 90 degrees of flexion. The clinician's thumbs are on the infant's medial thigh and the fingers on the infant's lateral thigh. Firmly traction the thigh while gently abducting the legs so that the femoral head is translated anterior into the acetabulum.

Interpretation: The test is positive if there is a reduction of the hip that produces a joint audible.

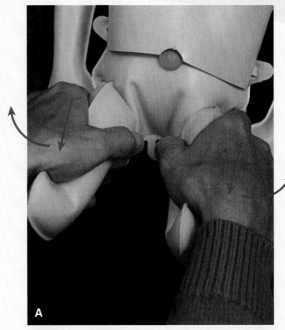

Barlow Test (Fig. 25-27B)

Purpose: To assess for congenital hip dislocation

Patient: Supine

Clinician: Standing at the patient's feet

Procedure: The patient is supine, with the hips and knees at 90 degrees of flexion. The clinician's thumbs are on the infant's medial thigh and fingers on the infant's lateral thigh. Apply a posterior force through the femur as the thigh is gently adducted.

Interpretation: The test is positive if the hip subluxes, which produces a joint audible.

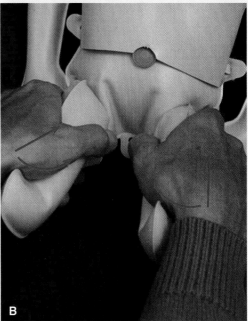

FIGURE 25–27 A. Ortolani test, and **B.** Barlow test. (Courtesy of Bob Wellmon Photography, BobWellmon.com.)

JOINT MOBILIZATION OF THE HIP

Note: The indications for the joint mobilization techniques described in this section are based on expected joint kinematics. Current evidence suggests that the indications for their use are multifactorial and may be based on direct assessment of mobility and an individual's symptomatic response.

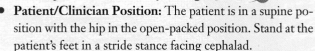

Hip Distraction

Indications:
- *Hip distractions* are indicated when there is a loss of mobility in all directions.

Accessory Motion Technique (Fig. 25-28)
- **Patient/Clinician Position:** The patient is in a supine position with the hip in the open-packed position. Stand at the patient's feet in a stride stance facing cephalad.
- **Hand Placement:** The patient's body weight provides stabilization, which can be enhanced by placing the foot of the contralateral leg on the table. A belt may be utilized at the patient's pelvis for additional stabilization. Both of your hands grasps the patient's distal tibia/fibula just proximal to the ankle (or above the knee if knee pathology exists). You may also use a mobilization belt around your gluteals and the patient's leg to reinforce your hand contacts.
- **Force Application:** While maintaining your hand contacts, shift your weight from your front to your back foot. You may also move the patient's hip in the direction of greatest restriction, while maintaining hand contacts and distraction force throughout the range of motion.

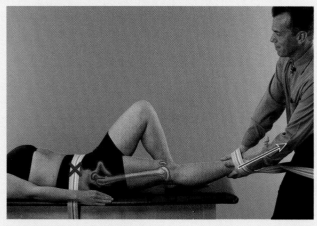

FIGURE 25–28 Hip distraction.

Accessory With Physiologic Motion Technique (Not pictured)
- **Patient/Clinician Position:** The patient and clinician are in the same position as described above.
- **Hand Placement:** Your hand placement is the same as that which is described above.
- **Force Application:** While maintaining force, move the hip in the direction of greatest restriction. Be prepared to move

during the mobilization to ensure correct force application. Force is maintained throughout the entire range of motion and sustained at end range.

Hip Inferior Glide

Indications:
- *Hip inferior glides* are indicated when there is a loss of hip flexion.

Accessory Motion Technique (Fig. 25-29)
- **Patient/Clinician Position:** The patient is in a supine position with the leg being mobilized placed over your shoulder with the knee flexed. You are standing to the side facing the patient. You may incorporate abduction/adduction or ER/IR to pre-position the hip in the direction of greatest restriction.
- **Hand Placement:** Stabilization is provided by the patient's body weight with assistance from a stabilization belt placed around the patient's pelvis. Your mobilization hands are clasped and placed over the anterior aspect of the proximal femur with your forearms in the direction in which force is applied. A mobilization belt may be used around your gluteals to reinforce hand contacts.
- **Force Application:** Apply an inferiorly directed mobilization force through your hand and belt contacts.

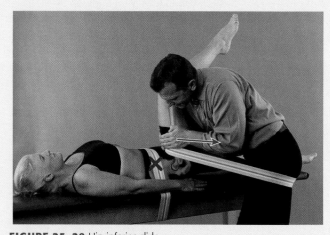

FIGURE 25–29 Hip inferior glide.

Accessory With Physiologic Motion Technique (Not pictured)
- **Patient/Clinician Position:** The patient and clinician are in the same position as described above.
- **Hand Placement:** Your hand placement is the same as that which is described above.
- **Force Application:** Apply an inferiorly directed mobilization force at the proximal femur as counterforce is elicited distally through your shoulder contact in a scooping-type motion as the hip is brought into progressively greater

ranges of hip flexion. The position of the hip may be altered slightly so that it is placed in the position of greatest restriction. Be prepared to move during the mobilization to ensure correct force application. Force is maintained throughout the entire range of motion and sustained at end range.

Hip Anterior Glide

Indications:
- *Hip anterior glides* are indicated when there is a loss of hip extension and ER.

Accessory Motion Technique (Fig. 25-30)
- **Patient/Clinician Position**: The patient is in a prone position near the edge of the table, with the hip in slight flexion, abduction, and external rotation (FABER), with the foot secured at the posterior aspect of the contralateral leg (figure-4 position). You may pre-position the hip at the point of restriction. You are standing contralateral to the side being mobilized with your leg securing the patient's foot against the table as needed.
- **Hand Placement:** Stabilization is provided by the patient's body weight and through securing the leg close to the surface of the table. A mobilization belt may also be used, around the patient's waist. Hand-over-hand contact is placed at the posterior aspect of the proximal femur just below the gluteal fold. Your elbows are extended and your forearms are positioned in line with the anterolateral direction of force. You may alternately place your stabilization hand at the anterior superior iliac spine on the side being mobilized with your mobilization hand is at the posterior aspect of the proximal femur.
- **Force Application:** An antero-laterally directed force is applied through your hand contacts.

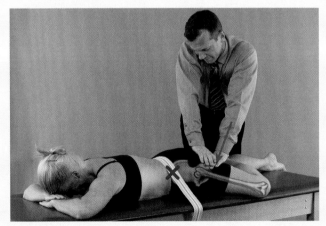

FIGURE 25–30 Hip anterior glide.

Accessory With Physiologic Motion Technique (Fig. 25-31)
- **Patient/Clinician Position:** The patient is in a prone position with the hip in neutral. Stand on the ipsilateral side of the hip being mobilized. Stabilization is provided by the patient's body weight or mobilization belt around the patient's

waist. The patient may be in a standing position. You are standing in front of the patient with a mobilization belt around the posterior aspect of the patient's proximal femur and your gluteals.
- **Hand Placement:** In prone, use one hand to grasp the anterior aspect of the patient's thigh to provide physiologic motion into hip extension. Place the other hand at the posterior aspect of the proximal femur, just inferior to the patient's gluteal fold with your forearm in line with the direction of force. In standing, both hands stabilize the patient's pelvis as the belt is placed over the proximal femur.
- **Force Application:** In prone, take up the slack in the joint and apply an anterior glide as the patient's hip is moved into progressively greater ranges of extension. In standing, the patient performs trunk backward bending or side-stepping, rotation, or lunging while anteriorly directed mobilizing force is provided through the belt contact. Be prepared to move during the mobilization to ensure correct force application. Force is maintained throughout the entire range of motion and sustained at end range.

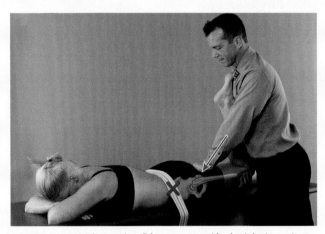

FIGURE 25–31 Hip anterior glide accessory with physiologic motion.

Hip Posterior Glide

Indications:
- *Hip posterior glides* are indicated for restrictions in hip flexion and IR.

Accessory Motion Technique (Fig. 25-32)
- **Patient/Clinician Position**: The patient is in a supine position with the hip flexed, slightly adducted, and internally rotated with the knee flexed. You are standing on the contralateral side of the hip being mobilized.
- **Hand Placement:** Stabilization is provided by the patient's body weight. Additionally, your stabilization hand or bolster is placed under the patient's posterior ischium just proximal to the patient's hip. Place your clasped mobilization hands or single mobilization hand over the patient's flexed knee with your forearms in line with the postero-lateral direction of force.

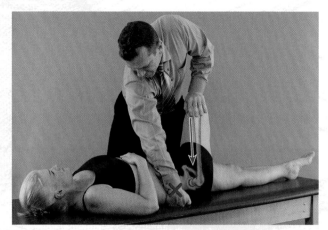

FIGURE 25–32 Hip Posterior glide.

- **Force Application:** With your hand contacts in place, take up the slack in the joint and apply a postero-lateral glide through the long axis of the femur. Alternately, you may apply a postero-lateral glide as you bring the patient's hip into progressively greater ranges of hip flexion.

Accessory With Physiologic Motion Technique (Fig. 25-33)
- **Patient/Clinician Position:** The patient and clinician are in the same position as that which is described above.
- **Hand Placement:** In supine, clasp your hands over the patient's flexed knee. In standing, the mobilization belt is placed from your gluteals to the anterior aspect of the patient's proximal femur.
- **Force Application:** In supine, patient moves into progressively greater ranges of hip flexion while clinician maintains

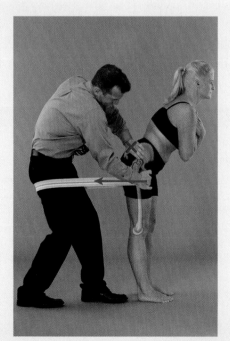

FIGURE 25–33 Hip posterior glide accessory with physiologic motion.

posteriorly directed mobilizing force. In standing, patient performs trunk forward bending or side-stepping rotation, or lunging while posteriorly directed mobilizing force is provided through the belt contact. The mobilization force is maintained throughout the entire range of motion and sustained at end range.

Hip Medial Glide

Indications:
- *Hip medial glides* are indicated for restrictions in hip abduction and ER.

Accessory Motion Technique (Fig. 25-34)
- **Patient/Clinician Position:** The patient is in a side-lying or supine position with the hip in neutral. You may pre-position the hip at the point of restriction. You are standing on the ipsilateral side of the hip being mobilized.
- **Hand Placement:** Your stabilization hand supports the leg at the medial aspect of the knee. Your open mobilization hand contacts the lateral aspect of the proximal femur. Your forearm is in line with the direction in which force is applied.
- **Force Application:** With your hand contacts in place, take up the slack in the joint and apply a medial glide to the proximal hip.

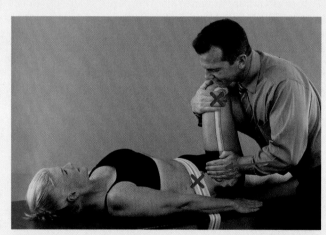

FIGURE 25–34 Hip medial glide.

Accessory With Physiologic Motion Technique (Not pictured)
- **Patient/Clinician Position:** The patient and clinician are in the same position as that which is described above.
- **Hand Placement:** The hand contacts are the same as that which is described above.
- **Force Application:** The patient moves into progressively greater ranges of hip abduction, ER, or flexion while you maintain your medially directed mobilization force. The mobilization force is maintained throughout the entire range of motion and sustained at end range.

Hip Lateral Glide

Indications:
- *Hip lateral glides* are indicated for restrictions in hip adduction and IR.

Accessory Motion Technique (Fig. 25-35)
- **Patient/Clinician Position:** The patient is in a supine position with the hip in neutral or with the hip flexed to 90 degrees and in varying degrees of ER/IR and abduction/adduction or standing. You may pre-position the hip at the point of restriction. You are standing on the ipsilateral side of the hip being mobilized.
- **Hand Placement:** Your stabilization hand is placed on the lateral aspect of the knee. A mobilization belt may also be used at the patient's pelvis for stabilization. If a mobilization belt is used, your stabilization hand is placed at the lateral aspect of the patient's pelvis. Your mobilization hand is placed on the medial aspect of the proximal femur with your forearm in the direction in which force is applied. If a mobilization belt is used, force is applied through the mobilization belt, which is placed between your gluteals and the medial aspect of the patient's proximal femur.
- **Force Application:** Apply a laterally directed force through either the mobilization hand contact at the medial aspect of the proximal femur or the mobilization belt while providing stabilization with your other hand.

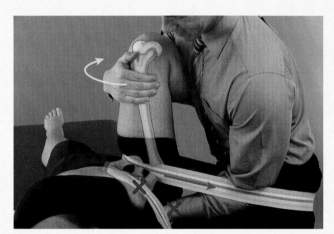

FIGURE 25–35 Hip lateral glide accessory motion and accessory with physiologic motion in supine.

Accessory With Physiologic Motion Technique (Figs. 25-35, 25-36)
- **Patient/Clinician Position:** For the supine technique, the patient is lying supine with the hip flexed to 90 degrees and in varying degrees of external or internal rotation. You may pre-position the hip at the point of restriction. You are standing in a straddle stance on the ipsilateral side of the hip being mobilized and facing the patient with the mobilization belt on the inner thigh at the proximal femur and around your gluteal folds. For the standing technique, the patient is standing in single leg stance position on the side being mobilized. You are standing on the side of the hip being mobilized.
- **Hand Placement:** In supine, your stabilization hand is placed on the lateral aspect of the patient's pelvis with the elbow of the stabilization arm placed at your anterior superior iliac spine (ASIS) and your forearm placed on the inner side of the mobilization belt. Your mobilization hand is placed over the patient's flexed knee and maintains the flexed knee in contact with your body. The mobilization belt is placed on the patient's inner thigh at the proximal femur and around your gluteal folds. In standing, both stabilization hands are placed over the lateral aspect of the patient's pelvis.
- **Force Application:** In supine, move the patient's hip into progressively greater ranges of hip internal or external rotation while you maintain a laterally directed force through the mobilization belt contact. In standing, with contacts in place, apply a laterally directed force through the mobilization belt while the patient rotates to the left or right, lunges forward or back, or performs a squatting motion.

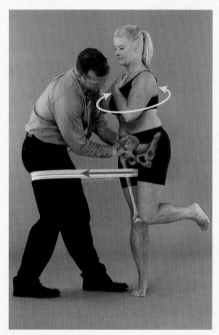

FIGURE 25–36 Hip lateral glide accessory with physiologic motion in standing.

CLINICAL CASE

CASE 1

Subjective Examination

History of Present Illness

A 45-year-old obese female presents to your facility today with chronic low back pain that she has had for years, with a more recent onset of right lateral hip pain along with right groin pain that began approximately 6 months ago. Since that time, her symptoms have progressively increased, with the hip pain now being her chief complaint. Her pain prohibits her from using the stairs at work, and it awakens her if she rolls onto the involved side during the night while sleeping.

Past Medical History: Chronic low back pain with insidious onset over 10 years ago for which she has received repeated bouts of chiropractic care; morbid obesity, hyperthyroidism, gout.

Social History: This patient is employed as a pharmacist, which requires her to stand most of the day in one position. Over the past 2 weeks, she has been unable to complete a full day of work without taking 400 mg of ibuprofen.

Objective Physical Examination

Examination of Structure

In standing, increased height of the left iliac crest, ASIS, and PSIS is noted. Increased lumbar lordosis, slight scoliotic C-curve with apex at right L3-4, bilateral genu recurvatum, and bilateral foot overpronation right greater than left noted. Toeing-in of the right foot is also noted. Measurement of leg length from ASIS to medial malleolus reveals right = 85 cm, left = 88.5 cm.

Lower Quarter Screen

AROM and break testing of the knee and ankle bilaterally are within normal limits (WNL) and symptom-free. Lumbar AROM reveals forward bending to be approximately 50% of normal, with poor curve reversal and pain at end range that does not peripheralize with single or repeated movements. Backward bending and rotation are approximately 75% of normal and pain-free, with end range stiffness only. Side bending right = 25%, with reversal of scoliosis and contralateral muscle pull; left = 75% symptom-free. No change in chief complaint of right hip pain with lumbar AROM.

Examination of Mobility

Physiologic Motion Testing

MOTION	AROM	PROM	END FEEL	PAIN REPRODUCTION	RELATIONSHIP OF R TO P*
Flexion	R = 46 degrees L = 60 degrees	R = 50 degrees L = 65 degrees	Soft tissue	Positive	R1 before P1 P2 before R2
Extension	R = −15 degrees L = −5 degrees	R = −15 degrees L = 0 degrees	Soft tissue	Negative	R1,2 before P1,2
External Rotation	R = 32 degrees L = 31 degrees	R = 40 degrees L = 35 degrees	Capsular	Negative	R1,2 before P1,2
Internal Rotation	R = 18 degrees L = 28 degrees	R = 20 degrees L = 35 degrees	Empty	Positive	P1,2 before R1,2
Abduction	R = 10 degrees L = 13 degrees	R = 10 degrees L = 15 degrees	Capsular	Negative	R1,2 without P
Adduction	R = 4 degrees L = 6 degrees	R = 5 degrees L = 8 degrees	Empty	Positive	P1,2 before R1,2

*R indicates onset of resistance; P indicates onset of pain, where R1,2 = first and final onset of tissue resistance and P1,2 = first and final onset of pain.

Accessory Motion Testing: Limited accessory mobility was noted for posterior glide and inferior glide, with R1,2 noted before P1,2.

Examination of Muscle Function: Left hip is grossly 4+/5 throughout, with the exception of internal and external rotation, which is 3+/5. On the right: Flexion = 4+/5, extension = 4/5; external rotation = 3+/5 with pain, internal rotation = 3/5 with pain; abduction = 3+/5 with pain; adduction = 4−/5. STT testing produces weakness and pain with hip abduction and internal rotation.

Neurological Testing: Light touch sensation and deep tendon reflexes are intact and symmetrical.

Palpation: Exquisite tenderness noted just posterior to the right greater trochanter. Anterior migration of the path of the instantaneous center of rotation (PICR) noted during active hip flexion in supine.

Functional Testing: Patient requires upper extremity assistance to squat to floor and return to standing, with groin pain noted. Step-down test reveals right hip internal rotation and adduction when stepping onto left foot. Gait reveals gluteus medius lurch with weight shift over right leg in single leg stance on right.

Special Testing: All testing is negative on the left. On the right: FABER = positive; femoral grind/Scour test = positive; Thomas test = positive, bilaterally; Trendelenburg = positive; sciatic nerve and femoral nerve neurodynamic testing = negative; Craig testing = negative; sacroiliac joint provocation testing = all negative.

1. Identify the structural impairments involved in this patient's case and differentiate them from the functional impairments that are present. How might these impairments contribute to this patient's condition?

2. Is there a relationship between chronic low back pain and lateral hip pain? Is there a relationship between this patient's obesity and her presenting condition? Describe these relationships.

3. How might this patient's work duties impact her condition? What strategies would you recommend to aid her in reducing stresses placed through her hip at work and during activities of daily living (ADLs)?

4. Do the deficits observed in accessory mobility correlate with those seen during physiologic mobility testing? What joint mobilization techniques would you use in the care of this patient? Perform each of them on a partner.

5. In addition to joint mobilization, what other manual and non-manual intervention strategies would you use in the care of this patient?

6. How does the relationship between resistance (R) and pain (P) that you observed during mobility testing dictate your intervention?

7. What is the role of progressive resistance exercise (PREs) in the care of this patient? Do you anticipate that PREs will address the patient's primary pain complaints or be better suited for addressing secondary impairments?

8. Based on the results of this examination, classify this patient based on an (1) impairment-based classification system, (2) movement impairment classification system, and (3) tissue-based classification system.

CASE 2

Subjective Examination

History of Present Illness

A 42-year-old truck driver presents to your facility today with chief complaint of right buttock pain, with paresthesia radiating into the posterior aspect of his right leg to his knee. He notes an overall increase in symptoms secondary to prolonged sitting, crossing his legs while sitting, and notes relief of his buttock pain with residual paresthesia when standing.

Past Medical History: Unremarkable with the exception of reporting the wearing of a Scottish Rite brace as an infant secondary to congenital hip dysplasia.

Objective Physical Examination

Examination of Structure: Observation in standing reveals a toeing-out of the right foot. All bony landmarks are equal in height and symmetrical bilaterally. Slight weight shift onto the left leg in static standing is noted.

Lower Quarter Screen: Range of motion and strength of bilateral knee, ankle, foot, and lumbar spine is WNL throughout. No reproduction of lower extremity symptoms with lumbar AROM.

Examination of Mobility

Physiologic Motion Testing

MOTION	AROM	PROM	END FEEL	PAIN REPRODUCTION	RELATIONSHIP OF R TO P
Flexion	46 degrees	R = 45 degrees L = 80 degrees	Soft tissue	Negative	R1,2 without P
Extension	70 degrees	R = 5 degrees L = 5 degrees	Capsular	Negative	R1,2 without P
External Rotation	15 degrees	R = 40 degrees L = 40 degrees	Normal capsular	Negative	R1,2 without P
Internal Rotation	11 degrees	R = 10 degrees L = 45 degrees	Empty	Positive	R1 before P1 R2 = P2
Abduction	27 degrees	R = 20 degrees L = 20 degrees	Normal capsular	Negative	R1,2 without P
Adduction	40 degrees	R = 10 degrees L = 15 degrees	Empty	Positive	R1 before P1 R2 = P2

*R indicates onset of resistance; P indicates onset of pain, where R1,2 = first and final onset of tissue resistance and P1,2 = first and final onset of pain.

Accessory Motion Testing: Accessory mobility testing of the hip is WNL throughout.

Examination of Muscle Function

MOTION	MMT	STT
Flexion	B = 5/5	Negative
Extension	B = 4/5	Positive
External Rotation	R = 3/5 L = 5/5	*Positive
Internal Rotation	B = 4+/5	Negative
Abduction	R = 3/5 L = 4+/5	Positive
Adduction	B = 4+/5	Negative

*Most painful
MMT indicates manual muscle testing; STT, selective tissue tension; B, bilateral.

Neurological Testing: No neurological signs present. Straight leg raise (SLR): R = positive at 65 degrees, L = negative.

Palpation: Exquisite tenderness to the touch and trigger points noted throughout palpation of the deep external rotator musculature of the hip on the right. Pain in the greater sciatic notch with extension of the knee with the hip flexed to 90 degrees.

Special Tests: On the right: FADIR = positive; FABER = negative; Craig test = positive for right femoral retroversion and confirmed by radiograph; lumbar quadrant = negative.

1. How significant of a role does this patient's occupation play in the pathogenesis of this condition? How significant of a role does this patient's previously diagnosed pediatric hip condition play in the pathogenesis of this condition?

2. Explain the relationship between this patient's condition and the structural and functional impairments that were identified. Are these impairments the result or the cause of this patient's presenting condition?

3. Describe the relationship between the findings from structural observation, mobility examination, and muscle function testing.

4. What do the results from physiologic and accessory mobility testing convey regarding the interventions that may be most effective?

5. Describe how you would confirm the efficacy of your interventions and make decisions regarding your plan of care. How would you determine your level of success?

6. What do the results of lumbar movement testing and the neurological examination tell you about the origin of these symptoms?

7. What is your prognosis for this patient? Describe the techniques that you believe would be most effective. How would you educate this patient regarding self-management and prophylaxis?

HANDS-ON

With a partner, perform the following activities:

1   Based on the pathoanatomic syndrome listed, identify the key historical indicators, examination findings, and prescribed intervention. Complete the grid.

PATHOANATOMIC SYNDROME	HISTORICAL INDICATORS	PHYSICAL EXAM FINDINGS	INTERVENTION
Osteoarthritis			
Rheumatoid Arthritis			
Avascular Necrosis			
Acetabular Labral Tears			
Legg-Calve-Perthes Disease			
Congenital Dysplasia			
Congenital Dislocation			
Slipped Capital Epiphysis			
Iliopsoas Strain			

Continued

PATHOANATOMIC SYNDROME	HISTORICAL INDICATORS	PHYSICAL EXAM FINDINGS	INTERVENTION
Adductor Muscle Strains			
Hip Flexion Contractures			
Ischial Bursitis			
Greater Trochanteric (GT) Bursitis			
Piriformis Syndrome			

2 Observe your partner as he or she performs active physiologic movements over single and repeated repetitions and single and multiplane directions and identify the quantity, quality, and any reproduction of symptoms that may be produced. Compare these active movements with performance of these same movements passively.

3 Perform passive physiologic movement testing in all directions, followed by passive accessory movement testing in all planes, and determine the relationship between the onset of pain (P1 and P2 if present) and stiffness or resistance (R1 and R2). Determine the end feel in each direction. Compare your findings bilaterally and on another partner.

4 Perform passive accessory movement testing in all planes with the wrist and hand in the neutral, or open-packed, position. Then perform the same tests with the hip in other nonneutral and close-packed positions. Identify any changes in the quantity and quality of available motion and report any reproduction of symptoms. Consider which anatomical structures are most responsible for limiting motion in each position. Complete the grid.

PASSIVE ACCESSORY MOVEMENT	QUANTITY, QUALITY, REPRODUCTION IN NEUTRAL	QUANTITY, QUALITY, REPRODUCTION IN NON-NEUTRAL	LIMITING STRUCTURES
Long Axis Distraction			
Inferior Glide			
Anterior Glide			
Posterior Glide			
Medial Glide			
Lateral Glide			

5 Perform procedures to identify the Reproduction of symptoms, Region of origin, and Reactivity level (3 R's) as described in this chapter and document your findings. What is the objective of performing these procedures?

6 Perform muscle testing for the key muscles about the hip using isometric break testing, static testing, and active testing based on the functional preference of each muscle during normal activity. Complete the grid.

MUSCLE TESTED	FUNCTIONAL PREFERENCE/ MANNER OF TESTING	RESULTS

7 Through palpation, attempt to identify the primary soft tissue and bony structures of the hip and compare tissue texture, tension, tone, and location bilaterally.

8 Based on your movement examination as identified above, choose two mobilizations. Perform these mobilizations on your partner and identify any immediate changes in mobility or symptoms in response to these procedures.

9 Perform each mobilization described in the intervention section of this chapter bilaterally on at least two individuals. Using each technique, practice Grades I to IV. Provide input to your partner regarding set-up, technique, comfort, and so on. When practicing these mobilization techniques, utilize the Sequential Partial Task Practice Method, in which students repeatedly practice one aspect of each technique (i.e., position, hand placement, force application) on multiple partners each time adding the next component until the technique is performed in real time from beginning to end. (Wise CH, Schenk RJ, Lattanzi JB. A model for teaching and learning spinal thrust manipulation and its effect on participant confidence in technique performance. *J. Man. Manip. Ther.*, August 2014.)

REFERENCES

1. Moore K, Dalley AI. *Clinically Oriented Anatomy*, 4th ed. Philadelphia, PA: Lippincott Williams & Wilkins; 1999.
2. Oatis CA. *Kinesiology: The Mechanics and Pathomechanics of Human Movement.* Philadelphia, PA: Lippincott Williams & Wilkins; 2004.
3. Konrath G, Hamel A, Olson S, et al. The role of the acetabular labrum and the transverse acetabular ligament in load transmission of the hip. *J Bone Joint Surg Am.* 1998;80:1781-1788.
4. Anda S, Svenningsen S, Dale LG, et al. The acetabulum sector angle of the adult hip determined by computed tomography. *Acta Radiol Diag.* 1986;27:443-447.
5. Levangie PK, Norkin CC. *Joint Structure and Function: A Comprehensive Analysis.* 4th ed. Philadelphia, PA: FA Davis; 2005.
6. Rosse C. *The Musculoskeletal System in Health and Disease.* Hagerstown, MD: Harper & Row; 1980.
7. Fischer P. Clinical measurement and significance of leg length & iliac crest height discrepancies. *J Man Manip Ther.* 1997:5;57-60.
8. Soukka A, Alaranta H, Tallroth K, Heliovarra M. Leg-length inequality in people of working age. *Spine.* 1991;16:429-431.
9. Rush WA, Steiner HA. A study of lower extremity length inequality. *Am J Radiol.* 1946;56:616-623.
10. Friberg O. Clinical symptoms and biomechanics of lumbar spine and hip joint in leg length inequality. *Spine.* 1983;8:643-651.
11. Kapandji I. *The Physiology of the Joints.* 5th ed. Baltimore, MD: Williams & Wilkins; 1987.
12. Arnold AS, Komattu AV, Delp SL. Internal rotation gait: a compensatory mechanism to restore abduction capacity decreased by bone deformity? *Dev Med Child Neurol.* 1997;39:40-44.
13. Williams P. *Gray's Anatomy.* 38th ed. New York, NY: Churchill Livingstone; 1999.
14. Escalante A, Lichtenstein MJ, Dhanda R, et al. Determinants of hip and knee flexion range: results from the San Antonio longitudinal study of aging. *Arthritis Care Res.* 1999;12:8-18.
15. Jerhardt J, Rippstein J. *Measuring and Recording of Joint Motion Instrumentation and Techniques.* Lewiston, NJ: Hogrefe & Huber; 1990.
16. MacConail MA, Basmajian JV. *Muscles and Movements: A Basis for Human Kinesiology.* Baltimore, MD: Williams & Wilkins; 1969.
17. Kaltenborn FM. *Mobilization of the Extremity Joints: Examination and Basic Treatment Techniques.* Oslo, Norway: Olaf Bokhandel; 1980.
18. Paris, SV, Loubert, PV. *Foundations of Clinical Orthopaedics, Course Notes.* St. Augustine, FL: Institute Press; 1990.
19. Patla CE, Paris, SV. *E1 Course Notes: Extremity Evaluation and Manipulation.* St. Augustine, FL: Institute of Physical Therapy; 1993.
20. Chesworth BM, Padfield BJ, Helewa A, Stitt LW. A comparison of hip mobility in patients with low back pain and matched healthy subjects. *Physiother Can.* 1994;46:267-274.
21. Cibulka MT, Sinacore DR, Cromer GS, Delitto A. Unilateral hip rotation range of motion asymmetry in patients with sacroiliac joint regional pain. *Spine.* 1998;23:1009-1015.
22. Delitto A, Erhard RE, Bowling RW. A treatment-based classification approach to low back syndrome: identifying and staging patients for conservative treatment. *Phys Ther.* 1995;75:470-489.
23. Cibulka MT. Low back pain and its relation to the hip and foot. *J Orthop Sports Phys Ther.* 1999;29:595-601.
24. Ellison JB, Rose SJ, Sahrmann SA. Patterns of hip rotation range of motion: comparison between healthy subjects and patients with low back pain. *Phys Ther.* 1990;70:537-541.
25. Perry J. *Gait Analysis: Normal and Pathological Function.* Thorofare, NJ: Slack; 1992.
26. Inman V, Ralston HJ, Todd F. *Human Walking.* Baltimore, MD: Williams & Wilkins; 1981.
27. Harris WH. Traumatic arthritis of the hip after dislocation and acetabular fractures: treatment by mold arthroplasty. An end-result study using a new method of result evaluation. *J Bone Joint Surg Am.* 1969;51:737-755.
28. Marchetti P, Binazzi R, Vaccari V, et al. Long-term results with cementless Fitek (or Fitmore) cups. *Arthroplasty.* 2005;20:730-737.
29. Klassbo M, Larsson E, Mannevik E. Hip disability and osteoarthritis outcome score. An extension of the Western Ontario and McMaster Universities Osteoarthritis Index. *Scand J Rheumatol.* 2003;32:46-51.
30. Dawson J, Fitzpatrick R, Carr A, Murray D. Questionnaire on the perceptions of patients about total hip replacement. *J Bone Joint Surg Br.* 1996;78:185-190.
31. Binkley J, Stratford P, Lott S, Riddle D., The North American Orthopaedic Rehabilitation Research Network. The Lower Extremity Functional Scale: scale development, measurement properties, and clinical application. *Phys Ther.* 1999;79:4371-4383.
32. Boissonnault WG. *Primary Care for the Physical Therapist: Examination and Triage.* St. Louis, MO: Elsevier Saunders; 2005.
33. Jemal A, Murray T, Samuels A, et al. Cancer statistics, 2003. *CA Cancer J Clin.* 2003;53:5-26.
34. Allen WC. Coxa saltans: the snapping hip revisited. *J Am Acad Orthop Surg.* 1995;3:303-308.
35. Fitzgerald RH. Acetabular labral tears-diagnosis and treatment. *Clin Orthop Relat Res.* 1995;311:60-68.
36. Magee DJ. *Orthopedic Physical Assessment.* 4th ed. Philadelphia, PA: WB Saunders; 2002.
37. Esola MA, McClure PW, Fitzgerald GK, Siegler S. Analysis of lumbar spine and hip motion during forward bending in subjects with and without a history of significant low back pain. *Spine.* 1996;21:71-78.
38. McClure PW, Esola M, Schreier R, Siegler S. Kinematic analysis of lumbar and hip motion while rising from a forward, flexed position in patients with and without a history of low back pain. *Spine.* 1997;22:552-558.
39. Cailliet R. *Low Back Pain Syndrome.* 5th ed. Philadelphia, PA: FA Davis; 1995.
40. McGill S. *Low Back Disorders: Evidence-Based Prevention and Rehabilitation.* Champaign, IL: Human Kinetics; 2002.
41. Nelson JM, Walmsley RPO, Stevenson JM. Relative lumbar and pelvic motion during loaded spinal flexion/extension. *Spine.* 1995;20:199.
42. Norkin CC, White DJ. *Measurement of Joint Motion: A Guide to Goniometry.* 3rd ed. Philadelphia, PA: FA Davis; 2003.
43. Chinkulprasert C, Vachalathiti R, Powers CM. Patellofemoral joint forces and stress during forward step-up, lateral step-up, and forward step-down exercises. *J Orthop Sports Phys Ther.* 2011;41:241-248.
44. Mascal CL, Landel R, Powers CM. Management of patellofemoral pain targeting hip, pelvis, and trunk muscle function: 2 case reports. *J Orthop Sports Phys Ther.* 2003;33:647-660.
45. Cyriax, J. *Textbook of Orthopaedic Medicine Volume One.* 8th ed. London, UK: Bailliere Tindall; 1982.
46. Delp SL, Hess WE, Hungerford DS, et al. Variation of rotation moment arms with hip flexion. *J Biomech.* 1999;32:493-501.

47. Murray MP, Sepic SB. Maximum isometric torque of hip abductor and adductor muscles. *Phys Ther.* 1968;48:1327-1335.
48. Tis LL, Perrin DH, Snead DB, Weltman A. Isokinetic strength of the trunk and hip in female runners. *Isok Exerc Sci.* 1991;1:22-25.
49. Donatelli R, Catlin PA, Backer GS, Drane DL, Slater SM. Isokinetic hip abductor to adductor torque ratio in normals. *Isok Exerc Sci.* 1991;1:103-111.
50. May WW. Maximum isometric force of the hip rotator muscles. *Phys Ther.* 1996;46:233-238.
51. Lindsay DM, Maitland ME, Lowe RC, Kane TJ. Comparison of isometric internal and external hip rotation torques using different testing positions. *J Orthop Sports Phys Ther.* 1992;16:43-50.
52. Cook G. *Movement: Functional Movement Systems: Screening, Assessment, Corrective Strategies.* Aptos, CA: On Target Publications; 2010.
53. Biel A. *Trail Guide to the Body.* Boulder, CO: Andrew Biel, LMP; 1997.
54. Dutton M. *Orthopaedic Examination, Evaluation, & Intervention.* New York, NY: McGraw-Hill; 2004.
55. Mitchell B, McCroy P, Brukner P, et al. Hip joint pathology: clinical presentation and correlation between magnetic resonance arthrography, ultrasound, and arthroscopic findings in 25 consecutive cases. *Clin J Sports Med.* 2003;13:152-156.
56. Cliborne A, Wainner R, Rhon D, et al. Clinical hip tests and a functional squat test in patients with knee osteoarthritis: reliability, prevalence of positive test findings, and short-term response to hip mobilization. *J Orthop Sports Phys Ther.* 2004;34:676-685.
57. Maslowski E, Sullivan W, Forster Harwood J, et al. The diagnostic validity of hip provocation maneuvers to detect intra-articular hip pathology. *Phys Med & Rehab.* 2010;2:174-181.
58. Martin RL, Sekiya JK. The interrater reliability of 4 clinical tests used to assess individuals with musculoskeletal hip pain. *J Orthop Sports Phys Ther.* 2008;38:71-77.
59. Dreyfuss P, Michaelsen M, Pauza K, McLarty J, Bogduk N. The value of medical history & physical examination in diagnosing sacroiliac joint pain. *Spine.* 1996;21:2594-2602.
60. Broadhurst NA, Bond MJ. Pain provocation tests for the assessment of sacroiliac joint dysfunction. *J Spinal Disorders.* 1998;11:341-345.
61. Flynn T, Fritz J, Whitman J, et al. A clinical prediction rule for classifying patients with low back pain who demonstrated short-term improvement with spinal manipulation. *Spine.* 2002;27:2835-2843.
62. Kokmeyer D, van der Wuff P, Aufdemkampe G, Fickenscher T. Reliability of multi-test regimens with sacroiliac pain provocation tests. *J Manipulative Physiol Ther.* 2002;25:42-48.
63. Fishman L, Dombi G, Michaelson C, et al. Piriformis syndrome: diagnosis, treatment and outcome: a 10 year study. *Arch Phys Med Rehabil.* 2002;83:295-301.
64. Maitland GD. *The Peripheral Joints: Examination & Recording Guide.* Adelaide, Australia: Virgo Press; 1973.
65. Narvani A, Tsiridis E, Kendall S, Chaudhuri R, Thomas P. A preliminary report on prevalence of acetabular labrum tears in sports patients with groin pain. *Knee Surg Traumatol Arthroscopy.* 2003;11:403-408.
66. Leuning M, Werlen S, Ungersbock A, Ito K, Ganz R. Evaluation of the acetabular labrum by MR arthroplasty. *J Bone Joint Surg.* 1997;79:230-234.
67. Fitzgerald RH Jr. Acetabular labrum tears: diagnosis & treatment. *Clin Orthop.* 1995;311:60-68.
68. Peeler JD, Anderson JE. Reliability limits of the modified Thomas test for assessing rectus femoris muscle flexibility about the knee joint. *J Athl Train.* 2008;43:470-476.
69. Browder D, Enseki K, Fritz J. Intertester reliability of hip range of motion measurements and special tests. *J Orthop Sports Phys Ther.* 2004;34:A1.
70. Trendelenburg F. Trendelenburg's test (1895). *Clin Orthop Relat Res.* 1998;355:3-7.
71. Bird PA, et al. Prospective evaluation of magnetic resonance imaging and physical examination findings in patients with greater trochanteric pain syndrome. *Arthritis Rheum.* 2001;44:2138-2145.
72. Peeler J, Anderson JE. Reliability of the Ely's test for assessing rectus femoris muscle flexibility and joint range of motion. *J Orthop Res.* 2008;26:793-799.
73. Offierski CM, MacNab IMB. Hip-spine syndrome. *Spine.* 1983;8:316-321.
74. Reynolds D, Lucas J, Klaue K. Retroversion of the acetabulum. *J Bone Joint Surg Br.* 1999;81:281-288.
75. Crane L. Femoral torsion and its relation to toeing-in and toeing-out. *J Bone Joint Surg Am.* 1959;41:421-428.
76. Ruwe PA, Gage JR, Ozonoff MB, DeLuca PA. Clinical determination of femoral anteversion. *J Bone Joint Surg Am.* 1992;74:820-830.
77. Staheli LT. Medial femoral torsion. *Orthop Clin North Am.* 1980;11:39-50.
78. Greenwood MJ, Erhard RE, Jones DL. Differential diagnosis of the hip vs. lumbar spine: five case reports. *J Orthop Sports Phys Ther.* 1998;27:308-315.
79. Burns SA, Burshteyn M, Mintken PE. Sign of the buttock following total hip arthroplasty. *J Orthop Sports Phys Ther.* 2010;40:377.
80. Ortolani M. The classic: congenital hip dysplasia in the light of early and very early diagnosis. *Clin Orthop Relat Res.* 1976;119:6-10.
81. Tachdjian MO. *Pediatric Orthopedics.* Philadelphia, PA: WB Saunders; 1972.
82. Baronciani D, Atti G, Andiloro F, et al. Screening for developmental dysplasia of the hip: from theory to practice. *Pediatrics.* 1997;99:e5.

Orthopaedic Manual Physical Therapy of the Knee

Christopher H. Wise, PT, DPT, OCS, FAAOMPT, MTC, ATC

Chapter Objectives

At the conclusion of this chapter, the reader will be able to:

- Identify the key anatomical and biomechanical features of the knee and their impact on examination and intervention.
- List and perform key procedures used in the orthopaedic manual physical therapy (OMPT) examination of the knee.
- Demonstrate sound clinical decision-making in evaluating the results of the OMPT examination.

- Use pertinent examination findings to reach a differential diagnosis and prognosis.
- Discuss issues related to the safe performance of OMPT interventions for the knee.
- Demonstrate basic competence in the performance of an essential skill set of joint mobilization techniques for the knee.

FUNCTIONAL ANATOMY AND KINEMATICS

Introduction

At first glance, the knee joint appears to be a simple hinge joint with two degrees of freedom that provides motion in the sagittal plane. Upon closer inspection, however, it is appreciated that motion is available within the other two cardinal planes as well. Further adding to its complexity is the fact that the knee is comprised of the *tibiofemoral joint*, or knee joint proper, and the *patellofemoral joint*, a planar joint that is involved in most cases of anterior knee pain (Fig. 26-1). Pain originating from the knee is present in approximately 20% of the population.[1]

The knee joint complex is uniquely positioned between the multiplanar hip and the equally mobile foot and ankle joints. Impairments of either the hip and/or the foot and ankle often contribute to the onset of knee pain and must routinely be considered in the management of these conditions. Likewise, pathology of the knee may lead to impairments both proximally and/or distally.

The Tibiofemoral Joint

The distal shaft of the femur culminates as two substantial condyles interposed by an intercondylar fossa, posteriorly. It

is within this fossa that the cruciate ligaments reside. The *lateral femoral condyle* extends more posteriorly than its medial counterpart.[2] The *medial femoral condyle* extends more distally and is curved in the transverse plane. Disparity in the size and shape of the femoral condyles contribute to the triplanar motion that is characteristic of this joint.

The proximal tibia consists of both a *medial* and *lateral plateau* corresponding to its respective femoral condyle. Both plateaus are concave from medial to lateral; however, the lateral plateau is slightly convex from anterior to posterior. These plateaus are generally considered to be only slightly concave, with a much larger radius of curvature than their corresponding condyles. Due to this incongruity, the knee lacks the stability that is required from osseous structures alone, thus requiring assistance, namely from the menisci, in order to achieve optimum stability. The larger articular surface contact area on the medial plateau functions to distribute loads, which is important since the medial plateau bears a greater extent of the forces in stance.[3] Like the femur, the two plateaus are divided by an intercondylar region, which includes the *intercondylar eminence*, serving as the attachment site for the menisci and cruciates. The most palpable osseous structure of the proximal tibia is the *tibial tuberosity*, which serves as the insertion for the patellar tendon. *Gerdy's tubercle* can be palpated just distal to

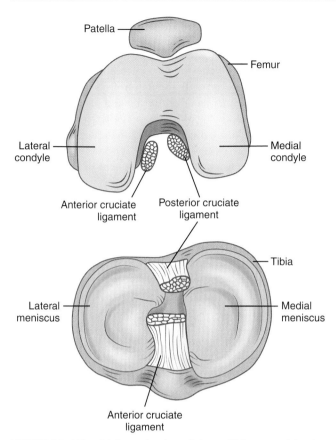

FIGURE 26–1 The tibiofemoral and patellofemoral joints comprising the knee joint complex including the cruciate ligaments and menisci.

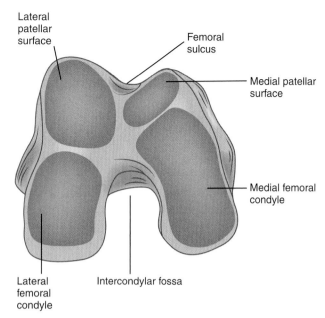

FIGURE 26–2 The articular surfaces of the patellofemoral and tibiofemoral joints. Note the difference in size between the articulating surfaces of the medial and lateral femoral condyles.

the lateral plateau and serves as the location to which the *lateral collateral ligament (LCL)* inserts.

The *tibiofemoral (TF) joint* is equipped with both a *medial* and a *lateral meniscus*, which disperse loads and enhance the congruency of the joint surfaces (Fig. 26-2).[4] The medial meniscus is C-shaped and is larger in diameter than the lateral O-shaped meniscus, yet covers a smaller percentage of the tibial plateau, thus subjecting the medial compartment to greater forces. The medial meniscus is securely attached to the tibia via the coronary ligaments as well as the TF joint capsule and *medial collateral ligament (MCL)*. The lateral meniscus is attached to the popliteus muscle and is more mobile, which may explain its relatively reduced incidence of injury.[4]

Stability of the Tibiofemoral Joint

The joint capsule and substantial ligamentous support system of the knee not only provides the necessary stabilization, but also serves to guide motion. The capsuloligamentous complex of the knee is quite extensive and, as expected, exerts its greatest effect at the end ranges of motion.[8] Unlike most joints, the two layers of the capsule are intermittently divided and serve different functions. The inner *synovial layer* of the capsule follows the femoral condyles, while the outer *fibrous layer* encapsulates the intercondylar notch and eminence. Therefore, the cruciate ligaments, which insert onto the eminence, are described as being intracapsular, yet extrasynovial. The *suprapatellar pouch* is located between the anterior aspect of the

femur and the quadriceps. This extension of the joint capsule is important for normal knee motion, much like the axillary folds of the glenohumeral joint capsule are necessary to allow full shoulder elevation. In the presence of trauma, this pouch may become engorged with effusion, particularly when the knee is in its fully extended position.[8] Folds in the synovial layer of the capsule form *plicae*, which may undergo inflammation and fibrosis resulting in the onset of medial knee pain.[8]

The well-known, and often injured, cruciate ligaments of the knee are vital both to the mobility and the stability of the knee joint. Each is named for the location of its insertion onto the tibia with the ACL inserting onto the anterior and lateral aspect of the tibia and the *posterior cruciate ligament (PCL)* inserting onto the posterior aspect of the tibia. The ACL courses posteriorly and inserts onto the medial aspect of the lateral femoral condyle as the more substantial PCL inserts onto the posterolateral aspect of the medial femoral condyle. The ACL is positioned more obliquely than the PCL which lends to its function in guiding knee joint arthrokinematics. Although the contributions of the ACL and PCL to knee joint stability are complex, these ligaments are generally responsible for limiting anterior and posterior tibial translation, respectively. The multibundle composition of the ACL and PCL suggests that these ligaments provide stability for the knee in a variety of planes. The ACL demonstrates its greatest tension at terminal extension and is least taut at the midrange of flexion.[9,10] The PCL develops greater tension as the knee flexes and is considered the primary restraint for knee flexion.[10] Both ligaments are important restraints, and therefore subject to injury, during transverse plane rotatory motion.

The MCL is broad and has extensive insertions into the medial meniscus and medial joint capsule. The narrower LCL inserts into the fibular head and is often easier to palpate across the lateral joint line of the knee. Although both the MCL and LCL develop their greatest degree of tension in full knee extension, they appear to play a greater role in stabilizing valgus and varus forces when the knee is in slight flexion.[11] Although the cruciate ligaments primarily restrict sagittal and transverse plane forces, the collateral ligaments also contribute to transverse plane stability.[11] Conversely, the cruciate ligaments assist the collaterals in their primary function as stabilizers of varus and valgus forces.[12] Dynamic stabilization resulting from muscle function is important throughout the midranges of knee motion.

Mobility of the Tibiofemoral Joint

Although the majority of motion within the TF joint occurs within the sagittal plane, this joint demonstrates six degrees of freedom about all three cardinal plane axes (Fig. 26-3). During open chain knee flexion, the tibia rolls posteriorly and glides posteriorly relative to the femur, with the reverse occurring during open chain knee extension (Fig. 26-4 A, B).[5] Closed chain kinematics reveals that the femur rolls anterior and glides posterior with extension and in the opposite direction during flexion (Fig. 26-4 C, D). The degree of translatory glide that accompanies this angular motion is minimal, particularly when performed in weight-bearing.[5] The normal range of knee flexion is documented as between *132 and 141 degrees* and normal knee extension, or more correctly stated, hyperextension is considered to be from *0 to 10 degrees*.[6,7]

Disparity in the geometric congruence between the medial and lateral aspects of the knee dictates that in addition to sagittal plane motion, transverse and frontal plane motion also readily occur. In open chain, up to *20 to 30 degrees* of medial,

or internal rotation, and *10 to 20 degrees* of adduction of the tibia on the femur occurs during movement from full extension to 90 degrees of flexion. Conversely, movement from flexion to extension involves *30 to 40 degrees* of lateral, or external rotation, and *10 to 20 degrees* of abduction.[2,5] When the knee is flexed, the amount of passive internal and external rotation greatly increases and may reach up to *80 degrees* (Fig. 26-5).[2,5] The term **screw home mechanism** is often used to define the final degree of tibial external rotation that occurs at the terminal range of knee extension, a useful component of knee stability. It is important to consider that the transverse and frontal plane motions that accompany sagittal plane motion occur throughout the entire range of motion and not at end range only. Transverse plane motion of the knee is the result of tension placed through the anterior cruciate ligament (ACL), the disparity in size and shape between the femoral condyles, and the oblique force vector of the quadriceps muscle group (Fig. 26-6).

The Patellofemoral Joint

The *patellofemoral (PF) joint* is comprised of the large sesamoid patella, which is contained within the quadriceps muscle tendon, and the concave trochlear groove formed between the two femoral condyles. The posterior articular surface of the patella is divided by a central ridge into a *medial facet* and larger *lateral facet*. The most medial aspect of the medial facet is occupied by the *odd facet*. Although the PF joint shares common structures with the TF joint, it functions quite uniquely and can be an independent source of pain and disability.

Several aberrations in PF joint alignment that may have an impact on both the mobility and stability of this articulation have been described clinically.[13] Normal medial/lateral alignment of the patella relative to the femur during motion, also referred to as **patellar medial/lateral tracking** or **glide**, is generally considered to reveal equidistance of the patella relative to the femoral condyles (Fig. 26-7).[14] A patella demonstrating excessive lateral tracking is common and may be a factor of either femoral or foot transverse or frontal plane malalignments. **Patellar tilt** describes the alignment of the patella about a superior-inferior axis. In full extension, the patella is normally in a small degree of lateral tilt.[8] Superior/inferior alignment of the patella is determined by a ratio of the distance between the length of the patella and the distance between the patella and the tibia.[8] **Patella alta** and **patella baja** are the terms used to describe a patella that is displaced superiorly and inferiorly, respectively. **Patellar medial** and **lateral rotations**, as determined by the inferior pole of the patella about an anterior-posterior axis may also be observed. Malalignment of the patella relative to the femur in any direction may place abnormal stresses through the PF joint or render the joint less stable.

Mobility of the Patellofemoral Joint

Under normal circumstances, the patella glides inferiorly *5 to 7 cm* on the femur during active knee flexion, which reverses during active knee extension.[15] The point of contact between the patella and femur changes as the knee moves (Fig. 26-8). Slight medial glide of the patella accompanies inferior translation from

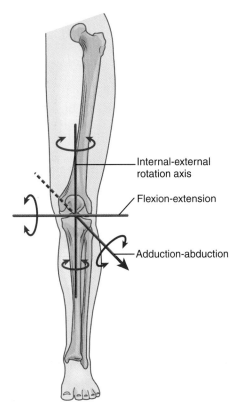

FIGURE 26–3 Axes of knee joint motion.

Internal-external rotation axis

Flexion-extension

Adduction-abduction

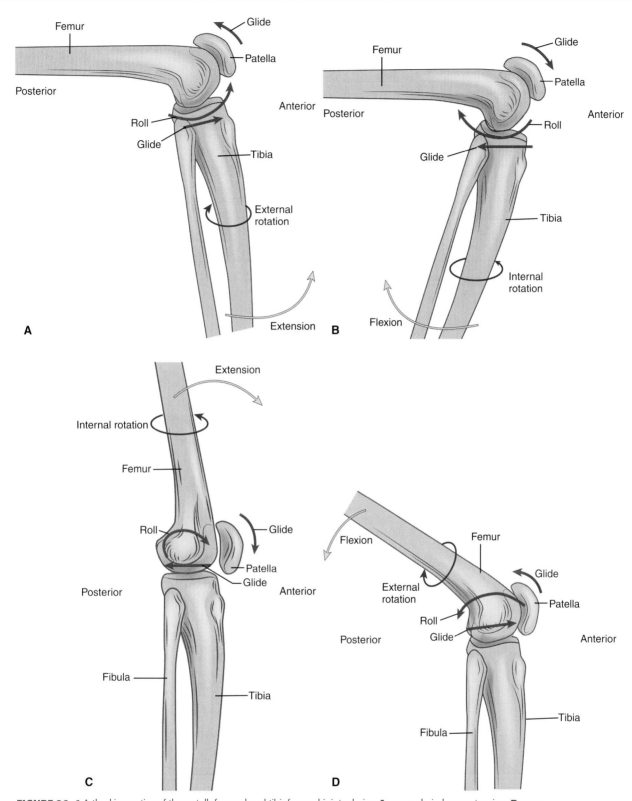

FIGURE 26–4 Arthrokinematics of the patellofemoral and tibiofemoral joints during **A.** open chain knee extension, **B.** open chain knee flexion, **C.** closed chain knee extension, and **D.** closed chain knee flexion.

0 to 30 degrees of flexion, after which lateral translation occurs, resulting in a C-curve translation.[16] In addition, the patella medially or laterally tilts around a superior/inferior axis, flexes and extends around a medial/lateral axis, and rotates around an anterior/posterior axis. From full knee extension to approximately

5 degrees of flexion, the PF joint is considered to be in its open-packed position.[16] During knee flexion, the patella becomes engaged within the trochlear notch of the femur, and PF motion becomes greatly reduced. Under normal circumstances the patella should passively glide approximately half of its width in

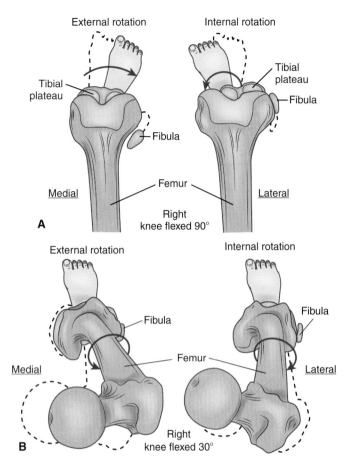

FIGURE 26-5 A. Transverse plane motion of the tibia/fibula on a fixed femur, with the knee flexed to 90 degrees produces internal and external rotation of the knee. **B.** Transverse plane motion of the femur on a fixed tibia/fibula with the knee flexed to 30 degrees in weight bearing. Because the tibia is fixed, the position of the knee in the transverse plane is opposite to the direction of femoral rotation. (Redrawn from: Neumann DA. *Kinesiology of the Musculoskeletal System: Foundations for Rehabilitation*, 2nd ed. St. Louis, MO: Mosby Elsevier; 2010, with permission.)

both medial and lateral directions when the PF joint is in its open-packed position.[17]

Stability of the Patellofemoral Joint

In the literature, six different configurations of the patellar facets have been described that relate to their size, concavity, convexity, and position.[18] These facets demonstrate a great degree of variability between individuals. The stability of the PF joint relates, in part, to the variability within the osseous configuration of the patella.

As previously described, the lateral femoral condyle projects farther anteriorly than the medial, thus contributing to the lateral stability of the PF joint. The central ridge that divides the facets at the posterior aspect of the patella is reciprocal with the concave sulcus formed between the two condyles of the femur. The **sulcus angle** is defined as the angle formed between the deepest part of the sulcus to the medial and lateral femoral condyles. Individuals with a shallow sulcus demonstrate a greater incidence of patellar subluxation.[19] The sulcus angle is best appreciated radiographically with the knee flexed, a projection known as the **sunrise view.**

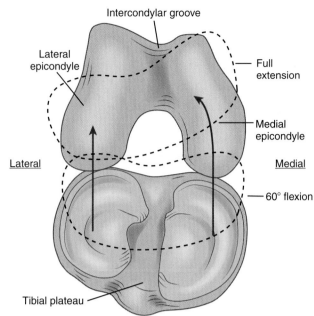

FIGURE 26-6 The screw home mechanism in open chain produces a translation of the tibial plateau within the transverse plane resulting in external rotation at terminal knee extension.

The Proximal Tibiofibular Joint

The proximal tibiofibular joint is located outside the knee joint proper and is mechanically linked with the distal tibiofibular joint, with the distal component exhibiting a greater degree of mobility. This planar synovial joint is supported by the *interosseous membrane* and the ligaments that attach to the head of the fibula. Motion between the tibia and fibula consists of gliding in all directions and rotation about a longitudinal axis.[8] These component motions seem to exist primarily for the purpose of enhancing ankle motion. Superior and inferior glide of the fibula relative to the tibia is presumed to occur during ankle dorsiflexion/eversion and plantarflexion/inversion, respectively. Rotation about the longitudinal axis serves to facilitate rotation of the tibia during knee and ankle motion.

EXAMINATION

The Subjective Examination

Self-Reported Disability Measures

The ***Lysholm Knee Scoring Scale***[20] is designed to determine the outcome of postsurgical rehabilitation and identify individuals with knee instability. Based on a perfect rating of 100, patients are assigned points for each disability reported. The ***Western Ontario and McMaster Universities Osteoarthritis Index (WOMAC)***[21] was initially developed to address individuals who were experiencing disability from osteoarthritis of the knee and was designed to obtain information regarding disability-related changes in response to intervention. The three individual dimensions of the WOMAC include pain, stiffness, and physical function. Each subscale may be individually summed or a total score of all three subscales may be

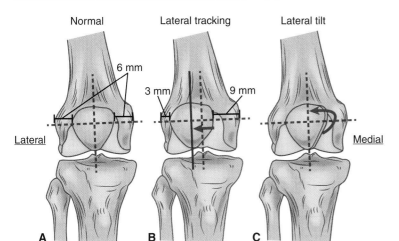

Normal   Lateral tracking   Lateral tilt

A   B   C

Lateral   Medial

Lateral rotation   Patella alta   Patella baja

D   E   F

Lateral   Medial

FIGURE 26–7 Alignment and malalignment of the patella.

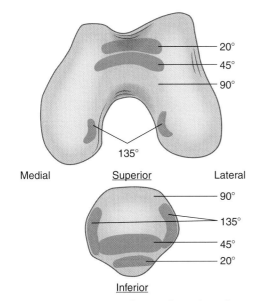

Medial   Superior   Lateral

Inferior

FIGURE 26–8 Kinematics of the patellofemoral joint during knee motion revealing points of contact on the femur and patella at various positions of the knee.

obtained.[22] Validity and test-retest reliability have been demonstrated in osteoarthritic patients undergoing joint replacement surgery or a regimen of anti-inflammatory medication.[21] The **Cincinnati Knee Rating System** is used as a means of measuring function in an active population. This tool is divided into two main sections, which are symptoms and function, totaling 100 points. The symptoms section includes the subcategories of pain, swelling, stability, and other symptoms, and the functional section includes the subcategories of overall activity level, walking, stairs, running, and jumping/twisting.[23] Lastly, the **Knee Outcome Survey** developed by Irrgang et al is divided into activity of daily living and sports activity subscales. The first section attempts to identify the full continuum of disability that may occur in response to knee pathology and has been found to possess good reliability.[25]

Review of Systems

Knee pain may be the result of *intermittent claudication*, which involves pain of the thigh and calf upon exertion that diminishes at rest. Individuals suffering from *peripheral vascular disease (PVD)* may exhibit such a pain pattern. In order to differentiate between vascular claudication and neurogenic claudication that is attributed to nerve root compression, the therapist may alter the patient's position during exertion to reduce compressive forces. Confirmation of the presence of PVD may involve diminished temperature of the distal extremity, the presence of vascular poorly healing wounds, diminished pedal pulses, the **ankle/brachial index (ABI)**, and the reactive **hyperemia test**. The ABI is obtained by dividing the systolic blood pressure of the ankle by the pressure of the brachial artery. An ABI of less than 0.97 confirms the presence of PVD.[26] The hyperemia test involves placing the extremity in a 45-degree straight leg raised position for 3 minutes and counting the time for venous return. Longer than 20 seconds suggests the presence of PVD. The clinician must be cognizant of the fact that the presence of PVD is often the product of cardiac ischemia, and measures must be taken to reduce additional stresses to the cardiac system.[27]

Septic arthritis, involving inflammation of the joint caused from bacterial infection, and *cellulitis*, which is an infection of the skin, may also lead to knee pain of nonmusculoskeletal origin. Septic arthritis involves throbbing pain, edema, increased temperature to the touch, as well as limitations in mobility. A variety of conditions may lead to an increased incidence of septic arthritis, including recent surgery, presence of rheumatoid or osteoarthritis, and an immunosuppressed host. Individuals with cellulitis present with pain, erythema, and swelling, along with fever and malaise. This condition is often the result of a recent wound or condition involving cardiac insufficiency.[27]

Among the most serious conditions that may mimic musculoskeletal knee pain is the presence of a *deep vein thrombosis (DVT)*. Therefore, patients must be routinely screened for the presence of DVTs. Those patients most susceptible to the onset of a DVT are those who are postsurgical, pregnant, or who have experienced prolonged immobilization.[27] Contrast venography is considered the gold standard for confirmation; however, the presence of a DVT should be considered in the presence of intense calf pain, along with tenderness and increased temperature to the touch over the calf. The *Homans sign*, which involves passive dorsiflexion of the ankle, will be positive in the presence of intense calf pain. An immediate course of anticoagulant therapy is necessary to avoid the occurrence of a pulmonary embolus. See Table 26-1 for a list of the medical red flags for individuals presenting with knee-related symptoms.

History of Present Illness

It is important to consider any previous impairments of the entire lower quarter that may or may not have previously required intervention. Recurrent injuries of the knee are common, and identifying the relationship between past and present impairments may be helpful in understanding the pathogenesis and etiology of the current condition.

Sharp, localized pain that is associated with joint clicking or catching and pain with overpressure at end range of knee flexion is suggestive of meniscal or ligamentous injury. Pain of degenerative origin is often associated with stiffness and is more severe in the morning and after long periods of immobility with improvement noted upon activity. Anterior knee pain is often associated with PF joint pathology and is often more severe after prolonged sitting. Severe anterior knee pain as a result of quick torsional movements in weight-bearing is often indicative of patellar subluxation or meniscal tears. Pain and locking from the position of extreme knee flexion may also be suggestive of meniscal injury. Ligamentous laxity may lead

Table 26-1	Medical Red Flags for the Knee	
MEDICAL CONDITION	**RED FLAGS**
Septic arthritis	Joint pain, edema, tenderness Recent injection, infection, surgery, open wound Compromised immunity
Deep vein thrombosis (DVT)	Positive Homans sign Calf is warm, erythemic, and exquisitely tender Recent surgery, period of immobilization, pregnancy, malignancy
Compartment syndrome	Overuse Cumulative trauma History of blunt trauma Firmness to palpation Exquisite tenderness Reduced pulse Paresthesia

to pain and inflammation along with joint sounds and the feeling of giving way during movement and activity. Giving way of the knee may also occur in response to the onset of pain during activity.

If edema is immediately present following injury, then ligamentous damage is suspected. Edema that occurs over hours and days following the injury is typically more capsular in nature or may suggest bursae pathology, especially in cases of a direct blow with localized edema.[28] Edema within the medial compartment is more easily visualized than edema of the lateral compartment or edema of the retro- and infrapatellar spaces.

Locking of the knee, typically in flexion with an inability to fully extend, is suggestive of internal derangement resulting from a plica syndrome or meniscal tear. Intra-articular crepitus of either the TF or the PF joint may be an indication of malalignment or osteoarticular degeneration, whereas extra-articular sounds may result from tendon snapping. The clinical significance of the common report of crepitus within the PF joint must be established prior to initiating intervention.

Mechanism of Injury

It is important to determine whether the knee-related symptoms gradually developed or whether they were the result of a single traumatic incident. When determining the specific mechanism of injury, it is important to also consider the impact of both proximal and distal components of the kinetic chain. Knee joint pathology may result from structural or functional aberrations that must be addressed in conjunction with management of the patient's primary complaint. In cases of traumatic injury, ascertaining such details as the direction of force, the position of the knee at the time of injury, as well as the weight-bearing status are all important. The ACL and meniscus are often injured from forces that hyperextend the knee, particularly if some degree of torsion is also involved. The MCL, along with the ACL, are often involved in traumatic valgus forces, whereas the LCL, along with the PCL, are often injured in response to excessive varus forces. Posterior translation of the knee when it is flexed, as often occurs during a motor vehicle accident (i.e., dashboard injury), may involve injury to the PCL. Sports that involve directional changes as well as acceleration and deceleration may challenge the stabilizing structures even in the absence of external forces. Jumping activities that involve landing in valgus, referred to as **ligament dominance**, asymmetrical landing, referred to as **leg dominance**, and dominant activation of the quadriceps relative to the hamstrings, known as **quadriceps dominance**, have all been shown to be predictive factors of injury to the ACL.[29]

The *Ottawa Knee Rules*[30,31] provide a list of criteria that suggests the need for radiographic examination if any one criterion is present. The criteria include the following: a (1) patient over 55 years old, (2) patellar tenderness without other bony tenderness, (3) tenderness over the fibular head, (4) an inability to actively flex the knee greater than 90 degrees, and (5) the inability to bear weight immediately following injury.

The Objective Physical Examination

Examination of Structure

Observation of increased temperature, using the dorsum of the hand, palpation of the medial and lateral joint lines, and the presence of a ballotable, or floating, patella may provide evidence of edema. *Circumferential measurements* using a cloth tape measurer is important to document changes in edema over time and may also be helpful to ascertain any degree of muscular atrophy resulting from injury. In the presence of swelling, the knee often assumes a position of approximately 30 degrees of flexion to accommodate for increased volume.

The patient is asked to march in place, then stand with feet apart in his or her preferred standing posture. Both frontal and transverse plane deformities often coexist and may be observed anteriorly as well as posteriorly. It is important, yet challenging, to determine the origin of any static deformities that may be observed at the knee. Observation of asymmetrical bony landmarks may suggest a *limb length discrepancy (LLD)*. A true structural LLD must be differentiated from a functional LLD resulting from positional faults of the pelvic girdle.[32–34] In the presence of a LLD, compensations may occur, which include foot overpronation, internal tibial torsion, and knee flexion on the longer side.[35,36]

In the frontal plane, the normal adult knee is postured in approximately 5 to 6 degrees of valgus, which is known as **genu valgum**. Until approximately 18 months, children demonstrate **genu varum**.[37] In the elderly, genu varum often returns as the medial compartment of the knee exhibits degenerative changes. This measurement varies considerably between individuals, and it is important to be aware of gender differences related to the **tibiofemoral shaft angle**, which is a frontal plane angle that is measured between the tibia and the femur. This angle is normally about 6 degrees on imaging.[38] Females

often have a greater angle, which may render them more susceptible to PF dysfunction or ligamentous instability, particularly for those involved in high impact sports.[39,40]

Since the patella is embedded within the tendinous insertion of the quadriceps muscle, its position is influenced by the force vector of the quadriceps muscle. The quadriceps angle, or **Q-angle**, is measured in supine with the quadriceps relaxed by drawing a line from the anterior inferior iliac spine (AIIS) to the midpoint of the patella and then a second intersecting line from the tibial tuberosity to the same point on the patella.[41] A normal Q-angle is considered to be 18 degrees for females and 13 degrees for males. An abnormal Q-angle suggests the presence of aberrant patellar tracking and PF dysfunction.[42,43] It is important to denote the difference between the tibiofemoral shaft angle, obtained from radiographs, and the Q-angle, which is a clinical measurement used to appreciate the force vector of the quadriceps.

Transverse plane alignment of the knee is considered normal when the femoral condyles and tibial plateaus are parallel with no degree of rotation.[44] There are a myriad of forces acting upon the patella that influence its relative position upon the femur (Fig. 26-9). Genu valgus and varus will contribute to patellar malalignment. **Femoral anteversion** has been correlated with aberrant mechanics of the PF joint and an increased Q-angle.[45] In addition, structural frontal plane deformities of the femur, such as **coxa valga** and **coxa vara**, may also contribute to observable knee malpositioning. Coxa valga, as evidenced by an increase in the femoral angle of inclination, may contribute to genu varus at the knee, and coxa vara, as evidenced by a decrease in the femoral angle of inclination, may contribute to genu valgus at the knee. See Chapter 25 for more information related to the contribution of the hip and femur to impairments of the knee.

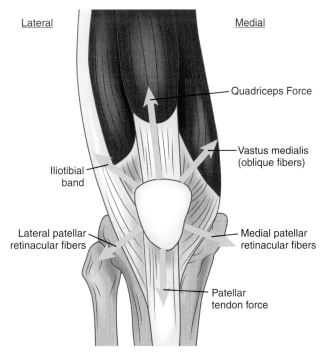

FIGURE 26–9 Forces that influence the alignment and tracking of the patella.

In addition to the femur's role in the onset of knee deformity, the tibia should also be considered. The tibia and the foot/ankle complex have an interdependent relationship.[46–48] Aberrant foot types have been found to contribute to altered mechanics and impairment throughout the lower quarter.[49–53] **External tibial torsion**, or **rotation** increases the Q-angle by moving the tibial tuberosity laterally, and **internal tibial torsion, or rotation** has the opposite effect.[45] The transverse plane position of the tibia is greatly influenced by the foot and ankle. A **pes planus**, or overpronated, foot leads to internal tibial torsion, and a **pes cavus**, or oversupinated, foot leads to external tibial torsion.[46–48] Therefore, a pes planus/cavus foot deformity, as determined by the relative height of the navicular from the floor in standing, may lead to genu valgus or varus, respectively, at the knee.[46–48] In addition, the position of the tibia in the frontal plane may also be considered by measuring the angle of the tibia relative to the horizontal. This measurement should be 0 degrees, indicating that the tibia is perpendicular to the floor. Before taking this measurement in standing, the foot must be placed in the **subtalar joint neutral (STJN)** position to minimize the effects of foot position on this measurement. A tibia that is in varus will require a greater degree of pronation to allow the metatarsal heads to contact the ground during gait.[54] The use of orthotics for the management of foot, knee, hip, and lumbar spine impairment is often considered.[55,56] Measurement of the STJN position and orthotic prescription will be covered in more detail in Chapter 27.

As the middle link of the closed kinetic chain, the knee may be the primary area of compensation, or the victim, of either hip and/or foot/ankle deformity or impairment. A typical presentation of genu valgus includes internal rotation of the hip or femoral anteversion, tibial internal torsion, and foot overpronation. The degree of femoral rotation often exceeds the degree of tibial rotation, thus causing the tibial tuberosity to be displaced laterally relative to the femur and thus increasing the Q-angle and contributing to lateral tracking of the patella. The opposite case may also occur in the case of genu varus which decreases the Q-angle and medial patellar tracking. It is often challenging for the clinician to determine if the primary impairment is occurring proximally leading to distal impairments or compensations or if the primary impairment is distal resulting in proximal impairments or compensations. In the case of "bottom down" impairments, femoral anteversion or retroversion may lead to tibial internal torsion and foot overpronation or tibial external torsion and foot oversupination, respectively (Fig. 26-10 A, B). In the case of "bottom up" impairments, foot overpronation or oversupination may lead to tibial internal torsion and hip internal rotation or tibial external torsion and hip external rotation, respectively. Compensations may occur distally or proximally to adapt for the primary impairment. Figure 26-10C demonstrates compensations that may occur distally in the presence of proximal impairments. Figure 26-10D demonstrates compensations that may occur proximally in the presence of distal impairments. Addressing both proximal and distal influences are critical in the management of the primary complaint of knee pain.

The line of gravity is expected to pass just anterior to the axis of the knee in an upright static posture, which denotes the role of the posterior knee joint capsule in providing passive support. Quadriceps or ankle dorsiflexor weakness, posterior capsular laxity, deficiency of the anterior cruciate ligament, or systemic conditions that produce joint laxity may result in a **genu recurvatum** deformity. Inability to achieve full knee extension may be the result of edema, as noted, or may be related to internal derangement or as a compensation for limitations in ankle dorsiflexion.

Examination of Mobility

Active Physiologic Movement Examination

The *active range of motion (AROM)* examination includes both single and repeated movements. These motions are performed best in the supine position with the extremity supported. In this position, the maximal amount of knee flexion can be ascertained in a manner that reduces the effects of passive insufficiency of the rectus femoris muscle. This supported position may also reduce the effects of pain or fear of pain associated with movement. These motions may also be assessed in the sitting position as well as standing in order to determine the effects of weight-bearing on mobility and symptoms. During the AROM examination, it is important to reliably measure the quantity of motion, the quality of motion, and any reproduction of symptoms.

During the AROM assessment, the clinician attempts to appreciate muscle function by observing the active contraction of the quadriceps and hamstrings. The quadriceps develop their greatest amount of force at approximately 60 degrees, and the hamstrings develop their greatest amount of force between 45 and 10 degrees.[43] Comparing the degree of active range with the degree of passive range serves to identify if the deficit is related to an impairment in muscle function or joint mobility. The presence of an **extensor lag**, which results in an inability to achieve full knee extension actively despite full passive range, may be observed.

The quadriceps and ACL have an antagonistic relationship during active terminal extension. During active tibia on femur knee extension, contraction of the quadriceps, in addition to producing a superior glide of the patella on the femur, also produces an anterior glide of the tibia relative to the femur. This anterior glide is resisted by most of the fibers of the ACL in addition to the hamstrings, posterior capsule, and collateral ligaments (Fig. 26-11). Conversely, during active tibia on femur knee flexion, the hamstrings and PCL are antagonists. As the hamstrings flex the knee, a posterior glide of the tibia on the femur is produced, which is chiefly resisted by the PCL as well as the quadriceps (Fig. 26-12).

The amount of motion available in the transverse and frontal planes is much less than that expected in the sagittal plane, and motion varies significantly depending on the position of the knee. Normal medial (internal) and lateral (external) torsion, or rotation of the tibia is substantial when the knee is flexed but greatly reduced when the knee is extended and during normal gait (see Fig. 26-5).[57,58] Frontal plane abduction/adduction of the tibia relative to the femur is estimated to be even less than transverse plane motion.[57] Most estimates of normal range of motion at the knee are based on measurements of passive range

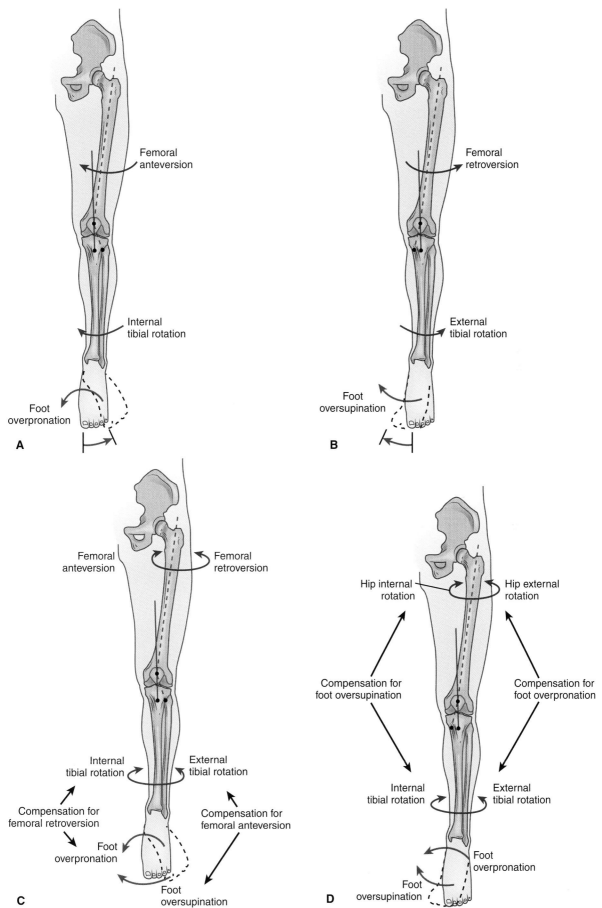

FIGURE 26–10 The impact of femoral torsion and tibial torsion on the lower extremity. **A.** and **B.** reveal structural deviations of the femur and their potential impact on the tibia and foot distally (i.e. bottom down impairments). **C.** reveals distal compensations resulting from proximal impairments and **D.** reveals proximal compensations resulting from distal impairments.

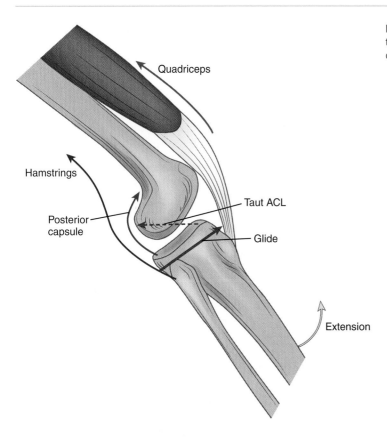

FIGURE 26–11 The relationship of the quadriceps muscle and the anterior cruciate ligament during active knee extension in open chain.

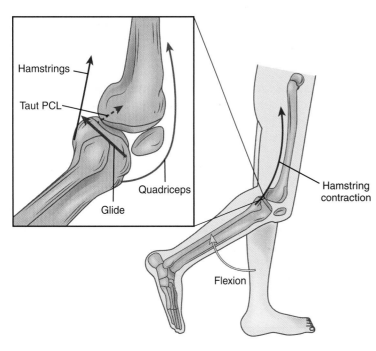

FIGURE 26–12 The relationship of the hamstrings muscle and the posterior cruciate ligament during active knee flexion in open chain.

and have been previously presented. Although specific quantification is challenging, these motions may be estimated by having the patient perform active knee extension and flexion in the seated position while palpating the tibial tuberosity. During active knee extension, lateral tibial rotation is perceived by palpating the lateral migration of the tuberosity and palpation of medial migration during active flexion.

Mobility restrictions of the PF joint may limit the overall motions of the knee. As previously described, superior and inferior gliding of the patella during active knee extension and flexion is required for normal TF extension and flexion, respectively (see Fig. 26-8). Likewise, medial and lateral gliding of the patella is an important component motion for medial and lateral rotation of the tibia relative to the femur. In sitting,

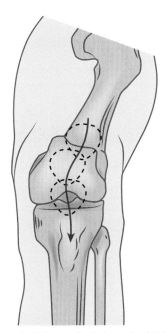

FIGURE 26–13 The path of the patella during active left knee flexion in open chain.

the clinician observes the C-curve path as the knee moves from extension to flexion, which reverses during movement from flexion to extension (Fig. 26-13).

The quantity of TF motion required to achieve normal gait ranges from approximately full extension at midstance to 75 degrees of flexion during the swing phase.[59] Because of higher demands for knee extension as opposed to knee flexion during gait, limitations in full knee extension more commonly lead to gait deviations and disability. Other activities of daily living, however, often require greater degrees of knee flexion. Ascending stairs, for example, requires approximately 90 to 100 degrees of knee flexion. Medial and lateral tibial rotation occurs to a minimal degree during normal gait, with external rotation occurring during the swing phase and internal rotation occurring in stance.[58] The least amount of motion during gait occurs in the frontal plane with abduction accompanying internal tibial rotation and adduction of the tibia accompanying external rotation.[58]

The presence of knee hypomobility is common, however, there are occasions where hypermobility, or instability, may be present. Such impairments are typical in the younger, female population or in those with systemic causes or congenital influences. Knee hypermobility may result in genu recurvatum in standing with PF hypermobility. A propensity toward ligamentous laxity may result in patellar subluxation, often laterally, during high-demand activities.

Passive Physiologic Movement Examination

When measuring *passive range of motion (PROM)* of the knee, the supine position is recommended for the reasons aforementioned. During measurement, efforts must be taken to avoid patient participation and any extraneous movement. The open-packed position for the TF joint is 10 to 20 degrees of flexion, and the close-packed position is maximal extension and

tibial external rotation.[60] The close- and open-packed positions for the PF joint are 30 to 60 degrees of flexion and 0 to 5 degrees of flexion, respectively.[60] In the presence of capsular restrictions, the capsular pattern of the knee has been described as flexion more limited than extension.[61] The end feels, or quality of resistance at end range, are soft tissue approximation for knee flexion as the lower leg contacts the hamstrings and capsular, or tissue stretch, for knee extension.[43]

As previously stated, the quantity of normal knee flexion is considered to range from *132 to 141 degrees*, and the degree of normal hyperextension is considered to range from *0 to 10 degrees*.[6,7] There is up to *20 to 30 degrees* of internal rotation with *10 to 20 degrees* of adduction and *30 to 40 degrees* of external rotation with *10 to 20 degrees* of abduction of the tibia on the femur.[2,5] With the knee in 90 degrees of flexion, *80 degrees* for both internal and external rotation may be noted passively. Table 26-2 displays the physiologic motions of the knee, including normal ranges of motion, open- and close-packed positions, normal end feels, and capsular pattern.

Passive Accessory Movement Examination

The primary criteria for determining the need to implement joint mobilization techniques that serve to enhance accessory motion are deficits that are identified during passive accessory mobility testing. Throughout this portion of the examination, the manual physical therapist endeavors to appreciate the relationship between the first and second onset of resistance (R1, R2) and the initial and final onset of pain (P1, P2). Understanding the nature of the relationship between tissue resistance and the presence of pain serves to guide subsequent intervention. During accessory motion testing, the therapist attempts to identify the excursion of motion, the nature and location of the end feel, as well as the onset of the patient's primary symptomatic complaint. Examination of accessory motion may be optimally performed by placing the joint in the position in which it is most likely to move, or the open-packed position. However, it is important for the manual physical therapist to also understand the nature of any restrictions that are present throughout the range of motion, particularly at end range. The therapist may bring the knee to its end range of both knee flexion and extension and test the degree of accessory motion, then compare that mobility with that experienced in the open-packed position. If restrictions are noted, the examination becomes the intervention. The mobilization techniques that follow later in this chapter will provide details regarding the performance of accessory glides and may be used for both examination and intervention of passive accessory movement. Table 26-3 displays the accessory motions of the knee.

Examination of Muscle Function

Examination of muscle function at the knee should constitute more than the standard assessment of strength. Subsumed within this portion of the examination is the assessment of endurance as well as muscle recruitment patterns. Isometric testing of each muscle within its maximally contracted position, known as *break testing*, only provides information regarding the status of the muscle at one specific position within the range of motion and is inadequate to provide all of the necessary information regarding

Table 26-2 Physiologic (Osteokinematic) Motions of the Knee						
JOINT	NORMAL ROM	OPP	CPP	NORMAL END FEEL(S)	CAPSULAR PATTERNS
Tibiofemoral	132-141° Flexion 0-10° Extension 20-30° Tibial internal torsion (rotation). 80° with knee flexed to 90° 30-40° Tibial external torsion (rotation). 80° with knee flexed to 90° 10-20° Adduction 10-20° Abduction	10-20° Flexion	Maximal extension and tibial ER	Flexion = soft tissue approximation Extension = elastic, capsular, tissue stretch	Flexion > Extension
Patellofemoral	5-7cm Inferior and Superior Glide with knee flexion and extension, respectively 50% width of patella Medial and Lateral Glide Medial and Lateral Tilt on superior-inferior axis Flexion and Extension on medial-lateral axis Rotation right and left on anterior-posterior axis	0-5° Flexion	30-60° Flexion	Soft in all directions	

ROM, range of motion; OPP, open-packed position; CPP, close-packed position.
(Adapted From: Wise CH, Gulick DT. *Mobilization Notes: A Rehabilitation Specialist's Pocket Guide.* Philadelphia, PA: F.A. Davis; 2009.)

Table 26-3 Accessory (Arthrokinematic) Motions of the Knee			
ARTHROLOGY	ARTHROKINEMATICS		
Tibiofemoral	**Concave surface:** Tibial plateau **Convex surface:** Femoral condyles	*To facilitate knee extension:* OKC = Tibia rolls and glides anterior on the femur. Medial tibial condyle glides anteriorly, lateral tibial condyle glides posteriorly. CKC = Femur rolls anterior and glides posterior on tibia. Medial femoral condyle glides posteriorly, lateral femoral condyle glides anteriorly.	*To facilitate knee flexion:* OKC = Tibia rolls and glides posterior on the femur. Medial tibial condyle glides posteriorly, lateral tibial condyle glides anteriorly. CKC = Femur rolls posterior and glides anterior on the tibia. Medial femoral condyle glides anteriorly, lateral femoral condyle glides posteriorly.
Patellofemoral	**Concave surface:** Trochlear groove of the femur **Convex surface:** Facets of the patella	*To facilitate knee extension:* Superior patellar glide To facilitate internal rotation: Medial patellar glide.	*To facilitate knee flexion:* Inferior patellar glide To facilitate external rotation: Lateral patellar glide.

OKC, open kinetic chain; CKC, closed kinetic chain.
(Adapted From: Wise CH, Gulick DT. *Mobilization Notes: A Rehabilitation Specialist's Pocket Guide.* Philadelphia, PA: F.A. Davis; 2009.)

muscle function. Muscle function testing must be performed over multiple repetitions in order to gain an appreciation of muscle endurance. Prior to returning the patient to full work or sport activity, it is also important to assess the ability of the muscles of the knee to function in a fashion that simulates their expected function. Testing should consider assessing the muscles using their dominant type of contraction, at their dominant length and in the dominant plane in which these muscles typically function. Muscle function testing should be performed in both closed- and open-chain positions, concentrically as well as eccentrically, within multiple planes, and over a series of repetitions. During muscle function testing, it is critical that each muscle is tested in isolation while disallowing any attempts at substitution.

At the knee, there is a predominance of multiarticulate muscles that provide important actions across adjacent joints. The *rectus femoris* is the central muscle of the quadriceps group that spans from the anterior inferior iliac spine (AIIS) to the common extensor tendon that inserts into the tibial tuberosity. This muscle is *actively insufficient* at the knee when it is performing maximal flexion at the hip, and it is *passively insufficient* at the knee when the hip is fully extended. A reduction in tension within the rectus is experienced when the hip is abducted, which results in an increase in knee flexion range of motion. Measurement of rectus femoris muscle function is best accomplished with the hip in neutral and may be differentiated from the remainder of the quadriceps, which are all one-joint muscles that are tested with the hip in flexion, thus reducing the contribution of the rectus. The rectus femoris seems to be involved in hip flexion primarily at the middle and end ranges of motion; however, its function increases with both external rotation and abduction of the hip.[62]

The remainder of the quadriceps consist of the *vastus intermedius*, *vastus medialis*, and *vastus lateralis*. The largest and most prominent of these muscles is the lateralis. The vastus medialis is divided into the oblique (VMO) and longus (VML) portions. Evidence reveals that the medialis is active throughout the entire range of knee extension and not only at terminal extension as once thought.[63] The collective action of the quadriceps results in a laterally oriented force vector through the patella. The medialis is one of the primary dynamic restraints serving to counterbalance these laterally oriented forces (see Fig. 26-9). The intermedius lies deep to the rectus, thus making it difficult to palpate.

The *tensor fascia latae (TFL)* muscle is a multijoint muscle that extends the knee but also functions at the hip as a flexor, abductor, and internal rotator. As a knee extensor, the TFL appears to be effected by transverse plane motion, or rotation, of the tibia.[64] In gait, the TFL advances the hip during swing and serves to advance the contralateral limb by producing internal rotation on the stance limb. As a hip abductor, the TFL assists the gluteus medius in controlling motion of the pelvis in the frontal plane in weight-bearing.

The hamstrings serve as the primary flexors of the knee. The medial head of the hamstrings is comprised of the *semimembranosus* and *semitendinosus*, and the lateral head is comprised of the *biceps femoris* muscle. In addition to knee flexion, this muscle group is also a prime extensor of the hip and, to a lesser extent, hip adductor and rotator. By virtue of its orientation, this muscle group is able to produce transverse plane rotation of the hip and rotation of the tibia relative to the femur. The role of the hamstrings in producing transverse plane motion is an important consideration in both identifying and treating weakness as well as tightness of this muscle group. Intervention designed to increase strength or flexibility of this muscle group may involve medial or lateral rotation of the hip or tibia in order to target the medial or lateral heads of the hamstrings. As a multijoint muscle that also crosses the hip, the hamstrings can become passively insufficient at the knee when the hip is flexed and actively insufficient at the knee when

the hamstrings are actively extending the hip. To isolate gluteal function from hamstring function during hip extension, the knee may be flexed. Although to a lesser extent, the hamstrings remain active as a hip extensor even when the knee is flexed.[8] During gait, the most important role of the hamstrings is to eccentrically control knee extension in late swing and to initiate hip extension in stance. The hamstrings have also been described as an important dynamic stabilizer of the knee, assisting the ACL with controlling anterior tibial translation.

In addition to the hamstrings, there are three synergistic muscles that also serve to flex the knee. The *sartorius* spans both the hip and knee, acting as a primary knee flexor by virtue of its orientation posterior to the axis of the knee joint as it courses toward its insertion at the medial aspect of the tibia serving to form the *pes anserine* along with the gracilis and semitendinosus. In addition, this muscle is also active as an external rotator and abductor of the hip. Of the three pes anserine muscles, the sartorius has the shortest moment arm for the production of knee flexion. The sartorius is most active as a flexor as the knee approaches 90 degrees.[65] The *gracilis* is primarily a hip adductor; however, as part of the pes anserine muscle group, this muscle also flexes the knee. Together, the sartorius and gracilis also contribute to internal rotation of the tibia during flexion. The final multijoint knee flexor is best known for its action as a talocrural joint plantar flexor. The biarticulate, two-headed *gastrocnemius* serves to flex the knee, differentiating it from its single joint counterpart, the *soleus*.

Because of the predominance of multijoint muscles at the knee, the relative positions of the hip and ankle must be considered when examining muscle function at the knee. As previously noted, alterations in the alignment of the femur and tibia resulting from structural or functional causes will influence the line of force and impact muscle function at the knee. With all things considered, the maximum strength of the knee flexors are approximately half of the maximum strength of the knee extensors. More specifically, the normal quadriceps-to-hamstring ratio is generally considered to be 5:3.

Examination of Function

For the acutely involved patient, functional testing may be delayed until a more appropriate time. Prior to discharge, however, it is important that the functional status of all patients be tested through the use of standardized testing, as will be described, or through activity-specific testing that assesses the patient's ability to perform the critical aspects of their daily life, sport, or work demands. The Functional Movement Screen (FMS) as described in Chapter 25 may be used to assess the functional capacity of the knee prior to sport participation.

Squat Test

The most basic of tests that allows assessment of hip, knee, and ankle mobility and strength is the full squat test. The patient is simply asked to touch the floor by squatting from an erect standing position. The patient is astutely observed that this activity is performed without compensation or onset of symptoms. It may be useful to ascertain the patient's response to this movement over the course of several repetitions.

Vertical Jump Test

The amount of muscular force production required to jump and land is substantial. The distance that an individual is able to jump can be quantified by putting chalk on the patient's fingertips and having them reach for a point on the wall. Change over time in response to intervention can be easily documented. The jump test, which assesses muscular power, a factor that considers the amount of force provided over a period of time, is particularly useful for individuals seeking to return to such sports as volleyball and basketball. As previously noted, observation of the manner in which the patient lands is critical in identifying potential predictors of injury.[29]

Running Tests

The *figure eight test* is useful in identifying an individual's ability to quickly change directions, particularly following an ACL reconstruction.[66] Two cones are placed 10 meters apart, and the individual is asked to perform a figure eight around both cones for a designated period of repetitions. Another commonly used running test is the *braiding test*, in which the individual is asked to run laterally alternately crossing each leg over the other for a distance of 8 feet.[67] This test assesses the individual's ability to perform lateral motions.

Hop Tests

The *single leg hop for distance test* involves hopping the greatest distance possible on the involved leg, which is then compared with the uninvolved leg and documented as a percentage. This test has demonstrated good reliability,[68] moderate sensitivity, and excellent specificity.[69] For the *crossover hop test*, the patient is asked to hop from the right to the left of a line three times as far as possible on one leg. The distance between take off and the third jump is calculated and compared from side to side. Good test-retest reliability has been identified for this test.[68] The *timed 6-meter hop test* is an excellent indicator of knee function because it tests balance, strength, and endurance, and this test has demonstrated moderate to good reliability.[68] The patient performs a single leg hop on the involved leg over a distance of 6 meters, which is compared to the uninvolved leg.

Palpation

Osseous Palpation

Careful palpation of the iliac crests, ASIS, AIIS, pubic tubercles, and ischial tuberosities should be performed and assessed for symmetry, a process that has been fully described in Chapter 25. These landmarks are confirmed by identifying each muscle through gentle resistance and tracing the muscle to its insertion site.

Palpation of the osseous structures of the knee is best accomplished in supine with the knee fully extended. Both medial and lateral femoral condyles and epicondyles are first identified and their anatomical variations appreciated. By first palpating the patella then gliding the patella to one side then the other, the examiner can identify the condyles that lie beneath and confirm them by moving the knee and identifying the tibiofemoral joint line. Just proximal to the medial epicondyle is the *adductor tubercle*, the insertion site for the adductor magnus muscle. This site is often tender upon palpation.

Both medial and lateral joint lines are then identified by moving the palpating finger from the femoral condyles distally. The joint line can be appreciated by moving the palpating finger vertically across the joint on either side. Placing varus or valgus force through the knee may assist in further opening the joint line (Fig. 26-14). The tibial plateaus are best palpated on either side of the patellar tendon in sitting with the knee flexed and confirmed as the knee is flexed and extended. All borders of the *patella* are palpated and its position relative to the condyles is appreciated. The patella's ability to move relative to the femur, as described above, is fully documented. Approximately 3 inches inferior to the patella is the prominent, and easily palpable, *tibial tuberosity*. The remainder of the *tibial shaft* with its central *tibial crest* can be palpated to its termination as the *medial malleolus* at the ankle (Fig. 26-15).

Soft Tissue Palpation

To palpate the muscles of the anterior thigh, the patient is seated. Knee extension is resisted, allowing the therapist to palpate the quadriceps as a group. The deep vastus intermedius may be palpated beneath the rectus, which is less active with the hip in flexion. To better palpate the rectus femoris, the patient is in supine and hip flexion, and knee extension is resisted. The proximal insertion of the rectus is best appreciated by resisting hip flexion and palpating over the AIIS. The vastus lateralis occupies the lateral compartment and can be differentiated from the bulk of the biceps femoris, which contracts with resistance to knee flexion. Alternating resistance from knee extension to flexion allows the therapist to identify the border between these two muscles. The tear-dropped shaped *vastus medialis oblique* is easily observed and palpated as it runs at an oblique angle of approximately 55 degrees from the patella. The insertion of this muscle group into the patella and the patellar tendon as it inserts into the tibial tuberosity is easily palpated.

The medial thigh is best palpated in side lying. The strap-like tendon of the *gracilis* is first palpated as it courses down the central portion of the medial thigh. The hip adductor muscle group can then be identified anterior and posterior to the gracilis. Palpation of the medial compartment of the thigh is described in Chapter 25 of this text. In supine with the leg to be palpated in the figure-four position, the *sartorius* can be palpated from the ASIS along its length as it obliquely crosses the anterior thigh with intermittent resistance for hip external rotation, abduction, and/or knee flexion (Fig. 26-16). Gentle resistance at the medial thigh is provided as the patient flexes thus allowing palpation of the two-finger-width sartorius muscle. The muscle belly of the sartorius runs toward its insertion at the ASIS, which allows differentiation from the gracilis that runs toward its insertion at the pubic tubercle. The tendons of the pes anserine are palpated with the sartorius most anterior, followed by the gracilis and then the semitendinosus. As the most posterior muscle of this group, it has the greatest moment arm to exert flexion forces through the knee.

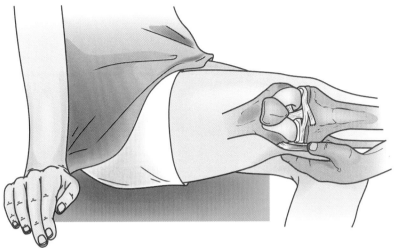

FIGURE 26–14 Palpation of the lateral joint line.

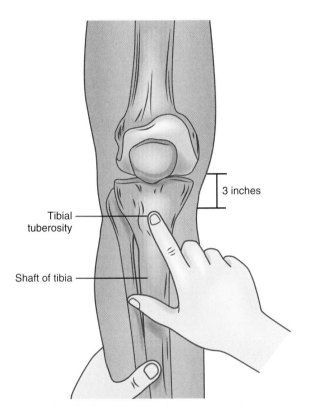

FIGURE 26–15 Palpation of the tibial tuberosity and tibial shaft.

3 inches

Tibial tuberosity

Shaft of tibia

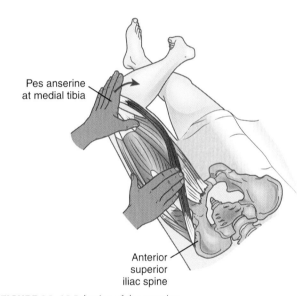

Pes anserine at medial tibia

Anterior superior iliac spine

FIGURE 26–16 Palpation of the sartorius.

Collectively, five individual tendons traverse the knee over its posterior aspect. The semitendinosus, gracilis, and sartorius occupy the medial aspect, and the biceps femoris and distal insertion of the *iltiotibial band (ITB)* occupy the lateral side (Fig. 26-17). Laterally, the biceps can be differentiated from the ITB, which is broad and has a more extensive insertion.

Posteriorly, the hamstrings are located between the vastus lateralis and the adductor magnus muscles. They may be palpated as a group in the prone position with the greatest differentiation possible distally as the muscles become tendinous. Beginning on the medial aspect of the posterior thigh, the already identified tendon-like semitendinosus is differentiated from the underlying broader semimembranosus muscle. Occupying the lateral aspect of the thigh is the biceps femoris, which inserts into the fibular head. These three muscles converge just proximal to the popliteal fossa, framing an inverted triangular-shaped space. All three muscles converge proximally at the ischial tuberosity.

Special Testing

Special tests for the knee have been clearly delineated in many other texts and in the literature. Therefore, only a brief description of selected special tests will be provided here. Table 26-4 provides an overview of the sensitivity, specificity, and likelihood ratios for the more commonly performed special tests used in the examination of the knee joint complex. The reader is encouraged to consult other sources for additional information regarding the performance of these useful confirmatory tests.

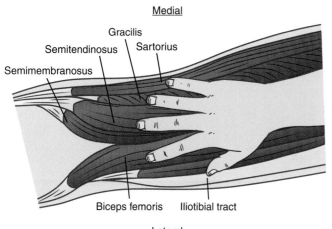

Medial

Gracilis

Semitendinosus — Sartorius

Semimembranosus

Posterior

Biceps femoris — Iliotibial tract

Lateral

FIGURE 26–17 Palpation of the flexor tendons at the posterior aspect of the knee.

Table 26-4	Special Tests for the Knee					
TEST	**SENSITIVITY**	**SPECIFICITY**	**+LR**	**−LR**	**RELIABILITY**	**REFERENCE**
Anterior drawer test	22%–95%	78%–97%	5.4–8.2	0.09–0.62	**0.34–0.54 (kappa)**	Jonsson et al.[70] Rosenberg et al.[71] Benjaminse et al.[72] Katz et al.[73] Malanga et al.[74] Lee et al.[75] Lui et al.[76] Mitsou et al.[77] Hardaker et al.[78] Tonino et al.[79] Boeree et al.[80] Cibere et al.[81] Rubinstein et al.[82]
Posterior drawer test	25%–90%	99%	90	0.10	0.82 (kappa)	Shelbourne et al.[83] Shino et al.[84] Ferrari et al.[85] Daniel et al.[86] Malanga et al.[74] Baker et al.[87] Loos et al.[88] Cibere et al.[81] Rubinstein et al.[82]
Posterior sag sign	46%–100%	100%	NA	NA	NA	Malanga et al.[74] Rubinstein et al.[82] Loos et al.[88] Fowler et al.[89] Staubi et al.[90]
Lachman test	63%–99%	42%–100%,	1.12–27.3	0.04–0.83	NA	Jonsson et al.[70] Katz et al.[73] Logan et al.[91] Lee et al.[75] Lui et al.[76] Mitsou et al.[77] Hardaker et al.[78] Tonino et al.[79] Boeree et al.[80] Rubinstein et al.[82] Paessler et al.[92] Cooperman et al.[93] Frank[94] Benjaminse et al.[72] Rosenberg et al.[71]

Table 26–4 Special Tests for the Knee—cont'd

TEST	SENSITIVITY	SPECIFICITY	+LR	−LR	RELIABILITY	REFERENCE
Lateral pivot-shift test	18%–98%, under anesthesia: 97%	97%–99%, under anesthesia: 93%	4.2–41	0.18–0.35	NA	Katz et al.[73] Lee et al.[75] Luiet al.[76] Mitsou et al.[77] Losee et al.[95] Tonino et al.[79] Boeree et al.[80] Rubinstein et al.[82] Malanga et al.[79] Benjaminse et al.[72] Ostrowski et al.[96] Bach et al.[97] Peterson et al.[98] Hardaker et al.[78]
Varus/valgus stress test	Varus: 25% Valgus: 86%–96%	Varus: NA Valgus: NA	NA	NA	Varus: 0–0.88 (kappa) Valgus: 0.02–0.66 (kappa)	Malanga et al.[74] Harilainen et al.[99] Dervin et al.[100] Jacobson et al.[101] Kurzweil et al.[102] Garvin et al.[103]
McMurray test	16%–95%	25%–98%,	0.39–8.0	0.83–2.84	0.35–0.95 (kappa)	Boeree et al.[80] Shelbourne et al.[104] McMurray[105] Evans et al.[106] Kim et al.[107] Fowler et al.[108] Karachalios et al.[109] Akseki et al.[110] Corea et al.[111]
Thessaly test	At 5 degrees: 66%–81% At 20 degrees: 89%–92%	At 5 degrees: 91%–96% At 20 degrees: 96%–97%	At 5 degrees: 6.8–16.5 At 20 degrees: 23–29.7	At 5 degrees: 0.21–0.76 At 20 degrees: 0.08–0.11	At 5 degrees: 0.95 At 20 degrees: 0.95	Konan et al.[112] Karachalios et al.[109] Pookarn-janamorakot et al.[113]
Apprehension test	7%–39%,	70%–92%,	0.87–2.3	0.79–1.0	NA	Hughston et al.[114] Fairbank[115] Haim et al.[116] Nijs et al.[117] Niskanen et al.[118]
Moving patella apprehension test	Under anesthesia: 100%	Under anesthesia: 88.4%	NA	NA	NA	Haim et al.[116] Ahmed et al.[119]
Ober test	NA	NA	NA	NA	0.90–0.94 (ICC)	Ober et al.[120] Reese et al.[121] Melchione et al.[122]
Noble test	NA	NA	NA	NA	NA	Gautam et al.[123] Noble et al.[124]
Renne test	NA	NA	NA	NA	NA	Magee [43]
Ottawa Knee Rules	Adults: 98%–100%, Children: 92%	Adults: 19%–54%, Children: 49%	NA	NA	NA	Vijayasankar et al.[125] Bachmann et al.[126] Emparanza et al.[127] Bulloch et al.[128] Stiell et al.[129] Richman et al.[130]

LR indicates likelihood ratios; ICC, intraclass correlation coefficient.

SPECIAL TESTS FOR THE KNEE

Special Tests for Ligamentous Dysfunction

Anterior Drawer Test (Fig. 26-18)

Purpose: To test the integrity of the anterior cruciate ligament

Patient: Supine with the hip and knee flexed to 90 degrees

Clinician: Sitting on the patient's involved foot with hand contact at the proximal tibia with thumbs over the anterior joint line to assess mobility.

Procedure: An anteriorly directed force is exerted through the hand contacts. Assessment of rotatory instability may be ascertained by performing the test by first prepositioning the tibia in external and then internal rotation and applying an anteriorly directed force. This test is known as the **Slocum test** and may be used to test additional structures such as the collateral ligaments and knee joint capsule, along with the ACL.

Interpretation: The test is positive if there is excessive anterior translation of the tibia or less than a firm, abrupt end feel.

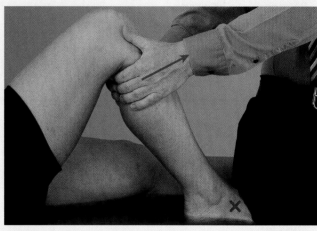

FIGURE 26–18 Anterior drawer test.

Posterior Drawer Test (Fig. 26-19):

Purpose: To test the integrity of the posterior cruciate ligament

Patient: Supine with the hip and knee flexed to 90 degrees

Clinician: Sitting on the patient's involved foot with hand contact at the proximal tibia with thumbs over the anterior joint line to assess mobility.

Procedure: A posteriorly directed force is exerted through the hand contacts. Performing the Slocum test with posteriorly directed force may also be done to assess the presence of rotatory instability.

Interpretation: The test is positive if there is excessive posterior translation of the tibia or less than a firm, abrupt end feel.

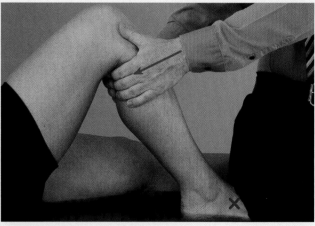

FIGURE 26–19 Posterior drawer test.

Posterior Sag Sign (Fig. 26-20)

Purpose: To test the integrity of the posterior cruciate ligament

Patient: Supine with the leg in an elevated straight leg raise position

Clinician: Standing to the side of the patient supporting the heel of the involved leg

Procedure: The patient is asked to relax as the clinician holds the heel with the leg in an elevated position.

Interpretation: The test is positive if there is posterior translation of the tibia relative to the femur.

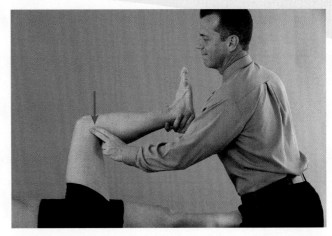

FIGURE 26–20 Posterior sag sign.

Lachman Test and Reverse Lachman Test
(Fig. 26-21 A, B)

Purpose: To test the integrity of the anterior cruciate ligament

Patient: Supine with the hip and knee flexed to 30 degrees

Clinician: Sitting at the foot of the table, one of the clinician's hands stabilizes the distal femur as the other hand grasps the posterior tibia.

Procedure: An anteriorly directed force is applied to the proximal tibia. Modifications have been recommended, including the prone Lachman test, in which force is directed anteriorly to test the ACL or posteriorly to test the PCL with the patient in prone and the knee in 30 degrees of flexion.

Interpretation: The test is positive if there is excessive anterior translation of the tibia or less than a firm, abrupt end feel.

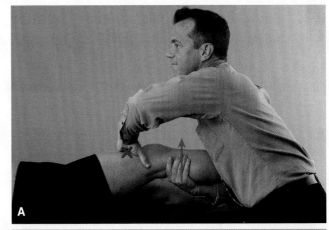

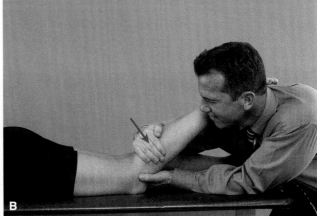

FIGURE 26–21 A. The standard Lachman test and **B.** the reverse Lachman test.

Lateral Pivot-Shift Test (Fig. 26-22)

Purpose: To test the integrity of the anterior cruciate ligament

Patient: Supine

Clinician: Standing to the side of the patient

Procedure: Beginning with the knee extended, valgus force is applied as the knee is internally rotated and flexed. The reverse pivot-shift test for posterolateral rotatory stability is performed with valgus stress and external tibial rotation as the knee is extended from a flexed position, which produces a subluxation.

Interpretation: The test is positive if there is reduction of the tibial plateau from an anteriorly translated position to its neutral position, which typically occurs at approximately 30 degrees of flexion. For the reverse pivot-shift test, as the knee is extended, the subluxation reduces as the lateral tibial plateau translates anteriorly.

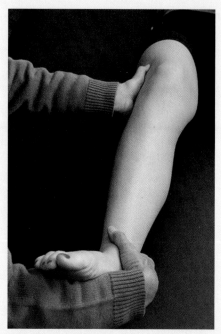

FIGURE 26–22 Lateral pivot-shift test. (Courtesy of Bob Wellmon Photography, BobWellmon.com.)

Varus/Valgus Stress Test (Fig. 26-23 A, B)

Purpose: To test the integrity of the lateral collateral and medial collateral ligaments, respectively

Patient: Supine, with the knee flexed to approximately 20 degrees

Clinician: Standing to the side of the patient

Procedure: A laterally directed, or varus, force followed by a medially directed, or valgus, force is applied to the knee at varying degrees of knee flexion.

Interpretation: The test is positive if there is lateral or medial joint line pain and/or laxity when compared bilaterally.

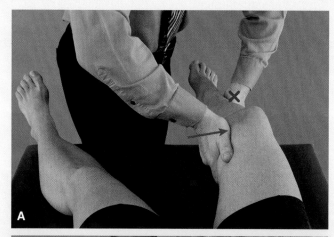

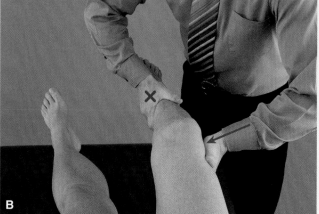

FIGURE 26–23 A. Varus stress test. **B.** Valgus stress test.

Special Tests for Meniscal Dysfunction

McMurray Test (Fig. 26-24 A, B)

Purpose: To test the integrity of the medial and lateral menisci

Patient: Supine

Clinician: Standing to the side of the patient grasping just proximal to the ankle with one hand as the other hand is positioned to apply force and palpate the medial and lateral tibiofemoral joint line.

Procedure: The tibia is externally rotated, and a valgus force is applied as the knee is passively brought into flexion and extension as the clinician palpates the medial joint line for the medial meniscus. Internal tibial rotation with varus stress as the knee is flexed and extended with palpation at the lateral joint line is performed to test the lateral meniscus.

Interpretation: The test is positive if there is a palpable click, joint audible, or pain over the joint line.

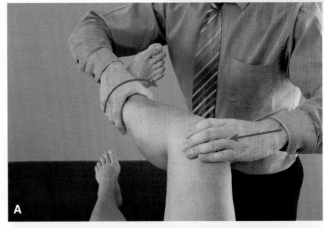
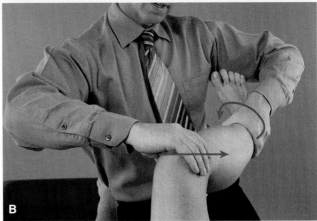

FIGURE 26–24 A. McMurray test for medial meniscus including valgus force and tibial external rotation. **B.** McMurray test for lateral meniscus including varus force and tibial internal rotation.

Thessaly Test (Fig. 26-25)

Purpose: To test the integrity of the medial and lateral menisci

Patient: Unilateral standing on the involved leg with the knee in 20 degrees of flexion

Clinician: Standing in front of the patient and holding the patient's arms

Procedure: The patient turns to the right and then left on the weightbearing leg as you guide the motion.

Interpretation: The test is positive if there is locking, catching, or pain at either the medial or lateral joint line.

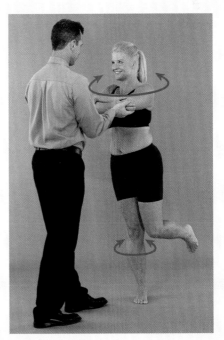

FIGURE 26–25 Thessaly test.

Special Tests for Patellofemoral Dysfunction

Apprehension Test (Fig. 26-26)

Purpose: To assess for patellofemoral hypermobility/instability

Patient: Supine with the patellofemoral joint in the open-packed position with quadriceps relaxed

Clinician: Standing to the side of the patient

Procedure: Gently move the patella in all planes but primarily in a lateral direction.

Interpretation: The test is positive if there is apprehension or contraction of the quadriceps to prevent lateral displacement of the patella.

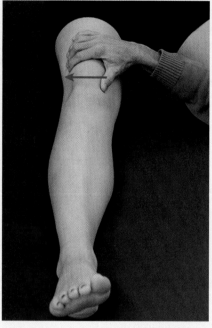

FIGURE 26–26 Apprehension test. (Courtesy of Bob Wellmon Photography, BobWellmon.com.)

Moving Patella Apprehension Test (Fig. 26-27)

Purpose: To assess for patellofemoral hypermobility/instability

Patient: Sitting

Clinician: Sitting in front of the patient

Procedure: Translate the patella laterally as the patient actively flexes and extends the knee.

Interpretation: The test is positive if there is apprehension and/or activation of the quadriceps during flexion and no apprehension during extension. Both parts of the test must be positive for the overall test to be positive.

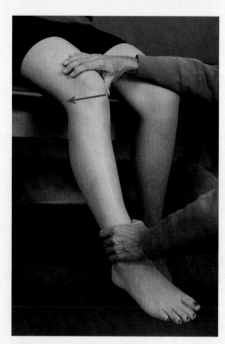

FIGURE 26–27 Moving patella apprehension test. (Courtesy of Bob Wellmon Photography, BobWellmon.com.)

Special Tests for Iliotibial Band (ITB) Dysfunction

Ober Test (Fig. 26-28)

Purpose: To assess for ITB tightness

Patient: Side lying with the involved side uppermost

Clinician: Standing behind the patient supporting the leg

Procedure: Extend the involved hip and allow the leg to move into adduction.

Interpretation: The test is positive if the leg fails to adduct past the midline of the body.

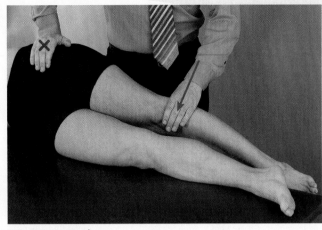

FIGURE 26–28 Ober test.

Noble Test (Fig. 26-29)

Purpose: To assess for ITB tightness and ITB friction.

Patient: Side lying with involved side uppermost, with the hip in extension and the knee in 90 degrees of flexion

Clinician: Standing behind the patient supporting the leg with the thumb over the lateral femoral condyle

Procedure: With the hip in extension and adduction, flex and extend the knee while applying pressure over the lateral femoral condyle.

Interpretation: The test is positive if there is pain or crepitus while the knee is being flexed and extended.

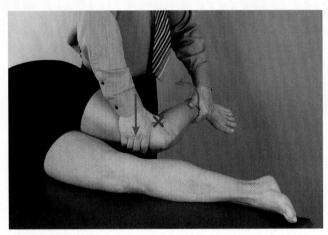

FIGURE 26–29 Noble test.

Renne Test (Fig. 26-30)

Purpose:	To assess ITB friction.
Patient:	Standing on the involved leg
Clinician:	Standing alongside the patient
Procedure:	Pressure is applied over the lateral femoral condyle while the patient flexes and extends the knee in standing.
Interpretation:	The test is positive if there is pain or crepitus at 30 degrees of knee flexion.

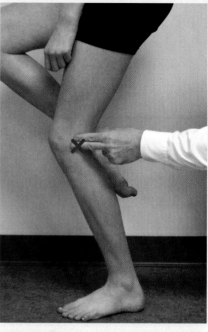

FIGURE 26–30 Renne test.

Special Tests for Fracture

Ottawa Knee Rules (Fig. 26-31)

Purpose:	To assess the need for plain film radiographs
Procedure:	Criteria: (1) Older than 55 years old, (2) isolated tenderness of the patella, (3) tenderness of the head of the fibula, (4) inability to flex more than 90 degrees, (5) inability to bear weight for four steps both immediately after injury and in the emergency department
Interpretation:	Radiographs are required if the client presents with any one of these criteria.

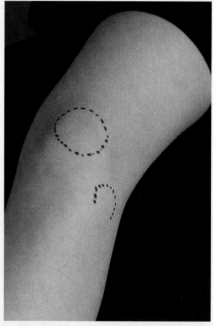

FIGURE 26–31 Ottawa Knee Rules. (Courtesy of Bob Wellmon Photography, BobWellmon.com.)

Joint Mobilization of the Knee

Note: The indications for the joint mobilization techniques described in this section are based on expected joint kinematics. Current evidence suggests that the indications for their use are multifactorial and may be based on direct assessment of mobility and an individual's symptomatic response.

Patellofemoral Joint Mobilizations

Patellofemoral Glide and Tilt

Indications:

- *Patellofemoral superior and inferior glides* are indicated for restrictions in knee extension and flexion, respectively. *Patellofemoral medial and lateral glides* are indicated for restrictions in knee internal torsion (rotation) and external torsion (rotation), respectively. *Patellofemoral tilts* are indicated for restrictions in all physiologic motions of the knee.

Accessory Motion Technique (Figs. 26-32, 26-33)

- **Patient/Clinician Position:** The patient is in the supine position with the patellofemoral joint in the open-packed position. The knee may be pre-positioned at the point of restriction. Stand to the side of the patient.
- **Hand Placement:** Stabilization is provided by the weight of the leg. Grasp the patella with the web space of your mobilization hand. For superior or inferior glides, place your hand at the inferior or superior poles of the patella, respectively. For medial or lateral glides, place your hand at the lateral or medial aspects of the patella, respectively. For tilts, place your thumbs over the superior, inferior, medial, or lateral aspects of the patella.

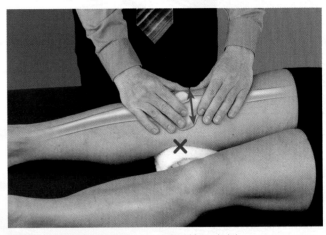

FIGURE 26-33 Patellofemoral medial and lateral glide.

- **Force Application:** For glides, your forearm is in line with the direction in which force is applied as your other hand provides reinforcement. For tilts, apply force in a posterior direction through the patellar contact with the objective of moving the opposing pole of the patella anteriorly.

Accessory With Physiologic Motion Technique (Not pictured)

- **Patient/Clinician Position:** The patient may be in an open chain sitting position or standing.
- **Hand Placement:** Utilize all hand contacts as described above.
- **Force Application:** Superior or inferior glides may be performed during open kinetic chain or closed kinetic chain active knee extension or flexion, respectively. Medial or lateral glides can be performed during closed kinetic chain tibial IR or ER, respectively, or during active knee extension and flexion. Mobilization force is maintained throughout the entire range of motion motion and sustained at end range.

Tibiofemoral Joint Mobilizations

Tibiofemoral Distraction

Indications:

- *Tibiofemoral distractions* are indicated for restrictions in all directions.

Accessory Motion Technique (Fig. 26-34)

- **Patient/Clinician Position:** The patient is in a supine position with the knee in the open-packed position or prone with

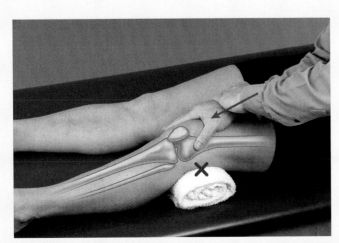

FIGURE 26-32 Patellofemoral inferior glide.

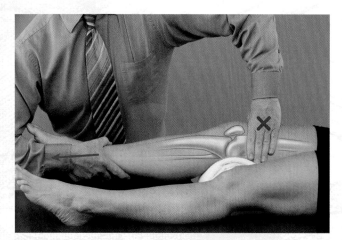

FIGURE 26–34 Tibiofemoral distraction.

the knee flexed to the point of the restriction. Stand at the foot of the patient on the side of the knee being mobilized.

- **Hand Placement:** Your stabilization hand stabilizes the distal thigh. A mobilization belt may be used to provide stabilization. Grasp the lower leg just proximal to the ankle with your mobilization hand(s). Your forearm is in line with the direction in which the force is applied.
- **Force Application:** Through your mobilization hand contact, apply a long-axis distraction force.

Accessory With Physiologic Motion Technique (Figs. 26-35, 26-36)

- **Patient/Clinician Position:** For knee extension, the patient is in a sitting position. You are sitting facing the patient. For knee flexion, the patient is prone with the knee flexed to the point of restriction. You are standing on the side of the knee being mobilized.
- **Hand Placement:** For knee extension, provide stabilization at the patient's anterior distal thigh. Grasp the lower leg just proximal to the ankle with your mobilization hand(s). For knee flexion, place your elbow over the patient's posterior thigh just proximal to the knee to provide stabilization. A towel may be

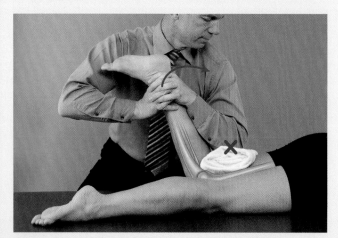

FIGURE 26–35 Tibiofemoral distraction accessory with physiologic motion into flexion technique.

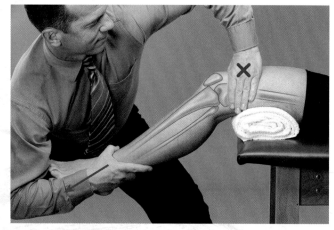

FIGURE 26–36 Tibiofemoral distraction accessory with physiologic motion into extension technique.

used to improve patient comfort. Your clasped mobilization hands grasp the patient's leg just proximal to the ankle.

- **Force Application:** For knee extension, apply a long axis distraction force through your mobilization hand contact as the patient actively moves into knee extension. Be prepared to move during motion in order to ensure that your forearm is in line with the direction in which force is applied. For knee flexion, maintain your mobilization hand contacts as the knee is passively flexed. As the length of the tibia effectively decreases relative to the length of your forearm, a distraction force is produced. There is no need to exert an additional distraction force during this procedure.

Tibiofemoral Anterior Glide

Indications:
- *Tibiofemoral anterior glides* are indicated for restrictions in knee extension.

Accessory Motion Technique (Fig. 26-37)

- **Patient/Clinician Position:** The patient is in a prone position with the knee in the open-packed position and bolster

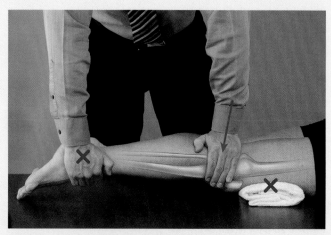

FIGURE 26–37 Tibiofemoral anterior glide in prone.

or wedge just proximal to the knee to eliminate pressure on the patella. You may pre-position the knee in varying degrees of flexion to the point of restriction with the bolster under the distal leg for support. Stand on the side of the knee being mobilized.

- **Hand Placement:**

Technique 1: Prone
- Provide stabilization just proximal to the patient's ankle to maintain knee position or stabilization is provided by placing the patient's lower leg on your shoulder if the knee is flexed 90 degrees or more. The heel of your hand contacts the posterior aspect of the patient's proximal tibia just below the knee, with your forearm in the direction in which force is applied, which may vary depending on the position of the knee. Both hands may contact the patient's proximal tibia if the knee is flexed 90 degrees or more.

Technique 2: Supine
- Provide stabilization to the anterior aspect of the patient's thigh, just proximal to the knee. Your mobilization hand contacts the posterior aspect of the proximal tibia.
- **Force Application:** Apply force through your mobilization hand contact in an anterior direction that is parallel to the treatment plane of the joint.

Accessory With Physiologic Motion Technique (Fig. 26-38)
- **Patient/Clinician Position:** The patient is standing with the knees flexed in a squat position. You are in a lunge position facing the patient.
- **Hand Placement:** The mobilization belt is positioned over the posterior aspect of the patient's proximal tibia and around your leg. One hand is used to reinforce the mobilization belt as the other hand assists in controlling motion into knee extension or both hands may be placed proximal to the knee anteriorly for stabilization.

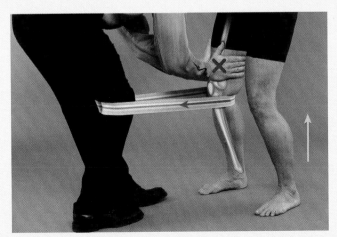

FIGURE 26–38 Tibiofemoral anterior glide accessory with physiologic motion into extension technique.

- **Force Application:** The patient actively moves from a squat position into an erect standing position moving the knee into extension as you apply an anterior glide through the mobilization belt as the femur is stabilized. Mobilization force is maintained throughout the entire range of motion motion and sustained at end range.

Tibiofemoral Posterior Glide

Indications:
- *Tibiofemoral posterior glides* are indicated for restrictions in knee flexion.

Accessory Motion Technique (Fig. 26-39)
- **Patient/Clinician Position:** The patient is in a supine position with the knee in an open-packed position with a bolster or wedge just proximal to the knee. You may pre-position the knee at the point of restriction. Stand on the side of the knee being mobilized.
- **Hand Placement:** To stabilize, contact the anterior thigh, just proximal to the knee against the bolster. Contact the anterior aspect of the patient's tibia just distal to the knee with your mobilization hand in line with the direction in which force is applied.
- **Force Application:** Apply force through your mobilization hand contact in a posterior direction that is parallel to the treatment plane of the joint.

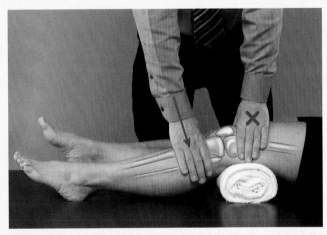

FIGURE 26–39 Tibiofemoral posterior glide.

Accessory With Physiologic Motion Technique (Fig. 26-40)
- **Patient/Clinician Position:** The patient is standing in an erect standing posture with his knees in extension. You are in a lunge position behind the patient.
- **Hand Placement:** The mobilization belt is positioned over the anterior aspect of the patient's proximal tibia and around your leg. Both hands are used to stabilize and control motion into knee flexion.

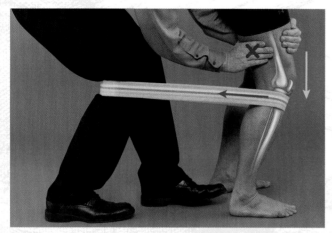

FIGURE 26–40 Tibiofemoral posterior glide accessory with physiologic motion into flexion technique.

- **Force Application:** The patient actively performs a squat moving the knee into flexion as you apply a posterior glide through the mobilization belt as the femur is stabilized. Mobilization force is maintained throughout the entire range of motion motion and sustained at end range.

Tibiofemoral Anterior Glide of Medial or Lateral Tibial Condyle

Indications:

- *Tibiofemoral anterior glides of the medial condyle* are indicated for restrictions in tibial external torsion (rotation) and knee extension. *Tibiofemoral anterior glides of the lateral condyle* are indicated for restrictions in tibial internal torsion (rotation) and knee flexion.

Accessory Motion Technique (Fig. 26-41)

- **Patient/Clinician Position:** The patient is in the prone position with the knee in the open-packed position with a bolster or wedge just proximal to knee and another bolster

supporting the lower leg. You may pre-position the knee in varying degrees of flexion to the point of restriction. Stand on the side of the knee being mobilized.

- **Hand Placement:** Provide stabilization just proximal to the patient's ankle to maintain knee position. Your mobilization hand contacts the posterior aspect of the patient's medial or lateral tibial plateau at the proximal tibia just below the knee, with your forearm in line with the direction in which force is applied. Both hands may be placed at the proximal tibia for mobilization. Force direction may vary depending on the position of the knee.
- **Force Application:** Apply force through your mobilization hand contact in an anterior direction that is parallel to the treatment plane of the joint. If both hands are used, one hand may provide mobilizing force anteriorly while the other hand provides posteriorly directed force as if opening a screw-top lid.

Accessory With Physiologic Motion Technique (Fig. 26-42)

- **Patient/Clinician Position:** The patient is standing in a lunge position with his or her involved foot placed on a stool. You are half-kneeling facing the patient.
- **Hand Placement:** Place one hand over the proximal medial tibial condyle and one hand over the proximal lateral tibial condyle and fibula just distal to the knee joint. Your forearms are in line with the direction in which force is applied, which varies during motion.
- **Force Application:** Apply an anteriorly directed force through the lateral tibial condyle and a posteriorly directed force through the medial tibial condyle as the patient lunges forward bringing the knee into greater ranges of flexion. Mobilization force is maintained throughout the entire range of motion motion and sustained at end range.

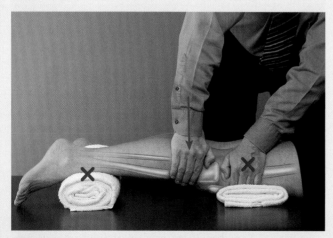

FIGURE 26–41 Tibiofemoral anterior glide of medial or lateral tibial condyle.

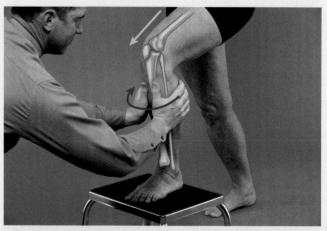

FIGURE 26–42 Tibiofemoral anterior glide of lateral tibial condyle and posterior glide of medial tibial condyle accessory with physiologic motion into flexion technique.

Tibiofemoral Posterior Glide of Medial or Lateral Tibial Condyle

Indications:

- *Tibiofemoral posterior glides of the medial condyle* are indicated for restrictions in tibial internal torsion (rotation) and knee flexion. *Tibiofemoral posterior glides of the lateral condyle* are indicated for restrictions in tibial external torsion (rotation) and knee extension.

Accessory Motion Technique (Fig. 26-43)

- **Patient/Clinician Position:** The patient is in a supine position with the knee in an open-packed position with a bolster or wedge just proximal to the knee. You may pre-position the knee at the point of restriction. Stand on the side of the knee being mobilized.
- **Hand Placement:** To stabilize, contact the anterior thigh, just proximal to the knee against the bolster. Contact the anterior aspect of the patient's tibia just distal to the knee with your mobilization hand. Your forearm is in line with the direction in which force is applied. Both hands may be placed at the proximal tibia for mobilization. Force direction may vary depending on the position of the knee.
- **Force Application:** Apply force through your mobilization hand contact in a posterior direction that is parallel to the treatment plane of the joint. If both hands are used, one hand may provide mobilizing force posteriorly while the other hand provides anteriorly directed force as if opening a screw-top lid.

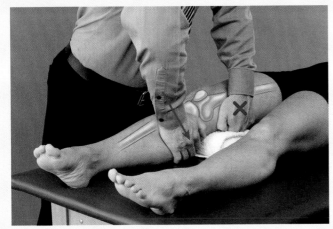

FIGURE 26–43 Tibiofemoral posterior glide of medial or lateral tibial condyle.

Accessory With Physiologic Motion Technique (Fig. 26-44)

- **Patient/Clinician Position:** The patient is standing in a lunge position with the involved foot placed on a stool. You are half-kneeling facing the patient.

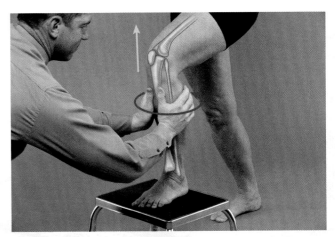

FIGURE 26–44 Tibiofemoral posterior glide of lateral tibial condyle and anterior glide of medial tibial condyle accessory with physiologic motion into extension technique.

- **Hand Placement:** Place one hand over the proximal medial tibial condyle and one hand over the proximal lateral tibial condyle and fibula just distal to the knee joint. Your forearms are in line with the direction in which force is applied, which varies during motion.
- **Force Application:** Apply a posteriorly directed force through the lateral tibial condyle and an anteriorly directed force through the medial tibial condyle as the patient extends the knee and steps up onto the stool. Mobilization force is maintained throughout the entire range of motion motion and sustained at end range.

Proximal Tibiofibular Joint Mobilizations

Proximal Tibiofibular Anterior and Posterior Glide

Indications:

- *Anterior fibular and posterior tibial glides* are indicated for restrictions in knee flexion and *posterior fibular and anterior tibial glides* are indicated for restrictions in knee extension.

Accessory Motion Technique (Fig. 26-45)

- **Patient/Clinician Position:** The patient is in a supine position with the knee in the open-packed position and a bolster or wedge just proximal to the knee. You may pre-position the knee in varying degrees of flexion to the point of restriction. Stand on the side of the knee being mobilized.
- **Hand Placement:** Stabilization is provided through the weight of the leg or through the use of a mobilization belt just proximal to the knee. Both hands contact the tibia and fibula just distal to the knee with the forearms in the direction in which force is applied.

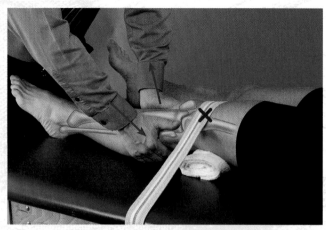

FIGURE 26-45 Proximal tibiofibular anterior and posterior glide to restore external tibial torsion (rotation).

- **Force Application:** One mobilizing hand exerts an antero-laterally directed force through the fibular head with simultaneous posteromedial force to tibia through the other mobilizing hand for flexion. One mobilizing hand exerts posteromedially directed force through the fibular head with anterolateral force to tibia through the other mobilizing hand for extension.

Accessory With Physiologic Motion Technique (Not pictured)

- **Patient/Clinician Position:** The patient is standing in a lunge position with the involved foot placed on a stool. You are half-kneeling facing the patient.
- **Hand Placement:** Place one hand over the proximal tibia and one hand over the fibula just distal to the knee joint. Your forearms are in line with the direction in which force is applied, which varies during motion.
- **Force Application:** Using both hand contacts, apply an anteriorly directed force through the fibular contact and posteriorly directed force through the tibial contact as the patient lunges forward bringing the knee into greater ranges of flexion. The patient may also step up onto the stool bringing the knee into greater ranges of knee extension as anteriorly directed force through the tibial contact and posteriorly

directed force through the fibular contact is applied. Mobilization force is maintained throughout the entire range of motion motion and sustained at end range.

Tibiofemoral Flexion High-Velocity Thrust (Fig. 26-46)

- **Indications:** *Tibiofemoral flexion high-velocity thrust* is indicated for restrictions in knee flexion range of motion.
- **Patient/Clinician Position:** The patient is lying supine with the knee in flexion and the foot resting on the table. You are standing on the ipsilateral side of the knee being mobilized.
- **Hand Placement:** Place the fingers of your stabilization hand within the popliteal crease forming a fulcrum. Grasp the distal aspect of the patient's leg, just proximal to the ankle with your mobilization hand.
- **Force Application:** As your stabilization hand maintains the fulcrum, your mobilization hand flexes the patient's knee to its maximum available range. Once resistance is engaged at end range, apply a high-velocity low-amplitude thrust by moving the patient's knee into further degrees of flexion against the fulcrum of your stabilization hand.

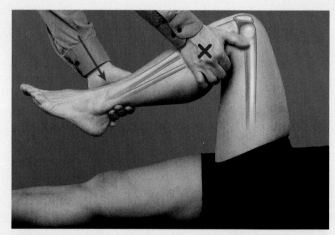

FIGURE 26-46 Tibiofemoral flexion high-velocity thrust.

CLINICAL CASE

CASE 1

Subjective Examination

History of Present Illness:

A 40-year-old self-employed carpet layer presents to your office today complaining of dull chronic pain in the anterior aspect of bilateral knees that increases upon prolonged sitting and attempts at kneeling and squatting. He is currently out of work because of his symptoms. He notes a progressive onset of symptoms without trauma beginning approximately 6 months ago. He has decided to seek care because his symptoms are affecting his ability to perform his regular work duties. His symptoms increase in severity secondary to performance of work duties, and he gets only minimal relief from the use of aspirin.

The patient's Western Ontario and McMaster Universities Osteoarthritis Index (WOMAC)[24] global score is a 65 (96 maximal score with higher score indicating a greater level of disability). His pain subscale = 15, stiffness subscale = 5, and physical function subscale = 45. His score on the Cincinnati Knee Rating System[26] index is 53 for both knees (100 maximal score with lower score indicating a greater level of disability).

Past Medical History

Patient reports intermittent knee pain over the years secondary to playing catcher on his high school baseball team.

Objective Physical Examination

Examination of Structure

Observation of the patient in standing reveals severe bilateral foot overpronation with calcaneal valgus and bilateral genu valgus. Bilateral patellae are noted to be displaced laterally, externally rotated, flexed, and medially tilted. Atrophy of bilateral VMOs is noted. The Q-angle, measured in supine is 23 degrees on the right and 20 degrees on the left. Circumferential measurements are equal bilaterally over the knee joint line, quadriceps, and calf. Structural foot assessment in non-weight-bearing subtalar joint neutral position reveals bilateral severe forefoot varus deformity, mild rear foot varus deformity, plantarflexed first ray, hallux limitus, with pinch callus at great toe, and pump bump at posterior calcaneus noted.

Examination of Mobility

Physiologic Mobility Testing: Knee (tibiofemoral) AROM and PROM are within normal limits (WNL) for both flexion and extension. Palpation of the PF joint during active knee extension reveals an increase in lateral migration of the patella and excessive flexion of the patella that is associated with crepitus and pain from approximately 30 degrees to end range extension. Less crepitus and pain noted with medially directed manual pressure within this range of motion. Passive patellofemoral mobility performed in the open-packed position reveals medial glide that is 25% the width of the patella, reduced lateral tilt (superior-inferior axis), reduced internal rotation (anterior-posterior axis), and reduced extension (medial-lateral axis).

Accessory Mobility Testing: All accessory motions of the tibiofemoral joint are WNL and pain free.

Examination of Flexibility

Increased stiffness and reduced flexibility is noted in bilateral hamstrings, gastrocnemius, and TFL musculature.

Examination of Muscle Function

Bilaterally, a reduction in VMO recruitment is noted during quadriceps maximal muscle contraction with the knee in open chain terminal extension. Manual muscle testing reveals quadriceps strength as a group to be 4/5 with a reduction to 4−/5 from 30 degrees of flexion to terminal extension, which is associated with the onset of pain upon testing. Hamstring strength is 5/5 and pain free. Bilateral gluteus medius strength is 3+/5, and bilateral hip external rotators, as a group, are also 3+/5 and pain free. Ankle muscle testing reveals 5/5 throughout.

Neurologic Testing

WNL throughout

Palpation

Bilateral retropatellar crepitus noted during active knee motion and passive PF glides with intermittent report of pain. Significant tightness noted within the ITB. Tenderness over the inferior pole and lateral facet of the patella. A moderate degree of noninflammatory thickening of the patellar tendon is noted. No edema is present.

Functional Testing

Moderate pain noted when transferring from sitting to standing with gluteus medius lurch present bilaterally. Severe overpronation is noted throughout the gait cycle with failure to resupinate in late stance. The squat test reveals significant pain over bilateral anterior knees most notable when approaching the full squat position and early during ascent. All other jump, running, and hop tests are inconclusive at this time.

Special Testing: Patellar lateral apprehension test = slightly positive bilaterally, Ober test = positive, Noble compression test = positive, Craig test = positive for bilateral femoral anteversion, Straight leg raising (SLR) = limited bilaterally at 45 degrees by hamstring tightness, All ligament and meniscal tests are negative.

1. Based on the information provided, what is your differential diagnosis? What additional information do you need to either refute or confirm your hypothesis?
2. What factors do you believe have predisposed this patient to this condition? Identify and explain any structural or functional impairments or behavioral factors that may have contributed to the onset of this condition and how you would go about addressing each of these factors.
3. Based on these findings, describe the plan of care for this patient. Provide specific information regarding both manual and nonmanual interventions and include specific procedures along with information regarding frequency, intensity, duration, and proper sequencing of interventions. In particular, highlight the manual interventions that are indicated, and perform each technique on your partner.
4. What role does muscle weakness and/or tightness play in the onset and perpetuation of this patient's condition?
5. Given the challenging nature of this patient's occupation, what advice would you give in regard to work modification, and what, if any, external support systems may be used to allow him to return to gainful employment? Do you believe that this condition would have occurred if work demands were less substantial?
6. Describe the kinematics of the patellofemoral joint. What is abnormal about the kinematics of this patient's patellofemoral joint, and what are the contributing factors?
7. Would diagnostic imaging be useful in the care of this patient? What particular tests and views would be most helpful? How would the results from diagnostic imaging impact your clinical decisions regarding this patient's care?

CASE 2

Subjective Examination

History of Present Illness

A 25-year-old female soccer player experienced an injury last evening during a game. She reports that her right foot was planted as she was cutting to the left, at which time another player, in an attempt to take the ball, was pushed, falling onto the posterolateral aspect of the planted foot. She reports a popping sound, immediate pain, and a giving way of the knee that required assistance off the field.

She presents to your office today as a direct access patient (having not yet been seen by a medical physician) noting severe pain, inability to bear weight on the leg, and a significant amount of edema that began several hours after the injury.

The patient's WOMAC[24] global score is a 65 (96 maximal score with higher score indicating a greater level of disability). Her pain subscale = 15, stiffness subscale = 5, and physical function subscale = 45. Her score on the Cincinnati Knee Rating System[26] index is 53 for both knees (100 maximal score, with lower score indicating a greater level of disability).

Past Medical History

The patient reports previous history of a left ACL tear with reconstruction using central third patellar tendon autograft performed 2 years ago, a sprained MCL on the right, left elbow ulnar collateral ligament sprain, and a lumbar spondylolisthesis secondary to performing gymnastics. She was also diagnosed 3 years ago with Marfan's syndrome. She reports intermittent cardiac arrhythmia.

Objective Physical Examination

Examination of Structure

Observation of the right knee reveals significant edema and quadriceps muscle atrophy. Knee is postured in approximately 30 degrees of flexion.

Examination of Mobility

Knee (Tibiofemoral) Physiologic Mobility Testing:

RIGHT KNEE MOTION	AROM	PROM	END FEEL	PAIN REPRODUCTION	RELATIONSHIP OF R TO P
Flexion	45 degrees	60 degrees	Empty	Positive	P1,2 only
Extension	−30 degrees	−15 degrees	Empty	Positive	P1,2 only
External tibial Rotation	N/A	15 degrees measured in −15 degrees extension	Soft	Positive	P1,2 before R1
Internal tibial rotation	N/A	10 degrees measured in 60 degrees flexion	Soft	Positive	P1,2 before R1
Tibial abduction	N/A	5 degrees measured in −15 degrees extension	Soft	Positive	P1,2 before R1
Tibial adduction	N/A	5 degrees measured in 60 degrees flexion	Soft	Positive	P1,2 before R1

AROM, active range of motion; PROM, passive range of motion; P1, initial onset of pain; P2, final onset of pain; R1, initial onset of resistance to motion; R2, final onset of resistance to motion.

PF joint mobility is WNL passively in all planes. Good pain-free mobility and tracking noted during active knee motion.

Accessory Mobility Testing: Tibiofemoral anterior glide is hypermobile with soft end feel. In addition, anterior glide of the medial tibial plateau is hypermobile with soft end feel. Distraction also reveals hypermobility.

Examination of Flexibility

Voluntary guarding noted within hamstrings and gastrocnemius during movement. Difficult to assess true flexibility due to voluntary guarding related to pain and fear of pain and joint motion limitations.

Examination of Muscle Function

A reduction in active right quadriceps recruitment and to a lesser extent hamstring recruitment. Formal knee manual muscle testing not performed secondary to pain and fear of pain. Hip and ankle muscle strength appears to be grossly 4+, 5/5 throughout.

Neurologic Testing

WNL throughout

Palpation

Increased temperature to the touch and edema present most notably within the medial TF joint compartment and within the popliteal fossa. Tenderness to the touch is noted to be significant over the MCL, medial joint line, and popliteal fossa.

Functional Testing

Patient is currently ambulating with bilateral axillary crutches 25% partial weight-bearing (PWB) on right using a swing-through gait pattern with an increase in pain with attempts to increase weight-bearing status.

Upon return to physical therapy, baseline functional testing is performed 6 weeks status post ACL reconstruction using allograft and medial meniscectomy, the patient presents with the following results of functional testing. The average of single leg hop for distance is 125 cm on the left and 75 cm on the right, revealing that the right knee is 60% of the capacity of the left. The crossover hop test reveals a score on the left of 300 cm and a score of 175 cm on the right, revealing a score of 58%. The timed 6 m hop test reveals 10.05 seconds on the left and 16.02 seconds on the right. Comparison of 10 m figure eight running to 10 m straight running reveals a ratio of 4.5:1.

Special Testing: Anterior drawer test = positive, Lachman test = positive, Lateral and reverse Pivot-Shift test = positive, Posterior drawer test = negative, McMurray test = positive, Apley compression test = positive

1. What is the value of self-reported disability measures when managing a patient of this kind? Discuss the parametric properties of the disability measures used in this case.
2. Discuss the impact of this patient's past medical history on the onset of her current injury. Given this past medical history, what measures might be taken to prevent reinjury?
3. Discuss the role of the muscles about the knee in providing dynamic stability to this joint. How are these muscles impacted by injury and pain? What is the value of their role in the rehabilitation of this injury?
4. Consider the various types of ACL reconstruction surgeries currently in use. What are the advantages/disadvantages to each? How might the type of reconstruction performed impact the course of intervention?
5. Discuss the role of the ACL in TF joint kinematics. How would the kinematics of the knee be altered in the presence of ACL deficiency?
6. What is the role of the MCL and meniscus in TF joint kinematics? How would the kinematics of the knee be altered in the presence of MCL and medial meniscal injury?

7. Why is the medial meniscus more susceptible to injury than the lateral meniscus? Why do medial meniscus tears often accompany injury to the ACL? How does involvement of the meniscus in this case make intervention for this patient more challenging? What are the criteria used to determine the course of conservative and surgical management of meniscal tears?
8. What do the results of functional testing 6 weeks post-ACL reconstruction tell us about this patient's current status and prognosis? What is the value of using functional testing in the care of this patient?
9. Discuss the value and limitations of the clinical tests used to confirm injury to the ACL and meniscus. What factors might lead to false-negative or false-positive results?
10. Describe your plan of care for this patient using the following grid.
11. How might manual therapy be used in the care of this patient? Perform the prescribed manual interventions on a partner.

INTERVENTION	PARAMETERS	WEEKS POST SURGERY	INDICATORS FOR PROGRESSION

HANDS-ON

With a partner, perform the following activities:

1 Palpate medial and lateral borders of the patella and follow the path of the patella as your partner flexes and extends his/her knee in open chain. Identify the presence of any aberrant motions, joint sounds, or pain. If present, provide manual force to either glide, rotate, tilt, or flex/extend the patella and observe any changes that may occur.

2 Palpate your partner during active knee flexion and extension in open chain and identify transverse and frontal plane motions. In standing, identify resultant changes in tibial and femoral position that occur in response to active pronation and supination of the foot.

3 Perform passive accessory mobility testing for TF distraction, anterior glides, and posterior glides, and identify the amount of motion, end feel, and onset of any symptoms. Compare to the other knee and with another partner. Perform these same procedures in open-packed, close-packed, as well as open chain and closed chain, and describe the differences.

4 Identify the positions of passive and active insufficiency for all multiarticulate muscles of the knee, and place these muscles in those positions on your partner. Complete the following grid.

MUSCLE	POSITION OF ACTIVE INSUFFICIENCY	POSITION OF PASSIVE INSUFFICIENCY

5 Perform each mobilization described in the intervention section of this chapter bilaterally on at least two individuals. Using each technique, practice Grades I through IV. Provide input to your partner regarding setup, technique, comfort, etc. When practicing these mobilization techniques, utilize the Sequential Partial Task Practice (SPTP) Method in which students repeatedly practice one aspect of each technique (ie. position, hand placement, force application) on multiple partners each time adding the next component until the technique is performed in real time from beginning to end. (Wise CH, Schenk RJ, Lattanzi JB. A model for teaching and learning spinal thrust manipulation and its effect on participant confidence in technique performance. *Journal of Manual & Manipulative Therapy*, August 2014.)

REFERENCES

1. Jackson JL, O'Malley PG, Kroenke K. Evaluation of acute knee pain in primary care. *Ann Intern Med*. 2003;139:575-588.
2. Churchill DL, Incavo SJ, Johnson CC, Beynnon BD. The transepicondylar axis approximates the optimal flexion axis of the knee. *Clin Orthop*. 1998;356:111-118.
3. Riegger-Krugh C, Gerhart TN, Powers WR, Hayes WC. Tibiofemoral contact pressures in degenerative joint disease. *Clin Orthop*. 1998;348:233-245.
4. Messner K, Gao J. The menisci of the knee joint. Anatomical and functional characteristics, and a rationale for clinical treatment. *J Anat*. 1998;193:61-78.
5. Wilson DR, Feikes JD, O'Connor JJ. Ligaments and articular contact guide passive knee flexion. *J Biomech*. 1998;31:1127-1136.
6. Roach KE, Miles TP. Normal hip and knee active range of motion: the relationship to age. *Phys Ther*. 1991;71:656-665.
7. Boone DC, Azen SP. Normal range of motion of joints in male subjects. *J Bone Joint Surg*. 1979;61:756-759.
8. Oatis CA. *Kinesiology: The Mechanics and Pathomechanics of Human Movement*. Philadelphia, PA: Lippincott Williams & Wilkins; 2004.
9. Kennedy JC, Weinberg HW, Wilson AS. The anatomy and function of the anterior cruciate ligament. *J Bone Joint Surg*. 1974;56A:223-235.
10. Fuss FK. The restraining function of the cruciate ligaments on hyperextension and hyperflexion of the human knee joint. *Anat Rec*. 1991;230:283-289.
11. Seering WR, Pizizli RL, Nagel DA, Schurman DJ. The function of the primary ligaments of the knee in varus-valgus and axial rotation. *J Biomech*. 1980;13:785-794.
12. Markolf KL, Gorek JF, Kabo JM, Shapiro MS. Direct measurement of resultant forces in the anterior cruciate ligament. An in vitro study performed with a new experimental technique. *J Bone Joint Surg*. 1990;72:557-567.
13. Tomsich DA, Nitz AJ, Threlkeld AJ, Shapiro R. Patellofemoral alignment: reliability. *J Orthop Sports Phys Ther*. 1996;23:200-215.
14. Powers CM, Mortenson S, Nishimoto D, Simon D. Criterion-related validity of a clinical measurement to determine the medial/lateral component of patellar orientation. *J Orthop Sports Phys Ther*. 1999;29:372-377.
15. Hehne JH. Biomechanics of the patellofemoral joint and its clinical relevance. *Clin Orthop*. 1990;258:73-85.
16. Grelsamer RP, Klein JR. The biomechanics of the patellofemoral joint. *J Orthop Sports Phys Ther*. 1998;28:286-298.
17. Carson WG, James SL, Larson RL. Patellofemoral disorders: physical and radiographic evaluation. Part I: physical examination. *Clin Orthop*. 1984;185:165-177.

18. Greenfield BH. *Rehabilitation of the Knee: A Problem-Solving Approach.* Philadelphia, PA: FA Davis; 1993.

19. Larson RL. The patellar compression syndrome: surgical treatment by lateral retinacular release. *Clin Orthop.* 1978;34:158.

20. Lysholm J, Gilquist J. Evaluation of knee ligament surgery results with special emphasis on the use of a scoring scale. *Am J Sports Med.* 1982;10:150-154.

21. Bellamy N, et al. Validation study of WOMAC: a health status instrument for measuring clinically important patient-relevant outcomes following total hip or knee arthroplasty in osteoarthritis. *J Orthop Rheumatol.* 1988;1:95-108.

22. McConnell S, Kolopack P, Davis AM. The Western Ontario and McMaster Universities Osteoarthritis Index (WOMAC): A review of its utility and measurement properties. *Arthritis Rheum.* 2001;45:453-461.

23. Noyes FR, McGinniss GH, Mooar LA. Functional disability in the anterior cruciate insufficient knee syndrome. *Sports Med.* 1984;1:287-288.

24. Irrgang JJ, Safran MR, Fu FH. The knee: ligamentous and meniscal injuries. In: Zachazewsji JE, Magee DJ, Quillen WS, eds. *Athletic Injuries and Rehabilitation.* Philadelphia, PA: WB Saunders; 1996:685.

25. Irrgang JJ, et al. Development of a patient-reported measure of function of the knee. *J Bone Joint Surg.* 1998;80A:1132-1145.

26. Boyko EJ, Ahroni JH, Davignon D, et al. Diagnostic utility of the history and physical examination for peripheral vascular disease among patients with diabetes mellitus. *J Clin Epidemiol.* 1997;50:659-668.

27. Boissonnault WG. *Primary Care for the Physical Therapist: Examination and Triage.* St. Louis, MO: Elsevier Saunders; 2005.

28. McFarland EG, Mamanee P, Queale WS, Cosgarea AJ. Olecranon and prepatellar bursitis. *Phys Sportsmed.* 2000;28:40-52.

29. Hewett TE, Myer GD, Ford KR, Heidt RS, et al. Biomechanical measures of neuromuscular control and valgus loading of the knee predict anterior cruciate ligament injury risk in female athletes: a prospective study. *Am J Sports Med.* 2005;33:492-501.

30. Stiell IG, Wells GA, McDowell I, et al. Use of radiography in acute knee injuries: need for clinical decision rules. *Acad Emerg Med.* 1995;2:966-973.

31. Stiell IG, Wells GA, Hoag RH, et al. Implementation of the Ottawa Knee Rule for the use of radiography in acute knee injuries. *JAMA.* 1997;278:2075-2079.

32. Friberg O, Nurminen M, Korhonen K. Accuracy and precision in clinical estimation of limb length inequality and lumbar lordosis. *Int Disabil Stud.* 1988;10:49-53.

33. Subotnick SI. Limb length discrepancies of the lower extremity (the short leg syndrome). *J Orthop Sports Phys Ther.* 1981;3:11-16.

34. McCaw ST. Leg length inequality. *Sports Med.* 1992;14:422-429.

35. McCaw ST, Bates BT. Biomechanical implications of leg length inequality. *Br J Sports Med.* 1991;25:10-13.

36. Blake RL, Ferguson HJ. Correlation between limb length discrepancy and asymmetrical rearfoot position. *J Am Podiatr Med Assoc.* 1993;83:625-633.

37. Kling JR. Angular deformities of the lower limbs in children. *Orthop Clin North Am.* 1987;18:513-527.

38. Fulkerson JP, Arendt EA. Anteiror knee pain in females. *Clin Orthop Relat Res.* 2000;372:69-73.

39. Chao EYS, Neluheni EVD, Hsu RWW, Paley D. Biomechanics of malalignment. *Orthop Clin North Am.* 1994;25:379-386.

40. Boden BP, Pearsall AW, Garrett WE, Feagin JA. Patellofemoral instability: evaluation and management. *J Am Acad Orthop Surg.* 1997;5:47-57.

41. Hughston JC, Walsh WM, Puddu G. *Patellar Subluxation and Dislocation.* Philadelphia, PA: WB Saunders; 1984.

42. Schulthies SS, Francis RS, Fisher AG, Van deGraaff KM. Does the Q-angle reflect the force on the patella in the frontal plane. *Phys Ther.* 1995;75:24-30.

43. Magee DJ. *Orthopedic Physical Assessment.* 5th ed. Philadelphia, PA: WB Saunders; 2006.

44. Eckhoff DG. Effect of limb malrotation on malalignment and osteoarthritis. *Orthop Clin North Am.* 1994;25:405-414.

45. Tria AJ, Palumbo RC, Alicia JA. Conservative care for patellofemoral pain. *Orthop Clin North Am.* 1992;23:545-554.

46. Reischl SF, Powers CM, Rao S, Perry J. Relationship between foot pronation and rotation of the tibia and femur during walking. *Foot Ankle Int.* 1999;20:513-520.

47. McClay I, Manal K. Coupling parameters in runners with normal and excessive pronation. *J Appl Biomech.* 1997;13:109-124.

48. Nigg BM, Cole GK, Nachbauer W. Effects of arch height of the foot on angular motion of the lower extremities in running. *Biomechanics.* 1993;26:909-916.

49. Rothbart BA, Estabrook L. Excessive pronation: a major biomechanical determinant in the development of chondromalacia and pelvic lists. *J Manipulative Physiol Ther.* 1988;11:373-379.

50. Nourbakhsh MR, Arab AM. Relationship between mechanical factors and incidence of low back pain. *J Orthop Sports Phys Ther.* 2002;32:447-460.

51. Dahle LK, Mueller M, Delitto A, Diamond JE. Visual assessment of foot type and relationship of foot type to lower extremity injury. *J Orthop Sports Phys Ther.* 1991;14:70-74.

52. Botte R. An interpretation of the pronation syndrome and foot types of patients with low back pain. *Am J Podiatr Med.* 1981;76-85.

53. Cibulka MT. Low back pain and its relation to the hip and foot. *J Orthop Sports Phys Ther.* 1999;29:595-601.

54. Carson WG. Diagnosis of extensor mechanism disorders. *Clin Sports Med.* 1985;4:231-246.

55. Larsen K, Keskula DR, Leboeuf-Yde C. Can custom-made biomechanic shoe orthoses prevent problems in the back and lower extremities? A randomized, controlled intervention trial of 147 military conscripts. *J Manipulative Physiol Ther.* 2002;25:326-331.

56. Dananberg HJ, Guiliano M. Chronic low-back pain and its response to custom-made foot orthoses. *J Am Podiatr Med Assoc.* 1999;89:109-117.

57. Mills OS, Hull ML. Rotational flexibility of the human knee due to varus/valgus and axial moments in vivo. *J Biomech.* 1991;24:673-690.

58. Lafortune MA, Cavanagh PR, Sommer HJ, Kalenak A. Three-dimensional kinematics of the human knee during walking. *J Biomech.* 1992;25:347-357.

59. Perry J, Burnfield JM. *Gait Analysis: Normal and Pathological Function.* 2nd ed. Thorofare, NJ: Slack; 2011.

60. Patla CE, Paris, SV. *E1 Course Notes: Extremity Evaluation and Manipulation.* St. Augustine, FL. Institute of Physical Therapy; 1993.

61. Fritz JM, Delitto A, Erhard RE, Roman M. An examination of the selective tissue tension scheme, with evidence for the concept of a capsular pattern of the knee. *Phys Ther.* 1998;78:1046-1061.

62. Carlsoo S. Fohlin L. The mechanics of the two-joint muscles rectus femris, sartorius, and tensor fascia latae in relation to their activity. *Scand J Rehabil Med.* 1969;1:107-111.

63. Mirzabeigi E, Jordan C, Gronley JK. Isolation of the vastus medialis oblique muscle during exercise. *Am J Sports Med.* 1999;27:50-53.

64. Kendall FP, McCreary EK, Provance PG. *Muscle Testing and Function.* Baltimore, MD: Williams & Wilkins; 1993.

65. Noyes FR, Sonstegard DA. Biomechanical function of the pes aanserinus at the knee and the effects of its transplantation. *J Bone Joint Surg.* 1973;55A:1241.

66. Fonseca ST, et al. Validation of a performance test for outcome evaluation of knee function. *Clin J Sports Med.* 1992;2:251-256.

67. Lephart SM, et al. Functional performance tests for the anterior cruciate ligament insufficient athlete. *Athl Train.* 1991;26:44-50.

68. Bolga LA, Keskula DR. Reliability of lower extremity functional performance tests. *J Orthop Sports Phys Ther.* 1997;26:138.

69. Noyes FR, Barber SD, Mangine RE. Abnormal lower limb asymmetry determined by function hop tests after anterior cruciate ligament rupture. *Am J Sports Med.* 1991;19:513-518.

70. Jonsson T, Althoff B, Peterson L, et al. Clinical diagnosis of ruptures of the anterior cruciate ligament: a comparative study of the Lachman test and the anterior drawer sign. *Am J Sports Med.* 1982;10:100-102.

71. Rosenberg TD, Rasmussen GL. The function of the anterior cruciate ligament during anterior drawer and Lachman's testing. *Am J Sports Med.* 1984;12:318-322.

72. Benjaminse A, Gokeler A, van der Schans CP. Clinical diagnosis of an anterior cruciate ligament rupture: a meta-analysis. *J Orthop Sports Phys Ther.* 2006;36:267-288.

73. Katz J, Fingeroth R. The diagnostic accuracy of ruptures of the anterior cruciate ligament comparing the Lachman test, the anterior drawer sign, & the pivot shift test in acute & chronic knee injuries. *Am J Sports Med.* 1986;14:88-91.

74. Malanga GA, Andrus S, Nadler SF, McLean J. Physical examination of the knee: A review of the original test description & scientific validity of common orthopedic tests. *Arch Phys Med Rehabil.* 2003;84:592-603.

75. Lee JK, Yao L, Phelps CT, Wirth CR, et al. Anterior cruciate ligament tears: MR imaging compared with arthroscopy & clinical tests. *Radiology.* 1988;166:861-864.

76. Lui SH, Osti L, Henry M, Bocchi L. The diagnosis of acute complete tears of the anterior cruciate ligament. *J Bone Joint Surg.* 1995;77:586-588.

77. Mitsou A, Vallianatos P. Clinical diagnosis of ruptures of the anterior cruciate ligament: a comparison between the Lachman test & the anterior drawer test. *Injury.* 1988;19:427-428.

78. Hardaker WT, Garrett WE, Bassett FH. Evaluation of acute traumatic hemarthrosis of the knee joint. *South Med J.* 1990; 83:640-646.

79. Tonino AJ, Huy J, Schaafsma J. The diagnostic accuracy of knee testing in the acutely injured knee. *ACTA Orthopedia.* 1986;52:479-487.

80. Boeree NR, Ackroyd CE. Assessment of the meniscus & cruciate ligaments: an audit of clinical practice. *Injury.* 1991;22:291-294.

81. Cibere J, Bellamy N, Thorne A, Esdaile JM, et al. Reliability of the knee examination in osteoarthritis: effect of standardization. *Arthritis Rheum*. 2004;50:458-468.

82. Rubinstein RA, Shelbourne KD, McCarroll JR, VanMeter CD, Rettig AC. The accuracy of the clinical examination in the setting of posterior cruciate ligament injuries. *Am J Sports Med*. 1994;22:550-557.

83. Shelbourne KD, Benedict F, McCarroll JR, et al. Dynamic posterior shift test: an adjuvant in evaluation of posterior tibial subluxation. *Am J Sports Med*. 1989;17:275-277.

84. Shino K, Horibe S, Ono K. The voluntary evoked posterolateral drawer sign in the knee with posterolateral instability. *Clin Orthop*. 1987;215:179-186.

85. Ferrari DA, Ferrari JD, Coumas J. Posterolateral instability of the knee. *J Bone Joint Surg Am*. 1994;76:187-192.

86. Daniel DM, Stone ML, Barnett P, Sachs R. Use of the quadriceps active test to diagnose posterior cruciate ligament disruption & measure posterior laxity of the knee. *J Bone Joint Surg*. 1988;70:386-391.

87. Baker CL, Norwood LA, Hughston JC. Acute combined posterior cruciate & posterolateral instability of the knee. *Am J Sports Med*. 1984;12:204-208.

88. Loos WC, Fox JM, Blazina ME, Del Pizzo W, Friedman MJ. Acute posterior cruciate ligament injuries. *Am J Sports Med*. 1981;8:86-92.

89. Fowler PJ, Messieh SS. Isolated posterior cruciate ligament injuries in athletes. *Am J Sports Med*. 1987;15:553-557.

90. Staubi H-U, Jakob RP. Posterior instability of the knee near extension. *J Bone Joint Surg*. 1990;72-B:225-230.

91. Logan MC, Williams A, Lavelle J, et al. What really happens during the Lachman test—a dynamic MRI analysis of tibiofemoral motion. *Am J Sports Med*. 2004;32:369-375.

92. Paessler HH, Michel D. How new is the Lachman test? *Am J Sports Med*. 1992;20:95-98.

93. Cooperman JM, Riddle DL, Rothstein JM. Reliability and validity of judgments of the integrity of the anterior cruciate ligament of the knee using the Lachman's test. *Phys Ther*. 1990;70:225-233.

94. Frank C. Accurate interpretation of the Lachman test. *Clin Orthop*. 1986;213:163-166.

95. Losee RE, Ennis TRJ, Southwick WO. Anterior subluxation of the lateral tibial plateau: a diagnostic test and operative review. *J Bone Joint Surg Am*. 1978;60:1015-1030.

96. Ostrowski JA. Accuracy of 3 diagnostic tests for anterior cruciate ligament tears. *J Athl Train*. 2006;41:120-121.

97. Bach BR, Warren RF, Wickiewitz TL. The pivot shift phenomenon: results and description of a modified clinical test for anterior cruciate ligament insufficiency. *Am J Sports Med*. 1988;16:571-576.

98. Peterson L, Pitman MI, Gold J. The active pivot shift: the role of the popliteus muscle. *Am J Sports Med*. 1984;12:313-317.

99. Harilainen A, Myllynen P, Rauste J, Silvennoinen E. Diagnosis of acute knee ligament injuries. *Ann Chir Gynaecol*. 1986;75:37-43.

100. Dervin GF, Stiell IG, Wells GA, et al. Physicians' accuracy & inter-rater reliability for the diagnosis of unstable meniscal tears in patients having osteoarthritis of the knee. *Can J Surg*. 2001;44:267-274.

101. Jacobson KE, Chi FS. Evaluation and treatment of medial collateral ligament and medial-sided injuries of the knee. *Sports Med Arthrosc Rev*. 2006;14:58-66.

102. Kurzweil PR, Kelley ST. Physical examination and imaging of the medial collateral ligament and posteromedial corner of the knee. *Sports Med Arthrosc Rev*. 2006;14:67-73.

103. Garvin GJ, Munk PL, Vellet AD. Tears of the medial collateral ligament. *Can Assoc Radiol J*. 1993;44:199-204.

104. Shelbourne KD, Martini DJ, McCarrell JR, et al. Correlation of joint line tenderness and meniscal lesions in patients with acute anterior cruciate ligament tears. *Am J Sports Med*. 1995;23:166-169.

105. McMurray TP. The semilunar cartilages. *Br J Surg*. 1942;29:407-414.

106. Evans PJ, Bell GD, Frank C. Prospective evaluation of the McMurray test. *Am J Sports Med*. 1993;21:604-608.

107. Kim SJ, Min BH, Han DY. Paradoxical phenomena of the McMurray test: an arthroscopic examination. *Am J Sports Med*. 1996;24:83-87.

108. Fowler PJ, Lubliner JA. The predictive value of five clinical signs in the evaluation of meniscal pathology. *Arthroscopy*. 1989;5:184-186.

109. Karachalios T, Hantes M, Zibis AH, Zachos V, et al. Diagnostic accuracy of a new clinical test (the Thessaly Test) for early detection of meniscal tears. *J Bone Joint Surg*. 2005;87A:955-962.

110. Akseki D, Ozcan O, Boya H, Pinar H. A new weight-bearing meniscal test & a comparison with McMurray & joint line tenderness. *Arthroscopy*. 2004;20:951-958.

111. Corea JR, Moussa M, Othman A. McMurray's test tested. *Knee Surg Sports Traumatol Arthrosc*. 1994;2:70-72.

112. Konan S, Rayan F, Haddad FS. Do physical diagnostic tests accurately detect meniscal tears? *Knee Surg Sports Traumatol Arthrosc*. 2009;17:806-811.

113. Pookarnjanamorakot C, Korsantirat T, Woratanarat P. Meniscal lesions in the anterior cruciate insufficient knee: the accuracy of clinical evaluation. *J Med Assoc Thailand*. 2004;87:618-623.

114. Hughston JC, Walsh WM, Puddu G. Patellar Subluxation and Dislocation. Philadelphia, PA: WB Saunders; 1984,

115. Fairbank HAT. Internal derangement of the knee in children and adolescents. *Proc R Soc Med*. 1937;30:427-432.

116. Haim A, Yaniv M, Dekel S, Amir H. Patellofemoral pain syndrome: validity of clinical & radiological features. *Clin Orthop*. 2006;451:223-228.

117. Nijs J, Van Geel C, Van der auwera D, Van de Velde B. Diagnostic value of five clinical tests in patellofemoral pain syndrome. *Man Ther*. 2006;11:69-77.

118. Niskanen RO, Paavilainen PJ, Jaakkola M, Korkala OL. Poor correlation of clinical signs with patellar cartilaginous changes. *Arthroscopy*. 2001;17:307-310.

119. Ahmed CS, McCarthy M, Gomez JA, Shubin Stein BE. The moving patellar apprehension test for lateral patellar instability. *Am J Sports Med*. 2009;37:791-796.

120. Ober FB. The role of the iliotibial and fascia lata as a factor in the causation of low-back disabilities and sciatica. *J Bone Joint Surg*. 1936;18:105-110.

121. Reese N, Bandy W. Use of an inclinometer to measure flexibility of the iliotibial band using the Ober test & Modified Ober test. *J Orthop Sports Phys Ther*. 2003;33:326-330.

122. Melchione W, Sullivan S. Reliability of measurements obtained by use of an instrument designed to measure iliotibial band length indirectly. *J Orthop Sports Phys Ther*. 1993;18:511-515.

123. Gautam VK, Anand S. A new test for estimating iliotibial band contracture. *J Bone Joint Surg Br*. 1998;80:474-475.

124. Noble HB, Hajek MR, Porter M. Diagnosis and treatment of iliotibial band tightness in runners. *Phys Sportsmed*. 1982;10:67-68,71-72, 74.

125. Vijayasankar D, Boyle AA, Atkinson P. Can the Ottawa knee rule be applied to children? A systematic review & meta-analysis of observational studies. *Emerg Med J*. 2009;26:250-253.

126. Bachmann LM, Haberzeth S, Steurer J, ter Riet G. The accuracy of the Ottawa Knee Rule to rule out knee fractures: a systematic review. *Ann Intern Med*. 2004;140:121-124.

127. Emparanza JI, Aginaga JR. Validation of the Ottawa knee rules. *Ann Emerg Med*. 2001;38:364-368.

128. Bulloch B, Neto G, Plint A, Lim R, et al. Validation of the Ottawa knee rules in children: a multicenter study. Ann Emerg Med. 2003;42:48-55.

129. Stiell IG. Clinical decision rules in the emergency department. *Can Med Assoc J*. 2000;163:1465-1466.

130. Richman PB. More on the Ottawa knee rules. *Ann Emerg Med*. 1999;33:476.

Orthopaedic Manual Physical Therapy of the Ankle and Foot

Christopher H. Wise, PT, DPT, OCS, FAAOMPT, MTC, ATC

Chapter Objectives

At the conclusion of this chapter, the reader will be able to:

- Identify the key anatomical and biomechanical features of the ankle and foot and their impact on examination and intervention.
- List and perform key procedures used in the orthopaedic manual physical therapy (OMPT) examination of the ankle and foot.
- Demonstrate sound clinical decision-making in evaluating the results of the OMPT examination.

- Use pertinent examination findings to reach a differential diagnosis and prognosis.
- Discuss issues related to the safe performance of OMPT interventions for the ankle and foot.
- Demonstrate basic competence in the performance of an essential skill set of joint mobilization techniques for the ankle and foot.

FUNCTIONAL ANATOMY AND KINEMATICS

Introduction

The ankle-foot complex performs a unique and complex role in bipedal gait and function. Throughout a typical gait pattern, this multijoint complex is responsible for performing two dichotomous roles. First, it serves as a mobile adapter upon initial heel strike and weight acceptance. Secondly, it functions as a rigid lever that facilitates forward propulsion. In addition to the challenge of accommodating the entire weight of the body to the underlying terrain, the ankle-foot complex is responsible for performing these roles efficiently, effectively, and reciprocally. The articulations that comprise the foot and ankle complex, each with its own axis of motion, provide triplanar mobility that is sufficient to allow normal function under a variety of conditions. The interdependence of this structure with proximal articulations renders it not only the source of accommodation but, as a result of both structural and functional impairments, a region that often demands compensatory strategies from its more proximal counterparts. As the most distal segment of the lower kinetic chain, the demands placed on it, coupled with its inherent complexity, render these structures a common locus of impairment and disability often requiring the specialized skills of the manual physical therapist.

The Distal Tibiofibular Joint

The *distal tibiofibular (TF) joint* has an interdependent relationship with its proximal counterpart, the *proximal tibiofibular (TF) joint*, and the impact of these articulations on ankle joint function is profound. This *syndesmotic joint* consists of a concave tibial joint surface that articulates with the convex fibula interposed with an *interosseous membrane* (Fig. 27-1). Although limited, motion within this joint is necessary for normal talocrural mobility. By virtue of its larger fibular facet on the talus, the distal fibula migrates through a greater arc of motion during dorsiflexion (DF) and plantar flexion (PF), which requires motion at both proximal and distal TF joints.

The Talocrural Joint

The ankle joint proper is often referred to as the mortise, or *talocrural (TC) joint*. The TC joint is considered to be a *synovial, hinge-type joint* allowing primarily sagittal plane motion about

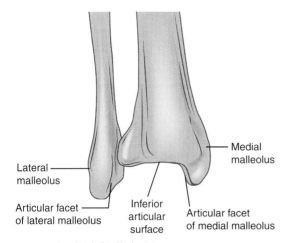

FIGURE 27–1 The distal tibiofibular joint.

a medial-lateral axis. The *medial malleolus, lateral malleolus,* and *posterior facet* of the tibia, often referred to as the third malleolus, compose the concave proximal aspect of the joint. The convex *dome* and *body* of the talus contain three distinct facets, which include a *trochlear facet* that is located superiorly, a large *fibular facet,* and a smaller *tibial facet,* all of which are enrobed in articular cartilage. The talus is wedge shaped, appearing broader anteriorly than posteriorly. Figure 27-2 displays the important landmarks of the talus and its articulation with the calcaneus.

The TC joint functions as an *adjustable mortise,* or wrench. The previously described distal TF joint is important in accommodating to the irregular, wedge-shaped talus as it moves in and out of the mortise during dorsiflexion and plantarflexion, respectively.

Mobility of the TC Joint

The terms typically used to denote triplanar motion of the foot and ankle are pronation and supination. **Pronation** consists of

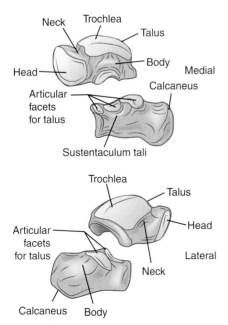

FIGURE 27–2 The talocalcaneal joint.

dorsiflexion in the sagittal plane, eversion in the frontal plane, and abduction in the transverse plane. **Supination** consists of plantarflexion in the sagittal plane, inversion in the frontal plane, and adduction in the transverse plane. Based on the oblique orientation of these joint axes, it is important to note that motions of the foot and ankle do not occur within a single plane. The relative contribution of each joint within the foot and ankle to the various components of pronation and supination varies depending on the independent axis of each joint.

The axis of the TC joint is considered to lie in the transverse plane between the medial and lateral malleoli.[1] However, due to the fact that the medial malleolus lies slightly anterior and superior to the lateral malleolus, the true joint axis for the TC joint is inclined 14 degrees from the transverse plane and 23 degrees from the frontal plane.[2] The oblique orientation of this axis mandates that motion at the TC joint occurs in a *triplanar fashion,* but that the majority of motion occurs within the sagittal plane (Fig. 27-3 A, B).[3]

This joint's primary contribution to pronation and supination is dorsiflexion and plantarflexion. Normal range of motion for *dorsiflexion (DF)* with the knee flexed is reported to range from *10 to 20 degrees*[4–6] and *34 to 50 degrees* for *plantarflexion (PF).*[4–6] The multiarticulate gastrocnemius may demonstrate passive insufficiency that limits the amount of available DF mobility at the TC joint. Minimizing the influence of this muscle by flexing the knee during passive measurement is important for directing appropriate intervention.

The talus glides anteriorly and posteriorly during open chain PF and DF, respectively (Fig. 27-4 A, B). During closed-chain DF, the concave mortise glides anteriorly over the fixed convex talus and posteriorly during PF. The open-packed position of the TC joint is considered to be 5 to 10 degrees of PF and the close-packed position is considered to be full DF.[7]

Stability of the TC Joint

The TC joint relies upon a complex system of passive restraints for its support. The *interosseous membrane* of the distal TF joint assists in supporting the TC joint as well. Supporting the medial aspect of the joint is the substantial *medial collateral ligamentous (MCL)* system, also known as the *deltoid ligament.* This structure courses from the medial malleolus to the navicular, talus, and calcaneus in a fan-shaped fashion and provides excellent support against valgus forces across both the TC and subtalar joints.

The ligaments supporting the ankle laterally are less robust and often considered as distinct structures. The most commonly injured ligament in the body is traditionally considered to be the *anterior talofibular (ATF) ligament.* This ligament runs horizontally from the anterior aspect of the lateral malleolus to the body of the talus. The *posterior talofibular (PTF) ligament* also runs horizontally but is longer than the ATF and runs posteriorly from the lateral malleolus to the talus and calcaneus. The PTF ligament is the strongest of the lateral ligaments and is, therefore, rarely damaged in isolation.[8] Sandwiched between the ATF and the PTF ligaments is the *calcaneofibular (CCF) ligament,* which is the longest of the lateral ligaments connecting the lateral malleolus to the lateral aspect of the

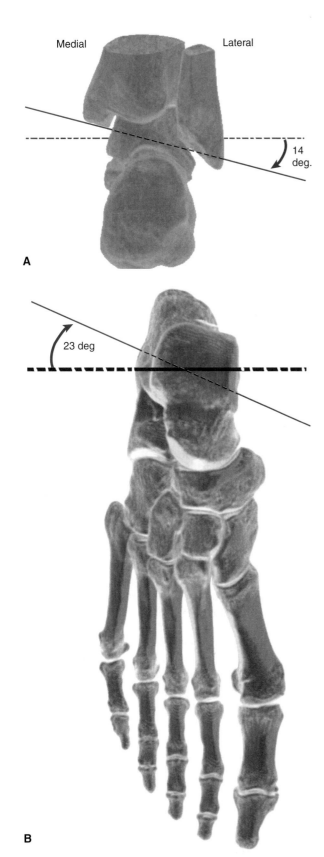

Medial   Lateral

14 deg.

A

23 deg

B

FIGURE 27–3 The axis of motion of the talocrural joint revealing **A.** 14 degrees inferior to the transverse plane and **B.** 23 posterior to the frontal plane. (From: Levangie PK, Norkin CC. *Joint Structure and Function: A Comprehensive Analysis*, 5th ed. Philadelphia, PA: FA Davis Company, 2011.)

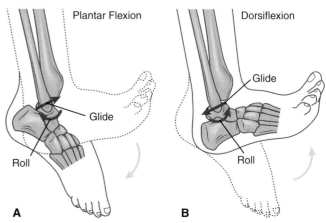

Plantar Flexion   Dorsiflexion

Glide   Glide

Glide   Roll

Roll

A   **B**

FIGURE 27–4 Accessory motions of the talocrural joint in open chain, which includes **A.** posterior roll and anterior glide during plantarflexion and **B.** anterior roll and posterior glide during dorsiflexion.

calcaneus. These ligaments are most commonly injured in response to varus forces when the ankle is in plantar flexion, the position in which the talus is less constrained by the osteological confines of the distal tibiofibular mortise.[8,9] Additional dynamic stability is provided through the large number of multijoint muscles that cross the ankle. The ligamentous constraints are most effective at providing uniplanar support at end range, either medially or laterally, while the muscles assist in midrange stability and support during multiplanar movement patterns.

The Subtalar Joint

The *subtalar joint (ST) joint* is sometimes referred to as the "coach" of the foot, alluding to its valuable role in dictating the manner in which motion occurs within the adjacent articulations. The ST joint is more specifically described as the*talocalcaneal joint*, or more accurately described, as the *talocalcaneonavicular joint*.

The inferior aspect, or underside, of the talus is observed to have three distinct facets for articulation with the calcaneus (Fig. 27-5). The large posterior facet is separated from the anterior and middle facets by a groove known as the *tarsal canal*. This orifice may be visualized on lateral radiographic images just anterior to the lateral malleolus where it emerges as the *sinus tarsi*. The anterior facet is located just anterior to the *sustentaculum tali*. The convex anterior and middle facets on the talus articulate with concave facets on the calcaneus and share a common joint capsule. These facets are distinctly smaller and distinguishable from the larger posterior facet, which bears the majority of superincumbent forces. The open-packed position of the ST joint is 0 to 5 degrees of pronation, and the close-packed position is full supination.[7]

From a mechanical perspective, it may be helpful to visualize the ST joint as a "mitered hinge" that effectively translates transverse plane rotational motions from the leg into frontal plane motions of the foot (Fig. 27-6). Conversely, this mitered hinge is also capable of translating frontal plane foot motion into transverse plane motion within the more proximal structures of the kinetic chain. In closed chain, the talus is thought to move upon the calcaneus, which is fixed from weight-bearing

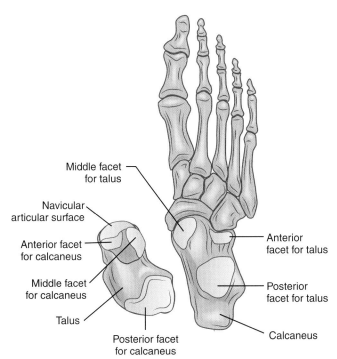

Middle facet for talus

Navicular articular surface

Anterior facet for calcaneus

Middle facet for calcaneus

Talus

Posterior facet for calcaneus

Anterior facet for talus

Posterior facet for talus

Calcaneus

FIGURE 27–5 The subtalar joint, also known as the talocalcaneo-navicular joint

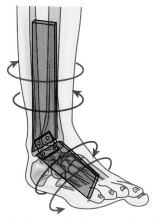

FIGURE 27–6 The subtalar joint functions as a mitered hinge. Transverse plane motion of the tibia is translated into frontal plane motion of the foot and vice versa. (Adapted from: Levangie PK, Norkin CC. *Joint Structure and Function: A Comprehensive Analysis*, 5th ed. Philadelphia, PA: FA Davis, 2011.)

forces. With the foot on the ground, external and internal rotation of the leg will cause supination and pronation of the foot, respectively, as the talus moves upon the fixed calcaneus. The ST joint, therefore, is important functionally in allowing the foot to accommodate to uneven terrain and in the transmission of weight-bearing forces.

There is much controversy that surrounds the validity, reliability, and clinical utility of considering the **subtalar joint neutral (STJN)** position.[10,11] Most clinicians attempt to find STJN in the manner described by Elveru et al,[12] who proposed palpation of the medial and lateral head of the talus while supinating and pronating the ST joint with the neutral position

described as that unique point where the talus is felt equally on both sides. This method of identifying STJN lacks reliability, therefore, explaining the variability of what is considered to be normal. Normal ranges for the STJN position have ranged from 1.5 degrees of calcaneal varus to 2 degrees of calcaneal valgus.[11,13] Because the foot rarely maintains the STJN position during gait, many clinicians and researchers have questioned the clinical significance of assessing and quantifying this position. Cornwall and McPoil[10] propose that the neutral position of the rearfoot may be better represented by the resting position of the calcaneus relative to the lower leg.

Without dispute, however, is the importance of the ST joint during gait and the cascade of impairments that may result from deficits in ST joint function. The ST joint is the primary articulation that enables this complex to perform its roles as mobile adapter and rigid lever throughout the gait cycle. Prior to heel strike, the foot is moving toward pronation. However, at the moment the heel strikes the ground, the foot is in supination and the rearfoot is inverted approximately 3 degrees. From heel strike to midstance, the foot behaves as a mobile adapter, rapidly pronating to absorb forces and to accommodate to terrain. The foot then resupinates, achieving a maximum of 5.5 degrees of calcaneal inversion just before push off.[10] Terminal stance supination increases stability and allows the foot to fulfill its role as a rigid lever, a condition ideal for the facilitation of forward propulsion. Aberrations in ST joint function may impact the manner in which this series of events takes place, resulting in compensation and impairment. As such, careful consideration of the ST joint in isolation and during closed chain function is necessary in order to understand the nature of any observed gait deviations.

Mobility of the ST Joint

The axis of ST joint motion is considered to be approximately 42 degrees superior to the transverse plane and 16 degrees medial to the sagittal plane (Fig. 27-7 A, B).[14] The ST joint axis most closely approximates a longitudinal axis, therefore contributing greatly to the frontal plane motions of inversion and eversion. Given its vertical orientation relative to the transverse plane, the ST joint contributes minimally to the transverse plane motions of abduction and adduction. Should the angle of the ST joint incline less than the normal 42 degrees, one may expect a greater degree of inversion/eversion available at this joint. Likewise, a more vertical axis would increase the degree of expected abduction and adduction.[14] The smallest contribution of the ST joint to triplanar pronation and supination is dorsiflexion and plantarflexion, respectively. ST joint sagittal plane and transverse plane motion is difficult to measure. ST joint abduction and adduction translates into tibial rotation in weight-bearing; therefore, the quantity of abduction and adduction of the talus on the calcaneus can be estimated by measuring the amount of tibial rotation observed in weight-bearing. Studies have demonstrated approximately 4 degrees of internal tibial rotation and 6 degrees of tibial external rotation during gait.[10]

The normal range of foot inversion and eversion is considered to be *18.7 to 32 degrees* and *3.9 to 12.2 degrees*, respectively.[13,15–17] It is important to note, however, that documented

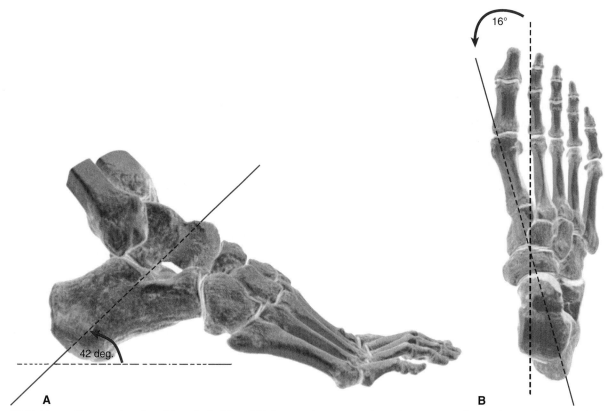

FIGURE 27–7 The axis of motion of the subtalar joint, which is **A.** 42 degrees superior to the transverse plane and **B.** 16 degrees medial to the sagittal plane. (From: Levangie PK, Norkin CC. *Joint Structure and Function: A Comprehensive Analysis*, 5th ed. Philadelphia, PA: FA Davis, 2011.)

normal ranges are used to describe compound motion of the foot and do not define motion of the ST joint in isolation.

Stability of the ST Joint

A variety of ligaments serve as the primary restraints for the ST joint. The *cervical ligament* courses between the neck of the talus and the neck of the calcaneus and is considered to be the strongest of the ST joint ligaments. Running obliquely and lying medial to the cervical ligament within the tarsal canal is the *interosseous ligament*, which consists of two bands. In addition to these ligaments that directly support the ST joint, the *calcaneofibular ligament*, which also provides support for the ankle joint, is an important secondary restraint. The myriad of muscles and their extensive insertions into the retinaculum of the foot provide additional support for the ST joint. This combination of ligamentous structures, in addition to the osteological features of this joint, make dislocation and instability of the ST joint rare.

The Midtarsal Joint

The *midtarsal (MT) joint* is also referred to as the *transverse tarsal joint* or the *Chopart joint*. The MT joint is a compound structure composed of both the *talonavicular joint*, medially and the *calcaneocuboid joint*, laterally, which creates an S-shaped joint line (Fig. 27-8). If the ST joint is the "coach" of the foot

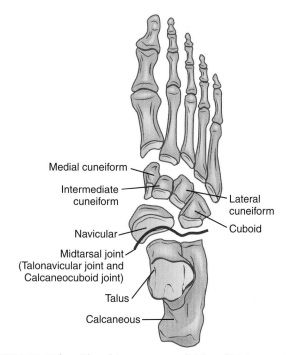

FIGURE 27–8 The midtarsal (transverse tarsal) joint, which is comprised of the medial and more mobile, talonavicular joint, and lateral and less mobile, calcaneocuboid joint.

dictating the functions of joints distal to it, then the MT joint may be considered to be the "star player" that responds to the function of the ST joint. The MT joint demarcates the transition from the rearfoot to the midfoot.

The talonavicular joint, between the convex head of the talus and the concave navicular, constitutes the medial compartment of the MT joint. This joint is a true ball-and-socket joint that shares a common capsule with the ST joint, providing the medial column of the foot with a relatively large amount of mobility. Functionally, medial mobility is important for force attenuation during gait as the foot pronates from heel strike to midstance. The intimate relationship between the ST joint and the MT joint in weight-bearing is revealed in the fact that ST joint motion of the talus on the calcaneus requires motion of the talus on the relatively fixed navicular as well.

The calcaneocuboid joint, located within the lateral column, is a saddle-type joint characterized by reciprocal topography between the anterior calcaneus and posterior cuboid, which renders this joint less mobile. Calcaneal movement at the ST joint in weight-bearing requires movement of the calcaneus on the relatively fixed cuboid.

In weight-bearing, the MT joint responds to, but works independently from, the ST joint. As the ST joint pronates in response to tibial internal rotation, the MT joint may also pronate, thus engaging the medial and more mobile column of the foot and providing the ability of the foot to attenuate forces at heel strike. Likewise, external tibial rotation will produce ST joint supination and subsequent MT joint supination, thus engaging the lateral and less mobile column of the foot and providing rigidity to the foot at push off. When the ST joint is pronated, weight is shifted to the medial column of the foot, thus engaging the more mobile talonavicular joint and creating a mobile foot as opposed to push off, where supination of the ST joint shifts weight laterally, creating a rigid lever for forward propulsion. As the link between the rearfoot and midfoot, the MT joint allows the forefoot to accommodate to uneven terrain. During excessive ST joint pronation or supination, for example, the MT joint may supinate or pronate, respectively, to provide accommodation.

Mobility of the MT Joint

Levangie and Norkin[14] have summarized the work of Manter[18] and Elftman[19] regarding the MT joint axes of motion. There is generally considered to be two axes within the MT joint around which motion occurs. The longitudinal axis, which provides inversion and eversion, is approximately 15 degrees superior to the transverse plane and 9 degrees medial to the sagittal plane (Fig. 27-9 A, B). The oblique axis of the MT joint is approximately 57 degrees medial to the sagittal plane and 52 degrees superior to the transverse plane (Fig. 27-10 A, B). About the oblique axis, dorsiflexion/plantarflexion and abduction/adduction are the primary motions. Motion about this oblique axis is enhanced when the foot is abducted. In cases where the TC joint is unable to provide adequate DF for function, the foot may be abducted in order to engage the oblique

axis of the MT joint in an effort to achieve greater ranges of motion. This subtle compensation within the MT joint although functionally desirable, may result in subsequent impairment including overpronation and **hallux abductovalgus (HAV)** deformity. Although influenced by the subtalar joint, the midtarsal joint is free to move in a manner that is functionally demanded by the forefoot (Fig. 27-11). Identification of MT joint compensation is critical in directing appropriate care.

Stability of the MT Joint

The *spring ligament* supports the inferior aspect of the talonavicular joint capsule and provides necessary support for the medial longitudinal arch. This ligament arises from the sustentaculum tali, is continuous with the deltoid ligament of the ankle, and supports the head of the talus medially. The *bifurcate ligament* supports the joint laterally. As noted, the joint capsule that is reinforced by these ligaments is continuous with the capsule of the ST joint.

The calcaneocuboid joint, possesses its own joint capsule that is reinforced plantarly and dorsally by the plantar and dorsal calcaneocuboid ligaments, respectively. The bifurcate ligament provides support for this joint laterally. The long plantar ligament supports the lateral longitudinal arch and extends distally beyond the MT joint.

The Tarsometatarsal Joint

The five *tarsometatarsal (TMT) joints* are planar synovial joints that form the articulations between the tarsal bones and their respective metatarsals. The base of the first, second, and third *metatarsals* articulate with the *medial (first) cuneiform, intermediate (second) cuneiform,* and *lateral (third) cuneiform,* respectively. The base of the fourth and fifth metatarsals both articulate with the *cuboid* along the lateral border of the foot. The second TMT joint is the most restricted, due in part to its relatively more proximal location. In addition to the TMT joint proper, small joint surfaces exist between each of the metatarsal bases, which allow motion intermetatarsally.

In the forefoot, the term **ray** is used to define each tarsal bone and its associated metatarsal. During examination, the mobility of each ray may be individually assessed and considered in regard to overall function of the foot and ankle.

Mobility of the TMT Joint

Subsumed within a consideration of TMT mobility is the negligible motion between the navicular and the three cuneiforms. The axis of motion for each of the TMT joints is triplanar and unique for each joint. The greatest degree of mobility occurs in the first followed by the fifth TMT joint. The axis of the first and fifth rays are oblique, allowing motion in all three planes (Fig. 27-12). The predominant motion of the third TMT joint is dorsiflexion and plantar flexion, and the axes of the second and fourth TMT joints are similar in orientation to the axes of the first and fifth TMTs, respectively. There is substantial individuality in TMT joint axes, and these axes can vary in response to the process of aging and following injury.

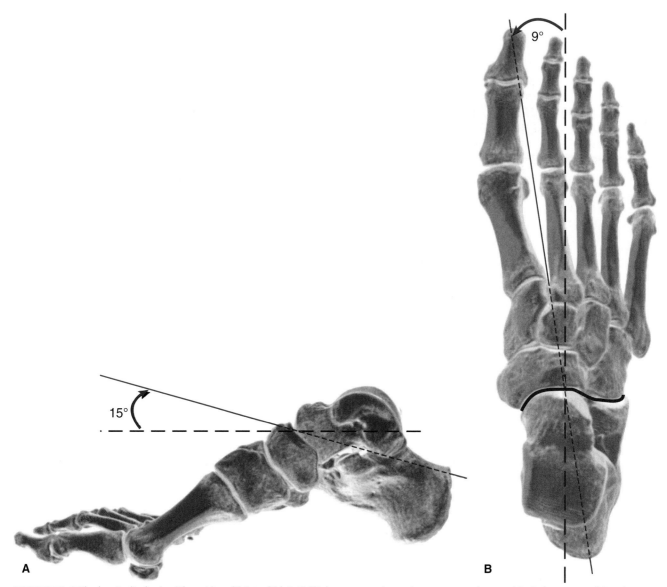

FIGURE 27–9 The longitudinal axis of the midtarsal joint, which is **A.**15 degrees superior to the transverse plane and **B.** 9 degrees medial to the sagittal plane. (From: Levangie PK, Norkin CC. *Joint Structure and Function: A Comprehensive Analysis*, 5th ed. Philadelphia, PA: FA Davis, 2011.)

The function of the TMT joints depend largely on the position and mobility of the ST and MT joints. In this regard, addressing impairments within the ST and MT joints often impact the function of the TMT joints.

Functionally, the five TMT joints work independently to achieve the primary role of bringing their respective metatarsal heads to the ground in weight-bearing. In so doing, these joints exert a profound impact on the position of the forefoot during gait. As the ST and MT joints perform their typical patterns of motion during the gait cycle as previously described, the TMT joints work independently to allow the forefoot to accommodate to the terrain. Functional or structural deviations of the ST and MT joints may require compensatory patterns of movement from the TMT joints.

Stability of the TMT Joint

As already described, metatarsals 1 through 3 articulate with the medial, intermediate, and lateral cuneiforms each having

their own individual joint capsule, which provides a fair amount of stability. The fourth and fifth TMT joints are formed between metatarsals 4 and 5 and share a common joint capsule as they articulate with the cuboid. The *deep transverse metatarsal ligament* serves the primary purpose of maintaining the close approximation of the metatarsals. This fibrous band of connective tissue, therefore, provides indirect stability to the TMT joints. The TMT joints are further reinforced by dorsal and plantar ligaments, which are continuous with the joint capsule and span each individual TMT joint.

The Metatarsophalangeal Joint

The five *metatarsophalangeal (MTP)* joints are formed by the convex head of the metatarsals and their respective concave proximal phalanges. The first MTP joint possesses two sesamoid bones that are located at the plantar aspect of the metatarsal head. These bones are kept in place by a band of ligaments but

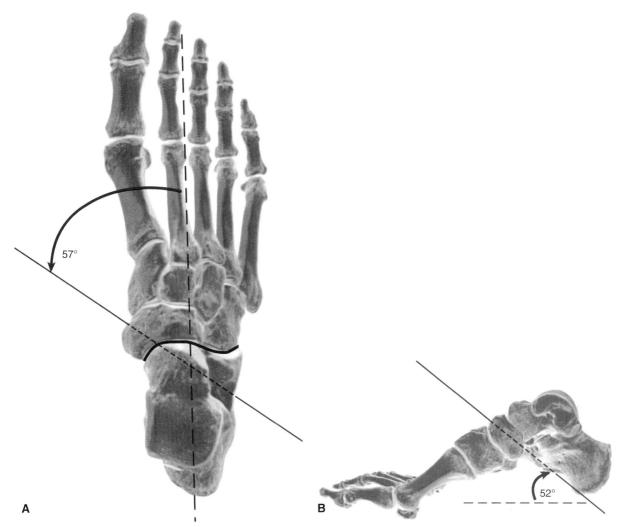

FIGURE 27–10 The oblique axis of the midtarsal joint, which is **A.** 57 degrees medial to the sagittal plane and **B.** 52 degrees superior to the transverse plane. (From: Levangie PK, Norkin CC. *Joint Structure and Function: A Comprehensive Analysis*, 5th ed. Philadelphia, PA: FA Davis, 2011.)

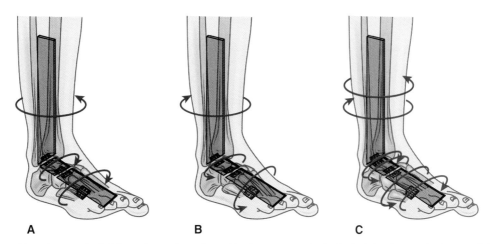

FIGURE 27–11 The midtarsal joint typically follows the motions dictated by the more proximal subtalar joint, thus moving into **A.** slight pronation in conjunction with tibial internal torsion (rotation) and subtalar joint pronation, **B.** slight supination in conjunction with tibial external torsion (rotation) and subtalar joint supination, **C.** the midtarsal joint may also compensate by pronating during excessive subtalar joint supination (red arrows) or supinating during excessive subtalar joint pronation (blue arrows) as determined by the functional demands of the forefoot. (Adapted from: Levangie PK, Norkin CC. *Joint Structure and Function: A Comprehensive Analysis*, 5th ed. Philadelphia, PA: FA Davis, 2011.)

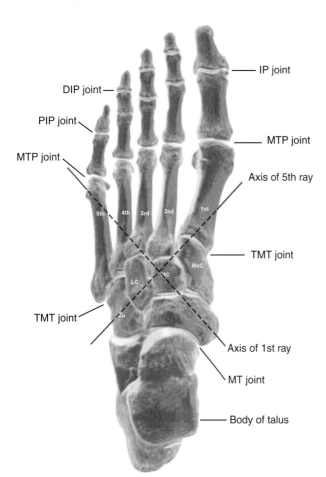

FIGURE 27–12 Axes of the first and fifth tarsometatarsal joints. (From: Levangie PK, Norkin CC. *Joint Structure and Function: A Comprehensive Analysis*, 5th ed. Philadelphia: FA Davis, 2011.)

maintain the ability to move. During terminal MTP extension, the sesamoids move distally. Functionally, the sesamoid bones share weight-bearing forces with the metatarsal head, which is most important in the late stages of stance. Additionally, these bones serve to protect and act as an anatomical pulley enhancing the function of the flexor hallucis longus and brevis muscles.

Mobility of the MTP Joint

Each MTP joint has two degrees of freedom consisting of both flexion/extension and abduction/adduction. During normal function, flexion and extension is, by far, the greatest, with extension being the predominant motion. The first MTP has been studied extensively, and mobility of this joint is a critical component of normal gait.[20-22] It is estimated that a minimum of 65 degrees of first MTP extension is required for normal ambulation, and 85 degrees is required to run.[22] Normal ranges of first MTP extension measured in non-weight-bearing may approach up to *96 degrees*.[20,21] There is a progressive decline in the amount of extension from the second to the fifth MTP, which averages *60 to 80 degrees*.[23] In the absence of normal first MTP extension, the foot behaves in a fashion similar to that observed when the foot is lacking dorsiflexion. Compensatory strategies such as steppage gait, vaulting, circumduction, or out-toeing may develop. Decreased first MTP

extension is termed **hallux limitus**. The term **hallux rigidus** is used to more specifically define a decrease in first MTP extension that is structural or nonreducible. Normal quantity for first MTP flexion is considered to range from *17 to 34 degrees*.[21] MTP abduction and adduction is valuable in allowing the foot to absorb forces during pronation and supination. Normal ranges for first MTP abduction/adduction are generally considered to be between *15 to 19 degrees*.

Based on the progressive decline in the length of the metatarsals from the first to the fifth, an obliquely orientated **metatarsal break** is formed (Fig. 27-13). As the heel rises during push off, MTP extension results in a metatarsal break that translates forces toward the lateral column of the foot, resulting in an inverted calcaneus and foot supination. The oblique orientation of the metatarsal break serves to distribute forces more evenly across all of the metatarsal heads and allows lateral weight translation that contributes to the close-packed position of foot supination, the preferred position for push off. The close-packed position of the MTP joints is considered to be full extension, where it is important for these joints to be stable for effective push off, and the open-packed position for the first MTP is 10 to 20 degrees of extension and 10 to 20 degrees of flexion for MTP joints 2 through 5.[9]

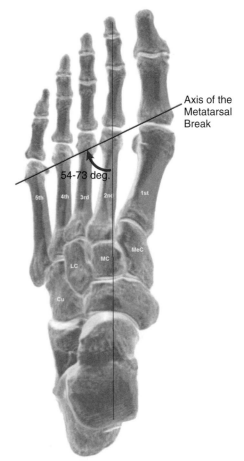

FIGURE 27–13 The metatarsal break of the metatarsophalangeal joints. (From: Levangie PK, Norkin CC. *Joint Structure and Function: A Comprehensive Analysis*, 5th ed. Philadelphia: FA Davis, 2011.)

In response to structural or functional impairments that typically result in foot overpronation, the first MTP may experience an increase in weight-bearing forces during push off. Over time, an increase in valgus stresses through the first MTP results in a deformity that was previously identified as an HAV, which is more commonly referred to as a bunion. This deformity consists of migration of the first metatarsal medially and proximal phalanx laterally, resulting in first MTP abduction. Pain, limited mobility, and degenerative changes can occur in the first MTP as a result of this deformity over time.

Stability of the MTP Joint

All five MTP joints possess collateral ligaments. In addition to the portion that spans the joint from metatarsal to phalanx, there is an oblique portion that connects the metatarsal head to a specialized fibrocartilage structure known as the *plantar plate*. This arrangement provides both weight-bearing protection for the metatarsal heads as well as substantial support for the MTP joints. The plantar plates are connected to one another through the *plantar aponeurosis*. They are continuous with the MTP joint capsule and are attached to the proximal phalanx distally. These plates also possess grooves that maintain the position of the long flexor tendons.

The Interphalangeal Joint

The great toe possesses only one *interphalangeal (IP) joint*, while each of the subsequent digits possess two. The *proximal IP joints (PIP)* are formed by the convex proximal phalanx and the concave middle phalanx, and the *distal IP joints (DIP)* are formed by the convex middle phalanx and the concave distal phalanx. Unlike the MTP joints, the IP joints only allow one degree of freedom into flexion and extension. In most cases, the great toe is the longest; however, in 22% of individuals the second toe is the longest, which is referred to as a **Morton's toe**.[24]

Mobility of the IP Joint

Under normal conditions, there is limited mobility of the IP joints, which display very limited extension and about 90 degrees of flexion.[23] In a sense, the IP joints operate in reverse of the MTP joints, which require a substantial amount of extension and limited flexion in order to function. The limited degree of extension mobility of the IP joints may be an important component that adds stability and enhances function of the foot in late stance. The degree of mobility diminishes from the second to the fifth digit. The close-packed position of the IP joints is considered to be full extension, and the open-packed position is 10 to 20 degrees of flexion.[9]

Stability of the IP Joint

Similar to those described for the MTP joints, the IP joints possess plantar plates that serve the function of protection for underlying structures. The IP joints also possess collateral ligaments that invest into the joint capsule. The joint capsule of the IP joints provides multidirectional stability that serves to disperse the significant loads experienced during ambulation.

EXAMINATION

The Subjective Examination

Self-Reported Disability Measures

Self-reported disability measures for the ankle and foot are sparse. The ***Foot Function Index*** studied by Budiman-Mak and colleagues[25] consists of three sections: pain, disability, and activity. The test-retest reliability of this tool has been found to be good (ICC = 0.87).[25] The ***Ankle Joint Functional Assessment Tool*** consists of 12 functionally relevant questions that are each scored on a scale from 0 to 4. This tool provides good insight into the individual's level of perceived disability related to important functional tasks.[26] The ***Lower Extremity Functional Scale***, as described in Chapter 25, may also be used for individuals presenting with ankle and foot dysfunction.

Review of Systems

Among the most deleterious conditions that may occur in the lower quarter is a *deep vein thrombosis (DVT)*. A patient who is reporting severe pain in the calf region that increases in response to active or passive dorsiflexion (known as the *Homan sign*) should be referred for further diagnostic testing. The therapist should be suspicious of such a condition, particularly in the postsurgical patient. Wells et al[27,28] developed a clinical prediction rule (CPR) to assist in differentially diagnosing patients presenting with a possible DVT. This CPR consists of the following seven criteria: (1) clinical symptoms of a DVT, (2) no alternative diagnosis, (3) heart rate greater than 100 bpm, (4) immobilization or surgery in the previous 4 weeks, (5) previous DVT or pulmonary embolus (PE), (6) hemoptysis, and (7) malignancy.[27,28] Probability of a DVT was based on the following scores: Low = less than 2, Moderate = 2 to 6, and High = more than 6. Individuals deemed as having low probability for the presence of a PE scored 4 and those with a high probability of a PE scored more than 4.[27,28] This CPR for prediction of a DVT was found to have median positive likelihood ratios of 6.62 for patients with high, 1 for moderate, and 0.22 for low pretest probability.[29] For detection of a PE, this CPR had a median positive likelihood ratios of 6.75 for high, 1.82 for moderate, and 0.13 for low pretest probability.[29] Wells et al[27,28] determined that the CPR may be used to identify patients at low risk of being diagnosed with a DVT, and the value of the rule was enhanced with the addition of a rapid latex D-dimer assay.[29]

Based on its anatomical location, it is not surprising that individuals with *peripheral vascular disease (PVD)* often demonstrate signs of vascular compromise in the foot and ankle. Signs of this condition include reduced pulses, decreased temperature, and wounds that fail to heal. An individual with PVD may also experience *intermittent claudication* that consists of leg pain upon exertion.

Within the lower leg, fascial sheaths form distinct compartments that may develop an increase in pressure in response to acute inflammation. Increased pressure within these compartments may cause neurovascular compromise, which requires immediate attention. The signs of *compartment syndrome* include extreme tenderness, edema, paresthesia, and diminished pedal pulses. Individuals experiencing compartment syndrome often report a history of direct trauma to the anterior lower leg or a history of repeated overuse.

History of Present Illness

For those involved in athletic participation, specific questions regarding the frequency and type of activity must be explored. The amount of running and the surfaces on which the patient is running must also be considered. Despite the presence of negative radiographs, a foot or ankle that remains symptomatic should be further investigated because false-negatives are not uncommon. Smaller fractures such as stress fractures of the metatarsals or small avulsion fractures of either malleoli may require *scintigraphy* for definitive diagnosis.

The location of symptoms is extremely valuable in the process of differential diagnosis. Lateral versus medial ankle pain allows the therapist to understand the direction of injury-producing forces and what structures may be involved. *Stress fractures* often result in specific areas of point tenderness. Pain or tenderness over specific tendons and pain with active motion and resistance suggests the presence of a *tendonopathy*. Pain into the anteromedial aspect of the lower leg is suggestive of *shin splints* or *compartment syndrome*.

Of critical importance to foot function is the patient's choice of footwear. The type of shoes worn must be commensurate with the patient's level of activity and the patient's foot type. The wear pattern of shoes provides valuable insight into an individual's foot function. Therefore, the shoes most commonly worn must accompany the patient to therapy.

Mechanism of Injury

When attempting to identify the specific mechanism of injury, the manual physical therapist must be careful to consider any antecedent contributors to the onset of symptoms. The interdependent nature of the lower quarter requires a detailed consideration of the hip and knee.

Most *lateral ankle sprains* occur with the foot in plantar flexion, the open-packed position of the talocrural joint. Damage to the anterior talofibular ligament and/or the other ligaments of the lateral ankle are often identified by a feeling of giving way, observation of a "popping sensation," and immediate edema. In cases of excessive varus or valgus stresses, compression on the medial or lateral aspects of the ankle may also occur, leading to compression fractures of the malleoli. Injuries with the ankle in extreme dorsiflexion may lead to compression fractures of the talar dome or damage to the interosseous membrane and distal tibiofibular joint, sometimes referred to as a high ankle sprain.

An individual's structural foot type or the presence of impairments may predispose an individual to certain conditions. A **pes planus** foot often leads to symptoms along the medial column of the foot resulting from pushing off of a foot that has failed to resupinate at terminal stance. Conditions such as plantar fasciitis, heel spurs, and bunions are common in this population. An individual with a **pes cavus** foot often develops symptoms along the lateral column of the foot that are associated with a diminished ability to attenuate forces at heel strike. In order to determine the need for further diagnostic imaging in the case of an acute ankle injury, the **Ottawa Ankle Rules** may be considered.[30] These guidelines will be discussed later in this chapter.

The Objective Physical Examination
Examination of Structure

Close inspection of static structure serves as the basis for understanding movement. The clinician, however, must be careful not to make direct correlations between the findings from the static exam and dynamic function.[16,31] During observation, it is important for the manual physical therapist to be aware of normal age-related changes. In the infant, the foot is typically pronated in the erect standing posture. As the foot begins to supinate, the medial longitudinal arch develops, and, in the adult, an observable arch is present.[32] When observing the ankle and foot, it is important to consider both open- and closed-chain positions.[33] What is observed in weight-bearing may vary considerably and in some cases may be in direct contrast to what is seen in non-weight-bearing.

Non-Weight-Bearing Examination

Clinical assessment of the *subtalar joint neutral (STJN)* position has undergone much debate in regard to its clinical utility, accuracy, and reproducibility.[10,11] With the patient lying prone, the STJN position is found by palpating the medial and lateral aspects of the dome of the talus while inverting and everting the rearfoot until the talus is felt equally on both sides. The foot is then dorsiflexed in order to lock the foot in this position. The clinician then measures the relative position of a bisection of the calcaneus to the tibia and documents the rearfoot position. A slight degree of rearfoot varus (2–4 degrees) is considered to be normal.[11,13,34] An individual with more or less than 4 degrees is considered to have a **rearfoot varus** or **rearfoot valgus** deformity, respectively. While in the STJN position, the therapist also assesses the forefoot position by measuring the angle between the plantar aspect of the calcaneus and a line formed by the metatarsal heads. Under normal conditions, the metatarsal heads should be aligned with the plantar aspect of the calcaneus with 0 degrees of either forefoot varus or valgus. If the forefoot is angled medially or laterally relative to the rearfoot, then the individual is considered to have a **forefoot varus** or **forefoot valgus** deformity, respectively.[35] Identification of a rearfoot and forefoot varus deformity, or the combination of both, are common among individuals, and the clinical relevance of their presence must be established (Fig. 27-14).

While holding the STJN position, the manual physical therapist may also assess the quantity of forefoot mobility, dorsiflexion range of motion, and first and fifth ray position and mobility. Although lacking evidence to support its validity, reliability, and generalizability to dynamic postures,[10,11] this method of assessing foot position provides baseline data of relative foot positions in non-weight-bearing that may have implications for weight-bearing function. Varus deformity of the rearfoot and/or forefoot measured in non-weight-bearing typically results in compensatory foot overpronation in weight bearing if the foot possesses adequate mobility.

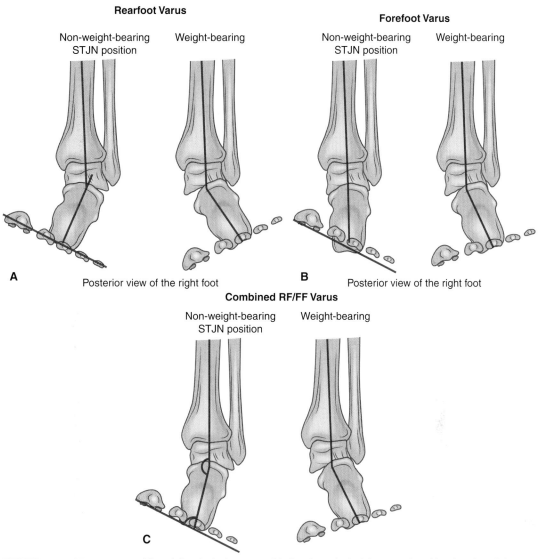

Rearfoot Varus

Non-weight-bearing STJN position   Weight-bearing

A   Posterior view of the right foot

Forefoot Varus

Non-weight-bearing STJN position   Weight-bearing

B   Posterior view of the right foot

Combined RF/FF Varus

Non-weight-bearing STJN position   Weight-bearing

C

FIGURE 27–14 Measurement of foot deformity in the non-weight-bearing subtalar joint neutral position (STJN) and the fully compensated weight bearing position. **A.** Rearfoot varus, **B.** forefoot varus, and **C.** combined rearfoot and forefoot varus may be identified with each having the effect, individually and collectively, of producing compensatory overpronation in weight-bearing.

The presence of a **plantar-flexed first ray**, characterized by a first metatarsal head positioned plantarly in reference to heads 2 through 5, often mimics a forefoot valgus deformity. Overpronation of the foot may alter the angle of pull for the peroneus longus, which becomes more lateral with less of a plantar vector as it inserts onto the first metatarsal, pulling it plantarly.[34] A rigid plantar-flexed first ray may lead to oversupination as the medial column contacts the ground during the midstance phase of gait and may require an orthotic in which the first ray is "cut out," thus allowing the first ray to remain plantar flexed. If the condition is flexible and the first metatarsal head is able to be moved so it is in line with metatarsals 2 through 5, then such a modification is not required.

Normal tibial alignment in the transverse plane reveals 12 to 18 degrees of external torsion, or rotation.[32,35] The clinician may estimate the degree of tibial rotation by observing the relative position of the medial and lateral malleoli to the tibial tuberosity

in sitting with the knee flexed to 90 degrees.[36] With the patient supine, the clinician may also first place the femur in neutral by palpating the medial and lateral condyles of the femur and placing them horizontally in the frontal plane. The medial and lateral malleoli are then palpated, and the angle of the line drawn between the two malleoli and the horizontal is measured.

Additional deformities that may be identified during non-weight-bearing observation includes **talipes equinovarus** deformity, also known as *clubfoot*. This results in limited dorsiflexion and is caused by a combination of congenital factors including neurological involvement. The rigid form of this disorder often requires surgery to maintain foot function. A *rocker bottom foot* is characterized by a forefoot that is dorsiflexed on the rearfoot, resulting in the absence of foot arches.

As already described, an *HAV* deformity is fairly common and often the result of overpronation, leading to medial migration of the metatarsal head and an increase in the **intermetatarsal**

angle and lateral deviation of the proximal phalanx. The result of an HAV is a bunion, which consists of exostosis of the first metatarsal head, callus formation, and a thickened bursa. A *tailor's bunion* occurs at the lateral aspect of the fifth metatarsal head and is also the result of overpronation. Resulting from the presence of a pes cavus foot, *claw toes* are fairly common and involve hyperextension of the MTP joints and flexion of the PIP and DIP joints. With claw toes, foot intrinsic muscle activity is altered, resulting in deformity. Similar in appearance is the *hammer toe* deformity, which involves extension of the MTP and flexion of the PIP with the DIP in variable positions. This condition may be the result of poorly fitting shoes or congenital factors and most commonly occurs in the second toe. A *mallet toe* consists of flexion of the DIP, which typically leads to callus formation on the dorsum of the DIP (Fig. 27-15). As mentioned, a *Morton's foot* is characterized by a second toe that is longer than the first. In such cases, increased stress is experienced by the second toe, thus leading to pain and functional limitations.

Individuals with an overpronatory foot type tend to experience forces through the medial column resulting in callus formation at the first metatarsal head and a callus on the medial aspect of the great toe, known as a *pinch callus*. Overpronators typically develop a *pump bump* that, when developed, becomes known as **Haglund's deformity**. This bony exostosis is located at the posterior aspect of the calcaneus as a result of shear-type forces as the foot rapidly pronates when going from heel strike to midstance and from excessive tensile forces at the insertion of the Achilles tendon. An oversupinating foot often results in callus formation on the plantar aspect of the fifth metatarsal head. Calluses and *plantar's warts*, which are located on the plantar aspect of the foot, may alter the typical weight-bearing forces experienced during gait due to pain.

Inversion ankle sprains often result in localized edema in the region of the anterior talofibular ligament which is just distal and anterior to the lateral malleolus. The presence of a *tendonopathy* suggests the presence of tendons that appear inflamed and/or fibrotic. Inflammation of the Achilles tendon, posterior tibialis tendon, and peroneus longus tendon may be easily observed and confirmed upon palpation.

Long-standing edema, pain, and immobility may result in *complex regional pain syndrome (CRPS)* resulting in the presence of vasomotor changes of the distal extremity. Such changes may include abnormal hair growth, shiny skin appearance, erythema, abnormal skin moisture or dryness, and brittle nails. A systematic assessment of the nailbeds must be performed to identify the color, shape, and level of brittleness. Astute observation of the nails and the underlying beds often yield useful information regarding the overall health of the individual. The *dorsal pedis artery* is a branch of the anterior tibial artery that is important for supplying the dorsum of the foot. This pulse can be palpated either over the talus or between the first and second metatarsals or medial and intermediate cuneiforms.

The value of astute observation of footwear cannot be overstated. Observation of shoe wear patterns provides valuable information regarding the routine forces experienced by the foot. Typically, the greatest wear is noted along the posterolateral edge of the heel which occurs in response to heel strike. Wear is also noted under the first metatarsal head as a result of push off in late stance. Overpronators may present with a heel that is collapsed medially. An oblique crease in the forefoot suggests the presence of a hallux rigidus condition.[32] Tight-fitting or narrow shoes may result in HAVs or a neuroma. Shoes with high heels have been associated with knee and back pain and are involved in the onset of ankle sprains, neuromas, and stress fractures.[37] Individuals who engage in extensive walking or running should be aware that shoes often break down at a much faster rate than they appear.

Weight-Bearing Examination

Moving proximally, the manual physical therapist observes the relationship between the position of the foot, knee, and hip. Structural deviations identified in non-weight-bearing impact proximal segments when the foot contacts the ground. Identifying the cause of postural deviations is challenging since compensations are common.

The presence of **tibial varum** or **tibial valgum** is ascertained by measuring the frontal plane angle formed between the tibia and the horizontal in weight-bearing and is synonymous with genu varum/valgum of the knee. To ascertain the true angle of the lower leg to the ground and reduce the effects of the foot on this measurement in a standing position, the foot is placed in the STJN position by palpating the talus while the individual inverts and everts. Under normal conditions, the tibia is perpendicular to the ground. The orientation of the lower leg to the ground may impact foot position and movement.[38,39] As previously described, a foot with adequate mobility, will compensate when the foot hits the ground. Therefore, it is important to consider the static non-weight-bearing positions of the foot only in light of the potential compensations that occur in closed chain.[34]

Combined foot deformities are common and lead to a cascade of complex compensations in the weight-bearing, mobile foot. For example, a combined *rearfoot varus-forefoot varus deformity* is commonly identified during the non-weight-bearing examination.[34] During gait, the ST joint will pronate in early stance to compensate for the rearfoot varus and continue to pronate through midstance to compensate for the forefoot varus. This foot will often display a limited capacity to resupinate during propulsion. In a combined *rearfoot varus-tibial varus deformity*, with the former observed in non-weight-bearing and the latter observed in weight-bearing, there is an increase in the total amount of varus that requires additional compensation in weight-bearing and gait.[34] If a sufficient amount of mobility is present, the ST joint may overpronate throughout midstance and fail to resupinate in

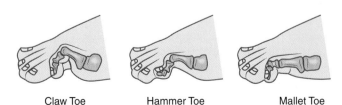

Claw Toe   Hammer Toe   Mallet Toe
FIGURE 27–15 Claw toe, hammer toe, mallet toe deformity.

the late stance phase. These compensations will place significant stress through the medial column of the foot, as well as compression of the lateral aspect of the ankle. A combined *rearfoot varus-flexible forefoot valgus deformity* that is observed in non-weight-bearing may result in ST joint overpronation and forefoot inversion in response to ground reaction forces.[34] This combined foot type often behaves much like a rearfoot varus deformity with excessive overpronation. There are occasions where the rearfoot may be mobile, but the forefoot may be rigid. A combined *rearfoot varus-forefoot valgus or plantar flexed first ray* may be present.[34] In early stance, the ST joint will overpronate, but in midstance the first ray contacts the ground prematurely, and due to its immobility, pronation will be limited. This foot type may result in an unstable, supinated foot.[34]

The presence of any toeing in or toeing out, also referred to as **foot adduction** and **foot abduction**, respectively, must also be noted in weight-bearing. The **Fick angle** defines the position of the foot relative to the sagittal plane with 12 to 18 degrees of toeing out, or abduction, considered to be normal.[32] Individuals with excessive forefoot abduction or external tibial rotation may present with the "too many toes sign" when viewed from behind.[40] An abnormal Fick angle may be caused by a transverse plane deviation of the tibia or may be the result of a structural abnormality elsewhere in the foot. If the primary structural or functional impairment is within the tibia, then the sufficiently mobile foot may exhibit compensatory strategies. For example, an internally rotated tibia may lead to compensatory oversupination and increased rigidity of the foot, whereas tibial external rotation may lead to compensatory overpronation of the foot in weight-bearing. Observing the position of the tibia when the foot is in STJN, although controversial, may assist in identifying whether the foot or the tibia is the origin of the primary structural impairment.

A general assessment of **medial longitudinal arch (MLA)** height can be ascertained by drawing an imaginary line, known as the **Feiss line**,[32] between the medial malleolus, navicular tubercle, and medial aspect of the first metatarsal head. A navicular that falls below or above this line is suggestive of a pes planus and pes cavus foot type, respectively (Fig. 27-16). Changes in arch height between weight-bearing and non-weight-bearing provides information regarding MLA mobility and the ability of the foot to accommodate for aberrant foot types. The **transverse tarsal arch**, with the middle cuneiform as the keystone, must also be considered. A loss of this arch is identified by callus formation at the second and third metatarsal heads. The arches of the foot are important for accommodation to uneven terrain.

Examination of Mobility

Active and Passive Physiologic Movement Examination

The interdependency among the joints of the lower quarter dictates that the primary role of the manual physical therapist during mobility testing is to differentiate the driving impairment from the secondary compensation(s). When considering mobility of the ankle/foot complex, both quantity and timing of these triplanar movements are important. Regions of hypo- or

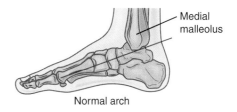

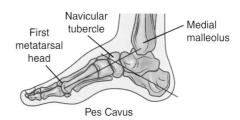

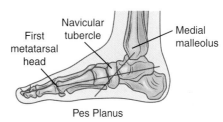

FIGURE 27-16 The Feiss line, which is drawn from the medial malleolus, through the navicular tubercle, to the first metatarsal head, is useful for determining a foot with a normal medial longitudinal arch (MLA), high MLA or pes cavus foot type, or low MLA or pes planus foot type.

hypermobility may compromise the ability of the foot to perform important functions, resulting in pain and disability.

Goniometric measurement of *dorsiflexion* is typically accomplished with the patient in prone with the knee flexed to reduce the effects of gastrocnemius **passive insufficiency**. A valuable method for distinguishing between true TC joint restrictions and gastrocnemius tightness is to compare the quantity of dorsiflexion with the knee flexed to the quantity of dorsiflexion with the knee extended. The amount of motion accomplished in weight-bearing that approximates true end range exceeds that which can be generated in non-weight-bearing, thus improving measurement reliability.[7] Therefore, measuring dorsiflexion in a weight-bearing position may be considered. Limitations in TC dorsiflexion pose significant functional limitations related to gait. If the tibia is unable to translate over the talus during normal gait, compensations will occur.

In the presence of limitations in inversion and eversion, the ST and MT joints are typically culpable. Measurement of rearfoot inversion/eversion is performed prone with the stationary arm in line with the tibia and the moveable arm in line with a bisection of the calcaneus. In sitting, forefoot inversion/eversion is assessed with the goniometer on the dorsum of the foot, with the stationary axis in line with the tibia and the moveable arm in approximate alignment with the third metatarsal.

The importance of great toe extension in gait and function has already been discussed. When measuring this motion, it is important to stabilize and disallow plantar migration of the first metatarsal head, a commonly occurring compensation.

The first metatarsal head may be stabilized manually or great toe extension may be performed in standing with stabilization provided by the weight-bearing surface.

Observation of a capsular pattern suggests restrictions within the noncontractile components of the foot and ankle complex. The capsular pattern of the TC joint is plantar flexion more limited than dorsiflexion (plantarflexion > dorsiflexion), the capsular pattern of the ST joint is inversion more limited than eversion (inversion > eversion), and the capsular pattern of first MTP joint is extension more limited than flexion (extension > flexion). As discussed elsewhere, the validity of clinically identifying capsular patterns is dubious, and its clinical relevance must be considered in the context of additional clinical information.

An appreciation of end feel is also useful in guiding subsequent intervention for the remediation of mobility impairments. An end feel is considered to be abnormal if it either occurs too early or too late within the range of motion or if it is contrary to that expected for the joint in question. Table 27-1 displays the physiologic motions of the ankle/foot, including

normal ranges of motion, open and closed-packed positions, normal end feels, and capsular patterns.

If symptoms are not reproduced during typical motion testing, then overpressure and counterpressure may be used. To isolate the primary locus of pathology, it may be useful to resist each of the single plane motions that compose the multiplane motions of pronation and supination. For example, if an individual complains of reproducible pain with pronation, the therapist may overpress dorsiflexion, eversion, and abduction individually. Reproduction of symptoms with dorsiflexion, for example, suggests the primary locus of pathology to be originating within the talocrural joint. In the case of painful pronation, where overpressure into dorsiflexion leads to symptom reproduction, counterpressure may then be used to inhibit dorsiflexion while eversion and abduction takes place. If the symptoms diminish, then involvement of the talocrural joint is confirmed. This process may also be used to identify involvement of proximal segments. For example, if an individual reports pain that is experienced when translating from heel strike to midstance during ambulation, then the examiner may

Table 27-1 Physiologic (Osteokinematic) Motions of the Ankle and Foot

JOINT	NORMAL ROM	OPP	CPP	NORMAL END FEEL(S)	CAPSULAR PATTERNS
Talocrural Joint	34–50° plantar flexion 10-20° dorsiflexion	5-10° PF	Maximal DF	Elastic for DF, PF, Inversion Hard for Eversion	PF > DF
Subtalar Joint	18.7-32° inversion/adduction 3.9-12.2° eversion/abduction	0-5° pronation	Maximal supination	Elastic (tissue stretch) for all planes	Inversion > Eversion
Midtarsal Joint	10° inversion/eversion 10° abduction/dorsiflexion 20° adduction/plantar flexion	Abduction, Eversion of the subtalar joint	Adduction, Inversion of the subtalar joint	Elastic for talonavicular joint Firm for calcaneocuboid joint	
Tarsometatarsal Joint	10°s dorsiflexion 10° plantar flexion	Pronation	Supination		
1st Metatarsophalangeal Joint	96° extension 17-34° flexion 15-19° abduction/adduction	10-20° extension	Maximal extension	Flexion/extension= capsular, elastic Abduction/adduction= ligamentous, firm	Extension > Flexion
2-5 Metatarsophalangeal Joint	60-80° flexion 35° extension	10-20° flexion	Maximal extension	Elastic	Extension >/= Flexion
Interphalangeal Joint	Minimal extension 90° flexion	10-20° flexion	Maximal extension	Flex/extension = capsular, elastic Abduction/adduction = ligamentous, firm	Flexion > Extension

OPP, open-packed position; CPP, close-packed position; PF, plantar flexion; DF, dorsiflexion (Adapted From: Wise CH, Gulick DT. *Mobilization Notes: A Rehabilitation Specialist's Pocket Guide.* Philadelphia, PA: FA Davis, 2009.)

use counterpressure to inhibit internal rotation of the tibia, thus reducing the contribution from proximal segments. If the reproducible pain diminishes, then the therapist may consider the proximal segments as contributory. This process may be referred to as **regional movement differentiation (RMD)**. (See "The Three Rs of the Examination/Evaluation Process" in Chapter 2.) Although RMD is considered anecdotal and should only be considered within the context of additional examination findings, it may serve to direct early intervention.

Passive Accessory Movement Examination

To minimize the influence of periarticular soft tissues passive accessory motion testing may best be performed in the open-packed position. It may be useful, however, for the examiner to assess accessory mobility throughout a range of physiologic motion as well. As with physiologic testing, end feel must also be assessed for each motion. Limitations and/or reproduction of symptoms during accessory motion testing serves as the primary criterion for initiation of joint mobilization, which is preferable to the extrapolation of accessory mobility, from the results of physiologic motion testing. The patient/clinician position, hand placement, stabilization, and mobilization contacts used for the accessory motion examination is often identical to that which is initially used for mobilization. The mobilization techniques that follow later in this chapter will provide details regarding patient and clinician position, hand contacts, and performance of accessory glides for the foot and ankle that may be used for both examination and intervention. Table 27-2 displays the accessory motions of the ankle and foot.

Examination of Muscle Function

Muscle function testing must be performed in a manner that is specific for the muscle in question and in a manner that simulates the typical function of the muscle. Each muscle must be tested using its dominant type of contraction (i.e., isometric, concentric, eccentric) and at the length (i.e., shortened, midrange, lengthened) and plane (i.e., frontal, sagittal, transverse) in which it typically functions.

Table 27-2	Accessory (Arthrokinematic) Motions of the Ankle and Foot		
	ARTHROLOGY	**ARTHROKINEMATICS**	
Distal Tibiofibular Joint	Concave surface: Tibia Convex surface: Fibula	*To facilitate dorsiflexion:* Tibia and fibula separate as the talus enters the joint, fibula glides superiorly	*To facilitate plantarflexion:* Tibia and fibula return to neutral
Talocrural Joint	Concave surface: Distal tibia/fibula Convex surface: Talus	*To facilitate dorsiflexion:* OKC-talus rolls anterior and glides posterior on tibia CKC-tibia rolls and glides anterior	*To facilitate plantarflexion:* OKC- talus rolls posterior and glides anterior on tibia CKC-tibia rolls and glides posterior
Subtalar Joint	Concave surface: Anterior calcaneal facet and posterior talus Convex surface: Posterior calcaneal facet and anterior talus	*To facilitate inversion:* OKC-anterior calcaneal facet rolls and glides medial while posterior calcaneal facet rolls and glides lateral CKC-talus rolls medial and glides lateral on anterior calcaneal facet while talus rolls and glides medial on posterior calcaneal facet	*To facilitate eversion:* OKC-anterior calcaneal facet rolls and glides lateral while posterior calcaneal facet rolls and glides medial CKC-talus rolls lateral and glides medial on anterior calcaneal facet while talus rolls and glides lateral on posterior calcaneal facet
Midtarsal (Talonavicular and Calcaneocuboid) Joint	Talonavicular Joint: Concave surface: Navicular Convex surface: Talus Calcaneocuboid Joint: Saddle joint	*To facilitate dorsiflexion and inversion:* Navicular and cuboid glide dorsally on talus and calcaneus, respectively	*To facilitate plantarflexion and eversion:* Navicular and cuboid glide plantarly on talus and calcaneus, respectively
Metatarsophalangeal Joint	Concave surface: Phalanx Convex surface: Metatarsal	*To facilitate flexion:* Phalanx rolls and glides plantarly on metatarsal	*To facilitate extension:* Phalanx rolls and glides dorsally on metatarsal
Interphalangeal Joint	Concave surface: Distal phalanx Convex surface: Proximal phalanx	*To facilitate flexion:* Distal phalanx rolls and glides plantarly on proximal phalanx	*To facilitate extension:* Distal phalanx rolls and glides dorsally on proximal phalanx

OKC, open kinetic chain; CKC, closed kinetic chain. (Adapted From: Wise CH, Gulick DT. *Mobilization Notes: A Rehabilitation Specialist's Pocket Guide.* Philadelphia, PA: FA Davis, 2009.)

Within the foot and ankle complex, the manual physical therapist must be aware of any multijoint muscles and the presence of **active insufficiency**. This most commonly occurs in relation to the large multiarticulate gastrocnemius muscle. The multijoint muscles of the ankle must be appreciated in regard to their location relative to the axis of motion across each of the joints that they traverse. By virtue of their location, each muscle often possesses more than one primary action (Fig. 27-17).

The intrinsic muscles of the foot function collectively during late stance, contributing to supination that is required to transform the foot into a rigid lever for push off.[41] Overpronation leads to increased activity of the foot intrinsics, presumably as an attempt to gain greater stability.[41] Enhancing the function of this muscle group will lead to improved function.

The function of the *anterior tibialis*, as the prime dorsiflexor of the foot, is indisputable. As an invertor of the foot, however, its role is less clear. The combined function of dorsiflexion and inversion is vital at heel strike where this muscle is active in eccentrically controlling pronation. By virtue of its insertion into the medial cuneiform, this muscle also supports the medial longitudinal arch.[42]

The *extensor digitorum longus (EDL)* and *extensor hallucis longus (EHL)* both assist with dorsiflexion. The broader EDL also contributes to eversion.[43] Perhaps its most valuable role, however, is extension of the MTP and IP joints of digits 2 through 5. The great toe is supplied by the EHL, which serves the primary role of great toe extension and contributes slightly to foot inversion.[43] Testing MTP and IP extension serves to differentiate the EHL and EDL from the anterior tibialis muscle.

The *triceps surae*, consisting of the *gastrocnemius, soleus,* and *plantaris* muscles, are the prime movers for ankle plantarflexion. Since the Achilles inserts slightly medial on the calcaneus,

it also contributes to inversion. Perhaps, a less considered role of the gastrocnemius is its role in controlling movement of the tibia over the foot during midstance and as a flexor of the knee, especially with knee flexion up to 90 degrees.[44] This muscle is differentiated from the others by testing plantarflexion with the knee flexed, which focuses on function of the soleus and plantaris. The soleus muscle is composed primarily of slow twitch fibers and is well-suited for activities of greater duration, such as upright standing.[45]

Contributing to plantarflexion, but serving to a greater extent as an invertor of the foot, is the posterior tibialis muscle that lies deep to the triceps surae. Assisting the posterior tibialis in its role as an invertor are the *flexor digitorum longus (FDL)* and the *flexor hallucis longus (FHL)* muscles. These muscles work closely with the anterior tibialis in providing inversion and dynamically supporting the medial longitudinal arch. The primary role of the FDL and FHL are as the prime movers for MTP and IP flexion and, more importantly, to stabilize the toes from ground reaction forces during the late stance phase of gait.

Foot eversion is primarily provided by the peroneal muscle group. The most substantial of the group, the *peroneus longus (PL)* has a unique and important relationship with the anterior tibialis muscle. The PL and anterior tibialis, both of which occupy the deep layer of the plantar foot, form a sling that supports the arches of the foot. The other two muscles of this group, the *peroneus brevis (PB) and peroneus tertius (PT)* assist with eversion and, as a group, collectively contribute to plantar flexion.

Selective tissue tension (STT) testing, as described in Chapter 5, may be performed in order to appreciate the onset of symptoms and used as a screening tool to target muscles that may require more specific testing.[46]

Examination of Function

Qualitative Gait Assessment

Generally speaking, the foot should be moving toward pronation at heel strike and continue to do so until mid- to late stance when the foot resupinates to prepare for push off. The proximal segments should be performing as expected relative to these motions. Such parameters as cadence, step/stride length, degree of weight-bearing, and quality of gait should be noted. If symptoms arise, it is important to identify the region of origin and at what specific point in the gait cycle they occur.

Heel Raise

As already described, as the plantar flexors exert their force upon the calcaneus via the Achilles tendon, the calcaneus will slightly invert, thus displaying the integrity of this muscle group and the contribution of the posterior tibialis, which is the prime invertor. The functional heel raise conveys the ability of the foot to supinate and shift weight onto the lateral column, thus developing the necessary rigidity.

Toe Walking

To assess the endurance of the plantar flexors, toe walking is then performed, and the distance traversed is measured as a

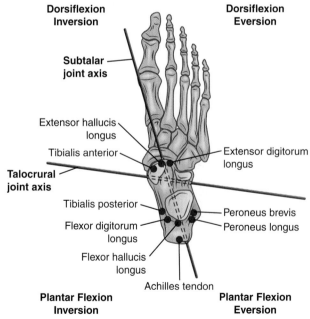

FIGURE 27–17 Locations of the multiarticulate muscles of the foot and ankle. Each muscle is able to perform a variety of actions based on the relationship of its insertion site to the talocrural and subtalar joint axes of motion.

baseline for future improvement. The onset of any symptoms during this activity are recorded.

Heel Walking

To test the function and endurance of the dorsiflexors, the patient is asked to walk on his or her heels over a given distance. Any symptoms and issues with loss of balance are recorded.

Supinated/Pronated Walking

To test the weight-bearing capacity of the foot to achieve certain positions and to determine the presence of symptoms, the patient is asked to ambulate on the lateral borders and then the medial borders of their feet. Observation of the impact that these patterns have on proximal segments must also be noted.

Lunge Walking

Asking the patient to take steps two to three times larger than normal may be useful in accentuating any deviations noted during normal gait. Lunge walking may confirm subtle deviations that were difficult to identify during normal walking.

Standing Rotation

In standing, with feet shoulder width apart, the patient is asked to rotate maximally in one direction followed by the other while keeping the feet in place. Rotation will cause ipsilateral supination and contralateral pronation. The patient's tolerance and mobility in each of these directions can be easily assessed.

Additional tests for the hip and knee described in Chapters 25 and 26 may also be considered.

Palpation

Osseous Palpation

Beginning at the distal-most aspect of the tibia and fibula, the *medial and lateral malleoli* are first palpated. These prominent landmarks are easily identifiable as the medial malleolus is observed superior and anterior to the lateral malleolus (Fig. 27-18).

Located directly within the mortise between the two malleoli is the *talus*. The dome of the talus is best palpated by first placing the ankle in plantar flexion. Confirmation may be obtained by passively inverting and everting the foot, which causes the talus to glide laterally and medially, respectively. The trochlea of the talus can be found on a line drawn between the medial malleolus and the tubercle of the navicular. Passive eversion of the foot will make the head more prominent. Lastly, the medial tubercle of the talus lies posterior and inferior to the medial malleolus. Passive dorsiflexion and plantar flexion will cause the tubercle to move around the medial malleolus.

The final component of the rearfoot that is palpated is the *calcaneus*. With the patient prone, the full extent of this prominent bone can be palpated, including the *calcaneal tuberosity*, which lies along the plantar surface, and the *sustentaculum tali*, which is located approximately 1 inch immediately distal to the medial malleolus (Fig. 27-19). The insertion of the *plantar fascia* into the proximal aspect of the calcaneus is palpated for tightness and tenderness.

The most prominent bony landmark on the medial aspect of the foot is the *navicular*, by virtue of its tubercle. The *navicular tubercle* will fall in line with the medial malleolus and the head of the talus (Fig. 27-20). The navicular occupies the medial compartment of the midfoot and articulates with all three cuneiforms. The lateral column of the midfoot is comprised of the *cuboid* and its articulations with the fourth and fifth metatarsals. To locate the cuboid, an imaginary line is drawn from the styloid process of the fifth metatarsal to the lateral malleolus, along which this bone can be palpated (Fig. 27-21).

After palpating the tubercle of the navicular, proceeding distally you will encounter the medial, or first, cuneiform. The cuneiforms are palpated by following each metatarsal up to its base, identifying the tarsometatarsal joint line, and moving onto each respective cuneiform (Fig. 27-22). To confirm, the medial cuneiform serves as the insertion site for the anterior tibialis

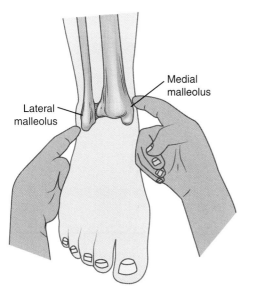

FIGURE 27–18 Palpation of the medial and lateral malleoli, which defines the talocrural joint axis of motion. The lateral malleolus is posterior and extends more distally than the medial malleolus.

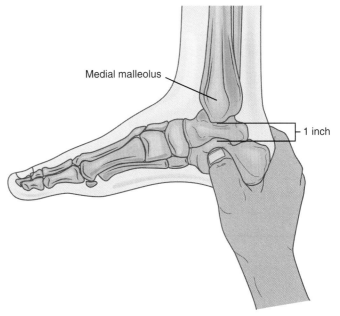

FIGURE 27–19 Palpation of the sustentaculum tali of the calcaneus.

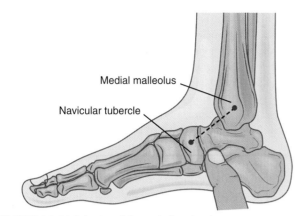

FIGURE 27–20 Palpation of the navicular tubercle.

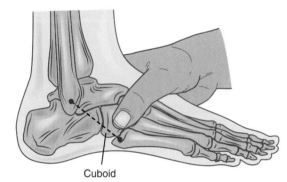

FIGURE 27–21 Palpation of the cuboid.

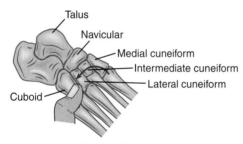

FIGURE 27–22 Palpation of the cuneiforms.

muscle, which can be easily identified in the anterior compartment of the leg and easily followed to its insertion onto this bone.

The metatarsals and phalanges are not difficult to visualize and palpate. The resting posture of each metatarsal head should be considered in reference to one another. The mobility of each metatarsal in reference to one another must also be determined. The length of each metatarsal and phalanx should be palpated. The styloid process at the base of the fifth metatarsal is easily palpated and is an important insertion site for the peroneus brevis muscle.

Soft Tissue Palpation

The largest and most easily palpated muscle of the lower leg is the *gastrocnemius*, spanning from the posterior condyles of the femur to the posterior calcaneus where it inserts along with the soleus as the Achilles tendon. Upon palpation, it is valuable

to identify both the medial as well as the lateral head of the gastrocnemius with the medial extending further distally. The broader single-joint soleus muscle is most easily palpated on either side of the gastrocnemius as this muscle begins to taper distally. For this palpation, the patient lies prone with the knee extended and the patient plantar flexes into the therapist's thigh isometrically. To isolate the soleus, the knee is flexed and plantar flexion is again elicited.

The tendons of the posterior tibialis, FDL, and FHL course around the medial malleolus before entering the foot (Fig. 27-23). It is difficult to palpate these tendons individually.

The tibial crest is first identified as the primary reference point to begin palpation of the dorsiflexors. The anterior tibialis can be palpated as it courses distally crossing midline and becoming tendinous before inserting onto the medial cuneiform (Fig. 27-24). Sandwiched between this muscle and the peroneals lies the EDL, which can be differentiated from

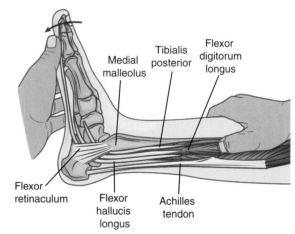

FIGURE 27–23 Palpation of the posterior tibialis, flexor digitorum longus (FDL), and the flexor hallucis longus (FHL) muscles.

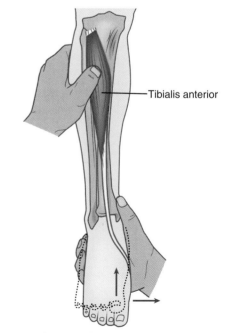

FIGURE 27–24 Palpation of the anterior tibialis muscle.

the anterior tibialis by eliciting toe extension. To identify the EHL, great toe extension is elicited and the tendon is followed proximally as the muscle belly of the EHL lies between the EDL and the anterior tibialis muscles.

Occupying the lateral compartment of the leg, the peroneus longus and brevis can be easily palpated and confirmed through resisting eversion (Fig. 27-25). These muscles are also effective plantar flexors by virtue of their posterior location relative to the axis of the ankle.

Due to their propensity toward injury, the ligamentous support structures of the ankle must also be palpated for signs of tenderness, inflammation, and integrity. The *anterior talofibular ligament* can be palpated just anterior and distal to the lateral malleolus. In the case of injury, it is common to observe localized edema and tenderness upon palpation. Moving posteriorly around the lateral malleolus, the *calcaneofibular ligament* is the next ligament to be palpated, followed by the *posterior talofibular ligament*. On the medial aspect of the ankle, the *deltoid ligament* can be palpated in its entirety between the medial malleolus and the sustentaculum tali. Strumming across the fibers of these ligaments assists with localization of these structures, and adding gentle inversion or eversion causes them to become taut and more easily identifiable.

Lastly, the blood supply to the foot can be appreciated by palpating the *posterior tibial artery*, which is located just posterior to the medial malleolus with the long flexor muscles. The *dorsal pedis artery* is superficial at the dorsum of the foot and can be palpated between the first and second metatarsals.

Special Testing

Special tests for the ankle and foot have been clearly delineated in many other texts and in the literature. Therefore, only a brief description of selected special tests will be provided here. Table 27-3 provides an overview of the sensitivity, specificity, and likelihood ratios for the more commonly performed special tests used in the examination of the ankle and foot complex. The reader is encouraged to consult other sources for additional information regarding the performance of these useful confirmatory tests.

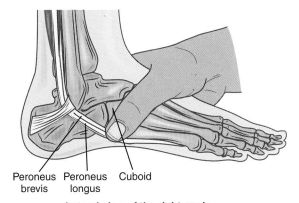

Peroneus   Peroneus   Cuboid
brevis   longus

Lateral view of the right angle

FIGURE 27–25 Palpation of the peroneal muscles.

Table 27-3 Special Tests for the Ankle and Foot

TEST	SENSITIVITY	SPECIFICITY	+LR	–LR	RELIABILITY	REFERENCE
Anterior Drawer Test	78%	75%	3.1	0.29	0.29	Lindstrand[47] Frost et al.[48] Birrer et al.[49] Tohyama et al.[50] Aradi et al.[51] Kjaersgaard-Andersen et al.[52] Colter[53] Hertel et al.[54]
Talar Tilt Test	67%	75%	2.7	0.44	0.44	Lindstrand[47] Birrer et al.[49] Aradi et al.[51] Kjaersgaard-Andersen et al.[52] Colter[53] Hertel et al.[54]
Squeeze Test	NA	NA	NA	NA	Kappa = 0.50	Hopkinson et al.[55] Alonso et al.[56] Norkus et al.[57] Peng[58] Brosky et al.[59] Nussbaum et al.[60] Boytim et al.[61] Wright et al.[62]

Continued

Table 27-3	Special Tests for the Ankle and Foot—cont'd					
TEST	**SENSITIVITY**	**SPECIFICITY**	**+LR**	**−LR**	**RELIABILITY**	**REFERENCE**
External Rotation Test	NA	95%	NA	NA	Kappa = 0.75	Alonso et al.[56] Lin et al[63] Beumer et al[64]
Thompson Test	40%–96%	NA	NA	NA	NA	Thompson[65] Scott et al.[66] Simmonds[67] Thompson et al.[68] Maffulli[69]
Impingement Sign	95%	88%	7.9	0.06	Kappa = 0.36	Alonso et al.[56]
Windlass Test	13.6%–31.8%	100%	NA	NA	ICC = 0.96–0.99	DeGarceau et al.[70]
Morton's Test	NA	NA	NA	NA	NA	Evans[71]
Tinel Sign	58%	NA	NA	NA	NA	Oloff et al.[72]
Ottawa Ankle Rules	Adults: 95%–100% Children: 83%–100%	Adults: 16% Children: 21%–50%	NA	NA	NA	Bachmann et al.[30] Stiell et al.[73] Stiell et al.[74] Auletta et al.[75] Auleley et al.[76] Kerr et al.[77]
Ottawa Foot Rules	Adults: 93%–100% Children: 100%	Adults: 12%–21% Children: 36%	NA	NA	NA	Stiell et al.[78]
Calcaneal Bump Test	NA	NA	NA	NA	NA	Cotton[79] Lindenfeld et al.[80]
Homans Sign	35%–48%	41%	0.81	1.27	NA	Cranley et al.[81] Knox[82]

LR, likelihood ratios; NA, not available; ICC, intraclass correlation.

SPECIAL TESTS FOR THE ANKLE AND FOOT

Special Tests for Ligamentous Laxity
Anterior Drawer Test (Fig. 27-26)

Purpose: To identify capsuloligamentous integrity of the ankle joint, in particular, the integrity of the ATF ligament

Patient: Supine with the ankle in 10 to 15 degrees of plantar flexion

Clinician: Standing at the foot of the patient

Procedure: The lower leg is stabilized while the calcaneus is grasped and translated anteriorly.

Interpretation: The test is positive if the talus translates anteriorly the extent to which is graded on a scale where 0 indicates no laxity and 3 indicates gross laxity.

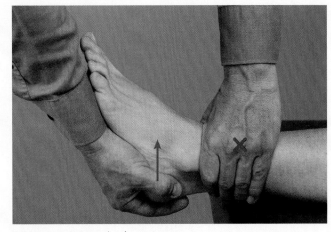

FIGURE 27–26 Anterior drawer test.

Talar Tilt Test (Fig. 27-27)

Purpose: To identify the lateral ligament integrity of the talocrural and subtalar joints

Patient: Supine or side lying with the ankle in 10 to 15 degrees of plantar flexion

Clinician: Sitting at the foot of the patient grasping the patient's ankle at the malleoli

Procedure: A medially directed thrust is applied to the calcaneus.

Interpretation: The test is positive if there is increased laxity when compared to the noninvolved side with a less firm end feel.

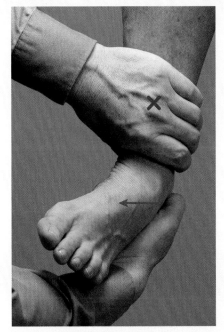

FIGURE 27–27 Talar tilt test.

Squeeze Test (Fig. 27-28)

Purpose: To identify the presence of a tibiofibular syndesmotic sprain, also known as a high ankle sprain

Patient: Supine, side lying, or sitting

Clinician: Standing at the foot of the patient with both hands grasping the lower leg

Procedure: A manual squeeze is applied by both hands to the lower leg.

Interpretation: The test is positive if there is an onset of pain proximal to the talocrural joint.

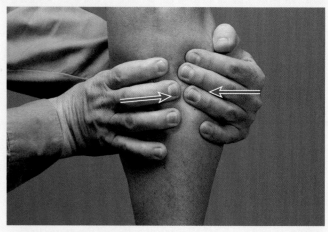

FIGURE 27–28 Squeeze test.

External Rotation Test (Fig. 27-29)

Purpose: To identify the presence of a tibiofibular syndesmotic sprain, also known as a high ankle sprain

Patient: Supine or sitting with the knee flexed to 90 degrees

Clinician: Standing to the side of the patient with one hand supporting the lower leg at the calf and the other supporting the foot

Procedure: Hold the talocrural joint in neutral and apply an external rotation force to the ankle.

Interpretation: The test is positive if there is a reproduction of pain proximal to the talocrural joint.

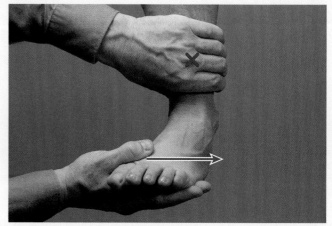

FIGURE 27–29 External rotation test.

Special Tests for Tendon Rupture
Thompson Test (Fig. 27-30)

Purpose: To identify the presence of an Achilles tendon rupture

Patient: Prone with the foot off the edge of the table

Clinician: Standing to the side of the patient

Procedure: While grasping the midbelly of the calf, a squeeze is applied.

Interpretation: The test is positive if the foot fails to plantar flex when the squeeze is applied.

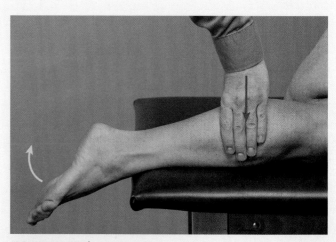

FIGURE 27–30 Thompson test.

Special Tests for Symptom Reproduction

Impingement Sign (Fig. 27-31)

Purpose:	To identify the presence of talocrural joint impingement
Patient:	Supine or sitting with knee flexed to 90 degrees
Clinician:	Standing to the side of the patient with one hand stabilizing the tibia with the thumb on the anterolateral aspect of the talus
Procedure:	Thumb pressure is applied as the ankle is brought into forceful dorsiflexion and eversion.
Interpretation:	The test is positive if there is a reproduction of pain at the anterolateral aspect of the ankle. Impingement is also suspected if more than five of the following criteria are present: (1) anterolateral tenderness, (2) anterolateral edema, (3) pain upon dorsiflexion and eversion, (4) pain with single leg squat, (5) pain with activity, and (6) ankle joint instability.

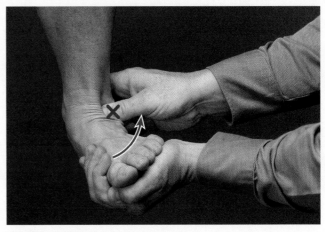

FIGURE 27–31 Impingement sign.

Windlass Test (Fig. 27-32 A, B):

Purpose: To assess for plantar fasciitis

Patient: Non-weight-bearing or weight-bearing

Clinician: Standing at patient's foot

Procedure: Stabilize ankle in neutral and extend the great toe.

Interpretation: The test is positive if there is pain along the medial longitudinal arch.

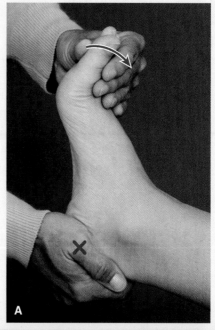

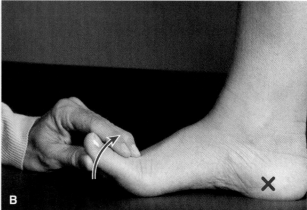

FIGURE 27–32 Windlass test, which can be performed in **A.** non-weight-bearing or **B.** weight-bearing. (Courtesy of Bob Wellmon Photography, BobWellmon.com.)

Morton Test (Fig. 27-33)

Purpose: To identify the presence of a neuroma of the digital nerves or the presence of a stress fracture

Patient: Supine or sitting

Clinician: Standing at the foot of the patient

Procedure: A manual squeeze is applied to the metatarsals of the forefoot.

Interpretation: The test is positive if there is a reproduction of pain, which may include paresthesias into the forefoot.

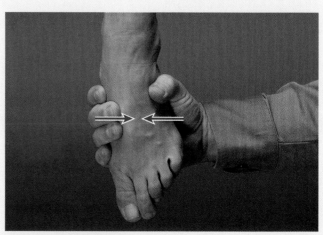

FIGURE 27–33 Morton test.

Tinel Sign (Fig. 27-34)

Purpose: To identify the presence of a tibial nerve entrapment at the tarsal tunnel

Patient: Supine or sitting

Clinician: Standing at the foot of the patient

Procedure: Gentle tapping is applied over the tarsal tunnel

Interpretation: The test is positive if there is a reproduction of pain and/or paresthesia

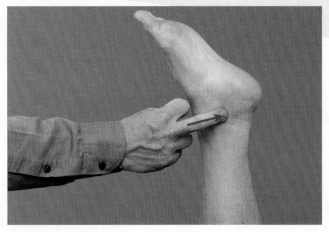

FIGURE 27–34 Tinel sign.

Special Tests for Fracture

Ottawa Ankle Rules (Fig. 27-35)

Purpose: To assess the need for the performance of plain film radiography

Procedure: Criteria: (1) bone tenderness at posterior edge of distal 6 cm of medial malleolus, (2) bone tenderness at posterior edge of distal 6 cm of lateral malleolus, (3) Totally unable to bear weight both immediately after injury and (for four steps) in emergency department

Interpretation: The test is positive if any of the criteria are present, suggesting the need for a plain film radiographic series of the ankle.

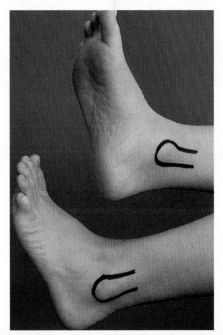

FIGURE 27–35 Ottawa ankle rules. (Courtesy of Bob Wellmon Photography, BobWellmon.com.)

Ottawa Foot Rules (Fig. 27-36)

Purpose: To assess the need for the performance of plain film radiography

Procedure: Criteria: (1) bone tenderness at navicular, (2) bone tenderness at base of fifth metatarsal, (3) totally unable to bear weight both immediately after injury and (for four steps) in emergency department.

Interpretation: The test is positive if any of the criteria are present, suggesting the need for a plain film radiographic series of the foot.

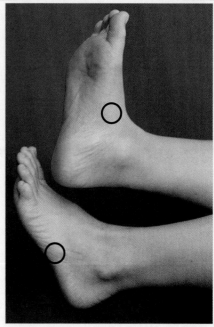

FIGURE 27–36 Ottawa foot rules. (Courtesy of Bob Wellmon Photography, BobWellmon.com.)

Calcaneal Bump Test (Fig. 27-37)

Purpose: To assess for the presence of a stress fracture

Patient: In non-weight-bearing with the ankle in neutral

Clinician: Sitting or standing at the patient's foot

Procedure: Apply a firm force with the thenar eminence to the patient's calcaneus.

Interpretation: The test is positive if there is pain.

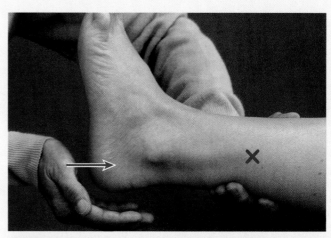

FIGURE 27–37 Calcaneal bump test. (Courtesy of Bob Wellmon Photography, BobWellmon.com.)

Special Tests for Vascular Compromise
Homans Sign (Fig. 27-38)

Purpose: To assess for the presence of a deep vein thrombosis (DVT) of the lower extremity

Patient: Supine

Clinician: Sitting or standing at the patient's foot

Procedure: Passively dorsiflex the foot and squeeze the calf.

Interpretation: The test is positive if exquisite pain is noted in the calf.

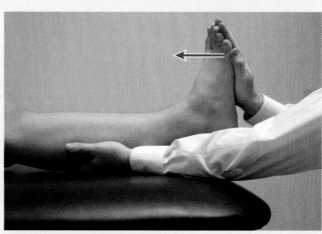

FIGURE 27–38 Homans sign

JOINT MOBILIZATION OF THE ANKLE AND FOOT

Note: The indications for the joint mobilization techniques described in this section are based on expected joint kinematics. Current evidence suggests that the indications for their use are multifactorial and may be based on direct assessment of mobility and an individual's symptomatic response.

Distal Tibiofibular Joint Mobilizations

Distal Tibiofibular Glides

Indications:
- *Distal tibiofibular glides* are indicated for restrictions in all motions of the talocrural joint

Accessory Motion Technique (Fig. 27-39)

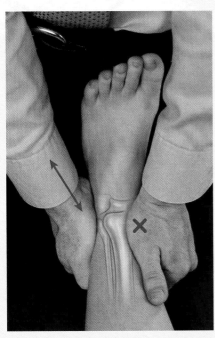

FIGURE 27–39 Distal tibiofibular glide. (From: Wise CH, Gulick DT. *Mobilization Notes: A Rehabilitation Specialist's Pocket Guide.* Philadelphia, PA: FA Davis, 2009.)

- **Patient/Clinician Position:** The patient is in the supine position with the foot supported on the table in the neutral position. Stand at the foot of the patient facing cephalad.
- **Hand Placement:** Stabilization is provided by the table and use of a lumbrical grip over the tibia or fibula. The heel of your mobilization hand contacts the distal aspect of the tibia or fibula.

- **Force Application:** While stabilizing the tibia, a posterior or anterior glide is imparted to the fibula. While stabilizing the fibula, a posterior or anterior glide is imparted to the tibia.

Accessory With Physiologic Motion Technique (Fig. 27-40)
- **Patient/Clinician Position:** Patient and clinician are in the same position as previously described.
- **Hand Placement:** Hand placement is the same as previously described.
- **Force Application:** Apply anterior or posterior glide at the tibia or fibula as active or passive dorsiflexion is elicited. Apply a posterior glide to the fibula as active or passive inversion is performed. Force is maintained throughout the entire range of motion and sustained at end range.

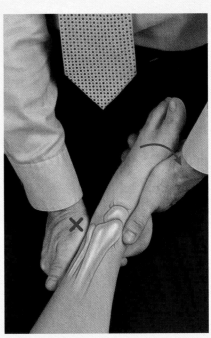

FIGURE 27–40 Distal tibiofibular glide accessory with physiologic motion technique. (From: Wise CH, Gulick DT. *Mobilization Notes: A Rehabilitation Specialist's Pocket Guide.* Philadelphia, PA: FA Davis, 2009.)

Talocrural Joint Mobilizations

Talocrural Distraction

Indications:
- *Talocrural distractions* is indicated for restrictions of motion in all directions.

Accessory Motion Technique (Fig. 27-41)

- **Patient/Clinician Position**: The patient is in the supine position with the foot over the edge of the table. Stand at the foot of the patient facing cephalad.
- **Hand Placement**: Stabilization is provided by the weight of the patient's body and a mobilization belt at the distal leg, as needed. The fingers of your hands are interlaced over the dorsum of the foot and anterior talus with your thumbs on the plantar aspect of the foot and your forearms parallel to one another in the direction of force.
- **Force Application**: Through your hand contacts over the talus, a distraction force is provided in the direction of the forearms by leaning back.

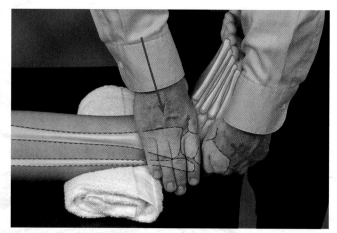

FIGURE 27–42 Talocrural posterior glide. (From: Wise CH, Gulick DT. *Mobilization Notes: A Rehabilitation Specialist's Pocket Guide*. Philadelphia, PA: FA Davis, 2009.)

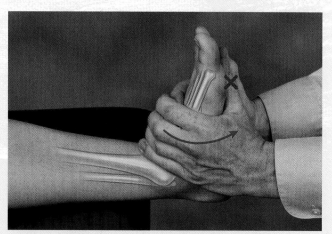

FIGURE 27–41 Talocrural distraction. (From: Wise CH, Gulick DT. *Mobilization Notes: A Rehabilitation Specialist's Pocket Guide*. Philadelphia, PA: FA Davis Company, 2009.)

Accessory With Physiologic Motion Technique (Not pictured)

- **Patient/Clinician Position**: The patient and clinician are in the same position as that previously described.
- **Hand Placement**: Hand placement is the same as that previously described.
- **Force Application**: Using your hand contacts, provide a fulcrum over the talus and apply a distraction force as the ankle is moved into greater ranges of dorsiflexion. Force is maintained throughout the entire range of motion and sustained at end range.

Talocrural Posterior Glide

Indications:

- *Talocrural posterior glides* are indicated for restrictions in talocrural dorsiflexion.

Accessory Motion Technique (Fig. 27-42)

- **Patient/Clinician Position**: The patient is in a supine position with the foot over the edge of the table. Stand at the foot of the patient facing cephalad.

- **Hand Position**: Provide stabilization by holding the patient's calcaneus with your hand. The web space of your mobilization hand is placed at the anterior aspect of the talus with your forearm in the direction in which force is applied.
- **Force Application**: Apply a posteriorly directed force through your hand contact at the anterior aspect of the talus. You may also apply a posteriorly directed force to the talus while actively or passively moving the ankle into progressively greater ranges of dorsiflexion. As an alternate accessory with physiologic motion technique, mobilization force is maintained throughout the entire range of motion and sustained at end range.

Accessory With Physiologic Motion Technique (Fig. 27-43)

- **Patient/Clinician Position**: The patient is standing in a lunge position with his or her foot on the side being mobilized on a stool. You are in a stride stance position facing

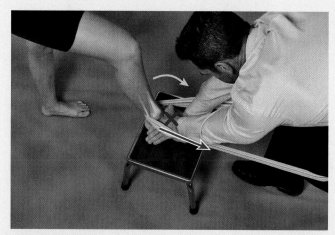

FIGURE 27–43 Talocrural posterior glide accessory with physiologic motion in standing technique. (From: Wise CH, Gulick DT. *Mobilization Notes: A Rehabilitation Specialist's Pocket Guide*. Philadelphia, PA: FA Davis, 2009.)

the patient. A mobilization belt may be used to provide additional force by placing it around the posterior aspect of the patient's distal leg.

- **Hand Placement:** The web space of both hands reinforce one another over the anterior aspect of the patient's talus. Your forearms are in line with the posterior direction of force.
- **Force Application:** The patient slowly shifts weight onto his or her front leg while maintaining the heel in contact with the ground as you apply a posteriorly directed force through the talus contact against the stabilization provided by the belt. Mobilization force is maintained throughout the entire range of motion and sustained at end range.

Talocrural Anterior Glide

Indications:

- *Talocrural anterior glides* are indicated for restrictions in talocrural plantar flexion.

Accessory Motion Technique (Fig. 27-44)

- **Patient/Clinician Position:** The patient is in a prone position with the foot over the edge of the table. Stand at the foot of the patient facing cephalad.

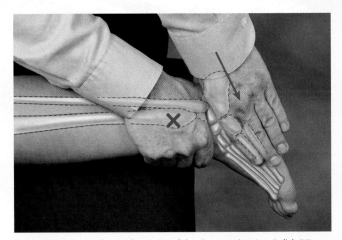

FIGURE 27–44 Talocrural anterior glide. (From: Wise CH, Gulick DT. *Mobilization Notes: A Rehabilitation Specialist's Pocket Guide*. Philadelphia, PA: FA Davis, 2009.)

- **Hand Placement:** Stabilize the distal leg against the table. The web space of the mobilization hand contacts the posterior aspect of the calcaneus with the forearm in the direction in which force is applied.
- **Force Application:** With the distal leg stabilized, apply an anteriorly directed force through the calcaneal contact, which mobilizes the talus in an anterior direction.

Accessory With Physiologic Motion Technique (Fig. 27-45)

- **Patient/Clinician Position:** The patient is in a supine position with the hip and knee flexed and the foot resting

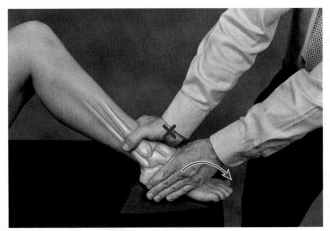

FIGURE 27–45 Talocrural anterior glide accessory with physiologic motion technique. (From: Wise CH, Gulick DT. *Mobilization Notes: A Rehabilitation Specialist's Pocket Guide.* Philadelphia: FA Davis, 2009.)

on the table or wedge. Stand at the foot of the patient facing cephalad.

- **Hand Placement:** Stabilize the distal leg against the wedge with the patient's foot in plantar flexion. Grasp the patient's talus with the web space of your mobilization hand with your forearm in the direction in which force is applied and prepared to move during the mobilization.
- **Force Application:** With the distal leg stabilized the mobilization hand applies an anteriorly-directed force through the talus. Mobilization force is maintained throughout the entire range of motion and sustained at end range.

Subtalar Joint Mobilizations

Subtalar (Talocalcaneal) Distraction, Medial, and Lateral Glide

Indications:

- *Subtalar (talocalcaneal) distractions* are indicated for restrictions in all motions of the subtalar joint. *Subtalar (talocalcaneal) medial and lateral glides* are indicated for restrictions in rearfoot eversion and inversion, respectively.

Accessory Motion Technique (Fig. 27-46)

- **Patient/Clinician Position:** The patient is in a prone position with the dorsum of the foot over the edge of the table. Alternately, the patient may be in a side lying position with the foot to be mobilized uppermost and the knee flexed. Stand on the ipsilateral side of the foot being mobilized facing caudally or sitting on the table with the patient's posterior thigh in contact with your back.
- **Hand Placement:** Provide stabilization by holding the patient's distal leg on the table or stabilize through the patient's flexed knee in contact with your back. With your

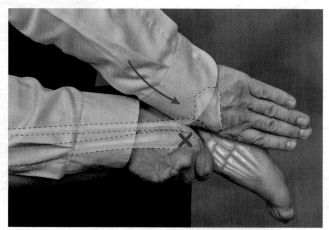

FIGURE 27–46 Subtalar (talocalcaneal) distraction, medial, and lateral glide. (From: Wise CH, Gulick DT. *Mobilization Notes: A Rehabilitation Specialist's Pocket Guide.* Philadelphia, PA: FA Davis, 2009.)

mobilization hand, grasp the patient's calcaneus or use both hands to grasp the calcaneus with your forearm(s) in line with the direction in which force is applied.

- **Force Application:** Impart a caudally directed force parallel to the long axis of the leg through your mobilization hand or hands.

Accessory With Physiologic Motion Technique (Calcaneal rocking) (Fig. 27-47)

- **Patient/Clinician Position:** The patient is sidelying with the foot being mobilized uppermost. The patient's knee is flexed and his posterior thigh is stabilized by your trunk. You are sitting on the table facing away from the patient.
- **Hand Placement:** Both of your hands are grasping the patient's calcaneus with the thumbs forming a "V" over the lateral aspect of the patient's calcaneus and your forearms in the direction in which force is applied. Stabilization is provided by your trunk.

- **Force Application:** Take up the slack in the joint and apply a distraction force through both hand contacts. Alternately, distraction in combination with a medial & lateral glide (known as rocking) may also be applied. Mobilization force is maintained throughout the entire range of motion and sustained at end range.

Midtarsal Joint Mobilizations

Midtarsal (Talonavicular and Calcaneocuboid) Glide

Indications:
- *Midtarsal (talonavicular and calcaneocuboid) dorsal glides* are indicated for restrictions in midtarsal joint dorsiflexion and inversion and *midtarsal (talonavicular and calcaneocuboid) plantar glides* are indicated for restrictions in midtarsal joint plantarflexion and eversion.

Accessory Motion Technique (Figs. 27-48, 27-49)

- **Patient/Clinician Position:** The patient is in a prone position with the foot on a wedge. Alternately, the patient is in a supine position with the foot over the edge of the table and a wedge supporting the distal leg. Stand at the foot of the patient facing cephalad.
- **Hand Placement:** Stabilization is provided by contacting the medial aspect of the patient's calcaneus and talus and fixating the foot onto the wedge for talonavicular mobilization or by contacting the lateral aspect of the calcaneus and fixating the foot on the wedge for calcaneocuboid mobilization. The mobilization hand uses a pinch grip or full hand grip over the medial aspect of the foot grasping the navicular for talonavicular mobilization or over the lateral aspect of the foot grasping the cuboid for calcaneocuboid mobilization.

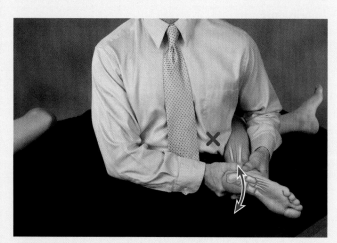

FIGURE 27–47 Subtalar (talocalcaneal) distraction, medial, and lateral glide accessory with physiologic motion technique (calcaneal rocking). (From: Wise CH, Gulick DT. *Mobilization Notes: A Rehabilitation Specialist's Pocket Guide.* Philadelphia, PA: FA Davis, 2009.)

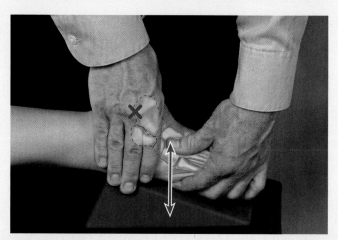

FIGURE 27–48 Midtarsal (talonavicular) glide. (From: Wise CH, Gulick DT. *Mobilization Notes: A Rehabilitation Specialist's Pocket Guide.* Philadelphia, PA: FA Davis, 2009.)

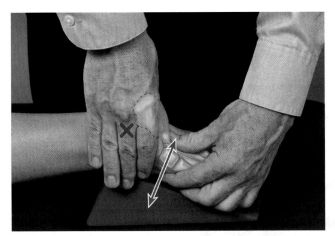

FIGURE 27–49 Midtarsal (calcaneocuboid) glide. (From: Wise CH, Gulick DT. *Mobilization Notes: A Rehabilitation Specialist's Pocket Guide.* Philadelphia, PA: FA Davis, 2009.)

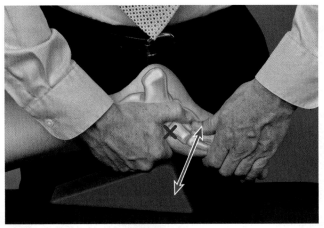

FIGURE 27–50 Intertarsal glide. (From: Wise CH, Gulick DT. *Mobilization Notes: A Rehabilitation Specialist's Pocket Guide.* Philadelphia, PA: FA Davis, 2009.)

- **Force Application:** Through your mobilization hand contact, apply a dorsal or plantar force through the navicular medially or cuboid laterally.

Accessory With Physiologic Motion Technique (Not pictured)
- **Patient/Clinician Position:** The patient and clinician are in the same position as previously described.
- **Hand Placement:** The same hand positions are used as previously described.
- **Force Application:** Apply a dorsal or plantar glide through the mobilization hand contact as active or passive ankle dorsiflexion and plantarflexion are performed, respectively.

Intertarsal Joint Mobilizations

Intertarsal Glide

Indications:
- *Intertarsal glides* are indicated for restrictions in all physiologic motions of the foot.

Accessory Motion Technique (Fig. 27-50)
- **Patient/Clinician Position**: The patient is in a prone position with the foot over the edge of the table and a wedge supporting the joint to be mobilized. Stand on the medial side to mobilize the lateral aspect of the foot and stand on the lateral side to mobilize the medial aspect of the foot.
- **Hand Placement:** Use a pinch grasp to stabilize the adjacent tarsal bone or use your open hand to fixate the foot on the underlying wedge. A pinch grasp of your mobilization hand contacts the tarsal bone to be mobilized with your forearm in the direction in which force is being applied.
- **Force Application:** Apply a plantar or dorsal glide as the adjacent tarsal bone is stabilized. Mobilization proceeds

sequentially from proximal to distal along the medial column beginning with mobilization of the navicular on the stabilized talus, followed by mobilization of the medial, intermediate, and lateral cuneiforms on the stabilized navicular, and mobilization of the medial cuneiform on the stabilized intermediate cuneiform. Mobilization is then performed sequentially from proximal to distal along the lateral column, beginning with mobilization of the cuboid on the stabilized calcaneus, followed by mobilization of the lateral cuneiform on the stabilized cuboid.

Accessory With Physiologic Motion Technique (Not pictured)
- **Patient/Clinician Position:** The patient and clinician are in the same position as previously described. The patient's foot is over the edge of the table.
- **Hand Placement:** The same hand positions are used as that which was previously described.
- **Force Application:** Apply glides to each tarsal bone while stabilizing each adjacent tarsal bone as passive or active motion in all directions is performed.

Tarsometatarsal Joint Mobilizations

Tarsometatarsal Distraction and Glide

Indications:
- *Tarsometatarsal distractions and glides* are indicated for restrictions in all physiologic motions of the tarsometatarsal joint and overall midfoot and forefoot mobility.

Accessory Motion Technique (Figs. 27-51, 27-52)
- **Patient/Clinician Position**: The patient is in the supine position with the knee in flexion and the foot resting on a wedge

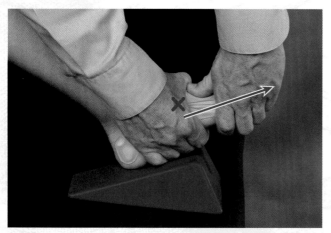

FIGURE 27–51 Tarsometatarsal distraction. (From: Wise CH, Gulick DT. *Mobilization Notes: A Rehabilitation Specialist's Pocket Guide*. Philadelphia, PA: FA Davis Company, 2009.)

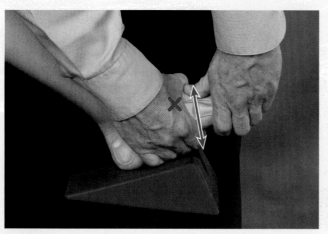

FIGURE 27–52 Tarsometatarsal glide. (From: Wise CH, Gulick DT. *Mobilization Notes: A Rehabilitation Specialist's Pocket Guide*. Philadelphia, PA: FA Davis, 2009.)

located at the joint to be mobilized. Stand on the medial side to mobilize the foot laterally and stand on the lateral side to mobilize the foot medially.

- **Hand Placement:** Use a pinch grasp to stabilize the adjacent tarsal bone or use your open hand to fixate the foot on the underlying wedge. Use a pinch grasp to contact the base of the metatarsal with your mobilization hand with your forearm in the direction in which force is applied.
- **Force Application:** While stabilizing the adjacent tarsal bone, apply a distraction force or glide in a plantar or dorsal direction through your mobilization contact to the base of the metatarsal. Metatarsals 1 through 3 are mobilized on the stabilized medial, intermediate, and lateral cuneiforms, respectively, and metatarsals 4 and 5 are mobilized upon the stabilized cuboid.

Intermetatarsal Joint Mobilizations

Intermetatarsal Sweep

Indications:
- *Intermetatarsal sweeps* are indicated for restrictions in mobility of the entire midfoot and forefoot, and will assist with all of the physiologic motions of the foot.

Accessory Motion Technique (Figs. 27-53, 27-54)
- **Patient/Clinician Position**: The patient is in the supine position with the foot over the edge of the table. Sit at the foot of the patient facing cephalad.

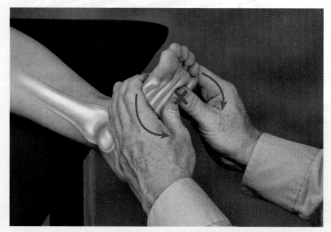

FIGURE 27–53 Intermetatarsal sweep with plantar fulcrum. (From: Wise CH, Gulick DT. *Mobilization Notes: A Rehabilitation Specialist's Pocket Guide*. Philadelphia, PA: FA Davis, 2009.)

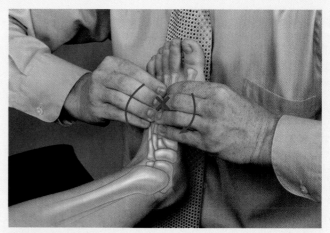

FIGURE 27–54 Intermetatarsal sweep with dorsal fulcrum. (From: Wise CH, Gulick DT. *Mobilization Notes: A Rehabilitation Specialist's Pocket Guide*. Philadelphia, PA: FA Davis, 2009.)

- **Hand Placement**: Your fingers are placed horizontally over the dorsal or plantar aspects of the forefoot and your thumbs are placed on the opposite side.
- **Force Application:** A sweeping motion is applied through your finger contacts which is designed to increase or decrease the plantar arch against the fulcrum of the opposing thumbs (Fig. 27-53). The process is then reversed and the thumbs provide a sweeping motion against the fulcrum of the opposing fingers (Fig. 27-54).

Accessory With Physiologic Motion Technique (Not pictured)

- **Patient/Clinician Position:** The patient and clinician are in the same position as previously described.
- **Hand Placement:** The hand contacts are the same as previously described.
- **Force Application:** The mobilization designed to increase the plantar arch is performed while the patient actively performs plantar flexion, and the mobilization designed to decrease the plantar arch is performed while the patient actively performs dorsiflexion. Mobilization force is maintained throughout the entire range of motion and sustained at end range.

Metatarsophalangeal Joint Mobilizations

Metatarsophalangeal Distraction and Glide

Indications:

- *Metatarsophalangeal distractions* are indicated for restrictions in motion in all directions. *Metatarsophalangeal dorsal and plantar glides* are indicated for restrictions in metatarsophalangeal extension and flexion, respectively.

Accessory Motion Technique (Figs. 27-55, 27-56)

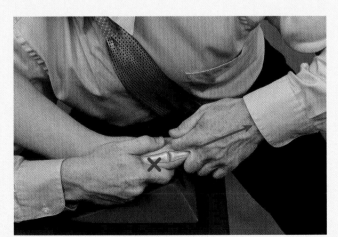

FIGURE 27–55 Metatarsophalangeal distraction. (From: Wise CH, Gulick DT. *Mobilization Notes: A Rehabilitation Specialist's Pocket Guide.* Philadelphia, PA: FA Davis, 2009.)

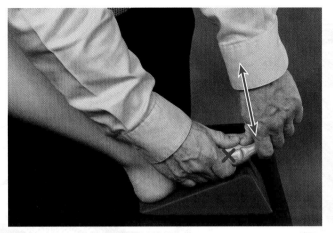

FIGURE 27–56 Metatarsophalangeal glide. (From: Wise CH, Gulick DT. *Mobilization Notes: A Rehabilitation Specialist's Pocket Guide.* Philadelphia, PA: FA Davis, 2009.)

- **Patient/Clinician Position**: The patient is in the supine position with the knee in flexion and the foot resting on a wedge. Stand at the foot of the patient facing cephalad.
- **Hand Placement**: Use a pinch grasp to stabilize the most distal aspect of the metatarsal head. Use a pinch or hook grasp to contact the most proximal aspect of the proximal phalanx with your mobilization hand with your forearm in the direction in which force is applied.
- **Force Application:** While stabilizing the adjacent metatarsal, apply a distraction force or glide in a plantar or dorsal direction through your mobilization contact to the base of the proximal phalanx.

Accessory With Physiologic Motion Technique (Not pictured)

- **Patient/Clinician Position:** The patient and clinician are in the same position as previously described.
- **Hand Placement:** The proximal phalanx is contacted medially and laterally with the mobilization hand.
- **Force Application:** Apply a distraction force during active or passive metatarsophalangeal flexion or extension. Apply a dorsal glide during active or passive extension or apply a plantar glide during active or passive flexion. A medial or, more commonly, lateral glide may also be applied during active extension or flexion depending on which is most limited and/or painful. Mobilization forces are maintained throughout the entire range of motion and sustained at end range.

Interphalangeal Joint Mobilizations

Interphalangeal Distraction and Glide

Indications:

- *Interphalangeal distractions* are indicated for restrictions in all directions. *Interphalangeal dorsal and plantar glides* are indicated for restrictions to improve interphalangeal extension and flexion, respectively.

Accessory Motion Technique (Figs. 27-57, 27-58)

- **Patient/Clinician Position**: The patient is in the supine position with the knee in flexion and the foot resting on a wedge. Stand at the foot of the patient facing cephalad.
- **Hand Placement**: Use a pinch grasp to stabilize the most distal aspect of the proximal or middle phalanx. Use a pinch or hook grasp to contact the most proximal aspect of the base of the middle (for PIP mobilization) or distal phalanx (for DIP mobilization) with your mobilization hand with your forearm in the direction in which force is applied.
- **Force Application**: While stabilizing the adjacent phalanx, apply a distraction force or glide in a plantar or dorsal direction through your mobilization contact to the base of the middle or distal phalanx. Unicondylar glides may be performed by directing forces through either the medial or lateral aspects of the most proximal aspect of the base of the middle (for PIP mobilization) or distal phalanx (for DIP mobilization).

Midtarsal High Velocity Thrust (Whip Manipulation) (Fig. 27-59)

- **Indications**: Midtarsal high velocity thrusts are indicated for restrictions in mobility of the calcaneocuboid or talonavicular joints.
- **Patient/Clinician Position**: The patient is lying prone near the edge of the table with his knee in 45 degrees to 60 degrees of flexion. You are standing at the foot of the patient facing cephalad.
- **Hand Placement:** Thumb-over-thumb contact is made over the plantar aspect of either the cuboid or the navicular and with the fingers of both hands wrapped around and resting on the dorsum of the patient's foot.
- **Force Application:** Apply force in a dorsal direction through both thumb contacts and maintain this force as you extend the patient's knee and plantarflex the ankle toward end range. Once tissue resistance is engaged, a high velocity, low amplitude thrust is applied through the thumb contacts as the foot is brought through an elliptical arc of motion that is produced by ulnar deviation of your wrists.

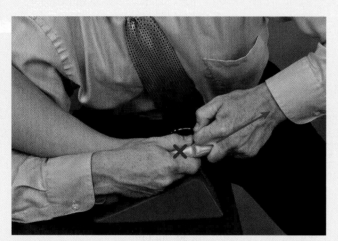

FIGURE 27–57 Interphalangeal distraction. (From: Wise CH, Gulick DT. *Mobilization Notes: A Rehabilitation Specialist's Pocket Guide.* Philadelphia, PA: FA Davis, 2009.)

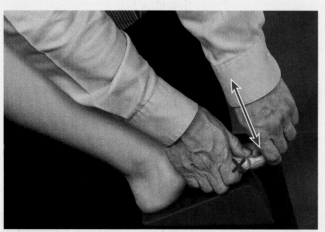

FIGURE 27–58 Interphalangeal glide. (From: Wise CH, Gulick DT. *Mobilization Notes: A Rehabilitation Specialist's Pocket Guide.* Philadelphia, PA: FA Davis, 2009.)

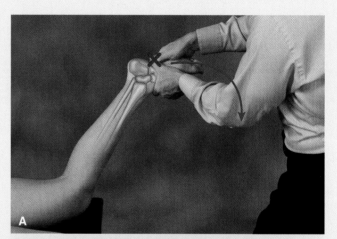

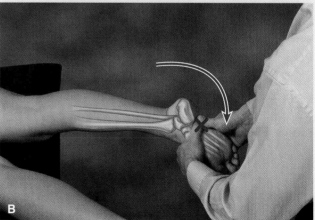

FIGURE 27–59 Midtarsal high velocity thrust (whip manipulation). **A.** Start position. **B.** End position. (From: Wise CH, Gulick DT. *Mobilization Notes: A Rehabilitation Specialist's Pocket Guide.* Philadelphia, PA: FA Davis, 2009.)

CLINICAL CASE

CASE 1

Subjective Examination

History of Present Illness

A 17-year-old female dancer presents with complaint of pain at the plantar aspect of the right foot. Her pain is most severe on taking the initial step when getting out of bed in the morning, when attempting to stand or ambulate after sitting for more than 20 minutes, and the day following extensive dance activities. At its worst, her pain is at a 7/10 level, and she reports constant pain at a 4/10 level, on average. She has not been seen by a physician and presents to your facility today with a worsening of symptoms since initial onset approximately 6 weeks ago. Patient's goal is to reduce symptoms to allow better tolerance for intensive practice in preparation for dance competition in 1 month.

Past Medical History

Several episodes of similar symptoms in the past that resolved with rest and over-the-counter medication. Previous history of recurrent ankle sprains bilaterally, patellofemoral pain syndrome with several episodes of patellar subluxation on the right, intermittent low back pain, and left shoulder pain.

Objective Physical Examination

Examination of Structure

In supine, Q-angle: right = 22 degrees, left = 20 degrees. Leg length: right= 68 cm, left = 72 cm. Bilateral hallux-abducto-valgus is noted right greater than left with exostosis and erythema on the right. In STJN the following was noted in prone: Right: 8 degrees of rearfoot varus, 14 degrees of forefoot varus, plantar flexed and hypomobile first ray, tibial varum = 3 degrees. Left: 5 degrees of rearfoot varus, 10 degrees of forefoot varus, plantar flexed and hypomobile first ray, tibial varum = 0 degrees.

In standing, bilateral pes planus noted with reduced Feiss line right greater than left. Bilateral rearfoot valgus, tibial internal torsion, and genu valgus. Observation of gait reveals bilateral overpronation right greater on left at heel strike and into midstance, with failure to resupinate at push off. Gait is antalgic with pain most notable at push off on the right.

Examination of Mobility

Passive Physiologic Mobility Testing: DF (knee flexed): right = 5 degrees, left = 10 degrees, decreased mobility with foot in STJN position; DF (knee extended): right = 0 degrees, left = 3 degrees; PF: bilateral = 40 degrees; Rearfoot Inversion: right = 40 degrees, left = 30 degrees; Rearfoot Eversion: bilateral = 10 degrees; Great toe extension: right = 15 degrees, left = 20 degrees; Hypermobile MTJ in rearfoot pronation and supination; Soft end feel for all without pain.

Passive Accessory Mobility Testing: Reduced glide of talus on right in all directions with stiffness dominance and capsular end feel. First MTP reduced dorsal and plantar glides with stiffness dominance and capsular end feel. Talonavicular and subtalar joint hypermobility.

Examination of Flexibility

Significant restrictions in gastrocnemius. See mobility testing.

Examination of Muscle Function

5/5 and pain-free throughout.

Neurological Testing

Lower quarter neurological screen intact and symmetrical for reflexes, dermatomes, myotomes.

Palpation

Exquisite tenderness to the touch at the medial calcaneal tubercle and within the medial longitudinal arch. Tenderness and edema are noted at the first MTP joint.

Functional Testing

Pain with single leg stance after 20 seconds and attempts at unilateral heel raises more than 5 repetitions on the right.

Special Testing

Windlass = positive Homan = negative, Tinel = negative, Thompson = negative, anterior drawer = slightly positive, talar tilt = slightly positive.

1. What is your diagnosis? Is further testing and/or imaging required to confirm your diagnostic hypothesis?
2. What is the significance of this patient's sport and age in the pathogenesis of this condition?
3. Describe the relationship between the findings from the structural and mobility examinations and the patient's presenting symptoms?
4. What is the prognosis for this patient? Describe the techniques that you believe would be most effective. How would you educate this patient regarding self-management and prophylaxis?

5. What joint mobilizations would you use? Describe the technique and grade that you would use, and perform them on a partner. In addition to manual physical therapy, what other interventions would you recommend? What type of external support and footwear would you recommend? Provide rationale for your choices.

CASE 2

Subjective Examination

History of Present Illness

A 53-year-old obese male presents with chief complaint of pain and paresthesia along the medial side of the right foot of 6 months duration. Symptoms are most severe when standing for more than 10 minutes and walking more than 100 feet. Paresthesia is most disabling and is primarily present along the medial and plantar aspects of the foot. His present symptoms are limiting him from performance of his regular duties as a truck driver, with increased symptoms from prolonged driving, most notably during manipulation of the clutch.

Past Medical History

The patient was diagnosed with insulin-dependent diabetes mellitus 7 years ago. In addition, he reports a positive cardiac history with a myocardial infarction 3 years ago. He has hypertension, which is controlled through medication.

Objective Physical Examination

Examination of Structure

Gait is antalgic with bilateral overpronation with gluteus medius lurch.

Examination of Mobility:

Passive Physiologic Mobility Testing: Limited in all directions with reproduction of pain upon rearfoot eversion.
Passive Accessory Mobility Testing: Hypomobility noted in calcaneocuboid mobility, subtalar joint mobility, and tarsometatarsal mobility digits 2 to 5.

Examination of Muscle Function

Foot intrinsic muscle weakness with reproduction of pain upon testing. Otherwise, unremarkable.

Neurological Testing

Reduced light touch sensation on the plantar aspect of the foot along the medial side.

Palpation

Tenderness along the tendons of the posterior tibialis and flexor digitorum.

Special Testing

Tinel = positive at tarsal tunnel, Morton test = positive, Homans sign = negative, squeeze test = negative.

1. What is your diagnosis? What additional diagnostic testing would you recommend to confirm your diagnosis?
2. Which aspect of the examination was most useful in coming to your conclusions? Perform each of the special tests used in this case on a partner and discuss the diagnostic value of these tests in light of their sensitivity and specificity.
3. How valuable is the use of manual physical therapy in this case? What techniques would you use? Perform your chosen techniques on a partner and provide rationale for your choices and expected outcomes from using these techniques.
4. What is your prognosis for this patient? To optimize outcomes, what recommendations would you make regarding activities of daily living and lifestyle changes?

HANDS-ON

With a partner, perform the following activities:

1 Observe your partner as he or she performs active physiologic movements over single and repeated repetitions and single and multiplane directions and identify the quantity, quality, and any reproduction of symptoms that may be produced. Compare these active movements with performance of these same movements passively.

2 Perform passive physiologic movement testing in all directions followed by passive accessory movement testing in all planes, and determine the relationship between the onset of pain (P1 and P2 if present) and stiffness or resistance (R1 and R2). Determine the end feel in each direction. Compare your findings bilaterally and on another partner.

3 Perform passive accessory movement testing in all planes with the ankle in the neutral, or open-packed, position. Then perform the same tests with the ankle in other non-neutral and close-packed positions. Identify any changes in the quantity and quality of available motion, and report any reproduction of symptoms.

4 Use overpressure and counterpressure to identify which of the joints within this multijoint system is the primary movement restriction and which may be the result of secondary compensation.

5 Through palpation, attempt to identify the primary soft tissue and bony structures of the ankle and foot and compare tissue texture, tension, tone, and location bilaterally.

6 Based on your movement examination as identified above, choose two mobilizations. Perform these mobilizations on your partner and identify any immediate changes in mobility or symptoms in response to these procedures.

7 Perform each mobilization described in the intervention section of this chapter bilaterally on at least two individuals. Using each technique, practice grades I to IV. Provide input to your partner regarding setup, technique, comfort, and so on. When practicing these mobilization techniques, utilize the Sequential Partial Task Practice (SPTP) Method in which students repeatedly practice one aspect of each technique (ie. position, hand placement, force application) on multiple partners each time adding the next component until the technique is performed in real time from beginning to end. (Wise CH, Schenk RJ, Lattanzi JB. A model for teaching and learning spinal thrust manipulation and its effect on participant confidence in technique performance. *Journal of Manual & Manipulative Therapy*, August 2014.)

REFERENCES

1. Rasmussen O, Tovberg-Jensen I, Hedeboe J. An analysis of the function of the posterior talofibular ligament. *Int Orthop.* 1983;7:41-48.
2. Masciocchi C, Barile A. Magnetic resonance imaging of the hindfoot with surgical correlations. *Skeletal Radiol.* 2002;31:131-142.
3. Lunberg A, Svensson OK, Nemeth G, et al. The axis of rotation of the ankle joint. *J Bone Joint Surg Br.* 1989;71:194-199.
4. Inman V, Mann R. Biomechanics of the foot and ankle. In: Mann R, ed. *DuVries Surgery of the Foot*, 4th ed. St. Louis, MO: CV Mosby; 1978.
5. Stiehl J. Biomechanics of the ankle joint. In: Stiehl J, ed. *Inman's Joints of the Ankle*, 2nd ed. Baltimore, MD: Williams & Wilkins; 1991.
6. Walker JM, Sue D, Miles-Elkousy N, et al. Active mobility of the extremities in older subjects. *Phys Ther.* 1984;64:919-923.
7. Roass A, Andersson GB. Normal range of motion of the hip, knee, and ankle joints in male subjects 30-40 years of age. *Acta Orthop Scand.* 1982;53:205-208.
8. Greene WB, Heckman JDE. *The Clinical Measurement of Joint Motion.* Rosemont, IL: American Academy of Orthopaedic Surgeons; 1994.
9. Patla CE, Paris SV. *E1 Course Notes: Extremity Evaluation and Manipulation.* St. Augustine, FL: Institute of Physical Therapy; 1993.
10. Cornwall MW, McPoil TG. Motion of the calcaneus, navicular, and first metatarsal during the stance phase of walking. *J Am Podiatr Med Assoc.* 2002;92:67-76.
11. McPoil TG, Cornwall MW. Relationship between neutral subtalar joint position and pattern of rearfoot motion during walking. *Foot Ankle.* 1994;15:141-145.
12. Elveru R, Rothstein J, Lamb R. Goniometric reliability in a clinical setting: subtalar and ankle joint measurements. *Phys Ther.* 1988;6:672-677.
13. Astrom M, Arvidson T. Alignment and joint motion in the normal foot. *J Orthop Sports Phys Ther.* 1995;22:216-222.
14. Levangie PK, Norkin CC. *Joint Structure and Function: A Comprehensive Analysis*, 5th ed. Philadelphia, PA: FA Davis; 2011.
15. Sarrafian S. Biomechanics of the subtalar joint. *Clin Orthop.* 1993;290:17-26.
16. McPoil TG, Cornwall MW. The relationship between static lower extremity measurements and rearfoot motion during walking. *J Orthop Sports Phys Ther.* 1996;24:309-314.
17. Milgrom C, Gilad M, Simkin A, et al. The normal range of subtalar inversion and eversion in young males as measured by three different techniques. *Foot Ankle Int.* 1985;6:143-145.
18. Manter J. Movements of the subtalar and transverse tarsal joints. *Anat Rec.* 1941;80:397.
19. Elftman H. The transverse tarsal joint and its control. *Clin Orthop.* 1960;16:41-45.
20. Hopson MM, McPoil TG, Cornwall MW. Motion of the first metatarsophalangeal joint. *J Am Podiatr Med Assoc.* 1995;85:198-204.
21. Shereff MJ, Bejjani FJ, Kummer FJ. Kinematics of the first metatarsophalangeal joint. *J Bone Joint Surg.* 1986;68A:392-398.
22. Mann RA, Hagy JL. The function of the toes in walking, jogging, and running. *Clin Orthop.* 1979;142:24-29.
23. Myerson MS, Sjereff MJ. The pathological anatomy of claw and hammer toes. *J Bone Joint Surg.* 1989;71:45-49.
24. Viladot A. Metatarsalgia due to biomechanical alterations of the forefoot. *Orthop Clin North Am.* 1973;4:165-178.
25. Budiman-Mak E, Conrad KJ, Roach KE. The foot function index: a measure of foot pain and disability. *J Clin Epidemiol.* 1991;44:561-570.
26. Rozzi SL, et al. Balance training for persons with functionally unstable ankles. *J Orthop Sports Phys Ther.* 1999;29:478-486.
27. Wells PS, Anderson DR, Rodger M, Ginsberg JS, et al. Derivation of a simple clinical model to categorize patients probability of pulmonary embolism: increasing the models utility with SimpliRED D-dimer. *Thromb Haemost Stuttgart.* 2000;83:416-420.
28. Wells PS, Owen C, Doucette S, Fergusson D, Tran H. The rational clinical examination: does this patient have deep vein thrombosis? *JAMA.* 2006;295:199-207.
29. Tamariz LJ, Eng J, Segal JB, Krishman JA, et al. Usefulness of clinical prediction rules for the diagnosis of venous thromboembolism: a systematic review. *Am J Med.* 2004;117:676-684.
30. Bachmann LM, Kolb E, Koller MT, et al. Accuracy of Ottawa ankle rules to exclude fractures of the ankle and mid-foot: systematic review. *BMJ.* 2003;326:417.
31. Knutzen KM, Price A. Lower extremity static and dynamic relationships with rearfoot motion in gait. *J Am Podiat Med Assn.* 1994;84:171-180.
32. Magee DJ. *Orthopedic Physical Assessment*, 5th ed. Philadelphia, PA: WB Saunders; 2008.
33. Lang LM, Volpe RG, Wernick J. Static biomechanical evaluation of the foot and lower limb: the podiatrist's perspective. *Man Ther.* 1997;2:58-66.
34. Sallade J. *Fitting Feet for Function: Course Notes.* Fleetwood, PA: John Sallade Seminars; 1994.
35. Hunt GC, Brocato RS. Gait and foot pathomechanics. In: Hunt GC, ed. *Physical Therapy of the Foot and Ankle.* Edinburgh, Scotland: Churchill Livingstone; 1988.
36. Dutton M. *Orthopaedic Examination, Evaluation, and Intervention.* New York, NY: McGraw-Hill; 2004.
37. Schon LC. Nerve entrapment neuropathy, and nerve dysfunction in athletes. *Orthop Clin North Am.* 1994;25:47-59.
38. Gross MT. Lower quarter screening for skeletal malalignment: suggestions for orthotics and shoewear. *J Orthop Sports Phys Ther.* 1995;21:389-405.
39. Mann RA. Biomechanical approach to the treatment of foot problems. *Foot Ankle.* 1982;2:205-212.
40. Hintermann B. Tibialis posterior dysfunction: a review of the problems and personal experience. *Foot Ankle Surg.* 1997;3:61-70.
41. Mann R, Inman VT. Phasic activity of intrinsic muscles of the foot. *J Bone Joint Surg.* 1964;46A:469-481.
42. Basmajian JV, DeLuca CJ. *Muscles Alive: Their Function Revealed by Electromyography.* Baltimore, MD: Williams & Wilkins; 1985.
43. Kendall FP, McCreary EK, Provance PG. *Muscle Testing and Function.* Baltimore, MD: Williams & Wilkins; 1993.
44. Klein P, Mattys S, Rooze M. Moment arm length variations of selected muscles acting on talocrural and subtalar joints during movement: an in vitro study. *J Biomech.* 1996;29:21-30.
45. Moss CL. Comparison of the histochemical and contractile properties of human gastrocnemius muscle. *J Orthop Sports Phys Ther.* 1991;13:322-327.
46. Cyriax, J. *Textbook of Orthopaedic Medicine Volume One*, 8th ed. London, England: Bailliere Tindall; 1982.
47. Lindstrand A. New aspects in the diagnosis of lateral ankle sprains. *Orthop Clin N Am.* 1976;7:247-249.
48. Frost HM, Hanson CA. Technique for testing the drawer sign in the ankle. *Clin Orthop.* 1977;123:49-51.
49. Birrer RB, Cartwright TJ, Denton JR. Immediate diagnosis of ankle trauma. *Phys Sport Med.* 1994;22:95-102.
50. Tohyama H, Yasuda K, Ohkoshi Y, et al. Anterior drawer test for acute anterior talofibular ligament injuries of the ankle: how much load should be applied during the test? *Am J Sports Med.* 2003;31:226-232.
51. Aradi AJ, Wong J, Walsh M. The dimple sign of a ruptured lateral ligament of the ankle: brief report. *J Bone Joint Surg Br.* 1988;70:327-328.
52. Kjaersgaard-Andersen P, Frich LH, Madsen F, et al. Instability of the hindfoot after lesion of the lateral ankle ligaments: investigations of the anterior drawer and adduction maneuvers in autopsy specimens. *Clin Orthop.* 1991;266:170-179.
53. Colter JM. Lateral ligamentous injuries of the ankle. In: Hamilton WC, ed. *Traumatic Disorders of the Ankle.* New York, NY: Springer-Verlag; 1984.
54. Hertel J, Denegar CR, Monroe MM, Stokes WL. Talocrural & subtalar joint instability after lateral ankle sprain. *Med Sci Sports Exerc.* 1999;31:1501-1508.
55. Hopkinson WJ, St Pierre P, Ryan JB, et al. Syndesmosis sprains of the ankle. *Foot Ankle.* 1990;10:325-330.
56. Alonso A, Khoury L, Adams R. Clinical tests for ankle syndesmosis injury: reliability and prediction of return to function. *J Orthop Sports Phys Ther.* 1998;27:276-284.
57. Norkus SA, Floyd RT. The anatomy and mechanisms of syndesmotic ankle sprains. *J Athletic Train.* 2001;36:68-73.
58. Peng JR. Solving the dilemma of the high ankle sprain in the athlete. *Sports Med Arthro Rev.* 2000;8:316-325.
59. Brosky T, Nyland J, Nitz A, et al. The ankle ligaments: consideration of syndesmotic injury and implications for rehabilitation. *J Orthop Sports Phys Ther.* 1995;21:197-205.
60. Nussbaum ED, Hosea TM, Sieler SD, et al. Prospective evaluation of syndesmotic ankle sprains without diastasis. *Am J Sports Med.* 2001;29:31-35.
61. Boytim MJ, Fischer DA, Neuman L. Syndesmotic ankle sprains. *Am J Sports Med.* 1991;19:294-298.
62. Wright RW, Barile RJ, Surprenant DA, et al. Ankle syndesmosis sprains in national hockey league players. *Am J Sports Med.* 2004;32:1941-1945.
63. Lin C-F, Gross MT, Weinfeld P. Ankle syndesmosis injuries: anatomy, biomechanics, mechanism of injury, and clinical guidelines for diagnosis and intervention. *J Orthop Sports Phys Ther.* 2006;36:372-384.

64. Beumer A, Swierstra BA, Mulder PG. Clinical diagnosis of syndesmotic ankle instability: evaluation of stress tests behind the curtains. *Acta Orthopedics Scand.* 2002;73:667-669.
65. Thompson T, Doherty J. Spontaneous rupture of the tendon of Achilles: a new clinical diagnostic test. *Anat Res.* 1967;158:126-129.
66. Scott BW, Al-Chalabi A. How the Simmonds-Thompson test works. *J Bone Joint Surg Br.* 1992;74:314-315.
67. Simmonds FA. The diagnosis of a ruptured Achilles tendon. *Practitioner.* 1957;179:56-58.
68. Thompson TC. A test for rupture of the tendoachilles. *Acta Orthop Scand.* 1962;32:461-465.
69. Maffulli N. The clinical diagnosis of subcutaneous tear of the Achilles tendon. A prospective study in 174 patients. *Am J Sports Med.* 1998;26:266-270.
70. DeGarceau D, Dean D, Reduejo SM, Thordarson DB. The association between diagnosis of plantarfascitis & Windlass test results. *Foot Ankle Int.* 2003;24:251-255.
71. Evans RC. *Illustrated Essentials in Orthopedic Physical Assessment.* St. Louis, MO: Mosby; 1994.
72. Oloff LM, et al. Flexor hallucis longus dysfunction. *J Foot Ankle Surg.* 1998;37:101-109.
73. Stiell IG, Greenberg GH, McKnight RD, Nair RC, et al. A study to develop clinical decision rules for the use of radiography in acute ankle injuries. *Ann Emerg Med.* 1992;21:384-390.
74. Stiell I, Wells G, Laupacis A, et al. for the Multicentre Ankle Rule Study Group. Multicentre trial to introduce the Ottawa ankle rules for use of radiography in acute ankle injuries. *Br Med J.* 1995; 311:594-597.
75. Auletta AG, Conway WF, Hayes WF, Guisto DF, Gervin AS. Indications for adiography in patients with acute ankle injuries: Role of the physical examination. *AJR.* 1991;157:789-791.
76. Auleley GR, Kerboull L, Durieux P, Courpied JP, Ravaud P. Validation of the Ottawa rules in France: A study in the surgical emergency departments of a teaching hospital. *Ann Emerg Med.* 1998;32:14-18.
77. Kerr L, Kelly AM, Grant J, et al. Failed validation of a clinical decision rule for the use of radiography in acute ankle injury. *NZ Med J.* 1994;107:294-295.
78. Stiell IG, McKnight RD, Greenberg GH, et al. Ottawa foot & ankle rules. *JAMA.* 1994;271:827.
79. Cotton FJ. Fractures and fracture-dislocations. Philadelphia, PA: WB Saunders; 1910.
80. Lindenfeld T, Parikh S. Clinical tip: heel-thump test for syndesmotic ankle sprain. *Foot Ankle Int.* 2005;26:406-408.
81. Cranley JJ, Canos AJ, Sull WJ. The diagnosis of deep venous thrombosis: fallibility of clinical symptoms & signs. *Arch Surg.* 1976;111:34-36.
82. Knox FW. The clinical diagnosis of deep vein thrombophebbitis. *Practitioner.* 1965;195:214-216.

Orthopaedic Manual Physical Therapy of the Lumbopelvic Spine

Christopher H. Wise, PT, DPT, OCS, FAAOMPT, MTC, ATC

Chapter Objectives

At the conclusion of this chapter, the reader will be able to:

- Identify the key anatomical and biomechanical features of the lumbopelvic spine and their impact on examination and intervention.
- List and perform key procedures used in the orthopaedic manual physical therapy (OMPT) examination of the lumbopelvic spine.
- Demonstrate sound clinical decision-making in evaluating the results of the OMPT examination.

- Use pertinent examination findings to reach a differential diagnosis and prognosis.
- Discuss issues related to the safe performance of OMPT interventions for the lumbopelvic spine.
- Demonstrate basic competence in the performance of a skill set of joint mobilization techniques for the lumbopelvic spine.

FUNCTIONAL ANATOMY AND KINEMATICS

Introduction

The human spine is a complex, complicated, and often confounding structure composed of *33 individual vertebrae* forming *25 mobile segments*. During typical function, the spine must move through a wide range of multiplanar motions while simultaneously serving as a stable base from which the muscles of the appendicular skeleton must perform their important functions.

The spine is divided into the *cervical (7)*, *thoracic (12)*, *lumbar (5)*, *sacral (5)*, and *coccygeal (3–5)* regions, each of which possess unique movement characteristics that allow the execution of a variety of functional demands (Fig. 28-1). In total, the spine was created with a variety of inherent engineering flaws that sacrifice stability for mobility. As a result, spinal dysfunction and subsequent disability has reached epidemic proportions in our society.

Lumbar Spine Arthrology and Kinematics

The **spinal motion segment** is considered to be the functional unit of the spine and is defined as the inferior aspect of the superior vertebra, the superior aspect of the inferior vertebra, and all of the structures in between (Fig. 28-2). Due to the interdependent nature of the spinal motion segment, impairment of any structure within the motion segment will eventually impact, to a greater or lesser degree, the other structures within the motion segment.

The Facet Joint

Within the spinal motion segment, the *articular facet joint*, sometimes referred to as the *interzygapophyseal or zygapophyseal joint*, plays a major role in dictating the direction and quantity of motion that occurs among adjacent vertebrae. As dictated by the sagittal plane orientation of the lumbar facet joints, the greatest extent of motion is in the sagittal plane (forward/backward bending), with less motion in the frontal plane (side bending), and the least amount of motion in the transverse plane (rotation).

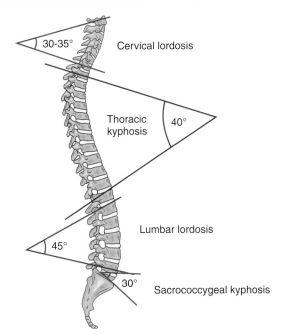

FIGURE 28–1 The regions of the vertebral column with their degree of spinal curvature.

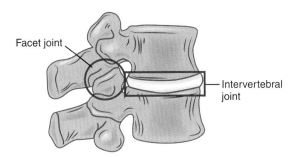

FIGURE 28–2 The spinal motion segment.

The facet joints are *synovial, planar joints* with a joint capsule that creates synovial fluid that occupies the intracapsular joint space between facets. The *capsuloligamentous complex (CLC)* of the facet joint is highly innervated, often sharing afferent innervation with the spinal segments above and below in an arrangement referred to as **triple innervation**.[1,2]

In addition to both directing and determining the extent of spinal motion, the facet joints also serve to resist shear and withstand superincumbent, compressive forces from the head, arms, and trunk (HAT). The presence of lordosis within the lumbar spine creates a moment that produces anterior shear among spinal segments when in erect standing, particularly at the L5-S1 motion segment. Although the facet joints bear a greater amount of compressive forces in the cervical spine, up to 20% of the overall compressive loads within the lumbar spine are experienced through the facet joints.[1]

The Intervertebral Joint and Disc

The *intervertebral (IV) joint* is a fibrocartilaginous joint that possesses substantially less mobility than the facet joint. It is composed of two adjacent vertebral bodies and an interposed fibrocartilaginous *intervertebral (IV) disc*. The IV joint, with its interposed disc, allows motion between adjacent vertebral bodies

through deformation of the disc, limits motion through annular fiber orientation, maintains the diameter of the *intervertebral foramen (IVF)* to allow for the passage of the nerve root, and transmits shock across the spinal segment from one vertebral body to the next.

The intervertebral disc is commonly considered to have two primary zones. The vastly hydrated and hydrophilic *nucleus pulposis* occupies the central portion of the disc. The perimeter of the disc is organized in concentric lamellae composed of Type I and Type II collagen, commonly known as the *annulus fibrosis*. On closer inspection, there are actually five zones of the IV disc, each with its own unique structure and function. The role of the IV disc in transmitting forces and facilitating movement is largely the result of its high water content and hydrophilic properties.[1] Compressive loads are distributed through the disc in a circumferential fashion in a process known as *radial expansion*.[3] The hydrated nucleus exerts a constant resting pressure on the annulus, which increases as load is applied and recoils when load is released. A reduction in the ability of the IV disc to function in this fashion is greatly compromised with a loss of fluid that results through injury or with aging. A continuous cycle of degeneration ensues that consists of the development of small fissures within the inner portions of the annulus leading to an inequitable distribution of forces that result in the migration of nuclear material toward the periphery of the disc. It is important to note that the pathogenesis of the commonly occurring herniated disc, begins with initial tissue damage within the type II collagen fibers of the annulus that lie toward the most central portion of the disc.

In general, IV discs that have a greater height-to-diameter ratio (i.e., thicker discs) will possess a greater ability to facilitate movement than discs with less height. With greater mobility, however, comes a greater potential for injury. The degree to which the disc remains hydrated depends largely on the extent to which the spinal segment moves throughout the course of a normal day. This normal cycle of disc hydration is commonly referred to as **diurnal change** and is an important consideration regarding the potential for injury. Nutrition of the disc depends largely on motion within the segment and the regular distribution of forces that occurs through motion (Fig. 28-3). Given the insufficient vascularity of the disc, segmental motion is an important prophylactic measure for the promotion of long-term disc health.

Nachemson[4] studied the intradiscal pressure of the L4-5 disc during certain postures and discovered that sitting in a forward bent position increased intradiscal pressure compared to erect standing. Conversely, supine lying reduced the intradiscal pressure by one half of that experienced in erect standing. Activities such as forward bending, lifting, in particular lifting with the arms extended, and coughing increased intradiscal pressure.[4] An awareness of the impact of specific positions and postures on intradiscal pressure is an important consideration in the prevention and management of disc pathology.

Lumbar Spine Ligaments

The two most substantial extrasegmental ligaments of the lumbar spine are the *anterior longitudinal ligament (ALL)* and the *posterior longitudinal ligament (PLL)*. These two ligaments vertically span the full length of the spine from the cranium to the

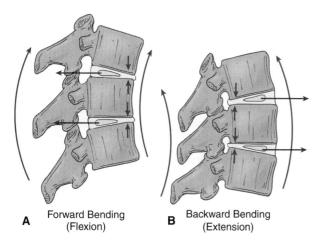

A Forward Bending (Flexion)   **B** Backward Bending (Extension)

FIGURE 28–3 Disc mechanics during sagittal plane motion revealing **A.** migration of the nucleus posteriorly and bulging of the annulus anteriorly with flexion and **B.** migration of the nucleus anteriorly and bulging of the annulus posteriorly with extension. (Adapted from: Levangie PK, Norkin CC. *Joint Structure and Function: A Comprehensive Analysis*, 5th ed. Philadelphia, PA: FA Davis Company, 2011.)

sacrum and serve as anterior and posterior restraints for the vertebral bodies at each level. The ALL is smaller in the cervical spine and becomes increasingly more substantial as it descends. The ALL is the primary restraint to the anterior migration of the lower lumbar vertebrae resulting from the presence of the lumbar lordotic curve. The PLL runs vertically along the posterior aspect or the vertebral bodies and IV discs and is more robust in the cervical spine, thus contributing to a relative reduction in the incidence of cervical disc herniations. The PLL is comprised of a thick central portion and smaller lateral slips. The larger central portion of the PLL may be contributory to the incidence of the more common posterolateral, rather than strictly posterior, disc herniation. The PLL forms the anterior boundary of the spinal canal. With degenerative changes, the PLL may buckle into the vertebral canal during backward bending, which may produce a transient central spinal stenosis with resultant spinal cord compression. The ALL and PLL serve as the primary restraints for backward bending and forward bending, respectively. Additional accessory restraints, which provide posterior stability, are the *supraspinous* and *interspinous ligaments* that run between adjacent spinous processes. The *intertransverse ligament*, between adjacent transverse processes, is uniquely positioned to resist contralateral side bending.

An important segmental ligament that prevents capsular impingement during the multiplanar motions of the spine is the *ligamentum flavum*. This paired ligament runs from lamina to lamina forming the posterior boundary of the vertebral canal resisting forward bending and releasing stored energy, by virtue of its highly elastic composition, to assist with the return of the motion segment to neutral.

The *iliolumbar ligament*, as its name implies, is a regional ligament that courses from the transverse processes of L4 and L5 obliquely to insert onto the ilium. This ligament unites the lumbar spine and pelvis restraining motion of both regions in all three cardinal planes.

Lumbar Spine Kinematics

To fully appreciate lumbar spine kinematics, it is vital to acknowledge the orientation of the lumbar facet joints, which largely direct and determine the manner in which segmental mobility occurs. The lumbar facet joints are aligned primarily in the sagittal plane and, to a lesser degree, in the frontal plane, with the exception of the inferior articular processes of L5, which lie in the frontal plane in order to articulate with the superior facets of S1. The superior articular facets are aligned such that they lie external and, therefore, enclose the inferior articular facets of the more superior vertebra. The cardinal plane motions of the lumbar spine consist of forward bending (FB) and backward bending (BB), also known as flexion and extension, in the sagittal plane, which range from *40 to 60 degrees* and *20 to 35 degrees*, respectively; side bending (SB), also known as lateral flexion, bilaterally in the frontal plane, which ranges from *15 to 20 degrees*; and rotation (ROT) bilaterally in the transverse plane, which ranges from *3 to 18 degrees* (Fig. 28-4).[5] Segmental motion is dictated by the three-joint complex just described (2 facet joints and 1 IV joint), allowing both linear (translatory) as well as angular (rotatory) motions, which possess six degrees of freedom (Fig. 28-5).

Observation of FB in standing reveals a reversal of the lordotic curve (Fig. 28-6). Once lumbar spinal segmental motion has been exhausted, the pelvic girdle engages and rotates anteriorly on the fixed femoral heads. During FB, the superior vertebra of the motion segment rotates and glides anteriorly, thus opening the IVF and producing a bilateral upglide and opening of the facet joints. If the annulus of the IV disc is intact, the anterior annulus will buckle anteriorly and the nucleus will migrate posteriorly. The interaction between the lumbar spine and pelvic girdle during FB and when returning from FB is referred to as **lumbopelvic rhythm**.[6,7] Hamstring flexibility may greatly impact the contribution from the pelvic girdle during FB. Esola et al[6] described the pattern of lumbar and hip motion during FB in 41 subjects with and without low back pain (LBP). For all subjects, the lumbar spine contributed more to early motion (2:1 L/H ratio), the lumbar spine and hips contributed equally to the middle phase of motion (1:1 L/H ratio), and the hips were primarily responsible for the late phase of motion (1:2 L/H ratio). [6]

BB typically occurs to a lesser degree than FB (Fig. 28-7). Segmental BB consists of a slight degree of posterior rotation and posterior glide, which is limited by the anterior longitudinal ligament, the approximation of posterior structures including compressive forces through the facet joints, and the spinous processes. During BB, the IVF closes and the facet joints experience bilateral downglide and closing as the annulus buckles posteriorly and the nucleus migrates anteriorly. In standing, the pelvic girdle will move into posterior rotation after lumbar mobility has been exhausted. The hip flexors have a powerful moment arm to resist the pelvic girdle contribution to BB.

Observation of lumbar SB should reveal equal contributions from all segments as performed from cephalad to caudal (Fig. 28-8). SB produces a slight segmental translation in the frontal plane leading to compression and closing of the IVF and downgliding and closing of the facet joint ipsilateral to the side to

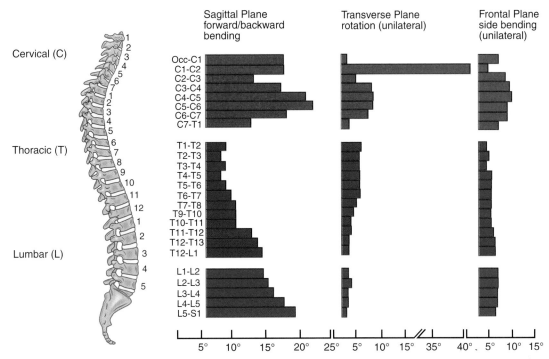

FIGURE 28–4 Segmental and total range of spinal motion in all three cardinal planes. (Adapted from: Neumann DA. *Kinesiology of the Musculoskeletal System: Foundations for Rehabilitation,* 2nd ed. St. Louis, MO: Mosby Elsevier, 2010, with permission.)

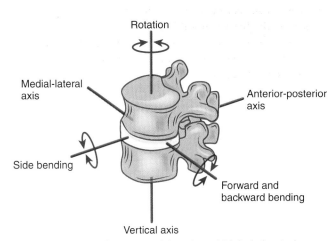

FIGURE 28–5 Osteokinematics of the spine, which includes six degrees of freedom. (Adapted from: Neumann DA. *Kinesiology of the Musculoskeletal System: Foundations for Rehabilitation*, 2nd ed. St. Louis, MO: Mosby Elsevier, 2010, with permission.)

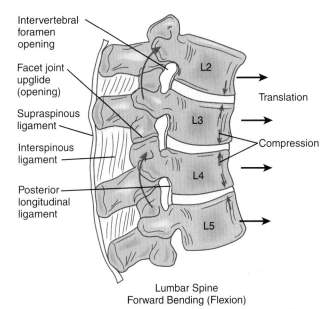

Lumbar Spine
Forward Bending (Flexion)

FIGURE 28–6 Kinematics of lumbar spine forward bending, which reveals upglide of the facet joints, anterior translation of the vertebra, opening of the intervertebral foramen, and tautness within the posterior ligamentous structures.

which SB has occurred. Opening of the IVF as well as upgliding and opening of the facet joint occurs on the contralateral side to which SB has occurred. Migration of the nuclear contents of the disc occurs opposite to the direction to which SB has occurred.

Due to the sagitally oriented facet joints, ROT occurs in a very limited fashion in the lumbar spine. Rotation produces an opening or gapping of the facet joint on the side to which ROT has occurred and closing or compression of the contralateral side (Fig. 28-9). Therefore, to maximally open a facet joint in a triplanar fashion, combined FB, contralateral SB, and ipsilateral ROT would be performed. Conversely, to maximally close a facet joint in a triplanar fashion, BB, ipsilateral SB, and contralateral ROT would be performed. An intimate understanding

of the manner in which facet joints guide segmental motion is valuable in directing the manual physical therapist toward differential diagnosis and optimal intervention strategies.

There is a plethora of discussion and controversy around the concept of *coupled motion* within the lumbar spine. Fryette, whose assertions were based on two-dimensional models, espoused that SB and ROT occur contralaterally when the lumbar spine is in neutral and ipsilaterally when the lumbar spine is in a non-neutral position. His contentions have been refuted

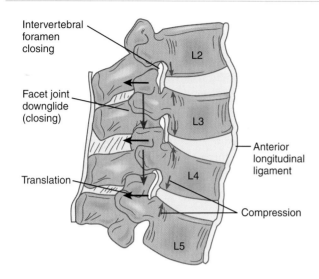

Lumbar Spine
Backward Bending (Extension)

FIGURE 28–7 Kinematics of lumbar spine backward bending, which reveals downglide of the facet joints, posterior translation of the vertebra, closing of the intervertebral foramen, and tautness within the anterior ligamentous structures.

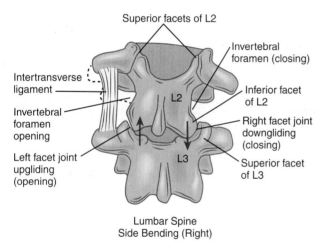

Lumbar Spine
Side Bending (Right)

FIGURE 28–8 Kinematics of lumbar spine side bending to the right, which reveals upglide of the left facet, downglide of the right facet, opening of the left intervertebral foramen, closing of the right intervertebral foramen.

in recent years with the advent of more sophisticated scientific analysis.[8-10] An appreciation of the six-degrees of freedom model has demonstrated significant variability in coupling at all spinal levels in both asymptomatic and symptomatic subjects. The current best evidence does not support a consistent coupling pattern in the lumbar spine and, therefore, brings into question paradigms that emphasize these concepts in the management of back pain through manual intervention.[8-10] Although an appreciation of coupling mechanics is helpful, recent evidence supports the use of an individual's symptomatic response to mechanical behavior as the preferred method for classification of LBP that may be effectively used to guide intervention.[8-10]

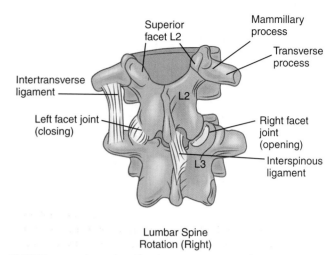

Lumbar Spine
Rotation (Right)

FIGURE 28–9 Kinematics of lumbar spine rotation to the right, which reveals opening of the right facet joint, closing of the left facet joint.

Pelvic Girdle Osteology

The Innominate Bone

The pelvic girdle is comprised of two innominate bones with an interposed sacrum and coccyx. The innominate bone is unfused until the second decade of life and is composed of the *ilium* superiorly, *ischium* posteriorly, and the *pubis* anteriorly and inferiorly. The female pelvis is broader, less dense, and possesses a steeper ilial slope, has a more cylindrical pelvic cavity, and a deeper sacral concavity when compared with the male pelvis. The male pelvis is characterized by denser bone, a longer sacrum, and less distance between the pubic tubercles.

The Sacrum

The sacrum is composed of five fused vertebrae, except in abnormal cases where movement may exist between the first and second sacral vertebra in a condition known as **lumbarization**. A related condition, known as **sacralization**, is present when L5 is fused to S1. There are several important bony landmarks on the sacrum that may be used to determine the mobility and position of the sacrum. The sacrum resembles an inverted pyramid with the *sacral base*, which articulates with L5 at the *lumbosacral junction*, comprising the cephalad-most aspect of the sacrum. The *sacral apex*, which articulates with the coccyx at the *sacrococcygeal junction*, is located caudally. Just medial to the sacrum's articulation with the ilium at about the level of S2 is an important landmark known as the *sacral sulcus*. Located along the lateral and inferior aspect of the sacrum just superior and lateral to the apex is the *inferior lateral angle (ILA)*. The first three sacral segments compose 87% of the total sacral articular surface.[11] There is general agreement that the joint surfaces of the SIJ are very irregular with a great degree of variability. The male sacrum possess greater irregularity, which increases with age.

Pelvic Girdle Arthrology and Kinematics

There are a total of 11 joints that compose the pelvic girdle. Jackson[12] has referred to this region as a *closed, osteoarticular ring* whose primary function is to efficiently transmit superincumbent forces while allowing appropriate force attenuation of ground reaction forces from the lower extremities. Erhard[13] refers to this region as the *lumbopelvic hip complex (LPHC)* and alludes to the functional interdependence that exists among each of these structures. These regions are linked neurophysiologically, biomechanically, and anatomically, and dysfunction in any one of these structures may lead to dysfunction in the others.[13]

Sacroiliac Joint

For centuries, confusion and controversy has surrounded the structure and function of the *sacroiliac joint (SIJ)*. This joint has been described as a diarthrodial/synovial joint anteriorly and as a synarthrosis/syndesmosis joint posteriorly.[14] This arrangement suggests that the majority of motion occurs in the anterior aspect of the joint. A small percentage of individuals exhibit fusion of the SIJ with increasing years. MacDonald[15] found less than 20% fusion rate in 59 sacroiliac joints. Among those found to have a fused SIJ, four different classes of joint fusion seem to exist.[15]

There is a great degree of variability among individuals. Using computed tomography (CT) for the purpose of identifying the presence of anatomical variants in 534 sacroiliac joints, *accessory joints* within the SIJ were the most common variant and were identified in 102 subjects (19.1%). Accessory joints were found unilaterally in 48 subjects and bilaterally in 54 subjects. Sixty-five of the 102 subjects with accessory joints were experiencing LBP.[16] Another study found that more than nine hundred sacroiliac joints revealed the presence of accessory joints, which increased with age, and had a higher incidence in males versus females.[17] The clinical significance of accessory joints within the SIJ is inconclusive.

A significant amount of controversy exists regarding the topography of the SIJ. To show the relationship between alterations in SIJ topography and function, friction coefficients were determined according to a statistical method using in vitro specimens. The highest coefficients were found in male specimens, the topography of which have coarse texture, ridges, and depressions.[18] SIJ joint surfaces are asymmetrical in size, shape, and direction, and lie in numerous planes, making radiographic imaging challenging.[14] A variety of in vitro and in vivo radiographic methods have revealed the surface orientation of the SIJ as complex and sinusoidal.[19] The topography of the SIJ resembles the corrugated pieces of a jigsaw puzzle. The structural features of the SIJ contribute to the relatively small degree of motion available at this joint.

Debate regarding the type of cartilage that lines the joint surfaces of the SIJ also exists. Some authors propose that the sacral articular surface is lined with hyaline cartilage that is 3 mm thick, with the ilial surface covered by fibrocartilage that is 1 mm thick.[19] Others contend that hyaline cartilage lines both surfaces.[15,20] More recent evidence suggests that both surfaces are lined with hyaline cartilage.[20] The cartilage on the sacral surface is typically thicker than that found on the ilial surface.

Stability of the SIJ

Under normal circumstances, the SIJ is considered to be a highly stable joint. In the vertical position, the SIJ derives its stability from superincumbent forces that force the sacrum, like a wedge, between the innominates. The stability that is provided in this manner is achieved through what is known as a **form-closure mechanism**. In the horizontal position, most stability is derived from ligamentous support, which has become known as a **force-closure mechanism**.

In the presence of higher friction coefficients and greater wedge angle, the stability of the SIJ is less reliant on ligamentous support.[18] Iliac graft harvesting for spinal fusion surgery may compromise the stability of the SIJ.[21] The CT findings of SIJs in patients who underwent iliac bone graft harvesting reveals that of 16 SIJs with ligamentous violation, 10 showed mild degenerative changes, and 6 showed moderate changes that may have occurred from compromised ligament integrity or from violation of the synovial aspect of the joint.[22]

The strongest SIJ ligament is the *interosseous ligament*, which is intra-articular, connecting the tuberosities of the sacrum and ilium. This substantial ligament is reinforced by the long dorsal ligament. The *long dorsal ligament* runs from the posterior superior iliac spine (PSIS) to S3,4. This ligament is superficial to the interosseous ligament. It invests into the sacrotuberous ligament, erector spinae, and thoracolumbar fascia. This ligament resists sacral backward bending.

The *sacrotuberous ligament* is quite extensive, with two extensions. This ligament forms the inferior border of the lesser sciatic foramen and is referred to as the antirotation ligament because it limits movement of the innominate relative to the sacrum in the sagittal plane. The *sacrospinous ligament* runs from the sacrum and coccyx to the ischial spine, where it forms the greater and lesser sciatic foramen. Both the sacrotuberous and sacrospinous ligaments resist forward bending of the sacrum.

Mobility of the SIJ

Although consensus exists that motion does occur within this joint, many still question whether there is enough motion to be considered clinically significant.[23] The contribution of the SIJ to the presence of LBP hinges on the nature and magnitude of motion that is available at this joint.[24] Bowen and Cassidy[25] proposed that SIJ motion in the young is more linear in nature while motion in older subjects is more rotatory in nature.[25] Using radiological technique with the ilia fixed, Weisl[26] found 6 degrees of rotation and 5.6 mm of translation of the sacrum.[26] Five millimeters of motion was found by Colachis et al[27] using implanted Kirschner wires with subjects in nine different positions.[27] A combination of rotation and translation up to 16 mm was identified by Grieve[28] using a three-dimensional technique.[28] Examination of SIJ movement during functional tasks was performed in 21 symptomatic and asymptomatic patients using roentgen stereophotogrammetric analysis (RSA), which involved the insertion of tantalum balls under fluoroscopy into the SIJ to identify motion. They found 1 to 2 degrees of motion when going from supine to standing or sitting; standing to hyperextension revealed 2 to 3 degrees of motion, with a mean translation of 0.5 mm, not exceeding 1.6 mm. They also identified decreased mobility with age and no difference in mobility between symptomatic and asymptomatic individuals, thus concluding that assessment of mobility is not a predictor of SIJ dysfunction.[29] The study that revealed the greatest degree of SIJ motion was one performed by Smidt et al.[24] In this study, five fresh cadaver specimens were evaluated using CT cross-sectional scans in five static positions with the subject in side-lying. When considering movement of the ilium about a fixed sacrum, the findings revealed that the hips in extreme positions caused a reduction in cranial and an increase in the caudal size of the joint with oblique, sagittal plane orientation. Extreme hip flexion to extension averaged 7 to 8 degrees of motion; total motion for reciprocal hip flexion and extension averaged 5 to 8 degrees; variability in sagittal plane motion between subjects was high, ranging from 3 to 17 degrees; and linear motion was from 4 to 8 mm, occurring in each of the cardinal planes. They confirmed the link between the hip and the SIJ and concluded that the SIJ possesses a significant degree of motion.[24] Using the RSA method, Sturesson et al[30] evaluated the magnitude of SIJ rotation in the reciprocal straddle position and compared these findings with those of Smidt.[24] Six women with pelvic pain were analyzed in standing, supine, and prone in a sustained straddle position with alternate right and left leg maximally flexed. They concluded that the motion of the SIJ does exist but to a much lesser degree than previously noted, adding that the amount of motion proposed by Smidt[24] would only occur upon subluxation of the joint.[30]

Motion within this joint was first appreciated in pregnant females through manual measurement of pelvic diameters.[3] Based on hormonal influences, this population represents those with the greatest degree of SIJ mobility. The release of the hormone *relaxin* during pregnancy alters the degree of mobility in the SIJ and may make pregnant individuals more vulnerable to SIJ dysfunction. MacLennan[31] identified a correlation between levels of relaxin present during pregnancy, pelvic instability, and pain. They further added that relaxin levels in the body may also increase during menstruation, thus provoking symptoms that are related to pelvic mobility.[31] Hagen[32] found pain upon stair climbing and position changes in a study with 23 pregnant women.[32] The population that represents those with the least amount of SIJ mobility appears to be older males. There was no decrease in mobility found in subjects ranging from 19 to 45 years old.[29] However, an increase in the incidence of intra-articular ankylosis of the SIJ after the age of 50 was identified more predominantly in males.[33,34] A microscopic analysis of the composition and topography of the SIJ revealed that mobility was present in the majority of cadavers until the age of 60 years. After 60 years, ankylosis occurred in 82% of males and 30% of females.[33,34] For a comprehensive review of SIJ kinematics, the reader is advised to consult the literature reviews performed by Walker[23] and Alderink.[35]

Movement of the ilium on a relatively fixed sacrum may be referred to as **iliosacral (IS) motion**. Movement of the sacrum on a relatively fixed ilium is known as **sacroilial (SI) motion**. Because there are two innominates that compose the pelvis,

iliosacral motion (i.e., motion of the ilium upon the sacrum) may occur symmetrically where both innominates, or ilia, are moving in the same direction, or they may occur asymmetrically, where both innominates are moving in different directions. Both IS and SI motions occur in a triplanar fashion, with the largest degree of mobility observed within the sagittal plane. For each SIJ motion, it is important to consider the axis of motion, the anatomical reference point, and the coupled relationships that exist between these motions and other structures within the lumbopelvic hip complex.

Iliosacral Mobility

IS motion is triplanar, and the anterior superior iliac spine (ASIS) serves as the anatomical reference point. IS sagittal plane motion is identified as anterior and posterior rotation (sometimes referred to as tilt). **Iliosacral anterior rotation** is defined as movement of the ASIS anteriorly and caudally, with simultaneous movement of the PSIS anteriorly and cranially. This motion is mechanically coupled with hip extension. **Iliosacral posterior rotation** is defined as movement of the ASIS posteriorly and cranially and movement of the PSIS posteriorly and caudally. Posterior rotation is mechanically coupled with hip flexion (Fig. 28-10). Iliosacral motion in the transverse plane is referred to as **iliosacral inflare** and **iliosacral outflare** and is defined as movement of the ASIS in a medial and lateral direction, respectively (Fig. 28-11). Inflare and outflare are mechanically coupled with hip internal rotation and external rotation, respectively. During gait, the innominate undergoes a motion identified as **iliosacral upslip** on the stance limb side. An upslip is defined as a cranial migration of both the ASIS and the PSIS. On the swing limb side, a relative caudal migration of both the ASIS and PSIS occurs and is defined as **iliosacral downslip** (Fig. 28-12).

Sacroilial Mobility

SI mobility refers to movement of the sacrum about a relatively fixed ilium. To understand SI mobility, one must first appreciate the axes around which motion is believed to occur, with an awareness that much debate surrounds this concept. Some have

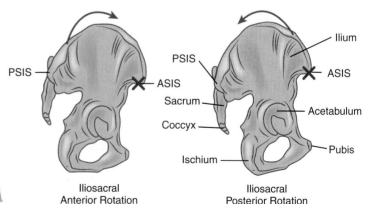

FIGURE 28–10 Iliosacral sagittal plane motion of anterior and posterior rotation as determined by the anterior superior iliac spine (ASIS), which is the reference point.

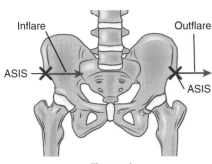

FIGURE 28–11 Iliosacral transverse plane motion of inflare and outflare as determined by the anterior superior iliac spine (ASIS), which is the reference point.

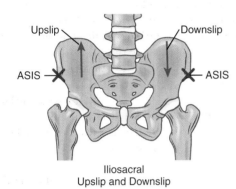

FIGURE 28–12 Iliosacral frontal plane motion of upslip and downslip as determined by the anterior superior iliac spine (ASIS), which is the reference point.

proposed an SIJ axis that is posterior to the pubic symphysis.[36] Others have stated that this horizontal axis is at the junction of the cranial and caudal aspects of the sacral joint surface and that around this axis rotation of the ilium and sacrum occurs in opposite directions. The traditional axes for SI motion was initially conjectured to consist of three transverse axes, the superior, middle, and inferior transverse axes. The anatomical reference point for sacral motion is the anterior aspect of the sacral base. Movement of the sacrum in the sagittal plane is referred to as **sacroilial forward bending**, or **flexion**, and **sacroilial backward bending**, or **extension**. Movement of the sacrum in the transverse plane is referred to as **sacroilial rotation** and movement in the frontal plane is referred to as **sacroilial side bending.** Sacral movement is mechanically linked to the lumbar spine. Although there is conflicting data regarding the direction of sacral motion relative to the lumbar spine, based on anecdotal clinical data it appears as though the sacrum moves in the direction opposite to L5 during initial movement, after which the sacrum follows movement of the lumbar spine in the sagittal plane. In the transverse plane, however, the sacrum appears to follow movement of the lumbar spine earlier in the range. Frontal plane motion of the sacrum is challenging to palpate and identify clinically and will be included as a potential component of sacral torsions.

More recently, sacral movement is considered to occur in a triplanar fashion around one of two oblique axes. The **right oblique axis (ROA)** courses from the left inferior lateral angle through the right SIJ. The **left oblique axis (LOA)** runs from the right inferior lateral angle through the left SIJ (Fig. 28-13). The motions that occur around these axes are referred to as **sacroilial torsions**. Smidt et al[24] have concluded that it is unlikely that a single set of mechanical axes can be identified to aid in our understanding of SI movement and function.[24]

There are two types of **sacroilial forward torsions**. A **sacroilial right on right oblique axis (right on right) forward torsion** consists of forward bending in the sagittal plane, rotation to the right in the transverse plane, and side bending to the right in the frontal plane. A **sacroilial left on left oblique axis (left on left) forward torsion** consists of forward bending in the sagittal plane, rotation to the left in the transverse plane, and side bending to the left in the frontal plane (Fig. 28-14). Conversely, there are two types of **sacroilial backward torsions**. A **sacroilial right on left oblique axis (right on left) backward torsion** consists of backward bending in the sagittal plane, rotation to the right in the transverse plane, and side bending to the right in the frontal plane. A **sacroilial left on right oblique axis (left on right) backward torsion** consists of backward bending in the sagittal plane, rotation to the left in the transverse plane, and side bending to the left in the frontal plane (Fig. 28-15).

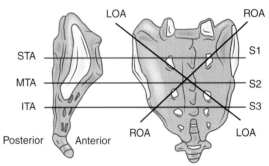

FIGURE 28–13 Axes of sacroilal motion showing the traditionally held superior (STA), middle (MTA), and inferior (ITA) transverse axes and the more commonly considered right (ROA) and left (LOA) oblique axes.

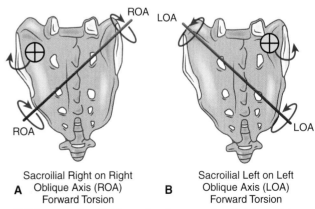

FIGURE 28–14 Sacroilial forward torsions, revealing **A.** right on right oblique axis (ROA) forward torsion and **B.** left on left oblique axis (LOA) forward torsion. The cross hairs denote the deeper sacral sulcus.

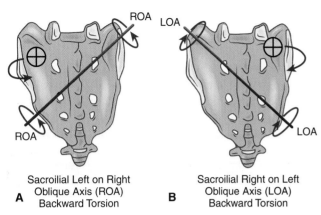

FIGURE 28–15 Sacroilial backward torsions, revealing **A.** left on right oblique axis (ROA) backward torsion and **B.** right on left oblique axis (LOA) backward torsion. The cross hairs denote the more superficial sacral sulcus.

Pubic Symphysis

The *pubic symphysis (PS)* is a critical joint in maintaining the closed, osteoarticular ring of the pelvic girdle. The PS absorbs, directs, controls, restricts, and stabilizes motion. PS is an amphiarthrodial, cartilaginous joint formed between the pubic rami and interposed fibrocartilaginous disc. This 3- to 5-mm disc is thicker anteriorly than posteriorly, with a longer vertical dimension in males, but it is wider in females. This joint resembles a "bushing" that permits tissue deformation as opposed to true joint excursion. The mean gap of the PS is 1 mm, anterior-posterior translation is 1.1 mm, rotation is 0.5 mm, and vertical translation is 2.5 mm.[37–39]

EXAMINATION

The Subjective Examination

Self-Reported Disability Measures

The Oswestry Disability Instrument

Among the most used disability measures in orthopaedic physical therapy is the ***Oswestry Disability Instrument (ODI)***.[40,41] The ODI is composed of 10 sections with questions assessing limitations of daily living which include: pain intensity, personal care, lifting, walking, standing, sleeping, sex life, social life, and travel. Each section has six statements that are assigned points in descending order from 0 to 5. To score the ODI, the scores from all checked statements are summed and doubled to obtain the final percentage score. A score of 0% to 20% suggests minimal disability, 20% to 40% reveals moderate disability, 40% to 60% is severe disability, 60% to 80% is crippled, and 80% to 100% denotes that the patient is either bed-bound or an exaggerator of symptoms.

The construct validity of the global rating of change scale as an external standard of meaningful change, used in assessing the responsiveness of the ODI, was studied. They compared measurement properties, reliability, and responsiveness of the ODI and the Quebec Back Pain Disability Scale (QBPDS). Sixty-seven patients with acute, work-related back pain completed both

scales initially and after 4 weeks of therapy. The modified ODI showed higher levels of test-retest reliability (ICC = 0.90, 95% CI = 0.78–0.96) as compared with the QBPDS (ICC = 0.55, 95% CI = 0.20–0.78). Responsiveness was 6 points for the ODI as compared with 15 points for the QBPDS.[42]

To determine whether self-reported disability was related to isokinetic performance of trunk musculature, 76 LBP patients were studied over 6 months. The relationship of each question on the ODI to isokinetic performance was studied as well as the total score. ODI scores were negatively correlated with isokinetic performance (– 0.47 to – 0.38). The ODI question regarding lifting most closely related to isokinetic performance, accounting for 21.5% to 28.4% of variation in performance. The authors concluded that the ODI may be useful in assisting clinicians with interpreting isokinetic performance values and in identifying patients who may be presenting with inappropriate illness behavior.[43]

In examining a series of available questionnaires on patient perception of symptomatology to determine those most appropriate for the given patient population, patients (n = 145) were asked to complete six individual disability questionnaires, of which the ODI was one. The ODI was one of three questionnaires that demonstrated sufficient reliability and responsiveness. Two-way analysis of variance showed the ODI to be responsive to time and gender (F = 7.706, p = 0.001 and F = 12.213, p = 0.001, respectively).[44]

Fifty-four patients with LBP were asked to complete the ODI along with three other disability questionnaires. Criterion-related validity showed that lifting tasks in regard to weight related most highly with the lifting category on the ODI, but in regard to lifting time, did not correlate. Sitting tasks correlated well with the sitting category on the ODI. In addition, the authors concluded that the ODI had some evidence of factorial validity, moderately high internal consistency, and good face validity.[45]

Another study compared the responsiveness of three different instruments used for evaluation of functional status and the severity of pain in 81 patients with nonspecific back pain for a duration of 6 weeks. The reference gold standard was a seven-point global perceived effect scale. By using effect size statistics and the receiver operating characteristic, all instruments (including the ODI) were able to discriminate between improvement and nonimprovement. The ODI was less sensitive to change and, for the patient's main complaint, was less specific to change.[46]

The Fear Avoidance Beliefs Questionnaire

The ***Fear Avoidance Beliefs Questionnaire*** has experienced increased attention in recent years.[47,48] The physical activity subscale consists of five statements related to the impact of activity on back pain on which the patient must rate their level of agreement on a six-point scale from completely disagree to completely agree. The work subscale consists of 11 statements related to the impact of work activity on the individual's back pain. Fear-avoidance scores for each section are based on calculations from selected items, and a total score is obtained by summing the responses on all items, with higher scores indicating the presence of fear-avoidance behaviors.

The McGill Pain Questionnaire

The *McGill Pain Questionnaire (MPQ)* consists of a list of adjectives that may be used to describe pain and the impact of intervention on the patient's experience of pain.[49] An individual is asked to circle all of the words that apply to the current situation, but only circle one word from each of the 20 groups of pain descriptors. To score, the words in each list are given a value that ranks from 1 to 6 beginning with the first word in each list. The total score for all words circled are summed as the total score. Administering this tool before and following intervention is useful at detecting change. A change in score is identified by calculating a percentage based on pre- and postintervention scores. Scores of greater than 30 suggest symptom exaggeration.[50] To ascertain the ability of the MPQ and ODI to enhance differential diagnosis of three broad categories of low back pain, individuals with low back pain underwent an examination that yielded the classification of back pain. Use of the MPQ, ODI, and combined MPQ/ODI were used to assess their correlation with the diagnosis obtained from the physical exam. Validity was deemed as agreement with the classification. The highest correlation was found when the MPQ/ODI was combined (90%) as opposed to the use of the MPQ (79%) or the ODI (74%) individually.[51]

The Ransford Pain Drawing

The *Ransford Pain Drawing* consists of both anterior and posterior views of the body on which the patient is asked to identify the location and type of symptoms currently experienced.[52] Ransford et al[52] developed a method called the *penalty point system*, which uses the standard pain drawing described by Mooney et al[53] to evaluate an individual's need for further psychological testing.[52] The patient is asked to identify the location and type of pain being experienced on the drawing. In order to score the pain drawing using this method, the therapist identifies "unreal" drawings, or drawings that represent an unlikely presentation of symptoms. Points ranging from 1 to 2 are assigned for each finding, and a total score of greater than 3 indicates a need for further psychological evaluation. This tool is deemed to be effective at quickly identifying approximately 93% of patients with poor psychosocial overlay.[50]

The Roland-Morris Disability Questionnaire

The *Roland-Morris Disability Questionnaire (RMDQ)* is a short test that is presumably better suited for the individual with acute pain. It is often used in concert with other tools to gauge progress.[54,55] In the RMDQ, the patient marks the statements that apply to their current situation, and the scores are summed and range from no disability (0) to severe disability.[13] The RMDQ has been found to correlate well with other tools such as the ODI and the 36-Item Short Form Health Survey.[56] The validity of the RMDQ has been established compared to a six-point scale, and its test-retest reliability was established in 20 patients with a correlation of 0.91.[54,55]

The Million Visual Analog Scale

The *Million Visual Analog Scale*, developed by Million et al,[57] is a self-assessment questionnaire that consists of 15 individual questions related to function. The individual is asked to mark his or her response on a 10 cm line. This scale is purported to have good reproducibility and can be used to document functional improvement.[57]

Review of Systems

At the time of the initial visit, it is of paramount importance that the manual physical therapist determine if the patient requires physical therapy (PT) services, if the patient requires PT in addition to a medical consultation, or if the patient requires an immediate referral to a physician with no further PT intervention until additional testing has ruled out an emergent condition. The chief indicator that the patient is experiencing a condition that is amenable to physical therapy is the patient's symptomatic response to movement or position. This information may be ascertained through the interview process or by direct observation at the time of the examination. Symptoms that do not change in response to movement or position are termed "nonmechanical" and may require further medical evaluation and are not likely to benefit from PT intervention alone.

The profile of individuals suspected as having cancer includes the following: males over 50 years old, a report of unexplained weight loss, a previous history of cancer, and failure to respond to conservative care.[58] Individuals presenting with this profile should be considered to have cancer until proven otherwise through additional medical testing.

Although cancer is among the most serious conditions that may mimic musculoskeletal pain, other disease processes must also be ruled out in patients presenting with back pain. Among the most serious conditions impacting the patient with low back pain is *cauda equina syndrome*, which consists of symptoms resulting from neurological compression that may or may not have a musculoskeletal etiology. Objective examination procedures used to identify the presence of this syndrome involve testing of the L4-S1 dermatomes, including sensory testing of the perianal region, and testing of the L4-S1 myotomes. Red flags suggesting the presence of cauda equina syndrome include sensory deficits in the L4-S1 dermatome and saddle region; progressive weakness of the lower extremities, particularly in ankle dorsiflexion, toe extension, and ankle plantarflexion; and report of urinary incontinence or retention.[59]

In cases of LBP, spinal *osteomyelitis* should also be ruled out. This condition may be suspected in the cases of immunosuppression, history of drug use, and a history of recent infection. An individual presenting with an increased body temperature and positive responses to these queries increases the suspicion of back pain secondary to the presence of an infection. Table 28-1 displays the medical red flags for the lumbar spine that must be ruled out before embarking on intervention directed toward a musculoskeletal cause.

History of Present Illness

Appreciating the specific *mechanism of injury* is of great relevance to the manual therapist when attempting to put together the pieces of the diagnostic puzzle. As described previously, Nachemson[60] identified the relationship between specific positions and intradiscal pressure. The amount of force experienced by the disc may be up to 10 times the amount of the

Table 28-1	Medical Red Flags for the Lumbopelvic Spine
MEDICAL CONDITION	**RED FLAGS**
Cauda Equina Syndrome	Saddle paresthesia
	Sensory and motor deficits in L4-S1 (ankle dorsiflexion, plantar flexion, and toe extension)
	Urinary and fecal incontinence
Spinal Tumor	Over 50 years old
	Unremitting pain
	Failure of conservative management
	History of cancer
	Unexplained weight loss
Spinal Fracture	Chronic use of steroids
	History of traumatic event
	Over 70 years old

(Adapted from: Boissonnault WG. *Primary Care for the Physical Therapist: Examination and Triage.* St. Louis, MO: Elsevier Saunders; 2005.)

weight that is being lifted, and the pressure through the disc is often greater in men compared to women because of the distribution of weight. Occupations that involve excessive material handling often precipitate the onset of low back pain.[61] Static, prolonged sitting postures with intermittent lifting and twisting may also lead to impairment.

Males between the ages of 25 and 50 years old are more likely to experience back pain of discogenic origin. Back pain from degenerative changes is often found in the population over the age of 45. As already noted, malignancy is most often associated with the population over the age of 50. Females exhibit low back pain more commonly than males. In such cases, the presence of gynecological conditions must be ruled out. Many females experience back pain while pregnant or during the postpartum period.

Centralization of symptoms serves as an indicator of favorable prognosis. In the presence of peripheral symptoms, the examiner must determine the specific location of neural compromise. An increase in symptoms with coughing or with performance of the *Valsalva maneuver* is suggestive of intrathecal pressure and often associated with disc pathology. *Central spinal stenosis*, often referred to simply as spinal stenosis, denotes compression on the spinal cord that results in neurological signs. *Lateral foraminal stenosis* denotes neurological signs and symptoms that occur as a result of encroachment on the mixed spinal nerve within the intervertebral foramen. The former typically involves bilateral symptoms, as well as a combination of both upper and lower motor neuron involvement. Those with lateral stenosis typically experience unilateral signs and symptoms that are primarily lower motor neuron in nature.

When considering the region of origin from which the symptoms arise, pain referral maps may be useful in determining involvement of the sacroiliac joint.[62,63] Pain maps of patients with

negative SIJ blocks revealed pain that was located cephalad to the L5 region. This finding suggests that individuals with low back pain that is cephalad to L5 are less likely to be experiencing pain that is originating from the SIJ. Sacral sulcus tenderness, pain over the SIJ, buttock pain, and pain in the region of the PSIS all demonstrated good sensitivity in determining SIJ involvement. However, performance of these tests in combination did not improve their diagnostic utility.[62] Fortin et al[63] determined that patients could be successfully screened for SIJ dysfunction based on comparison with a pain referral map. They found 100% correlation between two examiners when choosing patients believed to be presenting with SIJ pain maps.[63]

The Objective Physical Examination
Examination of Structure

The literature has not supported the relationship between structural aberrations and the severity of symptoms.[64] The clinical relevance of structural findings is determined by their relationship with the patient's chief complaint. A **lateral shift** is suggestive of a disc derangement. Most commonly, the upper body is laterally displaced, in reference to the lower body, away from the symptomatic side.[65] A lateral shift may be subtle and difficult to identify and, therefore, may be a contributor to an individual's poor tolerance for backward bending. See Chapter 9 of this text for a complete description of the lateral shift, including principles of management, clinical relevance, and its impact on prognosis. A band of hypertrophy or the presence of a unilateral or segmental increase in muscle tonicity may suggest the presence of segmental instability. Levangie[66] revealed that there was no evidence that any one of four SIJ-specific tests could be used to identify subjects with "positional faults" of the SIJ. Furthermore, the use of two or more tests did not improve their diagnostic accuracy.[66]

Neurovascular Examination

When performing the neurovascular examination, the manual physical therapist must make the distinction between the presence of *neurological symptoms* and *neurological signs*. The presence of signs increases the urgency for timely and appropriate care above that which is considered in the presence of neurological symptoms alone.

For *dermatomal* testing, a variety of modalities may be employed. A quick screen using light touch sensation testing may be initially performed. If positive findings are noted, more specific testing including such modalities as vibration, sharp/dull, hot/cold, and monofilament testing, among others may be used. *Deep tendon reflex (DTR)* testing must also be performed during the neurologic screen. The primary indicator of impairment is reflex asymmetry upon bilateral comparison. The DTRs performed during the lower quarter exam are the patellar tendon (L3-4), semitendinosis (L4), posterior tibialis (L4-5), biceps femoris (L5), and the Achilles tendon (S1-2). *Myotomal* testing, which assesses muscle function of the lower extremities should also be performed to screen for nerve involvement, may be performed in the following sequence bilaterally: hip flexion (L1,2), knee extension (L3), ankle dorsiflexion (L4), great toe extension (L5), ankle plantarflexion (S1), knee flexion (S2).

Examination of Mobility

Active Physiologic Movement Examination of the Lumbopelvic-Hip Complex

There are a variety of methods advocated for reliably quantifying spinal mobility. Such methods include the *back range of motion* device, *goniometry, single and double inclinometry, flexible ruler, and tape measurer.*[67-69] The primary limitation with each of these methods is failure to provide information about the relative contribution of each motion segment to the total amount of available motion. The *capsular pattern* of the lumbar spine is a limitation in backward bending, with rotation and side bending equally limited (BB > ROT = SB), according to Cyriax.[70] Others describe the capsular pattern as a limitation of forward bending with deviation toward the side of restriction, side bending that is contralateral to the side of the culpable segment, and rotation that is ipsilateral to the side of the culpable segment (FB with SB > contralateral SB > ipsilateral ROT). By virtue of the fact that this pattern of motion restriction represents the triplanar position in which the culpable facet joint is maximally opened, or decompressed, it is sometimes referred to as an **opening restriction**. A **closing restriction** is identified when the motion pattern reveals a restriction into backward bending, side bending that is ipsilateral to the side of the culpable segment, and rotation that is contralateral to the side of the culpable segment.

The normal extent of total active motion in the lumbar spine is *40 to 60 degrees* of FB, *20 to 35 degrees* of BB, *15 to 20 degrees* of SB, and *3 to 18 degrees* of ROT. A substantial degree of individual variability exists in lumbar spine mobility. During FB, gross observation should reveal a reversal of the lumbar lordotic curve.[71]

Iliosacral Active Physiologic Movement Examination

Iliosacral Anterior Rotation

The *forward-bending-PSIS (FB-PSIS) test* may be used to assess the amount of anterior IS rotation (Fig. 28-16). This test is sometimes performed in sitting; however, as a result of weight-bearing through the ischial tuberosities, less motion is anticipated in this position compared to standing. The seated FB-PSIS test has an ICC = 0.25.[47] During this test, impairment is identified on the side of the PSIS that moves first, fastest, and furthest compared to the contralateral side. Since this judgment is based on bilateral comparison, a variable that may confound the results is the presence of hypermobility. Reproduction of the patient's primary complaint during the test elevates its clinical relevance.

Iliosacral Posterior Rotation

The *Gillet,* or *march, test* may be used to ascertain the quantity of posterior IS rotation (Fig. 28-17). The Gillet test has been found to have an ICC of 0.59.[47] A positive finding is identified on the side that moves the least. The patient is asked to actively flex the hip above 90 degrees as the therapist monitors motion of the PSIS. The degree of normal mobility has been documented to be 4.5 to 9 mm of motion inferiorly and 2.5 to 6.5 mm medially. Reproduction of the patient's primary complaint during the test elevates its clinical relevance.

Iliosacral Inflare and Outflare

IS inflare and *outflare* mobility are both assessed using the *flare test* (Fig. 28-18). While palpating the PSIS, the patient externally and internally rotates his or her hip in standing with the heel of the foot on the ground. Normal movement is expected to be approximately 2.5 mm of both medial and lateral translation. Reproduction of the patient's primary complaint during the test elevates its clinical relevance.

Iliosacral Upslip and Downslip

To assess *IS upslip* and *downslip* mobility the *weight shift test* is used (Fig. 28-19). The therapist palpates bilateral PSIS and compares motion while the patient shifts weight from side to side. Superior translation, or upslip, should occur on the weight-bearing side, with relative inferior translation, or downslip, ocurring on the non-weight-bearing side. When compared bilaterally, asymmetrical motion suggests the presence of either hypomobility, hypermobility, or a combination of both. Reproduction of the patient's primary complaint during the test elevates its clinical relevance.

Iliosacral Versus Hip Regional Movement Differentiation

Once each of the iliosacral motions is actively tested and any reproduction of the patient's chief complaint has been

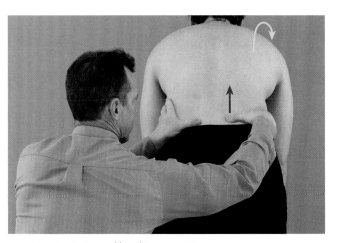

FIGURE 28–16 Forward-bending PSIS test.

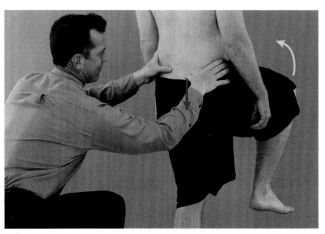

FIGURE 28–17 March/Gillet test.

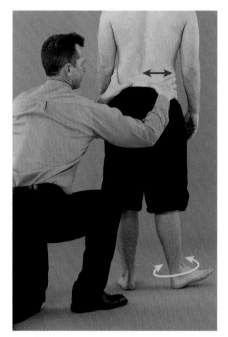

FIGURE 28–18 Flare test.

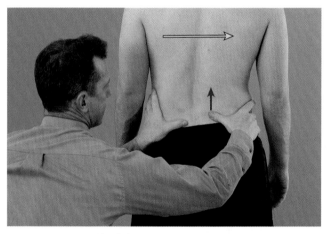

FIGURE 28–19 Weight shift test.

recorded, **regional movement differentiation (RMD)** testing can be initiated in an attempt to ascertain the primary region of symptomatic origin. In standing, explore the coupled relationship between the hip and IS motion by having the patient actively perform hip flexion with associated posterior IS rotation in the march position (ASIS moving posterior/superior), hip extension with anterior IS rotation in the lunge position (ASIS moving anterior/inferior), hip external rotation with IS outflare in the flare test position (ASIS moving laterally), and hip internal rotation with IS inflare in the flare test position (ASIS moving medially). Single and repeated movements are performed, and baseline symptoms are documented. If one of these combined movement patterns results in a reproduction of the patient's chief complaint, then **overpressure and counterpressure** may be used to isolate the origin of symptoms.

First, IS overpressure is provided in the symptomatic direction, which is expected to increase the chief complaint. This is

followed by IS counterpressure, which seeks to limit pelvic mobility in the direction of symptom reproduction with an expected decrease in the patient's chief complaint. As the patient flexes the hip and creates IS posterior rotation, overpressure is provided through the ASIS, followed by counterpressure, which is provided at the PSIS (Fig. 28-20). As the patient lunges, producing hip extension and anterior IS rotation, overpressure is provided at the PSIS followed by counterpressure at the ASIS (Fig. 28-21). In standing, the patient then externally and internally

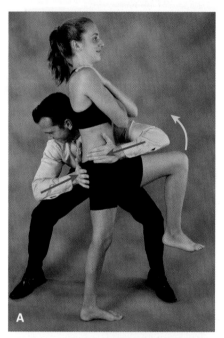

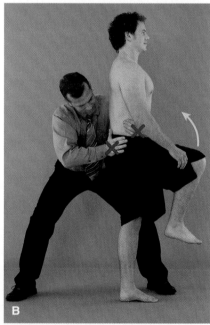

FIGURE 28–20 Regional movement differentiation (RMD) testing for iliosacral posterior rotation/hip flexion including **A.** overpressure and **B.** counterpressure (A. from: Wise CH, Gulick DT. *Mobilization Notes: A Rehabilitation Specialist's Pocket Guide.* Philadelphia, PA: FA Davis Company, 2009.)

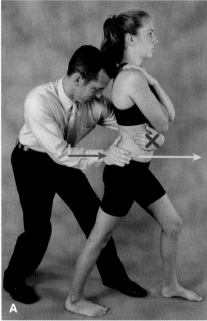

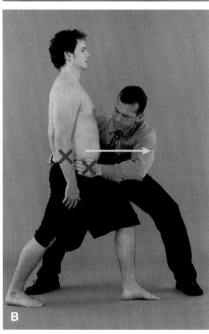

FIGURE 28–21 Regional movement differentiation (RMD) testing for iliosacral anterior rotation/hip extension including **A.** overpressure and **B.** counterpressure. (A. from: Wise CH, Gulick DT. *Mobilization Notes: A Rehabilitation Specialist's Pocket Guide.* Philadelphia, PA: FA Davis Company, 2009.)

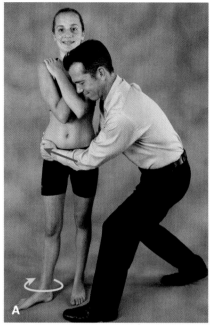

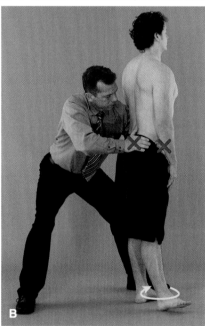

FIGURE 28–22 Regional movement differentiation (RMD) testing for iliosacral outflare/hip external rotation including **A.** overpressure and **B.** counterpressure (A. from: Wise CH, Gulick DT. *Mobilization Notes: A Rehabilitation Specialist's Pocket Guide.* Philadelphia, PA: FA Davis Company, 2009.)

rotates the hip, producing IS outflare and inflare, respectively. Overpressures followed by counterpressures are then provided over the ASIS and PSIS during these motions (Fig. 28-22 and Fig. 28-23). The IS region is considered to be involved as either the primary or secondary locus of pathology if the chief complaint is either increased or decreased in response to the application of manual pressure at the innominate.

Specific pressures provided at the pelvis are presumed to target movement of the ilium on the sacrum, or iliosacral motion. Therefore, any change in the initial reproducible sign is

due to external forces placed through the pelvis, thus suggesting the iliosacral region, rather than the hip, as the locus of pathology. If there was no symptomatic change in response to these forces, the hip, by default, would be suspected to be the region of symptomatic origin. Although clinical efficacy of this process has been observed, it has yet to be subjected to scientific scrutiny. However, this process is driven by the identification of the patient's symptomatic response to mechanical behavior, which, as noted, is advocated in the literature. If a reduction in the chief complaint is noted during testing, this

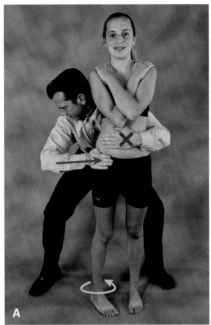

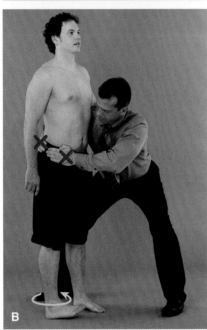

FIGURE 28–23 Regional movement differentiation (RMD) testing for iliosacral inflare/hip internal rotation including **A.** overpressure and **B.** counterpressure. (A. from: Wise CH, Gulick DT. *Mobilization Notes: A Rehabilitation Specialist's Pocket Guide.* Philadelphia, PA: FA Davis Company, 2009.)

examination procedure becomes the intervention. Such procedures, referred to as *accessory with physiologic motion* mobilizations, will be discussed later in this chapter.

Sacroilial Active Physiologic Movement Examination

Sacroilial Forward and Backward Bending

SI motion is coupled with lumbar motion and, although debate exists, appears to move in the opposite direction during early lumbar motion in the sagittal plane and in the same direction to lumbar motion in the transverse plane. The *sit-slump test* is used to explore the mechanical relationship between motion of the lumbar spine and SI motion (Fig. 28-24). With the patient in a seated position, the manual physical therapist palpates bilateral sacral sulci as the patient rolls the pelvis forward to sit erect, then backward to assume a slumped sitting posture. With lumbar FB and BB, the sacrum should initially move into BB and FB, respectively. This is evidenced by the sacral sulci becoming more prominent during SI BB and less prominent during SI FB. A positive test is indicated by a reduction in mobility compared with normal, asymmetric movement, or any reproduction of symptoms. The reliability of determining the movement or position of the sacrum is poor, therefore, reproduction of the patient's primary complaint during the test elevates its clinical relevance.

Sacroilial Rotation

SI rotation is assessed in sitting. The patient is asked to rotate bilaterally as the therapist palpates bilateral sacral sulci and assesses the quantity of motion from side to side. The sacrum should rotate in the same direction as the lumbar spine. For example, lumbar rotation to the right, is thought to produce SI rotation to the right as evidenced by an increase in the prominence of the right sacral sulcus and an increase in the depth of the left sacral sulcus. Symmetrical

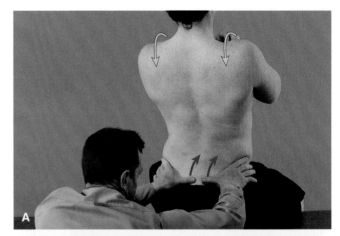

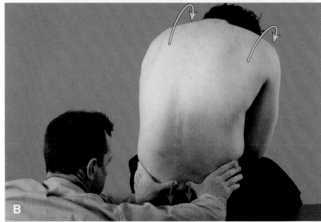

FIGURE 28–24 The sacroilial sit to slump test to assess **A.** sacroilial flexion/lumbar backward bending and **B.** sacroilial extension/lumbar forward bending.

movement or reproduction of symptoms suggests dysfunction. The reliability of determining the movement or position of the sacrum is poor, therefore, reproduction of the
patient's primary complaint during the test elevates its clinical relevance.

Sacroilial Versus Lumbar Regional Movement Differentiation
As in the exam of IS mobility, the concepts of RMD may also
be applied to assessment of SI motion. Once the patient's reproducible sign has been elicited through active motion in
the seated position, overpressure followed by counterpressure
may be systematically applied. As the patient slumps, thus
producing lumbar FB and SI BB, overpressure is applied
over the sacral apex followed by counterpressure over the
sacral base (Fig. 28-25). During active lumbar BB, SI FB is

produced, during which overpressure followed by counterpressure is applied over the sacral base and apex, respectively
(Fig. 28-26).

Specific pressures provided at the sacrum are presumed
to target movement of the sacrum on the ilium, or sacroilial
motion. Therefore, any change in the initial reproducible sign
is due to external forces placed through the sacrum, thus suggesting the sacroilial region, rather than the lumbar spine, as
the locus of pathology. If there was no symptomatic change in
response to these forces, the lumbar spine, by default, would
be suspected to be the region of symptomatic origin. Overpressure and counterpressure may also be used during testing
of sacroilial transverse plane motion that involves lumbar
and SI rotation in a seated position, as previously described
(Fig. 28-27).

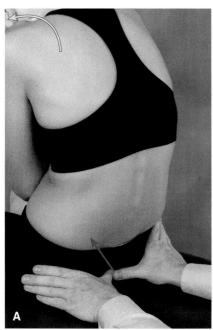
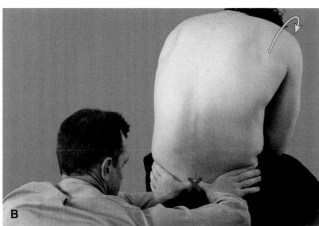

FIGURE 28–25 Regional movement differentiation (RMD) testing for sacroilial extension/lumbar flexion including **A.** overpressure at the sacral apex and **B.** counterpressure at the sacral base. (A. from: Wise CH, Gulick DT. *Mobilization Notes: A Rehabilitation Specialist's Pocket Guide.* Philadelphia, PA: FA Davis Company, 2009.)

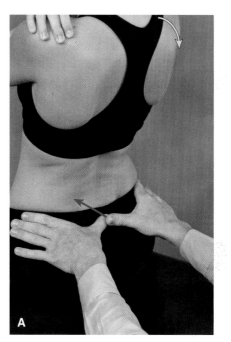
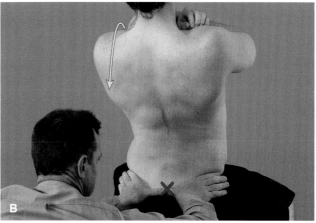

FIGURE 28–26 Regional movement differentiation (RMD) testing for sacroilial flexion/lumbar extension including **A.** overpressure at the sacral base and **B.** counterpressure at the sacral apex. (A. from: Wise CH, Gulick DT. *Mobilization Notes: A Rehabilitation Specialist's Pocket Guide.* Philadelphia, PA: FA Davis Company, 2009.)

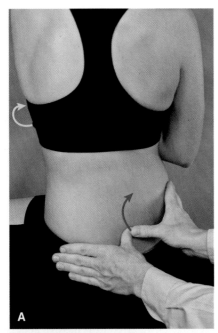

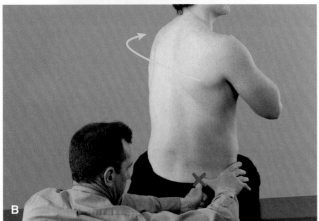

FIGURE 28–27 Regional movement differentiation (RMD) testing for sacroilial and lumbar rotation including **A.** overpressure at the left sacral sulcus with right lumbar rotation, **B.** counterpressure at the right sacral sulcus with right lumbar rotation. (A. from: Wise CH, Gulick DT. *Mobilization Notes: A Rehabilitation Specialist's Pocket Guide.* Philadelphia: FA Davis Company, 2009.)

Lumbar Spine Passive Physiologic Intervertebral Mobility Examination

Passive testing of physiologic mobility is accomplished through a series of testing identified as **passive physiologic intervertebral mobility (PPIVM)** testing (Figs. 28-28, 28-29, 28-30, 28-31). PPIVM testing is used to assess segmental physiologic motion. For ease of performance, this testing, in most cases, involves recruitment of motion from caudal to cephalad through passive movement of the lower extremities. In order to ascertain the degree of segmental mobility, palpation of the interspinous space is performed during passive motion recruitment. Table 28-2 displays the physiologic motions of the lumbar spine, including normal ranges of motion, open and closed-packed positions, normal end feels, and capsular patterns. The reader is referred to Chapter 7 of this text for a more detailed description of lumbar PPIVM testing.

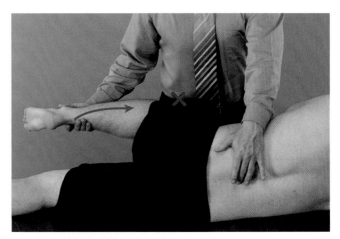

FIGURE 28–28 Lumbar forward-bending passive physiologic intervertebral mobility (PPIVM) examination.

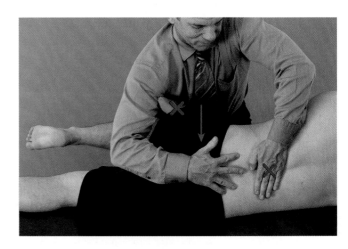

FIGURE 28–29 Lumbar backward-bending passive physiologic intervertebral mobility (PPIVM) examination.

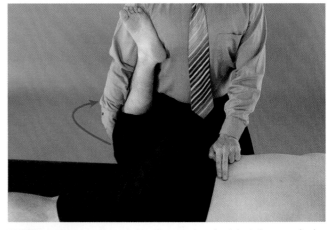

FIGURE 28–30 Lumbar side-bending passive physiologic intervertebral mobility (PPIVM) examination.

Iliosacral Passive Physiologic Mobility Examination

IS physiologic mobility may be passively assessed by directly contacting the innominates and moving them individually through each plane of motion to further refine the results of active range of motion (AROM) testing (Fig. 28-32). Anterior

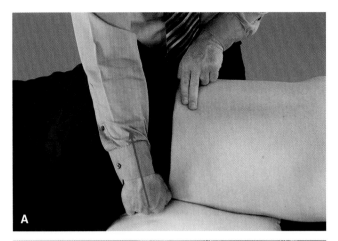

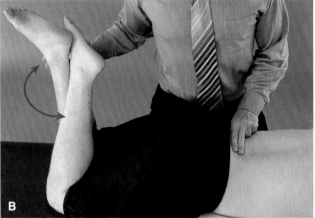

FIGURE 28–31 Lumbar rotation passive physiologic intervertebral mobility (PPIVM) examination using **A.** ilial lift technique and **B.** hip rotation technique.

and posterior rotation is performed with the patient in side-lying with hand contacts at the ASIS and ischial tuberosities. Inflare and outflare is assessed with the patient in the supine or prone position and hand contacts at the ASIS and PSIS. Upslip and downslip is tested most easily with the patient in side-lying with hand contacts at the iliac crest and ischial

tuberosities. Assessment of end feel and its relationship to symptom reproduction in each specific direction in which IS motion occurs may be valuable in identifying the dysfunctional region and, therefore, guide subsequent intervention.

Sacroilial Passive Physiologic Movement Examination

In order to assess passive physiologic SI mobility, the therapist may perform the *six step sacral spring technique* (Fig. 28-33). Spring testing assesses SI movement potential in all planes in a systematic fashion. The patient is placed in prone, and the therapist contacts six distinct regions of the sacrum: the base, the apex, bilateral sulci, and bilateral inferior lateral angles. Anteriorly directed force is imparted for the purpose of assessing the quantity and quality of end feel while noting any reproduction of symptoms. Isolation of which motion most closely reproduces the patient's chief complaint may assist in guiding intervention and determining outcomes.

Passive Accessory Movement Examination

In the spine, procedures designed to passively assess accessory motion are collectively referred to as **passive accessory intervertebral mobility (PAIVM)** testing. The primary goal of PAIVM testing is to gain an appreciation of the relationship between mobility and the onset of symptoms within each spinal segment. In addition to the perception of tissue resistance, the manual therapist must also note the initial onset of any symptoms. Fair to good intratester reliability, but poor intertester reliability, was found for judging passive segmental mobility in the lumbar spine.[72] Maher and Adams[73] identified that judgments of pain provocation were better than assessment of mobility for determining the dysfunctional segment in the lumbar spine.[73]

The PAIVM techniques used for examination are described in more detail in the intervention section of this chapter as mobilizations. The primary indicator for the use of these mobilizations lies in their use as examination procedures that serve to identify the hypomobile, or more reliably, the segment that reproduces symptoms. PAIVM testing and subsequent mobilization for each motion is described in the intervention section of this chapter. PAIVM testing has demonstrated

	Physiologic (Osteokinematic) Motions of the Lumbopelvic Spine				
JOINT	**NORMAL ROM**	**OPP**	**CPP**	**NORMAL END FEEL(S)**	**CAPSULAR PATTERN**
Lumbar	FB= 40– 60° BB =20–35° SB = 15–20° ROT= 3–18°	FB, contralateral SB and ipsilateral ROT	BB, ipsilateral SB and contralateral ROT	Elastic	FB with deviation > contralateral SB > ipsilateral ROT BB > ROT = SB (Cyriax[70])
Iliosacral Sacroilial	Angular motion = 3–20° Translatory motion = 0.5–8.0 mm Triplanar 0.5–8°	Maximum hip ER	Maximum hip IR	Firm	NA

Table 28–2

ROM, range of motion; OPP, open packed position; CPP, close packed position; FB, forward bending; BB, backward bending; SB, side bending; ROT, rotation; NA, not available.
(Adapted From: Wise CH, Gulick DT. *Mobilization Notes: A Rehabilitation Specialist's Pocket Guide.* Philadelphia, PA: FA Davis Company, 2009.)

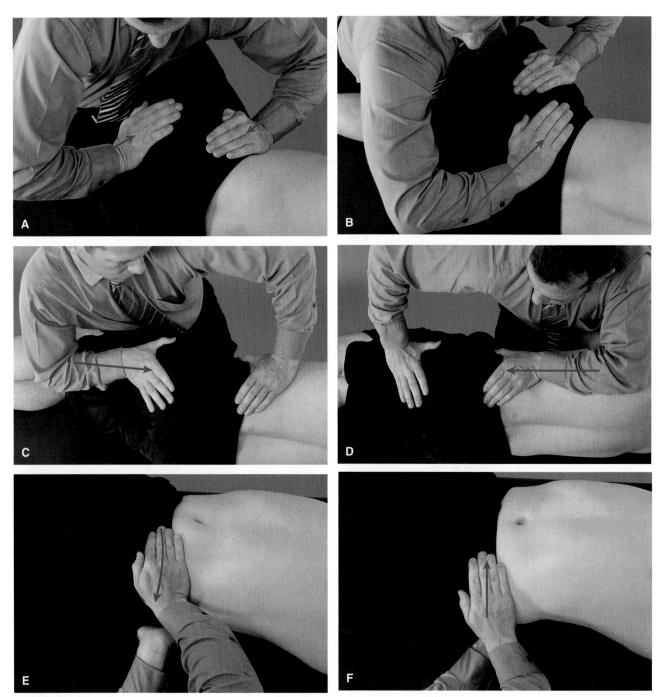

FIGURE 28–32 Iliosacral passive physiologic mobility examination including **A.** posterior rotation, **B.** anterior rotation, **C.** upslip, **D.** downslip, **E.** outflare, and **F.** inflare.

sensitivity = 0.43, –likelihood ratio = 0.60, specificity = 0.95, +likelihood ratio = 8.6. Reliability of these procedures is 0.25 to 0.57(kappa) for pain and ICC = 0.25 to 0.77 for mobility.[74,75] Table 28-3 displays the accessory motions of the lumbar spine.

Examination of Muscle Function

When considering the function of both the superficial and deep muscles of the spine, Bergmark[76] has adopted the terms **global stabilizing system** and **local stabilizing system** to refer to the superficial and deep musculature, respectively. Within this paradigm, the deep local muscles are best suited

to provide neutral zone control of spinal stability through monitoring and adjusting the degree of stiffness between segments. The reader is referred to Chapter 17 of this text for a detailed description of testing and training of the global and local muscle systems of the spine.

Palpation

Osseous Palpation

From the posterior view, the *iliac crests* are first palpated using the hands and are then visualized to assess their relative position. With the hands remaining on the iliac crests, the thumbs

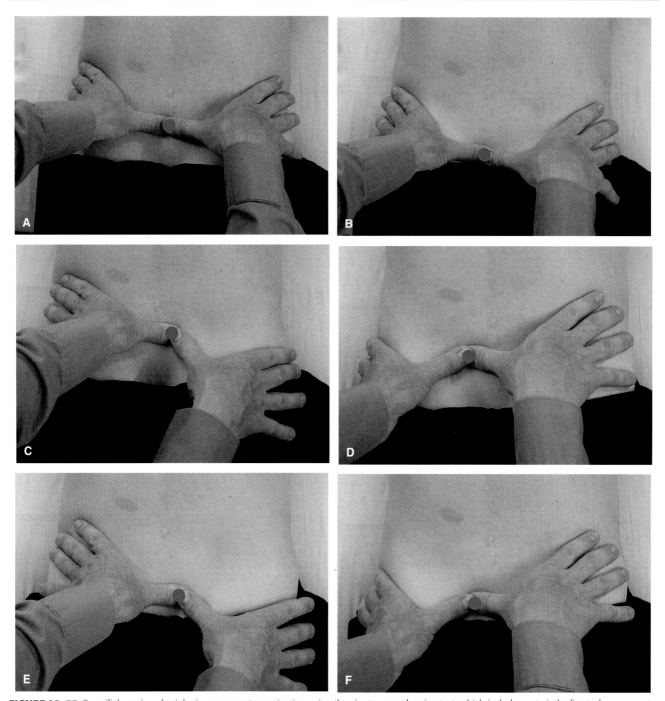

FIGURE 28–33 Sacroilial passive physiologic movement examination using the six-step sacral spring test, which includes anteriorly directed pressure at the **A.** sacral base, **B.** sacral apex, **C.** right sacral sulcus, **D.** left sacral sulcus, **E.** right inferior lateral angle, and **F.** left inferior lateral angle.

are then moved inferiorly to locate the *posterior superior iliac spines* on either side and are also visualized for relative position (Fig. 28-34). Moving farther inferiorly, the *ischial tuberosities* are identified for relative position. Asymmetry in the position of these landmarks in standing that diminish in non-weightbearing denotes the possibility of a limb length discrepancy but does not rule out other conditions. From the anterior perspective, the iliac crests are again palpated, this time the thumbs are moved inferiorly and medially to gain purchase on the *anterior superior iliac spines (ASIS)* and *anterior inferior iliac spines (AIIS)* (Fig. 28-35). The relative position of each of these structures is

noted and compared with identical palpations performed in non-weight-bearing. When viewed laterally, the PSIS should be approximately 15 degrees superior to the ASIS. An increase or decrease in the relative position of these landmarks suggests the presence of an anteriorly or posteriorly rotated innominate, respectively. During the palpation of bony landmarks, the manual therapist must be cognizant of the fact that the reliability of such procedures is poor and that such findings may not yield clinically relevant information.

In prone, the iliac crests are palpated to provide a reference point for locating the *L4 spinous process*, which is directly

Table 28–3	Accessory (Arthrokinematic) Motions of the Lumbopelvic Spine	
	ARTHROLOGY	**ARTHROKINEMATICS**
Lumbar Spine	Facet joint: Synovial joint primarily sagittal plane orientation with superior facets of interior vertebra facing medially and inferior facets of superior vertebra facing laterally. Intervertebral joint: Cartilaginous joint composed of two adjacent vertebral bodies and interposed fibrocartilaginous disc	***To facilitate forward bending:*** • Inferior facet of superior vertebra glides up and forward on superior facet of inferior vertebra • Nucleus pulposus migrates posteriorly, annulus fibrosis bulges anteriorly • Spinal canal and intervertebral foramen lengthen and open ***To facilitate backward bending:*** • Inferior facet of superior vertebra glides down and backward on superior facet of inferior vertebra • Nucleus pulposus migrates anteriorly, annulus fibrosis bulges posteriorly • Spinal canal and intervertebral foramen close ***To facilitate side bending (right):*** • Inferior facet of superior vertebra upglides on left and downglides on right • Right intervertebral foramen closes, left intervertebral foramen opens • Coupled with contralateral ROT in neutral and ipsilateral ROT out of neutral ***To facilitate rotation (right):*** • Inferior facets of superior vertebra open on right and closes on left • Right intervertebral foramen opens, left intervertebral foramen closes • Coupled with contralateral SB in neutral and ipsilateral SB out of neutral
Sacroiliac Joint	• Synovial joint anteriorly, syndesmosis joint posteriorly • Highly variable, irregular joint surfaces Controversy exists regarding topography, type of cartilage, and axis of joint motion	• Limited amount of motion, which occurs primarily in sagittal plane • Motion occurs around an oblique axis, which allows triplanar motion • Minimal amount of combined rotatory and translatory motion, which is less in males and reduces with age.
Pubic Symphysis	Amphiarthrodial, cartilaginous joint formed between the pubic rami and interposed fibrocartilaginous disc.	This joint resembles a "bushing" that permits tissue deformation. The mean gap is 1 mm, anterior-posterior translation is 1.1 mm, rotation is 0.5 mm, and vertical translation is 2.5 mm.

SB, side bending; ROT, rotation (Adapted From: Wise CH, Gulick DT. *Mobilization Notes: A Rehabilitation Specialist's Pocket Guide.* Philadelphia, PA: FA Davis Company, 2009.)

horizontal from the apex of the crests. Upon finding the spinous process of L4, the therapist moves inferiorly to identify the interspinous space between L4 and L5, then the *spinous process of L5*. To differentiate between L5 and S1, the hip is passively moved into extension or abduction, which produces motion at L5, but S1 as a fused vertebral segment remains immobile. The superior aspect of S1, known as the *sacral base*, may then be palpated in its entirety. Moving laterally, the *sacral sulci* are palpated as a flattened region just medial to the SIJ (Fig. 28-36). Lying directly horizontal from the PSIS is the *spinous process of S2*. Once identified, the therapist continues to palpate inferiorly, identifying the *central median crest* formed by the sacral spinous processes. This

palpation proceeds to the *apex of the sacrum* and then the *sacrococcygeal junction* and *coccyx*, which lies just superior to the *gluteal cleft*. Located at the inferior lateral aspect of the sacrum on either side is the region known as the *inferior lateral angle (ILA)*. From here, the therapist can palpate the borders of the sacrum into which the *sacrospinous* and *sacrotuberous* ligaments insert.

Once again relocating L4, the therapist can then move cephalad to palpate each subsequent spinous process within the lumbar spine and into the thoracic region. An effective way of considering the relative position of each respective spinous process is to perform a *pinch test*, in which the spinous process at each level is pinched between the therapist's fingers.

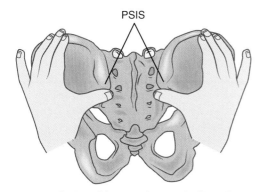

FIGURE 28–34 Palpation of the posterior superior iliac spines.

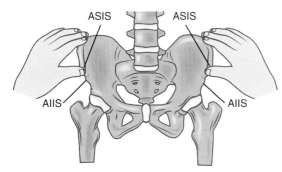

FIGURE 28–35 Palpation of the anterior superior iliac spines (ASIS) and anterior inferior iliac spines (AIIS).

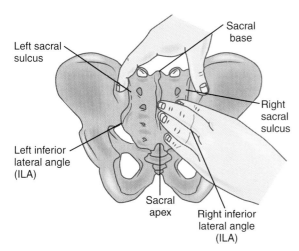

FIGURE 28–36 Palpation of the sacrum.

Each spinous process is held in this fashion as the next adjacent spinous process is palpated, and their relative positions are appreciated. A variation in the position of the spinous processes may suggest the presence of a rotated, flexed, or extended segment.

With the patient now lying supine, palpation of the *pubic crest* and *tubercles* is performed. Using a towel, the patient is asked to place their hand over their genitals forming a border of allowable space in which the therapist may palpate. The pubic tubercles are palpated for relative position. Beginning at the ASIS, the inguinal ligament is followed as it inserts onto the pubic tubercles on either side.

Soft Tissue Palpation

Beginning in prone, with a pillow under the abdomen, the *erector spinae*, as a group, are palpated. From central to lateral, the muscles that comprise this group consist of the *spinalis*, *longissimus*, and the *iliocostalis*. These muscles are best appreciated and differentiated from surrounding tissues by gently asking the patient to perform an isometric contraction for hip extension against manual resistance. Running vertically between the tenth rib and iliac crest and just lateral to the most lateral border of the erector spinae, is the *quadratus lumborum* muscle. Confirmation can be achieved through asking the patient to hike the hip. The *transversospinalis* muscle group lies deep to the erector spinae and is, therefore, less palpable. The muscles of this group consist of the *multifidi*, which span two to four spinal segments, and the *rotatores*, which span one to two segments. Palpation of these deep muscles is achieved by first identifying the spinous process and the transverse process at adjacent levels. A swelling of the multifidus can be felt under the palpating finger and a contraction can be noted in conjunction with the transverse abdominis muscle.[77] The multifidus may be most easily palpated over the posterior sacrum, and confirmation may be obtained by gentle isometric resistance of trunk rotation. See Chapter 17 for methods used to palpate the multifidus and transverse abdominis.

In supine, the muscles composing the abdominal wall are palpated. These are best palpated with the patient's hips and knees flexed. To palpate the *rectus abdominis*, the xiphoid process of the sternum and pubic tubercle are palpated. Gentle isometric resistance for trunk flexion is provided and the long, parallel rectus is palpated. The patient is asked to flex and rotate away from the therapist's palpating hand against gentle isometric resistance in order to palpate the *external oblique* muscle, which is oriented in a "hands in the pocket" direction. The patient then rotates toward the therapist as the palpating hand remains in place in order to identify the *internal oblique* muscle, which lies beneath and is oriented perpendicular to the external oblique (Fig. 28-37).

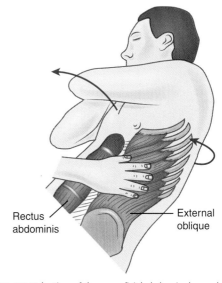

FIGURE 28–37 Palpation of the superficial abdominal muscles.

Special Testing

Potter and Rothstein[78] found that the interrater reliability was poor for all SIJ tests except sacroiliac gapping and compression, which achieved 90% and 70% agreement, respectively. Provocation tests for the SIJ were shown to have interrater reliability, and the authors concluded that tests focusing on which rely on the reproduction of symptoms should be the focus of further research regarding their role in classification and directing care.[78] Laslett and Williams[79] found good interrater reliability for both gapping/compression, pelvic torsion, and thigh thrust pain provocation tests.

In an effort to enhance the predictive value of these tests, Cibulka et al[80] discovered that a cluster of tests was more discriminating than using any single test in isolation when examining the SIJ. They suggested that a cluster of tests may serve to compensate for the limitations of any one specific test, the skill of the examiner, and for the diversity of the patient population. Sensitivity for the cluster of SIJ tests was 0.82, specificity was 0.88, and prevalence was 0.48. Positive predictive value was 0.86, and the negative predictive value was 0.84.[80] Table 28-4 provides an overview of the sensitivity, specificity, and likelihood ratios for the more commonly performed special tests used in the examination of the lumbopelvic spine. The reader is encouraged to consult other sources for additional information regarding the performance of these useful confirmatory tests.

Table 28–4	**Special Tests for the Lumbopelvic Spine**					
TEST	**SENSITIVITY**	**SPECIFICITY**	**+LR**	**−LR**	**RELIABILITY**	**REFERENCE**
Quadrant Test	NA	NA	NA	NA	NA	Lyle et al[81] Jensen[82]
Straight Leg Raise (SLR) Test	40%–97%	10%–57%	1.0–1.98	0.05–0.86	0.32–0.86 (kappa)	Kuo et al.[83] Breig and Troup[84] Charnley[85] Edgar and Park[86] Fahrni[87] Goddard and Reid[88] Scham and Taylor[89] Urban[90] Wilkins[91] Viikari-Juntura et al[92] Vroomen et al.[93] Rose[94] Mens et al.[95] DeVille et al.[96] Jonsson and Stromqvist[97] **Kosteljanetz et al[98]**
Bowstring Test	NA	NA	NA	NA	NA	Cram[99] Evans[100] Brudzinski[101] Meadows[102]
Prone Knee Bend (PKB) Test	NA	84%	NA	NA	0.21–0.26 (kappa)	Riddle and Freburger[103] Postacchini et al[104] Flynn et al[105] Potter and Rothstein[106] Vincent-Smith and Gibbons[107] Toussaint et al[108]
Slump Test	82.6%	54.7%	1.82	0.32	NA	Philip et al[109] Butler[110] Fidel et al[111] Johnson and Chiarello[112] Gabbe et al[113] Stankovic et al[114]

Table 28-4	**Special Tests for the Lumbopelvic Spine—cont'd**					
TEST	**SENSITIVITY**	**SPECIFICITY**	**+LR**	**-LR**	**RELIABILITY**	**REFERENCE**
Brudzinski-Kernig Test	NA	NA	NA	NA	NA	Cipriano[115]
Bike Test	NA	NA	NA	NA	NA	Dyck and Doyle[116]
Prone Instability Test	61%–72%	57%–58%	1.41	0.69	0.69–0.87 (kappa)	Hicks et al[117] Hicks et al[118] Schneider et al[119] Fritz et al[120]
Spine Torsion Test	NA	NA	NA	NA	NA	Meadows[102] Dobbs[121]
Pheasant Test	NA	NA	NA	NA	NA	Kirkaldy-Willis[122]
Anterior Instability Test	NA	NA	NA	NA	NA	Dobbs[121]
Posterior Instability Test	NA	NA	NA	NA	NA	Dobbs[121]
Farfan Torsion Test	NA	NA	NA	NA	NA	Farfan[123] Young and Aprill[124]
Supine to Long Sit Test	44%–62%,	64%–83%	1.37–3.6	0.46–0.88	0.06–0.19 (kappa)	Riddle and Freburger[103] Potter and Rothstein[106] Palmer and Epler[125] Bemis and Daniel[126] Levangie[127] Albert et al[128]
Sacroiliac Compression (C) and Distraction (D) Test	C: 7%–69% D: 4%–60%,	C: 63%–100% D: 74%–100%	C: 0.7 D: 1.1–3.2	C: 0.33–1.03 D: 0.5–0.98	C: 0.16–0.79 (kappa) D: 0.26–0.84 (kappa)	Albert et al[128] Flynn et al[105] Freburger and Riddle[129] van der Wurff et al[130] van der Wurff et al[131] Cibulka and Koldehoff[132] Blower and Griffin[133] Russell et al[134] Laslett and Williams[135] Kokmeyer et al[136] Ham et al[137] Laslett et al[138]
Gaenslen Test	21%–71%,	26%–72%,	0.75–2.2	0.65–1.12	0.54–0.76 (kappa)	Flynn et al[105] Laslett and Williams[135] Kokmeyer et al[136] Laslett et al[138] Broadhurst and Bond[140] Dreyfuss et al[141]
Posterior Shear (POSH) Test	80%	100%	NA	0.2	0.64–0.88 (kappa)	Flynn et al[105] Broadhurst and Bond[140] Laslett an Wililams[135]
Active Straight Leg Raise Test	87%	94%	14.5	0.13	0.82 (ICC)	Mens et al[95] Mens et al[142]

LR, likelihood ratio, NA, not available; ICC, intraclass correlation.

SPECIAL TESTING FOR THE LUMBOPELVIC SPINE

Special Tests for Symptom Reproduction
Quadrant Test (Fig. 28-38)

Purpose: To assess for closing dysfunction and intervertebral foramen pathology

Patient: Sitting in neutral

Clinician: Standing behind the patient

Procedure: The patient moves into extension, ipsilateral side bending and contralateral rotation with the assistance of the clinician. Overpressure is applied at end range.

Interpretation: The test is positive if there is a reproduction of radicular symptoms or local pain.

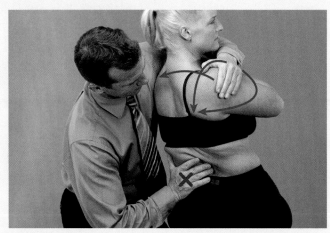

FIGURE 28–38 Quadrant test.

Special Tests for Neural Provocation
Straight Leg Raise Test

Purpose: To assess deficits in neural mobility and irritability of the sciatic nerve and its branches

Interpretation: The test is positive if there is a reproduction of neurological symptoms. From 0 to 35 degrees of hip flexion slack is taken up within the sciatic nerve, 35 to 70 degrees of hip flexion suggests limited neural mobility, and greater than 70 degrees denotes sacroiliac joint–related symptoms.

Straight Leg Raise-Sciatic Nerve Bias (Fig. 28-39)

Patient: Supine

Clinician: Standing at the patient's feet

Procedure: The clinician passively moves the patient into hip flexion, adduction, internal rotation, knee extension, followed by dorsiflexion of the ankle.

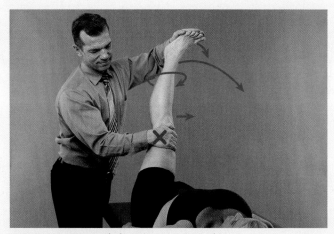

FIGURE 28–39 Straight leg raise-sciatic nerve bias.

Straight Leg Raise-Tibial Nerve Bias (Fig. 28-40)

Patient: Supine

Clinician: Standing at the patient's feet

Procedure: The clinician passively moves the patient into hip flexion, adduction, internal rotation, knee extentsion, followed by dorsiflexion and eversion of the ankle and extension of the toes.

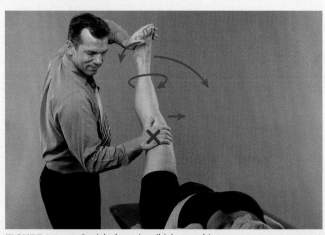

FIGURE 28–40 Straight leg raise-tibial nerve bias.

Straight Leg Raise-Common Peroneal Nerve Bias (Fig. 28-41)

Patient: Supine

Clinician: Standing at the patient's feet

Procedure: The clinician passively moves the patient into hip flexion, adduction, internal rotation, knee extension, followed by plantarflexion and inversion of the ankle.

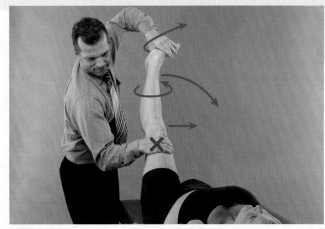

FIGURE 28–41 Straight leg raise-common peroneal nerve bias.

Straight Leg Raise-Sural Nerve Bias (Fig. 28-42)

Patient: Supine

Clinician: Standing at the patient's feet

Procedure: The clinician passively moves the patient into hip flexion, adduction, internal rotation, knee extension, followed by dorsiflexion and inversion of the ankle.

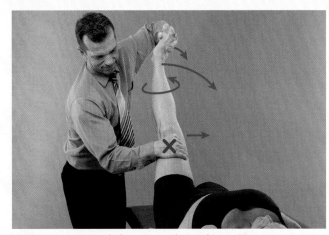

FIGURE 28–42 Straight leg raise-sural nerve bias.

Bowstring Test (Fig. 28-43)

Purpose: To assess deficits in neural mobility and irritability

Patient: Supine

Clinician: Standing at the patient's feet

Procedure: Perform a SLR to the point of discomfort, then flex the knee approximately 20 degrees to relieve symptoms then pressure is applied with the clinician's thumb to the popliteal area

Interpretation: The test is positive if there is a reproduction of radicular symptoms upon palpation of the popliteal fossa.

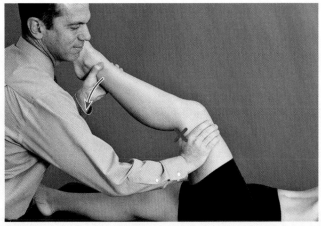

FIGURE 28–43 Bowstring test.

Prone Knee Bend

Purpose: To assess deficits in neural mobility and irritability of the femoral nerve and its branches

Interpretation: The test is positive if there is a reproduction of neurological symptoms.

Prone Knee Bend-Femoral Nerve Bias (Fig. 28-44)

Patient: Prone

Clinician: Standing at the patient's feet

Procedure: With the hip in neutral, the clinician passively flexes the knee.

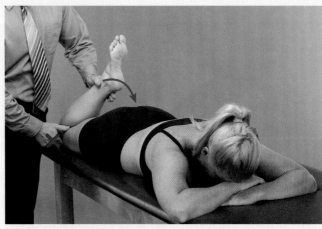

FIGURE 28–44 Prone knee bend-femoral nerve bias.

Prone Knee Bend-Lateral Femoral Cutaneous Nerve Bias (Fig. 28-45)

Patient: Prone

Clinician: Standing at the patient's feet

Procedure: The clinician passively extends and adducts the patient's hip and flexes the knee.

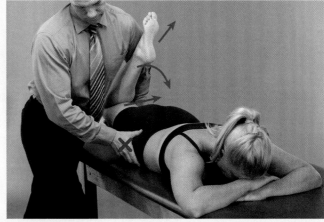

FIGURE 28–45 Prone knee bend-lateral femoral cutaneous nerve bias.

Prone Knee Bend-Saphenous Nerve Bias (Fig. 28-46)

Patient: Prone

Clinician: Standing at the patient's feet

Procedure: The clinician passively extends, abducts, and externally rotates the hip, extends the knee, and dorsiflexes and everts the ankle.

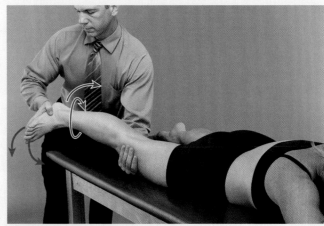

FIGURE 28–46 Prone knee bend-saphenous nerve bias.

Slump Test (Fig. 28-47)

Purpose: To assess deficits in neural mobility and irritability

Patient: Sitting

Clinician: Standing to the side of the patient.

Procedure: The patient moves into trunk flexion, cervical flexion, knee extension, and ankle dorsiflexion with the assistance of the clinician. Should symptoms arise, the exact position of each segment within the reproducible position is documented. While holding the reproducible position, the cervical spine is released and moved out of flexion. The impact of the change in the cervical position on the patient's symptoms is noted.

Interpretation: The test is positive if there is a reproduction of neurological symptoms, particularly if the symptoms diminish when the cervical component is released.

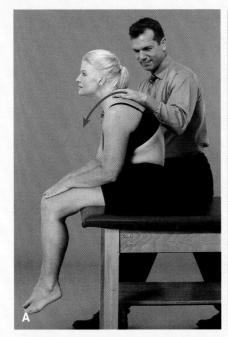
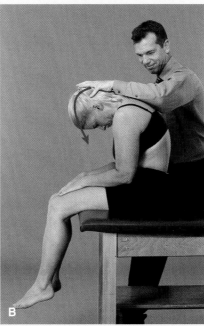
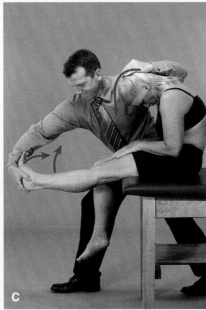
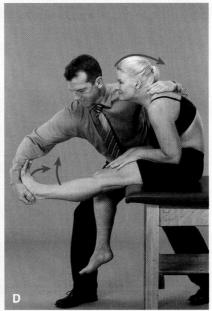

FIGURE 28–47 Slump test including **A.** trunk flexion, **B.** add neck flexion, **C.** add knee extension and ankle dorsiflexion, and **D.** release neck flexion while maintaining knee extension and ankle dorsiflexion.

Brudzinski-Kernig Test (Fig. 28-48)

Purpose: To assess meningeal irritation, dural irritation, nerve root involvement

Patient: Supine, with hands behind the head

Clinician: Standing at the patient's feet

Procedure: The patient flexes the neck and actively performs an SLR. If symptoms emerge, the knee is flexed, and changes in symptoms are monitored. Neck flexion and hip flexion may be performed individually.

Interpretation: The test is positive if there is a reduction in symptoms upon flexing the knee.

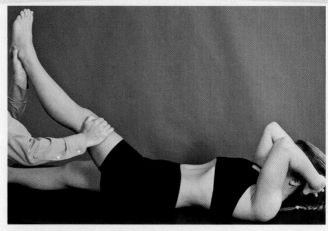

FIGURE 28–48 Brudzinski-Kernig test. (Courtesy of Bob Wellmon Photography, BobWellmon.com.)

Bike Test (Fig. 28-49)

Purpose: To distinguish between the presence of neurogenic versus intermittent claudication.

Patient: Sitting on the bike

Clinician: Standing and monitoring symptoms

Procedure: The patient is in an erect sitting posture while pedaling on an upright bike followed by pedaling in a slumped position, while the patient's response to each position is monitored.

Interpretation: Neurogenic claudication is suspected if there is a reproduction of leg pain and/or paresthesia upon pedaling that reduces when the patient slumps. Intermittent vascular claudication is suspected if there is no change in symptoms when the patient slumps.

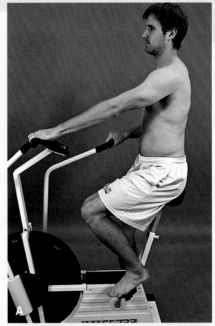

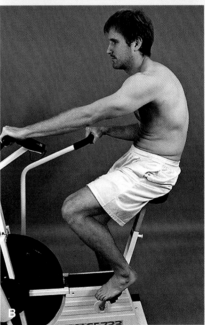

FIGURE 28–49 A, B Bike test. (Courtesy of Bob Wellmon Photography, BobWellmon.com.)

Special Tests for Segmental Instability
Prone Instability Test (Fig. 28-50)

Purpose: To assess lumbar segmental stability

Patient: Forward bent over the table with feet on the floor

Clinician: Standing to the side of the patient

Procedure: The clinician performs central anterior glides over the lumbar vertebrae with and without the patient's feet on the floor.

Interpretation: The test is positive if there is increased mobility and reproduction of symptoms with the feet on the floor, which subsides when the feet are lifted.

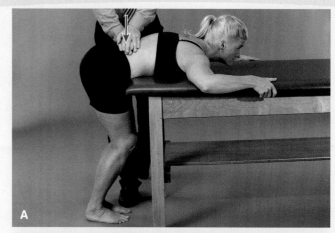
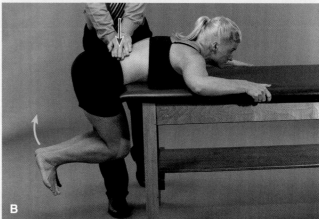

FIGURE 28–50 Prone instability test with **A.** feet on the floor and **B.** feet off the floor.

Spine Torsion Test (Fig. 28-51)

Purpose: To assess lumbar segmental stability

Patient: Side-lying

Clinician: Standing facing the patient

Procedure: The clinician produces rotation of the spine from above down to the segment to be tested, then provides overpressure while the pelvis is stabilized to localize force to the desired segment.

Interpretation: The test is positive if there is tissue laxity while providing overpressure into rotation and a reproduction of the chief complaint.

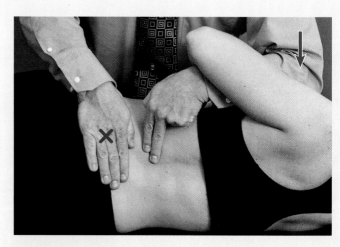

FIGURE 28–51 Spine torsion test. (Courtesy of Bob Wellmon Photography, BobWellmon.com.)

Pheasant Test (Fig. 28-52)

Purpose: To assess lumbar segmental stability

Patient: Prone

Clinician: Standing to side of patient

Procedure: The clinician passively flexes the patient's knee while anterior pressure is applied to the spinal segment.

Interpretation: The test is positive if there is a reproduction of symptoms over the tested segment.

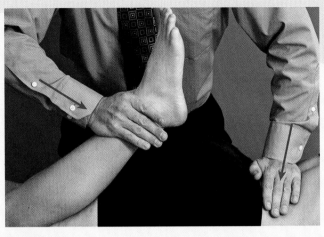

FIGURE 28–52 Pheasant test. (Courtesy of Bob Wellmon Photography, BobWellmon.com.)

Anterior Instability Test (Fig. 28-53):

Purpose: To assess lumbar segmental stability

Patient: Side-lying with the hips and knees flexed to 90 degrees

Clinician: The clinician stands in front of the patient with the patient's knees at the ASIS

Procedure: The clinician applies force through the long axis of the femurs as the superior vertebra of the tested segment is palpated for motion.

Interpretation: The test is positive if there is increased mobility between adjacent vertebrae and reproduction of symptoms upon testing.

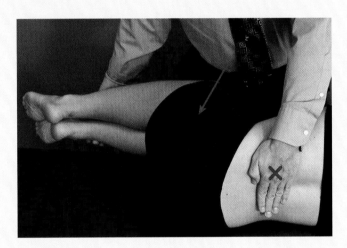

FIGURE 28–53 Anterior instability test. (Courtesy of Bob Wellmon Photography, BobWellmon.com.)

Posterior Instability Test (Fig. 28-54)

Purpose: To assess lumbar segmental stability

Patient: Sitting, with the elbows flexed on the clinician's chest

Clinician: Standing in front of the patient

Procedure: Pressure is applied through the patient's flexed elbows while stabilizing the caudal segment with both hands.

Interpretation: The test is positive if there is increased mobility between adjacent vertebrae and reproduction of symptoms upon testing.

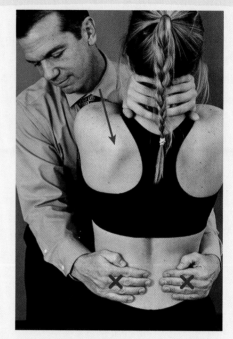

FIGURE 28–54 Posterior instability test. (Courtesy of Bob Wellmon Photography, BobWellmon.com.)

Farfan Torsion Test (Fig. 28-55)

Purpose: To assess lumbar segmental stability

Patient: Prone

Clinician: Standing to the side of the patient with one hand stabilizing the trunk, the other hand holding the anterior aspect of the ilium

Procedure: While stabilizing trunk, the clinician moves the contralateral ilium into rotation.

Interpretation: The test is positive if there is laxity while providing overpressure into rotation and reproduction of symptoms upon testing.

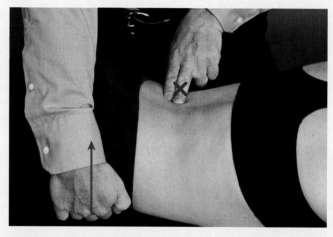

FIGURE 28–55 Farfan torsion test. (Courtesy of Bob Wellmon Photography, BobWellmon.com.)

Special Tests for Sacroiliac Joint Dysfunction:

Supine to Long Sit Test (Fig. 28-56)

Purpose: To assess for true leg length discrepancy versus a positional impairment of the sacroiliac joint(s)

Patient: Supine, then long sitting

Clinician: Standing at the patient's feet with hand contact at the patient's bilateral medial malleoli

Procedure: The clinician palpates the medial malleoli while the patient moves from supine to long sitting

Interpretation: Short-to-long leg position = posterior ilial rotation; long-to-short leg position = anterior ilial rotation; short leg with no change = length discrepancy or ilial upslip.

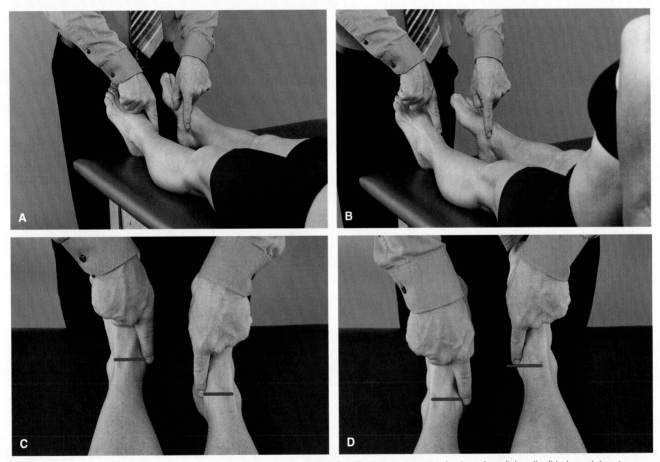

FIGURE 28–56 Supine to long sit test, which includes **A.** palpation of medial malleoli in supine, **B.** palpation of medial malleoli in long sitting. An appreciation of the medial malleoli relative to one another reveals **C.** right leg shorter/left leg longer in supine compared with **D.** right leg longer/left leg sorter in long sitting. A change in relative malleoli position between supine and sitting suggests the presence of a sagittal plane iliosacral positional fault.

Sacroiliac Compression and Distraction Test
(Fig. 28-57)

Purpose: To assess for the presence of sacroiliac joint dysfunction

Patient: Supine or side-lying

Clinician: Standing to the side of the patient with hands on the patient's iliac crests

Procedure: For compression, patient is supine or side-lying as an inward/downward force through the lateral aspect of the iliac crests is applied. For distraction, the patient is supine as an outward force is applied through the iliac crests.

Interpretation: The test is positive if there is reproduction of sacroiliac joint pain.

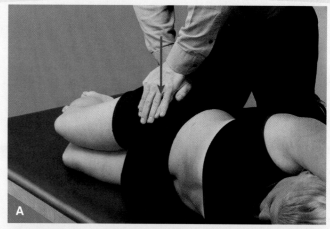
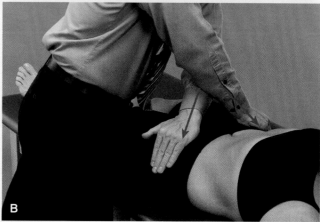

FIGURE 28–57 Sacroiliac **A.** compression test and **B.** distraction test.

Gaenslen Test (Fig. 28-58)

Purpose: To assess for the presence of sacroiliac joint dysfunction

Patient: Supine

Clinician: Standing to the side of the patient

Procedure: A single knee to chest maneuver is performed passively while the other leg remains extended over the edge of the table. Gentle overpressure is provided at end range.

Interpretation: The test is positive if there is reproduction of sacroiliac joint pain.

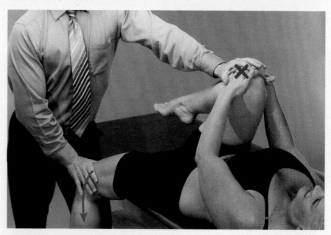

FIGURE 28–58 Gaenslen test.

Posterior Shear (POSH) Test (Fig. 28-59)

Purpose: To assess for the presence of sacroiliac joint dysfunction

Patient: Supine with the hip in flexion, slight abduction, and external rotation

Clinician: Standing to side of the patient and supporting the leg

Procedure: Force is applied through the long axis of the femur.

Interpretation: The test is positive if there is reproduction of sacroiliac joint pain.

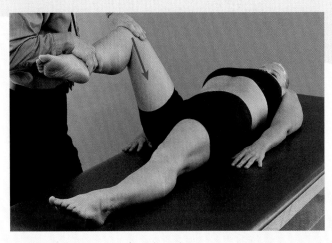

FIGURE 28–59 Posterior shear (POSH) test.

Active Straight Leg Raise Test (Fig. 28-60)

Purpose: To assess for pelvic instability

Patient: Supine

Clinician: Standing to side of the patient

Procedure: The patient performs an active SLR. If symptoms are noted, the clinician exerts a medially directed force through bilateral ilia and monitors for any change in symptoms.

Interpretation: The test is positive if there is pain with the active SLR that abolishes when external force is applied.

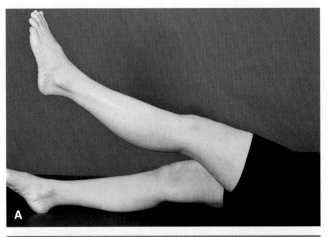

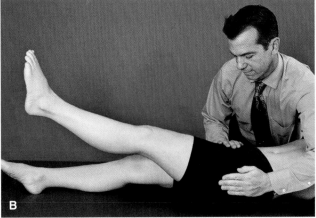

FIGURE 28–60 Active straight leg raise test. **A. B.** (Courtesy of Bob Wellmon Photography, BobWellmon.com.)

JOINT MOBILIZATION OF THE LUMBOPELVIC SPINE

Note: The indications for the joint mobilization techniques described in this section are based on expected joint kinematics. Current evidence suggests that the indications for their use are multifactorial and may be based on direct assessment of mobility and an individual's symptomatic response.

Lumbar Spine Joint Mobilizations

Central and Unilateral Anterior Glides

Indications:

- *Central and unilateral anterior glides* are indicated for restrictions in segmental mobility in all directions. Central glides assist primarily with sagittal plane motion of forward and backward bending while unilateral glides enhance rotation and side bending.

Accessory Motion Technique (Fig. 28-61, Fig. 28-62, Fig. 28-63)

- **Patient/Clinician Position:** The patient is in a prone position with a pillow supporting the lumbar spine. Stand to the side of the patient.
- **Hand Placement:** As a general technique, stabilization is not required. The region of the hand just distal to the pisiform contacts the spinous process for central glides and the transverse process for unilateral glides while the mobilizing hand lies over the contact hand. The elbows are extended, and the forearms are in the direction in which force is applied. Alternate hand placement includes thumb-over-thumb pressure, or split finger contacts over

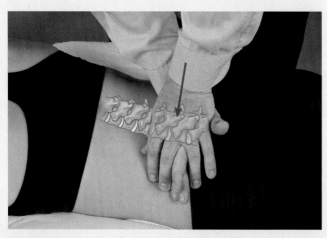

FIGURE 28–61 Central anterior glide with pisiform contact. (From: Wise CH, Gulick DT. *Mobilization Notes: A Rehabilitation Specialist's Pocket Guide.* Philadelphia, PA: FA Davis Company, 2009.)

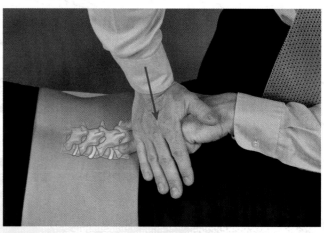

FIGURE 28–62 Central anterior glide with split finger contact. (From: Wise CH, Gulick DT. *Mobilization Notes: A Rehabilitation Specialist's Pocket Guide.* Philadelphia, PA: FA Davis Company, 2009.)

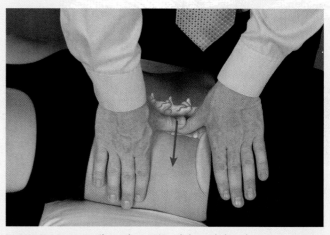

FIGURE 28–63 Unilateral anterior glide with hand contact over transverse process. (From: Wise CH, Gulick DT. *Mobilization Notes: A Rehabilitation Specialist's Pocket Guide.* Philadelphia, PA: FA Davis Company, 2009.)

the transverse processes of the same segment or the transverse processes of adjacent segments.

- **Force Application:** Anteriorly directed pressure is applied through hand contacts at either the spinous or transverse processes. Slight changes in force direction can be provided to improve specificity.

Accessory With Physiologic Motion Technique (Figs. 28-64, 28-65, 28-66, 28-67, 28-68)

- **Patient/Clinician Position:** The patient is sitting with the arms across the chest and a mobilization belt secured at the anterior aspect of the pelvis. You are standing behind the patient with the mobilization belt secured at your

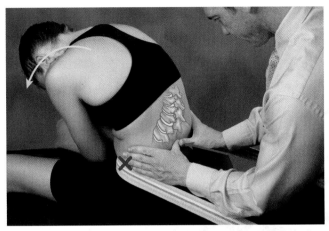

FIGURE 28–64 Central and unilateral anterior glide accessory with physiologic motion technique for forward-bending in sitting. (From: Wise CH, Gulick DT. *Mobilization Notes: A Rehabilitation Specialist's Pocket Guide*. Philadelphia, PA: FA Davis Company, 2009.)

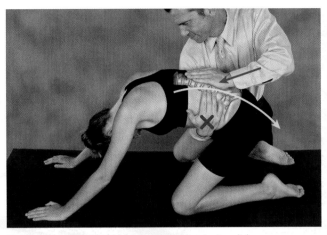

FIGURE 28–67 Central and unilateral anterior glide accessory with physiologic motion technique for forward-bending in quadruped. (From: Wise CH, Gulick DT. *Mobilization Notes: A Rehabilitation Specialist's Pocket Guide*. Philadelphia, PA: FA Davis Company, 2009.)

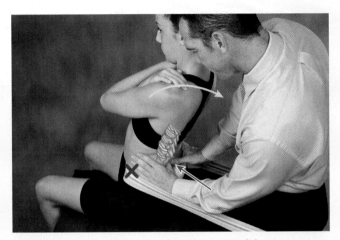

FIGURE 28–65 Central and unilateral anterior glide accessory with physiologic motion technique for backward-bending in sitting. (From: Wise CH, Gulick DT. *Mobilization Notes: A Rehabilitation Specialist's Pocket Guide*. Philadelphia, PA: FA Davis Company, 2009.)

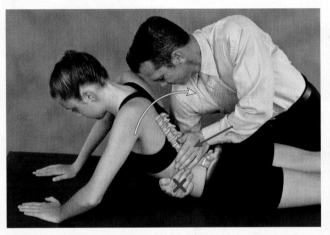

FIGURE 28–68 Central and unilateral anterior glide accessory with physiologic motion technique for backward-bending in prone. (From: Wise CH, Gulick DT. *Mobilization Notes: A Rehabilitation Specialist's Pocket Guide*. Philadelphia, PA: FA Davis Company, 2009.)

gluteal folds. An alternate position for forward bending involves the patient in a quadruped position such that the knees are far enough apart to allow for full range of motion. You are in a straddle stance position at the side of the patient. An alternate position for backward bending involves the patient in a prone press-up position. You are in a straddle stance position at the side of the patient.

- **Hand Placement:** Place thumb over thumb contact or hypothenar eminence contact at the transverse process or spinous process of the segment to be mobilized with your forearm in line with the direction in which force is applied. For the quadruped forward-bending technique and the prone backward-bending technique, the region just distal to the pisiform of your mobilization hand is in contact with the transverse process or spinous process of the segment to be mobilized with your forearm in line with the direction in which force is applied. Your stabilizing arm is placed around the patient's abdomen.

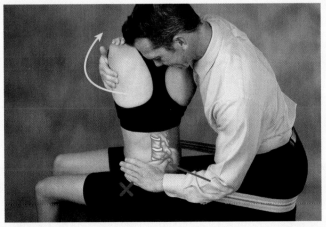

FIGURE 28–66 Central and unilateral anterior glide accessory with physiologic motion technique for rotation in sitting. (From: Wise CH, Gulick DT. *Mobilization Notes: A Rehabilitation Specialist's Pocket Guide*. Philadelphia, PA: FA Davis Company, 2009.)

- **Force Application:** As the patient actively moves into forward bending, backward bending, or rotation, apply force through your hand contacts in an anterior direction as the patient's pelvis is stabilized by the mobilization belt. You move as the patient moves in order to maintain the proper force direction throughout the motion. Force is maintained throughout the range of motion and sustained at end range. For the quadruped forward bending technique, as the patient actively moves into forward bending by bringing the buttocks to the heels, apply an antero-superior force through your mobilization hand as your stabilization arm supports the abdomen. Shift your weight from one foot to the other as the patient moves in order to maintain the proper force direction throughout the motion. Force is maintained throughout the range of motion and sustained at end range. For the prone backward-bending technique, as the patient actively moves into backward bending by performing a prone press-up, apply an antero-superior force through your mobilization hand as your stabilization arm supports the abdomen. Shift your weight from one foot to the other as the patient moves in order to maintain the proper force direction throughout the motion. Force is maintained throughout the entire range of motion and sustained at end range. Self-mobilization is performed using mobilization strap or towel placed over the segment to be mobilized, and force is applied while the patient performs active physiologic motion.

Physiologic Forward Bending

Indications:

- *Physiologic forward-bending mobilization* is indicated for restrictions in physiologic segmental forward bending and/or to improve facet joint opening.

Accessory Motion Technique (Figs. 28-69, 28-70)

- **Patient/Clinician Position:** The patient is supine in a double knee to chest position. You are standing in a straddle stance position at the side of the patient. An alternate position consists of the patient in a side-lying position with one third of the thigh over the edge of the table and the tibial tuberosity of the uppermost leg or both legs resting on your ASIS.
- **Hand Placement:** Your cephalad arm is placed at the anterior aspect of the patient's bilateral knees in order to control motion and keep the patient's knees close to the patient's chest. Your caudal hand is placed over the inferior vertebra of the segment being mobilized. In side-lying, the cephalad hand stabilizes at the spinous or transverse processes of the superior aspect of the segment being mobilized. The caudal hand is placed across the sacrum with fingers contacting the spinous or transverse processes of the inferior aspect of the segment to be mobilized.
- **Force Application:** Both of your hand contacts work together to produce a scooping motion that brings the

segment to be mobilized into forward bending. Your cephalad arm contact may resist the patient's hip extension force followed by further mobilization into forward bending. In the side-lying position, the clinician shifts weight from the caudal to the cephalad leg, creating physiologic forward bending. Your stabilization hand maintains constant force as the mobilization hand localizes forward-bending forces to the segment being mobilized.

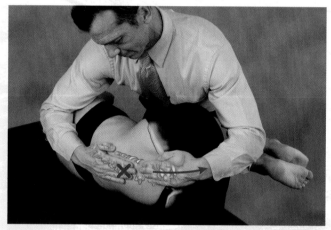

FIGURE 28–69 Physiologic forward-bending in side-lying. (From: Wise CH, Gulick DT. *Mobilization Notes: A Rehabilitation Specialist's Pocket Guide.* Philadelphia, PA: FA Davis Company, 2009.)

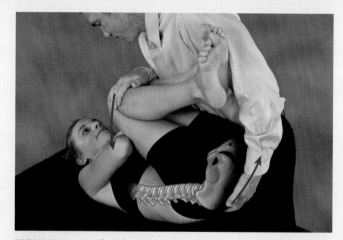

FIGURE 28–70 Physiologic forward-bending in supine. (From: Wise CH, Gulick DT. *Mobilization Notes: A Rehabilitation Specialist's Pocket Guide.* Philadelphia, PA: FA Davis Company, 2009.)

Accessory With Physiologic Motion Technique

- **Patient/Clinician Position:** The patient is in a seated position to stabilize the pelvis. Quadruped or standing positions may also be used. Stand behind or to the side of the patient. A mobilization belt may be placed from the clinician to the anterior aspect of the patient's pelvis to provide stabilization during force application.

- **Hand Placement:** Hand placement is the same as that which was described for the Central and Unilateral Anterior Glides Accessory With Physiologic Motion Technique
- **Force Application:** Force application is the same as that which was described for the Central and Unilateral Anterior Glides Accessory With Physiologic Motion Technique

Physiologic Backward Bending

Indications:

- *Physiologic backward bending mobilization* is indicated for restrictions in physiologic segmental backward bending and/or to improve facet joint closing.

Accessory Motion Technique (Fig. 28-71)

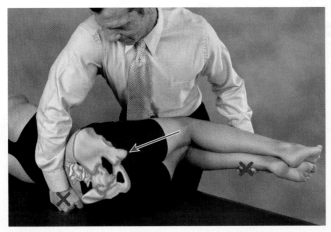

FIGURE 28–71 Physiologic backward-bending in side-lying. (From: Wise CH, Gulick DT. *Mobilization Notes: A Rehabilitation Specialist's Pocket Guide.* Philadelphia, PA: FA Davis Company, 2009.)

- **Patient/Clinician Position:** The patient is in a side-lying position with the hips and knees flexed to the segment to be mobilized with one third of the patient's thighs over the edge of the table and fixed on your ASIS. Stand in a straddle stance position facing the patient.
- **Hand Placement:** The cephalad hand provides stabilization at the spinous or transverse processes of the superior aspect of the segment to be mobilized. The caudal hand maintains the patient's flexed knees against the clinician's ASIS.
- **Force Application:** Apply force through the long axis of the patient's thigh as you stabilize the superior aspect of the segment to which mobilization force is being directed.

Accessory With Physiologic Motion Technique

- **Patient/Clinician Position:** The patient is in a sitting position to stabilize the pelvis. Prone or standing positions may also be used. You are standing behind or to the side of the patient. A mobilization belt may be placed from the

clinician to the anterior aspect of the patient's pelvis to provide stabilization during force application.

- **Hand Placement:** Hand placement is the same as that which was described for the Central and Unilateral Anterior Glides Accessory With Physiologic Motion Technique.
- **Force Application:** Force application is the same as that which was described for the Central and Unilateral Anterior Glides Accessory With Physiologic Motion Technique.

Physiologic Side Bending With Finger Block

Indications:

- *Physiologic side-bending mobilization with finger block* is indicated for restrictions in physiologic segmental side bending and/or to improve facet joint opening or closing.

Accessory Motion Technique (Figs. 28-72, 28-73)

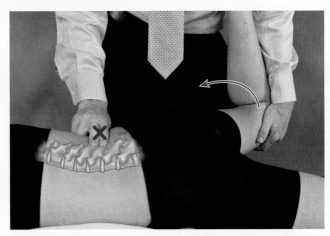

FIGURE 28–72 Physiologic side bending with finger block in prone (From: Wise CH, Gulick DT. *Mobilization Notes: A Rehabilitation Specialist's Pocket Guide.* Philadelphia, PA: FA Davis Company, 2009.)

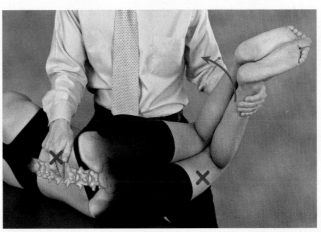

FIGURE 28–73 Physiologic side bending with finger block in side-lying. (From: Wise CH, Gulick DT. *Mobilization Notes: A Rehabilitation Specialist's Pocket Guide.* Philadelphia, PA: FA Davis Company, 2009.)

- **Clinician/Patient Position:** The patient is in a prone position with a pillow supporting the lumbar spine. You are in a straddle stance position at the side of the patient. Alternately, the patient is in a side-lying position with one third of the thighs over edge of table and resting on your anterior leg.
- **Hand Placement:** Your mobilization hand grasps the patient's closest leg just proximal to the knee with the patient's knee flexed or extended. Digits 2 and 3 or the thumb of your stabilization hand is placed along the side of the spinous process of the superior vertebra of the segment being mobilized on the side that you are standing. In the sidelying position, digits 2 and 3 or the thumb of your stabilization hand is placed at the upper side of the spinous process of the superior vertebra of the segment being mobilized and your other hand grasps the patient's ankles, which support the patient's flexed knees against your leg.
- **Force Application:** Move the patient's leg into abduction until movement arrives at the segment being mobilized. Force is localized by providing a finger block to the superior aspect of the target segment. In the sidelying position, move the patient's legs up or down creating rotation of the hips and subsequent sidebending of the lumbar spine. Recruit motion to the segment being mobilized and block movement with your stabilization hand for the purpose of localizing forces. Force is delivered to the segment to be mobilized by imparting motion to the lumbar spine through the leg. A prolonged stretch or oscillations are performed by moving the patient's leg against the blocked segment.

Accessory With Physiologic Motion Technique (Fig. 28-74)

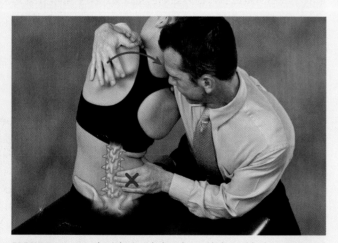

FIGURE 28–74 Physiologic side bending with finger block accessory with physiologic motion technique in sitting. (From: Wise CH, Gulick DT. *Mobilization Notes: A Rehabilitation Specialist's Pocket Guide.* Philadelphia, PA: FA Davis Company, 2009.)

- **Patient/Clinician Position:** The patient is in a sitting position to stabilize the pelvis with arms crossed. You are standing at the side of the patient.
- **Hand Placement:** With one arm woven through the patient's folded arms to control trunk movement into side bending, the other hand provides the finger block. A mobilization belt may be placed from the clinician to the anterior aspect of the patient's pelvis to provide stabilization during force application. Your finger or thumb is placed to the side of the spinous process immediately inferior to the segment to be mobilized on the side ipsilateral to the direction of side bending.
- **Force Application:** The finger block is maintained while the patient performs active side bending as you control and assist this motion down to the segment to be mobilized. Force is maintained throughout the entire range of motion and sustained at end range. A sustained hold and/or oscillations may be performed at end range.

Physiologic Rotation With Finger Block

Indications:

- *Physiologic rotation mobilization with finger block* is indicated for restrictions in physiologic segmental rotation and/or to improve facet joint opening or closing.

Accessory Motion Technique (Fig. 28-75)

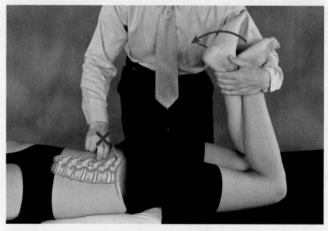

FIGURE 28–75 Physiologic rotation with finger block in prone. (From: Wise CH, Gulick DT. *Mobilization Notes: A Rehabilitation Specialist's Pocket Guide.* Philadelphia, PA: FA Davis Company, 2009.)

- **Patient/Clinician Position:** The patient is in a prone position, with a pillow supporting the lumbar spine with the knees extended or flexed. Stand to the side of the patient.
- **Hand Placement:** A finger or thumb block is provided at the side of the superior spinous process of the segment to

be mobilized as with the side-bending mobilization. With the patient's knees extended, your mobilizing forearm moves the gluteals aside as the hand grasps the patient's ASIS. Alternately, with the patient's knees flexed, grasp the patient's ankles in order to induce movement.

- **Force Application:** Your mobilization hand contact at the patient's ASIS imparts an upward force through the pelvis, which creates lumbar rotation at the segment to be mobilized. Alternately, lumbar rotational forces are produced through movement of the legs from side to side. A sustained hold and/or oscillations are performed by moving the pelvis or legs against the blocked segment.

Accessory With Physiologic Motion Technique (Fig. 28-76)

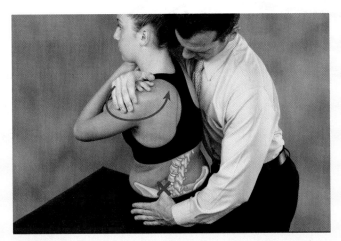

FIGURE 28–76 Physiologic rotation with finger block accessory with physiologic motion technique in sitting. (From: Wise CH, Gulick DT. *Mobilization Notes: A Rehabilitation Specialist's Pocket Guide*, PA. Philadelphia: FA Davis Company, 2009.)

- **Patient/Clinician Position:** The patient is in a sitting position to stabilize the pelvis with arms crossed. You are standing at the side of the patient.
- **Hand Placement:** With one arm woven through the patient's folded arms to control trunk movement into rotation, the other hand provides the finger block. A mobilization belt may be placed from the clinician to the anterior aspect of the patient's pelvis to provide stabilization during force application. Your finger or thumb is placed to the side of the spinous process immediately inferior to the segment to be mobilized on the side contralateral to the direction of rotation or on the transverse process on the side ipsilateral to the direction of rotation.
- **Force Application:** The finger block is maintained while the patient performs active rotation as you control and assist this motion down to the segment to be mobilized. Force is maintained throughout the entire range of motion and sustained at end range. A sustained hold and/or oscillations may be performed at end range.

Sacroiliac Joint Mobilizations

Iliosacral Anterior/Posterior Rotation Isometric Mobilization (Fig. 28-77)

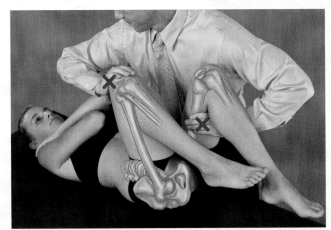

FIGURE 28–77 Iliosacral anterior/posterior rotation isometric mobilization. (From: Wise CH, Gulick DT. *Mobilization Notes: A Rehabilitation Specialist's Pocket Guide*. Philadelphia, PA: FA Davis Company, 2009.)

- **Indications:** *Iliosacral anterior rotation mobilization* is indicated for restrictions in IS anterior rotation or in the presence of a posteriorly rotated innominate positional fault. *Iliosacral posterior rotation mobilization* is indicated for restrictions in IS posterior rotation or in the presence of an anteriorly rotated innominate positional fault.
- **Patient/Clinician Position:** The patient is in a supine position with the hips in a variable degree of flexion. Stand at the side of the patient.
- **Hand Placement:** Your mobilization hand is placed at the anterior aspect of the distal thigh to mobilize the pelvis into anterior rotation and at the posterior aspect of the distal thigh to mobilize the pelvis into posterior rotation. Your stabilization hand provides counterforce on the alternate side of the contralateral thigh.
- **Force Application:** Use simultaneous force/counterforce by applying equal force through both hand contacts, simultaneously. Resisted isometric contraction of the hip flexors imparts an anterior rotation force to the pelvis, and resisted isometric contraction of the hip extensors imparts a posterior rotation force.

Iliosacral Anterior Rotation

- **Indications:** *Iliosacral anterior rotation mobilization* is indicated for restrictions in IS anterior rotation or in the presence of a posteriorly rotated innominate positional fault.

Accessory Motion Technique (Fig. 28-78)

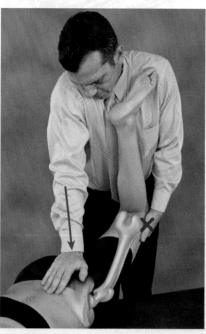

FIGURE 28-78 Iliosacral anterior rotation. (From: Wise CH, Gulick DT. *Mobilization Notes: A Rehabilitation Specialist's Pocket Guide.* Philadelphia, PA: FA Davis Company, 2009.)

- **Patient/Clinician Position:** The patient is in a prone position in a diagonal orientation on the table with one foot on the floor. You are in a stride stance position facing the same direction as the patient.
- **Hand Placement:** Stabilization of the contralateral pelvis is provided through the patient's foot in contact with the floor. Your caudal hand grasps the distal aspect of the patient's anterior thigh just proximal to the knee as the hypothenar eminence of your cephalad hand contacts the posterior superior iliac spine on the side being mobilized with your forearm in line with the direction in which force is applied.
- **Force Application:** Your caudal hand moves the patient's hip into extension as your cephalad hand applies an anterosuperior force through the posterior superior iliac spine. Between each progression, the patient may impart an isometric hip flexion force into your caudal hand contact at the anterior thigh for the purpose of utilizing the hip flexors to impart an additional anterior rotatory force followed by further movement of the hip into extension with simultaneous anterosuperior mobilization force provided by your cephalad hand.

Accessory With Physiologic Motion Technique (Fig. 28-79) 🌐

- **Patient/Clinician Position:** The patient is standing in a lunge or half-kneeling position with the leg on the side being mobilized placed behind the other leg. You are standing contralateral to the side being mobilized in a straddle stance position prepared to move as the patient moves.
- **Hand Placement:** Your stabilization arm and hand is placed over the patient's abdomen and your mobilization

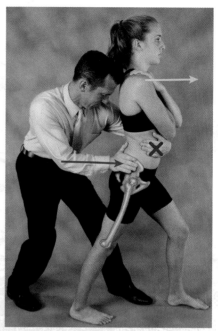

FIGURE 28-79 Iliosacral anterior rotation accessory with physiologic motion technique. (From: Wise CH, Gulick DT. *Mobilization Notes: A Rehabilitation Specialist's Pocket Guide.* Philadelphia, PA: FA Davis Company, 2009.)

hand is placed at the PSIS with your arm in line with the direction of force.
- **Force Application:** The patient gently shifts weight from the back leg to the front leg producing hip extension on the side being mobilized. This motion is performed as you impart an anteriorly-directed force through your PSIS contact while maintaining stabilization at the abdomen. Force is maintained throughout the entire range of motion and sustained at end range.

Iliosacral Posterior Rotation

Indications:
- *Iliosacral posterior rotation mobilization* is indicated for restrictions in IS posterior rotation or in the presence of an anteriorly rotated innominate positional fault.

Accessory Motion Technique (Fig. 28-80)
- **Patient/Clinician Position:** The patient is in a side-lying position facing you with the side to be mobilized uppermost and the hip flexed to 90 degress. You are standing in a straddle stance position facing the patient with the posterior aspect of the uppermost thigh against your trunk.
- **Hand Placement:** Stabilization is provided by maintaining the patient's contralateral hip in neutral and in contact with the table. The palm of your cephalad hand contacts the patient's ASIS and the palm of your caudal hand contacts the patient's ischial tuberosity on the side being mobilized, with your forearms in opposite directions in line with the direction in which force is applied.
- **Force Application:** Move the patient's hip into flexion. After taking up the slack in the joint, apply equal and opposite forces

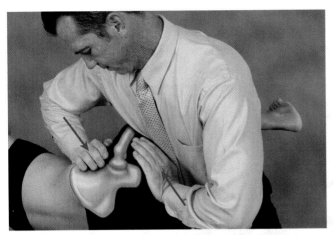

FIGURE 28-80 Iliosacral posterior rotation. (From: Wise CH, Gulick DT. *Mobilization Notes: A Rehabilitation Specialist's Pocket Guide.* Philadelphia, PA: FA Davis Company, 2009.)

through both of your hand contacts. Between each progression, the patient may impart an isometric hip extension force into your trunk for the purpose of utilizing the hip extensors to impart an additional posterior rotatory force followed by further movement of the hip into flexion with simultaneous mobilization force provided through your hand contacts.

Accessory With Physiologic Motion Technique (Fig. 28-81)

- **Patient/Clinician Position:** The patient is in a standing position. You are standing contralateral to the side being mobilized in a straddle stance position prepared to move as the patient moves.

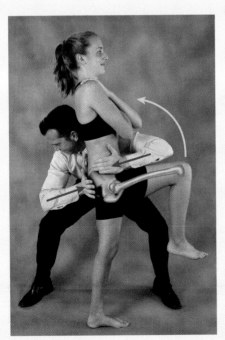

FIGURE 28-81 Iliosacral posterior rotation accessory with physiologic motion technique (From: Wise CH, Gulick DT. *Mobilization Notes: A Rehabilitation Specialist's Pocket Guide.* Philadelphia, PA: FA Davis Company, 2009.)

- **Hand Placement:** Your stabilization hand is placed over the patient's sacrum and your mobilization hand is placed at the ASIS with your arm in line with the direction of force.
- **Force Application:** The patient actively flexes the hip on the side being mobilized. This motion is performed as you impart a posteriorly directed force through your ASIS contact while maintaining stabilization at the sacrum. Force is maintained throughout the entire range of motion and sustained at end range.

Iliosacral Downslip

Indications:

- *Iliosacral downslip mobilization* is indicated for restrictions in mobility or in the presence of an upslip positional fault of the innominate.

Accessory Motion Technique (Fig. 28-82)

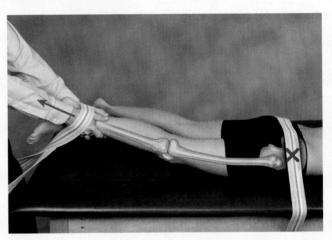

FIGURE 28-82 Iliosacral downslip. (From: Wise CH, Gulick DT. *Mobilization Notes: A Rehabilitation Specialist's Pocket Guide.* Philadelphia, PA: FA Davis Company, 2009.)

- **Patient/Clinician Position:** The patient is in a supine position when mobilization into posterior rotation is also being performed, or prone when mobilization into anterior rotation is also being performed. The hip is pre-positioned in adduction and internal rotation. Alternately, the patient is side-lying with the side being mobilized uppermost. Stand in a straddle stance position at the foot of the patient facing cephalad.
- **Hand Placement:** Stabilization is provided by the patient's weight. Both of your hands grasp the distal leg just proximal to the ankle or proximal to the knee as required with your forearms in the direction in which force is applied. Your hand contacts may be reinforced by placing the mobilization belt in a figure eight. When the patient is side-lying, your cephalad hand grasps the uppermost iliac crest.

- **Force Application:** Shift your weight from the front leg to the back leg while maintaining your hand contacts. With patient side-lying, impart a caudal force through the hand contact. Perform sustained hold and/or oscillations as indicated.

Accessory With Physiologic Motion Technique

- **Patient/Clinician Position:** The patient is standing on a step with leg on the side being mobilized off of the step. Kneel at the front, back, or side of the patient.
- **Hand Placement:** With both hands, grasp the distal aspect of the leg on the side being mobilized.
- **Force Application:** Apply a caudally directed force through the leg on the side being mobilized and subsequently through the pelvis. An alternate technique involves the patient in a side-lying position with the patient actively producing pelvic downslip during application of force by the clinician through the iliac crest. Force is maintained throughout the entire range of motion and sustained at end range.

Iliosacral Outflare/Inflare

Indications:

- *Iliosacral outflare and inflare mobilization* is indicated for restrictions in mobility or a positional fault of the innominate.

Accessory Motion Technique (Figs. 28-83, 28-84)

- **Patient/Clinician Position:** The patient is in a supine position with the hips in neutral. Stand on the side of the patient being mobilized for outflare and on the contralataral side for inflare.
- **Hand Placement:** Stabilization is provided by the patient's weight. For outflare, one hand grasps the medial aspect of the patient's ASIS as the other grasps the PSIS. For inflare, one hand grasps the lateral aspect of the ASIS as the other hand grasps the PSIS. Your forearms are in the direction in which force is applied.

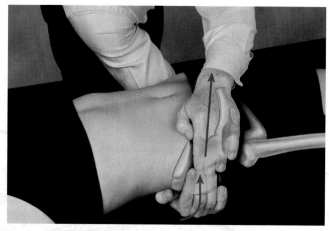

FIGURE 28–84 Iliosacral inflare. (From: Wise CH, Gulick DT. *Mobilization Notes: A Rehabilitation Specialist's Pocket Guide.* Philadelphia, PA: FA Davis Company, 2009.)

- **Force Application:** Apply force through both hand contacts moving the ASIS laterally and PSIS medially for outflare or moving the ASIS medially and PSIS laterally for inflare.

Accessory With Physiologic Motion Technique (Figs. 28-85, 28-86)

- **Patient/Clinician Position:** The patient is in a standing position. Stand contralateral to the side being mobilized.
  Hand Placement: For outflare, the stabilization hand contacts the PSIS or sacrum, and the mobilization hand contacts the medial aspect of ASIS. For inflare, the stabilization arm is placed across the abdomen, and the mobilization hand contacts the lateral aspect of the ASIS.

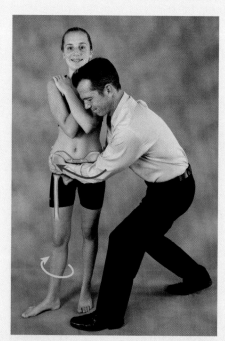

FIGURE 28–85 Iliosacral outflare accessory with physiologic motion technique in standing. (From: Wise CH, Gulick DT. *Mobilization Notes: A Rehabilitation Specialist's Pocket Guide.* Philadelphia, PA: FA Davis Company, 2009.)

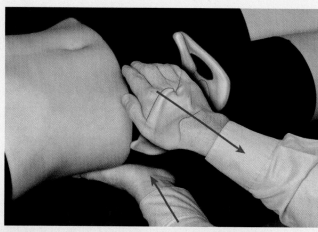

FIGURE 28–83 Iliosacral outflare. (From: Wise CH, Gulick DT. *Mobilization Notes: A Rehabilitation Specialist's Pocket Guide.* Philadelphia, PA: FA Davis Company, 2009.)

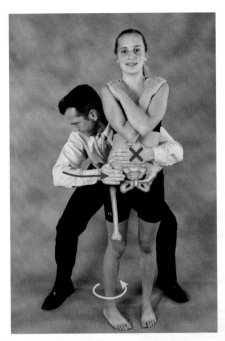

FIGURE 28–86 Iliosacral inflare accessory with physiologic motion technique in standing. (From: Wise CH, Gulick DT. *Mobilization Notes: A Rehabilitation Specialist's Pocket Guide.* Philadelphia, PA: FA Davis Company, 2009.)

- **Force Application:** For outflare, the patient performs hip ER as force is applied through the ASIS in a posterolateral direction with sacral stabilization. For inflare, the patient performs hip IR as force is applied through the ASIS in an anteromedial direction with abdominal stabilization.

Sacroilial Forward and Backward Bending

Indications:
- *Sacroilial forward and backwardbending mobilization* is indicated for restrictions in mobility or a positional fault of the sacrum.

Accessory Motion Technique (Figs. 28-87, 28-88)

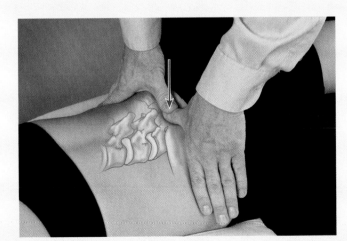

FIGURE 28–87 Sacroilial forward-bending in prone. (From: Wise CH, Gulick DT. *Mobilization Notes: A Rehabilitation Specialist's Pocket Guide.* Philadelphia, PA: FA Davis Company, 2009.)

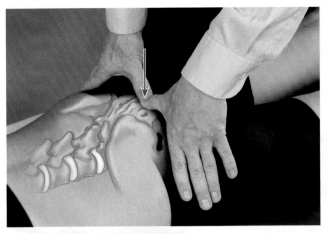

FIGURE 28–88 Sacroilial backward-bending in prone. (From: Wise CH, Gulick DT. *Mobilization Notes: A Rehabilitation Specialist's Pocket Guide.* Philadelphia, PA: FA Davis Company, 2009.)

- **Patient/Clinician Position:** The patient is in a prone position, with the hips in ER for sacroilial forward bending and IR for sacroilial backward bending. Stand at the side of the patient.
- **Hand Placement:** Stabilization is provided by patient's weight. For sacroilial forward bending, the aspect of the hand just distal to your pisiform or thumb over thumb contacts the base of the sacrum. For sacroilial backward bending, the aspect of the hand just distal to your pisiform or thumb over thumb contacts the apex of the sacrum. Your forearms are in the direction in which force is applied.
- **Force Application:** Apply force through your hand contacts. Sacroilial forward bending mobilization may be timed with expiration and sacroilial backward bending mobilization may be timed with inspiration.

Accessory With Physiologic Motion Technique (Figs. 28-89, 28-90)
- **Patient/Clinician Position:** The patient is in a sitting or standing position. You are standing or squatting behind the patient.
- **Hand Placement:** Stabilization is provided to the ilium as the patient is in a sitting position. Stabilization may also be provided by placing your arm across the patient's abdomen. Thumb over thumb contact or the region just distal to the pisiform is placed at the sacral base for overpressure into sacroilial forward bending or counterpressure for sacroilial backward bending or at the sacral apex for overpressure into sacroilial backward bending or counterpressure for sacroilial forward bending.
- **Force Application:** For sacroilial forward bending, the patient actively moves into lumbar backward bending as you impart force through your contact at the base of the sacrum for overpressure or at the apex of the sacrum for counterpressure. For sacroilial backward bending, the

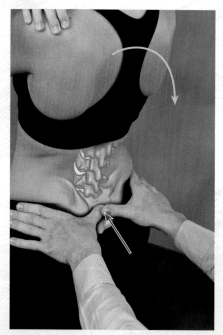

FIGURE 28–89 Sacroilial forward-bending accessory with physiologic motion technique in sitting. (From: Wise CH, Gulick DT. *Mobilization Notes: A Rehabilitation Specialist's Pocket Guide.* Philadelphia, PA: FA Davis Company, 2009.)

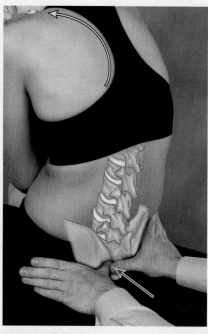

FIGURE 28–90 Sacroilial backward-bending accessory with physiologic motion technique in sitting. (From: Wise CH, Gulick DT. *Mobilization Notes: A Rehabilitation Specialist's Pocket Guide.* Philadelphia, PA: FA Davis Company, 2009.)

patient actively moves into lumbar forward bending as force is imparted through your contact at the apex of the sacrum for overpressure or at the base of the sacrum for counterpressure. Force is maintained throughout the entire range of motion and sustained at end range. Self-mobilization for sacroilial forward bending or backward

bending may be performed using fist pressure or ball and mobilization strap.

Sacroilial Forward and Backward Torsion

Indications:
- *Sacroilial forward and backward torsion mobilization* is indicated for restrictions in mobility or a positional fault of the sacrum.

Accessory Motion Technique (Figs. 28-91, 28-92)

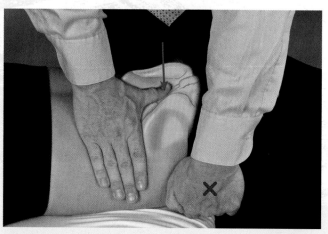

FIGURE 28–91 Sacroilial forward torsion in prone. (From: Wise CH, Gulick DT. *Mobilization Notes: A Rehabilitation Specialist's Pocket Guide.* Philadelphia, PA: FA Davis Company, 2009.)

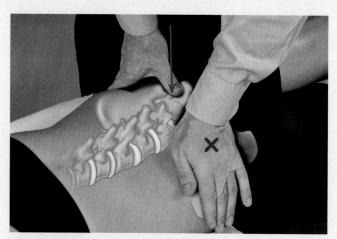

FIGURE 28–92 Sacroilial backward torsion in prone. (From: Wise CH, Gulick DT. *Mobilization Notes: A Rehabilitation Specialist's Pocket Guide.* Philadelphia, PA: FA Davis Company, 2009.)

- **Patient/Clinician Position:** The patient is in a prone position with the hip in ER on the side to which a forward torsion mobilization is being performed and with the hip in IR on the side to which a backward torsion mobilization is being performed. Stand behind or contralateral to the side being mobilized.

- **Hand Placement:** For sacroilial forward torsion, your stabilization hand contacts the ASIS on the side being mobilized. For sacroilial backward torsion, your stabilization hand contacts the PSIS on the side being mobilized. For sacroilial forward torsion, the aspect of the hand just distal to your pisiform or thumb of your mobilization hand contacts the sacral sulcus on the side being mobilized. For sacroilial backward torsion, the aspect of the hand just distal to your pisiform or thumb contacts the sacral inferior lateral angle contralateral to the side being mobilized.
- **Force Application:** Apply force through your mobilization hand contact while maintaining stabilization. Sacroilial forward torsion mobilizations may be timed with expiration and sacroilial backward torsion mobilizations may be timed with inspiration.

Accessory With Physiologic Motion Technique (Figs. 28-93, 28-94)

- **Patient/Clinician Position:** The patient is in a sitting or standing position. You are standing or squatting behind the patient.
- **Hand Placement:** Stabilization is provided to the ilium as the patient is in a sitting position. Stabilization may also be provided by placing your arm across the patient's abdomen. Thumb over thumb contact or the region just distal to your pisiform is placed at the right or left sacral sulcus for overpressure into left or right sacroilial forward torsion, respectively, or counterpressure for right or left sacroilial forward torsion, respectively. Thumb over thumb contact or the

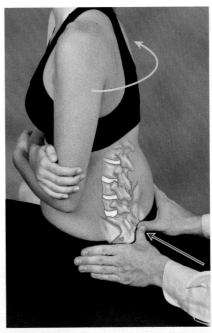

FIGURE 28-94 Sacroilial backward torsion accessory with physiologic motion technique in sitting. (From: Wise CH, Gulick DT. *Mobilization Notes: A Rehabilitation Specialist's Pocket Guide.* Philadelphia, PA: FA Davis Company, 2009.)

region just distal to your pisiform is placed at the right or left sacral inferior lateral angle for overpressure into left or right sacroilial backward torsion, respectively, or counterpressure for right or left sacroilial backward torsion, respectively. Your forearm is in line with the direction in which force is applied.

- **Force Application:** For sacroilial forward torsion, the patient actively moves into rotation as you impart force through your contact at the contralateral sacral sulcus for overpressure or at the ipsilateral sacral sulcus for counterpressure. For sacroilial backward torsion, the patient actively moves into rotation as you impart force through your contact at the contralateral inferior lateral angle of the sacrum for overpressure or at the ipsilateral inferior lateral angle of the sacrum for counterpressure. Force is maintained throughout the entire range of motion and sustained at end range.

Lumbar Rotation Mobilization With Ligamentous Tension Locking High-Velocity Thrust (Fig. 28-95) 🌐

- **Indications:** *Lumbar rotation mobilization high-velocity thrust* is indicated for restrictions in unilateral opening of a segment, to provide symptomatic relief, or to restore a segment to a neutral position. Ligamentous tension locking increases the specificity of this procedure. *Clinical prediction* rules are available to guide clinical decision-making in the use of this procedure. See Chapter 18 for more

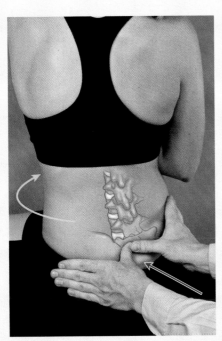

FIGURE 28-93 Sacroilial forward torsion accessory with physiologic motion technique in sitting. (From: Wise CH, Gulick DT. *Mobilization Notes: A Rehabilitation Specialist's Pocket Guide.* Philadelphia, PA: FA Davis Company, 2009.)

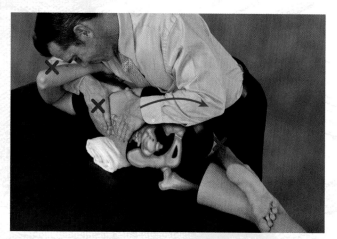

FIGURE 28–95 Lumbar rotation mobilization with ligamentous tension locking high-velocity thrust. (From: Wise CH, Gulick DT. *Mobilization Notes: A Rehabilitation Specialist's Pocket Guide.* Philadelphia, PA: FA Davis Company, 2009.)

information related to clinical prediction rules for the use of high-velocity thrust.

- **Patient/Clinician Position:** The patient is in a right side-lying position facing you with both hips and knees flexed. The patient is close enough to you to allow 1/3 of the thighs to be placed over the edge of the table. You are in a straddle stance position facing the patient. The patient set-up is as follows:
  1. You place the patient's knee of the upper leg in contact with your ASIS.
  2. Supporting the patient's upper leg with your caudal hand, move from left to right while palpating with your cephalad hand for motion to arrive at the lumbar interspinous space of the segment being mobilized.
  3. Once motion is felt to arrive at the desired segment, the patient's foot of the upper leg is placed behind the knee of the lower leg for stabilization.
  4. Your caudal hand is now moved to the interspinous space to monitor motion as your cephalad hand grasps the patient's lower arm and gently pulls toward the ceiling thus producing rotation down to the desired segment.
- **Hand Placement:** Your caudal hand is placed at the patient's posterior buttock and your cephalad hand weaves through the patient's upper arm in order to allow your cephalad hand to produce a skin lock with the caudal hand as your cephalad hand fingers are placed at the upper side of the spinous process of the superior vertebra of the segment being mobilized and the fingers of your caudal hand block the underside of the spinous process of the inferior vertebra of the segment being mobilized. An alternate hand contact uses the caudal forearm at the gluteals.
- **Force Application:** With all hand contacts in place, the patient is rotated toward you to place the trunk in a position that is perpendicular to the table. Slack is taken up until the ligamentous tension lock is engaged. Force is then applied

by either your cephalad arm contact through the patient's trunk while the cadual arm blocks at the pelvis or vice versa. The patient takes a deep breath and as they slowly exhale, slack is taken up and a high-velocity low amplitude thrust is delivered at end range. Alternately, using the gluteal contact, force is delivered superiorly and anteriorly in order to close the involved segment.

Lumbopelvic Regional High-Velocity Thrust (Fig. 28-96)

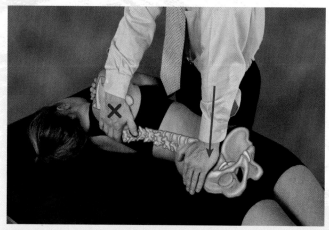

FIGURE 28–96 Lumbopelvic regional high-velocity thrust. (From: Wise CH, Gulick DT. *Mobilization Notes: A Rehabilitation Specialist's Pocket Guide.* Philadelphia, PA: FA Davis Company, 2009.)

- **Indications:** The *lumbopelvic regional high-velocity thrust* is indicated for restrictions in the lumbopelvic region and for symptomatic relief of low back pain. *Clinical prediction rules are* available to guide clinical decision-making in the use of this procedure. See Chapter 18 for more information related to clinical prediction rules for the use of high-velocity thrust.
- **Patient/Clinician Position:** The patient is in a supine position with hands clasped behind the neck. You are standing contralateral to the side being mobilized. Create sidebending away from you by bringing the patient's hips toward you.
- **Hand Placement:** Your caudal hand contact is placed at the patient's contralateral ASIS with your forearm in the direction of force and your cephalad hand is weaved through the patient's arms or contacts the posterior aspect of the patient's contralateral scapula.
- **Force Application:** Your hand contact at the patient's arms or scapula rotates the patient's trunk toward you until you feel motion arrive at the patient's ASIS. Once motion arrives at the ASIS, cease further rotation. While maintaining this position, impart a high-velocity low-amplitude thrust in a posterior direction through your hand contact at the patient's ASIS.

CLINICAL CASE

CASE 1

History of Present Illness (HPI)

A 28-year-old male reports to your office noting an incident that occurred 2 weeks ago involving twisting to the left and forceful hyperflexion secondary to being struck with a large rock. He intermittently reports tingling into the posterior aspect of his right leg to his knee primarily noted with prolonged sitting and unilateral weight bearing on the right. He reports a previous experience of tripping into a ditch at work approximately 6 months ago. He notes that since his injury, he has been inactive and spends much of his time sitting and playing video games. His pain is at a 3/10 level of intensity.

Self-Assessed Disability: Fear Avoidance Beliefs Questionnaire (FABQ) (work subscale) = 21

Inspection: Antalgic gait with decreased heel strike on the right

Neurological Screen: All within normal limits (WNL)

AROM

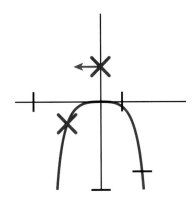

PPIVM: Hypomobile with FB, SB right, ROT left.

PAIVM: Hypomobility with central anterior glides over L2-3 region and unilateral anterior glides over the right transverse process of L2. R1 and R2 identified before onset of pain.

IS Mobility Tests: PSIS-FB test is positive.

SI Mobility Tests: Sit-slump = positive during slump; sacral spring = positive at sacral apex.

Strength: 4/5 strength in gluteus medius with pain, upper abdominals = 4/5, lower abdominals = 3+/5, prone transverse abdominis drawing-in = 3 mm Hg pressure decrease held for maximum of 5 sec for 2 repetitions

Palpation: Tenderness to the touch at the right midbuttock and right PSIS with increased lower extremity symptoms upon palpation, tenderness to the touch at the right greater trochanter, and significant guarding noted at bilateral paravertebral musculature.

Special Tests: SLR (sural nerve bias) = positive, Gaenslen test = positive, POSH = positive, supine to long sit = positive (right leg short in supine, long in sitting), quadrant = positive, Pheasant test = negative, Waddell test = positive on 4/5.

1. Perform each component of the exam on a partner.
2. Develop a problem list of impairments.
3. Establish a pathoanatomically based diagnosis.
4. Establish an impairment-based diagnosis.

5. Create a plan of care that includes three mobilizations, three stretching exercises, three progressive resistance exercises. Perform each on your partner.

CASE 2

HPI

A 15-year-old female reports to your clinic today with LBP at 8/10 level of intensity. She reports onset of symptoms over the past year due to increased competitive participation in gymnastics. Despite her symptoms, she has continued to participate and compete, which requires training 2 to 3 hours, 5 days/week. She is preparing for pre-Olympic tryouts. She currently reports paresthesia that occurs intermittently into the posterior aspect of the left leg and into the plantar aspect of her foot.

Self-Assessed Disability: Oswestry Disability Index = 42%

AROM

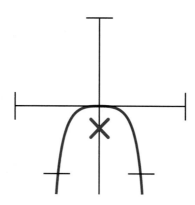

PPIVM: Hypomobility FB, SB bilateral, ROT bilateral L1-L4

PAIVM: Central anterior glides: L1-L4: RI/R2 before P1/P2, L5: positive for reproduction of symptoms, including left LE paresthesia.

Hip PROM: Bilateral hip extension = 5 degrees, right hip IR = 25 degrees, left hip IR = 15 degrees.

Strength: Prone transverse abdominis drawing in: 6 mm Hg for 5 sec hold x 5 repetitions until form fatigue. Segmental multifidus testing reveals erector spinae dominance.

Neurological Screen: Myotomes: left plantar flexion = 3/5 with inability to perform toe walking without assistance; all else = 5/5. Dermatomes and DTRs = WNL.

Palpation: Increased tissue tension and tone over the thoracolumbar paraspinal musculature. A palpable band of hypertrophy is noted over the L5-S1 segment. Increased guarding over this segment is noted in standing compared to prone lying with support.

Special Tests: SLR (tibial nerve bias) = positive at 20 degrees, slump test = positive with knee at 20 degrees, SI gap/compression = negative, FABER = negative, prone instability test = positive, anterior instability test = positive.

1. Perform each component of the exam on a partner.
2. Develop a problem list of impairments.
3. Establish a pathoanatomically based diagnosis.
4. Establish an impairment-based diagnosis.

5. Create a plan of care that includes three mobilizations, three stretching exercises, three progressive resistance exercises. Perform each on your partner.

CASE 3

HPI

T.J. is a 27-year-old male who presents to your facility today with complaint of severe right lumbosacral pain at an 8/10+ level of intensity, which occurred 2 days ago while performing repetitive lifting activities at work involving lifting 50-pound boxes from the floor to overhead. Upon further questioning, he describes radiating pain and numbness into the posterior aspect of his right leg and into his foot. His symptoms are constant in nature, and he has been unable to find significant relief with movement or position. Increased symptoms are noted with all motions, particularly when he attempts to stand erect. You notice his inability to sit in the waiting room, and when he is standing you observe a moderate left lateral shift and forward bent posture. He is currently out of work and on Workers'

Compensation until further notice. Diagnostic tests have been ordered but not yet performed. Self-Assessed Disability: Roland-Morris score is 18.

AROM: FB and repeated FB (flexion) in standing (RFIS) (5×) is approximately 25%, with an increase in his right LE symptoms, BB and repeated BB (extension) in standing (REIS) (5×) is 50% with pain in the lumbosacral region only.

Neurological Screen: DTRs: Right Achilles =3+, all else is WNL. Light touch sensation is diminished at the plantar aspect of the right foot only. Myotomal scan reveals weakness for ankle plantar flexion.

1. Perform each component of the exam on a partner.
2. Develop a problem list of impairments.
3. Establish a pathoanatomically based diagnosis.
4. Establish an impairment-based diagnosis.
5. Create a plan of care that includes three mobilizations, three stretching exercises, and three strengthening exercises. Perform each on your partner.

HANDS-ON

With a partner, perform the following activities:

1 Discuss the value of using self-assessment disability questionnaires during the examination of individuals with low back pain. What is the minimal clinically important difference (MCID) that must occur for each of the questionnaires to reveal a clinically significant change in an individual's status.

2 With the spine adequately exposed, observe your partner as he or she performs active lumbopelvic motion in standing for 5-10 repetitions in each plane. Appreciate both the quality and quantity of available motion. Identify any areas of hypo- or hypermobility and any motions that produce pain, any motions that feel restricted, and any motions that feel unstable. Assess whether or not your partner is demonstrating normal lumbopelvic rhythm during forward and backward bending, as described. Perform an active motion assessment on another individual as they stand side by side and identify any differences in each individual's movement pattern.

3 Perform the process of PPIVM and PAIVM testing for the lumbar spine, as described above. Determine the relationship between the onset of pain (P1 and P2), if present, and stiffness or resistance (R1 and R2), if present during PPIVM and PAIVM testing. Compare your findings during the active movement assessment with your findings during PPIVM and PAIVM testing. Perform PPIVM and PAIVM on at least one other individual and record any differences. Solicit feedback from your partner regarding your performance of these procedures.

4 If your partner presents with low back discomfort or pain, attempt to identify your partner's reproducible sign, region of origin, and reactivity level (the 3 R's). Perform regional movement differentiation (RMD) on your partner, which uses both overpressure and counterpressure to identify the most likely anatomic origin of your partner's discomfort. Classify the primary region of origin as either a lumbar spine, sacroilial, iliosacral, hip, or hybrid syndrome.

5 Through palpation, attempt to identify the primary soft tissue and bony structures of the lumbopelvic spine and compare tissue texture, tension, tone, and location bilaterally.

6 Perform each of the special tests used for identification of lumbar segmental instability on your partner. What is the sensitivity and specificity of these procedures? Perform each of the special tests used for identification of sacroiliac joint dysfunction (SJD) on your partner. What is the sensitivity and specificity of these procedures? What are some methods that you could use to identify further evidence that the SIJ is a component in an individual's low back complaints?

7 Based on your movement examination as identified above, choose 2 non-thrust mobilizations and 2 thrust mobilizations. Perform these mobilizations on your partner and, after reassessment, identify any immediate changes in mobility or symptoms in response to these procedures. If possible, video yourself performing these procedures and self-assess your performance. Solicit feedback from your partner regarding your performance of these procedures.

8 Perform each mobilization described in the intervention section of this chapter on at least two individuals. Using each technique, practice grades I to IV. Solicit input from your partner regarding position, hand placement, force application, comfort, etc. If possible, video yourself performing these procedures and self-assess your performance. When practicing these mobilization techniques, utilize the Sequential Partial Task Practice Method, in which students repeatedly practice one aspect of each technique (i.e., position, hand placement, force application) on multiple partners each time, adding the next component until the technique is performed in real time from beginning to end. (Wise CH, Schenk RJ, Lattanzi JB. A model for teaching and learning spinal thrust manipulation and its effect on participant confidence in technique performance. *J Manual & Manipulative Ther*, August 2014.)

9 Refer to Chapter 17 and discuss each of the systems for the classification of low back pain that are currently in use. Identify which system(s) are most evidence-based. Discuss the use of impairment-based models of classification and why they may be preferable over other models for the diagnosis and classification of low back pain. Describe how you might use each system to determine the differential diagnosis for each of the cases described above. How will the use of impairment-based models of classification impact or change your management of individuals with low back pain.

REFERENCES

1. Bogduk N, Twomey LT. *Clinical Anatomy of the Lumbar Spine*, 2nd ed. New York, NY: Churchill Livingstone; 1991.
2. Paris S, Loubert P. *FCO: Foundations of Clinical Orthopaedics*. St. Augustine, FL: Institute Press; 1990.
3. Oatis CA. *Kinesiology: The Mechanics and Pathomechanics of Human Movement*. Philadelphia, PA: Lippincott Williams & Wilkins; 2004.
4. Nachemson AL. Advances in low back pain. *Clin Orthop*. 1985;200:266-278.
5. Magee DJ. *Orthopedic Physical Assessment*, 4th ed. Philadelphia, PA: WB Saunders; 1992.
6. Esola MA, McClure PW, Fitzgerald GK, Siegler S. Analysis of lumbar spine and hip motion during forward bending in subjects with and without a history of low back pain. *Spine*. 1996;21:71-78.
7. McClure PW, Esola M, Schreier R, Siegler S. Kinematic analysis of lumbar and hip motion while rising from a forward, flexed position in patients with and without a history of low back pain. *Spine*. 1997;22:552-558.
8. Mellin G, Harkapaa K, Hurri H. Asymmetry of lumbar lateral flexion and treatment outcome in chronic low back pain patients. *J Spinal Disorders*. 1995;8:15-19.
9. Gertzbein S, Seligman J, Holthy R. Centrode patterns and segmental instability in degenerative disc disease. *Spine*. 1986;14:594-601.
10. Cook C. Lumbar coupling biomechanics-a literature review. *J Man Manip Ther*. 2003;11;137-145.
11. Solonen KA. The sacroiliac joint in the light of anatomical, roentgenological and clinical studies. *Acta Orthop Scand*. 1957;28(suppl):1-127.
12. Jackson R. *Pelvic Girdle Seminar Syllabus*. Middleburg, VA: Richard Jackson Seminars; 1995.
13. Erhard RE. *Manual Therapy in the Cervical Spine: Orthopaedic Physical Therapy Home Study Course 96-1*. Orthopaedic Section APTA; 1996.
14. Gray H. *Gray's Anatomy*. Philadelphia, PA: Lea and Febinger; 1995.
15. MacDonald GR, Hunt TE. Sacroiliac joints: observations on the gross and histological changes in the various age groups. *Can Med Assoc J*. 1952;66:157-163.
16. Prassopoulos PK, Faflia CP, Voloudaki AE, Gourtsoyiannis NC. Sacroiliac joints: anatomical variants on CT. *J Comput Assist Tomogr*. 1999;23:323-327.
17. Trotter M. Accessory sacroiliac articulations. *J Phys Anthropol*. 1937;22:247.
18. Vleeming A, Volkers ACW, Stoekart R, Snidjers CJ. Relation between form and function of the sacroiliac belt, pt II, biomechanical aspects. *Spine*. 1990.
19. Dijkstra PF, Vleeming A, Stoeckart R. Complex motion tomography of the sacroiliac joint. An anatomical and roentgenological study. *RöFo*. 1989;150:635-642.
20. Paquin JD, van der Rest M, Marie PJ, et al. Biochemical and morphologic studies of cartilage from the adult human sacroiliac joint. *Arthritis Rheum*. 1983;26:887-895.
21. Xu R, Ebraheim NA, Yeasting RA, Jackson WT. Anatomic considerations for posterior iliac bone harvesting. *Spine*. 1996;21:1017-1020.
22. Ebraheim NA, Elgafy H, Semaan HB. Computed tomographic findings in patients with persistent sacroiliac pain after posterior iliac graft harvesting. *Spine*. 2000;25:2047-2051.
23. Walker BF. Chronic low back pain: a summary and review. *COMSIG Rev*. 1992;1;9-11.
24. Smidt GL, Wei SH, McQuade K, Barakatt E, et al. Sacroiliac motion for extreme hip positions: a fresh cadaver study. *Spine*. 1997;22:2073-2082.
25. Bowen V, Cassidy JD. Macroscopic ad microscopic anatomy of the sacroiliac joint from embryonic life until the eighth decade. *Spine*. 1981;6:620-628.
26. Weisl H. The movements of the sacroiliac joint. *Acta Anat (Basel)*. 1955;23:80-91.
27. Colachis SC, Worden RE, Bechtol CO, Strohm BR. Movement of the sacroiliac joint in the adult male: a preliminary report. *Arch Phys Med Rehabil*. 1963;44:490-498.
28. Grieve EF. Mechanical dysfunction of the sacro-iliac joint. *Int Rehabil Med*. 1983;5:46-52.
29. Sturesson B, Selvik G, Uden A. Movements of the sacroiliac joints a roentgen stereophotogrammetric analysis. *Spine*. 1989;14:162-165.
30. Sturesson B, Uden A, Vleeming A. A radiostereometric anaylsis of the movements of the sacroiliac joints in the reciprocal straddle position. *Spine*. 2000;25:214-217.
31. MacLennan AH. The role of the hormone relaxin in human reproduction and pelvic girdle relaxation. *Scand J Rheumatol Suppl*. 1991;88:7-15.
32. Hagen R. Pelvic girdle relaxation from an orthopaedic point of view. *Acta Orthop Scand*. 1974;45:550-563.
33. Brooke R. The sacro-iliac joint. *J Anat*. 1924;58:299-305.
34. Resnick D, Niwayama G, Goergen TG. Degenerative disease of the sacroiliac joint. *Invest Radiol*. 1975;10:608-621.
35. Alderink GJ. The sacroiliac joint: review of anatomy, mechanics, and function. *J Orthop Sports Phys Ther*. 1991;13:71-84.
36. Lavignolle B, Vital JM, Senegas J, Destandau J, et al. An approach to the functional anatomy of the sacroiliac joints in vivo. *Anat Clin*. 1983;5:169-176.
37. Walheim GG, Olerud S, Ribbe T. Motion of the pubic symphysis in pelvic instability. *Scand J Rehabil Med*. 1984;16:163-169.
38. Walheim GG, Selvik G. Mobility of the pubic symphysis. In vivo measurements with an electromechanic method and a roentgen stereophotogrammetric method. *Clin Orthop Relat Res*. 1984;191:129-135.
39. Walheim G, Olerud S, Ribbe T. Mobility of the pubic symphysis. Measures by an electromechanical method. *Acta Orthop Scand*. 1984;55:203-208.
40. Fairbanks JC, Couper J, Davies JB, O'Brien JP. The oswestry low back pain disability questionnaire. *Physiotherapy*. 1980;66:271-273.
41. Fairbank J, Pynsent PB. The Oswestry Disability Index. *Spine*. 2000;25:2940-2953.
42. Fritz J, George S. The use of a classification approach to identify subgroups of patients with acute low back pain. *Spine*. 2000;25:106-114.
43. Ohnmeiss DD, Vanharanta H, Estlander AM, Jämsén A. The relationship of disability (Oswestry) and pain drawings to functional testing. *Eur Spine J*. 2000;9:208-212.

44. Triano JJ, McGregor M, Cramer GD, Emde DL. A comparison of outcome measures for use with back pain patients: results of a feasibility study. *J Manip Physiol Ther*. 1993;16:67-73.

45. Fisher K, Johnston M. Validation of the Oswestry Low Back Pain Disability Questionnaire, its sensitivity as a measure of change following treatment and its relationship with other aspects of the chronic pain experience. *Physiother Theory Pract*. 1997;13:67-80.

46. Beurskens AJHM, de Vet HCW, Koke AJA. Responsiveness of functional status in low back pain: a comparison of different instruments. *Pain*. 1996;65:71-76.

47. Flynn T, Fritz J, et al. A clinical prediction rule for classifying patients with low back pain who demonstrate short-term improvement with spinal manipulation. *Spine*. 2002;27:2835-2843.

48. Cleland JA, Fritz JM, Whitman JM, Childs JD, Palmer JA. The use of a lumbar spine manipulation technique by physical therapists in patients who satisfy a clinical prediction rule: a case series. *J Orthop Sports Phys Ther*. 2006;36:209-214.

49. Melzack R. The McGill Pain Questionnaire: major properties and scoring methods. *Pain*. 1975;1:277-299.

50. Blankenship KL. *Industrial Rehabilitation: The Basic Seminar: A Seminar Syllabus*. American Therapeutics; 1989.

51. Haas M, Nyiendo J. Diagnostic utility of the McGill Pain Questionaire and the Oswestry Disability Questionnaire for classification of low back pain syndromes. *J Man Physiol Ther*. 1992;15:90-98.

52. Ransford AO, Cairns D, Mooney V. The pain drawing as an aid to the psychological evaluation of patients with low-back pain. *Spine*. 1976;127:134.

53. Mooney V, Cairns D, Robertson J. A system for evaluation and treatment of chronic back disability. *West J Med*. 1976;124:370-376.

54. Roland M, Morris R. A study of the natural history of back pain, part I: the development of a reliable and sensitive measure of disability of low back pain. *Spine*. 1983;8:141-144.

55. Roland M, Morris R. A study of the natural history of low-back pain. Part II: development of guidelines for trials of treatment in primary care. *Spine*. 1983;8:145-150.

56. Roland M, Fairbank J. The Roland-Morris Disability Questionnaire and the Oswestry Disability Questionnaire. *Spine*. 2000;25:3115-3124.

57. Million R, Haavik Nilsen K, Jayson MIV, Baker RD. Evaluation of low back pain and assessment of lumbar corsets with and without back supports. *Ann Rheum Dis*. 1981;40:449-454.

58. Deyo RA, Diehl AK. Cancer as a cause of back pain: frequency, clinical presentation, and diagnostic strategies. *J Gen Intern Med*. 1988;3:230-238.

59. Boissonnault WG. *Primary Care for the Physical Therapist: Examination and Triage*. St. Louis, MO: Elsevier Saunders; 2005.

60. Nachemson A. The load on lumbar discs in different positions of the body. *Clin Rel Res*. 1966;45:107-112.

61. Wilder DG, Pope MH, Frymoyer FW. The biomechanics of lumbar disc herniation and the effect of overload and instability. *J Spinal Dis*. 1988;1:16-32.

62. Dreyfuss P, Michaelson M, Pauza K, McLarty J, Bogduk N. The value of medical history and physical examination in diagnosing sacroiliac joint pain. *Spine*. 1996;21:2594-2602.

63. Fortin JD, et al. Sacroiliac joint: pain referral maps upon applying a new injection/arthrography technique, part II: clinical evaluation. *Spine*. 1994;19:1483-1489.

64. Griegel-Morris P, Larson K, Mueller-Klaus K, Oatis CA. Incidence of common postural abnormalities in the cervical, shoulder, and thoracic regions and their association with pain in two age groups of healthy subjects. *Phys Ther*. 1992;72:425-431.

65. Matsui H, et al. Significance of sciatic scoliotic list in operated patients with lumbar disc herniation. *Spine*. 1998;23:338-342.

66. Levangie PK. The association between static pelvic asymmetry and low back pain. *Spine*. 1999;24:1234-1242.

67. Hart FD, Strickland D, Cliffe P. Measurement of spinal mobility. *Ann Rheum Dis*. 1974;33:136-139.

68. Mayer TG, Kondraske G, Beals SB, et al. Spinal range of motion: accuracy and sources of error with inclinometric measurement. *Spine*. 1997;22:1976-1984.

69. Moll JMH, Wright V. Measurement of spinal movement. In: Jason M, ed. *The Lumbar Spine and Back Pain*. New York, NY: Pitman Medical; 1976:93-112.

70. Cyriax JH, Cyriax PJ. *Cyriax's Illustrated Manual of Orthopaedic Medicine*, 2nd ed. Woburn, MA: Butterworth-Heinemann; 1993.

71. Okawa A, Shinomiya K, Komori H, Muneta T, et al. Dynamic motion study of the whole lumbar spine by videofluoroscopy. *Spine*. 23;1998:1743-1749.

72. Gonella C, Paris SV. Reliability in evaluating passive intervertebral motion. *Phys Ther*. 1982;62:436-444.

73. Maher C, Adams R. Reliability of pain and stiffness assessments in clinical manual lumbar spine examination. *Phys Ther*. 1995;74:801-811.

74. Binkley J, Stratford P, Gill C. Interrater reliability of lumbar accessory motion mobility testing. *Phys Ther*. 1995;75:786-795.

75. Maher C, Latimer J, Adams R. An investigation of the reliability and validity of posteroanterior spinal stiffness judgments made using a reference-based protocol. *Phys Ther*. 1998;78:829-837.

76. Bergmark A. Stability of the lumbar spine. A study in mechanical engineering. *Acta Orthop Scand*. 1989;230(suppl):20-24.

77. Richardson C, Jull G, Hodges P, Hides J. *Therapeutic Exercise for Spinal Segmental Stabilization in Low Back Pain. A Scientific Basis and Clinical Approach*. London, England: Churchill Livingston; 1999.

78. Potter NA, Rothstein JM. Intertester reliability for selected clinical tests of the sacroiliac joint. *Phys Ther*. 1985;65:1671-1675.

79. Laslett M, Williams M. The reliability of selected pain provocation tests for sacroiliac joint pathology. *Spine*. 1994;19:1243-1249.

80. Cibulka MT, Koldehoff R. Clinical usefulness of a cluster of sacroiliac joint tests in patients with and without low back pain. *J Orthop Sports Phys Ther*. 1999;29:83-92.

81. Lyle MA, Manes S, McGuinness M, et al. Relationship of physical examination findings & self-reported symptoms severity & physical function in patients with degenerative lumbar conditions. *Phys Ther*. 2005;85:120-133.

82. Jensen S. Back pain–clinical assessment. *Aus Fam Physician*. 2004;33.

83. Kuo L, Chung W, Bates E, Stephen J. The hamstring index. *J Pediatr Ortho*. 1997;17:78-88.

84. Breig A, Troup JDG. Biomechanical considerations in straight-leg-raising test: cadaveric & clinical studies of the effects of medical hip rotation. *Spine*. 1979;4:242-250.

85. Charnley J. Orthopedic signs in the diagnosis of disc protrusion with special reference to the straight-leg-raising test. *Lancet*. 1951;1:186-192.

86. Edgar MA, Park WM. Induced pain patterns on passive straight-leg-raising in lower lumbar disc protrusion. *J Bone Joint Surg Br*. 1974;56:658-667.

87. Fahrni WH. Observations on straight-leg-raising with special reference to nerve root adhesions. *Can J Surg*. 1966;9:44-48.

88. Goddard BS, JD Reid. Movements induced by straight-leg-raising in the lumbosacral roots, nerves, & plexus and in the intrapelvic section of the sciatic nerve. *J Neurol Neurosurg Psychiatry*. 1965;28:12-18.

89. Scham SM, Taylor TKF. Tension signs in lumbar disc prolapse. *Clin Orthop*. 1971;75:195-204.

90. Urban LM. The straight-leg-raising test: a review. *J Orthop Sports Phys Ther*. 1981;2:117-133.

91. Wilkins RH, Brody IA. Lasègue's sign. *Arch Neurol*. 1969;21:219-220.

92. Viikari-Juntura E, Porras M, Laasonen EM. Validity of clinical tests in the diagnosis of root compression in cervical disc disease. *Spine*. 1989;14:253-257.

93. Vroomen P, deKrom M, Knottnerus J. Consistency of history taking & physical examination in patients with suspected nerve root involvement. *Spine*. 2000;25:91-97.

94. Rose M. The statistical analysis of the intra-observer repeatability of four clinical measurement techniques. *Physiotherapy*. 1991;77:89-91.

95. Mens J, Vleeming A, Snijders C, Koes B, Stam H. Reliability & validity of the active straight leg raise test in posterior pelvic pain since pregnancy. *Spine*. 2003;26:1167-1171.

96. DeVille W, van der Windt D, Dzaferagic A, Bezemer P, Bouter L. The test of Lasegue Systemic: review of the accuracy in diagnosing herniated discs. *Spine*. 2000;25:1140-1147.

97. Jonsson B, Stromqvist B. The straight leg raising test & the severity of symptoms in lumbar disc herniation. *Spine*. 1995;20:27-30.

98. Kosteljanetz M, Espersen J, Halaburt H, Miletec T. Predictive value of clinical & surgical findings in patients with lumbago-sciatica. *Acta Neurochir*. 1984;73:67-76.

99. Cram RH. A sign of sciatic nerve root pressure. *J Bone Joint Surg Br*. 1953;35:192-195.

100. Evans RC. *Illustrated Essentials in Orthopedic Physical Assessment*. St. Louis, MO: Mosby; 1994.

101. Brudzinski J. A new sign of the lower extremities in meningitis of children (neck sign). *Arch Neurol*. 1969;21:217.

102. Meadows J. *Orthopedic Differential Diagnosis in Physical Therapy*. New York, NY: McGraw-Hill; 1999.

103. Riddle D, Freburger J. Evaluation of the presence of sacroiliac joint dysfunction using a combination of tests: a multicenter intertester reliability study. *Phys Ther*. 2002;82:772-781.

104. Postacchini F, Cinotti G, Gumina S. The knee flexion test: a new test for lumbosacral root tension. *J Bone Joint Surg Br*. 1993;75:834-835.

105. Flynn T, Fritz J, Whitman J, et al. A clinical prediction rule for classifying patients with low back pain who demonstrated short-term improvement with spinal manipulation. *Spine*. 2002;27:2835-2843.

106. Potter N, Rothstein J. Intertester reliability for selected clinical tests of the sacroiliac joint. *Phys Ther*. 1985;65:1671-1675.

107. Vincent-Smith B, Gibbons P. Inter-examiner & intra-examiner reliability of the standing flexion test. *Man Ther*. 1999;4:87-93.

108. Toussaint R, Gawlik C, Rehder U, Ruther W. Sacroiliac dysfunction in construction workers. *J Man Physiol Ther*. 1999;22:134-139.

109. Philip K, Lwe P, Matyas TA. The inter-therapist reliability of the slump test. *Aus J Phys Ther*. 1989;35:89-94.

110. Butler DA. *Mobilisation of the Nervous System*. Melbourne, Australia: Churchill Livingstone; 1991.

111. Fidel C, Martin E, Dankaerts W, et al. Cervical spine sensitizing maneuvers during the slump test. *J Man Manip Ther*. 1996;4:16-21.

112. Johnson EK, Chiarello CM. The slump test: the effects of head & lower extremity position on knee extension. *J Orthop Sports Phys Ther*. 1997;26:310-317.

113. Gabbe BJ, Bennell KL, Majswelner H, et al. Reliability of common lower extremity musculoskeletal screening tests. *J Phys Ther Sports*. 2004;5:90-97.

114. Stankovic R, Johnell O, Maly P, Willner S. Use of lumbar extension, slump test, physical & neurological examination in the evaluation of patients with suspected herniated nucleus pulposus. *Man Ther*. 1999;4:25-32.

115. Cipriano JJ. *Photographic Manual of Regional Orthopedic Tests*. Baltimore, MD: Williams & Wilkins; 1985.

116. Dyck P, Doyle JB. "Bicycle test" of van Gelderen in diagnosis of intermittent cauda equina compression syndrome. *J Neurosurg*. 1977;46:667-670.

117. Hicks GE, Fritz JM, Delitto A, Mishock J. Interrater reliability of clinical examination measures for identification of lumbar segmental instability. *Arch Phys Med Rehabil*. 2003;84:1858-1864.

118. Hicks GE, Fritz JM, Delitto A, McGill SM. Preliminary development of a clinical prediction rule for determining which patients with low back pain will respond to a stabilization exercise program. *Arch Phys Med Rehabil*. 2005;86:1753-1762.

119. Schneider M, Erhard R, Brach J, et al. Spinal palpation for lumbar segmental mobility & pain provocation: an interexaminer reliability study. *J Manipulative Physiol Ther*. 2008;31:465-473.

120. Fritz JM, Piva S, Childs J. Accuracy of the clinical examination to predict radiographic instability of the lumbar spine. *Eur Spine J*. 2005;14:743-750.

121. Dobbs AC. Evaluation of instabilities of the lumbar spine. *Ortho Phys Ther Clin N Am*. 1999;8:387-400.

122. Kirkaldy-Willis WH. *Managing Low Back Pain*. Edinburgh, Scotland: Churchill Livingstone; 1983.

123. Farfan HF. *Mechanical Disorders of the Low Back*. Philadelphia, PA: Lea & Febiger; 1973.

124. Young S, Aprill C. Characteristics of a mechanical assessment for chronic lumbar facet joint pain. *J Man Manip Ther*. 2000;8:78-84.

125. Palmer MC, Epler M. *Clinical Assessment Procedures in Physical Therapy*. Philadelphia, PA: JB Lippincott; 1990.

126. Bemis T, Daniel M. Validation of the long sitting test on subjects with iliosacral dysfunction. *J Orthop Sports Phys Ther*. 1987;8:336-345.

127. Levangie PK. Four clinical test of sacroiliac joint dysfunction; the association of test results with innominate torsion among patients with & without low back pain. *Phys Ther*. 1999;79:1043-1057.

128. Albert H, Godskesen M, Westergaard J. Evaluation of clinical tests used in classification procedures in pregnancy-related pelvic joint pain. *Eur Spine J*. 2000;9:161-166.

129. Freburger JK, Riddle DL. Measurement of sacroiliac joint dysfunction: a multicenter intertester reliability study. *Phys Ther*. 1999;79:1135-1141.

130. van der Wurff P, Hagmeijer RH, Meijne W. Clinical tests of the sacroiliac joint-a systematic methodological review, part 1-reliability. *Man Ther*. 2000;5:30-36.

131. van der Wurff P, Meijne W, Hagmeijer RH. Clinical tests of the sacroiliac joint-a systematic methodological review, part 2-validity. *Man Ther*. 2000;5:89-96.

132. Cibulka MT, Koldehoff R. Clinical usefulness of a cluster of sacroiliac joint tests in patients with and without low back pain. *J Orthop Sports Phys Ther*. 1999;29:83-92.

133. Blower P, Griffin A. Clinical sacroiliac tests in ankylosing spondylitis & other causes of low back pain. *Ann of Rheum Dis*. 1984;43:192-195.

134. Russell A, Maksymovich W, LeClerq S. Clinical examination of the sacroiliac joints. *Arthritis Rheum*. 1981;24:1575-1577.

135. Laslett M, Williams M. The reliability of selected pain provocation tests for sacroiliac joint pathology. *Spine*. 1994;19:1243-1249.

136. Kokmeyer D, van der Wuff P, Aufdemkampe G, Fickenscher T. Reliability of multi-test regimens with sacroiliac pain provocation tests. *J Manipulative Physiol Ther*. 2002;25:42-48.

137. Ham SJ, Walsum DP, Vierhout PAM. Predictive value of the hip flexion test for fractures of the pelvis. *Injury*. 1996;27:543-544.

138. Laslett M, April C, McDonald B, Young S. Diagnosis of sacroiliac joint pain: validity of individual provocation tests & composites of tests. *Man Ther*. 2005;10:207-218.

139. Russell A, Maksymovich W, LeClerq S. Clinical examination of the sacroiliac joints. *Arthritis Rheum*. 1981;24:1575-1577.

140. Broadhurst N, Bond M. Pain provocation tests for the assessment of sacroiliac joint dysfunction. *J Spinal Disorders*. 1998;11:341-345.

141. Dreyfuss P, Michaelsen M, Pauza K, McLarty J, Bogduk N. The value of medical history & physical examination in diagnosing sacroiliac joint pain. *Spine*. 1996;21:2594-2602.

142. Mens JM, et al. Validity of the active straight leg raise test for measuring disease severity in patients with posterior pelvic pain after pregnancy. *Spine*. 2002;27:196-200.

Orthopaedic Manual Physical Therapy of the Thoracic Spine and Costal Cage

Christopher H. Wise, PT, DPT, OCS, FAAOMPT, MTC, ATC

Chapter Objectives

At the conclusion of this chapter, the reader will be able to:

- Identify the key anatomical and biomechanical features of the thoracic spine and costal cage and their impact on examination and intervention.
- List and perform key procedures used in the orthopaedic manual physical therapy (OMPT) examination of the thoracic spine and costal cage.
- Demonstrate sound clinical decision-making in evaluating the results of the OMPT examination.

- Use pertinent examination findings to reach a differential diagnosis and prognosis.
- Discuss issues related to the safe performance of OMPT interventions for the thoracic spine and costal cage.
- Demonstrate basic competence in the performance of a skill set of joint mobilization techniques for the thoracic spine and costal cage.

FUNCTIONAL ANATOMY AND KINEMATICS

Introduction

The *thoracic spine* and its associated *costal cage* is comprised of 12 vertebrae and 12 paired costal segments and is sometimes referred to collectively as the *thorax*. The thoracic spine is mechanically stiffer and less mobile than either the cervical or lumbar regions and, therefore, a less common cause of spine-related impairment. The relative reduction in mobility that is characteristic of this region is related to the orientation of the thoracic articular processes, the ratio between intervertebral disc height and vertebral body height, and the intimate relationship that the thoracic spine shares with the costal cage. The thoracic spine and associated costal cage provide rigid support and protection for the vital organs that lie beneath. This structure also provides a stable foundation that facilitates optimal function of the diaphragm during respiration. Impairment of the thorax, therefore, may impact not only the musculoskeletal

system, but, by virtue of its functional demands, may also influence the respiratory, nervous, and circulatory systems as well. The 12 segments of the thoracic spine are configured to create a posterior convexity in the sagittal plane, known as **kyphosis.** This kyphosis is referred to as the primary spinal curve since it is the first to develop in utero. It serves to counterbalance the lordotic curves that are present in both the cervical and lumbar regions. Although less mobile than the remainder of the spine, the upper thoracic (T1-T4) and lower thoracic (T9-T12) segments often resemble adjacent spinal regions and possess an inclination toward greater degrees of mobility. The cervicothoracic and thoracolumbar regions are referred to as transitional vertebrae and have important clinical implications for the manual physical therapist.

Thoracic Spine Osteology

The kyphotic arrangement of the thoracic spine is due largely to the shape of the vertebral bodies, which possess greater height posteriorly. The magnitude of this posterior convexity increases with age and often becomes pathological primarily in older, postmenopausal females with osteoporosis, sometimes resulting in compression fractures of the vertebral body from relatively benign forces. The vertebral bodies of the thoracic spine are wider when measured anterior-posteriorly than medial-laterally and increase in size and density as they move toward the lumbar spine where the majority of super-incumbent forces are experienced.[1] Each vertebral body possesses a **demifacet** located at the posterolateral aspect of each vertebral body that provides an articulation for the head of each corresponding rib with the demifacet of each adjacent vertebra (Fig. 29-1). The superior articular facets of the thoracic spine are oriented posteriorly and slightly superolaterally, thus matching the inferior facets of the vertebra above, and generally reside in the *frontal plane.*

As with the vertebra of the cervical and lumbar spine, the posterior component of a typical thoracic vertebra is composed of the *neural arch*, which is formed by the paired *pedicles* and *laminae*. The thoracic neural arch, which contains the spinal cord, has a smaller diameter than elsewhere in the spine. The spinal canal in both the cervical and lumbar regions possesses a greater diameter in order to accommodate for enlargements of the cord, which result from the originations of the brachial and lumbosacral plexi.

Emanating from the neural arch posteriorly on either side are the slender, inferiorly-sloping *transverse processes.* Each thoracic transverse process contains a *costotubercular facet* that forms the *costotransverse* articulation with the *tubercle* of each corresponding rib. The *spinous processes* of the midthoracic spine are the longest within the spine and slope inferiorly, making them challenging for the manual physical therapist to palpate. Appreciating this feature is best accomplished by understanding the **rule of threes**. Simply stated, T1-3 spinous processes are level with the vertebral body at the same spinal level; T4-6 spinous processes are level with the vertebral bodies at one-half level below; T7-9 spinous processes are level with the vertebral bodies a full level below; the T10 spinous process remains a full level below; the T11 spinous process is a half

level below; and T12 spinous process is level with the vertebral body at the same level (Fig. 29-2). Understanding this osteologic feature of the thoracic vertebrae serves to guide the manual therapist through accurate palpation of these important landmarks.

Costal Cage Osteology

The *costal cage complex* is formed by the sternum anteriorly, the thoracic vertebrae posteriorly, and the interconnecting ribs. This osteoarticular configuration is uniquely designed to provide protection for the heart and lungs and serves to facilitate the act of respiration.

The *sternum* is composed of three main sections, with a joint located between each. The *manubrium*, with its *jugular notch*, is located at the level of T3. On either side of the manubrium are the facets for the articulation with the clavicular heads. The *body of the sternum* is the largest portion that joins the manubrium at the *manubriosternal junction*. This articulation is at an angle of 160 degrees, and movement occurs during respiration up until the fifth decade of life when it fuses in approximately 10% of the population.[2] The xiphoid process is an inferiorly and posteriorly sloping projection of bone. The *xiphosternal junction* also moves during respiration and fuses later in life.

Each of the 12 paired *ribs* consists of a *body, head,* and *tubercle* and is denoted by the prefix *costo-*. The head and tubercles are located posteriorly and form the articulations with the thoracic vertebrae, while the body of each rib curves anteriorly and inferiorly to insert into cartilage before attaching to the sternum either directly or indirectly. The *angle* of the rib is the most laterally projecting portion of the body, which, due to its prominence, is often the most easily palpated. Ribs 1 through 7 are referred to as the true ribs since they articulate directly with the sternum. Ribs 8 through 10 attach to the sternum via the costal cartilage, and ribs 11 and 12 are referred to as floating ribs since they possess no sternal articulation. The head of each rib articulates with the demifacets of two adjacent vertebrae as the costal tubercle articulates with the transverse process of the vertebra at the same level.[3]

Thoracic Spine Arthrology and Kinematics

The Facet Joint

As noted elsewhere in the spine, the facet joints of the thoracic spine are synovial joints that include all of the features characteristic of synovial joints. This includes a synovial joint capsule, hyaline cartilage-lined joint surfaces, and menisci, at some levels. The general orientation of the thoracic facet joints, with the exception of the upper and lower thoracic regions, which resemble the cervical and lumbar spines, respectively, is within the frontal plane. Although motion in all planes is much less within the thoracic spine than that noted elsewhere, sagittal plane and frontal plane motion is most limited.

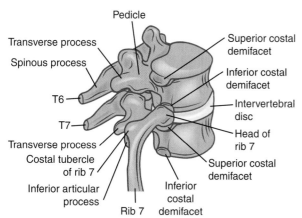

FIGURE 29–1 Demifacets of the costovertebral joint.

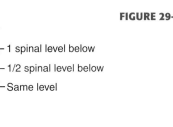

FIGURE 29–2 The thoracic spine "rule of threes."

1 spinal level below

1/2 spinal level below

Same level

Same level | 1/2 spinal level below | 1 spinal level below | Gradual decrease

Distance of spinous process from corresponding spinal level and transverse process

Thoracic Spine Kinematics

Normal ranges of motion for the thoracic spine have not been well documented. Combined forward/backward bending is reported to be *63 degrees*, the total amount of rotation is *62 degrees*, and the total amount of side bending is *68 degrees*.[4] The greatest degree of segmental mobility occurs in the transverse plane, with up to nearly 10 degrees of rotation present at T1-2 with a progressive decrease to 2 to 3 degrees at T9-12. Except for the lower thoracic region, thoracic rotation occurs to a much greater extent than that experienced in the lumbar spine where there is a minimal amount of motion. For this reason, thoracic rotation often serves as a compensation for lumbar immobility in the transverse plane. Frontal and sagittal plane motion is greatest at the lower thoracic segments, with up to 9 degrees of side bending and 13 degrees of combined forward/backward bending occurring at T11-12. Both side bending and combined forward/backward bending reach their minimum at T1-7.[5] Perhaps, the primary reason for an increase in the amount of mobility in the lower thoracic segments is related to the fact that the floating ribs 11 and 12 do not restrict mobility to the same extent as ribs 1 through 10.

As identified elsewhere within this text, **coupled movement** denotes the concept that when motion in one plane occurs within the spine, motion in another plane is mechanically forced to occur. Within the upper thoracic spine (T1-4), side bending is typically coupled with ipsilateral rotation, which reflects the kinematics of the cervical spine. The mid- to lower thoracic spine functions kinematically in a fashion that is similar to the lumbar spine. There is a significant degree of variation in coupled motion in the thoracolumbar spine, which challenges the clinical significance of these considerations.

Costal Cage Arthrology and Kinematics

Costovertebral Joints

Posteriorly, each rib articulates with the vertebral bodies of the spine via the *costovertebral joint (CV)*. This articulation is formed between the convex head of the rib, the concave demifacets formed by two adjacent vertebral bodies, and the intervertebral disc. The convex head of each rib articulates with the demifacet of the vertebra at the same thoracic level, as well as the level above. For example, rib 7 articulates with the vertebral

bodies of T6 and T7. The CV joints possess joint capsules that are reinforced by ligaments that insert into the outermost fibers of the intervertebral discs. This structural organization implies that impairments of the ribs may result in intervertebral disc derangement and vice versa. Derangement of the thoracic intervertebral discs are rare but when present may result in symptoms that follow the path of the rib as it angles around the thorax.

Costotransverse Joints

The *costotransverse (CT)* joints are formed between the *costal tubercle* of the rib and the *costal facet*, which is located on the anterior aspect of the transverse process of the corresponding vertebra (Fig. 29-3). For example, rib 7 articulates with the transverse process of T7. As with the CV joints, the CT joints have substantial capsular and ligamentous support. These joints are considered to be planar joints that allow both linear and torsional motions. Collectively, the CV and CT joints create an intimate relationship between the ribs and vertebrae. Consequently, traumatic forces to the costal cage may impact the position and mobility of the thoracic vertebrae and vice versa.

Costochondral, Chondrosternal, and Interchondral Joints

When appreciating the mobility of the thorax, the joints that compose the anterior aspect of the costal cage must be considered. As noted, ribs 1 through 7 articulate directly with the sternum. The first pair of ribs are the only ribs attaching the

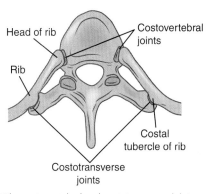

Head of rib

Costovertebral joints

Rib

Costal tubercle of rib

Costotransverse joints

FIGURE 29–3 The costovertebral and costotransverse joints.

manubrium. The second pair of ribs connects to the sternum at the manubriosternal junction. Ribs 3 through 7 attach to the body of the sternum. Each of the articulations between the ribs and the sternum are interposed with costal cartilage forming a *costochondral joint* between the rib and the costal cartilage and a *chondrosternal joint* between the costal cartilage and the concave facets of the sternum. The costochondral joints are surrounded by periosteum and lack ligamentous support. Ribs 8 to 10 connect to the sternum indirectly by first connecting to the costal cartilage of rib 7. These joints are referred to as the *interchondral joints.* These are synovial joints supported by ligaments that fuse with age.[6]

Costal Cage Kinematics

Although motion of the costal cage during respiration occurs in all three planes, depending on the rib, movement within a distinct plane predominates.[7] Due to the osteologic features of each rib and its articulation at both ends, motion of each rib is often described as a "hinge-type" movement. Posteriorly, the axis of motion passes through the neck of the rib, the CT joint, and the CV joint.[8]

Several authors have attempted to describe the kinematics of the thorax.[9,10] Rotation of the thoracic vertebral segments with their corresponding ribs are coupled with simultaneous translation in each of the cardinal planes. For example, forward bending occurs with simultaneous anterior linear translation (glide) of one vertebral segment and its corresponding ribs on the segment below. Sagittal plane motion of the thorax does not include motion in either the frontal or transverse plane.[11] Due to incomplete development of the superior demifacet of the CV joint, mobility of the thorax occurs to a much greater extent in the young.[11]

Although each rib has the capacity to move independently, the limited mobility in these joints often facilitates the movement of each pair of ribs together. *Pump handle* movement occurs in the sagittal plane and describes movement of the upper ribs during inspiration.[7] *Bucket handle* movement that occurs in the frontal plane takes place within the mid- to lower ribs during inspiration (Fig. 29-4).[7] During expiration the ribs return to their neutral position passively. Since the 11th and 12th ribs do not possess anterior articulations, their movement is best described as *caliper motion*, which occurs in the transverse plane. For the most part, the mid- to lower ribs have greater mobility than do the upper ribs.[7] Another, more subtle, movement, identified as *torsion*, also occurs during respiration about the long axis of the rib. The reference point for torsions is the anterior aspect of the rib. *External torsion* occurs when the anterior border rotates upward during inspiration. *Internal torsion* occurs when the anterior border rotates downward during expiration. Arm elevation has also been found to produce external torsion.

When considering mobility and position of each rib individually, the ribs at adjacent levels must be considered. Although each rib may move and/or exhibit a positional fault, or state of being malpositioned, in any of the three planes, assessment of individual ribs is often stated as either a frontal or transverse plane condition. A rib that moves superiorly or inferiorly in the frontal plane is known as *elevation* and *depression*, respectively. Elevation and depression of the ribs occur in conjunction with thoracic spine backward and forward bending, respectively, as does external and internal torsion (Fig. 29-5, Fig. 29-6) (Table 29-1, Table 29-2).[8,11] During these movements, the anterior aspect of the rib moves inferiorly while the posterior aspect moves superiorly during forward bending and

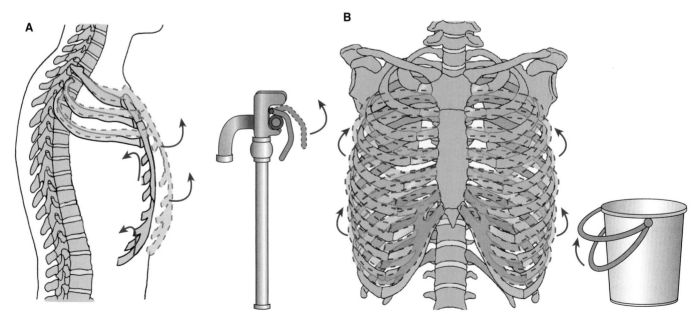

FIGURE 29–4 A. Pump handle motion of the upper ribs, which produce sagittal plane expansion of the costal cage and **B.** bucket handle motion of the mid- to lower ribs, which produces frontal plane expansion of the costal cage. (Adapted From: Levangie PK, Norkin CC. *Joint structure and function: A comprehensive analysis,* 5th ed. Philadelphia: F.A. Davis Company, 2011.)

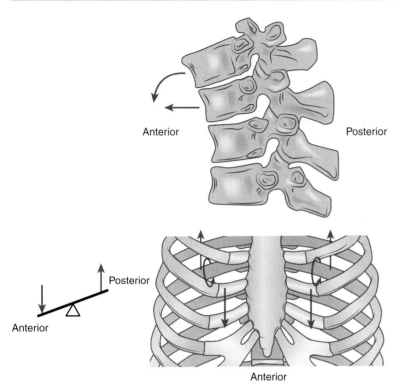

FIGURE 29–5 Thoracic-costal cage mobility into forward bending. Accessory anterior glide (red arrow) of each spinal segment accompanies angular motion (green arrow) into forward bending. During forward bending, the anterior aspect of the costal cage glides inferiorly (green arrow) and the CT joints glide superiorly with internal torsion (red arrows).

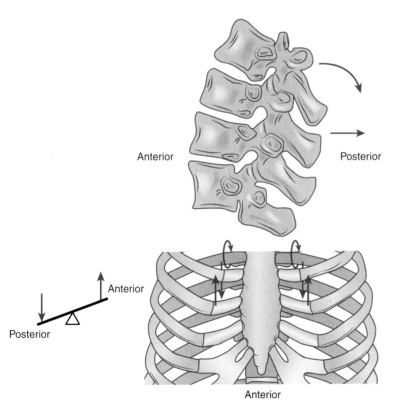

FIGURE 29–6 Thoracic-costal cage mobility into backward bending. Accessory posterior glide (red arrow) of each spinal segment accompanies angular motion (green arrow) into backward bending. During backward bending, the anterior aspect of the costal cage glides superiorly (green arrow) and the CT joints glide inferiorly with external torsion (red arrows).

Table 29–1	Thoracic Spine-Costal Cage Complex Mobility Into Forward Bending			
	FRONTAL PLANE	**SAGITTAL PLANE**	**TRANSVERSE PLANE**	**ACCESSORY MOTIONS**
Spinal Motions		• Anterior rotation		• Anterior translation (glide)
Costal Cage Motions		• Anterior costal cage depression, posterior costal cage elevation • Rib motion continues beyond spinal segmental motion		• Bilateral costotransverse superior glide and internal torsion • Rib motion continues beyond spinal segmental motion

Table 29–2	Thoracic Spine-Costal Cage Complex Mobility Into Backward Bending			
	FRONTAL PLANE	**SAGITTAL PLANE**	**TRANSVERSE PLANE**	**ACCESSORY MOTIONS**
Spinal Motions		• Posterior rotation		• Posterior translation (glide)
Costal Cage Motions		• Posterior costal cage depression, anterior costal cage elevation • Rib motion continues beyond spinal segmental motion		• Bilateral costotransverse inferior glide and external torsion • Rib motion continues beyond spinal segmental motion

in the opposite direction during backward bending. In the mobile costal cage, the rib will continue to rotate after spinal segmental motion has reached end range. Along with an anterior glide, which occurs as the inferior facet of the superior vertebra of the segment forward bends on the superior facet of the inferior vertebra, superior glide and internal torsion of the tubercle of the rib at the CT joint occurs with inferior glide and external torsion taking place with backward bending.

Midthoracic spine side bending produces rib depression and internal torsion on the side to which side bending has occurred and elevation and external torsion on the contralateral side (Fig. 29-7) (Table 29-3). Rib motion typically stops before vertebral motion, causing additional side bending of the vertebrae on the fixed ribs.[12] This produces a relative superior glide of the rib tubercle on the transverse process on the side to which side bending has occurred and a relative inferior glide of the rib tubercle on the contralateral side.[12] Accompanying the gliding of the tubercles is an anterior roll on the side that glides superior and a posterior roll on the contralateral side, thus producing internal and external torsion, respectively.[12] Arthrokinematics of the ribs are considered to be responsible for the coupled rotation that accompanies side bending in the midthoracic region.[12]

When rotation is the primary motion, a great deal of variability exists, with thoracic side bending occurring either ipsilaterally or contralaterally (Fig. 29-8) (Table 29-4). As the superior vertebra of a movement segment rotates, it also undergoes linear translation in the opposite direction.[12] For

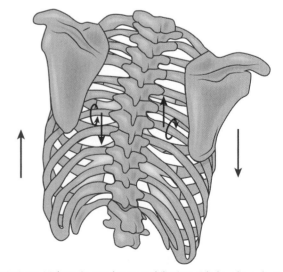

FIGURE 29–7 Thoracic-costal cage mobility into side bending where rib motion (green arrows) typically stops before vertebral motion, which produces a superior glide and internal torsion of the CT joint on the side to which side bending has occurred and a relative inferior glide and external torsion of the CT joint on the contralateral side (red arrows).

Table 29–3	Thoracic Spine-Costal Cage Complex Mobility Into Right Side Bending (in neutral)			
	FRONTAL PLANE	**SAGITTAL PLANE**	**TRANSVERSE PLANE**	**ACCESSORY MOTIONS**
Spinal Motions	• Right side bending		• Left rotation (end range, variable)	• Left facet joint glides superior • Right facet joint glides inferior • Translation (glide) to the right
Costal Cage Motions	• Left costal cage elevation • Right costal cage depression	• Left costal cage posterior rotation (roll) • Right costal cage anterior rotation (roll)	• Left costal cage posterior • Right costal cage anterior	• Right costotransverse superior glide and internal torsion • Left costotransverse inferior glide and external torsion

example, as T4 rotates to the right on T5, it also translates to the left. During this motion, rib 5 on the left translates superiorly in relation to the left transverse process at the CT joint and anteriorly rotates, or undergoes internal torsion.[12] The opposite motions occur with rib 5 on the right. Thoracic spine rotation produces movement of the ribs posteriorly on the side of rotation and anteriorly on the contralateral side. Inferior glide and external torsion of the CT joints takes place on the side to which rotation occurs as superior glide and internal torsion occurs on the contralateral side. The relationship between thoracic movement and

position and the costal cage is most evident when considering the presence of a rib hump on the side of convexity in the presence of a scoliosis.

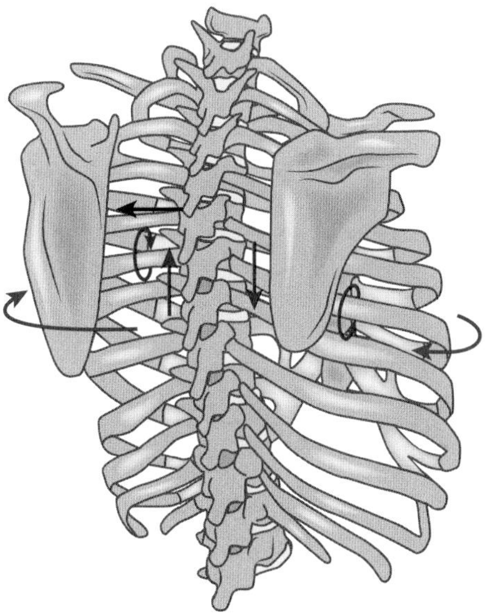

It is important to appreciate that the kinematics of the costal cage changes in the lower ribs. This change is primarily due to the fact that the CT joints of the lower thoracic spine are more planar in orientation, the head of the rib is not as closely associated with the demifacet of the superior vertebra, and the ribs attach more loosely to the sternum anteriorly.[12] During forward and backward bending, the ribs move in a sagittal plane with extensive motion occurring at the CV joints, especially at ribs 9 and 10 where the heads are only loosely associated with their superior demifacets. With side bending, the ribs will compress on the side of movement and further motion will occur as the ribs glide at the CT joints. Rotation in the lower thoracic region occurs with only minimal limitation from the costal cage.[12] The absence of a facet joint plane and the small CV joints that are present within these segments results in variability in the direction to which coupled side bending occurs.[12]

Ribs 1 and 2 are typically less mobile than T1 and T2. The head of the first rib does not articulate with C7; therefore, the glide and rotation of the ribs in the upper thoracic region are not able to influence spinal motion.[12] As noted, the upper thoracic spine functions like the midcervical spine by side bending and rotating ipsilaterally. At the end range of these motions, the more mobile vertebral segments continue to glide at the CT joints after the ribs have reached end range.[12]

EXAMINATION

The Subjective Examination

Self-Reported Disability Measures

When examining the upper thoracic spine, the self-reported disability instruments used during examination of the cervical spine are often implemented (see Chapter 30). Likewise,

FIGURE 29–8 Thoracic-costal cage mobility into rotation. During right rotation, vertebral segments sequentially rotate to the right (green arrows) and translate to the left (black arrow). During this motion, inferior glide and external torsion of the CT joint takes place on the side to which rotation occurs as superior glide and internal torsion of the CT joint occurs on the contralateral side (red arrows).

Table 29–4	Thoracic Spine-Costal Cage Complex Mobility Into Right Rotation (in neutral)			
	FRONTAL PLANE	**SAGITTAL PLANE**	**TRANSVERSE PLANE**	**ACCESSORY MOTIONS**
Spinal Motions	• Right side bending (intact ribs, variable)		• Right rotation	• Left facet joint glides superior • Right facet joint glides inferior • Left translation
Costal Cage Motions	• Left costal cage elevation • Right costal cage depression	• Left costal cage anterior rotation (roll) • Right costal cage posterior rotation (roll)	• Left costal cage anterior • Right costal cage posterior	• Right costotransverse superior glide and internal torsion • Left costotransverse inferior glide and external torsion

examination of the mid- to lower thoracic spine often includes disability measures that are used in cases of low back pain (see Chapter 28).

Systems Review

Due to the close proximity of vital organs to the thoracic spine and costal cage, nonmusculoskeletal causes of impairment must be ruled out in cases of symptoms arising from this region. One of the most serious conditions that must be ruled out in cases of thoracic impairment is the presence of a *pulmonary embolus*. This condition may result insidiously from routine surgery of the lower extremity or from periods of immobility.[13] Symptoms include severe substernal angina, dyspnea, and an abrupt reduction in blood pressure.[13] Additional pulmonary conditions, such as *pneumonia*, may result in chest pain that is most profound upon deep inspiration and may contribute to altered mobility of the costal cage.[13] Systemic signs of infection such as fever, chills, and malaise may also be present. A significant reduction in chest wall expansion is commonly observed in individuals with a *pneumothorax*.[13] Such a condition often occurs in the presence of trauma or intense episodes of coughing.[13] Sharp pain within the thorax may result from a condition known as *pleurisy*, an irritation of the pleural membranes between the lungs and the costal cage.[13] This pain is often present upon deep breathing, coughing, or mobility testing of the ribs or thoracic spine.[13]

An equally serious condition, *myocardial infarction*, also requires immediate referral if its presence is suspected. The classic sign of a myocardial infarction is angina with the potential for referral into either the left or right upper extremity, neck, and jaw.[13] This condition is often accompanied by nausea, syncope, or dyspnea, which may be the primary presenting features.[13] Another cardiac condition that may result in chest pain with referral of symptoms into the left arm is *pericarditis*.[13] Inflammation of the pericardium, which surrounds the heart, prevents chest expansion, leading to tachycardia and cardiac tamponade, a condition in which blood pressure drops during inhalation and is accompanied

by heavy breathing.[13] Pericarditis is usually accompanied by a fever, worsens upon lying, and improves with forward leaning.[13]

Kidney stones are a fairly common occurrence impacting a substantial portion of the population. Pain from kidney stones is often present in the lateral upper lumbar/lower thoracic region unilaterally. Men are typically more likely to develop kidney stones, and a past history that reflects the presence of kidney stones increase the likelihood of their reoccurrence. *Pyelonephritis*, or kidney infection, is often the result of a lower urinary tract infection and is common in females following intercourse. Both conditions often include typical signs of infection such as fever, malaise, and vomiting.

Lastly, a gastrointestinal condition that may refer symptoms to the shoulder or thorax is *cholecystitis*, or inflammation of the gall bladder.[13] An initial symptom of this condition is referred pain to the right scapula or upper abdominal quadrant with a positive *Murphy's sign*, difficulty with inspiration upon palpation of the right upper quadrant.[13] Table 29-5 displays the medical red flags that should be ruled out in patients with thoracic and costal cage symptoms.

History of Present Illness

In cases of neck or low back pain, the thoracic region must also be screened for its potential contribution. The specific *mechanism of injury (MOI)* is of great importance in distinguishing the nature of the condition. A delineation is made between symptoms that have occurred insidiously or from cumulative trauma over time versus those that are subsequent to a single traumatic event. Establishing the MOI is important for deciding whether further medical evaluation is necessary, including the need to obtain diagnostic images to rule out pathology.

Obtaining a symptomatic profile that attempts to ascertain the frequency and severity of symptoms throughout the course of a typical day and in response to ADL using a *numeric pain rating scale (NPRS)* is vital to the therapist's understanding of the condition. Detailed interrogation related to the patient's

Table 29–5	Medical Red Flags for the Thoracic Spine and Costal Cage	
MEDICAL CONDITION	**RED FLAGS**	
Pulmonary Embolus	Shoulder and/or chest pain Dyspnea	
Pneumonia	Fever, malaise, chills, nausea Reduced breath sounds	
Pneumothorax	Chest pain upon inspiration Reduced chest expansion Reduced breath sounds Recent history of trauma or respiratory disorder	
Pleurisy	Severe pain upon inspiration Dyspnea Recent history of respiratory disorder	

Pericarditis	Sharp pain in neck or shoulder
	  and relieved with leaning forward
	  or rest	

Myocardial Infarction	Angina
	Dyspnea, pallor
	History of coronary artery disease,
	  hypertension, diabetes, tobacco,
	  increased cholesterol
	Men over age 40, women over
	  age 50	

(Adapted from: Boissonnault WG. *Primary Care for the Physical Therapist: Examination and Triage.* St. Louis, MO: Elsevier Saunders; 2005.)

symptomatic response to thoracic spine movements and postures as well as the patient's tolerance for respiration must be obtained. Interscapular pain may be related to a thoracic condition; however, such symptoms are often associated with a cervical spinal lesion.[14] Anterior cervical disc lesions at C3-4, C4-5, C5-6, and C6-7 may cause interscapular pain at the suprascapular, superior angle, midvertebral border, and inferior angle levels, respectively.[15] Likewise, a posterolateral or central cervical disc lesion at C4-5 may refer symptoms to the interscapular region at the level of the root of the spine of the scapula.[15] Although less common, thoracic intervertebral disc lesions may result in "through the chest" type pain or pain that follows the path of the rib from posterior to anterior.[16,17] These regions of pain referral have been referred to as *Cloward signs*, or areas, after their originator.[16] It is often difficult to ascertain the presence of radicular symptoms related to thoracic intervertebral disc lesions. The posterior thoracic region may exhibit sensory changes in response to *posterior primary ramus* involvement.[16] Symptoms that arise from coughing or sneezing is suggestive of dural root pain. Pain upon respiration may signal a pulmonary or cardiac condition, as described above, or may occur in the presence of an impairment in any of the articulations that make up the thoracic-costal cage complex.

The Objective Physical Examination

Examination of Structure

Palpation of key bony landmarks may assist in appreciating the relative positions of anatomical structures. The superior and inferior angles of the scapula are at the level of T2 and T7, respectively. The medial border of the scapula normally rests approximately 5 cm lateral to the thoracic spinous processes on either side. While observing static structure, information related to the patient's quiet breathing pattern is also obtained.

Common postures often observed are the kypholordotic and flat back postures.[18] The typical **kypholordotic posture** involves an increased thoracic kyphosis with rounded shoulders and forward head,[18] whereas individuals with **flat back posture** have a reduction in their thoracic kyphotic curve with scapular medial winging.[18] The average degree of thoracic kyphosis is estimated to be approximately 40 degrees.[19] A reduction in upper thoracic kyphosis (T3-5) has been identified as one of six criteria that, if present, suggests the likelihood of immediate improvement in neck pain in response to thoracic spine thrust manipulation.[20] Screening procedures for identification of scoliosis often focus on observation of a *rib hump* upon forward bending, resulting from transverse plane deformity that is associated with this condition. Costal cage asymmetry that results in a rib hump may also be present in the absence of scoliosis.

Due to a variety of intrinsic or extrinsic factors, a rib may become displaced, which is confirmed through palpation. For example, if rib 6 is superiorly displaced, there will be a palpable reduction in the intercostal space between rib 5 and rib 6 and greater than normal intercostal space between rib 6 and rib 7. The same may be identified for displacements in the transverse plane. A rib displacement may impact thoracic spine mobility or vice versa and may result in a multitude of symptoms, including pain, reduced mobility, and respiratory impairment.

Through astute observation, the manual therapist attempts to relate the patient's reported symptoms to movement aberrations of the ribs during respiration. Observation of quiet breathing should be accomplished during the structural exam, which may include palpation of the upper, middle, and lower costal cage to assess the pattern of breathing and symmetry. The rate of breathing, expected to be *12 to 15 breaths/minute* during quiet respiration, and the presence of wheezes, rales, or coughing should also be documented.

The presence of chest deformities may also contribute to impairments in mobility and symptoms. *Pigeon-chested* individuals are characterized by a sternum that projects forward, which increases the sagittal plane dimension of the chest cavity and may impact volume during respiration.[21] *Cavus-chested* individuals have a reduced chest cavity volume that may also effect respiration and increased kyphosis.[21] A *barrel chest* deformity often occurs in the presence of chronic pulmonary conditions, such as *emphysema*.[21]

Neurovascular Examination

Testing of dermatomal sensation is performed as in other areas through the use of light touch, sharp/dull, vibration, monofilaments, and hot/cold modalities. In the thoracic spine, there is a substantial degree of dermatomal overlap. As aforementioned, thoracic radicular symptoms often follow the path of the ribs.[17] The following patterns of referral have been documented: **T5,** referral around the areola; **T7,8,** referral to the epigastric region; **T10,11,** referral to the umbilicus; **T12,** referral to the groin.[17] Symptomatic referral that does not follow a particular path is suggestive of pain referral from a myofascial trigger point, which must be confirmed through palpation.[22]

Examination of Mobility

Active Physiologic Movement Examination of the Thoracic Spine and Costal Cage

Quantity of Movement

Respiration

Observation in conjunction with palpation of the costal cage during respiration serves as a screening procedure designed to identify mobility impairments that can be further tested through passive procedures. As described, movement varies from region to region as previously described. All of the ribs move into external torsion during inspiration and internal torsion during expiration. For assessment, it may be best for the examiner to stand behind the seated patient. For assessment of the upper ribs, the therapist places his or her hands over the patient's clavicles to gently rest over the upper ribs while the patient performs quiet respiration. For assessment of ribs 5 to 10, the therapist places his or her hands on either side of the thorax and assesses the degree of expansion in the frontal plane. The patient is asked to inhale and exhale taking deep breaths while regional rib mobility is assessed. Costal cage mobility upon exertion may also be assessed following aerobic activity such as bike riding or treadmill ambulation.

To quantify regional costal cage mobility, a tape measure may be used to document chest circumference at distinct locations within the thorax, such as the *sternomanubrial junction,* the *xiphosternal junction,* and along the *inferior border of the 10th ribs.* Testing at each location provides the examiner with an overall profile of costal cage mobility.

Thoracic Regional Mobility Examination

To reliably quantify thoracic spine–costal cage regional motion, similar methods to those used elsewhere in the spine may be employed. Such methods may include *goniometry, tape measurement, single or double inclinometry,* or use of the *back range of motion (BROM)* device.[23–25] Normal values for regional thoracic spine range of motion are as follows: *63 degrees* of total forward bending (FB)/backward bending (BB), *68 degrees* of unilateral side bending (SB), and *62 degrees* of unilateral rotation (ROT).[26]

The upper thoracic spine is best tested in sitting, and the lower thoracic region is tested in standing. Motion is recruited from the cervical and into the thoracic spine in a cephalad-to-caudal fashion. The patient is asked to bring the chin to the chest and slowly bend forward, then look up toward the ceiling while being viewed from behind, for forward and backward bending, respectively. Upper thoracic backward bending may be best accomplished by asking the patient to perform bilateral shoulder flexion. With arms folded, side bending and rotation

in both directions are tested. As in other regions of the spine, both single and repeated motions are performed.

Thoracic Segmental Mobility Examination

Due to the large number of articulations and moving parts within this complex, the expediency of isolating a segmental lesion is increased by using active physiologic motion of the entire complex as a screening tool. Careful observation of active physiologic complex motion may allow the manual therapist to know where to begin segmental mobility testing. The following procedures related to the assessment of thoracic-costal cage mobility have been adapted from those previously described by Lee.[12]

Segmental mobility is assessed by using the same motions as those used for regional mobility testing, along with palpation to further isolate the lesion. Prior to movement, the therapist places the index finger and thumb on the transverse processes of two adjacent vertebrae bilaterally. These contacts are maintained as the patient performs motion in each of the planes described above. The original starting and final end position of each vertebra is identified, as well as the manner in which each segment moves. During side bending, palpation may reveal increased prominence of the transverse process on the ipsilateral side for upper thoracic and contralateral side for the lower thoracic region.

In addition to vertebral segmental motion, it is also vital to assess the mobility of each rib relative to its respective vertebra. This is accomplished by palpating the transverse process and its corresponding rib. For example, the thumb is placed on the transverse process of T7, and the thumb and finger of the other hand is placed along the shaft of the rib just medial to the angle of rib 7 during motion in all planes. The relative motion between each vertebra and its corresponding rib is assessed. As noted, in the mobile thorax, there is an additional glide of the transverse process that may be palpated once rib motion has ceased. In this fashion, the relative mobility of each vertebral segment and its corresponding rib may be tested in all planes.

Segmental differentiation may be accomplished through the use of counterpressure or blocking techniques. These procedures are predicated on using the motion that reproduces the patient's chief complaint, which must first be identified. Counterpressures are then sequentially elicited over each member of the motion segment, and changes in the patient's reproducible symptoms are noted, for example, if a patient presents with a reproduction of symptoms with thoracic left side bending in the upper thoracic region. Beginning at the most caudal segment of the movement chain, counterpressure is elicited, in this case along the left side of the T5 spinous process in an effort to restrict movement into left side bending. If this procedure alters the patient's complaint of pain in any way, the T5-6 segment is believed to be a contributing segment. Symptoms that reduce in response to this examination procedure provide immediate efficacy for the use of the same procedure for intervention. In this way, the efficiency of isolating the dysfunctional segment and the effectiveness of addressing the patient's chief complaint is greatly increased.

Evjenth and Gloeck[27] have developed a similar system of symptom localization. Others have used these methods in the literature.[28] Jull et al[29] showed that these methods are as reliable as diagnostic blocks performed with imaging in diagnosing cervical spine syndromes when performed by trained therapists. This method uses *"rotational symptom localization"* to isolate the impaired segment.[28] If active rotation to the left reproduces the symptoms, then the patient is brought into left rotation until the onset of pain and then slowly moved out of the pain into rotation right. This position is maintained while segmental pressures are applied over the right TP to produce left rotation at each level, beginning with the most caudal segment of the movement chain. When reproduction of the patient's chief complaint is brought on by segmental pressures, the impaired segment, or segments, are believed to have been identified.[28] Table 29-6 displays the physiologic motions of the thoracic spine, including normal ranges of motion, open- and closed-packed positions, and normal and abnormal end feels.

Thoracic-Costal Cage Passive Physiologic Movement Examination

Passive testing of physiologic mobility is accomplished through a series of testing identified as *passive physiologic intervertebral mobility (PPIVM)* testing. In order to ascertain the degree of segmental mobility, palpation of the interspinous space is performed during motion recruitment. Although described as passive, these techniques often involve assistance from the patient. In the thoracic spine, these tests are best accomplished in sitting. PPIVM testing is described in greater detail in Chapter 7 of this text.

When assessing passive physiologic motion into forward and backward bending of the upper thoracic spine, the patient is sitting with hands clasped behind his or her neck and elbows pointing forward (Fig. 29-9). The examiner controls upper thoracic motion through the patient's arms while palpating the interspinous space at each level from cephalad to caudal, beginning with recruitment of motion through

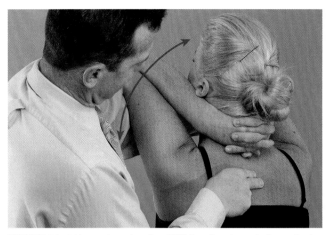

FIGURE 29–9 Upper thoracic spine PPIVM testing. Arrow indicates both upper thoracic forward bending and upper thoracic backward bending.

the cervical spine. An oscillating rhythm is used to allow better palpation of motion at each level. A progressive increase in motion is required to recruit motion at the more caudal levels.

For the mid- to lower thoracic region, the patient places his or her arms across the chest with hands resting on opposite shoulders. The examiner grasps the patient across the folded arms or weaves an arm through the patient's folded arms, eventually resting on the opposite shoulder. The interspinous space is palpated using the other hand, and motion in all planes is invoked (Fig. 29-10). In addition to eliciting physiologic motion in the cardinal planes, therapists may choose to also test the multiplanar motion capability of the thoracic spine. Some have suggested motion testing in four distinct quadrants (see Chapter 11) as a method of assessing the ability of spinal segments to move into patterns that are routinely used during functional activities.

In order to assess the passive physiologic motion of the ribs, the patient is passively moved into all planes in the same manner as described above, while the other hand palpates rib

Table 29–6	Physiologic (Osteokinematic) Motions of the Mid-Thoracic Spine				
JOINT	NORMAL ROM	OPP	CPP	NORMAL END FEEL(S)	CAPSULAR PATTERN
Mid-Thoracic Spine (T4-T12)	FB/BB = 4°(T4-6), 6°(T7-9), 12° (T10-12), 30°(total) SB = 6°(T4-6), 8° (T7-9), 8°(T10-12), 25-40°(total) ROT = 9°(T4-6), 9°(T6-9), 9° (T10-12), 30-50°(total)	FB, contralateral SB and ipsilateral ROT	BB, ipsilateral SB and contralateral ROT	Elastic	FB with deviation > contralateral SB, ipsilateral ROT

ROM, range of motion; OPP, open packed position; CPP, close packed position; FB, forward bending; BB, backward bending; SB, side bending; ROT, rotation. (Adapted From: Wise CH, Gulick DT. *Mobilization Notes: A Rehabilitation Specialist's Pocket Guide.* Philadelphia, PA: FA Davis Company, 2009.)

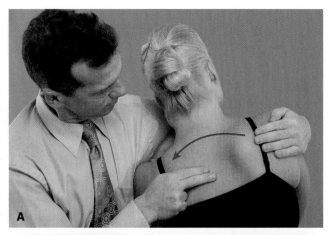

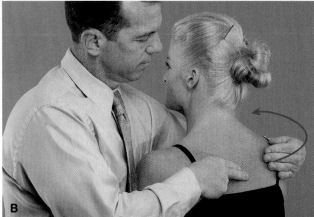

FIGURE 29–10 Mid thoracic spine PPIVM testing. **A.** Midthoracic side bending. **B.** Midthoracic rotation.

motion at the shaft of the rib, just medial to the angle. With the patient sitting, mobility assessment is best accomplished by palpating the contralateral side of the costal cage. Anterior translation and roll may be palpated during forward bending while posterior translation and roll may be observed during backward bending. Side bending produces rib elevation on the side contralateral to motion with simultaneous depression on the ipsilateral side. Rotation produces movement of the ribs in the transverse plane. The motion of each rib in reference to the next adjacent rib is noted. Any rib positional faults are noted since starting position may alter its movement capacity. During passive testing, end feel is noted in all planes.

Thoracic-Costal Cage Passive Accessory Movement Examination

Accessory motion testing allows the therapist to gain an understanding of the arthrokinematic motions that are taking place within each spinal segment. In the spine, these procedures are collectively referred to as *passive accessory intervertebral mobility (PAIVM)* testing. During PAIVM testing, an individual's symptomatic response to accessory glides have been found to be a more reliable indicator than stiffness in determining the pathologic segment.[30]

As described in Chapter 28, the primary goal of PAIVM testing is to gain an appreciation of the relationship between mobility and the onset of symptoms within each spinal segment.

As force is applied through the tested segment, the first and final onset of tissue resistance, defined as ***R1 and R2***, is appreciated in relation to the first and final onset of pain, defined as ***P1 and P2***. This process of identifying the primary restraints to motion has been fully described by Maitland et al[17] (see Chapter 8).

Thoracic Spine PAIVM Testing

PAIVM testing is performed with the patient in prone with appropriate pillow support. Preferably, the patient's arms are at his or her sides so that myofascial restrictions do not limit segmental mobility. To improve patient comfort and engender relaxation, ¼ to ½ inch compressible foam, referred to as mobilization foam, may be used. The mobilizing force may be applied using various methods. The spinous or transverse processes are contacted for central or unilateral glides, respectively, using the area just distal to the pisiform or thumb. Once contact has been made, either the contralateral hand or thumb places force through the *dumby-hand* or *dumby-thumb* contact to elicit the necessary motion.

Due to the orientation of the facet joints of the upper thoracic spine, which are approximately 45 degrees between the frontal and horizontal planes, PAIVM testing of this region is best accomplished with the examiner standing at the patient's side, with thumb over thumb contact at the transverse process on the side to which the therapist is standing, at which time force is applied through the thumb contact in a superoanterior direction.

A mobility impairment is identified when a reduction in the degree of expected mobility or a reproduction of symptoms occurs in response to PAIVM testing at a specific level. The challenge of detecting mobility impairments through PAIVM testing lies in the examiner's ability to assess restrictions, which has not been found to be reliable. The patient's symptomatic response to accessory motion testing may be a more reliable method for assessment and classification. If a restriction has been identified or the presence of a stiffness-dominant disorder during PAIVM testing has been noted, then the same procedure used for examination may be employed for intervention. The PAIVM techniques used for examination will be described in more detail in the mobilization section of this chapter. Table 29-7 displays the accessory motions of the thoracic spine.

Costal Cage Accessory Motion Testing

Accessory mobility of the costal cage as described by Lee[13] will be summarized here with modifications. Segmental testing of the CT joints is best performed using blocking procedures. With the patient prone with appropriate pillow support, one thumb contacts the inferior aspect of the selected transverse process to provide blocking as the other thumb contacts the superior aspect of the corresponding rib just lateral to the tubercle (Fig. 29-11).[12] Inferiorly directed force is applied through the rib contact as the transverse process is blocked.[12] The degree of inferior glide and reproduction of any symptoms is noted. Superior glide is tested by now moving the blocking thumb to the superior aspect of the transverse process and the mobilizing thumb to the inferior aspect of the rib, after which a superiorly directed

Table 29-7	Accessory (Arthrokinematic) Motions of the Mid-Lower Thoracic Spine and Costal Cage		
	ARTHROLOGY	**ARTHROKINEMATICS**	
Mid-Lower Thoracic Spine (T4-T12)	**Facet Joints:** Synovial joints with frontal plane orientation **Intervertebral Joints:** Fibrocartilaginous joints with interposed disc	*To facilitate FB/BB:* Inferior facets of superior vertebra upglide on superior facets of inferior vertebra. Nucleus pulposis migrates posteriorly, annulus fibrosis bulges anteriorly. Spinal canal and IV foramen lengthen and open. *To facilitate SB(right):* Right inferior facet of superior vertebra downglides, left inferior facet upglides. Right IV foramen closes, left opens. Coupled with contralateral ROT (neutral), ipsilateral ROT (non-neutral).	*To facilitate ROT(right):* Right inferior facet of superior vertebra downglides, left inferior facet upglides. Right IV foramen closes, left opens. Coupled with ipsilateral SB if ROT occurs first and when in non-neutral position. Coupled with contralateral SB if SB occurs first (neutral).
Costal Cage	**Manubriosternal and Xiphosternal Joints:** Synchondrosis joints with fibrocartilage disc **Chondrosternal, Costochondral, Interchondral Joints:** Cartilaginous joints **Costovertebral Joints:** Convex head of rib with 2 concave vertebral body demifacets and IV disc (ie. Rib 7 with T6-7) **Costotransverse Joints:** Costal tubercle of rib with costal facet on transverse process (ie. Rib 7 with T7)	*To facilitate pump handle (upper ribs):* Sagittal plane motion of upper ribs *To facilitate bucket handle (middle ribs):* Frontal plane motion of middle ribs	*To facilitate caliper motion:* Transverse plane motion of ribs 11 and 12 *To facilitate internal/external torsion:* Anterior border of rib moves internally during expiration and externally during inspiration

FB, forward bending; BB, backward bending; SB, side bending; ROT, rotation; IV, intervertebral. (Adapted From: Wise CH, Gulick DT. *Mobilization Notes: A Rehabilitation Specialist's Pocket Guide.* Philadelphia, PA: FA Davis Company, 2009.)

force is applied (Fig. 29-12).[12] As orientation of the CT joint plane changes in the lower thorax region, the force is directed in a more lateral direction through application of force along the shaft of the rib.[12] Both inferior glide and superior glide of the CT joints, if found to be impaired, become the intervention. These procedures are more fully delineated within the mobilization section of this chapter.

Of particular importance when examining accessory motion of the costal cage is the relative position and mobility of the first rib and the presence of a cervical rib. To test for the

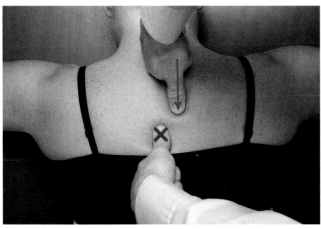

FIGURE 29–11 Costotransverse joint accessory motion testing inferiorly with transverse process blocking.

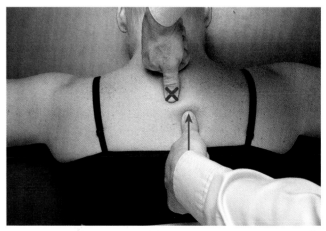

FIGURE 29–12 Costotransverse joint accessory motion testing superiorly with transverse process blocking.

presence of an elevated first rib or for limited inferior mobility of ribs 1 and 2, the patient lies supine with the head slightly side-bent and rotated toward the side to be tested in an effort to place the scaleni in a relaxed, shortened position. The second metacarpophalangeal (MCP) is placed midway between the neck and the shoulder at the slope formed by the upper trapezius. The hand applies inferior force toward the patient's contralateral hip, then moves slightly posterior as if to work around the upper trapezius and then finally inferior again to contact the posterior portion of the first rib. The relative position is compared bilaterally by determining the point of first contact as well as the mobility by determining the end feel and ease with which the rib can be glided inferiorly. These pressures are timed with the patient's normal breathing patterns. A similar process is described later in this chapter wherein this procedure may be used for mobilization of the first rib.

Examination of Muscle Function

The critical issue in determining muscle function throughout the thorax is often as much a factor of identifying motor recruitment patterns and issues related to the timing of contractions as it is related to the force-generating capabilities of these muscles. The deep muscles of the posterior spine consist of the *transversospinalis* muscles, which consist of single or multisegmental muscles. This group consists of the *rotatores* and the *multifidi*.[31,32] As opposed to other regions of the spine, in the thoracic region, the intercostals are also included in this local, or deep muscle, stabilizing system.[31,32]

Lee[12] describes the **prone arm lift test** (Fig. 29-13), which may be used to determine the strategy that is adopted to stabilize the thorax during arm-raising activities.[12] This test is based on the same premise as that used in the development of the **active straight leg raise (ASLR) test**,[33,34] but thus far this test has not been validated. With the patient prone, the examiner closely examines the pattern of muscle activation and the presence of pain as the patient raises his or her arm into flexion. During the initial movement, the scapula should remain in contact with the thorax, and no thoracic movement should be detected. The examiner then applies circumferential pressure over the costal cage as the patient lifts again. The impact of external support provided by the therapist on the patient's symptoms and ease of performance is then evaluated. Improved function with external support suggests the presence of deficits in the stabilizing system of the thorax and the need to enhance local muscle function. This concept may be applied to the performance of muscles during other functional tasks. Symptoms or difficulty in the performance of an activity that is enhanced with external support suggests the need to focus intervention toward dynamic stabilization of the local muscle system. Painful conditions that impact the upper extremity, such as shoulder impingement syndrome, may actually be the result of a poorly functioning muscular-stabilizing system within the thorax. Immediate changes in function and symptoms may result when external support is provided. Such suggestions remain anecdotal and require validation testing in order to support their use.

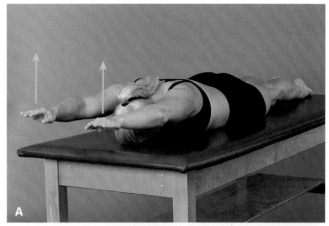
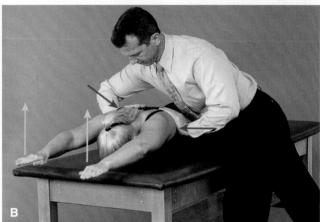

FIGURE 29–13 (A, B) The prone arm lift test.

Palpation

Osseous Palpation

Palpation of bony structures may begin anteriorly with palpation of the sternum. With the patient in supine, the therapist first identifies the *jugular notch* located between the clavicular heads. The *sternoclavicular (SC) joints* are palpated bilaterally for relative position. Moving caudally, the *manubrium* demarcates the superior portion of the sternum that articulates with the clavicles, as well as ribs 1 and 2, followed by the entirety of the sternum from *body* to *xiphoid process*.

When palpating the costal cage, it is important to keep in mind the orientation of the ribs and how they angle superiorly as they go from anterior to posterior. Palpation of ribs 1 and 2 are best accomplished by moving laterally from the manubrium on either side. As noted, rib 1 can be accessed through the posterior triangle of the neck posteriorly and just inferior to the medial clavicle anteriorly (Fig. 29-14). Confirmation of correct palpation is accomplished by assessing rib motion upon deep breathing. To palpate ribs 3 through 10, it may be easiest to palpate along the lateral thorax where there is less soft tissue and muscle. To palpate rib 11 and 12, one can move caudally over the edge of the tenth rib posteriorly to identify the tips of these floating ribs. To confirm correct palpation, one may identify T11 and T12 and follow the ribs as they project from these vertebrae.

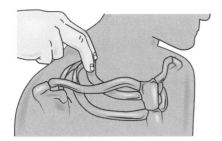

FIGURE 29–14 Palpation of the first rib.

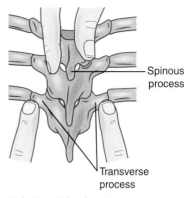

FIGURE 29–16 Palpation of the thoracic spine transverse processes at the same level and the thoracic spinous process using the "pinch" test to assess position.

With the patient in prone and a pillow placed lengthwise at the chest, the thoracic vertebrae are palpated. T2 and T8 are approximately level with the superior and inferior angles of the scapula, respectively (Fig. 29-15). T10 can be identified by following rib 10 into its posterior insertion. Perhaps the most reliable method for establishing the thoracic level is to first differentiate between C6, C7, and T1 in sitting. The first prominent spinous process is that of C6, however, C7 represents the most prominent, spinous process. To distinguish between levels, the spinous process of C6 is will move anteriorly as the patient actively or passively moves into cervical backward bending, whereas C7 and T1 will move to a lesser extent. Once T1 has been confirmed, the examiner may palpate caudally along the full extent of the spine.

To assess the relative position of each vertebra with the next adjacent vertebra, the examiner may perform the "pinch test," in which the *spinous processes (SPs)* are pinched between the finger and thumb at adjacent levels and observed for their relative position. If, for example, the spinous process of T5 is located to the right relative to T6, a left-rotated segment is suspected.

Moving just off the spinous process on either side are the slender *transverse processes (TPs)* (Fig. 29-16). These important landmarks are often challenging to palpate through the paravertebral musculature but can be identified as a firm region through gliding of the fingers vertically. The TPs are an important landmark when attempting to identify segmental positional faults in the thoracic spine. During palpation of

spinous and transverse processes, the examiner must be aware of the *rule of threes*, as previously defined.

Often performed in sitting, palpation of the TPs at each level is performed in erect sitting, slumped sitting, and backward-bent sitting. The relative change in the position of the TP in each position serves to identify the presence of a triplanar positional fault. In neutral, if the T6 TP on the right is more prominent than the TP on the left, it is not possible to verify if the left side is held forward or if the right side is held back. Upon slumped sitting, if the TPs on both sides become equally prominent, then clearly the right TP has moved as evidenced by its forward translation during forward bending, so the examiner may deduce that the left TP is simply stuck forward. Confirmation may be obtained as backward-bent sitting now reveals that there is even greater disparity between the TPs, since the left side is unable to translate posteriorly during backward bending. According to the osteopathic literature (see Chapter 4), such faults are present in a triplanar fashion. In the previous scenario, this fault would be identified as a *flexed* (left TP is forward or flexed), *rotated* (left TP is forward and right TP is backward thus producing rotation), and *side-bent* (side bending accompanies rotation). Since this fault was confirmed out of the neutral position (i.e., confirmed with patient extended), then side bending and rotation are believed to be coupled ipsilaterally, thus leading to the identification of this condition as a Flexed(F), Rotated(R), Sidebent(S) Right positional diagnosis (ie. FRS right). A positional fault of fewer than three segments is termed a *type II, non-neutral fault*, whereas a fault that extends into three or more spinal segments is defined as a *type I, neutral fault*. Type II faults follow non-neutral mechanics, namely side bending and rotation, which occur ipsilaterally, and type I faults follow neutral mechanics, where side bending and rotation occur contralaterally.

There are two faults found in neutral, which are identified as *neutral side-bent right (NSR)* (implying rotation left) and *neutral side-bent left (NSL)* (implying rotation right) deformities. There are four faults that may be identified when the spine is out of neutral, identified as *flexion rotation side-bent right (FRSR)* (Fig. 29-17) and *flexion rotation side-bent*

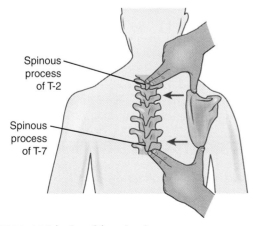

Spinous process of T-2

Spinous process of T-7

FIGURE 29–15 Palpation of thoracic spinous processes.

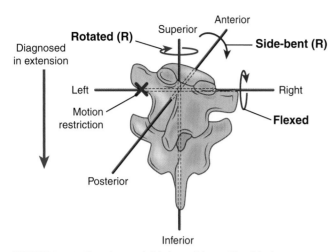

FIGURE 29–17 Flexed rotated side bent, right positional fault.

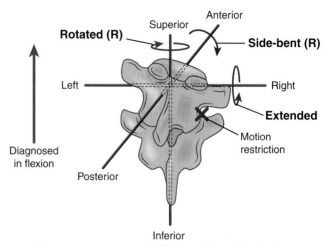

FIGURE 29–19 Extended rotated side bent, right positional fault.

left (FRSL) (Fig. 29-18), which are diagnosed when the patient is extended, and *extension rotation side-bent right (ERSR)* (Fig. 29-19) and *extension rotation side-bent left (ERSL)* (Fig. 29-20), which are diagnosed when the patient is flexed. These diagnoses are positional in nature. Mobility impairments believed to result from these faults are expected to be in the direction opposite to that which is described for the positional diagnosis. For example, an ERSL positional diagnosis would be presumed to possess mobility impairments into flexion rotation side bending to the right. Intervention then would focus on techniques designed to flex and rotate and side bend the involved segment to the right (Table 29-8). This method of triplanar positional diagnosis and intervention used for correction have been largely developed, advocated, and popularized through the osteopathic approach to OMPT, the details of which are covered in Chapter 4 of this text. Limitations in reliably identifying the static position of bony landmarks is well reported. Therefore, an emphasis on correlating the patient's chief complaint with motion limitations is advocated.

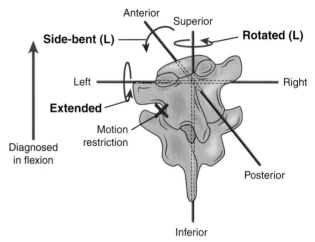

FIGURE 29–20 Extended rotated side bent, left positional fault.

Soft Tissue Palpation

Palpation of the soft tissues of the thorax is best accomplished with the patient in a supported non-weight-bearing position. Muscle tone, temperature, and the presence of palpable tenderness are all documented. The *erector spinae* group can be palpated along the entire length of the spine from lumbar to the thoracic region. This muscle group is divided from central to lateral into the *spinalis, longissimus,* and *iliocostalis* muscles. Confirmation of these muscles may be accomplished through gently lifting the head or leg from the prone-lying position, at which time these muscles should engage.

Lying deep to the erector spinae muscles is the transversospinalis muscle group, including the *multifidi* and *rotatores.* Due to their size and their depth, these muscles are challenging to palpate. These muscles are palpated in the laminar groove between the spinous and transverse processes. With contraction, a fullness is felt within the muscle.

Another muscle that is of great importance to the function of the thorax is the muscle that is considered the

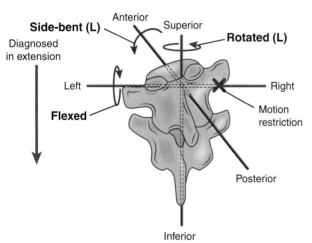

FIGURE 29–18 Flexed rotated side bent, left positional fault.

Table 29-8	Triplanar Positional Faults With Positional Diagnosis, Movement Diagnosis, and the Position for Treatment			
DIAGNOSIS	**DIAGNOSE IN:**	**PD**	**MD (OPPOSITE)**	**PT (SAME)**
FRS Right	Extension	Flexed, rotated, SB to the right	Extension, rotation. SB to the left	Extension, rotation, SB left
ERS Right	Flexion	Extended, rotated, SB to the right	Flexion, rotation, SB to the left	Flexion, rotation, SB to the left
FRS Left	Extension	Flexed, rotated, SB to the left	Extension, rotation, SB to the right	Extension, rotation, SB to the right
ERS Left	Flexion	Extended, rotated, SB to the left	Flexion, rotation, SB to the right	Flexion, rotation, SB to the right

PD positional diagnosis; MD, movement diagnosis; PT, position for treatment; FRS, flexed, rotated, and side bent; SB, side bending; ERS, extended, rotated, and side bent.

primary muscle of respiration, the *diaphragm*. This broad extensive dome-shaped muscle inserts onto the inner surface of the costal cage. Restrictions in rib mobility may limit respiration by disallowing the abdominal cavity to expand in the required fashion. Furthermore, a reduction in costal cage mobility may influence the length-tension relationship of the diaphragm, leading to a reduction in force output. This muscle is palpated on the underside of the costal cage by curling the fingertips up and under the ribs during inhalation.

Located between each adjacent rib are the external and internal intercostal muscles. Like the oblique muscles, the *external intercostal* runs obliquely in a "hands-in-pocket" direction, and the *internal intercostals* run perpendicularly in the opposite direction. Although debatable, the external intercostals are involved in rib elevation during inhalation. To palpate, simply identify the ribs and intercostal spaces and confirm through engaging the patient in deep breathing.

Special Tests

The reader is encouraged to consult other sources for additional information regarding the performance of these useful confirmatory tests. Examination of this region may also involve ruling out the presence of conditions in the cervical and lumbar spine, therefore, the reader is encouraged to consult Chapters 28 and 30 for additional special tests that may be used in the examination of the thorax. Special tests for the thorax have been clearly delineated in many other texts and in the literature. Therefore, only a brief description of selected special tests will be provided here. The reader is encouraged to consult other sources for additional information regarding the performance of these useful confirmatory tests.

SPECIAL TESTS FOR THE THORACIC SPINE AND COSTAL CAGE

Thoracic Slump Test (Fig. 29-21)

Purpose: To identify the presence of a nerve root or dural root adhesion

Patient: In a long sitting position, the patient flexes the knees 45 degrees, with arms behind the back, at which time baseline symptoms are assessed.

Clinician: Standing to the side of the patient

Procedure: While applying pressure over the shoulders, the patient is asked to flex the neck and extend the head on neck with overpressure as needed. Lastly, the examiner passively extends the knee and dorsiflexes the ankle on the symptomatic side and again reassesses symptoms.

Interpretation: The test is positive if reproduction of the patient's chief presenting symptoms occurs.

Lhermitte Sign

Purpose: To test for the presence of a cervical upper motor neuron lesion

Patient: Sitting

Clinician: Assess baseline symptoms

Procedure: Patient performs lower cervical flexion and extension

Interpretation: The test is positive if there is a neurological-type response typically into the extremities or in midline.

Beevor Sign

Purpose: To identify deficits in abdominal strength or the presence of a T7-12 spinal nerve root palsy

Patient: Hooklying

Clinician: Observing at the patient's side

Procedure: The patient is asked to sit up or cough.

Interpretation: The test is positive if there is a deviation of the umbilicus suggesting abdominal muscle weakness. The deviation will occur in a direction opposite from the area of weakness and may suggest nerve root compromise

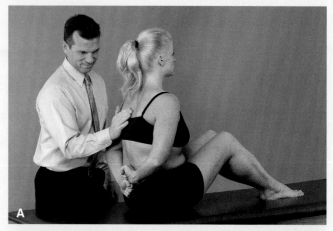
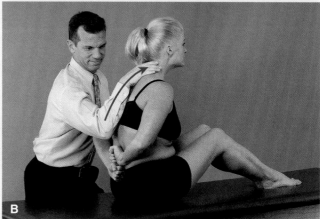
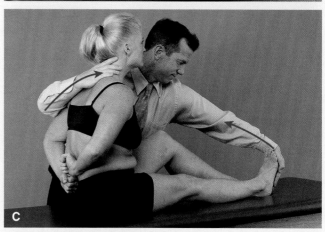

FIGURE 29–21 (A, B, C) Thoracic slump test.

MOBILIZATION OF THE THORACIC SPINE AND COSTAL CAGE

Note: The indications for the joint mobilization techniques described in this section are based on expected joint kinematics. Current evidence suggests that the indications for their use are multifactorial and may be based on direct assessment of mobility and an individual's symptomatic response.

Thoracic Spine Joint Mobilizations

Mid-Lower Thoracic Central and Unilateral Anterior Glides

Indications:
- *Mid-lower thoracic central and unilateral anterior glides* are indicated for restrictions in segmental mobility for all physiologic motions of the thoracic spine.

Accessory Motion Technique (Fig. 29-22)
- **Patient/Clinician Position:** The patient is in a prone position with the neck and head in neutral with the head supported and a pillow under the thoracic spine. The patient's head, neck, and thoracic spine may be prepositioned in flexion, extension, side bending, or rotation to facilitate or localize the mobilization. Stand to the side of the patient.
- **Hand Placement:** Stabilization is provided by pillow support. With your forearm in the direction in which force is applied, your mobilization hand may use any of the following hand contacts: 1.) the region just distal to the pisiform with thumb directed caudally contacting the spinous or transverse process, 2.) thumb-over-thumb or hypothenar eminence-over-thumb contacting the spinous or transverse process, 3.) split finger with digits 2 and 3 each contacting the transverse processes of the same vertebra, 3.) split finger with digits 2 and 3 each contacting the transverse processes of adjacent vertebrae on different sides (i.e., one contact on transverse process of T5 on left and other on transverse process of T6 on right).
- **Force Application:** Apply an anteriorly directed force through your mobilization hand contact(s). For the upper thoracic spine (T1-T4), force is applied in a superior and anterior direction.

Accessory With Physiologic Motion Technique (Figs. 29-23, 29-24, 29-25, 29-26)
- **Patient/Clinician Position:** The patient is in a sitting position. Stand to the side and/or behind the patient and be prepared to move in order to facilitate the application of forces in the proper direction.
- **Hand Placement:** The following hand contacts are used:
  - *Forward bending:* The patient is in a sitting position with arms folded across the chest, grasp the patient across his or her folded arms or weave through the folded arms to rest upon the contralateral shoulder or hold patient across the folded arms. The hypothenar eminence of the other hand is on the spinous process of the segment being mobilized (Fig. 29-23).
  - *Backward bending:* The patient is in a sitting position with folded arms raised and his or her forehead resting on the arms, support the weight of the folded arms and head. The

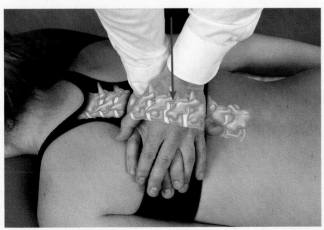

FIGURE 29–22 Mid-lower thoracic central and unilateral anterior glide. (From: Wise CH, Gulick DT. *Mobilization Notes: A Rehabilitation Specialist's Pocket Guide.* Philadelphia, PA: FA Davis Company, 2009.)

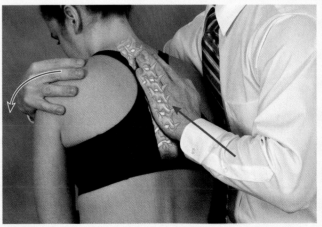

FIGURE 29–23 Mid-lower thoracic central and unilateral anterior glide: accessory with physiologic motion for forward bending in sitting. (From: Wise CH, Gulick DT. *Mobilization Notes: A Rehabilitation Specialist's Pocket Guide.* Philadelphia, PA: FA Davis Company, 2009.)

hypothenar eminence of the other hand is on the spinous process of the segment being mobilized (Fig. 29-24).

- *Side bending:* The patient is in a sitting position with the arms folded across the chest. For side bending toward you, place your axilla on the patient's ipsilateral shoulder. For side bending away from you, weave your hand through the patient's folded arms to rest upon the contralateral shoulder. The hypothenar eminence of the other hand is on the spinous process of the segment being mobilized (Fig. 29-25).
- *Rotation:* The patient is in a sitting position with arms folded across the chest. Weave your hand through the folded arms to rest upon the contralateral shoulder or hold patient across the folded arms. The hypothenar eminence of the other hand is on the transverse process of the segment being mobilized (Fig. 29-26).
- **Force Application:** Provide assistance and control as the patient moves through the desired motion while applying

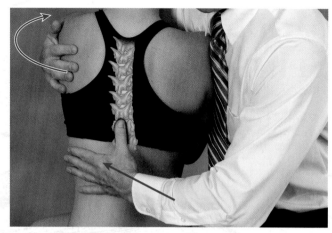

FIGURE 29–26 Mid-lower thoracic central and unilateral anterior glide: accessory with physiologic motion for rotation in sitting. (From: Wise CH, Gulick DT. *Mobilization Notes: A Rehabilitation Specialist's Pocket Guide.* Philadelphia, PA: FA Davis Company, 2009.)

force through the mobilization hand contacts. Force is maintained throughout the entire range of motion and sustained at end range.

Upper Thoracic Upglide "Scoop" Mobilization

Indications:

- *Upper thoracic upglide "scoop" mobilizations* are indicated for restrictions in upper thoracic upglide, which is an accessory motion of forward bending, side bending, and rotation and/or for restrictions in cervical spine mobility.

Accessory with Physiologic Motion Technique (Fig 29-27)

- **Patient/Clinician Position:** The patient is sitting in a low chair with his or her forehead placed on the folded arms. Stand in front of the patient in a stride stance position with your front leg between the patient's legs.

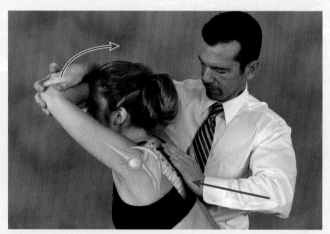

FIGURE 29–24 Mid-lower thoracic central and unilateral anterior glide: accessory with physiologic motion for backward bending in sitting. (From: Wise CH, Gulick DT. *Mobilization Notes: A Rehabilitation Specialist's Pocket Guide.* Philadelphia, PA: FA Davis Company, 2009.)

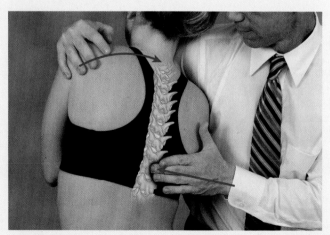

FIGURE 29–25 Mid-lower thoracic central and unilateral anterior glide: accessory with physiologic motion for side bending in sitting. (From: Wise CH, Gulick DT. *Mobilization Notes: A Rehabilitation Specialist's Pocket Guide.* Philadelphia, PA: FA Davis Company, 2009.)

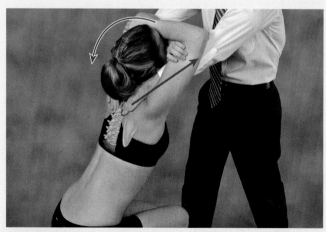

FIGURE 29–27 Upper thoracic upglide "scoop" mobilization. (From: Wise CH, Gulick DT. *Mobilization Notes: A Rehabilitation Specialist's Pocket Guide.* Philadelphia, PA: FA Davis Company, 2009.)

- **Hand Placement:** Stabilization is provided by the patient's weight. The second and third fingers of both hands are placed over the articular pillars of the superior vertebra of the segment being mobilized. Your fingers may be placed bilaterally for bilateral upglide (i.e., forward bending) or unilaterally to facilitate unilateral upglide (i.e., side bending or rotation). To achieve these contacts, your arms are threaded through patient's folded arms.
- **Force Application:** Using the patient's arms as counter-pressure, a supero-anterior force is provided through your finger contacts. To achieve greater ranges of upglide, the therapist may move the patient into side bending and/or rotation contralateral to the side in which force is being applied. The spectrum of oscillations may be used including a high velocity low amplitude thrust.

Thoracic Physiologic Side Bending With Finger Block

Indications:
- *Thoracic physiologic side bending with finger block mobilizations* are indicated for restrictions in mid-lower thoracic side bending and opening restrictions contralateral to the direction in which side bending occurs.

Accessory With Physiologic Motion Technique (Fig. 29-28)
- **Patient/Clinician Position:** The patient is in a sitting position with his or her arms folded across the chest. Stand to the side and/or behind the patient and be prepared to move in order to facilitate the application of forces in the proper direction.
- **Hand Placement:** For side bending in the direction ipsilateral to where you are standing, place your axilla on the

patient's ipsilateral shoulder. For side bending contralateral to where you are standing, weave your arm through the patient's folded arms to rest upon the patient's contralateral shoulder. The thumb or fingers of the stabilization hand are placed at the spinous process of the inferior vertebra of the segment being mobilized on the side ipsilateral to the direction in which the patient is side bending.
- **Force Application:** The patient actively sidebends with your guidance and assistance. Once motion is felt to arrive at the desired segment to be mobilized, the inferior vertebra of the desired segment is blocked by the stabilization hand.

Thoracic Physiologic Rotation With Finger Block

Indications:
- *Thoracic physiologic rotation with finger block mobilizations* are indicated for restrictions in mid-lower thoracic rotation and opening restrictions ipsilateral to the direction in which side bending occurs.

Accessory With Physiologic Motion Technique (Fig. 29-29)
- **Patient/Clinician Position:** The patient is in a sitting position with his or her arms folded across the chest. Stand to the side and/or behind the patient and be prepared to move in order to facilitate the application of forces in the proper direction.
- **Hand Placement:** Grasp the patient across his or her folded arms. Place the area just distal to your pisiform, thumb, or fingers of the stabilization hand in contact with the transverse process of the inferior vertebra of the segment being mobilized on the ipsilateral side to which

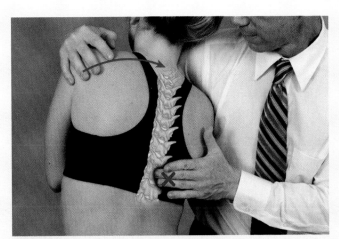

FIGURE 29–28 Thoracic physiologic side bending with finger block. (From: Wise CH, Gulick DT. *Mobilization Notes: A Rehabilitation Specialist's Pocket Guide.* Philadelphia, PA: FA Davis Company, 2009.)

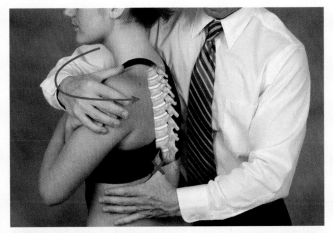

FIGURE 29–29 Thoracic physiologic rotation with finger block. (From: Wise CH, Gulick DT. *Mobilization Notes: A Rehabilitation Specialist's Pocket Guide.* Philadelphia, PA: FA Davis Company, 2009.)

rotation occurs or at the spinous process of the inferior vertebra of the segment being mobilized on the contralateral side. Your forearm is in line with the direction in which force is applied.

- **Force Application:** The patient actively rotates with your guidance and assistance. Once motion is felt to arrive at the desired segment to be mobilized, the inferior vertebra of the desired segment is blocked by the stabilization hand.

Thoracic Anterior Glide With Rotation "Screw" High-Velocity Thrust (Fig. 29-30)

- **Indications:** *Thoracic anterior glide with rotation "screw" high-velocity thrusts* are indicated for restrictions in segmental mobility throughout the mid-lower thoracic spine and for symptomatic relief of musculosekeletal pain in the thoracic region.
- **Patient/Clinician Position:** The patient is in a prone position with his or her neck and head in neutral and the trunk supported with a pillow under the thoracic spine. Stand to the side of the patient.
- **Hand Placement:** Stabilization is provided by the table and the patient's body weight. With your shoulders directly over the thoracic segment being mobilized and your elbows flexed, the hypothenar aspect of both hands are placed at the transverse processes of the same segment for anterior glide or at the transverse processes on opposite sides of adjacent segments for anterior glide with rotation.
- **Force Application:** Soft tissue slack is taken up as hand contacts move in equal and opposite directions to create a skin lock. As the patient slowly exhales, an anteriorly-directed force is applied through your hand contacts until end range is achieved at which time a high velocity low amplitude thrust is applied.

Thoracic Segmental Anterior Glide With Rotation "Pistol" High-Velocity Thrust (Fig. 29-31)

- **Indications:** *Thoracic segmental anterior glide with rotation "pistol" high-velocity thrusts* are indicated for restrictions in segmental mobility throughout the mid thoracic spine and for symptomatic relief of musculosekeletal pain in the thoracic region.
- **Patient/Clinician Position:** The patient is in a hooklying position with his or her hands folded and clasped behind the neck. Stand to the side of the patient. An alternate position involves the patient in a hooklying position with the arms folded in a "W" configuration across the chest.
- **Hand Placement:** Your cephalad arm is placed over the patient's flexed elbows and forearms to control motion. Your caudal hand assumes a pistol grip hand position with your thenar eminence and flexed 3rd, 4th, and 5th digits placed over the transverse processes of the segment being mobilized with the spinous process positioned within the space formed between the thenar eminence and your flexed fingers. Alternately, your hand may be ulnarly or radially deviated to position the hand contacts at the transverse processes on the opposite sides of adjacent vertebrae for the purpose of producing rotatory force. An alternate hand placement involves placing your cephalad hand under the patient's head and neck for the purpose of controlling the patient's trunk and your caudal hand forming the same pistol grip hand position, as described.
- **Force Application:** The patient is pre-positioned in forward bending and side bending, as desired, until motion arrives at the segment being mobilized. To accomplish this, the patient is slowly lowered by controlling the patient's trunk with your forearm that lies across the patient's flexed elbows and is reinforced by your chest until motion is recruited to the desired segment where your pistol hand is

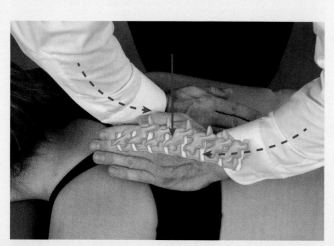

FIGURE 29–30 Thoracic anterior glide with rotation "screw" high velocity thrust. (From: Wise CH, Gulick DT. *Mobilization Notes: A Rehabilitation Specialist's Pocket Guide*. Philadelphia, PA: FA Davis Company, 2009.)

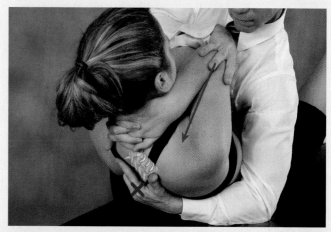

FIGURE 29–31 Thoracic segmental anterior glide with rotation "pistol" high-velocity thrust. (From: Wise CH, Gulick DT. *Mobilization Notes: A Rehabilitation Specialist's Pocket Guide*. Philadelphia, PA: FA Davis Company, 2009.)

positioned. Alternately, the patient is slowly lowered down to the segment being mobilized by controlling motion through with your cephalad hand, which is supporting the patient's head and neck. Be careful not to move the patient beyond the segment being mobilized. As the patient exhales, slack is taken up through all hand contacts and a high velocity low amplitude thrust is applied posteriorly through the long axis of the patient's humeri by your chest over forearm contact at the patient's flexed elbows.

Upper/Midthoracic Distraction High-Velocity Thrust (Fig. 29-32 A, B)

- **Indications:** *Upper/midthoracic distraction high-velocity thrusts* are indicated for restrictions in segmental mobility throughout the upper-mid thoracic spine and for symptomatic relief of musculosekeletal pain in the cervicothoracic region.
- **Patient/Clinician Position:** The patient is in a sitting position on the table with his or her fingers clasped behind the head and not the cervical spine. The patient is prepositioned in variable degrees of flexion or extension designed to localize forces with greater flexion required when mobilizing more caudal levels. Stand behind the patient on a stool as needed.
- **Hand Placement:** Stabilization is provided by the patient's body weight. For the upper thoracic region (T1-4), your arms are threaded through the patient's flexed arms with your hands resting over the patient's hands behind the head. For the mid thoracic region (T5-8), your hands grasp the patient's flexed elbows.
- **Force Application:** While maintaining hand contacts, lean back in order to produce a distraction force within the patient's upper or mid thoracic spine. To localize forces to the segment being mobilized, you may flex or extend the patient to the desired level. Once motion is recruited to the desired segment and slack is taken up within the segment, the patient pushes their arms into your arms. This serves to reduce upper extremity mobility and localizes forces to the spine. Upon exhalation, a high velocity low amplitude thrust is applied in a superior and posterior direction.

Upper Thoracic Facet Opposition Lock High-Velocity Thrust (Fig. 29-33)

- **Indications:** *Upper thoracic facet opposition lock high-velocity thrusts* are indicated for restrictions in unilateral opening of a segment in the lower cervical or upper thoracic spine when specificity is required, which is facilitated through facet opposition locking. This technique is also indicated for symptomatic relief of musculosekeletal pain in the cervicothoracic region.
- **Patient/Clinician Position:** The patient is in a sitting position with the patient's head and neck in neutral. Stand on

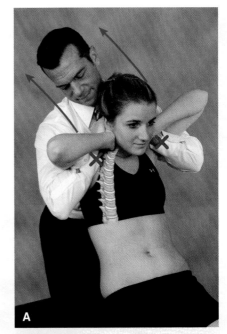

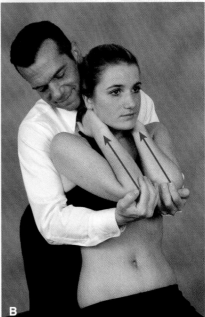

FIGURE 29–32 Upper/midthoracic distraction high-velocity thrust. **A.** Upper thoracic mobilization. **B.** Midthoracic mobilization. (From: Wise CH, Gulick DT. *Mobilization Notes: A Rehabilitation Specialist's Pocket Guide*. Philadelphia, PA: FA Davis Company, 2009.)

the contralateral side from where your finger block is being applied.

- **Hand Placement:** The thumb of your mobilization hand contacts the side of the spinous process of the inferior vertebra of the segment being mobilized contralateral to the side on which you are standing. Your stabilization hand moves the patient's head and cervical/upper thoracic spine into side bending away from you then rotation toward you until motion arrives at your mobilization thumb contact. Be sure to maintain both positions while performing the technique, which is achieved by holding the patient's head between your stabilization arm and your chest with your stabilization hand at the superior vertebra of the segment being mobilized. Pre-positioning the patient in side bending and rotation creates a facet-opposition lock of the superior segments designed to localize force to the segment being mobilized.

- **Force Application:** While maintaining all hand contacts and recruitment down to the desired segment, a gentle distraction force is provided by standing erect from a slightly squatted position while maintaining your stabilization arm and hand contacts. Once the slack is taken up within the segments, a high velocity low amplitude thrust is applied through the mobilizing thumb contact at the side of the spinous process in a transverse direction.

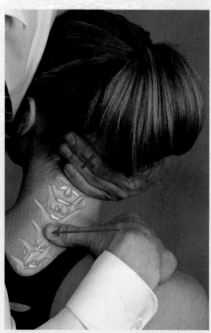

FIGURE 29–33 Upper thoracic facet opposition lock high-velocity thrust. (From: Wise CH, Gulick DT. *Mobilization Notes: A Rehabilitation Specialist's Pocket Guide*. Philadelphia, PA: FA Davis Company, 2009.)

Costal Cage Joint Mobilizations

First Rib Depression (Exhalation) Mobilization

Indications:

- *First rib depression (exhalation) mobilizations* are indicated for restoration of normal position and motion to an elevated rib.

Accessory Motion Technique (Not pictured)

- **Patient/Clinician Position:** The patient is in a supine position with the cervical spine pre-positioned in side bending

and rotation toward the side being mobilized in order to reduce tension of the lateral cervical musculature. Stand or sit at the head of the patient facing caudally.

- **Hand Placement:** Stabilization is provided by the patient's body weight. With the radial aspect of your 2nd metacarpophalangeal joint in contact with the superior aspect of the 1st rib with your forearm in the direction in which force is applied toward the patient's contralateral hip. Your elbow is held at your ASIS. Your other hand supports the patient's head in ipsilateral side bending and rotation.
- **Force Application:** As the patient exhales, slack is taken up and force is applied in the direction that is toward the patient's contralateral hip. The rib may be held in a depressed position as the patient inhales, which provides a stretch to the accessory muscles of respiration.

Accessory With Physiologic Motion Technique (Fig. 29-34 A)

- **Patient/Clinician Position:** Assume a half-kneeling position on the table behind the patient. The patient is in a sitting position on the table with the arm on the side being mobilized placed over your anterior thigh. The patient's head is sidebent and rotated toward the side being mobilized to reduce the tension of the lateral cervical musculature.
- **Hand Placement:** Your stabilization arm maintains the patient's cervical spine in side bending and slight rotation toward the side being mobilized. With the radial aspect of your 2nd metacarpophalangeal joint contact the superior aspect of the 1st rib with your forearm in the direction in which force is applied toward the patient's contralateral hip.
- **Force Application:** Using your flexed knee and stabilization arm, move the patient toward the side of mobilization and side bend the cervical spine slightly over the mobilization hand, take up the slack and apply a caudal and medially directed force to the superior aspect of the 1st rib as the patient exhales. The patient may also inhale as the first rib is maintained with caudal pressure with further mobilization into depression upon exhalation. Self-mobilization of the first rib into depression may be performed by placing a towel across the rib being mobilized with one end secured under patient's axilla and the other held by the patient. Downward force is applied to the first rib through the towel contact as the patient exhales and side bends his or her cervical spine contralaterally. Caudal force may be maintained by the towel as the patient inhales in order to stretch the accessory muscles of respiration (Fig. 29-34 B).

Rib Elevation (Inhalation) Mobilization

Indications:

- *Rib elevation (inhalation) mobilizations* are indicated for restrictions in rib elevation and to restore the normal position

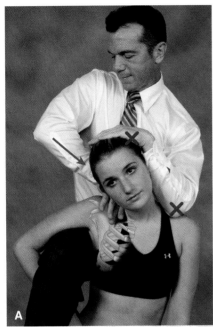

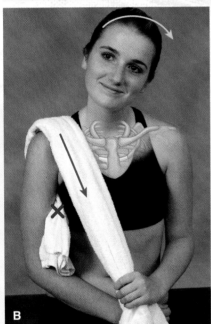

FIGURE 29–34 First rib depression mobilization. **A.** First rib depression accessory with physiologic motion. **B.** First rib depression self-mobilization. (From: Wise CH, Gulick DT. *Mobilization Notes: A Rehabilitation Specialist's Pocket Guide.* Philadelphia, PA: FA Davis Company, 2009.)

of a depressed rib. It is most effective for improving bucket handle elevation of ribs 3-10.

Accessory Motion Technique (Fig. 29-35 A)

- **Patient/Clinician Position:** The patient is in a side lying position with the uppermost arm overhead.
- **Hand Placement:** The web space of your stabilization hand contacts the rib below that which is being mobilized. Hold his or her arm in an overhead position.

- **Force Application:** Move the patient's arm into greater degrees of elevation while rib contact is maintained by your stabilization hand, which blocks motion and produces rib separation. Force may be coordinated with the patient's breathing with mobilization force elicited during inhalation.

Accessory With Physiologic Motion Technique (Fig 29-35 B)

- **Patient/Clinician Position:** The patient is in a sitting position with the arms across the chest. Stand to the side and in front of the patient on the side that is being mobilized.
- **Hand Placement:** The web space of your stabilization hand contacts the rib below being mobilized. Weave your mobilization arm through the patient's folded arms with your hand resting on the contralateral shoulder.
- **Force Application:** Side bend the patient away from the side being mobilized while rib contact is maintained by your stabilization hand, which blocks motion and produces rib separation. Force may be coordinated with the patient's breathing with mobilization force elicited during inhalation. Force is maintained throughout the entire range of motion and sustained at end range.

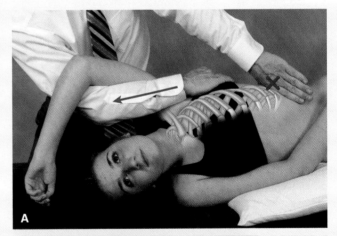

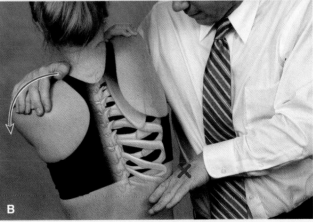

FIGURE 29–35 Rib elevation (inhalation) mobilization. **A.** Rib elevation in side lying. **B.** Rib elevation in sitting accessory with physiologic motion.

Rib Depression (Exhalation) Mobilization

Indications:

- *Rib depression (exhalation) mobilizations* are indicated for restrictions in rib depression and to restore the normal position of an elevated rib. It is most effective for improving bucket handle depression of ribs 3-10.

Accessory Motion Technique (Not pictured)

- **Patient/Clinician Position:** The patient is in a sitting position with the arms across the chest. Stand to the side and in front of the patient on the same side which is being mobilized.
- **Hand Placement:** The web space of your mobilization hand contacts the rib being mobilized. Your stabilization arm is placed across the patient's folded arms.
- **Force Application:** While stabilizing the patient's torso, apply a downward force through the rib contact. Force may be coordinated with the patient's breathing, which is elicited during exhalation.

Accessory With Physiologic Motion Technique (Fig. 29-36)

- **Patient/Clinician Position:** The patient is in a sitting position with the arms across the chest. Stand to the side and in front of the patient on the same side which is being mobilized.
- **Hand Placement:** The web space of your mobilization hand contacts the rib being mobilized. Your axilla is placed over the patient's ipsilateral shoulder as your arm is weaved through the patient's folded arms, with your hand contacting the patient's contralateral torso.
- **Force Application:** Move the patient into side bending toward the side being mobilized as you apply downward force

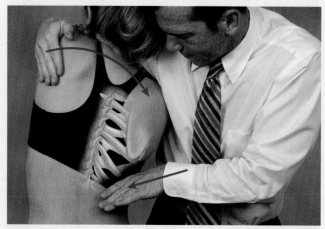

FIGURE 29–36 Rib depression (exhalation) mobilization accessory with physiologic motion.

through the rib contact. Force may be coordinated with the patient's breathing, which is elicited during exhalation. Force is maintained throughout the entire range of motion and sustained at end range.

Rib Anterior Mobilization

Indications:

- *Rib anterior mobilizations* are indicated for restrictions in motion of the ribs in an anterior direction in the transverse plane and to restore the normal position of a rib that is positioned posteriorly. It is most effective for ribs 3-10.

Accessory With Physiologic Motion Technique (Fig. 29-37 A)

- **Patient/Clinician Position:** The patient is in a sitting position with the arms across the chest. Stand to the side and behind of the patient on the opposite side from that which is being mobilized.
- **Hand Placement:** The web space of your mobilization hand contacts the posterior aspect of the rib being mobilized. Your other arm is placed across the patient's folded arms with your hand resting on the patient's posterior shoulder.
- **Force Application:** Rotate the patient toward you and away from the side being mobilized. Once motion arrives at the rib being mobilized, apply an anteriorly directed force through your mobilization hand at the posterior aspect of the rib. Force is maintained throughout the entire range of motion and sustained at end range.

Accessory With Physiologic Motion Technique With Blocking (Fig. 29-37 B)

- **Patient/Clinician Position:** The patient is in a sitting position with the arms across the chest. Stand to the side and in front of the patient on the opposite side from that which is being mobilized.
- **Hand Placement:** The web space of your blocking hand contacts the anterior aspect of the rib just inferior to the rib being mobilized. Your other arm is placed across the patient's upper back with your hand resting on the patient's posterior shoulder.
- **Force Application:** Move the patient into rotation toward you and away from the side being mobilized. Once motion arrives at the rib being mobilized, use your blocking hand contact at the anterior aspect of the rib to block motion as the involved rib and ribs superior are brought further anteriorly. Force is maintained throughout the entire range of motion and sustained at end range.

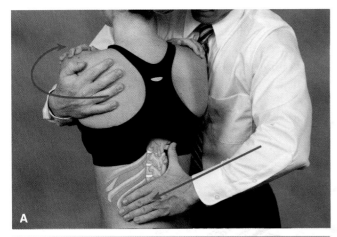

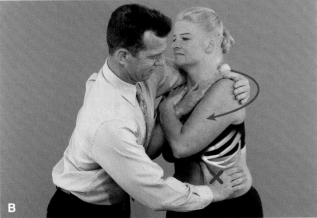

FIGURE 29–37 A. Rib anterior mobilization accessory with physiologic motion. **B.** Rib anterior accessory with physiologic motion with blocking.

Rib Posterior Mobilization

Indications:

- *Rib posterior mobilizations* are indicated for restrictions in motion of the ribs in a posterior direction in the transverse plane and to restore the normal position of a rib that is positioned anteriorly. It is most effective for ribs 3–10.

Accessory With Physiologic Motion Technique (Fig. 29-38 A)

- **Patient/Clinician Position:** The patient is in a sitting position with the arms across the chest. Stand to the side and behind the patient on the opposite side from that being mobilized.
- **Hand Placement:** The web space of your mobilization hand contacts the anterior aspect of the rib being mobilized. Your other arm is placed across the patient's folded arms with your hand resting on the patient's anterior shoulder.
- **Force Application:** Rotate the patient away from you and toward the side being mobilized. Once motion arrives at the rib being mobilized, apply a posteriorly directed force

through your mobilization hand at the anterior aspect of the rib. Force is maintained throughout the entire range of motion and sustained at end range.

Accessory With Physiologic Motion Technique with Blocking (Fig. 29-38 B)

- **Patient/Clinician Position:** The patient is in a sitting position with the arms across the chest. Stand to the side and behind the patient on the opposite side from that which is being mobilized.
- **Hand Placement:** The web space of your blocking hand contacts the posterior aspect of the rib just inferior to the rib being mobilized. Your other arm is placed across the patient's folded arms with your hand resting on the patient's anterior shoulder.
- **Force Application:** Move the patient into rotation away from you and toward the side being mobilized. Once motion arrives at the rib being mobilized, use your blocking hand contact at the posterior aspect of the rib to block motion as the involved rib and ribs superior are brought further posteriorly. Force is maintained throughout the entire range of motion and sustained at end range.

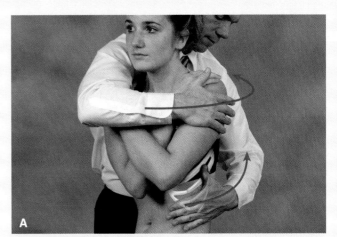

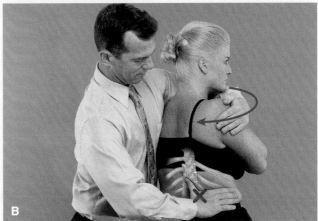

FIGURE 29–38 A. Rib posterior mobilization accessory with physiologic motion. **B.** Rib posterior accessory with physiologic motion with blocking.

Type I Neutral Dysfunction Muscle Energy Technique (Fig. 29-39 A, B)

- **Indications:** *Type I neutral dysfunction muscle energy techniques* are indicated for restoration of normal position and mobility of a type I positional fault

- **Patient/Clinician Position:** The patient is in a sitting position with the arms folded across the chest in a neutral, erect sitting posture without either flexion or extension. Stand to the side and behind the patient.

- **Hand Placement:** One arm is placed across the patient's folded arms to control biplanar motion and resist patient-generated forces. The fingers of the other hand palpate the segment being mobilized to ensure localization of forces.

- **Force Application:**
  - For a *neutral, rotated, side-bent right (NRS right)* lesion, stack the involved segment in the frontal and transverse planes by *side bending left* and *rotating right* while the palpating hand ensures localization of forces to the desired segment. Upon achieving this position, move the patient into the *interbarrier zone*. The patient then performs a gentle 6-second isometric hold in any plane against your resistance. Following the hold, move the patient further

into each plane being careful not to move beyond the desired segment to be mobilized. Repeat this process for 3-5 repetitions (Fig. 29-39 A).

- For *neutral, rotated, side-bent left (NRS left)* lesion, stack the involved segment in the frontal and transverse planes by *side bending right* and *rotating left* while the palpating hand ensures localization of forces to the desired segment. On achieving this position, move the patient into the *interbarrier zone*. The patient then performs a gentle 6-second isometric hold in any plane against your resistance. Following the hold, move the patient further into each plane being careful not to move beyond the desired segment to be mobilized. Repeat this process for 3-5 repetitions (Fig. 29-39 B).

Type II Flexion Dysfunction Muscle Energy Technique (Fig. 29-40 A, B)

- **Indications:** *Type II flexion dysfunction muscle energy techniques* are indicated for restoration of normal position and mobility of a type II flexion positional fault.

- **Patient/Clinician Position:** The patient is in a sitting position with the arms folded across the chest in a neutral,

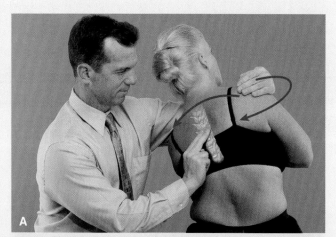

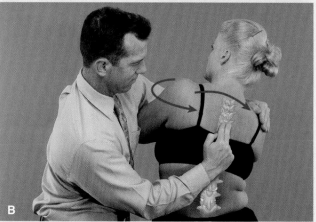

FIGURE 29–39 Type I neutral dysfunction muscle energy technique, for **A.** neutral, rotated, side-bent right lesion and **B.** neutral, rotated, side-bent left lesion.

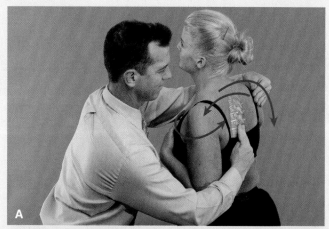

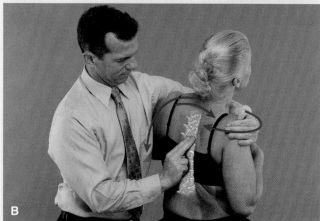

FIGURE 29–40 Type II flexion dysfunction muscle energy technique for **A.** flexed, rotated, side-bent right lesion and **B.** flexed, rotated, side-bent left lesion.

erect sitting posture without either flexion or extension. Stand to the side and behind the patient.

- **Hand Placement:** One arm is placed across the patient's folded arms to control triplanar motion and resist patient-generated forces. The fingers of the other hand palpate the segment being mobilized to ensure localization of forces.
- **Force Application:**
  - For a *flexed, rotated, side-bent right (FRS right)* lesion, stack the involved segment in the sagittal, frontal, and transverse planes by *extending, side bending left*, and *rotating left* while the palpating hand ensures localization of forces to the desired segment. On achieving this position, move the patient into the *interbarrier zone*. The patient then performs a gentle 6-second isometric hold in any plane against your resistance. Following the hold, move the patient further into each plane being careful not to move beyond the desired segment to be mobilized. Repeat this process for 3-5 repetitions (Fig. 29-40 A).
  - For *flexed, rotated, side-bent left (FRS left)* lesion, stack the involved segment in the sagittal, frontal, and transverse planes by *extending, side bending right*, and *rotating right* while the palpating hand ensures localization of forces to the desired segment. Upon achieving this position, move the patient into the *interbarrier zone*. The patient then performs a gentle 6-second isometric hold in any plane against your resistance. Following the hold, move the patient further into each plane being careful not to move beyond the desired segment to be mobilized. Repeat this process for 3-5 repetitions (Fig. 29-40 B).

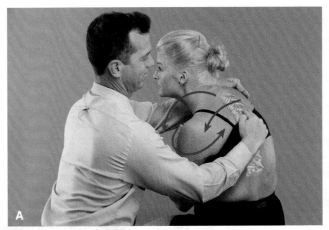

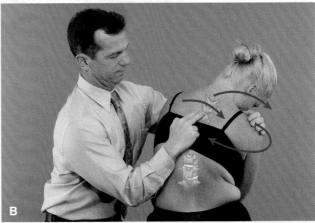

FIGURE 29–41 Type II extension dysfunction muscle energy technique for **A.** extended, rotated, side-bent right lesion and **B.** extended, rotated, side-bent left lesion.

Type II Extension Dysfunction Muscle Energy Technique (Fig. 29-41 A, B)

- **Indications:** *Type II extension dysfunction muscle energy techniques* are indicated for restore of normal position and mobility of a type II extension positional fault
- **Patient/Clinician Position:** The patient is in a sitting position with the arms folded across the chest in a neutral, erect sitting posture without either flexion or extension. Stand to the side and behind the patient.
- **Hand Placement:** One arm is placed across the patient's folded arms to control triplanar motion and resist patient-generated forces. The fingers of the other hand palpate the segment being mobilized to ensure localization of forces.
- **Force Application:**
  - For an *extended, rotated, side-bent right (ERS right)* lesion, stack the involved segment in the sagittal, frontal, and transverse planes by *flexing, side bending left*, and *rotating left* while the palpating hand ensures localization of forces to the desired segment. On achieving this position, move the patient into the *interbarrier zone*. The patient then performs a gentle 6-second isometric hold in any plane against your resistance. Following the hold, move the patient further into each plane being careful not to move beyond the desired segment to be mobilized. Repeat this process for 3–5 repetitions (Fig. 29-41 A).
  - For an *extended, rotated, side-bent left (ERS left)* lesion, stack the involved segment in the sagittal, frontal, and transverse planes by *flexing, side bending right*, and *rotating right* while the palpating hand ensures localization of forces to the desired segment. Upon achieving this position, move the patient into the *interbarrier zone*. The patient then performs a gentle 6-second isometric hold in any plane against your resistance. Following the hold, move the patient further into each plane being careful not to move beyond the desired segment to be mobilized. Repeat this process for 3–5 repetitions (Fig. 29-41 B).

CLINICAL CASE STUDY

History of Present Illness (HPI)

Harry presents to your clinic today with a long history of midthoracic spine pain with intermittent radiating symptoms into the lateral and anterior costal cage regions bilaterally. He notes onset of symptoms approximately 2 years ago, at which time he was performing a slide tackle while playing soccer that resulted in extreme trunk rotation. Harry reports significant pain upon inspiration on the right with a reduction in his ability to fully inspire. Reproduction of symptoms is also noted with trunk movement, primarily when twisting to look behind him when backing up in his car.

Posture/Observation: In standing the following is observed: left convexity with apex at T7, right convexity with apex at L3, and increased height of the left shoulder. Observation of his respiratory pattern reveals that the patient is an upper chest breather at a rate of 12 breaths/minute.

AROM: FB = 90% pain free with left rib hump; BB = 75% pain free; SB right = 90% pain free; SB left = inability to achieve curve reversal, pain; ROT right = 50% pain; ROT left = 90% pain free.

PPIVM: Spring testing reveals hypomobility throughout the thoracic spine, most notable T5-T9; Costal cage mobility: Hypomobile ribs 4 to 8 for bucket-handle on the right.

Neurological Screen: Within normal limits throughout

Strength Testing: Grossly 5/5 throughout

Special Tests: Poor segmental breathing at the lower lobe on the right

Palpation: Tenderness to the touch at the thoracic paravertebral musculature and along the intercostal spaces of ribs 5 through 10 on the right as well as over the sternocostal joints anteriorly, right greater than left, hyperactive scaleni are noted. Increased height of the left iliac crest.

Perform each component of the exam on a partner.

1. Develop a problem list of impairments.
2. Establish a pathoanatomical-based diagnosis.
3. Establish an impairment-based diagnosis.

4. Create a plan of care that includes three mobilizations, three stretching exercises, three strengthening exercises. Perform each on your partner.

HANDS-ON

With a partner, perform the following activities:

1 With the spine adequately exposed, observe your partner as he or she performs active thoracic spine motion in standing for 5-10 repetitions in each plane. Appreciate both the quality and quantity of available motion. Identify any areas of hypo- or hypermobility and any motions that produce pain, any motions that feel restricted, and any motions that feel unstable. Perform an active motion assessment on another individual as they stand side by side and identify any differences in each individual's movement pattern.

2 Perform motion testing of the thoracic spine-costal cage complex using active physiologic mobility testing as a screening tool to identify any potential areas of hypo- or hypermobilty. Attempt to use overpressure and counterpressure to isolate the suspected region of symptomatic origin, if present. Follow the process of rotational symptom localization, as described in this chapter, to further isolate the origin.

3 Perform passive physiologic movement of the thoracic spine and ribs in sitting as described in this chapter. Attempt to identify any specific areas of hypo- or hypermobility. If identified, test these specific areas through accessory mobility testing.

4 Perform a general respiration screen on your partner for the upper ribs and mid to lower ribs as described in this chapter. Identify any areas of hypo- or hypermobility. Attempt to identify any ribs that need further assessment.

5 Perform accessory mobility testing of the costal cage including blocking techniques for the CT joint and assessment of first rib mobility and position.

6 Perform PAIVM testing of the thoracic spine. Determine the relationship between the onset of pain (P1 and P2), if present, and stiffness or resistance (R1 and R2), if present. Compare your findings during the active movement assessment with your findings during PAIVM testing. Perform PAIVM testing on at least one other individual and record any differences. Solicit feedback from your partner regarding your performance of these procedures.

7 Through palpation, attempt to identify the primary soft tissue and bony structures of the thoracic spine-costal cage complex, including the entire costal cage from anterior to posterior. Compare tissue texture, tension, tone, and location of each structure.

8 Based on your movement examination as identified above, choose 2 non-thrust mobilizations and 2 thrust mobilizations. Perform these mobilizations on your partner and, after reassessment, identify any immediate changes in mobility or symptoms in response to these procedures. If possible, video yourself performing these procedures and self-assess your performance. Solicit feedback from your partner regarding your performance of these procedures.

9 Perform each mobilization described in the intervention section of this chapter on at least two individuals. Using each technique, practice grades I to IV. Solicit input from your partner regarding position, hand placement, force application, comfort, etc. If possible, video yourself performing these procedures and self-assess your performance. When practicing these mobilization techniques, utilize the Sequential Partial Task Practice Method, in which students repeatedly practice one aspect of each technique (i.e., position, hand placement, force application) on multiple partners each time, adding the next component until the technique is performed in real time from beginning to end. (Wise CH, Schenk RJ, Lattanzi JB. A model for teaching and learning spinal thrust manipulation and its effect on participant confidence in technique performance. *J Manual & Manipulative Ther*, August 2014.)

REFERENCES

1. Resnick DK, Weller SJ, Benzel EC. Biomechanics of the thoracolumbar spine. *Neuro Surg Clin North Am*. 1997;8:455-469.
2. Saumarez RC. An analysis of possible movements of human upper rib cage. *J Appl Physiol*. 1986;60:678-689.
3. Kapandji IA. *The Physiology of the Joint. Vol. 3, The Trunk and the Vertebral Column*. Edinburgh, Scotland: Churchill Livingstone; 1974.
4. Greene WB, Heckman JD. *The Clinical Measurement of Joint Motion*. Rosemont, IL: American Academy of Orthopaedic Surgeons; 1994.
5. White AA III, Panjabi MM. Kinematics of the spine. In: White AA III, Panjabi MM, eds. *Clinical Biomechanics of the Spine*, 2nd ed. Philadelphia, PA: JB Lippincott; 1990.
6. Paris SV, Loubert PV. *Foundations of Clinical Orthopaedics, Course Notes*. St. Augustine, FL: Institute Press; 1990.
7. Wilson TA, Rehder K, Krayer S, et al. Geometry and respiratory displacement of human ribs. *J Appl Physiol*. 1987;62:1872-1877.
8. Oatis CA. *Kinesiology: The Mechanics and Pathomechanics of Human Movement*. Philadelphia, PA: Lippincott Williams and Wilkins; 2004.
9. Panjabi MM, Brand RA, White AA. Mechanical properties of the human thoracic spine. *J Bone Joint Surg*. 1976;58:642.
10. Willems JM, Jull GA, Ng JKF. An in vivo study of the primary and coupled rotations of the thoracic spine. *Clin Biomechanics*. 1996;2:311.
11. Lee DG. *Manual Therapy for the Thorax-A Biomechanical Approach*. Delta, British Columbia: Delta Orthopedic Physiotherapy Clinic; 1994.
12. Lee D. *The Thorax: An Integrated Approach*. White Rock, British Columbia: Diane G. Lee Physiotherapist Corporation; 2003.
13. Boissonnault WG. *Primary Care for the Physical Therapist: Examination and Triage*. St. Louis, MO: Elsevier Saunders; 2005.
14. Henderson JM. Ruling out danger: differential diagnosis of thoracic spine. *Phys Sports Med*. 1992;20:124-132.
15. McKenzie R, May S. *The Lumbar Spine Mechanical Diagnosis and Therapy Volume One*. Waikanae, New Zealand: Spinal Publications; 2003.
16. Cloward RB. Cervical discography: a contribution to the etiology and mechanism of neck, shoulder, arm pain. *Ann of Surg*. 1959;150:1052-1064.
17. Maitland GD, Hengeveld E, Banks K, English K. *Maitland's Vertebral Manipulation*, 6th ed. Woburn, MA: Butterworth-Heinemann; 2001.
18. Kendall F, McCreary E, Provance P. *Muscles: Testing and Function with Posture and Pain*, 4th ed. Baltimore, MD: Lippincott Williams and Wilkins; 1993.
19. Levangie PK, Norkin CC. Joint structure and function: a comprehensive analysis, 4th ed. Philadelphia, PA: FA Davis Company; 2005.
20. Cleland JA, Glynn P, Whitman JM, Eberhart SL, et al. Short-term effects of thrust versus nonthrust mobilization/manipulation directed at the thoracic spine in patients with neck pain: a randomized clinical trial. *Phys Ther*. 2007;87:431-440.

21. Magee DJ. *Orthopedic Physical Assessment*, 4th ed. Philadelphia, PA: WB Saunders; 1992.
22. Simons DG, Travell JG, Simons LS. *Travell and Simons' Myofascial Pain and Dysfunction: The Trigger Point Manual, Vol. 1*, 2nd ed. Baltimore, MD: Williams Wilkins; 1999.
23. Hart FD, Strickland D, Cliffe P. Measurement of spinal mobility. *Ann Rheum Dis.* 1974;33:136-139.
24. Mayer TG, Kondraske G, Beals SB, et al. Spinal range of motion: accuracy and sources of error with inclinometric measurement. *Spine.* 1997;22:1976-1984.
25. Moll JMH, Wright V. Measurement of spinal movement. In: Jason M, ed. *The Lumbar Spine and Back Pain*. New York, NY: Pitman Medical; 1976;93-112.
26. Greene WB, Heckman JD. *The Clinical Measurement of Joint Motion*. Rosemont, IL: American Academy of Orthopaedic Surgeons; 1994.
27. Gloeck C, Evjenth O. *Symptom Localization in the Spine and Extremity Joints*. Seehausen, Germany: eBooks Central; 1997.
28. Krauss J, Creighton D, Ely JD, Podlewsks-Ely J. The immediate effects of upper thoracic translatoric spinal manipulation on cervical pain and range of motion: a randomized clinical trial. *J Manual Manip Ther.* 2008;16:93-99.
29. Jull G, Bogduk N, Marsland A. The accuracy of manual diagnosis for cervical zygapophyseal joint pain syndromes. *Med J Aust.* 1988;148:233-236.
30. Mahar C, Adams R. Reliability of pain and stiffness assessments in clinical manual lumbar spine examination. *Phys Ther.* 1994;74:801-811.
31. Richardson C, Jull G, Hodges P, Hides J. *Therapeutic Exercise for Spinal Segmental Stabilization in Low Back Pain. A Scientific Basis and Clinical Approach*. London, England: Churchill Livingston; 1999.
32. Bergmark A. Stability of the lumbar spine. A study in mechanical engineering. *Acta Orthop Scand.* 1989;230(suppl):20-24.
33. Mens JMA, Vleeming A, Snijders CJ, Koes BJ, Stam HJ. Reliability and validity of the active straight leg raise test in posterior pelvic pain since pregnancy. *Spine.* 2001;26:1167.
34. Mens JMA, Vleeming A, Snijders CJ, Stam HJ, Ginai AZ. The active straight leg raising test and mobility of the pelvic joints. *Eur Spine.* 1999;8:468.

Orthopaedic Manual Physical Therapy of the Cervical Spine and Temporomandibular Joint

Christopher H. Wise, PT, DPT, OCS, FAAOMPT, MTC, ATC

Chapter Objectives

At the conclusion of this chapter, the reader will be able to:

- Identify the key anatomical and biomechanical features of the cervical spine and temporomandibular joint (TMJ) and their impact on examination and intervention.
- List and perform key procedures used in the orthopaedic manual physical therapy (OMPT) examination of the cervical spine and TMJ.
- Demonstrate sound clinical decision-making in evaluating the results of the OMPT examination.

- Use pertinent examination findings to reach a differential diagnosis and prognosis.
- Discuss issues related to the safe performance of OMPT interventions for the cervical spine and TMJ.
- Demonstrate basic competence in the performance of a skill set of joint mobilization techniques for the cervical spine and TMJ.

INTRODUCTION

Neck-related disorders (NRD) impact an estimated 10% to 15% of the general population.[1] Some estimate that 70% of individuals will experience mechanical neck pain at some point in their lives.[2] Twenty-five percent of all individuals seeking outpatient physical therapy services present with primary complaint of neck pain.[2] These conditions are more common in women, and their prevalence increases over the age of 50 years.[1] In addition to personal hardship, neck pain places a substantial financial burden on society, with one-third of those reporting neck pain requiring long-term medical care.

FUNCTIONAL ANATOMY AND KINEMATICS

Cervical Spine Arthrology and Kinematics

Largely due to its anatomical complexity, differential diagnosis of neck-related disorders is challenging. The cervical spine is comprised of two distinct regions. The **subcranial**, or **suboccipital**, region consists of the *occiput*, the *atlas (C1)*, and the *axis (C2)*. The **midcervical to lower cervical** region is defined as the inferior aspect of C2 to C7. Due to its facet joint orientation and subsequent kinematics, which resembles that of the cervical spine, the first three or four thoracic vertebral segments (T1–T4) are often considered in the management of NRD.

The Subcranial Articulations

The cervical vertebra possessing the greatest breadth is the *atlas (C1)*. Its prominently projecting lateral masses, which provide protection for the vertebral arteries, may be palpated between the angle of the mandible and the mastoid process bilaterally (Fig. 30-1). The anterior arch of C1 forms a bony buttress and an important articulation with the *odontoid process, or dens*, which projects superiorly and posteriorly from the body of C2. C1 is without a vertebral body, and its spinal canal is divided by the *transverse ligament*, which is the horizontal component of the *cruciform ligament*. The axis (C2) is located approximately three finger-widths inferior to the greater

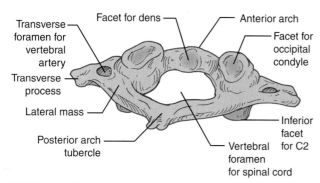

FIGURE 30–1 The atlas (C1).

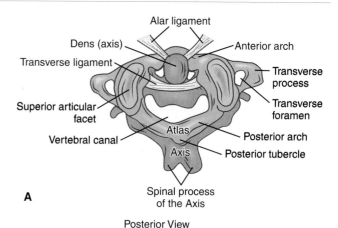

A

Posterior View

B

FIGURE 30–4 The atlantoaxial complex.

occipital protuberance (Fig. 30-2). C2 represents the first vertebra with a body and spinous process, the latter of which can be easily palpated upon cervical flexion.

The superior articular condyles of C1 are concave, slightly ellipsoidal, face medially, and are congruent with the large convex condyles of the *occiput*.[3] The *occipitoatlantal* complex, referred to as *OA* (Fig. 30-3), primarily allows movement in the sagittal and frontal planes. Three distinct articulations form the *atlantoaxial* complex, which is referred to as *AA* (Fig. 30-4). The two laterally positioned facet joints consist of convex-on-convex articular surfaces and slope inferiorly in a medial to lateral direction. Some authors describe the atlantal surfaces

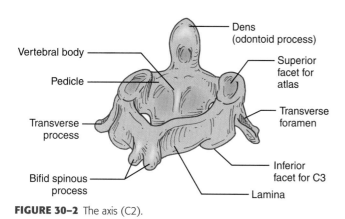

FIGURE 30–2 The axis (C2).

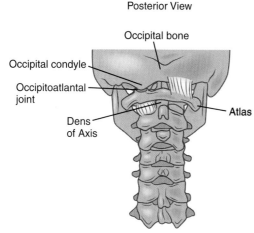

FIGURE 30–3 The occipitoatlantal complex.

as concave, and the axial surfaces as convex.[3] The central pivot joint is formed between the odontoid process of C2 and the anterior arch of C1, anteriorly, and transverse ligament, posteriorly.

The unique mobility demands required from the subcranial spine renders this region susceptible to instability. The transverse ligament, by virtue of its relationship with the dens, restrains anterior migration of C1 during upper cervical flexion. Likewise, the anterior arch of C1 limits posterior migration of C1 during extension. The paired *alar ligaments* run from the apex of the dens superiorly, laterally, and anteriorly to insert onto the occipital condyles and rim of the *foramen magnum*.[4] This ligament is important in limiting rotation of the occiput and atlas on the axis.[5] Side bending produces immediate ipsilateral rotation of C2, which is largely the result of tension that develops within the alar ligament. The small *apical ligament*, running from the apex of the dens vertically to insert on the anterior precipice of the foramen magnum, offers only scant stability.[4]

The Mid to Lower Cervical Articulations (C3-C7)

The anterior component of a typical midcervical vertebra is composed of the *vertebral body*, which is comparatively less robust than in other regions of the spine. The pedicles and lamina form the triangular *spinal canal*. The *transverse processes* possess a *transverse foramen* for the passage of the *vertebral artery*, and the *spinous processes* are bifid and irregular, with the second, sixth, and seventh being most prominent (Fig. 30-5 A).

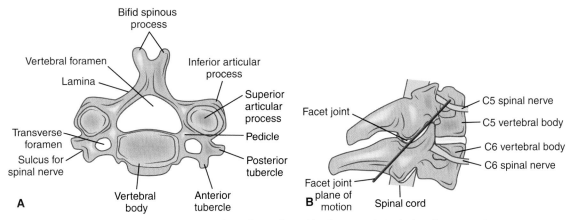

FIGURE 30–5 A. The mid to lower cervical spinal vertebra and **B.** mid to lower cervical spinal motion segment.

Of particular note is the orientation of the synovial *zygapophyseal facet joints*, which are at a 45-degree angle between the transverse and frontal planes with the superior facets facing superiorly and posteriorly and the corresponding inferior facets directed inferiorly and anteriorly (Fig. 30-5 B). The highly elastic and paired *ligamentum flavum* serves a role in the avoidance of capsular impingement during motion.[6] The *anterior longitudinal ligament (ALL)*, which spans the space between anterior vertebral bodies at each adjacent level, becomes more substantial as it descends. The *posterior longitudinal ligament (PLL)*, which forms the anterior wall of the spinal canal, spans from vertebral body and disc at each adjacent spinal level. The PLL is most robust in the cervical spine and may play a role in supporting the intervertebral disc. The *ligamentum nuchae*, which plays a passive role in supporting the head, spans from the greater occipital protuberance to C7, firmly inserting into the spinous processes at each level and interdigitating with the posterior spinal musculature.[7]

Forming fibrous cartilaginous articulations between each adjacent vertebral body, with the exception of C1-2, are the *intervertebral discs*. Like elsewhere in the spine, the intervertebral discs are composed of incomplete rings of fibrous connective tissue, known as the *annulus fibrosis* on the periphery, and the hydrophilic *nucleus pulposis*, which occupies the central portion of the disc. In the cervical spine, the nucleus makes up a much smaller percentage of the total area of the disc compared to adjacent spinal regions.[7] The *uncinate processes*, located on the lateral, superior aspect of the vertebral bodies, form lateral interbody joints, known as the *uncovertebral joints*, or the *joints of Von Luschka*.

Cervical Spine Kinematics

Based on its inherent structure, the cervical spine sacrifices stability for mobility. Variability in motion exists between each spinal segment; therefore, determining mobility of the head and neck as a single structure, which is routinely done in the clinic, should be reconsidered in favor of appreciating segmental mobility.

Subcranial Segmental Kinematics

The *occipitoatlantal (OA)* articulation is often referred to as the "yes" or "maybe" joint because it primarily allows sagittal plane and frontal plane motion. *Forward nodding* and *backward nodding* are the terms used to refer to sagittal plane motion that occurs subcranially. As the head flexes (forward nods) on the neck, the occipital condyles roll anteriorly and glide posteriorly, with the opposite occurring during extension (backward nods) in order to maintain the axis of rotation in a neutral position (Fig. 30-6, Fig. 30-7). In the literature, total forward to backward nodding OA range of motion is reported to be approximately *14 to 35 degrees*.[8,9] OA side nodding considered by some to not be a physiologic motion but rather a motion that may occur as a coupled motion in response to external forces (Fig. 30-8).[7] OA side nodding has been reported to range up to *11 degrees* when manually induced[10] but only *5 degrees* during active physiologic motion.[3] There is a negligible amount of rotation available at the OA articulation.[3]

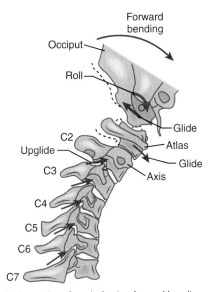

FIGURE 30–6 Kinematics of cervical spine forward bending.

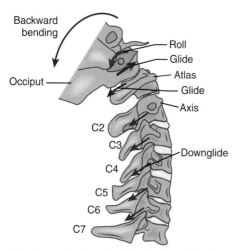

FIGURE 30–7 Kinematics of cervical spine backward bending.

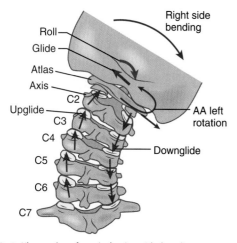

FIGURE 30–8 Kinematics of cervical spine side bending.

The majority of motion available at the *atlantoaxial (AA)* segment occurs in the transverse plane, which provides approximately *40 degrees* of rotation (Fig. 30-9 A).[3] This joint is, therefore, often referred to as the "no" joint. More than half of all rotation available in the cervical spine occurs at this

articulation. It is important to note that AAs contribution to rotation occurs first, and rotation below this level takes place only after motion at AA has been fully exhausted. During rotation, the occiput rotates, for example, to the right, producing immediate rotation of the atlas in the same direction. The left inferior facet joint of C1 glides anteriorly as the right facet of C1 glides posteriorly, while each slides down their respective slope formed by the convex superior facet of C2.[7] As more motion is required, right rotation then extends into the midcervical spine, where subcranial side bending to the left is needed to allow the eyes to be maintained in a level position. This motion creates a gliding of the atlas to the left as it follows the occiput. Therefore, at end range of right rotation, the atlas has rotated to the right and glided to the left on the axis (Fig. 30-9 B). The alar ligament and facet joint capsules provide primary and secondary restraints at end ranges of rotation.[7]

Although to a lesser degree than rotation, flexion (forward nodding) and extension (backward nodding) is also available at the AA segment providing approximately *20 degrees* of combined forward and backward nodding.[3] This motion is directed by the odontoid process, which slopes posteriorly, thus allowing the atlas to move up and back during extension and down and forward during flexion. As the occiput rolls and glides, the atlas, by virtue of its intimate relationship with the occiput, will follow. The atlas glides anteriorly and posteriorly during OA forward and backward nodding, respectively, and also follows the occiput in the direction to which side bending occurs.

The quantity of AA side nodding is minimal and estimated to be approximately *5 degrees*.[3] During side bending right, the occiput rolls to the right and glides to the left on the atlas, after which the atlas follows the occiput and glides to the right. With continued right side bending, the left alar ligament is engaged, which brings the axis into right rotation. The atlas is now in left rotation relative to the axis, thus allowing the head to remain facing forward. As side bending proceeds into the midcervical spine, additional right rotation will occur, thus requiring a greater degree of left AA rotation to allow the head

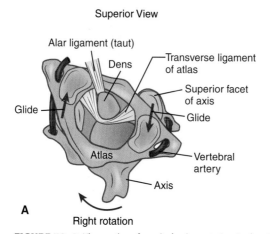

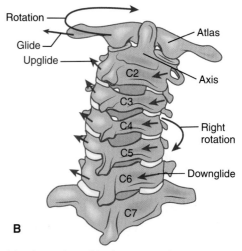

FIGURE 30–9 Kinematics of cervical spine rotation in the **A.** subcranial region and **B.** mid to lower cervical region.

to remain facing forward (see Fig. 30-8). Both cervical side bending and rotation involve a complex interaction between the subcranial and midcervical spinal regions, and either region may contribute to identified limitations.

Mid to Lower Cervical Segmental Kinematics (C2-C7)

Based on the orientation of the facet joints, which are 45 degrees between the transverse and frontal planes, segmental motion involves movement up and forward, referred to as **upglide**, or down and backward, referred to as **downglide**. During forward bending and backward bending, bilateral upglide with anterior translation and downglide with posterior translation occurs, respectively (see Figs. 30-6 and 30-7). Combined forward-backward bending range of motion has been measured to range from *9 to 28 degrees* and is greater in the more cephalad segments.[7]

In the midcervical spine, side bending and rotation are coupled movements that are mechanically forced to occur ipsilaterally.[11] This coupled movement is sometimes referred to as type II, physiologic, or functional, side bending/rotation. The atlas will invariably follow the occiput during motion. During midcervical motion, the subcranial region will enable the head to remain facing forward, via the AA segment, and the eyes to remain level, via the OA segment. Rotation to the left at AA, for example, may accompany mid-cervical side bending to the right when keeping the head facing forward is functionally desirable. Likewise, side bending to the left at OA, may accompany mid-cervical rotation right for the purpose of keeping the eyes in a level position. These complex motions are referred to as nonphysiologic or nonfunctional motions. Nonphysiologic motions are more complex and require motion at both the subcranial and midcervical regions, whereas physiologic or functional motions are midcervical dominant and do not require subcranial motion. A comparison between these motions during the movement examination may assist the therapist in identifying the area of primary segmental restriction.[11] For example, if functional side bending, which primarily occurs within the midcervical region, is full and pain free but nonfunctional side bending, which requires subcranial motion to enable the head to remain facing forward, is limited and/or painful, the therapist may suspect the subcranial

segments as the culpable region and direct intervention accordingly. Side bending has been measured to range from *2 to 6 degrees* segmentally (*35 degrees* total) and rotation from *2.1 to 6.9 degrees* segmentally (*45 degrees* total), depending on the level.[7] Another method that may be used for isolating subcranial from midcervical motion is to engage the patient in active, active assisted or passive cervical retraction and protraction. Cervical retraction represents the combined motions of upper cervical flexion (forward bending) and lower cervical extension (backward bending). Conversely, cervical protraction includes the combined motions of upper cervical extension (backward bending) and lower cervical flexion (forward bending) (Fig. 30-10). Figs. 30-6 to 30-10 display both subcranial and mid to lower cervical kinematics during physiologic motion.

Temporomandibular Arthrology and Kinematics

Temporomandibular Arthrology

The *temporomandibular joint (TMJ)* is classified as a synovial joint possessing articular surfaces lined with fibrocartilage rather than hyaline cartilage (Fig. 30-11). The requirements placed on this joint in regard to frequency of motion and applied forces are substantial and render this joint susceptible to dysfunction. Each TMJ is inextricably linked to its contralateral counterpart, and mobility impairments in one of these joints will invariably impact function of the other. In addition, the muscles acting across the TMJ have the capacity to impart exceptional forces over a relatively small surface area.

At rest, the convex *mandibular condyle* is seated securely within the concave *glenoid fossa* of the temporal bone. After the initial phase of opening, the majority of motion occurs between the convex condyle and the convex *articular eminence* of the temporal bone, thus creating an incongruent and less stable articular relationship.

Each TMJ has two distinct joint spaces that are divided by the *articular disc*, which serves to enhance congruency. The *inferior joint space*, between the condyle and inferior disc, is a hinge joint that allows angular motion within the sagittal plane.

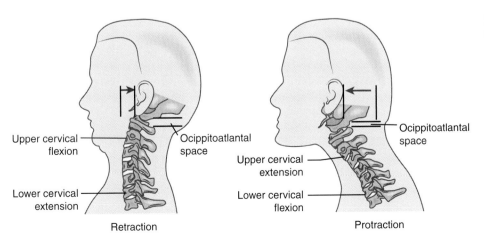

FIGURE 30–10 Kinematics of cervical retraction and protraction.

Upper cervical flexion

Ocippitoatlantal space

Lower cervical extension

Retraction

Ocippitoatlantal space

Upper cervical extension

Lower cervical flexion

Protraction

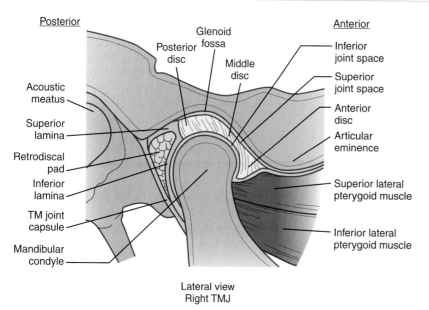

Posterior — Glenoid fossa — Anterior

Posterior disc — Middle disc

Inferior joint space
Superior joint space
Anterior disc
Articular eminence
Superior lateral pterygoid muscle
Inferior lateral pterygoid muscle

Acoustic meatus
Superior lamina
Retrodiscal pad
Inferior lamina
TM joint capsule
Mandibular condyle

Lateral view
Right TMJ

FIGURE 30–11 The temporomandibular joint.

The *superior joint space* is a planar joint in which linear translation occurs between the articular eminence and the superior disc. The biconcave disc accommodates for the convexity of both the eminence and the condyle, thus adding to joint stability.[12] Normal function of the disc is predicated on the ability of the disc to move in concert with the condyle. This feature is accomplished by the lateral pterygoid, whose superior and inferior heads insert into the disc and condyle, respectively.

The capsuloligamentous complex (CLC) of the TMJ is thin and permits triplanar motion. The greatest degree of laxity is within the superior joint space where the greatest degree of motion occurs. This capsular arrangement allows the disc to be more firmly attached to the condyle with greater freedom of movement relative to the temporal bone.[13] Capsular laxity is most evident anteriorly, precipitating anterior subluxations of the condyle.[14] Due to the highly vascular nature of the CLC, damage to this structure results in a cycle of edema and fibrosis, ultimately resulting in mobility impairments. Mechanoreceptors present within the CLC are important for enhancing the precision of TMJ motion and are important to consider during intervention.

The *TM ligament* with its oblique and horizontal portions serve as suspensory ligaments with the *oblique portion*, tethering the neck of the condyle, and the *horizontal portion* attaching to the lateral pole of the condyle, posterior disc, and articular eminence. The oblique portion limits posterior and inferior migration of the mandible and rotation while the horizontal portion primarily limits posterior translation.[12,13] Collectively, the TM ligament serves as the primary restraint to posterior and lateral translation of the condyle and is important for protecting the structures of the retrodiscal region.

The *sphenomandibular ligament* and the *stylomandibular ligament* sandwich the ramus of the mandible as they course anteriorly and inferiorly from their respective sphenoid bone and styloid process origins. Because of their location, these ligaments are suspensory ligaments most involved in limiting anterior translation of the mandible.[12,14] These ligaments may also utilize stored energy that was developed during opening to assist in the return of the condyle posteriorly during mouth closing.

Temporomandibular Kinematics

Mandibular depression and *elevation*, or mouth opening and closing, requires precise and symmetrical motion of four distinct joints. Full mouth opening requires both roll or rotation and anterior glide or translation of the condyle that equals approximately *40 to 50 mm*. A quick assessment of mobility may be ascertained in the ability of the TMJ to open the width of three-knuckles. The disc's more intimate association with the condyle suggests less mobility within the inferior joint space. Under ideal conditions, the disc closely follows the condyle through its excursion of motion. Controversy exists regarding the timing of superior and inferior joint motion. Some consider initial mouth opening to consist of angular motion of the condyle relative to the disc occurring as a hinge around an axis that extends through both poles of the condyle within the inferior joint space (Fig. 30-12 A). This is followed by full mouth opening, which is achieved through anterior glide or translation of both the disc and condyle within the superior joint space (Fig. 30-12 B).[15] Others believe that motions of each joint space, although unique, occur simultaneously during mouth opening.[16,17] In cases where anterior migration of the condyle is prohibited, an opening of only *10 to 25 mm* is possible, suggesting normal function of the inferior joint space.

Motion of the disc along with the condyle during opening and closing is critical and controlled through a fine interplay between the elastic properties of the retrodiscal pad and the superior head of the lateral pterygoid muscle. This muscle intends to translate the disc along with the condyle anteriorly during opening and eccentrically control posterior translation of the disc-condyle complex during closing while the condyle completes its final motion into posterior rotation.[18] Motion of the disc in this fashion is dependent on the extensibility of the bilaminar retrodiscal pad, which inserts into the posterior

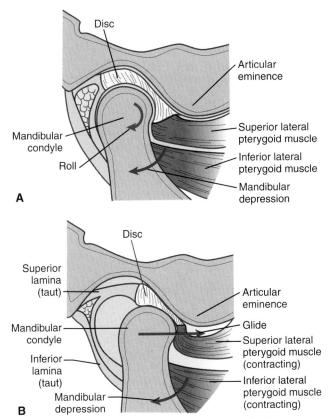

FIGURE 30–12 Mandibular depression revealing **A.** early phase rotation which occurs in the inferior joint space and **B.** late phase translation which occurs in the superior joint space.

disc, thereby restraining anterior translation with opening and retrieving the disc upon closing. A variety of factors may alter the kinematics of the disc, resulting in reduced mobility and symptoms.

Mandibular protrusion and *retrusion* involves linear translation without rotation, requiring isolated motion within the superior joint space. Protrusion involves anterior glide or translation of both condyles equally up to *6 to 9 mm* (Fig. 30-13 A). Retrusion involves posterior glide or translation back to the resting position and up to *3 mm* beyond (Fig. 30-13 B). The retrodiscal pad and TM ligament must possess adequate elasticity to allow the normal excursion of protrusion and retrusion, respectively. A

comparison of protrusion and depression allows the therapist to isolate which joint space is most involved. For example, if mandibular depression and protrusion are equally limited, then impairment within the superior joint space is suspected.

Lateral deviation consists of rotation or roll of the condyle about a vertical axis ipsilaterally and anterior glide or translation of the condyle contralaterally, resulting in deviation of the mandible in the transverse plane (Fig. 30-14). Normal excursion is considered to be *8 mm* to either side.[14] This transverse plane motion is necessary for normal mastication and for speech. Its asymmetrical movements allow the examiner to test anterior translation unilaterally. If opening is limited, for example, and right lateral deviation is equally limited but left deviation is normal, then impairment of the superior joint space of the left TMJ is suspected.

EXAMINATION

The Subjective Examination

Self-Reported Disability Measures

For individuals with neck-related disorders, a variety of self-reported disability instruments have been found to be reliable and valid.[19–21] The presence of high levels of fear avoidance beliefs combined with anxiety over movement has been found to be an important factor in determining a patient's immediate response to a specific intervention for both the cervical spine and the lumbar spine.[22–25]

Neck Disability Index

Perhaps, the most commonly used self-assessment questionnaire in the management of neck-related disorders is the **Neck Disability Index (NDI)**, an adaptation of the Oswestry Disability Instrument (see Chapter 28). The NDI has been widely used both clinically and in the literature. The patient is asked to place a mark in each of the 10 sections next to the statement that most closely applies to his or her current condition. The test-retest reliability of the NDI is 0.89.[19] Most importantly, the NDI provides valuable information regarding the patient's ability to engage in functionally relevant activities and serves as a valid measure of progress throughout intervention.

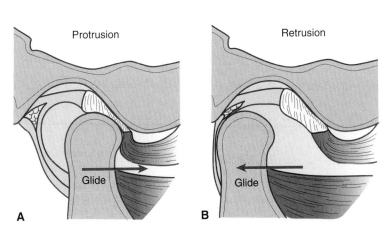

FIGURE 30–13 A. Mandibular protrusion and **B.** Mandibular retrusion.

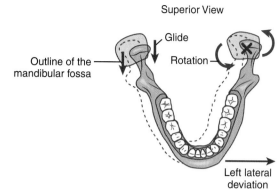

FIGURE 30-14 Mandibular lateral deviation.

Table 30-1	Medical Red Flags for the Cervical Spine
MEDICAL CONDITION	**RED FLAGS**
Cervical Segmental Instability	Recent history of trauma
	Use of oral contraceptives
	History of spondyloarthropathy (i.e., rheumatoid arthritis)
	Upper motor neuron signs/symptoms
	Bilateral extremity involvement
Cervical Neuropathy	Pain and paresthesia into the upper extremity
	Symptoms are influenced by cervical motion
	Lower motor neuron signs/symptoms
	With or without history of recent trauma
Myocardial Infarction	Angina
	Dyspnea, pallor
	History of coronary artery disease, hypertension, diabetes, tobacco, increased cholesterol
	Men over age 40, women over age 50

(Adapted from: Boissonnault *WG. Primary Care for the Physical Therapist: Examination and Triage.* St. Louis, MO: Elsevier Saunders; 2005.)

Northwick Park Disability Questionnaire

To complete the ***Northwick Park Disability Questionnaire (NPQ)***, the patient responds to nine individual categories of functional activities, and points are assigned based on patient response to specific phrases that describe their function. For scoring, the sum is divided by 36 and multiplied by 100 to provide a percentage (Score/36 × 100%), with a higher percentage representing greater disability. This instrument has been found to possess good short-term repeatability and internal consistency.[21]

Review of Systems

Metastasis does not occur nearly as often in the cervical spine as in other regions of the spine.[26] An individual with a history, diagnosis, or suspected presence of cancer must be referred for further evaluation and closely monitored. Unremitting night pain that is disassociated from movement or position often serves as a red flag that signals the presence of malignancy. Deyo et al[27] suggest that cancer should be routinely suspected in the population of males over the age of 50 with a previous history of cancer accompanied by recent unexplained weight loss and failure to respond to conservative intervention.[27] A malignant tumor of the superior sulcus of the lung, known as *Pancoast's tumor,* may appear initially as shoulder pain causing entrapment of the brachial plexus, most notably, the C8-T1 nerve roots. Symptoms consist of vertebral border of scapula pain and neurological symptoms that radiate distally along the ulnar nerve distribution of the hand.[28] Those most at risk are men older than 50 years who smoke.[28] Table 30-1[28] displays the cervical spine red flags requiring a medical referral that must be identified during the initial examination.[28]

History of Present Illness

The association between the patient's chief complaint and movement or position is the first criterion for establishing the existence of a mechanical movement disorder. Of particular importance is establishing the patient's *symptomatic profile* and *level of reactivity.* A *numeric pain rating scale (NPRS)* score greater than a 5 or 6/10, a significant increase in the NPRS score with motion, an extended amount of time in return of

symptoms to the baseline level, the presence of an empty end feel, and peripheralization of symptoms are all suggestive of a highly reactive state.

Capsular impingement is suspected in cases of a recent, sudden onset of sharp, localized neck pain brought on by a minor incident such as suddenly turning the head and looking up. Neck stiffness is a common complaint in individuals who are experiencing *spondylosis,* especially during the morning waking hours in those over 40 years of age. The occurrence of *cumulative trauma disorders (CTD)* are common in the cervical spine and result from individuals spending prolonged periods of time in poor, static postures. *Myofascial syndromes* often result insidiously and may represent the primary impairment or occur secondary to an underlying condition, such as injury to the facet joint or disc.

The presence of peripheral symptoms must be further explored for the purpose of ascertaining their origin. A true *cervical radiculopathy* must be differentiated from a *peripheral nerve entrapment syndrome* or referred symptoms from some other source such as an active, muscular *trigger point.* Wainner et al[29] have proposed a clinical prediction rule (CPR) that may be used to rule in the presence of a cervical radiculopathy. They identified that a cervical radiculopathy is suspected if the following criteria are present: positive Spurling test, positive upper limb tension test, positive neck distraction test, and less than 60 degrees of cervical spine rotation toward the involved side. If three of the four criteria are present the positive likelihood ratio (+LR) is 6.1, if all four criteria are present the +LR is 30.3.[29]

If bilateral neurological signs or symptoms are present, a *central spinal stenosis, or myelopathy,* is suspected. In such cases, a combination of both upper and lower motor neuron symptoms are reported bilaterally. In addition to the neurological signs and symptoms just described, the patient may also present with hypertonicity, hyperreflexia, clonus, bowel and bladder dysfunction, sexual disturbances, as well as balance and coordination disturbances. Neuropathies from systemic disorders, such as alcohol use or diabetes, may also present with bilateral extremity involvement (see Chapter 19).

An additional consideration when examining the cervical spine is the presence of headaches. *Cervicogenic headaches* are defined as "a unilateral headache associated with evidence of cervical involvement through provocation of pain by movement of the neck or by pressing the neck; concurrent pain in the neck, shoulder, and arm; and reduced range of motion of the neck with or without other features."[30] Current evidence, however, reveals that these features were not pathognomonic to this population.[31] The most reliable features were pain that begins in the neck with radiation to the frontal and temporal regions into the ipsilateral extremity and reproduction with neck movement.[32] The ***International Headache Society*** has proposed criteria that may be used to diagnose cervicogenic headaches (Table 30-2).[33] Current evidence using fluoroscopically guided diagnostic blocks reveal that 70% of these cervicogenic headaches emanate from the C2-3 facet joints,[34] and the C3-4 segment appears to be only occasionally involved.[35] There were, however, no distinctive clinical features, including loss of motion or tenderness, that were found to be specific to the involved segment.[36] The mechanism underlying cervicogenic headaches has been proposed to involve the *trigeminocervical nucleus* (Fig. 30-15), which receives afferents from C1-3 that

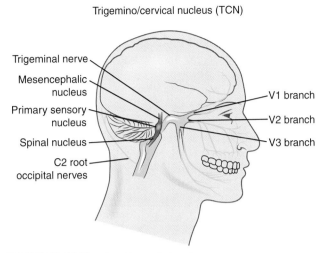

Trigemino/cervical nucleus (TCN)

FIGURE 30-15 The trigeminocervical nucleus.

converge on second-order neurons that also receive afferents from the trigeminal nerve.[37] Consequently, upper cervical pain can be referred to regions of the head innervated by cervical nerves or the trigeminal nerve. Noxious stimulation studies reveal that the OA, C1-2, and C2-3 segments can refer pain to the occipital region.[34,38,39] Diagnostic block studies reveal that C1-2 refers pain to the occiput, vertex, orbit, and ear. The C2-3 segment spreads into the occipital, parietal, frontal regions, and orbit, and the C3-4 segment primarily refers symptoms to the upper neck.[35]

Vertigo, tinnitus, seizures, and visual disturbances should be differentiated from headaches. Cervicogenic dizziness may result from suboccipital restrictions. Dizziness may also result from central nervous system or inner ear disorders such as *Meniere's disease, vestibular neuritis, vestibular labyrinthitis,* or *benign paroxysmal positional vertigo.* Visual disturbances may include nystagmus, diplopia, and loss of acuity. *Vertebrobasilar insufficiency (VBI)* often results in symptoms that include vertigo, nausea, diplopia, tinnitus, dysarthria, and nystagmus, which typically commence or increase upon performance of cervical extension.[11] Clinical screening tests for identification of VBI will be described later in this chapter. Such symptoms may also be suggestive of a sympathetic nervous system disorder.

Among the most challenging musculoskeletal conditions to manage are *whiplash associated disorders (WAD).* As defined by Spitzer et al,[40] a WAD is "an acceleration-deceleration mechanism of energy transfer to the neck which may result from rear-end or side-impact, predominantly in motor vehicle collisions, but also from diving accidents. . . . The energy transfer may result in bony or soft-tissue injuries, which in turn may lead to a variety of clinical manifestations." Symptoms typically consist of dizziness, deafness, tinnitus, headache, memory loss, dysphagia, and temporomandibular joint pain, among others.[40] The cervical facet joints have been implicated as the source of neck pain after whiplash.[41] WAD victims may not experience immediate symptoms; however, 27% of subjects still report pain 6 months after initial injury.[42] Fifteen percent to 20% of subjects develop persistent pain and disability.[43] The U.S.

Table 30-2	The International Headache Society Criteria for Classification of Cervicogenic Headaches

A. Pain localized to neck and occipital region. May project to forehead, orbital region, temples, vertex or ears.

B. Pain is precipitated or aggravated by neck movements or sustained neck posture.

C. At least one of the following:
  1. Resistance to or limitation of passive neck movements
  2. Changes in neck muscle contour, texture, tone, or response to active and passive stretching and contraction
  3. Abnormal tenderness of neck muscles

D. Radiological examination reveals at least one of the following:
  1. Movement abnormalities in flexion/extension
  2. Abnormal posture
  3. Fractures, congenital abnormalities, bone tumors, rheumatoid arthritis or other distinct pathology (not spondylosis or osteochondrosis)

(Classification from Headache Classification Subcommittee of the International Headache Society. The International Classification of Headache Disorders: 2nd ed. *Cephalalgia* 2004;24(Suppl 1):8-151.)

annual costs associated with WAD are $29 billion.[40] To assist in diagnosis and management, several systems of classification for WAD exist. The *Quebec Task Force* classification system is presented in Table 30-3.[40] This system is based primarily on the severity of signs and symptoms at the time of the injury. More recently, Sterling[44] developed a system for classification of WAD revealing that those who experience chronic pain and disability are characterized by widespread sensory hypersensitivity suggestive of disturbances in central pain processing as well as an acute posttraumatic stress reaction. This classification system incorporates measurable motor, sensory and psychological impairments (Table 30-4).[44]

Patients presenting with a chronic history of symptoms suggestive of cervical instability must also be tested prior to initiating manual interventions. Cook et al[45] used a Delphi survey method to establish consensus among orthopaedic manual physical therapy experts on the signs and symptoms for classification of clinical cervical spine instability and reported the following symptoms as reaching the highest consensus: "intolerance to prolonged static postures, fatigue and inability to hold head up, better with external support, including hands and collar, frequent need for self-manipulation, feeling of instability, shaking, or lack of control, frequent episodes of acute attacks, and sharp pain, possibly with sudden movements." [45] The physical examination findings related to cervical instability that reached highest consensus among the clinical OMPT experts were "poor coordination/neuromuscular control, including poor recruitment and dissociation of cervical segments with movement, abnormal joint play, motion that is not smooth throughout range of motion, including segmental hinging, pivoting, and fulcruming, and aberrant movement."[45] Due to the inherent risks associated with stability screening procedures,

Table 30-3	The Quebec Task Force Classification System for Whiplash Associated Disorders

QUEBEC TASK FORCE GRADE	PRESENTATION
0	No complaint of neck pain No physical signs
I	Neck pain, stiffness, and tenderness No physical signs
II	Neck pain Musculoskeletal signs including tenderness to the touch and decreased range of motion
III	Neck pain Musculoskeletal signs including tenderness to the touch and decreased range of motion Neuromuscular signs including diminished deep tendon reflexes, muscle weakness, sensory loss
IV	Neck pain Fracture or dislocation confirmed by imaging

(Report of the Quebec Task Force on Spinal Disorders. *Spine.* 1987;12(7 Suppl):1-59.)

Table 30-4	Classification for Whiplash-Associated Disorders as Proposed by Sterling[44]

STERLING CLASSIFICATION	PRESENTATION
WAD 0	No complaint of neck pain No physical signs
WAD I	Neck pain, stiffness, and tenderness No physical signs
WAD IIA	Neck pain Motor impairment Decreased range of motion Altered muscle recruitment patterns (CCFT) Sensory impairment Local cervical mechanical hyperalgesia
WAD IIB	Neck pain Motor impairment Decreased range of motion Altered muscle recruitment patterns (CCFT) Sensory impairment Local cervical mechanical hyperalgesia Psychological impairment Elevated psychological distress
WAD IIC	Neck pain Motor impairment Decreased range of motion Altered muscle recruitment patterns (CCFT) Sensory impairment Local cervical mechanical hyperalgesia Generalized sensory hypersensitivity Sympathetic nervous system involvement Psychological impairment Elevated psychological distress Elevated acute posttraumatic stress

WAD III	Neck pain
	Motor impairment
	Decreased range of motion
	Altered muscle recruitment patterns (CCFT)
	Sensory impairment
	Local cervical mechanical hyperalgesia
	Generalized sensory hypersensitivity
	Sympathetic nervous system involvement
	Psychological impairment
	Elevated psychological distress
	Elevated acute posttraumatic stress
	Neurological signs of conduction loss including:
	  Decreased or absent deep tendon reflexes
	  Muscle weakness
	  Sensory deficits

WAD IV	Fracture or dislocation

CCFT, craniocervical flexion test; WAD, whiplash-associated disorder.

if the historical interview raises suspicion of instability, it is recommended to forego formal screening procedures and manual interventions and refer the patient for further medical testing.[46]

Determining the nature of an individual's TMJ complaints must also be explored during the historical interview. The specific activities or motions that produce or relieve symptoms, the intensity, location, and duration of symptoms, as well as the relationship between pain and other symptoms such as clicking or joint crepitus are all important pieces of the diagnostic puzzle. Jaw pain, stiffness, and temporal headaches in the morning are often caused by **bruxism** during sleep. Compressive forces through the TMJ and hyperactivity of the masticatory muscles result in such symptoms, which are often best controlled through the use of dental appliances, behavioral interventions, and anxiety medications, all of which fall outside of the purview of the manual physical therapist. The incidence of pain when eating firm or chewy foods, such as steak, nuts, raw vegetables, salad, or gum chewing is a common complaint of individuals with temporomandibular dysfunction (TMD). Pain within the dentitia as a result of dental caries or gum disease should be differentiated from pain emanating from the TMJ.

A differentiation must be made between patient complaints of clicking versus crepitus. An *opening click* occurs as the condyle reduces by moving over the posterior aspect of the anteriorly displaced disc during opening. A *closing click* occurs in the final phase of closing as the disc migrates anteriorly, causing the condyle to once again sublux over the posterior margin of the disc. A *reciprocal click* occurs on both opening and closing.

The presence of an *open-locked* (mouth stuck open) or *closed-locked* (mouth stuck closed) condition suggests a disc that has migrated so far posteriorly or anteriorly, respectively, that full jaw mobility is inhibited. Locking of the TMJ from disc displacement is often associated with joint clicking. For example, an open-locked condition includes a reciprocal click, with the second click representing migration of the disc posterior to the condyle, thus limiting terminal posterior translation during closing.

Secondary features often associated with TMD include complaints of hearing loss, ear pain, blockage, tinnitus, or vertigo. Headaches of TMJ origin should be differentiated from other causes, such as those previously discussed. Headaches that are associated with the TMJ often occur in the morning after a night of bruxism or eating and are unrelated to cervical spine motion. Consultation with the patient's dentist, orthodontist, endodontist, or periodontist may be necessary for the achievement of optimal outcomes in individuals with TMD.

Medical Testing and Diagnostic Imaging

Information regarding the patient's laboratory test values and the results of any diagnostic imaging performed serves as the second tier in the premanipulative screening process. This information may be vital in determining the impact of preexisting comorbidities and the status of spinal structures following a traumatic event.

The **Canadian Cervical Spine Rules**[47,48] (Fig. 30-16) were developed to guide decisions regarding when radiographs may

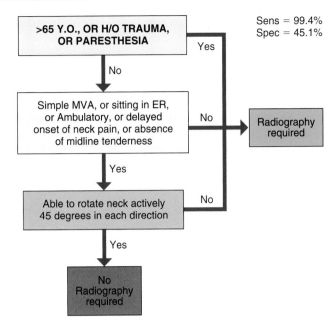

FIGURE 30–16 The Canadian Cervical Spine Rules. (Data from: Steill, IG, Clement CM, McKnight RD, et al. The Canadian c-spine rule vs. the Nexus low-risk criteria in patients with trauma. *N Engl J Med.* 2003; 2510-2518; Steig IG, Wells GA, Vandemheem KL, et al. The Canadian c-spine rule for radiography in alert and stable trauma patients. *JAMA.* 2001;286: 1841-1848.)

be indicated in a patient who is alert with a cervical injury. The sensitivity and specificity for identifying the target condition of a cervical spine injury, which includes dislocation, fracture, or instability, diagnosed through imaging is 99.4% and 45.1%, respectively.[47,48]

Plain Film Radiography

In the case of a precipitating traumatic event, a standard series of plain film radiographs, including *anteroposterior*, *lateral*, *oblique*, and *open-mouth* views, must be performed prior to embarking on manual intervention.[49] Lateral views and *stress views*, which are lateral views taken with the spine in either flexion or extension, are helpful in determining the presence of instability.[50] Three parallel lines are drawn on the radiograph along the anterior vertebral bodies, posterior vertebral bodies, and spinolaminar junction. Instability is detected if there is an interruption in this three parallel line relationship. On the lateral view, the **atlantodental interface**, or space between the odontoid process and the anterior arch of the atlas, can be appreciated. An interface of greater than 3 mm suggests disruption of the transverse ligament or odontoid fracture.[50] The oblique view, which consists of four distinct views, provides visualization of the intervertebral foramina.[50] The open-mouth view provides information regarding the integrity of the subcranial region. When considering the results of diagnostic imaging, the examiner must be aware of the high incidence of false-positive findings in the asymptomatic population.[39,51,52]

Rocabado[53] describes cranioverteberal centric relation as the "three-dimensional articular ligamentous position of the cranium over the upper cervical spine, where the condyles of the occiput adopt a stable position over the atlas which maintains a stable anteroposterior and lateral position with the odontoid process and a horizontal alignment over the shoulders of the axis."[53] The midline position is determined by the spinous process of C2, which should be in line with the dens as determined by the open mouth view.[53]

When determining the static posture of the head and neck, a particular lateral plain film radiograph, called the *lateral cephalometric view*, may be useful.[53] Normal distance on lateral films should reveal 20 mm, or two to three finger widths, between the occiput and C2.[53] A reduction in the occipitoatlantal space suggests a posteriorly rotated occiput, thus increasing the potential for greater occipital nerve entrapment.[53] This view may also be used to assess **McGregor's plane,** which is defined as a line drawn on radiographs from the inferior border of the occiput to the hard palate.[53] Under normal conditions, this plane should be horizontal, with alterations noted as the head is flexed or extended.[53] This plane is also used to assess the *odontoid plane*, which under normal conditions, positions the odontoid at 101 degrees to the McGregor plane.[53] On this view, a C2-C7 vertical line may also be drawn through the facet joints at each level.[53] In the presence of normal lordosis, the vertebral bodies should lie anterior to this vertical line.[53] A patient is deemed to have a reduced lordosis if the posterior vertebral body is in contact or posterior to this line.[54] These findings not only define cervical posture, but may be used to describe dental occlusion and TMJ position as well.[53]

Doppler Ultrasound

The paired vertebral arteries, along with the internal carotid arteries, are responsible for the entire supply of oxygenated blood to the brain. The importance of these arteries in maintaining brain function and sustaining life cannot be underestimated. The diagnostic gold standard used to screen for vertebrobasilar ischemia (VBI) is the *Doppler ultrasound (DUS).*[54,55] However, some studies have shown *magnetic resonance angiography* and *computed tomographic angiography* to be more sensitive in diagnosing vertebral artery stenosis than DUS.[56] DUS is used to measure blood flow through the vertebrobasilar arterial system. This procedure should be performed prior to the use of cervical thrust following trauma when other screening procedures suggest compromise. Patients with VBI often present with poor tolerance for cervical extension.[32] A patient presenting clinically with such symptoms should be referred for administration of a DUS prior to the performance of any clinical premanipulative screening and prior to the utilization of cervical thrust, particularly to the upper cervical segments.

The Objective Physical Examination

Examination of Structure

Observation of the patient begins without the patient's knowledge from the time they enter the facility. Formal observation of static posture is typically performed with the patient seated and adequately disrobed and requires careful observation that is enhanced through astute surface palpation. From the *anterior view,*

the relative position of the head on neck and head and neck on the torso are determined. Displacement of head on neck, or lateral shift, may be the result of disc derangement[57] or myofascial restrictions. Cervical transverse plane deformities will result in asymmetrical distribution of forces through the TMJs.[53] From this view, relative shoulder heights are noted, with the expectation that depression is common on the dominant side. The relative contour of the superior border of the upper trapezius and general resting tone of all musculature should be symmetrical.

Vertical dimension is considered normal if the distance between the corner of the eye and the corner of the mouth is equal to the distance between the nose and the chin.[58] In a cohort of individuals with observed vertical facial asymmetry, 42% exhibited headaches of musculoskeletal origin.[53] These headaches were most often found to be on the side to which the chin was deviated.[53] *Panoramic view radiographs* may be taken, which include bilateral TMJs.[53] Asymmetry in the height of the mandibular condyles may result in ischemia within the TMJs as a result of asymmetrical force distribution resulting in headaches.[53]

Dental malocclusions should also be noted for their potential role in TMD.[58] A **class I occlusion** refers to the normal relationship of the maxillary and mandibular teeth in the anterior-posterior dimension.[58] A **class II overbite** or **class III underbite** consists of mandibular teeth that are positioned posterior and anterior to their normal position, respectively.[58] With the mouth closed, the maxillary incisors should close over the mandibular incisors by approximately 2 to 3 mm.[58] The presence of a *crossbite* or *occlusal interference*, defined as premature contact of the dentitia on one side, may increase compression and lead to uneven dental wear patterns.[58] If the occiput is anteriorly or posteriorly rotated on the atlas, as in cases of postural deviations, dental occlusion is altered.[53] The resting position of the tongue should be on the anterior aspect of the hard palate and the resting position of the TMJ, known as **freeway** or *interocclusal space*, should be approximately *2 to 4 mm* between the central incisors at rest.[58]

At rest, individuals are typically diaphragmatic breathers. In the presence of upper respiratory disorders, individuals may become mouth-dominant breathers. Mouth breathing changes the resting position of the TMJ leading to increased compressive forces. Upper respiratory breathers may also use accessory muscles resulting in increased tone.

The status of the muscles of facial expression may also be observed. Evidence of facial droop as seen with *ptosis*, or drooping of the eyelid, or drooping of the mouth on one side may be a sign of a *cerebrovascular accident* or *Bell's palsy*.

From the lateral view, the common presence of a forward head posture, consisting of lower cervical flexion and upper cervical extension, and rounded shoulders may be observed. Such a posture results in elevated forces in the subcranial region and TMJ. Evidence reveals that the frequency of neck-related pain increases in the presence of poor posture; however, the severity of cervical symptoms is unrelated to posture.[59]

Neurovascular Examination

The *dermatomal sensation scan* is first performed using the handle of the reflex hammer or light touch from the examiner's fingers. Modalities such as light touch, sharp/dull, hot/cold, vibration, two-point discrimination, and proprioception may all be screened.

Deep tendon reflexes (DTR) for the biceps (C5-6), brachioradialis (C6), and triceps (C7-8) should also be tested. A grade of 0 or 1+ suggests the presence of a complete or partial lower motor neuron lesion, whereas a score of 3+ or 4+ suggests a partial or complete upper motor neuron lesion.

Lastly, a complete myotomal scan is performed. With the patient sitting in neutral, gentle submaximal isometric resistance is provided to test the following motions and nerve root derivations which consist of, *C1-2:* cervical flexion, *C3:* cervical side bending, *C4:* shoulder shrug, *C5:* shoulder abduction, external rotation, *C6:* elbow flexion, wrist extension, *C7:* elbow extension, wrist flexion, *C8:* thumb extension, ulnar deviation, *T1:* hand intrinsics.[58] Identification of weakness with break testing of any of these motions warrants more formal manual muscle testing in both gravity eliminated and antigravity positions as needed.

The Babinski reflex is tested by taking the blunt end of the reflex hammer or finger and running it along the plantar aspect of the foot beginning at the calcaneus and moving along the lateral edge of the foot to the metatarsals.[58] Normally, the toes should go into slight flexion. A positive test is identified by the great toe extending and abducting at the metatarsophalangeal joint.[58] Another reflex, the Hoffmann sign, is also used to screen for upper motor neuron lesions in the upper extremity.[58] This test is performed by holding the middle finger and quickly flicking the distal phalanx.[58] This test is positive if the interphalangeal joint of the thumb on the same hand flexes.[58]

Examination of Mobility

Active Physiologic Movement Examination of the Cervical Spine

Quantity of Movement

As previously described, the orientation of the facet joints of the midcervical spine provide either upglide or downglide. In addition, it is important to remember that midcervical side bending and rotation are coupled movements that occur ipsilaterally during functional motion (Fig. 30-17). However, when desirable the head may face forward or eyes remain level. In such a situation, the suboccipital spine will produce contralateral rotation or side bending at the AA and OA articulations, respectively, in what is referred to as nonfunctional motion (Fig. 30-18). Therefore, astute observation of functional versus nonfunctional active motion may guide the therapist in further investigation. For example, if nonfunctional right side bending, which involves midcervical right side bending with right rotation as well as left AA rotation to keep the head facing forward, is limited, but functional side bending, which involves right midcervical side bending and rotation without suboccipital motion, is normal, the culpable region is the AA segment. In particular, a left AA rotation restriction is suspected. If both nonfunctional and functional right side bending is equally limited, then either the subcranial or midcervical region may be culpable. In such cases, a restriction may be present in

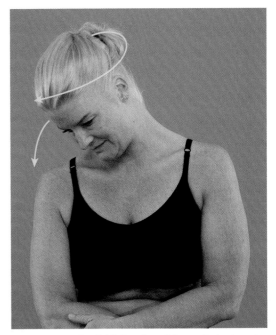

FIGURE 30–17 Functional side bending of the cervical spine where side bending and rotation occur ipsilaterally at the midcervical spine without subcranial motion.

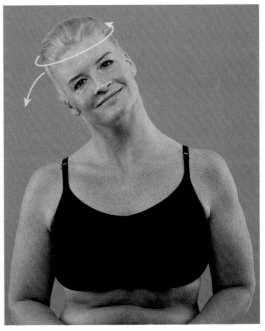

FIGURE 30–18 Nonfunctional side bending of the cervical spine where side bending and rotation occur ipsilaterally at the midcervical spine to the right in addition to subcranial atlantoaxial rotation to the left.

downglide on the right and/or upglide on the left at the midcervical region and/or rotation to the left at AA. Figure 30-19, which was adapted from Paris and Rot,[60] provides an algorithmic approach to differentiating between midcervical and subcranial regional mobility restrictions.

To more closely isolate subcranial motion, the patient may perform active, followed by passive, forward nodding

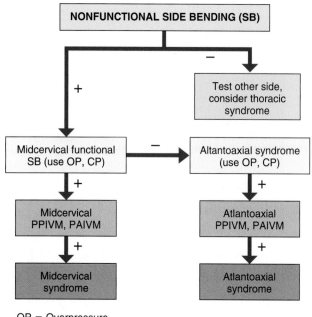

OP = Overpressure
CP = Counterpressure
+ = Reproducible symptom and/or mobility restriction
– = No reproduction of symptoms or mobility restriction

FIGURE 30–19 Algorithmic approach to differentiate between midcervical and subcranial regional mobility restrictions. OP, overpressure; CP, counterpressure; +, reproducible symptom and/or mobility restriction; -, no reproduction of symptoms or mobility restriction; SB, side bending; PAIVM, passive accessory intervertebral mobility testing; PPIVM, passive physiologic intervertebral mobility testing.

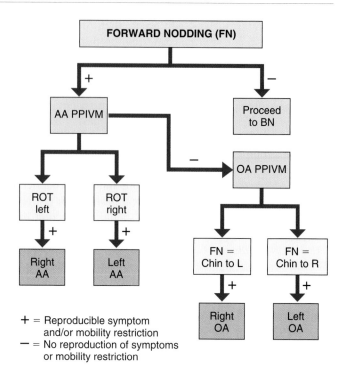

+ = Reproducible symptom
  and/or mobility restriction
– = No reproduction of symptoms
  or mobility restriction

FIGURE 30–20 Algorithmic approach to differentiate the specific segment and side of subcranial mobility restrictions through forward nodding. AA, atlantoaxial; OA, occipitoatlantal; BN, backward nodding; FN, forward nodding; PPIVM, passive physiologic intervertebral mobility testing; PAIVM, passive accessory intervertebral mobility testing; +, reproducible symptom and/or mobility restriction; -, no reproduction of symptoms or mobility restriction; ROT, rotation; L, left; R, right. (Adapted with permission from Paris SV, Rot J. 125 Course Notes: Examination, Evaluation, and Nonthrust Manipulation with Emphasis on the Upper Cervical Spine and Cervical Syndromes. American Academy of Orthopaedic and Manual Physical Therapists; 2007.)

(Fig. 30-20), backward nodding (Fig. 30-21), and side nodding, bilaterally (Table 30-5). To isolate motion to the subcranial region, gentle cueing may be provided by the therapist. During testing, the therapist is cognizant of any deviations of the chin toward one side or the other. The patient is then placed in supine, and nodding is performed passively. If the chin is observed to deviate during active motion testing, the therapist may place the chin in the deviated position during passive testing to ascertain the path of least of restriction. Passive end feel through the use of overpressure is performed in all directions.

There are a variety of methods advocated for reliably quantifying spinal mobility. Such methods include the *cervical range of motion (CROM)* device, *goniometry*, *inclinometry*, and *tape measure*. Evidence suggests that both the CROM and goniometry possess intrarater reliability; however, only the CROM has demonstrated interrater reliability.[61] Visual estimation, which is commonly used, has been found to be unreliable for quantifying motion.[61]

The normal extent of total active motion in the cervical spine is *80 to 90 degrees* of forward bending, *70 degrees* of backward bending, *20 to 45 degrees* of side bending to each side, and *45 degrees* of rotation to each side. Table 30-6 displays the physiologic motions of the cervical spine, including normal ranges of motion, open- and closed-packed positions, and normal and abnormal end feels.

Regional Movement Differentiation

If the reproduction of symptoms is brought on with a particular motion, localization may be performed using segmental overpressure or counterpressure in an attempt to identify the involved segment through the process of *regional movement differentiation*. For example, if rotation reproduced the patient's primary symptom, the patient would rotate until the symptoms are reproduced, after which the examiner would slowly rotate the patient in the opposite direction until the reproducible symptom subsides. In this position, gentle unilateral anterior pressures would be elicited over the transverse processes contralateral to the direction in which rotation occurs (i.e., pressure on the left TP for right rotation) beginning in the lower cervical region in an attempt to once again reproduce the symptom segmentally (Fig. 30-22 A).[62] Similarly, the patient may actively rotate while segmental counterpressure is applied to the transverse processes ipsilateral to the direction in which rotation occurs (i.e., pressure on the left TP for left rotation) (Fig. 30-22 B). A reduction in the reproducible pain on counterpressure identifies the segment that is most culpable and suggests a useful procedure for intervention. Several approaches advocate the use of symptomatic response to movement in diagnosis and intervention of spinal disorders.[57,63]

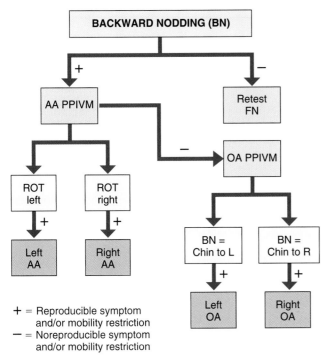

+ = Reproducible symptom
   and/or mobility restriction
− = Noreproducible symptom
   and/or mobility restriction

FIGURE 30–21 Algorithmic approach to differentiating the specific segment and side of subcranial mobility restrictions through backward nodding. AA, atlantoaxial; OA, occipitoatlantal; BN, backward nodding; FN, forward nodding; PPIVM, passive physiologic intervertebral mobility testing; PAIVM, passive accessory intervertebral mobility testing; +, reproducible symptom and/or mobility restriction; -, no reproduction of symptoms or mobility restriction; ROT, rotation; L, left; R, right. (Adapted with permission from Paris SV, Rot J. 125 Course Notes: Examination, Evaluation, and Nonthrust Manipulation with Emphasis on the Upper Cervical Spine and Cervical Syndromes: American Academy of Orthopaedic and Manual Physical Therapists; 2007.)

Active Physiologic Movement Examination of the Temporomandibular Joint

Quantity of Movement

Quantifying TMJ physiologic motion is best documented in millimeters using a ruler. It is sometimes more helpful to mark the range using a tongue depressor, after which a ruler can be used to obtain the measurements. Normal *mandibular depression (opening)* is considered *35 to 50 mm, elevation (closing)* is the return of the mandible to allow *incisor contact, protrusion* is *6 to 9 mm, retrusion* is *3 to 4 mm,* and *lateral deviation* is *10 to 15 mm* to either side. For ease of documentation and easy reference, a *T diagram* may be used (Fig. 30-23). The diagram is arranged as if the patient is facing the examiner. On the horizontal axis, lateral deviation to either side is documented, and on the vertical axis opening and protrusion is documented. Each axis is divided into 1 mm increments on which the amount of available motion is documented.

Quality of Movement

The quality of TMJ motion is best appreciated through performance of repeated movements while both TMJs are palpated just anterior to the tragus or anteriorly within the external auditory meatus (Fig. 30-24). It is not uncommon for individuals to adopt a C-curve or S-curve pattern of deviation in response to capsular restrictions or a subluxed disc, respectively. Palpation of the TMJ may reveal increased joint excursion on the side opposite to the side of deviation. Under normal conditions, joint excursion should be equal bilaterally during opening and protrusion. During lateral deviation, joint excursion occurs on the contralateral side. In addition to an appreciation of movement aberrations, identification of joint sounds, such as clicking or crepitus, may also suggest the presence of a mobility impairment.

Table 30–5	Subcranial Mobility Differentiation		
SUB-OCCIPITAL IMPAIRMENT	**AROM/PROM FINDINGS**	**PPIVM FINDINGS**	**PAIVM FINDINGS**
Right OA (Atlas to R)	Non-Fxn ROT Left FN chin to Left BN chin to Right SN to Right	Atlas limited during SB Right and ROT Left	OA central PA pressures and Right unilateral PA pressures
Left OA (Atlas to L)	Non-Fxn ROT Right FN chin to Right BN chin to Left SN to Left	Atlas limited during SB Left and ROT Right	OA central PA pressures and Left unilateral PA pressures
Right AA Rotation	Non-Fxn SB Left + FN ⟶ + BN ⟶	AA ROT Left AA ROT Right	AA central PA and Left unilateral PA pressures
Left AA Rotation	Non-Fxn SB Right + FN ⟶ + BN ⟶ FN, BN, SN=Nod	AA ROT Right AA ROT Left	AA central PA and Right unilateral PA pressures

Table 30-6	Physiologic (Osteokinematic) Motions of the Cervical Spine				
JOINT	**NORMAL ROM**	**OPP**	**CPP**	**NORMAL END FEEL(S)**	**CAPSULAR PATTERN**
OA	FN/BN = 14– 35° SN = 5°	Slight FN	BN	Elastic	Limited BN and ipsilateral deviation
AA	ROT = 40° FB/BN = 20° SN = 5°	Slight FN	BN	Firm	Limited FN and contralateral deviation
Mid to lower cervical (C2-T3)	FB/BB = 9–28° SB = 35° ROT = 45°	FB and contralateral SB and ROT	BB and ipsilateral SB and ROT	Elastic	Limited FB, contralateral SB and ROT
Temporomandibular Joint	Depression = 40–50 mm Elevation = return to fully closed Protrusion = 6–9 mm Retrusion = 3 mm beyond neutral Lateral Deviation = 8 mm	Freeway Space = 2–4 mm	Full dental occlusion	Elastic	Limited depression, protrusion, laterally deviate to side of restriction,

ROM, range of motion; OPP, open packed position; CPP, close packed position; OA, occipitoatlantal; AA, atlantoaxial; FN, forward nodding; BN, backward nodding; SN, side nodding; FB, forward bending; BB, backward bending; SB, side bending; ROT, rotation; NA, not available. (Adapted from: Wise CH, Gulick DT. *Mobilization Notes: A Rehabilitation Specialist's Pocket Guide.* Philadelphia, PA: FA Davis Company, 2009.)

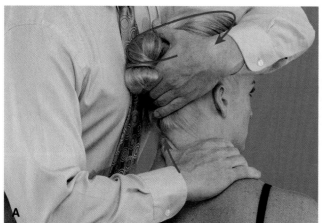 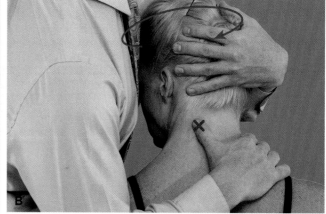

FIGURE 30–22 Regional movement differentiation of the cervical spine. **A.** Overpressure into right rotation. **B.** Counterpressure into left rotation.

Cervical Spine Passive Physiologic Intervertebral Mobility Examination

Passive physiologic intervertebral mobility (PPIVM) testing is used to assess the movement characteristics of intervertebral segments. These procedures are done to refine the diagnosis and isolate the culpable segment. Cervical spine PPIVM testing may be conducted in weight-bearing and/or non-weight-bearing positions. Reliability of testing intervertebral motion of the cervical spine has been found to be poor to moderate by Fjellner et al[64] and Smedmark et al.[65] Gonella and Paris[66] found good intrarater reliability but poor interrater reliability when using PPIVM testing to assess segmental motion, and Maher and Adams[67] found that the provocation of symptoms was a more reliable method of identifying segmental dysfunction when compared with assessment of mobility in the lumbar spine.

PPIVM testing for the midcervical spine is best accomplished by testing upglide and downglide as opposed to individual physiologic motions (Fig. 30-25). PPIVM testing for the subcranial region should include testing of forward nodding (FN) backward nodding (BN). To test, the clinician ulnarly and radially deviates his or her wrists to perform passive flexion and extension, respectively, of the patient's head on neck around an axis drawn through the patient's ear (Fig. 30-26 A). The quantity of motion, end feel, and any reproduction of symptoms is evaluated. The patient's head may be prepositioned in slight right or left side nodding for bilateral differentiation. Side nodding (SN) bilaterally should also be tested. To test, the clinician passively side bends the patient's head on neck around an axis drawn through the patient's nose (Fig. 30-26 B). The quantity of motion, end feel, and any

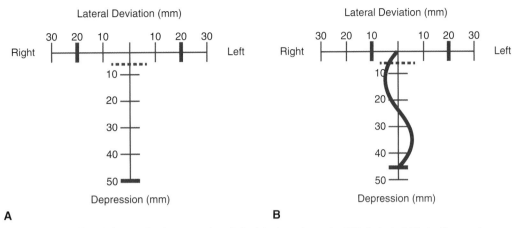

FIGURE 30–23 The "T" diagram for documentation of physiologic motion at the TMJ. **A.** An individual with normal mobility and the following motion profile: depression=50mm, protrusion=6-9mm, right lateral deviation=20mm, left lateral deviation=20mm. **B.** An individual with abnormal mobility and the following motion profile: depression=45mm with S-curve on opening, protrusion=6-9mm, right lateral deviation=10mm, left lateral deviation=20mm.

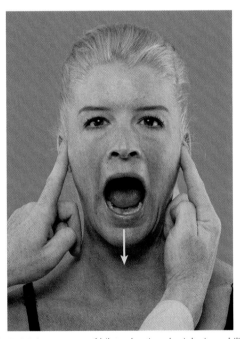

FIGURE 30–24 Assessment of bilateral active physiologic mobility testing of the TMJ.

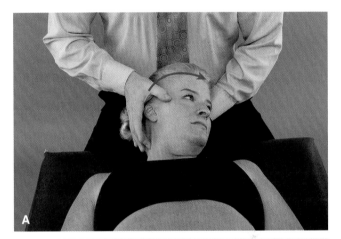

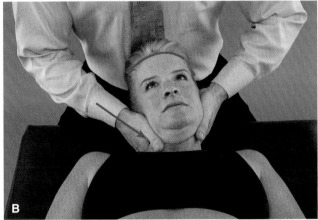

FIGURE 30–25 Midcervical PPIVM examination. **A.** Upglide. **B.** Downglide.

reproduction of symptoms is again evaluated. Both FN/BN and SN PPIVM testing are designed to assess motion of the subcranial region in the sagittal and frontal planes, which are motions primarily provided by the OA segment. When testing subcranial nodding, it is critical that motion is isolated to the subcranial region and is disallowed from occurring in more caudal levels.

To provide differentiation between the OA and AA segments, individual testing of the OA and AA articulations may also be performed. Mobility impairments are based on bilateral comparison, segmental comparison, and comparison with a hypothetical normal. During each PPIVM test, the quantity of motion, quality of motion, and any reproduction

of symptoms is appreciated. This process of PPIVM testing has been most clearly defined by Paris.[11,60] The midcervical techniques used for examination can be modified to become intervention, descriptions of which may be found later in this chapter. Subcranial PPIVM techniques are described below.

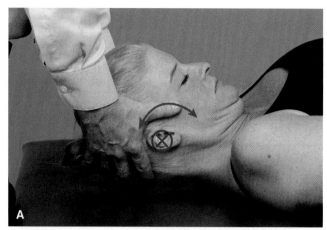

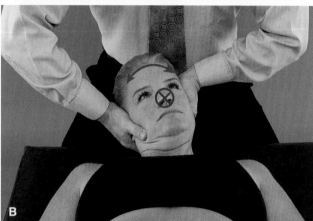

FIGURE 30–26 PPIVM examination of the occipitoatlantal segment including **A.** forward nodding and backward nodding, and **B.** side nodding.

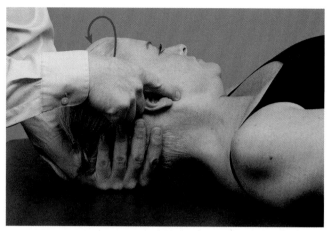

FIGURE 30–27 PPIVM examination of the occipitoatlantal segment, which involves palpation of the lateral mass of C1 that occurs at end range of rotation to the contralateral side.

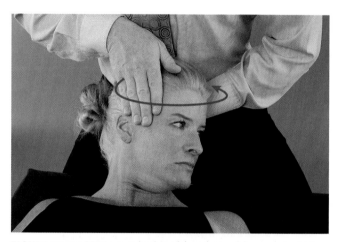

FIGURE 30–28 PPIVM examination of the atlantoaxial segment, which involves prepositioning in maximal cervical flexion and rotation bilaterally.

Occipitoatlantal PPIVM Examination (Fig. 30-27)
Patient: Supine with the head and neck in neutral
Clinician: Standing at the head of the patient, one hand supporting the occiput and the other on the lateral mass of C1, which is located between the mastoid process and the angle of the mandible
Technique: The occipital hand rhythmically creates rotation as the lateral mass is palpated and compared bilaterally.

Atlantoaxial PPIVM Examination (Fig. 30-28)
Patient: Supine with the head and neck maximally flexed
Clinician: Standing at the head of the patient, with both hands supporting the patient's head and neck in the flexed position
Technique: The head is rotated on the neck maximally in one direction then the other as the amount of rotation is perceived and compared bilaterally.

Passive Accessory Movement Examination

Cervical PAIVM Examination

As defined by Maitland et al,[63] the primary goal of cervical PAIVM testing is to identify the relationship between the onset of pain and the onset of tissue resistance.[63] The manual physical therapist must endeavor to identify the first and final onset of resistance (R1 and R2, respectively), as well as the first and

final onset of pain (P1 and P2, respectively). Based on these relationships, the segment may be classified as possessing either *symptom-dominant* behavior, where pain predominates, or *stiffness-dominant* behavior, where intra-articular stiffness predominates.[63] The cervical spine PAIVM examination techniques, if impairment is revealed, becomes the intervention. In addition to the techniques that are described in detail later in this chapter under intervention which may be used to identify segmental impairment, the following PAIVM techniques may also be used. Table 30-7 displays the accessory motions of the cervical spine.

Midcervical Transverse PAIVM Testing/Mobilization (Fig. 30-29)
Patient: Prone with the head and neck in neutral
Clinician: Standing to the side of the patient with the thumb at the side of the spinous process being mobilized
Technique: Apply transverse force through the thumbs

Midcervical Posterior PAIVM Testing/Mobilization (Fig. 30-30)
Patient: Supine with the head and neck in neutral
Clinician: Stand to side, thumb contact at anterior transverse process away from carotid pulse
Technique: Apply a posterior force through the thumb

Table 30-7	**Accessory (Arthrokinematic) Motions of the Cervical Spine**		
ARTHROLOGY		**ARTHROKINEMATICS**	
Occipitoatlantal (OA) Joint	Concave surface: Superior atlas facet Convex surface: Occiput	*To facilitate flexion:* Occiput rolls anterior & glides posterior	*To facilitate extension:* Occiput rolls posterior & glides anterior
Atlantoaxial (AA) Joint	Convex surface: Superior and Inferior axis facet	*To facilitate flexion:* Atlas pivots anterior on axis	*To facilitate extension:* Atlas pivots posterior on axis
Mid to lower cervical (C2-T3)	Facets are oriented at 45° between the transverse and frontal planes	*To facilitate flexion:* Inferior facet of superior vertebra glides up and forward on superior facet of inferior vertebra *To facilitate rotation:* Inferior facet of superior vertebra glides posterior & inferior on ipsilateral side & anterior & superior on contralateral side	*To facilitate extension:* Inferior facet of superior vertebra glides down and back on superior facet of inferior vertebra *To facilitate SB:* Inferior facet of superior vertebra glides inferior & posterior & on ipsilateral side & superior & anterior on contralateral side
		To facilitate protraction: Craniocervical segments extend while mid-low cervical segments flex	*To facilitate retraction:* Craniocervical segments flex while mid-low cervical segments extend

FB, forward bending; BB, backward bending; SB, side bending; ROT, rotation; IV, intervertebral. (Adapted From: Wise CH, Gulick DT. *Mobilization Notes: A Rehabilitation Specialist's Pocket Guide*. Philadelphia, PA: FA Davis Company, 2009.)

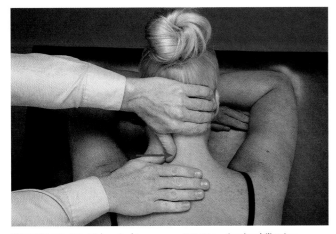

FIGURE 30-29 Midcervical transverse PAIVM testing/mobilization.

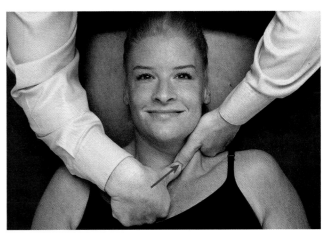

FIGURE 30-30 Midcervical posterior PAIVM testing/mobilization.

Occipitoatlantal Unilateral Anterior PAIVM Testing/Mobilization (Fig. 30-31)
Patient: Prone with head and neck in neutral
Clinician: Standing at the head, thumb contact at lateral mass of C1
Technique: Apply anterior force toward patient's ipsilateral eye

Atlantoaxial Unilateral Anterior PAIVM Testing/Mobilization (Fig. 30-32)
Patient: Prone with head and neck rotated 30 degrees toward side to be tested
Clinician: Standing at the head, thumb contact at transverse process of C2
Technique: Apply anterior force toward patient's mouth

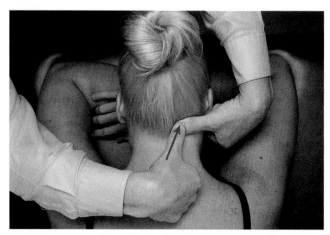

FIGURE 30–31 Occipitoatlantal unilateral anterior PAIVM testing/mobilization.

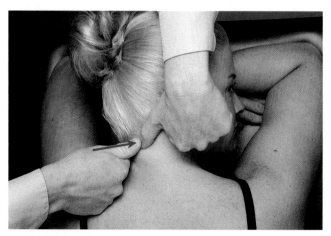

FIGURE 30–32 Atlantoaxial unilateral anterior PAIVM testing/mobilization.

Temporomandibular Accessory Movement Examination

Similar to accessory motion testing in the spine, accessory testing of the TMJ allows the examiner to more specifically isolate the lesion and better understand the origins of any presenting mobility impairments. During accessory testing, the examiner assesses the quantity of motion, the end feel, as well as the onset of any symptoms. When assessing accessory glide of the TMJ, applying a slight distraction force prior to the glide is often better tolerated. The examination procedures described here become the intervention and are, therefore, described in the intervention section of this chapter.

Examination of Muscle Function

Based on normal functional demands, muscle endurance, as opposed to strength, may be a more important variable to consider. Formal muscle testing is well defined in a variety of other texts.

Cervical spinal muscles may be divided into both deep and superficial groups. The deep group serves primarily as stabilizers, as the more superficial muscles serve as prime movers. In recent years, the deep stabilizing muscular system of the

cervical spine has undergone critical analysis, and training of this group has been found to be effective in reducing neck pain and headaches.[68–73]

The *deep neck flexors* are comprised of the *longus capitis* and *longus colli* muscles. In addition, the *deep neck extensors*, consisting of the *multifidus* and *rotatores*, are also important stabilizers. The middle layer is comprised of the *semispinalis cervicis* and *capitis*. The deep and middle layers primarily serve as force transducers that function in midrange to provide proprioceptive feedback regarding movement and position of the associated segments.

The deep stabilizing system is tested and trained using the *craniocervical flexion test* and the *craniocervical flexion exercise* regimen (Fig. 30-33). The process of testing and training using this approach is fully described in Chapter 17 of this text.

When considering muscle function of the TMJ, it is important to appreciate the function of these muscles both bilaterally, as well as unilaterally. The "rule of the mandible" states that the muscles that insert to the outer and inner surface of the mandible produce lateral deviation to the ipsilateral and contralateral sides, respectively.

The muscles that contribute to mouth opening include both the *infrahyoid* muscles, which act isometrically to stabilize the hyoid bone, and the *suprahyoid* muscles, which act concentrically to depress the mandible. In addition, the *lateral pterygoid*, with its superior head inserting into the disc and its inferior head inserting into the mandibular condyle, is active in terminal opening.

Perhaps, the most powerful muscle per square inch in the body is the *masseter* muscle. Mirroring the orientation of the masseter, yet positioned on the inner surface of the mandible, is the *medial pterygoid* muscle.

Assisting in closing is the superficial *temporalis* muscle. Its posterior, horizontally oriented fibers reveal its role, not only in closing, but retrusion as well. Considering its role in lateral deviation, of particular note is the force couple created with the lateral pterygoid.

Palpation

Osseous Palpation

With the patient prone, the examiner may explore the large, centrally located, *greater occipital protuberance* as well as the

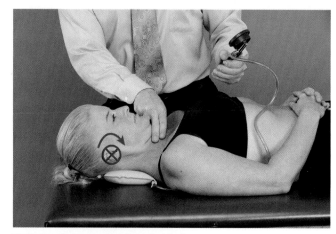

FIGURE 30–33 The craniocervical flexion test.

superior and *inferior nuchal lines*, which serve as important insertion sites for muscles and ligaments. Laterally, the *mastoid processes*, which serve as important muscular insertion sites, are palpated.

The lateral mass of C1 is best palpated in the space between the angle of the mandible and the mastoid process (Fig. 30-34). Confirmation of its location and OA mobility is achieved by palpating the degree of lateral translation of this landmark during contralateral rotation. The first, and fairly prominent, *spinous process* is that of C2, located three finger widths inferior to the greater occipital protuberance (Fig. 30-35). To confirm, the head may be slightly flexed or side bent resulting in greater prominence and motion of this landmark. Each subsequent spinous process may be palpated in midline by using the

pinch test, where each process is contacted between finger and thumb, to assess the position of each segment relative to adjacent segments. Lying just lateral to each spinous process are the *articular pillars*, identified as ridges when moving vertically. The spinous processes of C6 and C7 are easily palpable, with C7 being most prominent (Fig. 30-36). To differentiate between the spinous processes of C6 and C7, the spine is extended, which translates the spinous process of C6 anteriorly while C7 remains in place.

Moving anteriorly, the facial bones are palpated with the patient supine. The horizontally oriented *zygomatic arch*, formed by the union of the temporal and zygomatic bones, can be easily identified. The full extent of the mandible is palpated beginning with the *body* and *submandibular fossa* then moving laterally to the angle and the posteriorly projecting *ramus*. Just anterior to the external auditory meatus is the *mandibular condyle*, the *lateral pole* of which translates anteriorly and inferiorly with opening (Fig. 30-37). The *coronoid process*, which lies 1 inch below the mid-zygomatic arch, is most easily palpated if the mouth is slightly open. The *hyoid bone* is palpated anteriorly at the level of C2. Confirmation is achieved by having the patient swallow, which produces elevation of the hyoid. Moving caudally from the hyoid, the *trachea* with its concentric rings of *cricoid cartilage* and the prominent *thyroid cartilage*, with its central tip, may be palpated.

Soft Tissue Palpation

The large *sternocleidomastoid (SCM)* serves as the lateral border of the anterior triangle of the neck (Fig. 30-38). It can be distinguished from the scalenes by resisting contralateral rotation. Above the clavicle and just lateral to the SCM lies the *anterior scalene* as it dives beneath the clavicle to arrive at the first rib. Moving laterally, the *middle scalene* and *posterior scalene*, which lies adjacent to the levator scapula, is palpated (Fig. 30-39). Prepositioning the head in slight contralateral rotation may

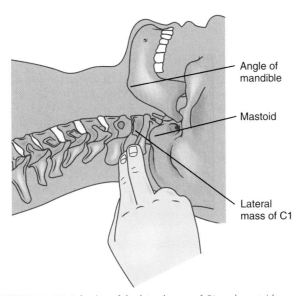

Angle of mandible

Mastoid

Lateral mass of C1

FIGURE 30-34 Palpation of the lateral mass of C1 and mastoid process.

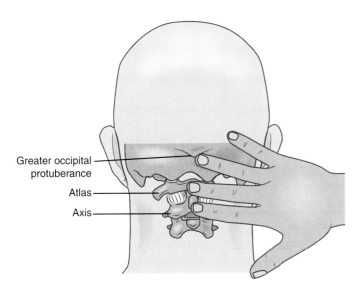

Greater occipital protuberance

Atlas

Axis

FIGURE 30-35 Palpation of the greater occipital protuberance, posterior tubercle of C1, and spinous process of C2.

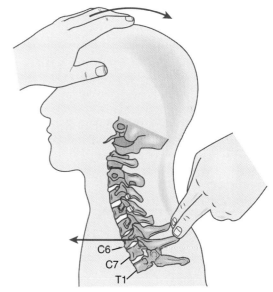

C6
C7
T1

FIGURE 30-36 Palpation of the spinous processes of C6, C7, and T1.

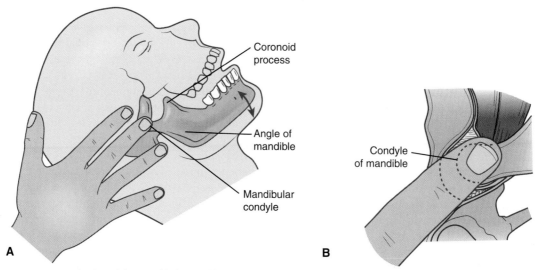

FIGURE 30–37 Palpation of the mandibular condyle, angle of the mandible, and coronoid process of the mandible.

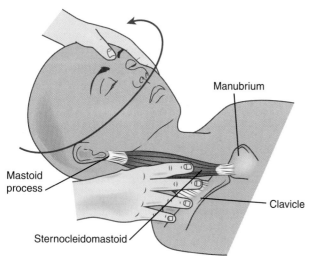

FIGURE 30–38 Palpation of the sternocleidomastoid.

provide greater exposure to facilitate palpation and gentle resistance of ipsilateral side bending will serve to recruit these muscles.

While the patient is in supine, the muscles of mastication may also be palpated. The most powerful and prominent muscle is the *masseter* (Fig. 30-40). Palpation of the zygomatic arch and angle of the mandible serves to demarcate its course. With a gloved hand, the examiner may place a finger intraorally along the inside aspect of the cheek as the thumb rests on the cheek externally. With the finger lateral to the dentitia, the patient bites as the examiner palpates the *medial pterygoid* muscle intraorally as the *masseter* muscle is palpated externally.

At the temporal aspect of the cranium, the thin belly of the *masseter* muscle can be palpated, with confirmation achieved through resistance of mouth closing, ipsilateral

FIGURE 30–39 Palpation of the anterior and middle scalenes.

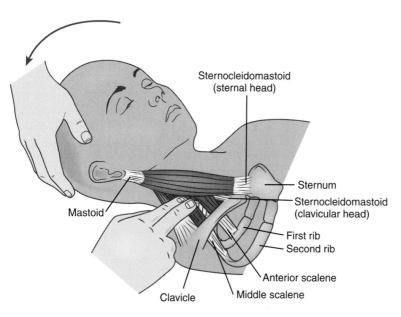

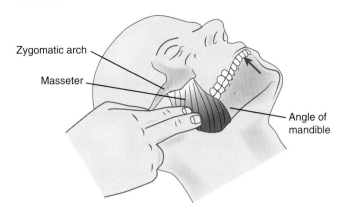

FIGURE 30–40 Palpation of the masseter.

lateral deviation, or retrusion. Although challenging, the *lateral pterygoid*, is palpated intraorally in the space just posterior to the last maxillary molar during resisted protrusion (Fig. 30-41).

The four *suboccipital muscles* lie deeply in the space between the occipital protuberance and C2. Palpatory differentiation is not possible, however, as a group these muscles swell under the fingers with gentle resistance into extension. The *semispinalis* muscle occupies a midline position and acts as the prime mover for cervical extension. It is differentiated from the *splenius* group, which departs from its midline origin to obliquely course toward its insertion on the mastoid process. They are differentiated from the *upper trapezius* which, in contrast to the splenii, produces contralateral rotation. In the same fashion, the ipsilaterally rotating *levator scapula* can be differentiated from the trapezius.

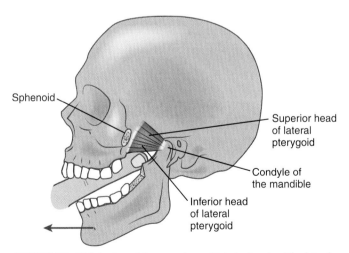

FIGURE 30–41 Palpation of the superior and inferior heads of the lateral pterygoid intraorally.

Special Testing

Due to the inherent risks associated with manual intervention of the cervical spine, premanipulative screening procedures may be recommended. Most physical therapists agree that all available screening tests should be performed prior to manipulation;[74] however, controversy regarding the usefulness and safety of these procedures exists. No single test or combination of screening tests has been found to reliably identify those who are at risk of injury from cervical thrust. Furthermore, the screening tests themselves possess inherent risk and may impart greater force than the thrust techniques themselves.[75] Some have suggested that a variety of attributes derived from the patient's history, such as body mass index (BMI), blood pressure, and history of cardiovascular or cerebrovascular compromise, may be better predictors and may help identify those for whom thrust should be withheld. Nevertheless, until agreement exists regarding the use of these tests, for medicolegal reasons, it may be most prudent to employ them, albeit judiciously. It has been proposed that prior to the implementation of cervical thrust manipulation, the manual physical therapist should engage in a four-tier premanipulative screening process that consists of (1) a detailed *historical interview*, (2) the results of *medical testing and diagnostic imaging*, (3) clinical examination procedures designed to assess the *structural stability* of the cervical spine, and (4) clinical examination procedures designed to assess the status of the *vertebrobasilar arterial system* (Table 30-8).[76] To assist in guiding clinical decisions in the use of thrust manipulation in the cervical spine, several clinical prediction rules (CPRs) have been developed. Tseng et al[77] developed a CPR to guide the use of cervical thrust for individuals with neck pain. Cleland et al[78] developed a CPR to guide the use of thoracic thrust for individuals with neck pain. Unfortunately, the latter has failed to achieve validity, and more recent evidence suggests that cervical thrust for neck-related disorders may have greater efficacy than thoracic thrust.[79] See Chapter 18 of this text for more information regarding CPRs for the use of thrust manipulation in the cervical spine.

Due to the inherent risks associated with these procedures and their lack of sensitivity and specificity,[80] it is recommended that they be used only in cases where the first two tiers of screening are negative and only in those who are about to immediately receive cervical thrust.

Special tests for the cervical spine have been clearly delineated in many other texts and in the literature. Therefore, only a brief description of selected special tests will be provided here. Table 30-9 provides an overview of the sensitivity, specificity, and likelihood ratios for the more commonly performed special tests used in the examination of the cervical spine. The reader is encouraged to consult other sources for additional information regarding the performance of these useful confirmatory tests.

Table 30-8 The Four-tier Premanipulative Screening Process for the Cervical Spine

Tier 1: Review of Systems
- Rheumatoid arthritis, Down syndrome, Ehrlos-Danios syndrome, Marfan syndrome, lupus erythematosus, ankylosing spondylitis, diffuse idiopathic skeletal hyperostosis, spondyloarthropathy, cancer (> 50 years old, failure to respond, unexplained weight loss, previous history), bone density concerns (osteporosis, steroid use, chronic renal failure, postmenopausal females)
- Pregnancy or immediately postpartum, oral contraceptives, anticoagulant therapy
- Recent trauma
- Intolerance for static postures[107]
- Acute pain with movement, improved with external support
- Extension brings on vertigo, nausea, diplopia, tinnitus, dysarthria, and mystagmus

Tier 2: Medical Testing and Diagnostic Imaging
- Lab values suggesting systemic disease (see tier 1)
- Plain film radiography including:
  - Open-mouth view: visualization of odontoid and C1-C2
  - Lateral view and lateral stress view: visualization of parallel line relationship and atlanto-dental interface (> 3mm)
  - Oblique view: visualization of defect in pars interaticlaris
- MRI, CT scans, scintigraphy for identification of subtle pathology
- Doppler ultrasound for detection of vertebrobasilar ischemia

Tier 3: Clinical Screening Procedures for Segmental Stability*
- Sharp-Purser test
- Aspinall test
- Transverse ligament stress test
- Test for Odontoid Fracture
- Alar ligament stress test
- Passive physiology intervertebral mobility testing(> Grade 5)
- Mobilization prepositioning
- Active range of motion assessment revealing poor movement quality

Tier 4: Clinical Screening Procedures for Vertebrobasilar Ischemia*
- Vertebral artery test
- Neck torsion test

Abbreviation: CT, computed tomography; MRI, magnetic resonance imaging.
*Tier 3 and tier 4 tests are described and figures are presented in the text.

Table 30-9 Special Tests of the Cervical Spine

TEST	SENSITIVITY	SPECIFICITY	+LR	–LR	RELIABILITY	REFERENCE
Sharp-Purser Test	69%	96%–98%	17.25	0.32	NA	Uitvlugt and Indenbaum[81]
Aspinall Test	NA	NA	NA	NA	NA	Aspinall[82]
Transverse Ligament Stress Test	9%–37%	86%–96%	NA	NA	NA	Meadows and Magee[83] Pettman[84]
Test for Odontoid Fracture	NA	NA	NA	NA	NA	Magee[60]
Alar Ligament Stress Test	NA	NA	NA	NA	NA	Meadows and Magee[83] Pettman[84] Olson et al[85]
Vertebral Artery Test	NA	NA	NA	NA	NA	Grant[86] Grant[87] Rivett[88] Keery and Taylor[89] Kunnasmaa and Thiel[90]
Neck Torsion Test	NA	NA	NA	NA	NA	Pettman[84] Vidal and Huijbregts[91] Norre[92]

Table 30-9	Special Tests of the Cervical Spine—cont'd					
TEST	**SENSITIVITY**	**SPECIFICITY**	**+LR**	**−LR**	**RELIABILITY**	**REFERENCE**
Foraminal Distraction Test	26%–43%*	90%–100%*	4.4*	0.62*	0.41–0.88 (kappa)	Wainner et al[29] Pettman[84] Spurling and Scoville[93] Viikari-Juntura et al[94]
Spurling Test (upper/lower quadrant sign)	30.5%–86% *	50%–100%*	1.92–4.87*	0.58–0.69*	0.60–0.62 (kappa)	Wainner et al[29] Spurling and Scoville[93] Viikari-Juntura et al[94] Tong et al[95] Bertilson et al[96]
Median Nerve Bias Neurodynamic Test	94%–97%*	22%*	1.3*	0.012*	0.76 (kappa)	Wainner et al[29] Butler[97] Coppieters et al[98] Coppieters et al[99] Keneally[100] McClellan and Swash[101] McClellan[102] Garmer et al[103] Kleinrensink et al[104]
Ulnar Nerve Bias Neurodynamic Test	NA	NA	NA	NA	NA	Wainner et al[29] Butler[97] Coppieters et al[98] Coppieters et al[99] Keneally[100] McClellan and Swash[101] McClellan[102] Garmer et al[103] Kleinrensink et al[104]
Radial Nerve Bias Neurodynamic Test	72%–97%	33%	1.1	0.85	0.83 (kappa)	Wainner et al.[29] Butler[97] Coppieters et al[98] Coppieters et al[99] Keneally[100] McClellan and Swash[101] McClellan[102] Garmer et al[103] Kleinrensink et al[104]
Shoulder Abduction (Bakody) Maneuver	17%–68%,	80%–100%	1.9–2.12	0.64–0.9	0.20–0.40 (kappa)	Wainner et al[29] Viikari-Juntura et al[93]

LR, likelihood ratio; Sn, sensitivity; Sp, specificity; NA, not assessed.
*Distraction, Spurling, median nerve bias, ipsilateral rotation <60 degrees:
2 of 4 tests +: Sn = 39%, Sp = 56%, (+)LR = 0.88
3 of 4 tests +: Sn = 39%, Sp = 94%, (+)LR = 6.1
4 of 4 tests +: Sn = 24%, Sp = 99%, (+)LR = 30.3

SPECIAL TESTS FOR THE CERVICAL SPINE

Segmental Stability Tests
Sharp-Purser Test (Fig. 30-42)[81]

Purpose: To identify a subluxation of C1 on C2, which may result from a reduction in the integrity of the transverse ligament

Patient: Sitting with the head and neck in neutral

Clinician: Standing to the side of the patient. One hand is on the patient's forehead and the "golf tee" hand position of the thumb and index finger of the other hand is at the spinous process of C2 to stabilize.

Procedure: The clinician flexes the patient's head on neck and applies a posteriorly-directed force through the forehead contact against the stabilized C2 vertebra.

Interpretation: The test is positive if reduction of C1 on C2 is noted, the end feel is soft, or patient reports symptoms including esophageal pressure and other neurologically related cord compression symptoms.

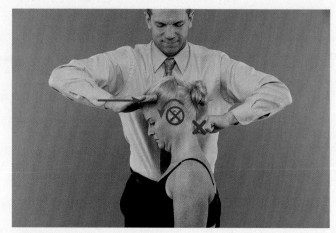

FIGURE 30–42 Sharp-Purser test.

Aspinall Test (Fig. 30-43)[82]

Purpose: To test the integrity of the transverse ligament when the Sharp-Purser test is negative

Patient: Supine with the head and neck in neutral

Clinician: Standing at the head of the patient. One hand at the patient's chin maintains head on neck flexion while the other hand is at C2.

Procedure: While maintaining the head on neck flexed position, an anteriorly directed force is applied to C2.

Interpretation: The test is positive if the end feel is soft or patient reports symptoms including esophageal pressure and other neurologically related cord compression symptoms.

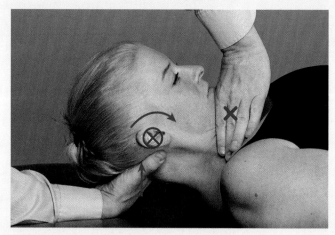

FIGURE 30–43 Aspinall test.

Transverse Ligament Stress Test (Fig. 30-44)[83,84]

Purpose: To test the integrity of the transverse ligament

Patient: Supine with the head and neck in neutral

Clinician: With both hands, support the occiput with the fingers over the atlas

Procedure: The occiput and atlas are translated anteriorly without flexion or extension and held for 15 seconds.

Interpretation: The test is positive if the end feel is soft or in the presence of muscle spasm, nausea, vertigo, paresthesia, nystagmus, or esophageal pressure.

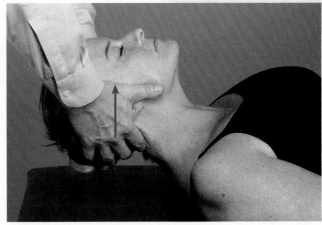

FIGURE 30–44 Transverse ligament stress test.

Test for Odontoid Fracture (Fig. 30-45)[58]

Purpose: To identify a loss of integrity of the odontoid process

Patient: Supine with the head and neck in neutral

Clinician: One hand supports the occiput, the other hand contacts the lateral mass of the atlas.

Procedure: Apply a medially directed force through the atlas contact as the other hand supports the occiput

Interpretation: The test is positive if there is increased translation of the lateral mass.

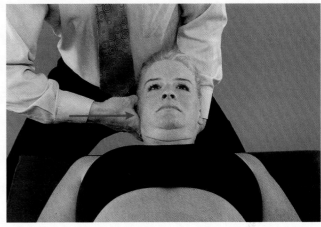

FIGURE 30–45 Test for odontoid fracture.

Alar Ligament Stress Test (Fig. 30-46)[83-85]

Purpose: To test the integrity of the alar ligament

Patient: Supine with the head and neck in neutral

Clinician: Support the occiput with both hands while the index fingers palpate the spinous process of the axis

Procedure: The occiput is side bent slightly to each side.

Interpretation: The test is positive if there is a delay in movement of the spinous process of the axis, which rotates ipsilateral to the direction of side bending.

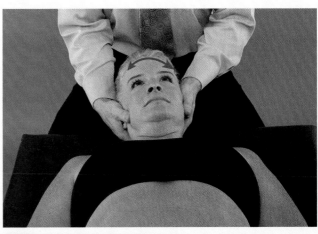

FIGURE 30–46 Alar ligament stress test.

Vascular Integrity Tests
Vertebral Artery Test (Fig. 30-47)[86-90]

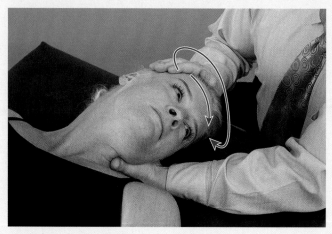

FIGURE 30–47 Vertebral artery test.

Purpose: To assess for vertebrobasilar ischemia/insufficiency

Patient: Supine with the head and neck in neutral

Clinician: Standing at the patient's head supporting the occiput with one hand as the other hand provides a fulcrum at the upper cervical region

Procedure: The clinician sequentially extends, side bends, then rotates the patient's head ipsilaterally until the maximum amount of motion is obtained in each plane. The patient is then engaged in simple conversation with eyes remaining open. This position is held for 15 to 30 seconds as the examiner determines the presence of any signs or symptoms. Following a 30-second to 1-minute rest period, this procedure is repeated contralaterally.

Interpretation: The following signs constitute a positive test result: nystagmus, pupil dilation, slurred speech, diminished responsiveness, apparent distress. The following symptoms also constitute a positive test result: dizziness, tinnitus, nausea, blurred vision, any additional unpleasant sensations.

Neck Torsion Test (Fig. 30-48)[84,91,92]

Purpose: To differentiate between vertebral artery compromise and positional vertigo when performed following the vertebral artery test

Patient: Sitting

Clinician: Standing in front of the patient with the hands on either side of the patient's head

Procedure: The head is held stable while the patient rotates his or her body to the left and to the right in sitting.

Interpretation: The test is positive if there are signs of vertebral artery compromise as noted above. If the test is negative, then the signs and/or symptoms found during vertebral artery testing are deemed to be the result of positional vertigo.

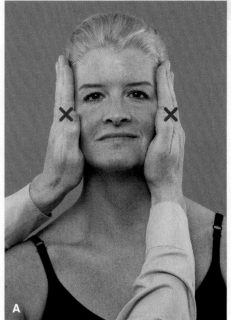

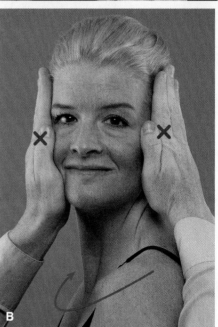

FIGURE 30–48 Neck torsion test.

Neural Provocation Tests
Foraminal Distraction Test (Fig. 30-49)[29,84,93,94]

Purpose: To test for the presence of a cervical radiculopathy

Patient: Sitting or supine

Clinician: Standing behind the patient or sitting at the head of the patient with the thenar eminence of both hands resting on the patient's mastoid processes.

Procedure: Gentle distraction force is applied through both hand contacts.

Interpretation: The test is positive if there is a reduction in the patient's presenting symptoms.

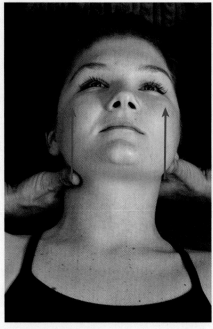

FIGURE 30–49 Foraminal distraction test.

Spurling Test (Upper/Lower Quadrant Sign) (Fig. 30-50 A, B)[29,93–96]

Purpose: To test for the presence of a cervical radiculopathy

Patient: Sitting with the neck passively pre-positioned into extension, ipsilateral side bending, and ipsilateral rotation. This is performed in neutral for the *lower quadrant sign*. For the *upper quadrant sign*, the patient first performs cervical protraction using a "chin poke" maneuver designed to isolate forces to the upper cervical segments.

Clinician: Standing behind the patient

Procedure: Gentle compression force is applied consisting of triplanar overpressure.

Interpretation: The test is positive if there is a reproduction in the patient's presenting symptoms.

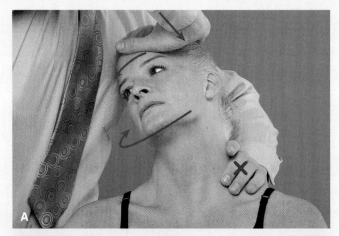

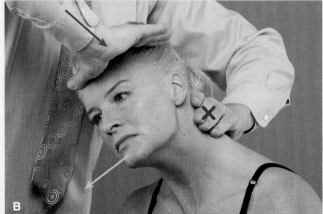

FIGURE 30–50 Spurling Quadrant Test. **A.** Lower quadrant. **B.** Upper quadrant.

Median Nerve Bias Neurodynamic Test
(Fig. 30-51)[29,97–104]

Purpose: To assess the neurodynamics of the median nerve

Patient: Supine with the head and neck in neutral

Clinician: Standing facing the head of the patient on the side being tested

Procedure: A closed fist is placed at the superior aspect of the shoulder to provide scapular depression. While maintaining this hand position, gently move the patient into the following positions: head and neck contralateral side bending, ipsilateral shoulder abduction and external rotation, elbow extension, forearm supination, and wrist/finger extension. Further differentiation may be determined by appreciating the effect of head and neck position on symptoms.

Interpretation: The test is positive if there is a reproduction of pain or paresthesia into the median nerve distribution of the upper extremity. The therapist documents the location at which the symptoms are produced.

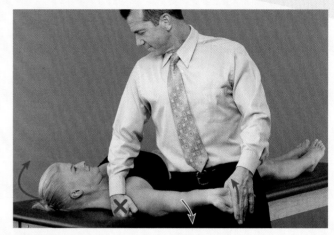

FIGURE 30–51 Median nerve bias neurodynamic test.

Ulnar Nerve Bias Neurodynamic Test
(Fig. 30-52)[29,97–104]

Purpose: To assess the neurodynamics of the ulnar nerve

Patient: Supine with the head and neck in neutral

Clinician: Standing facing the head of the patient on the side being tested

Procedure: A closed fist is placed at the superior aspect of the shoulder to provide scapular depression. While maintaining this hand position, gently move the patient into the following positions: head and neck contralateral sidebending, ipsilateral shoulder abduction and external rotation, elbow flexion, forearm pronation, and wrist/finger extension. Further differentiation may be determined by appreciating the effect of head and neck position on symptoms.

Interpretation: The test is positive if there is a reproduction of pain or paresthesia into the ulnar nerve distribution of the upper extremity. The therapist documents the location at which the symptoms are produced.

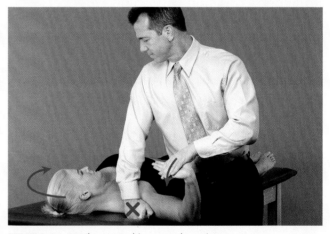

FIGURE 30–52 Ulnar nerve bias neurodynamic test.

Radial Nerve Bias Neurodynamic Test

(Fig. 30-53)[29,97–104]

Purpose: To assess the neurodynamics of the radial nerve

Patient: Supine with the head and neck in neutral with the shoulder over the edge of the table

Clinician: Standing facing the feet of the patient on the side being tested

Procedure: The clinician's leg maintains scapular depression throughout the procedure. While maintaining depression, gently move the patient into the following positions: head and neck contralateral side bending, ipsilateral shoulder abduction and internal rotation, elbow extension, forearm pronation, and wrist/finger flexion. Further differentiation may be determined by appreciating the effect of head and neck position on symptoms.

Interpretation: The test is positive if there is a reproduction of pain or paresthesia into the ulnar nerve distribution of the upper extremity. The therapist documents the location at which the symptoms are produced.

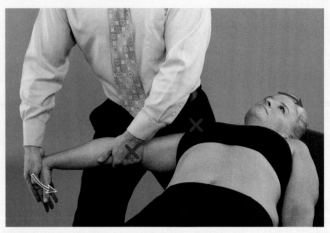

FIGURE 30–53 Radial nerve bias neurodynamic test.

Shoulder Abduction (Bakody) Maneuver

(Fig. 30-54)[29,94]

Purpose: To test for the presence of a cervical radiculopathy

Patient: Sitting

Clinician: Assess baseline symptoms and monitors performance

Procedure: Patient abducts the shoulder and places the dorsum of the hand on the top of his or her head.

Interpretation: The test is positive if there is a reduction in the patient's presenting symptoms, which typically involve the upper extremities.

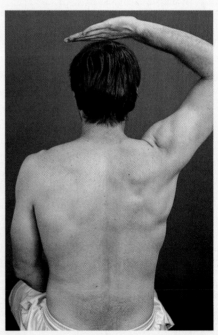

FIGURE 30–54 Shoulder abduction (Bakody) maneuver. (Courtesy of Bob Wellmon Photography, BobWellmon.com)

JOINT MOBILIZATION OF THE CERVICAL SPINE AND TEMPOROMANDIBULAR JOINT

Note: The indications for the joint mobilization techniques described in this section are based on expected joint kinematics. Current evidence suggests that the indications for their use are multifactorial and may be based on direct assessment of mobility and an individual's symptomatic response.

Temporomandibular Joint Mobilizations

Temporomandibular Distraction

Indications:

- *Temporomandibular distractions* are indicated for restrictions of the temporomandibular joint in all directions.

Accessory Motion Technique (Fig. 30-55)

- **Patient/Clinician Position:** The patient is in a sitting position with the head and neck in neutral. Stand to the side of the patient.
- **Hand Placement:** Your arm cradles the patient's head, keeping it close to your chest for stabilization. The thumb of your mobilization hand contacts the mandibular molars as the flexed second digit contacts the submandibular region.
- **Force Application:** A distraction force is applied in a downward direction through your thumb contact.

Accessory With Physiologic Motion Technique (Not pictured)

- **Patient/Clinician Position:** The patient and clinician are in the same position as that which was described above.
- **Hand Placement:** Your hand placement is the same as that which was described above.
- **Force Application:** The patient actively opens the mouth while downward force is applied through the thumb contact.

Temporomandibular Anterior Glide

Indications:

- *Temporomandibular anterior glides* are indicated for restrictions in mandibular depression, protrusion, and contralateral lateral deviation of the temporomandibular joint.

Accessory Motion Technique (Fig. 30-56) (Not pictured)

- **Patient/Clinician Position:** The patient is in a sitting position with the head and neck in neutral. Stand to the side of the patient.
- **Hand Placement:** Your arm cradles the patient's head, keeping it close to your chest for stabilization. The thumb of your mobilization hand contacts the mandibular molars as the flexed second digit contacts the submandibular region.
- **Force Application:** Slight distraction force followed by anterior glide is applied through your thumb contact.

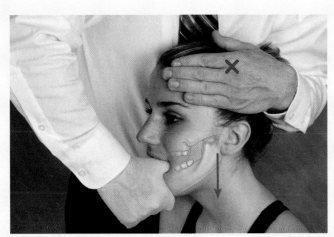

FIGURE 30–55 Temporomandibular distraction. (From: Wise CH, Gulick DT. *Mobilization Notes: A Rehabilitation Specialist's Pocket Guide.* Philadelphia, PA: FA Davis Company; 2009.)

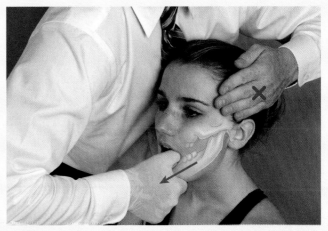

FIGURE 30–56 Temporomandibular anterior glide. (From: Wise CH, Gulick DT. *Mobilization Notes: A Rehabilitation Specialist's Pocket Guide.* Philadelphia, PA: FA Davis Company; 2009.)

Accessory With Physiologic Motion Technique (Not pictured)

- **Patient/Clinician Position:** The patient and clinician are in the same position as that which was described above.
- **Hand Placement:** Your hand placement is the same as that which was described above.
- **Force Application:** The patient actively protrudes the mandible while an anterior glide is applied through the thumb contact.

Temporomandibular Lateral Glide

Indications:

- *Temporomandibular lateral glides* are indicated for restrictions in lateral deviation of the temporomandibular joint.

Accessory Motion Technique (Fig. 30-57)

- **Patient/Clinician Position:** The patient is in a sitting position with the head and neck in neutral. Stand to the side of the patient.

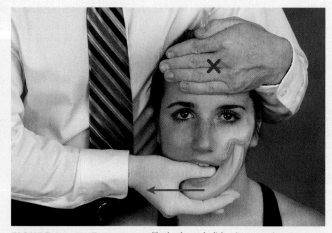

FIGURE 30–57 Temporomandibular lateral glide. (From: Wise CH, Gulick DT. *Mobilization Notes: A Rehabilitation Specialist's Pocket Guide.* Philadelphia, PA: FA Davis Company; 2009.)

- **Hand Placement:** Your arm cradles the patient's head, keeping it close to your chest for stabilization. The thumb of your mobilization hand contacts the mandibular molars as the flexed second digit contacts the submandibular region on the contralateral side to which you are standing.
- **Force Application:** A distraction force followed by lateral glide is applied through the thumb contact toward the side to which you are standing.

Accessory With Physiologic Motion Technique (Fig. 30-58)

- **Patient/Clinician Position:** The patient and clinician are in the same position as that which was described above.
- **Hand Placement:** Your stabilization hand contacts the patient's head. Your mobilization hand contacts the patient's mandible externally, or intraorally.

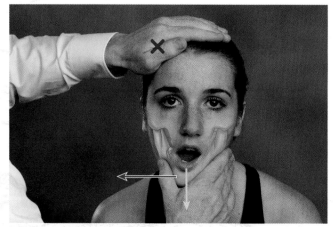

FIGURE 30–58 Temporomandiblar lateral glide: accessory with physiologic motion technique. (From: Wise CH, Gulick DT. *Mobilization Notes: A Rehabilitation Specialist's Pocket Guide.* Philadelphia, PA: FA Davis Company; 2009.)

- **Force Application:** The patient actively opens and closes the mouth, laterally deviates the mandible, or protrudes the mandible in the direction of restriction or symptoms as gentle force is applied through the mobilization hand contact. Force is maintained throughout the entire motion and sustained at end range.

Cervical Spine Joint Mobilizations

Cervical Central and Unilateral Anterior Glides

Indications:

- *Cervical central and unilateral anterior glides* are indicated for restrictions in segmental mobility in all directions and to reduce symptoms. Central pressures assist primarily with restoring sagittal plane motion of forward and backward bending while unilateral pressures enhance rotation and side bending.

Accessory Motion Technique (Fig. 30-59)

- **Patient/Clinician Position:** The patient is in a prone lying position with the head in neutral with the folded arms supporting the head or with the arms at the side and a bolster supporting the head. You are standing at the head of the patient.
- **Hand Placement:** As a general technique, stabilization is not required. Prior to thumb placement, a mobilization gutter is formed by using the fingers to gather the soft tissues along the lateral aspect of the neck thus allowing better mobilization contact. For central glides, both of your thumbs are placed side by side or thumb over thumb contact is made over the spinous process on the superior vertebra of the segment being mobilized or at bilateral transverse processes of the same vertebra. For unilateral glides, thumb over thumb contact is

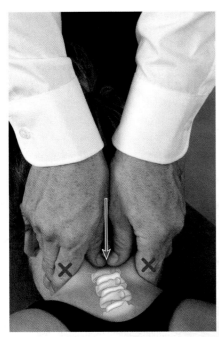

FIGURE 30–59 Cervical central and unilateral anterior glide. (From: Wise CH, Gulick DT. *Mobilization Notes: A Rehabilitation Specialist's Pocket Guide*. Philadelphia, PA: FA Davis Company; 2009.)

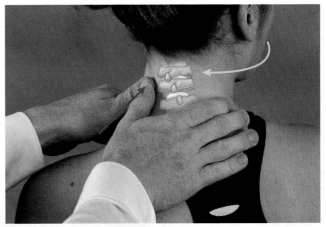

FIGURE 30–60 Cervical unilateral anterior glide: rotation accessory with physiologic motion technique. (From: Wise CH, Gulick DT. *Mobilization Notes: A Rehabilitation Specialist's Pocket Guide*. Philadelphia, PA: FA Davis Company; 2009.)

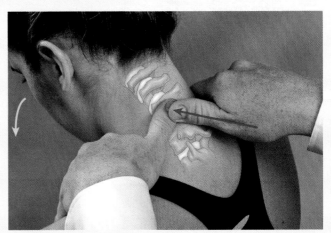

FIGURE 30–61 Cervical unilateral anterior glide: forward bending accessory with physiologic motion technique. (From: Wise CH, Gulick DT. *Mobilization Notes: A Rehabilitation Specialist's Pocket Guide*. Philadelphia, PA: FA Davis Company; 2009.)

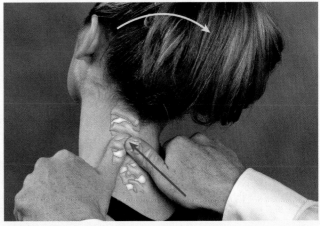

FIGURE 30–62 Cervical unilateral anterior glide: side bending accessory with physiologic motion technique. (From: Wise CH, Gulick DT. *Mobilization Notes: A Rehabilitation Specialist's Pocket Guide*. Philadelphia, PA: FA Davis Company; 2009.)

made over the transverse process of the segment being mobilized. Your forearms are in line with the direction of force.

- **Force Application:** The location and direction of force varies depending on the target segment. (1) When mobilizing C3-T4, apply gentle force in an anterior direction through the thumb contacts (Fig. 30-59). (2) When mobilizing the OA segment, gentle force is applied through your thumb contacts at the lateral mass of C1 in an anterior direction toward the patient's ipsilateral eye (Fig. 30-31). (3) When mobilizing the AA segment, the patient's head is rotated ipsilaterally approximately 30 degrees, and gentle force is applied through your thumb contacts at the articular pillar of C2 in an anterior direction toward the patient's mouth (Fig. 30-32).

Accessory With Physiologic Motion Technique (Figs. 30-60, 30-61, 30-62, 30-63)

- **Patient/Clinician Position:** The patient is in a seated position. You are standing behind or to the side of the patient and prepared to change position throughout the mobilization to ensure proper force direction.
- **Hand Placement:** Your thumb over thumb contact is applied at the transverse or spinous processes of the desired segment being mobilized. Your forearms are in the superoanterior direction in which force is applied. Your fingers grasp the musculature at the anterior aspect of the cervical spine to provide stabilization.
- **Force Application:** Apply force through your thumb contacts in a superoanterior direction while the patient performs the movement that reproduces the symptoms and/or is restricted, which includes either rotation, forward bending, side bending, or backward bending. Force is maintained throughout the entire motion and sustained at end range.

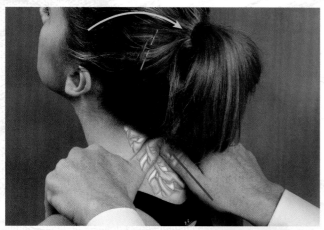

FIGURE 30–63 Cervical unilateral anterior glide: backward bending accessory with physiologic motion technique. (From: Wise CH, Gulick DT. *Mobilization Notes: A Rehabilitation Specialist's Pocket Guide.* Philadelphia: FA Davis Company; 2009.)

Midcervical Opening Upglide Mobilization (Fig. 30-64)
- **Indications:** *Cervical opening upglide mobilizations* are indicated for restrictions in segmental opening and upgliding, which is an important accessory motion for forward bending, contralateral side bending, and contralateral rotation.
- **Patient/Clinician Position:** The patient is in a supine position with the head and neck in neutral. Stand at the head of the patient.
- **Hand Placement:** Your stabilization hand supports the patient's occiput allowing it to move into contralateral rotation as the segment is being mobilized. The metacarpophalangeal joint of the second digit of your mobilization hand

contacts the articular pillar of the desired segment being mobilized with your finger placed across the vertebra being mobilized. An alternate hand placement consists of utilizing a chin cradle hold to control and support head movement.
- **Force Application:** Your mobilization hand contact applies force along the treatment plane of the facet joint which is toward the patient's ipsilateral eye as the occiput remains supported. Oscillations are provided and force is maintained throughout the entire motion and sustained at end range. Varying degrees of flexion and extension may be utilized to isolate force to the desired segment. Alternately, rotation of the head and neck is produced via the chin cradle hold while force is elicited through your thumb or finger contact at the articular pillar.

Midcervical Closing Downglide Mobilization
Indications:
- *Cervical closing downglide mobilizations* are indicated for restrictions in segmental closing and downgliding, which is an important accessory motion for backward bending, ipsilateral side bending, and ipsilateral rotation.

Accessory Motion Technique (Fig. 30-65)
- **Patient/Clinician Position:** The patient is in a supine position with the head and neck in neutral. Stand at the head of the patient.
- **Hand Placement:** Your stabilization hand supports the patient's occiput allowing it to move during mobilization. The metacarpophalangeal joint of the second digit of your mobilization hand contacts the articular pillar of the desired segment with the forearm in line with the treatment plane

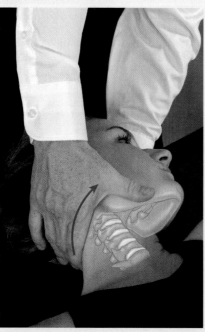

FIGURE 30–64 Midcervical opening upglide mobilization. (From: Wise CH, Gulick DT. *Mobilization Notes: A Rehabilitation Specialist's Pocket Guide.* Philadelphia, PA: FA Davis Company; 2009.)

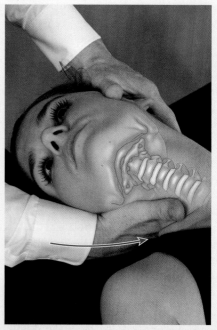

FIGURE 30–65 Midcervical closing downglide mobilization. (From: Wise CH, Gulick DT. *Mobilization Notes: A Rehabilitation Specialist's Pocket Guide.* Philadelphia, PA: FA Davis Company; 2009.)

of the facet joint, which is directed toward the patient's contralateral hip with the elbow braced against your anterior superior iliac spine.

- **Force Application:** Apply force through your mobilization hand contact in an inferoposterior direction toward the patient's contralateral hip while the stabilization hand supports the patient's occiput as it backward bends, side bends, and rotates ipsilaterally. An alternate technique consists of placing the patient's occiput on your abdomen for support as the second metacarpophalangeal joints of both hands are placed at the articular pillars being mobilized. Inferoposteriorly directed force is delivered alternately on each side of the spine.

Accessory With Physiologic Motion Technique (Fig. 30-66)

- **Patient/Clinician Position:** The patient is in a sitting position. Stand behind the patient.
- **Hand Placement:** The metacarpophalangeal joint of the second digit contacts the articular pillar of the desired segment with the forearm in line with the treatment plane of the facet joint.
- **Force Application:** Inferoposterior force is applied as the patient actively performs ipsilateral side bending and rotation as you apply gentle overpressure. Force is maintained throughout the range of motion and sustained at end range.

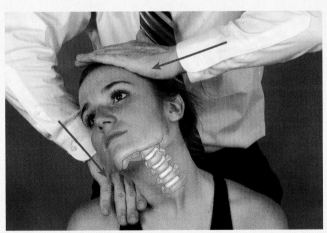

FIGURE 30–66 Midcervical closing downglide mobilization: accessory with physiologic motion technique. (From: Wise CH, Gulick DT. *Mobilization Notes: A Rehabilitation Specialist's Pocket Guide.* Philadelphia, PA: FA Davis Company; 2009.)

Cervical Physiologic Forward Bending With Finger Block

Indications:

- *Physiologic forward bending with finger block mobilizations* are indicated for restrictions in forward bending and bilateral upglide and opening throughout the cervical spine.

Accessory With Physiologic Motion Technique (Fig. 30-67)

- **Patient/Clinician Position:** The patient is in a sitting position with the head and neck in neutral. Stand at the side of the patient.
- **Hand Placement:** The thumb and flexed second digit of your stabilization hand forms a "golf-tee" hand position that is placed at the spinous process of the inferior vertebra of the segment being mobilized to block motion as it arrives. The arm of your mobilization hand cradles the patient's head and maintains contact with your chest as the fifth digit of your mobilization hand is placed across the spinous process of the superior vertebra of the segment being mobilized.
- **Force Application:** The patient's head and neck are passively moved into forward bending by the mobilization hand contact down to the desired level as the inferior vertebra of the segment is stabilized by the stabilization hand contact. Oscillations and sustained holds may be performed at end range.

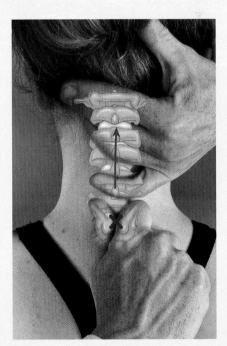

FIGURE 30–67 Cervical physiologic forward bending with finger block. (From: Wise CH, Gulick DT. *Mobilization Notes: A Rehabilitation Specialist's Pocket Guide.* Philadelphia, PA: FA Davis Company; 2009.)

Cervical Physiologic Side Bending With Finger Block

Indications:

- *Cervical physiologic side bending with finger block mobilizations* are indicated for restrictions in side bending and opening mobility on the contralateral side to which motion occurs throughout the cervical spine.

Accessory With Physiologic Motion Technique (Fig. 30-68)

- **Patient/Clinician Position:** The patient is in a sitting position with the head and neck in neutral. Stand behind the patient.
- **Hand Placement:** The thumb of your stabilization hand is placed to the side of the spinous process of the inferior vertebra of the segment being mobilized on the ipsilateral side to which motion occurs to block motion as it arrives. Your mobilization hand is placed on the patient's head to assist in controlling motion into side bending.
- **Force Application:** The patient's head and neck are passively moved into side bending by the mobilization hand down to the desired level as the inferior vertebra of the segment is stabilized by the stabilization hand contact. Oscillations and sustained holds may be performed at end range.

Accessory With Physiologic Motion Technique (Fig. 30-69)

- **Patient/Clinician Position:** The patient is in a sitting position with the head and neck in neutral. Stand on the side to which rotation will occur.
- **Hand Placement:** The thumb of your stabilization hand is placed on the articular pillar of the inferior vertebra of the segment being mobilized, on the side to which you are standing to block motion as it arrives. The arm of your mobilization hand cradles the patient's head and maintains contact with your chest as your fifth digit is placed across the spinous process of the superior vertebra of the segment being mobilized as your hand supports the occiput.
- **Force Application:** Your mobilization hand moves the head and neck into rotation toward the side on which you are standing with assistance from the patient to the desired level as the inferior vertebra of the segment being mobilized is blocked by the stabilization hand contact. Oscillations and sustained holds may be performed at end range.

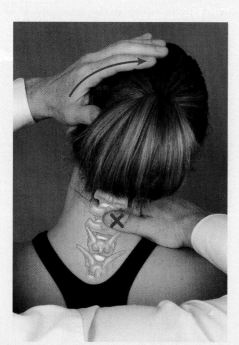

FIGURE 30–68 Cervical physiologic side bending with finger block. (From: Wise CH, Gulick DT. *Mobilization Notes: A Rehabilitation Specialist's Pocket Guide.* Philadelphia, PA: FA Davis Company; 2009.)

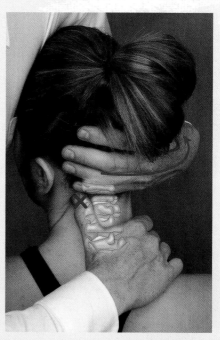

FIGURE 30–69 Cervical physiologic rotation with finger block. (From: Wise CH, Gulick DT. *Mobilization Notes: A Rehabilitation Specialist's Pocket Guide.* Philadelphia, PA: FA Davis Company; 2009.)

Cervical Physiologic Rotation With Finger Block

Indications:

- *Cervical physiologic rotation with finger block mobilizations* are indicated for restrictions in rotation and opening mobility on the contralateral side to which motion occurs throughout the cervical spine.

Subcranial Distraction

Indications:

- *Subcranial distractions* are indicated for soft tissue and joint restrictions in the subcranial region, which are designed to enhance all physiologic movement of the head on neck.

Accessory Motion Technique (Fig. 30-70)

- **Patient/Clinician Position:** The patient is in a supine position with the head and neck in neutral. Stand at the head of the patient.
- **Hand Placement:** The fingertips of both hands contact the occiput just inferior to the inferior nuchal line as your anterior shoulder contacts the patient's forehead and provides a fulcrum as distraction force is applied through the fingers.
- **Force Application:** Apply gentle distraction force through your hand contacts against the resistance created by your shoulder at the patient's forehead. For increased distraction, forward nodding is added around an axis that is in line with the patient's ears. Increased localization is provided by adding slight side bending.

Accessory With Physiologic Motion Technique (Not pictured)

- **Patient/Clinician Position:** The patient and clinician are in same position as that which was described above.
- **Hand Placement:** The clinician's hands are in the same position as that which was described above.
- **Force Application:** The patient gently forward nods his or her head on neck as the clinician provides a gentle distraction force using the finger contacts and counterpressure at the patient's forehead. You may precede force application by gently resisting isometric backward bending, to create a hold-relax stretch.

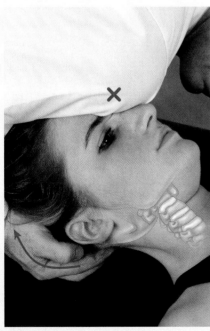

FIGURE 30–70 Subcranial distraction. (From: Wise CH, Gulick DT. *Mobilization Notes: A Rehabilitation Specialist's Pocket Guide.* Philadelphia, PA: FA Davis Company; 2009.)

Occipitoatlantal Unilateral Nod

Indications:

- *Occipitoatlantal unilateral nods* are indicated for restrictions in subcranial forward bending and anterior translation of the atlas.

Accessory Motion Technique (Fig. 30-71)

- **Patient/Clinician Position:** The patient is in a supine position with the head and neck in neutral. Sitting at the head and to the side of the patient.
- **Hand Placement:** The third digit of the stabilization hand is placed under the patient's neck and on the posterior arch or lateral mass of the atlas (C1) on the contralateral side to which you are sitting. Your other hand is placed on the patient's epicranium and over the forehead.
- **Force Application:** The hand at the patient's head gently guides the patient into forward nodding of the head on neck against the counterpressure of the finger contact at the atlas, which applies a gentle force anteriorly. The patient may be prepositioned in slight side bending to either side to assist in isolating the mobilization force.

Accessory With Physiologic Motion Technique (Not pictured)

- **Patient/Clinician Position:** The patient and clinician are in the same position as that which was described above. Alternately, the patient may be in a sitting position with the clinician standing behind them.
- **Hand Placement:** Your hands are in the same position as that which was described above. When performed in sitting, use your thumb to apply force to the atlas.
- **Force Application:** The patient gently forward nods his or her head on neck as you gently guide this motion against your finger or thumb contact at the atlas. The patient may

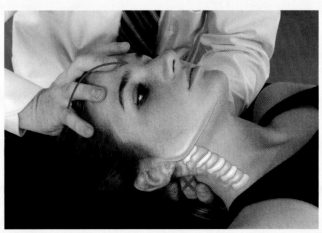

FIGURE 30–71 Occipitoatlantal unilateral nod. (From: Wise CH, Gulick DT. *Mobilization Notes: A Rehabilitation Specialist's Pocket Guide.* Philadelphia, PA: FA Davis Company; 2009.)

be prepositioned in slight side bending to either side to assist in isolating the mobilization force. You may precede force application by gently resisting isometric backward bending, to create a hold-relax stretch.

Occipitoatlantal Lateral Glide

Indications:

- *Occipitoatlantal lateral glides* are indicated for restrictions in subcranial side bending and lateral translation of the atlas.

Accessory Motion Technique (Fig. 30-72)

- **Patient/Clinician Position:** The patient is in a supine position with the head and neck in neutral. Sit at the head of the patient.
- **Hand Placement:** The stabilization hand provides a chin cradle hold that places the patient's head and neck in side bending in the direction in which the mobilization force is applied. The radial aspect of the second MCP joint of the mobilization hand is placed at the lateral mass of the atlas.
- **Force Application:** The head is slightly sidebent on the neck in the direction in which the mobilization force is applied. The chin cradle hold is maintained as the mobilization hand applies a laterally directed force through the mobilization hand contact at the lateral mass of the atlas.

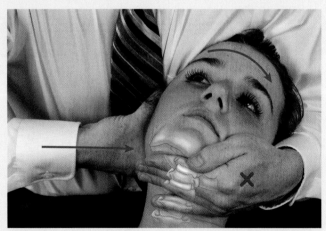

FIGURE 30–72 Atlantoaxial lateral glide: accessory motion technique. (From: Wise CH, Gulick DT. *Mobilization Notes: A Rehabilitation Specialist's Pocket Guide.* Philadelphia, PA: FA Davis Company; 2009.)

Accessory With Physiologic Motion Technique (Fig. 30-73)

- **Patient/Clinician Position:** The patient is in a sitting position. Sit or stand behind the patient.
- **Hand Placement:** One hand is placed on the patient's epicranium. The radial aspect of the second MCP joint is placed at the lateral mass of the atlas as the thumb extends across the posterior arch of the atlas.

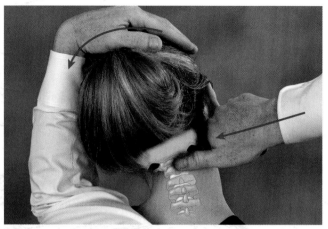

FIGURE 30–73 Occipitoatlantal lateral glide: accessory with physiologic motion technique. (From: Wise CH, Gulick DT. *Mobilization Notes: A Rehabilitation Specialist's Pocket Guide.* Philadelphia, PA: FA Davis Company; 2009.)

- **Force Application:** Guide the patient as he or she actively side bends in the direction in which the mobilization force is applied, as you apply a laterally directed force through the mobilization hand contact at the lateral mass of the atlas.

Occipitoatlantal Distraction High-Velocity Thrust (Fig. 30-74)

- **Indications:** *Occipitoatlantal distraction high-velocity thrust mobilizations* are indicated for restrictions in mobility in all directions and symptoms within the subcranial region and more specifically within the occipitoatlantal segment.
- **Patient/Clinician Position:** The patient is in a supine position with the head and neck in neutral. Stand at the head and to the side of the patient.

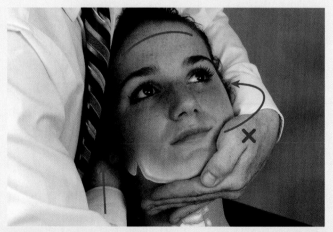

FIGURE 30–74 Occipitoatlantal distraction high-velocity thrust. (From: Wise CH, Gulick DT. *Mobilization Notes: A Rehabilitation Specialist's Pocket Guide.* Philadelphia, PA: FA Davis Company; 2009.)

- **Hand Placement:** Your stabilization hand creates a chin cradle hold over the patient's occiput and mandible. The radial side of the second MCP joint of your mobilization hand contacts the patient's mastoid process on the ipsilateral side to which you are standing.
- **Force Application:** Using the chin cradle hold, the patient's head and neck is prepositioned in forward bending, ipsilateral side bending, and contralateral rotation until tissue resistance is experienced after which slight OA backward nodding is produced. Once motion has been engaged in all three planes, a gentle squeeze is applied through all hand contacts followed by a high velocity low amplitude thrust in a cephalad direction through the mastoid hand contact.

Midcervical Nonrotatory Closing High-Velocity Thrust (Fig. 30-75)

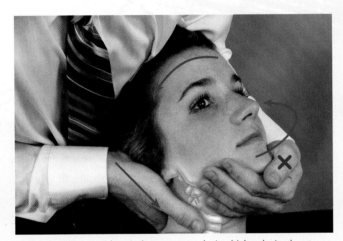

FIGURE 30–75 Midcervical nonrotatory closing high-velocity thrust. (From: Wise CH, Gulick DT. *Mobilization Notes: A Rehabilitation Specialist's Pocket Guide.* Philadelphia, PA: FA Davis Company; 2009.)

- **Indications:** *Midcervical nonrotatory closing high-velocity thrust mobilizations* are indicated for restrictions in downgliding, or closing, and symptoms within the midcervical spine.
- **Patient/Clinician Position:** The patient is in a supine position with the head and neck in neutral. Stand at the head of the patient.
- **Hand Placement:** Your stabilization hand creates a chin cradle hold over the patient's occiput and mandible or the occiput and neck are supported by both hands. The radial side of the second MCP joint of your mobilization hand contacts the articular pillar of the segment being mobilized.
- **Force Application:** The patient's head and neck are prepositioned in backward bending, contralateral rotation, and ipsilateral side bending to the segment being mobilized until end range is achieved in each plane. Once end range is achieved in all three planes, apply a high velocity low amplitude thrust in the direction of downglide toward the patient's opposite hip. Adding slight distraction may assist in making the technique more effective.

CLINICAL CASE STUDIES

CASE 1

History of Present Illness

A 45-year-old female presents with neck and right arm pain beginning 2 years ago when she suffered a whiplash injury due to a motor vehicle accident. Her symptoms completely resolved about 1 year ago. However, she reports that last week while playing tennis there was a return of symptoms secondary to forcefully serving the ball. Her symptoms progressively increased over the next several hours. On subsequent days, her symptoms were worse on awakening in the morning and eased after a warm shower with stretching. Her symptoms consist of cervical pain with occasional paresthesia into the medial border of the scapula and distally into the upper extremity to the elbow on the right. An increase in symptoms was also noted following more than 2 hours of sitting, which she does approximately 8 hours daily at work. On the average her pain is at a 2/10 level.

Neck Disability Index (NDI): 40%

Observation: Increased muscle tone in the right scalene and sternocleidomastoid; forward head and rounded shoulder posture noted.

AROM: Forward bending (FB) = 75%; backward bending (BB) = 25% with peripheralization and pain increase to 3/10; nonfunctional side bending (SB) right = 10% with peripheralization and pain increase to 3/10; nonfunctional SB left = 75%; functional SB = within normal limits (WNL) bilaterally; rotation (ROT) right = 25% with peripheralization and pain increase to 3/10; ROT left = 75%.

PPIVM: Positive AA ROT left

PAIVM: Resistance before pain at bilateral OA and right AA

Strength: 4-/5 noted at cervical flexion without pain, otherwise 5/5.

Neurological: Intact and symmetrical DTR and light touch; sharp/dull sensation

Special Tests: Upper quadrant right = positive, all with peripheralization of symptoms; vertebral artery = negative; alar ligament = negative; transverse ligament = negative; Sharp-Purser = negative.

Radiographs: Oblique views reveal multilevel narrowed IVF, with osteophytes at the articular facets C1-5 right greater than left.

1. Perform each component of the exam on a partner.
2. Develop a problem list of impairments.
3. Establish a pathoanatomically based diagnosis.
4. Establish an impairment-based diagnosis.

5. Create a plan of care that includes: three mobilizations, three stretching exercises, three strengthening exercises. Perform each on your partner.

CASE 2

History of Present Illness

Bobbi presents to your facility today with a gradual onset of cervical pain, dizziness, and constant occipital headaches with initial onset approximately 3 months ago. Bobbi also complains of intermittent right upper extremity (UE) symptoms consisting of pain and paresthesia along the radial side of her right arm. She was initially seen 2 weeks ago by her physician, who referred her to your facility for evaluation and treatment.

Cervical pain increases from 2/10 to 4/10 only after performing her secretarial job at the end of the day. Her headache is noted only in the morning and after dinner. Her dizziness is most notable when lying prone or when looking back when driving. Right UE paresthesia is present when reaching behind to buckle her daughter in the car seat.

Posture: Rounded shoulders, head forward and deviated left.

AROM: FB = WNL and reduction in right UE paresthesia; BB = 25% and increase in UE paresthesia; SB right = 25% and increase in UE paresthesia; SB left = 50% and decrease in UE paresthesia; ROT right = 75% and increase in paresthesia; ROT left = 90% and decrease in UE paresthesia.

Joint Scan: TMJ AROM reveals reciprocal click on 8 out of 10 repetitions, 25 mm opening, C-curve deviation to right.

PAIVM: Hypomobility noted with central anterior pressures at C4-C6, with resistance noted before pain at each level and reproduction of right UE paresthesia with unilateral anterior pressures at C5 on the left.

Neurological: Right biceps DTR = 1+; light sensation = decrease C6 dermatome on right.

Manual Muscle Testing: Grossly 5/5

Special Tests: Alar ligament = negative; transverse ligament = negative; vertebral artery = negative; lower and upper quadrant = positive on right with reproduction of headache and upper extremity paresthesia; foraminal compression/distraction = positive; median nerve bias upper limb tension test (ULTT) = positive; radial/ulnar nerve bias ULTT = negative.

Palpation: Hyperactive scaleni, suboccipital musculature.

1. Perform each component of the exam on a partner.
2. Develop a problem list of impairments.
3. Establish a pathoanatomically based diagnosis.
4. Establish an impairment-based diagnosis.

5. Create a plan of care that includes: three mobilizations, three stretching exercises, three strengthening exercises. Perform each on your partner.

HANDS-ON

With a partner, perform the following activities:

1 Discuss the value of using self-assessment disability questionnaires during the examination of individuals with low back pain. What is the minimal clinically important difference that must occur for each of the questionnaires to reveal a clinically significant change in an individual's status.

2 Observe your partner as he or she performs active functional side bending followed by active non-functional side bending. Appreciate and compare the quantity and quality of these motions and identify any reproduction of symptoms. If a difference in motion is noted between these two motions, discuss with your partner some of the potential reasons for this difference. How would you confirm your hypothesis regarding the primary origin of these observed motion impairments? Perform an active motion assessment on at least one other individual and compare your findings.

3 Perform PPIVM testing of the subcranial and midcervical spine and attempt to identify any motion restrictions or motions that reproduce symptoms. If a motion restriction is identified, use PAIVM testing to confirm your hypothesis. Ask at least one other individual to perform PPIVM and PAIVM testing on your partner and see if your findings correlate. When testing, determine the relationship between the onset of pain (P1 and P2) and stiffness or resistance (R1 and R2), if present. Compare your findings during the active movement assessment with your findings during PPIVM and PAIVM testing. Solicit feedback from your partner regarding your performance of these procedures.

4 Based on the findings from AROM, PPIVM, and PAIVM testing, identify three joint-mobilization techniques that would be most appropriate for your partner. Perform these techniques on your partner. Retest your partner's mobility immediately following each technique and identify any changes. What other manual and non-manual interventions would you include either before or following your joint mobilization techniques?

5 Through palpation, attempt to identify the primary soft tissue and bony structures of the cervical spine and TMJ and compare the tissue texture, tension, tone, and location of these structures bilaterally.

6 Perform the premanipulative screening process on your partner including both vascular integrity testing and spinal segmental stability testing. Perform each of these special tests on your partner. What is the sensitivity and specificity of these procedures? What other methods should be employed to ensure safety prior to initiating cervical spine high velocity low amplitude thrust procedures? Perform these tests on your partner. If appropriate and with their consent, perform the cervical spine thrust techniques presented in this chapter on your partner.

7 Perform each mobilization described in the intervention section of this chapter on at least two individuals. Using each technique, practice grades I to IV. Solicit input from your partner regarding position, hand placement, force application, comfort, etc. If possible, video yourself performing these procedures and self-assess your performance.

8 Refer to Chapter 17 and discuss each of the systems for the classification of neck pain that are currently in use. Identify which system(s) are most evidence-based. Discuss the use of impairment-based models of classification and why they may be preferable over other models for the diagnosis and classification of neck pain. Describe how you might use each system to determine the differential diagnosis for each of the cases described above. How will the use of impairment-based models of classification impact or change your management of individuals with neck pain. When practicing these mobilization techniques, utilize the Sequential Partial Task Practice Method, in which students repeatedly practice one aspect of each technique (i.e., position, hand placement, force application) on multiple partners each time, adding the next component until the technique is performed in real time from beginning to end. (Wise CH, Schenk RJ, Lattanzi JB. A model for teaching and learning spinal thrust manipulation and its effect on participant confidence in technique performance. *J Manual & Manipulative Ther*, August 2014.)

REFERENCES

1. Hoving JL, Koes B, DeVet HCW, VanDerWindt DA, et al. Manual therapy, physical therapy, or continued care by a general practitioner for patients with neck pain: a randomized, controlled trial. *Annals of Int Med.* 2002;10:713-722.
2. Cote P, Cassidy JD, Carroll L. The factors associated with neck pain and its related disability in the Saskatchewan population. *Spine.* 2000;25:1109-1117.
3. Herzog W. *Clinical Biomechanics of Spinal Manipulation.* New York, NY: Churchill Livingstone; 2000.
4. Romanes GJ. *Cunningham's Textbook of Anatomy.* Oxford, UK: Oxford University Press; 1981.
5. Dvorak J, Schneider E, Saldinger P, Rahn B. Biomechanics of the craniocervical region: the alar and transverse ligaments. *J Orthop Res.* 1988;6:452-461.
6. Paris SV, Loubert PV. *Foundations of Clinical Orthopaedics, Course Notes.* St. Augustine, FL: Institute Press; 1990.
7. Mercer SR. Structure and function of the bones and joints of the cervical spine. In: Oatis CA, ed. *Kinesiology: The Mechanics and Pathomechanics of Human Movement.* Philadelphia, PA: Lippincott Williams & Wilkins; 2004.
8. Lind B, Sihlbom H, Nordwall A, Malchau H. Normal range of motion of the cervical spine. *Arch Phys Med Rehabil.* 1989;70:692-695.
9. Fielding JW, Cochran GVB, Lawsing JF, Hohl M. Tears of the transverse ligament of the atlas. *J Bone Joint Surg.* 1974;56A:1683-1691.
10. Worth DR, Selvik G. Movements of the craniovertebral joints. In: Grieve G, ed. *Modern Manual Therapy of the Vertebral Column.* Edinburgh: Churchill Livingstone; 1994:53-68.
11. Paris SV. *S3 Course Notes.* St. Augustine, FL: Institute of Graduate Physical Therapy; 1992.
12. Eggleton TL, Langton DM. Clinical anatomy of the TMJ complex. In: Krauss SL, ed. *Temporomandibular Disorders*, 2nd ed. New York, NY: Churchill Livingstone; 1994.
13. Sommer O, Aigner F, Rudisch A, et al. Cross-sectional and functional imaging of the temporomandibular joint: radiology, pathology, and basic biomechanics of the jaw. *Radiographics.* 23:e14; 2003.
14. Levangie PK, Norkin CC. *Joint Structure and Function: A Comprehensive Analysis*, 4th ed. Philadelphia, PA: FA Davis; 2005.
15. Helland M. Anaotmy and function of the temporomandibular joint. *J Orthop Sports Phys Ther.* 1980;1:145-152.
16. Isberg A, Westesson P. Steepness of articular eminence and movement of the condyle and disc in asymptomatic temporomandibular joints. *Oral Surg Oral Med Oral Pathol Oral Radiol Endod.* 1998;86:152-157.
17. Ferrario VF, Sforza C, Miani A Jr, et al. Open-close movements in the human temporomandibular joint: does a pure rotation around the intercondylar hinge axis exist? *J Oral Rehabil.* 1996;23:401-408.
18. Yang X, Pernu H, Pyhtinen J, et al. MR abnormalities of the lateral pterygoid muscle in patients with nonreducing disc displacement of the TMJ *Cranio.* 2002;20:209-221.
19. Vernon H, Minor S. The neck disability index: a study of reliability and validity. *J Manipulative Physiol Ther.* 1991;14:409-415.
20. Fritz JM, George SZ, Delitto A. The role of fear-avoidance beliefs in acute low back pain: relationships with current and future disability and work status. *Pain.* 2001;94:7-125.
21. Leak AM, Cooper J, et al. The Northwick Park Neck Pain questionnaire, devised to measure neck pain and disability. *Br J Rheumatol.* 1994;33:469-474.
22. Fritz JM, George SZ. Identifying specific psychosocial factors in patients with acute, work-related low back pain; the importance of fear-avoidance beliefs. *Phys Ther.* 2002;82:973-983.
23. Cleland JA, Fritz JM, Whitman JM, et al. The use of a lumbar spine manipulation technique by physical therapists in patients who satisfy a clinical prediction rule: a case series. *J Orthop Sports Phys Ther.* 2006;36:209-214.
24. Childs JD, Fritz JM, Flynn TW, et al. A clinical prediction rule to identify patients with low back pain most likely to benefit from spinal manipulation: a validation study. *Annals Int Med.* 2004;141:920-928.
25. Flynn T, Fritz J, Whitman J, et al. A clinical prediction rule for classifying patients with low back pain who demonstrate short-term improvement with spinal manipulation. *Spine.* 2002;27:2835-2843.
26. Weinstein JN, McLain RF. Primary tumors of the spine. *Spine.* 1987; 12:843-851.
27. Deyo RA, Rainville J, Kent DL. What can the history and physical examination tell us about low back pain? *JAMA.* 1992;268:760-765.
28. Boissonnault WG. *Primary Care for the Physical Therapist: Examination and Triage.* St. Louis, MO: Elsevier Saunders; 2005.
29. Wainner RS, Fritz JM, Irrgang JJ, et al. Reliability and diagnostic accuracy of the clinical examination and patient self-report measures for cervical radiculopathy. *Spine.* 2003;28:52-62.
30. Sjaastad O, Fredriksen TA, Pfaffenrath V. Cervicogenic headache: diagnostic criteria. *Headache.* 1998;38:442-445.
31. Leone M, D'Amico D, Frediani F, Torri W, et al. Clinical considerations on side-locked unilaterally in long-lasting primary headaches. *Headache.* 1993;33:381-384.
32. van Suijlekom JA, de Vet HCW, van den Berg SGM, Weber WEJ. Intraobserver reliability of diagnostic criteria for cervicogenic headache. *Cephalgia.* 1999;19:817-823.
33. International Headache Society. The International Classification of Headache Disorders, 2nd ed. *Cephalgia.* 2004;24(Suppl 1): 115-116.
34. Dwyer A, Aprill C, Bogduk N. Cervical zygapophyseal joint pain patterns I: a study in normal volunteers. *Spine.* 1990;15:453-457.
35. Cooper G, Bailey B, Bogduk N. Cervical zygapophyseal joint pain maps. *Pain Med.* 2007;8:344-353.
36. Lord S, Barnsley L, Wallis B, Bogduk N. Third occipital headache: a prevalence study. *J Neurol Neurosurg Psychiatr.* 1994;57:1187-1190.
37. Bogduk N. The neck and headaches. *Neurol Clin N Am.* 2004;22:151-171.
38. Dreyfuss P, Michaelson M, Fletcher D. Atlanto-occipital and lateral atlanto-axial joint pain patterns. *Spine.* 1994;19:1125-1131.
39. Schellhas KP, Smith MD, Gundry CR, Pollei SR. Cervical discogenic pain: prospective correlation of magnetic resonance imaging and discography in asymptomatic subjects and pain sufferers. *Spine.* 1996;21:300-301.
40. Spitzer WO, Skovron ML, Salmi LR, et al. Scientific monograph of the Quebec Task Force on Whiplash-Associated Disorders: redefining "whiplash" and its management. *Spine.* 1995;20(8 Suppl):1S-73S.
41. Sapir DA, Gorup JM. Radiofrequency medial branch neurotomy in litigant and nonlitigant patients with cervical whiplash: a prospective study. *Spine.* 2001;15:268-273.
42. Fernandez de las Penas C, Fernandez-Carnero J, Fernandez A, Lomas-Vega R, Miangolarra-Page J. Dorsal manipulation in whiplash treatment: a randomized controlled trial. *Journal of Whiplash and Related Disorders.* 2004;3:55-72.
43. Sullivan MJ, Adams H, Rhodenizer T, Stanish WD. A psychosocial risk factor-targeted intervention for the prevention of chronic pain and disability following whiplash injury. *Phys Ther.* 2006;86:8-18.
44. Sterling M. A proposed new classification system for whiplash associated disorders-implications for assessment and management. *Man Ther.* 2004;9:60-70.
45. Cook C, Brismee J-M, Fleming R, Sizer PS. Identifiers suggestive of clinical cervical spine instability: Delphi Study of Physical Therapists. *Phys Ther.* 2005;85:895-906.
46. Symons BP, Leonard T, Herzog W. Internal forces sustained by the vertebral artery during spinal manipulative therapy. *J Manipulative Physiol Ther.* 2002;25:504-510.
47. Stiell IG, Clement CM, McKnight RD, et al. The Canadian C-Spine rule vs. the NEXUS low-risk criteria in patients with trauma. *N Engl J Med.* 2003:2510-2518.

48. Stiell IG, Wells GA, Vandemheen KL, et al. The Canadian cervical spine rule for radiography in alert and stable trauma patients. *JAMA.* 2001;286:1841-1848.

49. Leong WK, Kermode AG. Acute deterioration in Chiari type 1 malformation after chiropractic cervical manipulation. *J Neurol Neurosur Psych.* 2001;70:816-817.

50. McKinnis LN. *Fundamentals of Musculoskeletal Imaging.* Philadelphia, PA: FA Davis; 2005.

51. Boden SD, Davis DO, Dina TS, et al. Abnormal magnetic-resonance scans of the lumbar spine in asymptomatic individuals: a prospective investigation. *J Bone Joint Surg Am.* 1990;72:403-408.

52. Wiesel S, Tsourmas N, Feffer HL, et al. A study of computer-assisted tomography, I: the incidence of positive CAT scans in an asymptomatic group of patients. *Spine.* 1984;9:549-551.

53. Rocabado M. *Cranioverterbal-Craniomandibular Disorders in Headache Patients.* AAOMPT Course Notes. St. Louis, MO: AAOMPT; 2007.

54. Haynes MJ, Cala LA, Melsom A, Mastaglia FL, et al. Posterior ponticles and rotational stenosis of vertebral arteries. A pilot study using Doppler ultrasound velocimetry and magnetic resonance angiography. *J Manipulative Physiol Ther.* 2005;28:323-329.

55. Montaner J, Molina C, Alvarez-Sabin J, Codina A. "Herald hemiparesis" of basilar artery occlusion: early recognition by transcranial Doppler ultrasound. *European J Neuro.* 2000;7:91-93.

56. Khan S, Cloud GC, Kerry S, Markus HS. Imaging of vertebral artery stenosis: a systematic review. *J Neurolo Neurosur & Psych.* 2007;78:1218-1225.

57. McKenzie R, May S. *The Lumbar Spine Mechanical Diagnosis and Therapy Volume One.* Waikanae, New Zealand: Spinal Publications; 2003.

58. Magee DJ. *Orthopedic Physical Assessment,* 5th ed. St Louis, MO: Saunders-Elsevier; 2008.

59. Griegel-Morris P, Oatis C. Incidence of common postural abnormalities in the cervical, shoulder, and thoracic regions and their association with pain in two age groups of healthy subjects. *Phys Ther.* 1992;72:426-430.

60. Paris SV, Rot J. *Examination, Evaluation, and Non-thrust Manipulation with Emphasis on the Upper Cervical Spine and Cervical Syndrome. AAOMPT Course Notes.* St. Louis, MO: AAOMPT; 2007.

61. Youdas JW, Carey JR, Garrett TR. Reliability of measurements of cervical spine range of motion: comparison of three methods. *Phys Ther.* 1991;72:98-104.

62. Krauss J, Creighton D, Ely JD, Podlewsks-Ely J. The immediate effects of upper thoracic translatoric spinal manipulation on cervical pain and range of motion: a randomized clinical trial. *J Man Manip Ther.* 2008;16:93-99.

63. Maitland G, Hengeveld E, Banks K, English K. *Maitland's Vertebral Manipulation,* 6th ed. Oxford, U.K.: Butterworth-Heinemann; 2001.

64. Fjellner A, Bexander C, Faleij R, Strender LE. Interexaminer reliability in physical examination of the cervical spine. *J Manipulative Physiol Ther.* 1999;22:511-516.

65. Smedmark V, Wallin M, Arvidsson I. Inter-examiner reliability in assessing passive intervertebral motion of the cervical spine. *Manual Ther.* 2000;5:97-101.

66. Gonella C, Paris SV. Reliability in evaluating passive intervertebral motion. *Phys Ther.* 1982;62:436-444.

67. Mahar C, Adams R. Reliability of pain and stiffness assessments in clinical manual lumbar spine examination. *Phys Ther.* 1994;74:801-811.

68. Kay TM, Gross A, Goldsmith C, et al. Exercises for mechanical neck disorders. *Cochrane Database Syst Rev.* 2005;CD004250.

69. Gross AR, Hoving JL, Haines TA, et al. A Cochrane Review of manipulation and mobilization for mechanical neck disorders. *Spine.* 2004;29:1541-1548.

70. Sarig-Bahat H. Evidence for exercise therapy in mechanical neck disorders. *Man Ther.* 2003;8:10-20.

71. O'Leary S, Falla D, Jull G. Recent advances in therapeutic exercise for the neck: implications for patients with head and neck pain. *Aust Endod J.* 2003;29:138-142.

72. Chui TTW, Law EYH, Chui THF. Performance of the craniocervical flexion test in subjects with and without chronic neck pain. *J Orthop Sports Phys Ther.* 2005;35:567-571.

73. Jull G, Trott P, Potter H, et al. A randomized controlled trial of exercise and manipulative therapy for cervicogenic headache. *Spine.* 2002;27:1835-1843.

74. Fullen BM, Maher T, Bury G, Tynan A, et al. Adherence of Irish general practitioners to European guidelines for acute low back pain: a prospective pilot study. *Eur J Pain.* 2007;11:614-623.

75. Symons BP, Leonard T, Herzog W. Internal forces sustained by the vertebral artery during spinal manipulative therapy. *J Manipulative Physiol Ther.* 2002;25:504-510.

76. Wise CH, Schenk RJ. Clinical decision-making in the application of cervical spine manipulation. In: Hughes C, ed. *Home Study Course 21.1.5, Cervical and Thoracic Pain: Evidence of Effectiveness in Physical Therapy.* La Crosse, WI: Orthopaedic Section American Physical Therapy Association; 2011.

77. Tseng YL, Wang WTF, Chen WY, Hou TJ, et al. Predictors for the immediate responders to cervical manipulation in patients with neck pain. *Man Ther.* 2006;11:306-315.

78. Cleland JA, Glynn P, Whitman JM, Eberhart SL, et al. Short-term effects of thrust versus nonthrust mobilization/manipulation directed at the thoracic spine in patients with neck pain: a randomized clinical trial. *Phys Ther.* 2007;87:431-440.

79. Puentedura EJ, Cleland JA, Landers MR, Mintken PE, Louw A, Fernández-de-Las-Peñas C. Development of a clinical prediction rule to identify patients with neck pain likely to benefit from thrust joint manipulation to the cervical spine. *J Orthop Sports Phys Ther.* 2012;42:577-92.

80. Flynn TW, Cleland JA, Whitman JM. *Users' Guide to the Musculoskeletal Examination.* Buckner, KY: Evidence in Motion; 2008.

81. Uitvlugt G, Indenbaum S. Clinical assessment of atlantoaxial instability using the Sharp-Purser test. *Arthritis Rheumatol.* 1988;31:918-922.

82. Aspinall W. Clinical testing for the craniovertebral hypermobility syndrome. *J Orthop Sports Phys Ther.* 1990;12:47-54.

83. Meadows JJ, Magee DJ. An overview of dizziness and vertigo for the orthopedic manual therapist. In: Boyling JD, Palastanga N, eds. *Grieve's Modern Manual Therapy: The Vertebral Column,* 2nd ed. Edinburgh, Scotland: Churchill Livingstone; 1994.

84. Pettman E. Stress tests of the craniovertebral joints. In: Boyling JD, Palastanga N, eds. *Grieve's Modern Manual Therapy: The Vertebral Column,* 2nd ed. Edinburgh, Scotland: Churchill Livingstone; 1994.

85. Olson KA, Paris SV, Spohr C, Gorniak G. Radiographic assessment and reliability study of the craniovertebral sidebending test. *J Man Manip Ther.* 1998;6:87-96.

86. Grant R. Vertebral artery insufficiency: A clinical protocol for pre-manipulative testing of the cervical spine. In: Boyling JD, Palastranga N, eds. *Grieve's Modern Manual Therapy: The Vertebral Column,* 2nd ed. Edinburgh, Scotland: Churchill Livingstone; 1994.

87. Grant R. Vertebral artery testing: the Australian Physiotherapy Association Protocol after 6 years. *Man Ther.* 1996;1:149-153.

88. Rivett DA. The premanipulative vertebral artery testing protocol. *NZ J Physiother.* 1995;23:9-12.

89. Keery R, Taylor AJ. Cervical artery dysfunction assessment and manual therapy. *Man Ther.* 2006;11:243-253.

90. Kunnasmaa KT, Thiel HW. Vertebral artery syndrome: a review of the literature. *J Orthop Med.* 1994;16:17-20.

91. Vidal P, Huijbregts P. Dizziness in orthopaedic physical therapy practice: history and physical examination. *J Mal Manip Ther.* 2005;13:221-250.

92. Norre ME. Cervical vertigo: diagnostic and semiological problem with special emphasis upon "cervical nystagmus." *Acta Otorhinolaryngol Belg.* 1987;41:436-452.

93. Spurling R, Scoville W. Lateral rupture of the cervical intervertebral discs. *N Engl J Med.* 1944;231:279-287.

94. Viikari-Juntura E, Porras M, Laasonen EM. Validity of clinical tests in the diagnosis of root compression in cervical disc disease. *Spine.* 1989;14:253-257.

95. Tong HC, Haig AJ, Yamakawa K. The Spurling test and cervical radiculopathy. *Spine.* 2002;27:156-159.

96. Bertilson BC, Grunnesjo M, Strender LE. Reliability of clinical tests in the assessment of patients with neck/shoulder problems-impact of history. *Spine.* 2003;28:2222-2231.

97. Butler, DS. Mobilisation of the nervous system. Singapore: Churchill Livingstone; 1991.

98. Coppieters MW, Stappaerts KH, Everaert DG, Staes FF. Addition of test components during neurodynamic testing: effect of ROM and sensory responses. *J Orthop Sports Phy Ther.* 2001;31:226-237.

99. Coppieters M, Stappaerts K, Janssens K. Reliability and detecting onset of pain and submaximal pain during neural provocation testing of the upper quadrant. *Phys Res Int.* 2002;7:34-42.

100. Keneally M. The upper limb tension test. In: *Proceedings, Manipulative Therapists Association of Australia,* 4th biennial conference, Brisbane; 1985.

101. McClellan DL, Swash M. Longitudinal sliding of the median nerve during movements of the upper limb. *J Neurol Neurosurg Psychiatr.* 1976;39:566-569.

102. McClellan DL. Longitudinal sliding of the median nerve during hand movements: a contributory factor in entrapment neuropath. *Lancet.* 1975;633:1843-1851.

103 Garmer DA, Jones A, McHorse KJ. The ulnar nerve bias upper limb neurodynamic tension test: an investigation of responses in asymptomatic subjects. Cincinnati, OH: APTA Conference Abstract: 2002.

104. Kleinrensink GJ, Stoeckart R, Mulder PGH, Hock GVD, et al. Upper limb tension tests as tools in the diagnosis of nerve and plexus lesions: anatomical and biomechanical aspects. *Clin Biomechanics.* 2000;15:9-14.

A

Abdominal Series: Performed to test if there is central inhibition related to weakness of the lower extremities. There are four separate components to the supine abdominal series.

Abnormal Rhythms: Movement patterns that do not follow the expected kinematics of the joint in question (i.e., poor scapulohumeral rhythm).

Accessory: Motions that are considered to be synonymous with arthrokinematic movement. They consist of motions that are available within a joint that may accompany the classical (osteokinematic) movements or those that may be passively produced apart from the classical movement. Accessory movements are necessary for normal kinematics and subsequent joint function. See *Arthrokinematic*.

Accessory Soft Tissue Movement Testing: Performed by passively moving soft tissues in all directions.

Acetabular Anteversion: The orientation of the acetabulum in an anterior direction. This structural feature is an important determinant of hip joint stability. Acetabular anteversion that is larger than the normal values of 18.5 degrees and 21.5 degrees for males and females, respectively, may render the hip susceptible to anterior dislocation.

Active Insufficiency: Occurs when a multijoint muscle reaches a length (shortened) where it can no longer apply an effective force.

Active Range of Motion (AROM): Motion occurring entirely through the volition of the individual, that is produced through active muscle contraction.

Active Movement: See *Active Range of Motion (AROM)*.

Active Myofascial Trigger Points (MTrPs): Trigger points that produce symptoms, including local tenderness and pain, referral of pain or other paresthesias to a distant site, with peripheral and central sensitization.

Active Subsystem: Relative to the spine, comprises contractile skeletal muscle and is most involved in contributing to stability within the neutral zone.

Actual Resting Position: Used when it is impossible, difficult, or impractical to achieve the true resting position. The therapist places the joint in the position in which the least amount of tension is elicited and where the patient reports the least discomfort.

Acture: A term that recognizes that posture is a dynamic neuromuscular state that allows a person to be prepared for action.

Acute Phase Response (APR): A nonspecific reaction that occurs when the inflammation that is produced by repetitive activity, trauma, or infection is sufficient to alter the capabilities of the humoral components of the immune system.

Acute Response Proteins (ARPs): Humoral defensive components whose concentration is depressed in response to a complex network of molecular and cellular responses.

Acute Stage: Stage characterized by a progressive increase in signs and symptoms. During this stage, it is critical that the therapist provide intervention only if it will aid in the reparative process.

Adaptive Shortening: May result from prolonged immobility. Muscles and their connective tissue structures reduce in length, leading to restricted movement that eventually impacts the joint over which the muscles lie.

Adherent Nerve Root (ANR) Syndrome: Created by adhesions that have formed around the spinal nerve root or dura preventing normal mobility. In contrast to the other types of dysfunction, which produce symptoms local to the spine, a lumbar ANR syndrome may include symptoms that radiate into the extremity. This syndrome may mimic a posterior derangement.

Adjustive Distraction: Manual techniques that typically involve the use of high-velocity thrust for the purpose of repositioning subluxed or dislocated joints. These techniques are not routinely used in the clinic, but are important for therapists engaged in the care of athletes.

Afferent Pathways: Neural pathways that direct primarily sensory information toward the spinal cord.

Alpha: The probability (as measured by a *p*-value) that any differences observed are due to chance.

Alpha Gain: The state of the reflex arc when the sarcomere becomes hyperinnervated, owing to an increase in nerve impulses that are carried along the alpha motor nerve from the anterior horn of the spinal cord to the involved muscle fibers.

AMBRI: A type of shoulder instability that is atraumatic, multidirectional with bilateral shoulder findings with rehabilitation as appropriate treatment, and rarely the need for inferior capsular shift surgery.

Amplitude: Excursion of movement that is used during joint mobilization.

Anatomical Movements: Bone rotational movements that are classified as *standard*, or *uniaxial* and are motions that occur around one axis in one plane.

Angle of Inclination (AI): The angle formed by a line drawn through the femoral head and neck and the long axis of the femoral shaft in the frontal plane.

Angle of Torsion (AT): This angle of the femur exists within the transverse plane. This angle is best visualized by placing the femoral condyles in the frontal plane and measuring the angle between the frontal plane and a line drawn through the femoral head and neck. A normal range for the AT in adults is 15 to 25 degrees.

Angle of Wiberg: See *Center Edge (CE) Angle.*

Ankle/Brachial Index (ABI): The measure obtained by dividing the systolic blood pressure of the ankle by the pressure of the brachial artery. An ABI of less than 0.97 confirms the presence of peripheral vascular disease.

Anterior Depression (AD): One of four pelvic girdle motions based on proprioceptive neuromuscular facilitation diagonals that occurs during gait. AD occurs as the pelvis assists the leg to elongate down and forward for initial contact with the ground. The ability for the right quadratus lumborum to elongate with good eccentric control is critical for proper deceleration of the limb.

Anterior Elevation (AE): One of four pelvic girdle motions based on proprioceptive neuromuscular facilitation diagonals that occurs during gait. AE is the most efficient when the iliopsoas and abdominals contract synergistically to promote trunk stabilization during the initial swing phase.

Anteriorly Rotated Pelvis: Typically accompanied by hyperextension of the knees, increased lumbar lordosis, a backward bent costal cage, an elevated sternum, and forward head.

Anteriorly Sheared Pelvis: Typically causes the sway back posture with the knees flexed, costal cage posterior, a depressed sternum, and forward head.

Ape Hand Deformity: Resulting from palsy of the median nerve alone may lead to the thumb falling into the frontal plane with the other digits, along with atrophy of the thenar eminence and the inability to engage in thumb opposition.

Arthrokinematic: Defined as the relative motion that occurs between joint surfaces and structures within a joint.

Articular Hypomobility: Motion limitations that lead to a decrease in range in both passive physiologic intervertebral movement (PPIVM) and passive arthrokinematic (accessory) intervertebral movement (PAIVM).

Asanas (ā·sa·nas): Physical postures used in yoga as a form of exercise promoting cardiovascular fitness, strength, and flexibility. Each posture contributes to increased body awareness and proper positioning of the body in space both at rest and during movement.

Ashtanga: Methods of hatha yoga that use fast, flowing asana movements.

Associated Oscillations: The oscillations used within the facilitated oscillatory approach derive their origin from the Trager method. Oscillatory movements are incorporated at various locations throughout the body. The use of repetitive movement induces relaxation of the muscles. Although no direct manual contact to the muscle occurs, these oscillations are effective in reducing tightness.

Asymmetrical Movement: Dysfunction, tests, and interventions that are combined/multiplanar or triplanar. In contrast to symmetrical dysfunctions, they are unequal bilaterally, or unilateral, in nature, thus indicating that the dysfunction is occurring on one side of the segment (i.e., asymmetrical).

Atlantodental Interface: Space between the odontoid process and the anterior arch of the atlas.

Attractors: Available patterns of movement that are well learned.

Autogenic Inhibition: Resistance that is applied to the restricted agonist prior to stretching when performing hold and contract-relax stretching.

Autonomic Nervous System (ANS): A division of the peripheral nervous system that is distributed to glands and smooth muscle, whose primary functions are carried out below the level of conscious input.

Awareness through Movement (ATM): A process in which the practitioner provides verbal guidance for the client to actively explore many facets of a movement, thereby discovering ways of doing things that may have never occurred to the client or a movement that he or she has not done for many years. Throughout ATM, the movement done by the client is entirely voluntary.

Axon: A single elongated protoplasmic neuronal process with the specialized function of moving impulses away from the dendritic zone and ending in a number of axon telodendria.

Axonotmesia: A loss of continuity of the nerve axons with maintenance of the continuity of the connective tissue sheaths.

Axoplasmic Transportation (AXT): A non-impulse-based condition along the core of the nerve fiber of trophic nutrients to the tissues innervated by the nerve, neurotransmitter substances to the synapses of the nerve, and metabolites back to the central nervous system.

B

Beau's Lines: Transverse ridges that reveal disruptions in nail growth secondary to nutritional deficiency or systemic disease.

Behavior of Symptoms Questions: A series of questioning, during which the therapist seeks to differentiate local pain from referred pain and to ascertain the patient's level of irritability.

Biomechanical Examination: One of two primary types of objective examination within the Canadian approach to OMPT. Designed to determine the movement characteristics of involved joints and associated structures.

Bishop's Hand Deformity: Injury to the ulnar nerve that leads to flexion of digits 4 and 5.

Body Tilt Test: An examination procedure that involves holding the head, neck, and trunk together so that they are moved as a single entity through tilting the seated trunk forward/backward and side to side. This maneuver is designed to stimulate the labyrinth, but not the cervical proprioceptors or the vertebral artery. Any dizziness produced, therefore, is likely to be generated by the vestibular system.

Bone Rotational Movement: Refers to movement that occurs around an axis.

Bone Translational Movements: Linear motions that occur parallel to an axis in one particular plane.

Bouchard's Nodes: PIP joint deformity resulting from osteoarthritis.

Boutonniere Deformity: A rupture of the central tendon of the extensor hood mechanism may result in a flexion deformity of the PIP and extension deformity of the DIP.

Bruxism: The act of grinding the teeth.

Bunnell-Littler Test: A test used to differentiate between hand intrinsic tightness and capsular restrictions. Tightness of the hand intrinsic muscles is suspected if the PIP joint moves better with the MCP in flexion, and joint capsular restrictions are suspected if the PIP joint is unable to flex in either position.

C

Capsular Pattern: Specific and characteristic patterns of joint motion loss that suggest restrictions that are present within the synovial capsule of the joint. Their presence is an indication for the use of joint mobilization techniques that are designed to mobilize restrictions and restore normal mobility. These patterns are often contrasted with the presence of myofascial patterns for the purpose of determining the primary cause of a motion restriction. Such patterns have been described for every joint and are named as the most restricted to the least restricted motion (i.e., capsular pattern of the glenohumeral joint is ER>Abduction>IR).

Capsuloligamentous Complex (CLC): The noncontractile soft tissue structures that surround the joint consisting collectively of the synovial joint capsule and the periarticular ligaments, which are often indistinguishable from one another.

Carrying Angle: The angle between the long axis of the humerus and the long axis of the ulna when the elbow is extended and fully supinated.

Causalgia: A prolonged dry, burning, itching type of pain that is usually recalcitrant even to narcotics, only yielding to antiseizure medications. Causalgia is rarely caused by nerve root damage but rather usually by central lesions, particularly those involving the thalamus and peripheral nerves.

Center Edge (CE) Angle: This angle is determined upon radiography by connecting a line drawn between the lateral rim of the acetabulum and the center of the femoral head, which forms an angle with the vertical.

Central Disorders: Space-occupying lesions within the spinal canal.

Centralization Phenomenon: Occurs when symptoms migrate from a distal location to a more proximal location often in responses to specific motions or positions. The inability to centralize symptoms has been reported as the strongest predictor of chronic pain and disability.

Chemical Muscle Guarding: When this form of guarding is present, individuals will present as having a heaviness or bogginess to the touch related to chemical responses to injury.

Chromatolysis: The process of degeneration of the cell body, axon, and synapse after axonal injury.

Chronic Stage: In reference to healing, this stage is typically applied to static conditions with a history of usually greater than three months. It is important for the therapist to appreciate that chronic conditions often involve a considerable degree of behavioral changes that lack a direct correlation to true organic pathology.

Circumferential Techniques: Typically performed on the extremities for the purpose of restoring muscle play so that soft tissue is able to move circumferentially around long bones.

Classic Claw Hand Deformity: Composed of MCP extension and PIP/DIP flexion in the presence of an intrinsic minus hand.

Class I Occlusion: Refers to the normal relationship of the maxillary and mandibular teeth in the anterior-posterior dimension.

Class II Overbite: Consists of mandibular teeth that are positioned posterior to their normal position.

Class III Underbite: Consists of mandibular teeth that are positioned anterior to their normal position.

Classical Movements: Are considered to be synonymous with osteokinematic movement. They consist of active movements, which are used to evaluate joint range and muscle function, and passive movements, which are used to determine the nature of the resistance at end range (i.e., flexion, abduction, etc.). See *Osteokinematic*.

Clinical Compartment: Within the Australian approach, this compartment contains information that is obtained during the course of the examination from direct interaction with the patient. It is imperative that during the course of the examination and reexamination process the therapist disallows the theoretical compartment from obstructing the search for clinical facts.

Clinical Guideline Index: A commonly used in classification system for spinal disorders, attempts to guide intervention that flows from the assigned diagnostic classification. The popular systems of McKenzie and Delitto are of this type.

Clinical Instability: Relative to the spine, a significant decrease in the capacity of the stabilizing system of the spine to maintain the intervertebral neutral zones within physiologic limits, which results in pain and disability.

Clinical Prediction Rule (CPR): A logistic regression analysis is used to identify findings from the historical and physical examination that could serve as predictors for a successful outcome in response to a specific intervention.

Clinician-Generated Forces: Manual techniques that involve assisting the patient with movement from midrange to end range with therapist overpressure.

Clonus: A repeated unidirectional joint movement caused by an involuntary muscle contraction of the agonist. This is assessed by a quick agonist stretch.

Closed Chain: Exercises with the distal end fixed.

Close-Packed Position: Also known as non-resting position. The articular surfaces of joints are incongruous except in this one special position of joint congruency. The position in which the least degree of mobility between articular surfaces is available.

Closing Restriction: A spinal classification syndrome where symptoms and/or limited motion is identified with movement toward the painful side or in the direction that produces approximation of the spinal facet joints and intervertebral foramen.

Collagen: The fiber best suited to resist tensile forces, in contrast to elastin and reticulin, which both have more resiliency and elasticity. Collagen is an adaptable material that can be as rigid as bone or as pliable as the integument. Recent evidence has identified as many as 12 different types of collagen.

Colle's Fracture: Fracture of the wrist that may present with a dorsal displacement of the distal radius, known as a "dinner fork deformity," secondary to falling on a hand with the wrist in extension.

Combination of Isotonics (COI): Facilitates the ability to perform controlled and purposeful movements and enhances mobility of joint and soft tissues. COI identifies the patient's capacity to transition between the three types of isotonic contractions.

Combined Accessory Movements: Manual techniques that involve two or more accessory movements (i.e., unilateral posteroanterior pressure produces a combination of PA glide and rotation).

Combined Movement Testing: Includes a combination of both accessory and physiologic movement. These tests may be used when neither physiologic movement testing (osteokinematic movements) nor accessory movement testing (arthrokinematic movements) reproduces the patient's symptoms individually.

Combined Physiologic Movements: Manual techniques that involve two or more physiologic movements (i.e., passive movement of the patient into combined lumbar right side bending and rotation).

Combined Physiologic with Accessory Movements: Manual techniques that involve the use of physiologic movements combined with accessory movements (i.e., cervical spine is passively moved into rotation while the therapist applies a unilateral posteroanterior glide).

Comfort Zone (CZ): As the position of comfort is attained, a reduction in tenderness as the manual physical therapist identifies a palpable reduction in the tone of the tender point.

Comorbidities: Conditions that accompany the primary condition for which the individual is seeking care. Symptoms from these other conditions may confound the results of the examination and impact patient outcome and prognosis.

Comparable Sign: A combination of pain, stiffness, and spasm that the examiner identifies upon examination and considers to be the exact reproduction of the signs and/or symptoms with which the patient has presented.

Competent Disc: The annular wall of the intervertebral disc is intact. In such cases, the derangement is considered to be reducible and lasting changes are often achieved.

Component: Are one type of accessory movement that takes place within a joint to enable a particular active movement to occur. Full, pain-free motion cannot occur in a joint without a normal degree of component motion. Examination of a joint's component motion assists with detecting dysfunctions that may interfere with normal active motion (i.e., roll, glide). See *Arthrokinematic.*

Compression: Manual techniques that involve the separation of two joint surfaces perpendicular to the treatment plane of the joint.

Compression Phenomenon: When pressure is applied to the portion of the nerve root that is not covered by the dural sheath, paresthesia rather than pain is typically reported.

Compression Testing: These tests involve the use of compressive forces that are placed through the joint to assess the patient's response in an effort to identify a comparable sign that may not have been identified otherwise.

Concentric: An active shortening of a muscle group.

Conduction Tissue: One of three types of tissues according to Cyriax. This type of tissue refers to nerve, which has the capability to become excitable and conduct a nerve impulse either refferently or afferently.

Confirmation Testing: Tests used to assist in identifying the primary site of dysfunction. These tests consist of a series of specific movements. Through stabilization of joints adjacent to the suspected dysfunctional joint, these tests attempt to differentiate which joint, within a multijoint movement system, is the primary source of the comparable sign.

Construct Validity: Describes the theoretic basis for using a measurement or judgment to make a clinical inference and is typically supported by research evidence.

Contract-Relax: Techniques that use either a concentric or a maintained isotonic contraction followed by a stretch that are designed to stretch the intrinsic muscular connective tissue elements.

Contractile Tissue: One of three types of tissues according to Cyriax. This type of tissue refers to muscle that has the ability to perform a contraction and is responsible for active movement of joints.

Convex-Concave Rule (Theory): When the convex joint surface moves upon a relatively fixed concave surface, the direction of joint glide is believed to be in the opposite direction to bone displacement. When the concave joint surface moves upon the fixed convex surface, the direction of joint glide is purported to be in the same direction as the bone displacement.

Corrective Interventions: Interventions that are often the reason why patients seek care. These are the interventions that facilitate achievement of the primary objectives as established during the examination. Manipulation to reduce restrictions, exercise to improve strength and endurance, and transverse friction massage to eliminate adhesions are all included within this domain.

Cortical Bone: Also known as compact bone.

Counterpressure: Manual application of external force for the purpose of eliminating or reducing motion at a particular joint during active motion that involves multiple joints. This may be used to assess the impact of reduced motion at a joint on an individual's chief complaint or to reduce the presence of an aberrant movement pattern that is observed during active movement. If the chief complaint is reduced, this technique may become the intervention.

Coupled Movements: Motions that are mechanically forced to occur together.

Cover Position: A patient position used by the therapist to perform a mobilization. For example, place the patient's right hand on the left shoulder and apply resistance through the elbow into the upper extremity extension-adduction pattern.

Coxa Valga: An angle of inclination that is greater than 125 degrees in an adult.

Coxa Vara: An angle of inclination that is less than 125 degrees in an adult.

Cranial Osteopathy: Founded by William Garner Sutherland. Current practitioners of craniosacral technique claim they can detect and treat cranial rhythm dysfunction through gentle touch.

Cranioverteberal Centric Relation: The three-dimensional articular ligamentous position of the cranium over the upper cervical spine, where the condyles of the occiput adopt a stable position over the atlas, which maintains a stable anteroposterior and lateral position with the odontoid process and a horizontal alignment over the shoulders of the axis.

Criterion-Referenced Validity: The comparison of the test result to some outside reference.

Cubitus Valgus: A carrying angle of the elbow that is greater than 15 degrees.

Cubitus Varus: A carrying angle of the elbow that is less than 5 to 10 degrees.

Cytokines: Effector neuropeptide molecules produced by many cells, including monocytes/macrophages and lymphocytes, in response to injury.

D

Deep Friction Massage (DFM): Soft tissue techniques in which the therapist's fingers and the patient's skin must move simultaneously to avoid injury to skin. DFM must be given perpendicular to the tissue fiber.

de Kleyn Test: An occlusive test for the neurovascular system of the neck and head. The full test is to position the neck in rotation and extension with the head overlying the edge of the plinth. A minimized de Kleyn (MdeK) consists of maintaining the same position on the bed, and a progressive minimized de Kleyn (PMdeK) consists of arriving at the minimized de Kleyn in stages, taking care that each stage is either symptom free or any symptoms that are provoked are investigated and cleared before progressing on to the next, more aggressive, position. Generally, the positive response for this test is dizziness, but it is rarely a true positive for vertebral basilar insufficiency (VBI).

Dendritic Zone: The term used to refer to the receptor membrane of a neuron.

Derangement Syndrome: The pathoanatomical model for the presence of a derangement that is an internal displacement of the intervertebral disc, which affects the normal resting position of the joint surfaces. Displacement of intradiscal material is presumed to obstruct normal segmental spinal motion to varying degrees. Derangements typically develop as a result of sustained or repetitive loading (often into flexion and/or rotation), chronic postural stresses (often into flexion and/or rotation), or trauma.

Dharana (Dhahruh-nah): Concentration used in yoga.

Dhyana (dhy·ān·a): Meditation used in yoga that is described as a conscious mental process that induces a set of integrated physiologic changes.

Diagnostic Accuracy: Determined by comparing the finding in question (usually a positive or negative clinical test result) to some gold standard, or criterion reference, that is an accepted indicator of the diagnosis in question.

Differential Diagnostic Examination: One of two primary types of objective examination within the Canadian approach to OMPT. It is designed to reach a definitive diagnosis, including identification of pathological conditions that are outside the purview of physical therapy.

Differentiation Testing: Tests that are designed to determine the source of the patient's symptoms by distinguishing between two or more potentially involved joints or structures. These tests are performed by facilitating active or passive movements simultaneously across at least two adjacent joints while attempting to reproduce symptoms.

Direct Oscillations: Performed through the treatment hand directly into the restriction. Although the technique is considered to be direct, the force is produced through the body and is simply transmitted through the hand. This technique is similar to a grade III or IV joint mobilization, and the patient's body should move along with the oscillation.

Direct Method: A method of determining restrictions in joint gliding that is employed by the clinician performing passive translatory glides in all directions. During performance of these procedures, the therapist ascertains the relationship between tissue resistance and the patient's report of pain, as well as the quality of resistance at end range, or end-feel, in each direction.

Direct Techniques: A setup that engages the somatic dysfunction barrier and an applies an activating force that moves through the barrier to reestablish motion. Manual interventions that involve the use of force that is applied in the same direction as the restriction (i.e., force that moves into the restriction).

Direction Susceptible to Movement (DSM): The path in which motion is least restricted. The DSM leads to musculoskeletal impairment through cumulative trauma of associated structures. Over time the DSM will produce wear in a characteristic pattern through repeated movement around an altered center of rotation.

Directional Preference: The term given to the direction of movement that causes the symptoms to centralize. This movement, or positional bias, gives the practitioner and patient a powerful tool that may be used to positively affect symptom behavior and guide intervention.

Disinhibition: Following a cerebrovascular accident (CVA), higher centers fail to check and "inhibit" muscle tone resulting in hypertonicity. This process forms the basis for the typical spastic synergic pattern present in individuals with hemiplegia.

Distraction: Manual techniques that involve the separation of two joint surfaces perpendicular and away from the treatment plane of the joint. Distraction may be used to unweight the joint, stretch the joint capsule, and reduce a dislocation.

Diurnal Change: The normal cycle of disc hydration.

Dominant Sign: A reproducible physical examination finding that relates to the patient's reported chief complaint.

Downglide: Used to refer to segmental spinal motion that is in a backward and downward direction.

Drop-Wrist Deformity: A condition in which not only wrist and hand extension is limited, but wrist and hand flexion may be limited as well.

Dupuytren's Contracture: Involves the atraumatic formation of nodules, primarily at digits 3 to 5, which impacts hand function.

Dysfunction: A state of altered mechanics manifesting itself as either an increase (hypermobility) or decrease (hypomobility) in the expected amount of motion, or as aberrant motion (i.e., poor motion quality).

Dysfunction Syndrome: The result of periarticular soft tissues surrounding one or more of their spinal segments are contracted, adhered, or adaptively shortened. Movement or prolonged positioning becomes painful when restricted soft tissues are brought to the end of their available motion. Pain with movement may lead to the avoidance of end-range positions, which results in greater restrictions and a more profound loss of movement. May result as a secondary complication of lumbar surgery, sciatica, trauma, or disc derangement, typically emerging at a minimum of 6 weeks following the insulting event. Accounts for 4% and 19% of patients with mechanical low back pain.

E

Eccentric: A controlled active lengthening of a muscle group.

Effect Size: Provides a ratio value that indicates how much of a difference, in terms of standard deviations, is present between groups.

Efferent Pathways: Neural pathways that direct primarily motor information away from the spinal cord.

Elastin: Found in the skin, tendons, lungs, and the linings of arteries. It is found in varying degrees within ligaments, most predominantly in the ligamentum nuchae, ligamentum flavum, and intervertebral discs.

Elbow Flexion Test (EFT): Performed through application of a slow and progressively applied vertical force through the forearms to assess the neuromuscular and motor control response to forearm loading.

Empty End-feel: Occurs in response to significant pain or spasm.

End-Feel: The quality of resistance at end range of a joint or soft tissue structure.

Endomysium: Loose connective tissue that encompasses each muscle fiber.

Endoneurium: With its longitudinally arranged collagen fibers, this is the membrane associated with the neural tube and maintains positive pressure around the neuron.

Epimysium: Surrounds the muscle and has additional fibers that connect to surrounding structures.

Epineurium: The outermost connective tissue of the fascicles. Collagen bundles are arranged longitudinally. External epineurium provides a definitive sheath among the fascicles. Internal epineurium helps keep the fascicles apart and assists gliding between fascicles, a necessary adjunct to movement, especially when the nerve must move about a joint.

Essentialist View: Ascribes to the belief that disease exists fully formed and is waiting to be identified.

Evidence-Based Practice (EBP): Using the best available research evidence interfaced with the patient's unique values and circumstances and the clinician's expertise to make clinical decisions.

Exaggeration Method: An exaggerated indirect method wherein the setup moves in the direction of freedom, past the balance point, to the normal physiologic barrier opposite the motion loss barrier. At this point, an activating force is applied.

Extended Rotated Side-Bent (ERS): A spinal segment that demonstrates a positional diagnosis in which it is extended, rotated, and side-bent relative to the next adjacent segment. Rotation and side bending are presumed to occur ipsilaterally. These positional disorders are believed to occur within one to three segments.

Extension Dysfunction Syndrome: Symptoms are produced at the end range of extension and abate as the patient moves away from this position.

Extension in Lying (EIL): Patient-generated exercises that involve extension in a prone lying position, often performed in a repetitive fashion in a range and fashion that is tolerated by the patient.

Extension in Standing (EIS): Patient-generated exercises that involve extension in a standing position, often performed in a repetitive fashion in a range and fashion that is tolerated by the patient.

Extension Principle: A series of specific exercises that involvement movement of the spine into extension.

Extension Sitting Test: Conducted on a table with the patient facing the therapist and feet suspended using a mobilization belt between the therapist's pelvis and patient's spine. The therapist segmentally moves the belt cephalad to maximize the anterior translation of each individual vertebra. While sustaining anterior pressure through the strap, increased neural tension is elicited through knee extension, dorsiflexion, and neck flexion/extension.

Extensor Lag: The inability to achieve full knee extension actively despite the fact that full passive range may be observed.

External Torsion: Movement of a rib along its long axis, resulting in palpable prominence at the superior border of the rib angle and the inferior border of the sternal end.

External Tibial Torsion: Sometimes referred to as rotation increases; the Q-angle by moving the tibial tuberosity laterally.

External Validity: Describes the generalizability of the findings, or to whom the results of a study may be applied.

Exteroceptors: Include those receptors affected by changes in the external environment.

Extra-articular Hypomobility: This type of motion restriction typically due to inextensibility of muscle secondary to scarring or adhesions or due to an increase in muscle tone. Extra-articular hypomobility results in a restriction during PPIVM testing without a decrease noted during PAIVM testing.

Extracellular Matrix (ECM): Consists primarily of fibers (elastin and collagen), proteoglycans (PGs), and glycoproteins.

Extrasegmentally: Referring of pain into more than one dermatomal distribution.

F

Facet-Opposition Locking: Procedures that involve the placement of facet joint surfaces in a maximally opposed position and are said to be in maximal apposition. They are used to reduce the amount of mobility available at regions adjacent to the target articulation for the purpose of localizing manual forces. Often used in the spine, these procedures involve movement of adjacent joints into a position that produces apposition of articular surfaces (i.e., cervical facet opposition locking technique).

Facilitated Spinal Segment: Central nervous system becomes overloaded with sensory input and becomes unable to selectively differentiate the specific origin of each individual stimulus, which leads to a misinterpretation of afferent information.

Fascia: More organized and has a greater amount of collagen than does loose connective tissue. Macroscopically, there are two distinct fascial systems.

Fascial Fulcrum Concept: By introducing stress in specific patterns, we can introduce forces down to the level of the cell and affect its functional capacity, thus moving us beyond a pathomechanical model to a pathophysiological/pathochemical model.

Fascicles: Bundles of muscle fibers.

Feiss Line: A line drawn between the medial malleolus, navicular tubercle, and medial aspect of the first metatarsal head. A navicular that falls below or above this line is suggestive of a pes planus and pes cavus foot type, respectively.

Femoral Anteversion: Anterior rotation of the femur in the transverse plane.

Femoral Retroversion: A femur with less than 15 degrees of anterior rotation in the transverse plane.

Fibronectin: A network-forming glycoprotein that functions to allow for intracellular and extracellular communication in order to achieve homeostasis.

Fibrosis: The laying down of fibrous tissue, normally considered pathological. Fibrosis, however, occurs as part of the normal wound-healing process. Fibrosis follows a similar pathway to normal wound healing except there is a chronic progression of the fibrotic process characterized by continuous insult or stimulus that is either chemical or mechanical in nature.

Fick Angle: Defines the position of the foot relative to the sagittal plane with 12 to 18 degrees of toeing out, or abduction, considered to be normal.

Finger-Flexed Position: A hand position for manual interventions which maintains the metacarpophalangeal and interphalangeal joints in a slight degree of flexion.

Finger Gliding: One finger along the skin normally reveals that the finger glides easily, creating a wave of skin in front of it. Dysfunctional tissues will cause a slowing down of the finger glide or resistance.

Firm End-Feel: The result of capsular or ligamentous stretching.

First Stop: Where marked resistance is felt toward the end of the Grade II motion.

Flat Back Posture: A reduction in their thoracic kyphotic curve with scapular medial winging

Flat Palpation: Consists of placing finger or thumb pressure perpendicular to the muscle fibers while compressing them against underlying tissue or bone.

Flexed Rotated Side-Bent (FRS): A spinal segment that demonstrates a positional diagnosis in which it is flexed, rotated, and side-bent relative to the next adjacent segment. Rotation and side bending are presumed to occur ipsilaterally. These positional disorders are believed to occur within one to three segments.

Flexion Dysfunction Syndrome: Symptoms produced at the end range of flexion that abate as the patient moves away from this position.

Foot Abduction: The presence of toeing out.

Foot Adduction: The presence of toeing in.

Force-Closure Mechanism: The method by which the SIJ derives its stability, most notably when in the horizontal position, from ligamentous support.

Forefoot Valgus: The forefoot is angled laterally relative to the rearfoot.

Forefoot Varus: The forefoot is angled medially relative to the rearfoot.

Form-Closure Mechanism: The method by which the SIJ derives its stability from superincumbent forces that force the sacrum, like a wedge, between the innominates.

Freeway Space: Open-packed position of the TMJ, which is 2 to 4 mm between the central incisors.

Full Articular Pattern: A capsular pattern that is observed within the facet joints of the spine. See *Capsular Pattern*.

Full Thickness Tear: A complete rupture of a muscle or tendon.

Functional Integration (FI): A process in which the practitioner uses his or her hands to produce gentle force vectors through the client's skeleton in a seemingly passive process. The client is asked to attend to sensory dimensions of this process and track the evolving movements using available kinesthetic and proprioceptive information.

Functional Joints: The interfaces between soft tissue structures that are separated by fascia (extracellular matrix) and lubricated by the ground substance.

Functional Movement: Active motions that occur in oblique planes and simulate the motions that individuals typically perform during normal functional tasks. They are sometimes referred to as physiologic movement.

Functional Movement Patterns (FMP): Provides a mechanism to efficiently identify mechanical, neuromuscular, and motor control dysfunctions. Based on the awareness through movement (ATM) approach and PNF diagonal patterns, FMPs include the pelvic clock, arm circles, trunk side bending, hip rotations, and shoulder girdle clocks.

Functional Palpation: Designed to identify the exact condition of the underlying joint, soft tissue, nerve, and organ during normal motions. Functional palpation uses passive, active, and resisted PNF patterns and normal functional motions to effectively examine the quantity and quality of the three dimensional motions of joints and soft tissues. Based on function, these tissues are examined during various postures and movements.

Functional Reproducing Movements: A particular movement routinely performed during daily activities that is known to reproduce symptoms.

Functional Soft Tissue Mobilization (FSTM): Seeks to identify the accessory mobility (muscle play), intrinsic tone, and functional excursion (ability of the muscle to lengthen and fold) of the myofascial structures.

Functional Squat (FS) Test: An excellent method to examine common functional movement patterns that involve the entire body. The patient stands with a normal base of support and squats as far as possible without pain while keeping the heels on the ground. During the squat, the patient's balance and sequence of motion are noted.

Functional Tests: Provide an objective measure of postural and structural integrity coupled with assessment of motor control capacity. These tests provide proprioceptive feedback that may be assessed before and after intervention.

G

Gamma Bias: In order to respond to changing demands, gamma motor neurons produce a steady resting tone within the muscle spindle.

Gamma Gain: In myofascial dysfunction, an increase in gamma bias. This process will result in changes within the extrafusal muscle fibers, namely hypertonicity and spasm.

General Resistance: Resistance applied to the cervical spine and chin to facilitate the short neck flexors during axial elongation.

Genu Recurvatum: An impairment of the knee in which the knee is in a position of increased hyperextension suggesting quadriceps or ankle dorsiflexor weakness, posterior capsular laxity, deficiency of the anterior cruciate ligament, or systemic conditions that produce joint laxity.

Genu Valgum: The normal degree of knee valgum that is present in a weight-bearing position. This is 5 to 6 degrees.

Genu Varum: The normal degree of knee varum that is present in a weight-bearing position that is greatest prior to 18 months of age.

Glide(ing): Occurs when joint surfaces are congruent and is defined as a single point on one joint surface repeatedly contacting new points on the other joint surface. A passive accessory movement in which force is elicited in a direction that is parallel to the treatment plane.

Global Stabilizing System: The superficial muscles of the spine that are best adapted to produce spinal motion.

Glycosaminoglycans (GAGs): Negatively charged molecules that create an osmotic imbalance resulting in the absorption of water that hydrates the matrix. There are six major GAGs, of which chondroitin sulfate 4 and 6 and hyaluronic acid (HA) are the most widely recognized.

Gold Standard: Criterion reference that is an accepted indicator of the diagnosis in question.

Golgi Tendon Organ: Mechanoreceptors found within tendons that respond to length changes in a muscle resulting from passive stretching or active muscle contraction. When facilitated, the GTO provides relaxation in the muscle to which it is associated.

Grade I: A mobilization that consists of small amplitude movement near the beginning of range and short of tissue resistance (R1).

Grade II: A mobilization that consists of large amplitude movement that goes well into the range, occupying any part of the range that is free of stiffness or muscle spasm and short of tissue resistance (R1).

Grade III: A mobilization that consists of large amplitude movement that moves into stiffness or muscle spasm. It consists of a large amplitude that occurs at approximately 50%, or halfway, between R1 and R2.

Grade III– – – and Grade IV– –: Mobilizations that occur at the onset of R1.

Grades III– and Grade IV–: Mobilizations that occur at approximately 25% between R1 and R2.

Grade III+ and Grade IV+: Mobilizations that occur at approximately 75% between R1 and R2.

Grade III++ and Grade IV++: Mobilizations that occur at R2.

Grade IV: A mobilization that consists of small amplitude movement moving into stiffness or muscle spasm. It occurs at 50% between R1 and R2.

Grade I-Grade II Traction-Mobilizations, within Slack: Short-term effects that are effective in controlling pain and promoting muscle relaxation. These techniques may impact range of motion through the introduction of low-level movement that serves to alter joint inflammation and reduce pain. These techniques are applied through the slow distraction of joint surfaces in the resting or actual resting position.

Grade III Stretch-Traction Mobilization: Techniques believed to alter positional relationships, which may have an impact on the presenting neurological symptoms. These techniques seek to improve motion in directions that are both parallel (joint glide) as well as perpendicular (joint distraction) to the treatment plane.

Grade III Stretch Mobilizations: Are effective in restoring joint play when hypomobility is associated with an abnormal end-feel that relates to the patient's symptoms.

Grade III Stretch-Glide Mobilizations: Attempt to introduce translator motions to the joint that are parallel to the joint's treatment plane while disallowing the rolling component that is associated with normal motion.

Ground Substance: The environment in which all connective tissue components exist.

Group V: Also known as a high-velocity thrust mobilization, is of small amplitude and high velocity that occurs at the end of available range of movement.

Group 1: Pain-Dominant Behavior Diagnostic Classification Grouping: Present when pain is the primary origin of the movement disorder.

Group 2: Stiffness-Dominant Behavior Diagnostic Classification Grouping: Present when joint restrictions are the primary origin of the movement disorder.

Group 3a and 3b: Pain and Stiffness Combined Behavior Diagnostic Classification Grouping: More common than other groupings and is present when both pain and stiffness are contributing to the movement disorder, with (a) denoting pain as the primary limitation and (b) denoting stiffness as the primary limitation.

Group 4: Momentary Pain Behavior Diagnostic Classification Grouping: No loss of joint range, but intermittent pain associated with certain movements. Most Group 4 patients do not seek intervention because their symptoms are not significant enough to impact their normal level of function.

H

Haglund's Deformity: A bony exostosis located at the posterior aspect of the calcaneus as a result of shear-type forces as the foot rapidly pronates when going from heel strike to mid-stance and from excessive tensile forces at the insertion of the Achilles tendon.

Hallux Abductovalgus (HAV): Deformity of the first metatar-sophalangeal joint of the foot, which results in medial migra-tion of the first metatarsal and lateral migration of the first proximal phalanx often in response to altered biomechanics.

Hallux Limitus: A decrease in first MTP extension.

Hallux Rigidus: A decrease in first MTP extension that is structural or nonreducible.

Hard Disc Lesion: A fissure beginning at the innermost por-tion of the annulus that develops with gradual extrusion of nuclear material along the path of the fissure. An annular disc lesion is believed to occur instantaneously.

Hard End-Feel: Experienced during elbow extension when there is normally occurring bone-to-bone contact.

Headache Sustained Natural Apophyseal Glides (SNAGs): Performed In a nonoscillatory, sustained fashion. Identical positioning and handling as described for cervical NAGs is adopted, however, the spinous process of C2 is contacted. A minimal degree of force is applied in a posteroanterior direction and sustained for a minimum of 10 seconds.

Heberden's Nodes: DIP joint deformity resulting from osteoarthritis.

Hemarthrosis: A joint impairment that involves inflammation related to bloody exudate within the joint that occurs within minutes following insult. The joint is typically hot to the touch with a significant degree of pain present.

High Reactivity: Characterized by pain that occurs prior to end range. The type of manual technique, grade of technique, sequencing of techniques, and decisions regarding the use of other procedures will all be governed by the patient's ob-served level of reactivity. The patient's level of reactivity may change on a daily basis, thus requiring intervention to be adjusted accordingly. Usually pain is above 6 with onset that occurs prior to tissue resistance.

High-Velocity Thrust: See *Thrust.*

High-Velocity Low-Amplitude (HVLA) Thrust: See *Thrust.*

Hold-Relax: Techniques that use an isometric contraction fol-lowed by a stretch that are designed to stretch the intrinsic muscular connective tissue elements.

Homans Sign: Used to identify the presence of a deep vein thrombosis, this test involves passive dorsiflexion of the ankle that produces intense calf pain.

Hypermobility: An increase in accessory or physiologic range of motion that is beyond the joint's normal range. If patho-logic, the joint is defined as possessing instability.

Hyperemia Test: Involves placing the extremity in a 45-degree straight leg raised position for 3 minutes and counting the time for venous return. Longer than 20 seconds suggests the presence of peripheral vascular disease.

Hypomobility: A decrease in accessory or physiologic range of motion.

I

Identification Phase: Phase of treatment progression within the FM approach that includes discovering three-dimensional joint or soft tissue dysfunction in static and dynamic pos-tures and movements.

Iliosacral Anterior Rotation: Defined as movement of the ASIS anteriorly and caudally, with simultaneous movement of the PSIS anteriorly and cranially. This motion is mechan-ically coupled with hip extension.

Iliosacral Downslip: Defined as a caudal migration of both the ASIS and the PSIS.

Iliosacral Inflare: Iliosacral motion in the transverse plane that is defined by movement of the ASIS medially, that accom-panies hip internal rotation.

Iliosacral (IS) Motion: Movement of the ilium on a relatively fixed sacrum.

Iliosacral Outflare: Iliosacral motion in the transverse plane that is defined by movement of the ASIS laterally, which ac-companies hip external rotation.

Iliosacral Posterior Rotation: Defined as movement of the ASIS posteriorly and cranially and movement of the PSIS posteriorly and caudally. Posterior rotation is mechanically coupled with hip flexion.

Iliosacral Upslip: Defined as a cranial migration of both the ASIS and the PSIS.

Immediate Stage: In reference to healing, this stage represents the first few minutes following the onset of the condition. During this phase, appropriate action could be taken to provide immediate correction of the condition or lessen its effects.

Impact Test: This test identifies aggravating activities or move-ment patterns that inhibit central and peripheral muscles. These findings assist the therapist in training the patient in more efficient body mechanics.

Incompetent Disc: An intervertebral disc in which the annular wall is compromised. Symptoms may appear to be central-ized in non-weight-bearing but do not remain centralized in standing. In such cases, a derangement is deemed as *irreducible.*

Indirect Method: A method of determining restrictions in joint glide predicated upon the convex-concave rule. As deficits are noted in an individual's physiologic movement, deficits in joint gliding are deduced. See *Convex-Concave Rule.*

Indirect Technique: The setup requires moving away from the barrier to a specific site (balance point) where various phys-iologic or inherent mechanisms cause the somatic dysfunc-tion barrier to dissipate.

Indirect Technique: Manual interventions that involve the use of force that is applied in the opposite direction of the restriction (i.e., force that moves away from the restriction). These are appropriate when direct techniques produce pain or are ineffective.

Inert Tissue: One of three types of tissues according to Cyriax. This type of tissue refers to noncontractile tissues such as ligaments. These tissues are mainly affected by passive movement and ligament stress testing. The most provocative tests for these tissues are passive movements, with concentration on end-feel and reproduction of pain.

Inherent Forces: Body's tendency toward balance and homeostasis.

Initial Evaluation: Evaluation made at the time of the first visit and designed to relate examination findings to symptom behavior while identifying the stage and irritability of the disorder.

Initial Working Hypothesis (H1): The provisional diagnosis that is subject to change as the hypothesis is tested against new information generated by the subjective and objective examination.

Injuring Movements: Movements that require the patient to actually reenact, if possible, the initial mechanism that led to their current symptoms in cases where symptoms can not otherwise be reproduced.

Instability: Defined as an increase in the range of the neutral zone of the joint. The neutral zone is the area within a range of motion in which there is no resistance to that motion. The presence of motion where no appreciable motion should exist.

Instantaneous Center of Rotation: The axis around which segments move throughout their path.

Internal Torsion: Movement of a rib along its long axis, resulting sharper inferior border palpated posteriorly and a sharper superior border palpated anteriorly.

Internal Tibial Torsion: Sometimes referred to as rotation decreases the Q-angle by moving the tibial tuberosity medially.

Interoceptors: Nerve receptors that are sensitive to changes within visceral tissues and blood vessels.

Intervention to Intervention Evaluation: Seeks to determine intervention effectiveness related to specific techniques during the course of the patient's care.

Intraclass Correlation Coefficient (ICC): Used for continuous measures such as degrees of motion or pain intensity.

Intrinsic Minus Hand: A condition that results in a loss of the hand arches, atrophy of the hand intrinsics, and unchecked extrinsic muscle activity causing in the classic claw hand deformity.

Involuntary Muscle Guarding: A form of guarding in which individuals will display a reduction in the degree of guarding when the joint is supported. This form of guarding may be the result of injury to the muscle or it may be occurring in response to underlying joint dysfunction.

Initial Evaluation: See *Initial Examination*.

Initial Examination: Performed at the time of the first visit and designed to relate examination findings to symptom behavior while identifying the stage and irritability of the disorder.

Internal Derangement: Refers to peripheral joint lesions, such as loose bodies or subluxed bones, which will cause a loss of motion in a partial articular pattern.

Internal Validity: Describes the degree to which the observed changes in the dependent variable (outcome of interest) are caused by the independent variable (the treatment).

Intervention to Intervention Evaluation: Seeks to determine intervention effectiveness related to specific techniques during the course of the patient's care.

Isometric Contraction: Characterized by a state in which the external force is equal to the internal force, thus preventing external movement. PNF defines an isometric contraction by the patient's intention to maintain a consistent position in space.

Irritability: One aspect of the S.I.N.S. process of examination. It is determined by the amount of activity required to produce and increase symptoms, the magnitude of symptoms, and the amount of time it takes for symptoms to return to a baseline.

Isometric without Locking: Manual techniques that involve using specifically localized isometric muscle contractions to mobilize joints. See *Muscle Energy Techniques (MET)*.

Isotonic Contraction: Characterized by a state in which motion occurs when the internal force of the contraction overcomes the external force. PNF defines it as a contraction in which the intention is to move.

Isotonic Reversals: One type of antagonist reversal that uses isotonic contractions performed on alternate sides of a joint for the purpose of restoring muscular reciprocation.

Iyengar: A form of yoga that uses poses held for longer durations, with attention to specific performance. Iyengar is one of the most popular styles of hatha in the West and uses props to accommodate the special needs of the practitioner.

J

Jendrassik Maneuver: During DTR testing, a maneuver in which the patient clenches the teeth, flexes both sets of fingers into a hook-like form, and interlocks fingers. The tendon is then hit with a reflex hammer to elicit the reflex. The elicited response is compared with the reflex result of the same action when the maneuver is not in use. A larger reflex response will often be observed when the patient is occupied with the maneuver.

Joint Play: Is considered to be one type of accessory movement that is not under voluntary control. These movements occur only in response to external forces that take place at the terminal range of normal joints. A movement that is not under voluntary control yet is essential to the painless performance of active movement.

Judgment: Made by an examiner who rates the quality of one or more patient characteristics, such as passive mobility of a joint.

Jump Sign: A quick twitch of muscle activity that is often used to confirm the presence of a tender point.

K

Kappa Coefficient (K): Useful for categorical data such as a positive versus negative test result.

Kinematics: The study of motion that does not account for the forces responsible for producing or influencing that motion.

Kinetics: The study of movement in relation to forces that are acting upon it.

Kundalini Yoga (KY): Includes a vast array of meditation techniques. Elements of the KY protocol may have applications for psycho-oncology patients.

Kypholordotic Posture: Involves an increased thoracic kyphosis with rounded shoulders and forward head.

Kyphosis: Posterior convexity of the spine in the sagittal plane that occurs in the thoracic spine.

L

Lancinating Pain: Short, sharp flash of pain that is intense and electrical in nature, which runs along the involved dermatome and is narrow banded, spanning only an inch or two in width. Such pain would be described as intolerable if it lasted more than a brief moment. This type of pain is typical of true nerve root pain.

Latent Myofascial Trigger Points (MTrPs): Trigger points that produce pain only when stimulated.

Lateral Shift: Defined as a frontal plane postural deviation in which the upper trunk is displaced laterally relative to the lower trunk and the upper trunk is unable to move past the midline. This postural deviation is nonstructural and is caused by pressure on a nerve root from a disc herniation or other space-occupying lesion. The lateral shift is named by the direction in which the upper torso is displaced. It is also known as an acute lumbosacral or sciatic scoliosis.

Laterally Displaced Derangement: A displacement of the disc in a lateral direction (i.e., posterolateral) that does not respond to sagittal plane motions. Repeated movement testing with a lateral bias is required, such as extension in lying position with the hips displaced laterally to one side, then the other, or side gliding in the standing position.

Law of the Artery: A law that states that the body is a unit; structure and function are reciprocally interrelated; and the body possesses self-regulatory mechanisms for rational therapies based on an understanding of body unity, self-regulatory mechanisms, and the interrelation of structure and function.

Law of the Nerve: A law that states that a vertebra may become subluxed; that this subluxation tends to impinge other structures (nerves, blood vessels, and lymphatics passing through the intervertebral foramen); that, as a result of impingement, the function of the corresponding segment of the spinal cord and its connecting spinal and automatic nerves are interfered with and the function of the nerve impulse impaired; that, as a result thereof, the innervation to certain parts of the organism is abnormally altered and such parts become functionally or organically diseased or predisposed; and that adjustment of a subluxed vertebra removes the impingement of the structure passing through the intervertebral foramen, thereby restoring to diseased parts their normal innervation and rehabilitating them functionally and organically.

Lazy Cobra: A patient position that involves placement of his or her hand behind the neck to assist with diagonal cervical flexion and extension.

Left Oblique Axis (LOA): A triplanar axis around which SIJ motion is believed to occur that courses from the right inferior lateral angle through the left SIJ.

Leg Dominance: Jumping activities that involve asymmetrical landing that places more weight on one leg than the other.

Leg Swing Mobility Test: In which the patient swings the leg from flexion to extension, and the therapist palpates the posterior superior iliac spine and anterior superior iliac spine. If there is an abrupt stop, the restriction correlates to the direction in which hip motion is limited.

Lengthening: Soft tissue mobilization technique that is usually performed along the direction of the restriction.

Ligament Dominance: Jumping activities that involve landing in valgus.

Ligamentous Instability: Results from rupture or laxity of the ligamentous support system, which is typically detected during the differential diagnostic examination.

Ligamentous-Tension Locking: A soft tissue method of restricting motion across a particular spinal segment. These techniques are predicated upon the concept that when motion is introduced within a spinal segment, movement of that same segment in all other directions will be limited. They are used to reduce the amount of mobility available at regions adjacent to the target articulation for the purpose of localizing manual forces. Often used in the spine, these procedures involve movement of adjacent joints into a position that engages the ligaments and therefore reduces undesired motion (i.e., lumbar ligamentous tension locking technique).

Likelihood Ratio (LR): Describes the likelihood that a patient who has the condition of interest would have a certain test result divided by the likelihood that a patient who does not have the condition of interest would have the same test result.

Local Stabilizing System: The deep muscles of the spine designed to provide spinal stability in the neutral zone.

Local Twitch Response (LTR): A spinal cord reflex, leading to involuntary sudden contractions of muscle fibers within a taut band.

Localization Phase: Phase of treatment progression within the FM approach, which includes determining the exact depth and direction of the barrier's hardest end-feel, accompanied by passive or active movements of the specific body part.

Lordosis: A sagittal plane spinal curvature with anterior convexity that is present in the lumbar and cervical spine.

Low-Velocity, Moderate-Amplitude (LVMA): See *Mobilization (nonthrust)*.

Low Reactivity: Indicated when there is no pain at end range or when pain occurs with overpressure only. The type of manual technique, grade of technique, sequencing of techniques, and decisions regarding the use of other procedures will all be governed by the patient's observed level of reactivity. The patient's level of reactivity may change on a daily basis, thus requiring intervention to be adjusted accordingly.

Usually consists of pain that is less than 3 on a scale of 1 to 10 or onset of pain at or after end range has been achieved.

Lower Motor Neuron: Consists of a cell body located in the anterior gray column of the spinal cord or brain stem and an axon passing via the peripheral nerves to the motor end plate within the muscle.

Lumbar Protective Mechanism (LPM): Refers to the trunk's ability to automatically stabilize against external force in the efficient state. To perform this test, the patient is positioned against a stable surface with the trunk unsupported or in a stride stance. A slow and progressive force is applied to the shoulders in anteroposterior and posteroanterior diagonal directions to reveal the patient's stabilizing response.

Lumbarization: Movement that exists between the first and second sacral vertebrae.

Lumbopelvic Rhythm: Interaction between the lumbar spine and pelvic girdle during FB and when returning from FB.

M

Maintained Contraction: Refers to a dynamic contraction in which the patient's intention to produce movement is limited by a greater external force.

Mallet Finger: A rupture of the extensor tendon at its insertion into the distal phalanx, may occur at any digit and is easily identified by observing the DIP resting in a flexed position.

Manipulation: The skilled passive movement to a joint. An accurately localized, single, quick, and decisive movement of small amplitude following careful positioning of the patient. This term is used synonymously with mobilization to define therapeutic maneuvers that are directed toward restoring accessory motion to a joint. They may take the form of distraction techniques, nonthrust techniques, or thrust techniques. See *Thrust.*

Manipulation Movements: See *Manipulation.*

Manual Muscle Testing (MMT): Involves the use of carefully delivered manual resistance for the purpose of ascertaining the ability of muscles to actively contract. MMT is routinely used during examination and reexamination for the purpose of guiding resistance training, determining progress and outcomes, and to assist in differential diagnosis and prognosis.

Mass Flexion Pattern: Initiated with pelvic anterior/elevation progressing to lower extremity flexion/adduction, scapular anterior depression, followed by upper extremity extension/adduction.

McGregor's Plane: A line drawn on radiographs from the inferior border of the occiput to the hard palate.

Measurement: Requires some form of tool and generates a quantity such as length (such as centimeters) from a tape measure, degrees from a goniometer, or a percentage score from a questionnaire.

Mechanical: A condition that is impacted by movement or position. Once determined, such conditions are often amenable to physical therapy management.

Mechanical Dysfunction: According to Cyriax, a term that is often used to define a lesion of the spine that will present as a loss of motion in a partial articular pattern.

Mechanical Effects: The impact that manual interventions may have upon the structures that contribute to a physiologic restriction to further motion that may or may not be associated with pain. Capsular restrictions, adhesions, fibrosis, and scarring may all pose an actual limitation to normal mobility toward which joint mobilization may be directed. One mechanism under which joint mobilization is believed to be effective is by stretching, breaking, or increasing the extensibility of joint restrictions. These restrictions are reduced through techniques that engage the joint barrier (Grades III-V).

Mechanical Locking: Typically, the result of a loose body or degeneration of joint surfaces. Patients typically present relatively pain-free, but with restricted motion that is sudden in onset. Intervention techniques include thrust manipulation, which is often in the direction of the restriction to release the mechanical block, much like closing a stuck drawer in order to release it.

Medial/Lateral Rotations: Determined by the inferior pole of the patella about an anterior-posterior axis.

Medial Longitudinal Arch (MLA): An arch of the foot that spans from medial to lateral and can be assessed using the Feiss Line.

Medicine Training Therapy (MTT): An approach that uses belts, stabilization benches, and pulley weights to stabilize spinal segments. In this approach, neighboring segments above and below the lesion are "locked out," while manual resistance and TE is used to stabilize hypermobile or hypomobile spinal segments.

Mesentery: A thin sheet of connective tissue with mesothelial surfaces that conduct blood and lymph vessels and nerves to other structures.

Mesoneurium: A loose areolar tissue that surrounds peripheral nerve trunks and provides friction relief between the nerve and adjacent structures.

Metatarsal Break: Based on the progressive decline in the length of the metatarsals from the first to the fifth, an obliquely orientated line of TMT joint extension is created.

Mindfulness-Based Stress Reduction: A clinically valuable, self-administered intervention for cancer patients with orthopaedic-related conditions.

Minimal Detectable Change (MDC): Indicates how much change is required to be certain that a true change has occurred (i.e., beyond the error).

Mitchell (muscle energy) Model: A series of postulated sacral axes are coupled with diagnoses of sacral torsions to reflect sacral motion, or restriction, relative to the lumbar spine and the mechanics of gait.

Mixed Index: A hybrid classification system that incorporates several, or all, of the other types. The Quebec Task Force is an example of this type of system.

Mixers: Chiropractors who mixes traditional chiropractic philosophy with modern physical therapy rehabilitation techniques.

Mobilization (nonthrust): Passive movement that is performed with a rhythm and a grade in a manner in which the patient is able to prevent the technique from being performed. This term is used synonymously with manipulation to define therapeutic maneuvers that are directed toward restoring accessory motion to a joint. They often include oscillations as described by Maitland as well as stretch and progressive oscillation, combining oscillation with stretch. These techniques may be used to mechanically elongate connective tissues and to fire muscle and joint receptors.

Mobilization Belts: Serve to enhance the force-producing capabilities of the therapist when mobilizing larger joints. These belts should be at least 3 to 6 inches in width and 72 inches in length to ensure a larger surface area for greater patient comfort.

Mobilization Foam: A 5- by 7-inch piece of medium-density foam 3/4- to 1-inch thick, which is extremely important for improving the comfort of mobilization that is performed over bony prominences or already tender areas and serves to enhance contact and disallow sliding over structures to be mobilized.

Mobilization Phase: Phase of treatment progression within the FM approach that includes maintaining pressure on the dysfunctional structure while performing passive techniques, patient active movements, and resisted patterns.

Mobilization with Movement (MWM): Active or passive physiologic movement occurs simultaneously with passive accessory mobilization.

Moderate Reactivity: Present when pain occurs simultaneous with achieving end range. The type of manual technique, grade of technique, sequencing of techniques, and decisions regarding the use of other procedures will all be governed by the patient's observed level of reactivity. The patient's level of reactivity may change on a daily basis, thus requiring intervention to be adjusted accordingly.

Monoarticular Steroid-Sensitive Arthritis: Occurs spontaneously without any signs of rheumatological involvement and is a diagnosis of exclusion. It most commonly occurs at the shoulder, elbow, hip, knee, or ankle and often resolves spontaneously over several months or years. The intervention of choice for this condition is steroid injection.

Morton's Toe: Individuals in which the second toe is the longest.

Motion Segment: The inferior half of the superior vertebra and the superior half of the inferior vertebra and all other structures between them, including muscle, nerve, disc, facet joint, and so on.

Motor Control Phase: Phase of treatment progression within the FM approach that includes using a combination of isotonics and isotonic reversal techniques to enhance local and global coordinated movement.

Motor Unit: Consists of all the muscle fibers innervated by the terminal branches of a single motor neuron.

Movement Diagnosis (MD): Segment currently restricted, which is opposite that of the positional diagnosis (PD).

Movement Diagram: Serves as a dynamic map that represents the quality and quantity of a patient's passive movement test findings. The movement diagram provides a visual depiction of the amount, behavior, and relationship between pain and range of motion.

Movement Systems Balance (MSB) Model: As espoused by Sahrmann and colleagues, is based on concepts first proposed by Kendall. The foundation of this approach includes the concept that movement imbalance results from the development of an altered path of the instantaneous center of rotation (PICR). Precise movement is the key to preventing impairment and pain results when the PICR becomes altered.

Multisegmental Motion: Gross movements of the spine.

Muscle Energy Techniques (MET): An active muscle contraction is performed for the purpose of restoring joints to a more normal positon and normal mobility. Postisometric relaxation, reciprocal inhibition, or rapid rhythmic resistive duction.

Muscle Spindle: Mechanoreceptors found within extrafusal muscle that responds to length changes in a muscle and is facilitated through performance of quick passive stretching. When facilitated, the spindle provides an increase in tension in the muscle to which it is associated.

Myelin: Composed of a lipoprotein complex arranged in many layers. The myelin sheath envelops the axon except at its ending and at periodic constrictions that are approximately 1 mm apart.

Multiaxial Movements: Bone rotational movements that occur simultaneously around more than one axis in more than one plane.

Muscle Play: Motion occurring between muscles, which highlights the ability of muscles to move freely in relationship to each other.

Muscle Spasm: Most appropriate to describe increased tone of a muscle that is of neurologic origin.

Muscle Tone Dysfunctions: Present as tight nodules or bands of sensitivity within a muscle belly.

Myofascial Pattern: Specific and characteristic patterns of motion loss that suggest restrictions that are present within myofascial structures. Their presence is an indication for the use of stretching and soft tissue mobilization techniques that are designed to improve myofascial extensibility and restore normal mobility. These patterns are often contrasted with the presence of capsular patterns for the purpose of determining the primary cause of a motion restriction.

Myofascial Trigger Points (MTrPs): Hyperirritable spots in skeletal muscle associated with a hypersensitive palpable nodule in a taut band.

Myositis Ossificans: Heterotopic bone formation.

Myotatic Reflex Arc: Also known as the stretch reflex arc, the monosynaptic reflex arc, or gamma motor neuron loop and is considered to be the basis of normal resting tone within muscle. The components of this reflex arc include the extrafusal muscle fiber, which has the ability to contract, relax, and elongate; the muscle spindle, with its intrafusal muscle fibers, which is responsive to the length and velocity of stretch; and the afferent and efferent nerves.

N

Natural Apophyseal Glides (NAGs): Techniques that do not include the combination of accessory and physiologic movement as used when performing SNAGs. Rather, they use oscillatory mobilization that is directed parallel to the treatment plane of the joint. The direction of force is critical and is dictated by the position of the therapist's mobilizing hand.

Nature: One aspect of the S.I.N.S. process of examination. It includes a consideration of the suspected pathology as well as patient characteristics such as personality, pain tolerance, and cultural components.

Nebulin: Spans the length of the actin filaments and acts as a stabilizing structure. Nebulin regulates muscle contractions by inhibiting cross-bridge formation until actin is activated by Ca2+.

Negative Predictive Value: Describes the number of true negatives/total number of negative findings. This describes the likelihood that a negative test is truly negative.

Nerve Entrapment Syndromes: Syndromes that may be caused by degenerative, postural, or myofascial restrictions. Symptoms often consist of paresthesia or pain that is nonspecific and intermittent and is affected by movement and position. The classic neurological signs may also be present, which include a change in sensation, reflexes, and myotomal strength. Intervention typically involves addressing the insulting factor, such as correcting posture or stretching tight muscle and neural mobilization.

Neural Control Subsystem: Relative to the spine, receives input from structures in the other two subsystems for the purpose of determining the requirements for stability and coordinated movement in any given task.

Neuromuscular Reeducation (NMR) (stabilization) Phase: Phase of treatment progression within the FM approach that includes using prolonged holds at the end of the newly gained range to assist in maintaining the new range and to protect the joint by stabilizing the segment.

Neuropathic Pain: Pain produced by most neurological tissues when they are damaged or seriously inflamed. It is described as lancinating or causalgic, and both are felt through the areas subserved by the injured nerve tissue.

Neurophysiologic Effects: The impact that manual interventions may have upon the neurological structures that are associated with a joint. One mechanism under which joint mobilization is believed to be effective is by stimulating joint neurological receptors that lead to reduced pain and improved mobility. These receptors are enacted through the use of all grades of mobilization (Grades I-V).

Negative Ulnar Variance: An ulna that is shorter than normal relative to the distal radius.

Neurapraxia: Defined as a segmental block of axonal conduction. The nerve can conduct an action potential above and below the blockage but not across the blockage. The conduction block is due to a physiologic process without histological change.

Neurotmesis: Like axonotmesis, involves destruction of the axons. In addition, the connective tissues are also injured. This is caused by a severe contusion, stretch, avulsion, or laceration. There are three basic types of neurotmesis.

Neutral Rotated Side-Bent (NRS): A spinal segment that demonstrates a positional diagnosis in which it is rotated and side-bent, typically in contralateral direction. These positional disorders are believed to occur within multiple segments.

Nodes of Ranvier: The manner in which myelin is arranged. The discontinuity in the myelin sheath allows rapid impulse conduction as the action potential leaps from one node to the next.

Nominalist View: A view of diagnosis, which now predominates, that does not require the cause to be known in order for intervention to be initiated.

Noncapsular Pattern: A movement pattern that does not display deficits in a characteristic pattern that is suggestive of capsular restriction. Motion deficits are attributed to some an extra-articular restriction.

Noncoupled Movements: Describe motions that do not invariably occur together, but rather may occur together depending on the condition.

Nonfunctional Movement: Active motions that occur within the cardinal planes of motion. They are sometimes referred to as nonphysiologic movement.

Nonmechanical: A condition that is *not* impacted by movement or position. Such conditions may require consultation and/or referral for additional medical management.

Nonphysiologic Movement: See *Nonfunctional Movement.*

Non-Resting Position: See *Close-Packed Position.*

Nonthrust: See *Mobilization.*

Number Needed to Treat (NNT): Describes the number of patients treated with one intervention before being certain that one patient improved who would not have improved without that intervention.

O

1 × 1 × 1 × 1 Rule: Calls for the manual physical therapist to use one hand to move one joint in one direction at one point in time.

Open Chain: Exercises without the distal end fixed.

Open-Packed Position: Also known as loose-packed or resting position. Defined as the position in which the greatest degree of mobility between articular surfaces is available.

Opening Restriction: A spinal classification syndrome where symptoms and/or limited motion is identified with movement away from the painful side or in the direction that produces decompression or distraction of the spinal facet joints and intervertebral foramen.

Oscillatory Movements: Manual intervention that includes a cycle of force delivered in intermittent bouts using more, then less force. A variety of rhythms may be used to provide oscillations, and these procedures may be performed prior to tissue resistance or into tissue resistance depending on the predetermined objective of the intervention.

Osteoarthritis: Degenerative process related to the joint and the structures about the joint that includes active joint inflammation.

Osteoarthrosis: Degenerative process related to the joint and the structures about the joint that does not include active joint inflammation.

Osteokinematic: The gross movement of limbs or body parts relative to one another and relative to environmental references.

Ottawa Ankle Rules: Provide a list of criteria that suggests the need for radiographic examination of the ankle if any one criterion is present.

Ottawa Knee Rules: Provide a list of criteria that suggests the need for radiographic examination of the knee if any one criterion is present.

Overpressure: Additional force provided to a joint and associated structures by the therapist or patient at the end range of available motion. This procedure is used to assess endfeel, joint play, and an individual's symptomatic response.

Overuse Syndromes: Common dysfunctions of the musculoskeletal system when the stress introduced to tissues is greater than the ability of the tissues to respond through repair or by an increase in their strength.

P

Pain-Dominant Behavior: An observed active or passive movement pattern in which pain serves as the primary limitation to normal mobility.

Pain Release Phenomenon (PRP): Techniques for individuals presenting with chronic conditions when the early stages of healing have occurred. These techniques involve reproduction of a patent's pain complaint through either an active contraction of the painful region or stretch of the involved structures. Typically, the painful activity is maintained for a maximum of 20 seconds, within which symptoms should resolve.

Painful Arc: Defined as a point, or points, within a range of motion in which a patient experiences discomfort.

Painful Entrapment: Response in synovial joints to an awkward movement performed in a rapid fashion, such as a quick turn of the cervical spine. The patient often presents with an inability to return the neck to the neutral, or fully erect, position. Intervention includes distraction to release the impingement followed by isometric recruitment of capsular muscles to retrieve the facet joint capsule from impingement.

Palliative Interventions: Interventions that are designed to provide relief of symptoms and are readily used in the case of an acute condition. Such procedures may include rest, ice, or electric stimulation.

Palpation for Condition: Includes the palpation of structures in an attempt to identify the level of involvement or status of various tissues in the region of dysfunction. By palpating the skin, subcutaneous tissue, muscle, and joint, the manual therapist attempts to identify the presence of tightness, tenderness, altered temperature, altered texture, the presence of trigger or tender points, and the level of involvement or status of various tissues in the region of dysfunction.

Palpation for Mobility: Includes the palpation of structures in an attempt to ascertain the degree of accessory motion within a joint and to identify end-feels.

Palpation for Position: Includes the palpation of structures in an attempt to identify the presence of positional faults or altered relationships between adjacent bony structures about a joint.

Parallel Technique: Technique performed by applying finger pressure parallel to the muscle, either between the bone and the muscle or between two adjacent muscles. The therapist slides his or her finger along the muscle, attempting to separate it from the surrounding tissues.

Partial Articular Pattern: See *Noncapsular Pattern.*

Passive Accessory Movement: Consist of arthrokinematic motions that accompany the osteokinematic motions (i.e., roll, glide).

Passive Accessory Intervertebral Mobility (PAIVM) Testing: Passive procedures that are used to specifically identify the quantity and quality of accessory intervertebral joint mobility and any associated reproduction of symptoms (i.e., glide).

Passive Insufficiency: The inability of a muscle that spans two or more joints to be stretched sufficiently to produce a full range of motion in all the joints simultaneously.

Passive Intervertebral Mobility (PIVM) Testing: See *Passive Physiologic Intervertebral Mobility (PPIVM) Testing.*

Passive Localization Tests: Used to identify the specific location of the lesion, to identify the direction that is symptomatic, and to measure the degree of restriction.

Passive Movement: Movement that is produced entirely by external forces, either manually or mechanically.

Passive Physiologic Movement: Consist of osteokinematic motions such as flexion, abduction, external rotation, and so on.

Passive Physiologic Intervertebral Mobility (PPIVM) Testing: Passive procedures that are used to specifically identify the quantity and quality of physiologic intervertebral joint mobility and any associated reproduction of symptoms (i.e., side bending, rotation).

Passive Subsystem: Relative to the spine, comprises spinal osteology, facet joint capsules, ligaments, and the passive tension of the musculotendinous unit. The passive subsystem is most involved in contributing to spinal stability at or near the end ranges of movement.

Patella Alta: Describes a patella that is displaced superiorly.

Patella Baja: Describes a patella that is displaced inferiorly.

Patellar Medial/Lateral Tracking (Glide): Alignment of the patella that, when normal, is generally considered to reveal equidistance of the patella relative to the femoral condyles.

Patellar Tilt: Describes the alignment of the patella about a superior-inferior axis.

Path of the Instantaneous Center of Rotation (PICR): See *Instantaneous Center of Rotation.*

Pathoanatomical Origin: A condition that has as its cause an impairment in the structural and anatomical aspects of a given body region (i.e., herniated nucleus pulposis).

Patient Cooperative Reflex Activities: Eye movements and activation of other specific muscles in specific directions and/or at a specific time.

Patient-Generated Forces: Techniques that take place in midrange with eventual progression to end range and end range with self-overpressure.

Pelvic Shear: Also known as side gliding, is a valuable examination tool as it involves the use of a complex movement pattern that requires efficient hip, pelvic, lumbar, and thoracic function. Any movement that is limited, inefficient, or painful can be performed following intervention to assess treatment efficacy.

Pericapsular Restrictions: One of the primary causes of articular hypomobility that is produced by inextensibility of the periarticular tissues and identified during the examination by the presence of a hard capsular end-feel.

Perimysium: Dense connective tissue sheath that surrounds fascicles.

Perineurium: A thin sheath of connective tissue that surrounds bundles of nerve fibers. The role of the perineurium as protecting the contents of the endoneural tubes, acting as mechanical barriers to external forces, and serving as a diffusion barrier. With a high ratio of elastin to collagen, it is thought to prevent neural damage from tensile forces.

Peripheralization: The process by which symptoms move from a proximal to a more distal location.

Perpendicular Deformation: The process in which heels of the hands are placed on one side of the spine, with the fingertips resting on the opposite side of the spine. Both hands come together to produce a single "tool," consisting of a row of fingertips that engages the border of the muscle.

Pes Cavus: A structural impairment of the foot revealing a foot that is oversupinated leading to external tibial torsion.

Pes Planus: A structural impairment of the foot revealing a foot that is overpronated leading to internal tibial torsion.

Phases: The concept of determining the relationship between pain and end-feel.

Phase One: Characterized by pain that is reproduced or exacerbated after the end-feel has been reached. The joint is, therefore, determined to be minimally irritable.

Phase Two: Characterized by pain that is reproduced or exacerbated at the same time that the end-feel is reached. This joint is therefore considered to be moderately irritable.

Phase Three: Consists of pain that is reproduced or exacerbated at some point before end-feel is reached. The joint is therefore considered to be severely irritable.

Phasic Shake: If the patient attempts to produce a stabilizing contraction with a phasic response, an oscillating contraction will occur secondary to fatigue.

Physiologic Movement: See *Functional Movement* and *Osteokinematic*.

Physiological Response Method Techniques: Technique that depends on careful patient positioning and movement to obtain a therapeutic result by creating conditions in which tissues must move in certain physiologically predetermined directions.

Physiological Soft Tissue Movement Testing: A test in which the muscle is moved into the maximally lengthened position, and careful assessment of end-feel may differentiate the presence of muscle shortening as opposed to restricted joint movement. These tests may also be used to examine neural tension and mobility.

Pincer Palpation: Includes use of a pincer grip where muscle fibers are placed between the clinician's fingers and thumb and rolled in a direction that is perpendicular to the muscle fibers.

Pisiform-Contact Position: A hand position for manual interventions in which the area of the hypothenar eminence just distal to the pisiform is placed over the region to be mobilized as the wrist is locked in terminal extension with the fingers extended.

Planar Joint: A joint with flat, or slightly reciprocal, joint surfaces such as the AC joint.

Plane of the Scapula (POS): Position of the shoulder determined by the resting position of the scapula on the thorax. This position may vary slightly between individuals but is generally thought to be 30 to 45 degrees anterior to the frontal plane.

Plantar-Flexed First Ray: Characterized by a first metatarsal head positioned plantarly in reference to heads 2 through 5.

Plastic Region: Portion of the stress-strain curve where permanent deformation occurs. In such a position, minimal force is required to mechanically influence the barrier.

Position of Comfort (POC): The triplanar position, which is passively achieved for the purpose of reducing tender point irritability and achieving normalization of tissues associated with the presenting myofascial impairment.

Position of Treatment (PT): Direction in which motion is to be restored, which is the same as the movement diagnosis (MD).

Position Four: For mobilization of the T1-T2 segment. In prone, on the elbows, with his or her hand on the opposite shoulder (cover position) and the forehead resting on the elbow with the face in the bend of the arm to prevent upper cervical extension. This position includes addition of anterior to posterior motion.

Position One: For mobilization of the T1-T2 segment. In prone, with the back of the patient's hand on the buttocks or lumbar spine. This position is used to examine the ability of the vertebrae to rotate superiorly.

Position Three: For mobilization of the T1-T2 segment. In prone, with the hand on the back of the head. This position tests the ability of the vertebrae to rotate inferiorly.

Position Two: For mobilization of the T1-T2 segment. In prone, with the hand placed flat on the table above the shoulder. This position tests vertebral movement into pure rotation.

Positional Diagnosis (PD): The asymmetric position of the segment.

Positional Distraction: Manual techniques that are most valuable when treating the spine. This technique involves careful patient positioning that provides maximal triplanar opening of an intervertebral foramen for the purpose of reducing nerve root pressure. The use of pillows or straps allows maintenance of this position for a period of time that the patient may independently perform several times each day.

Positional Fault Theory: Suggests that joints having less than optimal positional relationships will adopt faulty movement patterns that lead to reduced function and/or pain. Mobilization is, therefore, performed in an attempt to restore normal articular relationships.

Positive Predictive Value: Describes the number of true positives/total number of positives. This describes the likelihood that a positive test is truly positive.

Positive Ulnar Variance: An ulna that is longer than normal relative to the distal radius.

Postural Syndrome: Syndromes that occur from prolonged positions that place undue stress on anatomical tissues. As with other overuse syndromes, dysfunction that results from prolonged poor posture is often insidious and takes a long time to occur. This occurs when normal soft tissues experience abnormal stresses, typically in response to prolonged static loading at end range.

Posterior Depression (PD): One of four pelvic girdle motions based on PNF diagonals that occurs during gait. PD is necessary for effective midstance and push off. The therapist should be able to palpate the gluteal muscles or observe plantar flexors firing in an efficient recruitment pattern during this phase.

Posterior Derangement: Injury to the disc that involves displacement of the disc in a posterior direction.

Posterior Elevation (PE): One of four pelvic girdle motions based on PNF diagonals that occurs during gait. PE promotes trunk stability in conjunction with contralateral anterior elevation.

Pranayama (prā·Nā·yā·ma): Regulated breathing used in yoga.

Prancing: Used to emphasize the initiation of hip flexion and involves taking high steps while walking.

Pratyahara (Prut-yahhah-ruh): Withdrawing of the senses used in yoga.

Predictive Validity: Describes the degree to which a finding can be used to predict a future event. Predictive validity is a major requirement of measures used to develop a patient prognosis.

Preparatory Interventions: Interventions that are used to engage the involved tissues so that they will respond more favorably to the primary intervention that is to follow. Massage, moist heat, and Grade I and II oscillations are examples.

Prescriptive Validity: Describes the degree to which a certain finding will be influenced by treatment. Prescriptive validity must be established by randomized clinical trials.

Primary Somatic Dysfunction: Somatic dysfunction site usually corresponds with the biomechanical history, site of specific trauma, or area of compensation.

Prognostic Index: A type of classification system that serves to predict the future status of the individual patient.

Progressive Oscillation without Locking: Manual techniques that involve a progressive series of three to five medium-amplitude oscillations that begin at midrange and gradually move toward end range.

Progressive Oscillations: Mobilizations that involve a series of oscillations that go into progressively greater ranges of motion.

Prolonged Stretch: Manual techniques that involve a slow and steady progression of manual force to end range where the force is maintained for a designated period of time.

Pronation: Motion of the foot that consists of dorsiflexion in the sagittal plane, eversion in the frontal plane, and abduction in the transverse plane.

Proprioceptors: Receive impulses directly from muscle spindles, Golgi tendon organs, tendons, and periarticular tissues.

Prospective: Research designs in which a specific purpose has been identified and a consistent plan for data collection is used prior to data collection.

Protective Muscle Spasm: An involuntary sustained contraction and shortening of muscle fibers at the level of the sarcomere.

Proteoglycan: A sugar protein complex with an electrocharge suitable for extensive water-binding capabilities.

Q

Q-angle: Standing for quadriceps angle, this is measured in supine with the quadriceps relaxed by drawing a line from the anterior inferior iliac spine (AIIS) to the midpoint of the patella and then a second intersecting line from the tibial tuberosity to the same point on the patella.

Quadriceps Dominance: Jumping activities that involve dominant activation of the quadriceps relative to the hamstrings.

R

Randomized Controlled Trials (RCT): Research designs that test hypotheses and provide the least biased approach to intervention research. Subjects are randomly assigned to receive a specific treatment (independent variable), and their outcomes (dependent variables) are compared to similar subjects who are randomly assigned to not receive the treatment (controlled designs) or who receive an alternative treatment of interest (noncontrolled designs).

Range-of-Motion Box: Originally designed to assist the therapist in visualizing changes in direction of the patient's head and neck during SCS of the cervical spine. This tool provides a visual depiction of the manner and direction in which the cervical spine may be smoothly transitioned from one quadrant to another in pursuit of the position of comfort.

Ray: Each tarsal bone and its associated metatarsal.

Reactivity: The level of irritability of a condition typically determined by level of pain, time for symptoms to return to baseline after insult, and/or the presence of symptoms peripheralization.

Reactivity and Relationship: Used during the initial examination and reexamination to determine the level of irritability and the relationship between the reproducible symptoms and movement.

Rearfoot Varus Deformity: An individual with more than 4 degrees of varus when the foot is in the subtalar joint neutral position.

Rearfoot Valgus Deformity: An individual with less than 4 degrees of varus when the foot is in the subtalar joint neutral position.

Reciprocal Inhibition: Resistance that is applied to the antagonist of the restricted agonist prior to stretching when performing hold and contract-relax stretching.

Reducible Derangement: A displaced disc that is able to be restored to its original position. It is presumed that the outer annulus is intact and therefore the disc follows normal disc mechanics. A reducible derangement is identified by a condition that centralizes and is often an indicator of a favorable prognosis.

Region of Origin: Used during the initial examination and re-examination to Identify the region, or regions, from which the symptoms have arisen. Identification allows the manual therapist to more efficiently and effectively address the origin of symptoms.

Regional Movement Differentiation (RMD): A process of motion assessment designed to identify the segment from which the symptoms arise within a multijoint system. The process begins with baseline testing designed to incite the chief complaint. Once this symptom is reproduced, over-pressure and counterpressure is specifically applied in an attempt to isolate the culpable segment.

Relative Flexibility: In a multisegmental system, movement will take the path of least resistance.

Release Phenomenon: According to Cyriax, pressure on the nerve trunk that typically produces paresthesia after the pressure has been released. Frequently, stroking the skin over the paresthetic region or performance of active motion of the involved extremity will produce a cascade of paresthesias. Within the strain-counterstrain paradigm, this represents a relaxation in hypertonic soft tissues allowing an increase in the range of motion that is beyond the original barrier.

Reliability: Describes the error in a measurement or judgment that occurs in repeated observations made by the same examiner (intrarater) or between different examiners (interrater).

Repeated Movement Testing: The use of multiple, consecutive movements in each direction during the examination for the purpose of ascertaining a patient's directional preference.

Reproducible Sign or Symptom: Used during the initial examination and reexamination to confirm the presence of a mechanical movement disorder and to identify the specific position, movement, or behavior that incites the patient's chief presenting complaint.

Resistance 1 (R1): Range of movement in which the first barrier to movement occurs.

Resistance 2 (R2): Range of movement in which the final barrier to movement occurs.

Respiratory Cooperation or Force: Inhalation causing spinal curves to straighten and extremities to externally rotate; exhalation causing spinal curves to accentuate and extremities to internally rotate.

Resting Position: See *Open-Packed Position.*

Reticulin: Fibers are glycoprotein, but less tensile than collagen or elastin. There is a slight variation in the combination of protein sequences within this tissue that allows it to form networks of durable, yet pliable, meshing.

Retrospective: Research that is designed and performed after data has been collected and are obviously more prone to bias than are prospective designs.

Retrospective Evaluation: Performed at distinct times throughout intervention and at the conclusion of intervention to determine overall effectiveness and future prognosis.

Reverse Headache Sustained Natural Apophyseal Glides (SNAGs): Manual techniques that are performed by the therapist supporting the occiput with one hand and using an open lumbrical grasp to hold C2. C2 is held in position as the occiput is moved anteriorly, thus producing a posteroanterior mobilization of the occiput and C1 relative to C2, which is the opposite effect of the headache SNAG.

Reverse Natural Apophyseal Glides (RNAGs): Downglide of the segment in question through application of force applied to the inferior vertebra of the segment. These techniques approximate the forces that occur during neck retraction (axial extension) exercises.

Rhythmic Distraction: Manual techniques performed with alternate periods of rest; is designed to "gate" the patient's perception of pain.

Right Oblique Axis (ROA): A triplanar axis around which SIJ motion is believed to occur that courses from the left inferior lateral angle through the right SIJ.

Rockette Walking: Emphasizes pelvic anterior elevation with the verbal cues of using a "long leg" walk from the thoracolumbar junction.

Rollerblading: This is used to emphasize push-off and propulsion. It involves initiating motion in the trunk through a subtle lean forward and then propelling the body forward through the lengthening of the hip and push-off through the foot.

Roll-Gliding: Occurs during bone rotational movements.

Rolling: An angular movement that involves approximation of new points on one joint surface with new points on the other joint surface. The direction of rolling is invariably in the direction in which the bone is being displaced.

Rotatory: Angular movement of a segment about an axis.

Rule of Threes: System for identifying the relationship between the spinous processes and vertebrae in the thoracic spine.

S

Sacralization: The fusion of L5 and S1.

Sacroilial Backward Bending: Movement of the sacrum relative to a fixed ilium in the sagittal plane where the base of the sacrum moves posteriorly.

Sacroilial Backward Torsions: Triplanar motion of the SIJ around an oblique axis in which the sagittal component of the motion moves in a posterior direction.

Sacroilial Forward Bending: Movement of the sacrum relative to a fixed ilium in the sagittal plane where the base of the sacrum moves anteriorly.

Sacroilial Forward Torsion: Triplanar motion of the SIJ around an oblique axis in which the sagittal component of the motion moves in an anterior direction.

Sacroilial Left on Left Oblique Axis (left on left) Forward Torsion: Triplanar SIJ motion that consists of forward bending in the sagittal plane, rotation to the left in the transverse plane, and side bending to the left in the frontal plane.

Sacroilial Left on Right Oblique Axis (left on right) Backward Torsion: Triplanar SIJ motion that consists of backward bending in the sagittal plane, rotation to the left in the transverse plane, and side bending to the left in the frontal plane.

Sacroilial (SI) Motion: Movement of the sacrum on a relatively fixed ilium.

Sacroilial Right on Left Oblique Axis (right on left) Backward Torsion: Triplanar SIJ motion that consists of backward bending in the sagittal plane, rotation to the right in the transverse plane, and side bending to the right in the frontal plane.

Sacroilial Right on Right Oblique Axis (right on right) Forward Torsion: Triplanar SIJ motion that consists of forward bending in the sagittal plane, rotation to the right in the transverse plane, and side bending to the right in the frontal plane.

Sacroilial Rotation: Movement of the sacrum relative to a fixed ilium in the transverse plane where the anterior aspect of the sacrum moves to the right or left.

Sacroilial Side Bending: Movement of the sacrum relative to a fixed ilium in the frontal plane where the anterior aspect of the sacrum moves to the right or left.

Sacroilial Torsions: Triplanar motions of the SIJ that occur around an oblique axis.

Saddle Joint: A joint that operates about three axes of motion. The SC joint is an example in which the sternal articular surface is concave in the frontal plane and convex in the sagittal plane, which corresponds to the medial articular surface of the clavicle.

Scalene Elongation: The first rib is stabilized with one hand as the cervical spine is passively side-bent contralaterally and the specific region of tightness is localized through cervical rotation.

Scanning Examination: An intermediate detailed examination of specific body regions that have been identified by findings emerging from the initial screen; the scan (for somatic dysfunction) focuses on segmental areas for further definition or diagnosis.

Scaption: Elevation of the shoulder that occurs within the plane of the scapula (POS).

Scapulohumeral Rhythm (SHR): In its ideal form, SHR has been defined as the "synchronous culmination of shoulder girdle joint harmony. SHT is used to define the relative amount of GH motion versus ST motion during active elevation.

Screening Examination: For the neuromusculoskeletal system, this answers the question, Is there a problem that deserves additional evaluation?

Screening Tests: Pretest screening procedures that may be used within the Canadian Approach prior to performance of formal movement testing and may be used to improve efficiency. These tests focus on a specific segment so that a more detailed examination can occur. These tests are not intended to be exhaustive and are inclusive rather than exclusive. The screening tests advocated by NAIOMT faculty include position tests, quadrant tests (both peripheral and spinal), and the H and I tests.

Screw Home Mechanism: The final degree of tibial external rotation that occurs at the terminal range of knee extension, a useful component of knee stability.

Secondary Somatic Dysfunction: Somatic dysfunction arising from a viscerosomatic or somatosomatic reflex.

Segmental Facilitation: A state of heightened excitation of the spinal cord segment resulting in a decreased response threshold caused by prolonged nociceptive input. The effect of segmental facilitation is segmentally distributed hypertonicity, increased deep tendon reflex briskness, vasoconstriction, and nonfatigable weakness due to neuromuscular incoordination.

Segmental Instability: Occurs as a result of degeneration of the zygapophyseal joint surfaces and intervertebral discs of the spine. This is determined from the biomechanical examination and the patient's history.

Segmental Motion: Movement of one vertebra relative to an adjacent vertebra.

Segmental Stability Test (SST): Identifies movements that are not expected to exist at an appreciable degree. The primary goal is to identify the presence of abnormal joint play in each direction.

Selective Tissue Tension (STT) Testing: According to Cyriax a healthy muscle contracting isometrically should be both strong and pain free. STT seeks to selectively facilitate an isometric contraction of the muscle in question and, in so doing, identify the muscle's strength and any provocation of symptoms. STT is designed to differentiate a contractile from an inert lesion and if contractile to further identify the specific muscle that is impaired.

Self-Headache Sustained Natural Apophyseal Glides (SNAGs): Techniques that involve performance of a chin tuck while using a towel to provide counterforce over C2 in a PA direction.

Self-Mobilization: Techniques that serve to provide lasting improvement, increase the efficiency of intervention, allow the patient to take a more active role in his or her care, and that may be used as preventative measures.

Self-Mobilization Straps: Nylon straps with handles and rubber that are used to localize forces during self-mobilization of the spine and extremities.

Self-Mobilization with Movement (MWM): Active or passive physiologic movement occurs simultaneously with passive accessory mobilization that is performed entirely by the patient, often using either a self-mobilization strap or towel to facilitate accessory glide during active movement. These techniques are designed to allow the patient to become an active participant in his or her own care and to maintain improvement between visits.

Sensitivity: Defined as the number of positive findings/number of people with the condition of interest. Tests with high degrees of sensitivity are generally useful to rule out a condition (i.e., a negative test is likely to indicate the absence of the condition).

Sensitizing Maneuver: A position that is used during neurodynamic testing that may be used to differentiate between the presence of neurological symptoms from symptoms of another origin. For example, during upper limb neurodynamic testing, the cervical flexion component may be altered by moving the patient in and out of flexion while ascertaining the effect of these altered positions on the patient's reported symptoms.

Septic Arthritis: Joint inflammation that requires antibiotic therapy.

Settled Stage: In reference to healing, the condition becomes more stable and the therapist is better able to appreciate the effects of intervention. During this stage, the patient is able to handle moderate stresses, including manipulation.

Severity: One aspect of the S.I.N.S. process of examination. It denotes the intensity of the patient's current symptoms. This determination is based on the degree to which symptoms limit the patient's activity and normal sleeping patterns.

Shortening: Soft tissue mobilization technique in which tissues can be applied in any direction around the restriction.

Side Gliding Dysfunction Syndrome: Symptoms are produced at the end range of side gliding in a particular direction and abate as the patient moves away from this position.

Side Gliding in Standing (SGIS): Frontal plane movement of the spine that involves translation of the trunk laterally upon the lower body.

S.I.N.S.: Stands for severity, irritability, nature, and stage. This acronym highlights the essence of the Australian Approach to OMPT view of the examination process.

Site of Symptoms Questions: Questions that are the first step toward clarifying the depth, nature, behavior, and chronology of symptoms. The objective of this line of questioning is to provide an indication regarding the pain-sensitive structures that are likely to be involved.

Skin Locking Techniques: A manual intervention procedure that allows the therapist to mobilize joints by using the mechanical advantage of placing tension through the overlying soft tissues.

Skin Sliding: The skin slides along the underlying tissues as hands are moved. This form of examination is performed around the image of a clockface.

Slack Zone (SZ): Located at the beginning of Grade II movement. Within the SZ, there is minimal resistance to movement.

Slouch-Overcorrect Exercise: Teaches patients how to find a good posture in sitting, and involves active movement from an exaggerated slouched to an exaggerated erect sitting position.

Slow Rhythms: Mobilizations that involve cycles of increased then decreased force that are indicated for painful joints.

Smith's Fracture: Fracture of the wrist that may present with volar displacement of the distal radius secondary to falling on a flexed wrist.

Smooth Oscillations: Characterized by steady, uninterrupted oscillations that may be performed at either high or low frequency. May be optimal for the patient who is experiencing substantial pain.

Soft Disc Lesion: Pathogenesis of this condition involves the nucleus (soft material) gradually becoming displaced.

Soft End-Feel: The result of soft tissue approximation or stretching.

Soft Tissue Passive Movement: Performed using physiologic soft tissue movements and accessory soft tissue movements.

Somatic: Referring to the neuromusculoskeletal system.

Somatic Dysfunction: Impaired or altered function of related components of the somatic (body framework) system: skeletal, arthrodial, and myofascial structures, and related vascular, lymphatic, and neural elements.

Special Questions: Those questions that must be asked in order to detect any inherent risks to the performance of manual therapy and to isolate any factors that may limit the effectiveness of intervention.

Specific Segmental Resistance: Applied to the articular pillars of the inhibited level during axial elongation. In a dysfunctional state, the patient is unable to effectively maintain the position.

Specificity: The number of negative findings/number of people who do not have the condition. Tests with high specificity are generally useful to rule in a condition (i.e., a positive test is likely to indicate the presence of the condition).

Spinal Mobilization with Arm Movement (SMWAM): Lateral force direction for this mobilization sustained as the patient actively performs the symptom-producing arm movement. The patient may perform any cardinal plane or combined plane shoulder motion that is provocative, and the elimination of symptoms is expected as the spinal mobilization force is provided and maintained throughout the motion. This technique is used to reduce radicular symptoms into the upper extremity.

Spinal Mobilization with Leg Movement (SMWLM): In sidelying position, the involved extremity is uppermost as the patient's hip is brought into a slight degree of abduction to tolerance. The therapist applies transverse pressure along the side of the spinous process of the superior aspect of the segment to be mobilized. This pressure is maintained as the patient actively moves his or her leg into SLR with support from an assistant. This technique is used to reduce radicular symptoms into the lower extremity.

Spinal Motion Segment: The inferior half of the superior vertebra and the superior half of the inferior vertebra and all other structures between them, including muscle, nerve, disc, facet joint, and so on.

Stabilization Wedge: Typically composed of firm rubber with a gutter for pressure relief, stabilization wedges are placed between the treatment table and the body part to be mobilized. These devices enhance performance of stabilization techniques by making the hands of the therapist more available to attend to other aspects of the technique.

Stabilizing Reversals: One type of antagonist reversal that uses static contractions performed on alternate sides of a joint for the purpose of promoting core control.

Stable Hypomobility: Limits the quadrant range of motion regardless of the manner in which the patient achieves this position.

Staccato Oscillations (Rhythms): Mobilizations that involve the use of unexpected frequency of delivery, varied rhythms, and changing the amplitude of rhythms in interrupted bursts for patients who have difficulty relaxing.

Stage: One aspect of the S.I.N.S. process of examination. This feature takes into consideration the length of time since onset (acute, subacute, chronic) and the stability of the condition (improving, stable, unstable).

Standard Error of Measurement (SEM): Allows the degree of error to be expressed in the same units as the measure of interest and is especially valuable when addressing individual patients.

STAR: Acronym used in the osteopathic approach that stands for sensation change, tissue texture change, asymmetry, restriction of motion.

Star Diagram: May be used to provide a visual description of spinal motion. This method of recording motion uses a combination of long and short lines and arrows. This diagram provides information regarding both the quality and quantity of spinal motion at a glance and expedites the often laborious task of documenting spinal motion.

Stationary Holding Rhythms: Mobilizations that involve applying movement slowly up to the motion limitation, which is then held for a period of time. When pain or limitation subsides, further movement into the restricted range is achieved.

Statistical Conclusion Validity: Addresses the possibly of a statistical error that results in a wrong conclusion.

Status Index: A type of classification system that defines the patient problem and is the most prevalent type used for patients with LBP. The ICD-10 classification system is a type of status index.

Still Point: Following strain-counterstrain, a slight wobble, or shift, in the joint followed by a point of smooth motion.

Strachan (high-velocity low-amplitude) Model: Diagnosis of the sacrum is named largely with respect to its motion, or restriction, relative to the innominates.

Straddle-Stance Position: The feet are in line and beyond shoulder-width apart with the knees slightly flexed.

Straight Leg Raise (SLR) with Traction: Patient brought into the SLR position short of the point of limitation or pain. The therapist then uses a flexed elbow and opposing hand to grasp just proximal to the ankle to provide a distraction force through the long axis of the extremity. As distraction is applied, the therapist will note an increase in the available range of SLR without symptoms or report of tightness.

Straights: Chiropractors who ascribe to traditional chiropractic theory.

Stretch without Locking Mobilizations: Applied at the end range for the purpose of moving the joint capsule into the plastic region of deformation, thus improving available motion.

Stride-Forward Lean Position: Position in which nearly all of the therapist's weight may be placed through the front leg as he or she leans into the table.

Stride-Stance Position: One foot in front of the other and the knees slightly flexed.

Structural Examination: Used to determine inefficiencies in the patient's structure that may lead to inefficiencies in function.

Strumming: Can be used both as an examination and mobilization technique for muscle play dysfunctions. The setup for strumming is the same as that for perpendicular mobilization. However, once the perpendicular deformation is performed, the therapist allows the fingers to slide over the muscle belly and then back to the starting position.

Stiffness-Dominant Behavior: An observed active or passive movement pattern in which restrictions within the articular and peri-articular structures serves as the primary limitation to normal mobility.

Stretch without Locking: Techniques that are applied at the end range for the purpose of moving the joint capsule into the plastic region of deformation, thus improving available motion.

Stride-Stance Position: One foot is in front of the other and the knees are slightly flexed.

Subacute Stage: In reference to healing, a plateau in signs and symptoms. Although intervention may provide intermittent relief for the patient in this stage, care must be taken so as not to interfere with the natural course of healing.

Subluxed Joint: One of the primary causes of articular hypomobility that is independent of tissue extensibility and identified during the examination by the presence of a jammed or pathomechanical end-feel.

Subtalar Joint Neutral (STJN): A position of the subtalar joint that is considered to be neither in varus (inversion) or valgus (eversion). This position is often used as a reference point for determining the alignment of the foot and ankle.

Sulcus Angle: Defined as the angle formed between the deepest part of the sulcus to the medial and lateral femoral condyles.

Sunrise View: A radiographic projection that is taken with the knee flexed.

Superficial Fascia: The loose connective tissue underlying the skin and infiltrated with adipose tissue. This tissue helps conserve body heat and is responsible for body contours. Because the fibers are loosely arranged, this tissue is able to deform without significant damage.

Supination: Motion of the foot consisting of plantarflexion in the sagittal plane, inversion in the frontal plane, and adduction in the transverse plane.

Supportive Interventions: Interventions that are those interventions used following corrective techniques for the purpose of maintaining the gains just achieved and reducing any negative secondary effects of such changes. Supportive techniques include patient education, home exercises, and modalities to relieve postactivity soreness.

Sustained Natural Apophyseal Glides (SNAGs): Manual techniques in which the therapist contacts the painful and/or restricted segment and applies thumb-over-thumb force in the direction of the treatment plane as the patient actively moves into the painful and/or restricted active movement.

Sutherland (craniosacral) Model: Motion, or restriction, of the sacrum described relative to the cranium.

Swan-Neck Deformity: Deformity involving PIP extension, DIP flexion, as well as MCP flexion; may result from tendon rupture or contracture of the intrinsic hand muscles.

Symmetrical Movement: Dysfunction, tests, and interventions that are uncombined and uniplanar. In contrast to asymmetrical dysfunctions, they are equal bilaterally, thus indicating that the dysfunction is occurring on both sides of the segment (i.e., symmetrical).

Symptom Alleviation Tests: Use joint traction and movement in a direction that attempts to alleviate symptoms.

Symptom Provocation Tests: Use joint compression and movement that is in a symptom-provoking direction.

Synergic Pattern: Onset of hypertonicity, or muscle spasm, that often occurs in a very characteristic pattern following a cerebrovascular accident (CVA).

Synovitis: A joint impairment that involves inflammation of synovial fluid which is typically warm to the touch and elicits a moderate amount of pain. The swelling is typically gradual in onset.

Systematic Reviews: Reviews produced by investigators who identify relevant studies and, using a series of decision rules, create reproducible summaries of the topic of interest. Systematic reviews are considered as secondary analyses and have the advantage of providing a quantitative estimate of the best available evidence.

T

Talipes Equinovarus: A foot deformity, also known as *clubfoot*. This results in limited dorsiflexion and is caused by a combination of congenital factors including neurological involvement.

Teleceptors: Receptors that are sensitive to distant stimuli.

Tender Point: Local regions within a muscle that are exquisitely painful upon palpation. Tender points identified in the extremities were not found in the muscle being strained or stretched, but rather in its antagonist. The mechanism by which these tender points are present is believed to be related to a sudden stretch placed on the muscle following insult. These points may be described as small areas (approximately 1 cm in diameter) of intense, tender, edematous muscle and fascial tissue.

Tenodesis Grip: Movement of the wrist into extension and the subsequent finger flexion that results. This may be used to grasp objects by individuals without volitional finger flexor function.

Tensegrity: Also known as tensional integrity. This term was used to describe a natural phenomenon whereby a system stabilizes itself mechanically via an intricate balance and distribution of compressional and tensional forces on the skeleton.

Theoretical Compartment: Within the Australian approach, contains information that the therapist either knows or speculates. This information is typically obtained through formal education or research. Included in this compartment is information related to pathology, biomedical engineering, neurophysiology, and anatomy, all of which contribute to the patient's formal diagnosis. During the course of the examination and reexamination process the therapist disallows the theoretical compartment from obstructing the search for clinical facts.

Therapeutic Pulse: A sensation of movement, filling of space, and a pulsation that occurs during myofascial release. The amplitude of this therapeutic pulse increases during the technique and subsides as the tissue tension release occurs.

Thoracic Outlet: The area between the intervertebral foramen and the insertion of the pectoralis minor muscle at the humerus.

Thoracic Outlet Syndrome (TOS): A condition that involves entrapment of the brachial plexus and subclavian artery and vein, which may lead to both neurological and/or vascular compromise.

Thoracobrachial Angle: The angle between the arm and the thorax that provides information related to an elevated shoulder, scoliosis, lateral shift, or trunk lean.

Three-Planar Fascial Fulcrum Approach: An approach to myofascial release that is always indirect. Based on its indirect nature, this form of MFR is considered to be more comfortable compared to direct methods, and resistance is less when the barriers are not engaged.

Three *R*'s: Reproducible sign or symptoms, region of origin, reactivity level. The primary objective of the initial examination is to determine these three *R*'s.

Thrust: An accurately localized, single, quick, and decisive movement of small amplitude following careful positioning of the patient. Techniques involve a sudden, high-velocity, short-amplitude motion that is delivered at the pathological limit of an accessory motion. These techniques are used to reduce positional faults, release an adhesion, or fire joint receptors. Sometimes used interchangeably with manipulation. See *Manipulation*.

Thumb-over-Thumb Position: A hand position for manual intervention in which the dumby-thumb makes contact upon the specific segment to be mobilized while the force-application thumb contacts the dumby-thumb and applies the mobilization force.

Tibial Valgum: Ascertained by measuring the frontal plane angle formed between the tibia and the horizontal in weight-bearing and is synonymous with genu valgum of the knee.

Tibial Varum: Ascertained by measuring the frontal plane angle formed between the tibia and the horizontal in weight-bearing and is synonymous with genu varum of the knee.

Tinel Sign: Elicited over an area of focal demyelination that accompanies nerve entrapment. A positive Tinel sign is noted when manual tapping over a suspected area of nerve entrapment produces paresthesia or reproduction of symptoms along the distal distribution of the culpable nerve.

Tissue Extensibility: The ability of tissues to optimally elongate and fold (shorten) while maintaining a springy end-feel.

Titin: The largest known vertebrate protein. Titin filaments are responsible for passive tension generation when sarcomeres are stretched and provide muscle stiffness by virtue of its spring mechanism in the I band.

Tonic Spread: Very slowly applied resistance designed to facilitate the core muscles.

Trabecular Bone: Also known as cancellous or spongy bone.

Tracing and Isolating Procedures: Use of passive and active movement with functional palpation to assist in localizing the specific peripheral and central adherences.

Traction: Occurs perpendicular to the treatment plane in a direction that is away from the joint.

Transition Zone (TZ): Tissues become taut and more resistance is appreciated.

Translatory: Movement of a body segment in a linear (straight) path. This rarely occurs in isolation in the body.

Translatory Joint Play: Occurs during bone translatory movements.

Transverse Tarsal Arch: An arch of the foot that spans the foot longitudinally and has the middle cuneiform as the keystone.

Traumatic Arthritis: Monoarticular steroid-sensitive arthritis, will often benefit from a steroid injection. Traumatic arthritis refers to joint inflammation secondary to trauma.

Treatment Plane (TP): Determined by the concave aspect of the joint and is at a right angle to a line drawn from the axis of rotation to the center of the concave articulating surface.

Trial Treatment: The use of a small, controlled dose of manual intervention that is used to ascertain patient response and overall effect. When initiating intervention or embarking on a new procedure, providing less than a full dose of the chosen intervention may assist in guiding future care. The dose may be varied by altering the number of sets/repetitions, reducing the intensity, grade, or location of the chosen procedure.

Trigger: Considered to be the immediate provoking agent and not the cause. For a trigger to cause symptoms for the first time, a predisposition in the form of an asymptomatic pathology must already be present. This word typically lacks usefulness when describing the aggravating factor of an already symptomatic condition.

Trigger Points (TrPs): See Myofascial Trigger Points (MTrPs).

Triple Innervation: Afferent innervation shared with the spinal segments above and below the segment from which the nerve arises.

TUBS: Type of shoulder instability that is of traumatic onset, unidirectional anterior, with a Bankart lesion responding to surgery.

Turtle Neck Test: Used to assess upper quadrant dural mobility. The therapist positions the patient in a hook-lying position and cradles the head with gentle traction.

Twenty-Four Hour Rule: May be applied to both the examination and subsequent interventions. This rule states that the symptoms that occur from any patient encounter should not last longer than 24 hours following the encounter and should only be mild in nature.

Type I Error: Occurs when the researcher wrongfully rejects the null hypothesis (i.e., concludes that there is a significant treatment effect when there actually is not). This represents a false-positive finding.

Type I Somatic Dysfunction: Occurs when the patient is in the neutral position and side bending and rotation occur to opposite sides, usually in groups

Type II Error: Occurs when the researcher wrongfully accepts the null hypothesis (concludes that there is no difference when actually there is). This represents a false-negative finding.

Type II Somatic Dysfunction: Occurs with significant flexion or extension, and rotation and side bending occur at a single segment and to the same side.

U

Ulnar Drift: Ulnar migration and deformity of the MCP and IP joints resulting from rheumatoid arthritis.

Unlocking Spiral: Soft tissue mobilization technique that is performed by maintaining pressure on the restriction and superimposing a clockwise or counterclockwise motion through the treatment hand. The rotation is produced by the therapist's forearm moving toward pronation or supination.

Unstable Hypomobility: Presents with restrictions in only one of the sequences for accessing end range of the quadrant position. This finding indicates an instability that fixates (subluxes) in response to compressive forces from weight-bearing.

Upglide: Used to refer to segmental spinal motion that is in an upward and forward direction.

V

Vasa Nervorum: The blood supply of the peripheral nervous system.

Vertical Compression Test (VCT): Performed through application of a slow and progressively applied vertical force to the patient's shoulders to assess the integrity of the structural system, which is measured by the attenuation of force through the segments to the base of support. An efficient system allows for force attenuation without any buckling or shear.

Viniyoga: A popular form of yoga that allows poses to be customized to the individual, thus proving useful for those with physical limitations.

Voluntary Muscle Guarding: Guarding in which individuals will display an increase in muscle tone owing to pain or fear of pain and is primarily revealed during active movement.

W

Weber-Fechner Principle: The idea that excessive effort interferes with our ability to detect small changes.

X, Y, Z

Zero Position: A term that is used synonymously with anatomical position. All range-of-motion measurements are taken from the zero starting position.

INDEX

Page numbers followed by *f* indicate figures; *t*, tables; *b*, boxes.